SECOND EDITION

Interventions in
Structural, Valvular, and Congenital Heart Disease

SECOND EDITION

Interventions in Structural, Valvular, and Congenital Heart Disease

EDITED BY

Horst Sievert, MD

CardioVascular Center Frankfurt;
Sankt Katharinen Hospital
Frankfurt, Germany

Shakeel A. Qureshi, FRCP

Evelina London Children's Hospital
Guy's & St Thomas Trust
London, United Kingdom

Neil Wilson, FRCP

Department of Paediatric Cardiology
John Radcliffe Hospital
Oxford, United Kingdom

Ziyad M. Hijazi, MD MPH FACC MSCAI

Rush Center for Congenital & Structural Heart Disease
Rush University Medical Center
Chicago, IL, United States

ASSOCIATE EDITORS

Jennifer Franke, MD

CardioVascular Center Frankfurt
Frankfurt, Germany;
University of Heidelberg
Heidelberg, Germany

Stefan Bertog, MD

CardioVascular Center Frankfurt
Frankfurt, Germany

Sameer Gafoor, MD

CardioVascular Center Frankfurt;
Sankt Katharinen Hospital
Frankfurt, Germany

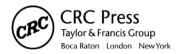

CRC Press
Taylor & Francis Group
Boca Raton London New York

CRC Press is an imprint of the
Taylor & Francis Group, an **informa** business

CRC Press
Taylor & Francis Group
6000 Broken Sound Parkway NW, Suite 300
Boca Raton, FL 33487-2742

Printed on acid-free paper
Version Date: 20141017

International Standard Book Number-13: 978-1-4822-1563-2 (Pack - Book and Ebook)

Visit the Taylor & Francis Web site at
http://www.taylorandfrancis.com

and the CRC Press Web site at
http://www.crcpress.com

Contents

Preface to the Second Edition

This book is intended as a practical guide for the interventional treatment of congenital, valvular, and structural heart disease for invasive cardiologists in the pediatric and adult fields. You will appreciate that this second edition gives us the opportunity to report consolidated results and increase the bibliography of established interventional procedures. In keeping with the explosion of structural interventions in adults and the huge increase in transcatheter aortic valve replacement we have recruited many new authors who are pioneers and leaders in those fields. We have also encouraged younger interventionists who we feel write well and who will become leaders in the future. We have also expanded the concept of the importance of imaging alongside the technical details of equipment and its safe and effective delivery.

Where possible we have tried to emphasize practical aspects of the procedures, including the important issues of indications and patient selection, potential pitfalls, and complications. Greater understanding, technical know-how, and wider availability of catheters, balloons, delivery systems, and devices have spread intervention into the realm of acquired valve disease, degenerative disease of the aorta, paravalve leakage, postinfarction ventricular septal defects, and closure of the left atrial appendage.

Some of the procedures covered in the book, such as fetal interventions, hybrid procedures, mitral valve repair, are emerging techniques representing the forefront of interventional treatment today, and will not be practiced in every catheter laboratory. We have collated contributions from a team of expert interventionists throughout the world in an effort to draw together, via the common link of catheter technology, an approach to congenital and structural heart disease that results in a new emerging specialist, the cardiovascular interventionist.

We hope this edition will go a little further than the first to provide guidance and in-depth education to personnel of all levels and disciplines involved in interventional cardiac catheterization. We see it as a tool of reference for all. Our aim is to see a well-thumbed copy in catheter lab viewing rooms and coffee rooms throughout the world. Please do send feedback to us if you perceive shortcomings or have interests and techniques that you feel should be included in future editions.

Horst Sievert
Shakeel A Qureshi
Neil Wilson
Ziyad M Hijazi

Foreword by Dr. Michael Tynan

This is the second edition of the book *Percutaneous Interventions for Congenital Heart Disease*, now with "Structural Heart Disease" preceding "Congenital Heart Disease." Thus, it encompasses almost everything that is not atherosclerotic, inflammatory, or metabolic. The new edition is considerably larger, with an additional 300 pages, which includes 41 chapters. The contributors come from all over the world representing rising talent as well as the "Old Guard." However, it still retains the essential "how to" philosophy of the first edition and of the annual Frankfurt CSI course, which gave birth to the book. The expansion is not just in pages but in concepts, such as the online video resources that are incorporated.

Having lived through this era of less invasive treatment for heart disease, from the introduction of balloon atrial septostomy by Bill Rashkind in 1966, perhaps I should not be astonished at the rapidity with which it has blossomed, but I am astonished. The slow start in the 1960s has given way to ever-increasing momentum. In the 1980s and 1990s, the ideas and practice of peripheral vascular interventionists were incorporated into pediatric cardiology and so balloon dilation of valves and vessels became routine. Stents and implantable occlusion devices were explored. Devices have come and gone with technology improvements so that defect closure is now effective and safe. Over these early years of the twenty-first century the rate of innovation appears almost exponential. What would the pioneers such as Rashkind, Gianturco, and Gruentzig make of the possibilities today? They would love it.

This rapid development has been made possible by the close cooperation between physicians and industry. It would be hard to overstate the importance of the contribution of our colleagues in industry. But the number and complexity of the procedures dealt with in this book pose problems for trainers and trainees alike. It is in this area that the book will be invaluable.

Michael Tynan, MD, FRCP
Emeritus Professor of Paediatric Cardiology
King's College
London

Foreword by Dr. Martin Leon

Most knowledgeable interventional historians would argue that the era of less-invasive nonsurgical cardiovascular therapy mushroomed when Andreas Gruentzig performed the first successful coronary angioplasty in 1977, fulfilling his dream to accomplish catheter-based percutaneous treatment of vascular disease in alert, awake patients. Undoubtedly, Andreas would have delighted in the astounding developments of the ensuing decades, as disciples of his "simple" procedure applied creativity, technical acumen, and scientific rigor to sculpt the burgeoning multidisciplinary subspecialty of interventional cardiovascular therapeutics.

Thus, a heritage has emerged within the interventional cardiovascular community. We believe that "less invasive" is preferred, certainly by patients and also by the healthcare system in general; and less-invasive means catheter-based, nonsurgical, whenever possible. We are technology addicts, especially new gizmos which can shorten procedures, improve outcomes, and expand treatment indications. We are passionate about experimental and clinical research and evidence-based medicine, which is fundamental to every important therapy change and to the interventional device development process. We rely heavily on adjunctive imaging—this is a visual subspecialty …echo/IVUS/OCT, MR/CT, "fusion" imaging, and other new invasive imaging modalities. We are passionate about the interface of clinical medicine and the rapid communication of ideas, including educational meetings and physician training initiatives. We have a vibrant entrepreneurial spirit, are risk-takers, and rapidly embrace new therapies. We strongly support and promote global and multidisciplinary collaborations. *In short, we have a cultural identity … innovation, strong industry partnerships, impatience leading to evolution and forward motion; we have a need to stimulate change and to continually reinvent ourselves, in pace with advances in biomedical science and technology!*

This second edition of *Interventions in Structural, Valvular, and Congenital Heart Disease* is the embodiment of our rapidly expanding subspecialty and now represents the definitive textbook covering all forms of nonvascular interventional therapies. The wastebasket term "structural" heart disease refers to the newest and most diverse branch of the interventional tree, embracing a potpourri of congenital, valvular, and acquired cardiovascular disorders, previously left untreated or relegated to surgical therapy alternatives. This newcomer on the interventional horizon

is unique for several reasons. First, the diversity and complexity of interventional skills required to safely and successfully treat both neonates and octogenarians with advanced cardiac lesions is unprecedented. Second, the intersecting physician groups are far-reaching, spanning pediatric and adult interventional cardiology, imaging specialists (not just angiography, but also echocardiography, MR imaging, and CT angiography), and hybrid surgical therapists. Finally, since many of the cardiac anomalies targeted for catheter-based treatment occur rarely, the focused interventionalists working in this rarified zone have clustered into a small, well-bonded fraternity. The purpose of this textbook is to highlight the practical teaching experiences of this congenital, valvular, and structural interventional fraternity.

This textbook serves as a comprehensive syllabus including a virtual "who's who" author list, representing the thought leaders from all allied fields under the umbrella of congenital, valvular, and structural heart disease. The organizational structure is both authoritative and intuitive with easy-to-navigate sections beginning with the catheterization laboratory environment, new imaging modalities for diagnosis and procedural guidance, vascular access, fetal and infant interventions, valvular interventions, and marching through an orderly progression of every conceivable congenital and structural lesion category, which has been managed using existing or proposed interventional therapies. Every section has been expanded and enhanced since the first edition with new contributors and topics, representing the absolute latest in new devices, interventional techniques, and clinical data descriptions. Clearly, the greatest area of expansion is in the breakthrough area of interventional valve therapies, especially transcatheter aortic valve implantation and new mitral regurgitation therapies. The textbook has a familiar stylistic consistency emphasizing clinical treatment indications and practical operator technique issues with helpful procedural "tips and tricks" and careful descriptions of potential complications. The breadth of this textbook is impressive extending from commonly recognized conditions (such as an expanded section on left atrial appendage closure methodologies for atrial fibrillation), to less well-established domains, including innovations in interventional heart failure diagnosis and therapy.

Lest one thinks that this textbook is merely a compendium of obscure interventional oddities, this segment of the subspecialty is exploding and the topics in this textbook represent the greatest potential growth area in all of interventional cardiovascular medicine. In 5 to 10 years it is entirely conceivable that this small fraternity of interventionalists focused on congenital, valvular, and structural therapies will multiply into an army of catheter-based therapists with specialized operator skills, an advanced appreciation of cardiac imaging modalities, and a thorough clinical understanding of multivaried cardiac disease states. This dramatically improved second edition of *Interventions in Structural, Valvular, and Congenital Heart Disease* fills a medical literature void and should be heartily embraced by all cardiovascular healthcare professionals, from the curious to the diehard interventional practitioner. I expect as this field continues to transform in the future that subsequent editions of this textbook will help to define the unpredictable progress of this unique subspecialty.

Martin B. Leon, MD
Professor of Medicine,
Columbia University Medical Center
Director, Center for Interventional Vascular Therapy
Chairman Emeritus, Cardiovascular Research Foundation
New York City

Video Contents

No.	Description	URL
Video 5.1	3D Jet.	http://goo.gl/3Xifcl
Video 7.1	Great vessel axial plane.	http://goo.gl/YXAgna
Video 7.2	Guide wire crossing the interatrial septum.	http://goo.gl/r4qnXR
Video 7.3	Parasagittal long axis four-chamber plane.	http://goo.gl/7CW38U
Video 7.4	Profile of Amplatzer septal occluder implanted.	http://goo.gl/gJRdXm
Video 13.1	The needle is directed medially, superiorly and posteriorly while small amount of dilute contrast is injected to outline the hepatic vein.	http://goo.gl/pQEwlw
Video 13.2	Contrast is injected outlining the hepatic vein.	http://goo.gl/DjDivW
Video 13.3	Hand injection outlines portal vein rather than the hepatic vein.	http://goo.gl/gIVGxu
Video 13.4	The needle is guided toward the hepatic vein while contrast is being injected.	http://goo.gl/85B9g9
Video 13.5	Hand injection demonstrates thrombosis of the inferior baffle of Fontan patient. Thus the hepatic route could not be used.	http://goo.gl/pgiclw
Video 13.6	The wire is manipulated along the hepatic vein to the heart.	http://goo.gl/I8CsxT
Video 13.7	Sheath advancement is facilitated by the straight wire course. The dilator may need to be separated from the sheath while advancing the sheath in small infants to avoid trauma to the heart.	http://goo.gl/3aSuf1
Video 13.8	Transhepatic stenting of stenosed RV to PA conduit.	http://goo.gl/cduQNG
Video 13.9	Balloon atrial septostomy is being performed in a 2-day-old newborn using the transhepatic approach.	http://goo.gl/BAxryP
Video 13.10	A pulmonary vein wedge angiogram using the transhepatic approach outlines the stenoses of Sano anastomosis in a patient with hypoplastic left heart syndrome.	http://goo.gl/zT62zR
Video 13.11	A pulmonary vein wedge angiogram using the transhepatic approach outlines the stenoses of Sano anastomosis in a patient with hypoplastic left heart syndrome.	http://goo.gl/mgd0Cx
Video 13.12	Dilated hepatic veins in a patient with single ventricle.	http://goo.gl/8Yf9xK
Video 13.13	The transhepatic approach allowed the use of a relatively larger sheath for balloon angioplasty of coarctation in a patient with single ventricle post-stage 1 palliation preserving the femoral artery.	http://goo.gl/hPMq8Q
Video 13.14	Transhepatic stenting of LPA in a Fontan patient with complex congenital heart disease consisting of heterotaxy syndrome, interrupted IVC, and left SVC with no right SVC.	http://goo.gl/mhguiO

(continued)

(continued)

Contributors

Tommaso Acquaviva
Department of Emergency and Organs Transplantation
University of Bari
Bari, Italy

Hitesh Agrawal
Department of Pediatrics
John H. Stroger Jr. Hospital of Cook County
Chicago, Illinois

Zaheer Ahmad
King Abdulaziz Cardiac Center
King Abdulaziz Medical City
National Guard Health Affairs
Riyadh, Saudi Arabia

Lishan Aklog
Pavilion Holdings Group
and
PAXmed Inc.
New York, New York

Mustafa Al-Qbandi
Department of Pediatric Cardiology
Chest Diseases Hospital
Kuwait City, Kuwait

Mazeni Alwi
Paediatric and Congenital Heart Centre
Institut Jantung Negara (National Heart Institute)
Kuala Lumpur, Malaysia

Rui Anjos
Department of Pediatric Cardiology
Hospital de Santa Cruz
Lisbon, Portugal

R. Arora
New Delhi, India

Jeremy Asnes
Pediatric Cardiology
Yale School of Medicine
New Haven, Connecticut

Nitish Badhwar
Department of Medicine
University of California–San Francisco
San Francisco, California

Jesus Damsky Barbosa
Catheterization Laboratory for Congenital Heart
    Disease
Hospital de Niños Pedro de Elizalde
Buenos Aires, Argentina

Krzysztof Bartus
Department of Cardiovascular Surgery and
    Transplantology
Jagiellonian University
John Paul II Hospital
Krakow, Poland

John L. Bass
University of Minnesota
Amplatz Children's Hospital
Minneapolis, Minnesota

Lee Benson
Department of Pediatrics
Hospital for Sick Children
University of Toronto School of Medicine
Toronto, Ontario, Canada

Jamie Bentham
Department of Paediatric Cardiology
John Radcliffe Hospital
Oxford, United Kingdom

Stefan Bertog
CardioVascular Center Frankfurt
Frankfurt, Germany

Peter C. Block
Emory University School of Medicine
Emory University Hospital
Atlanta, Georgia

Philipp Bonhoeffer
Department of Cardiology
Fondazione G. Monasterio
Pisa, Italy

Alessandro Santo Bortone
Department of Emergency and Organs
 Transplantation
University of Bari
Bari, Italy

I. Bozdag-Turan
Department of Cardiology
University Hospital Rostock
Rostock, Germany

Andras Bratincsak
Department of Pediatrics
University of Hawaii
Honolulu, Hawaii

Annkathrin Braut
CardioVascular Center Frankfurt
Frankfurt, Germany

Grazyna Brzezinska-Rajszys
The Heart Catheterization Laboratory
Department of Pediatric Cardiology
Children's Memorial Health Institute
Warsaw, Poland

Lutz Buellesfeld
Department of Cardiology
Bern University Hospital
Bern, Switzerland

Franziska Buescheck
CardioVascular Center Frankfurt
Frankfurt, Germany

Haran Burri
Department of Medical Specialties
University Hospital of Geneva
Geneva, Switzerland

Carla Canniffe
Mater Misericordiae Hospital
Dublin, Ireland

Qi-Ling Cao
Rush Center for Congenital and Structural Heart
 Disease
Rush University Medical Center
Chicago, Illinois

Massimo Caputo
University of Bristol
Bristol, United Kingdom

Francesco Casilli
Emodinamica e Radiologia Cardiovascolare
Policlinico San Donato IRCCS
Milan, Italy

John P. Cheatham
Nationwide Children's Hospital
and
Cardiology Division
The Ohio State University
Columbus, Ohio

Jonathan M. Chen
Seattle Children's Hospital
and
University of Washington School of Medicine
Seattle, Washington

Albert K. Chin
Pavilion Medical Innovations
Norwell, Massachusetts

Antonio Colombo
San Raffaele Scientific Institute
and
EMO-GVM Centro Cuore Columbus
Milan, Italy

Rodrigo N. Costa
Catheterization Laboratory for Congenital Heart Disease
Instituto Dante Pazzanese de Cardiologia and Hospital do
 Coração
São Paulo, Brazil

Matt Daniels
Radcliffe Department of Medicine
John Radcliffe Hospital
Oxford, United Kingdom

Ryan R. Davies
Nemours Cardiac Center
Alfred I. DuPont Hospital for Children
Wilmington, Delaware

Emanuela de Cillis
Institute of Cardiac Surgery
Department of Emergency and Organs Transplantation
University of Bari
Bari, Italy

Joseph DeGiovanni
Birmingham Children's and Queen Elizabeth Hospitals
Birmingham, United Kingdom

Brian J. deGuzman
Pavilion Holdings Group
and
Kaleidoscope Medical LLC
Paradise Valley, Arizona

Mirko Doss
Department of Thoracic and Cardiovascular Surgery
Kerckhoff Clinic
Bad Nauheim, Germany

Makram R. Ebeid
University of Mississippi Medical Center
Jackson, Mississippi

Tina Edwards-Lehr
CardioVascular Center Frankfurt
Sankt Katharinen Hospital
Frankfurt, Germany

Neal Eigler
Heart Institute
Cedars-Sinai Medical Center
Los Angeles, California

Howaida El Said
Department of Pediatrics
Rady Children's Hospital
University of California San Diego
San Diego, California

Ted Feldman
Cardiology Division
Evanston Hospital
NorthShore University Health System
Evanston, Illinois

Hans Reiner Figulla
Department of Internal Medicine I
(Cardiology, Angiology, Pneumology and Intensive Care
    Medicine)
University Hospital Jena
Friedrich-Schiller University
Jena, Germany

Jennifer Franke
CardioVascular Center Frankfurt
Frankfurt, Germany

and

Department of Cardiology
University Hospital Heidelberg
Heidelberg, Germany

Christian Frerker
Division of Cardiology
Asklepios Klinik St. Georg
Hamburg, Germany

Sameer Gafoor
CardioVascular Center Frankfurt
and
Sankt Katharinen Hospital
Frankfurt, Germany

Mark Galantowicz
Department of Cardiothoracic Surgery
The Heart Center
Nationwide Children's Hospital
Columbus, Ohio

Wei Gao
Department of Cardiology
Shanghai Jiaotong University School of Medicine
Shanghai, People's Republic of China

Marc Gewillig
Pediatric Cardiology
University Hospital Gasthuisberg
Leuven, Belgium

Alexander Ghanem
Department of Cardiology
Asklepios Klinik St. Georg
Hamburg, Germany

Sebastian Goreczny
Evelina London Children's Hospital
London, United Kingdom

Miguel A. Granja
Catheterization Laboratory for Congenital Heart Disease
Hospital Italiano de Buenos Aires
Buenos Aires, Argentina

David Gregg
Division of Cardiology
Medical University of South Carolina
Charleston, South Carolina

Eberhard Grube
Department of Medicine/Cardiology
University Hospital Bonn
Bonn, Germany

Alexandra Heath
Pediatric Cardiology Section
Kardiocentrum
La Paz, Bolivia

William E. Hellenbrand
Pediatric Cardiology Department
Yale University Medical Center
New Haven, Connecticut

Ziyad M. Hijazi
Department of Pediatrics
Sidra Medical and Research Center
Doha, Qatar

and

Pediatrics and Internal Medicine
James A.Hunter, MD, University
Rush University Medical Center
Chicago, Illinois

Ilona Hofmann
Cardiovascular Center Frankfurt
Frankfurt, Germany

Noa Holoshitz
Rush Center for Congenital and Structural Heart Disease
Rush University Medical Center
Chicago, Illinois

H. Ince
Department of Cardiology
Vivantes Klinikum Am Urban und im Friedrichshain
Berlin, Germany

Frank F. Ing
Children's Hospital–Los Angeles
and
University of Southern California
Los Angeles, California

Vladimir Jelnin
Lenox Hill Heart and Vascular Institute
North Shore/LIJ Health System
New York, New York

Saibal Kar
Heart Institute
Cedars-Sinai Medical Center
Los Angeles, California

Damien Kenny
Rush Center for Congenital and Structural Heart
    Disease
Rush University Medical Center
Chicago, Illinois

Prafulla Kerkar
Department of Cardiology
King Edward VII Memorial Hospital
Mumbai, India

Sachin Khambadkone
Paediatric and Adolescent Cardiology
Great Ormond Street Hospital
London, United Kingdom

S. Kische
Department of Cardiology
Vivantes Klinikum Am Urban und im
    Friedrichshain
Berlin, Germany

Chad Kliger
Lenox Hill Heart and Vascular Institute
North Shore/LIJ Health System
New York, New York

Miltiadis Krokidis
Department of Radiology
Addenbrooke's University Hospital
Cambridge, United Kingdom

Karl-Heinz Kuck
Division of Cardiology
Asklepios Klinik St. Georg
Hamburg, Germany

R. Krishna Kumar
Amrita Institute of Medical Sciences and
    Research Centre
Kerala, India

Robert Kumar
Lenox Hill Heart and Vascular Institute
North Shore/LIJ Health System
New York, New York

Simon Lam
Cardiovascular Center Frankfurt
Frankfurt, Germany

Azeem Latib
San Raffaele Scientific Institute
and
EMO-GVM Centro Cuore Columbus
Milan, Italy

Larry Latson
Pediatric and Adult Congenital Cardiology
Joe DiMaggio Children's Hospital
Memorial Healthcare System
Hollywood, Florida

Alexander Lauten
Department of Internal Medicine I
(Cardiology, Angiology, Pneumology and Intensive Care
    Medicine)
University Hospital Jena
Friedrich-Schiller University
Jena, Germany

Trong-Phi Le
Department of Structural and Congenital Heart Disease
Klinikum Links der Weser
Bremen, Germany

Randall J. Lee
Department of Medicine
University of California–San Francisco
San Francisco, California

Ting-Liang Liu
Department of Cardiology
Shanghai Children's Medical Center
Shanghai, People's Republic of China

Kiran K. Mallula
Rush Center for Congenital and Structural Heart
    Disease
Rush University Medical Center
Chicago, Illinois

Katharina Malsch
Klinikum Hanau
Hanau, Germany

Takashi Matsumoto
Heart Institute
Cedars-Sinai Medical Center
Los Angeles, California

Bernhard Meier
Department of Cardiology
Bern University Hospital
Bern, Switzerland

Inês Carmo Mendes
Department of Pediatric Cardiology
Hospital de Santa Cruz
Lisbon, Portugal

Haverj Mikailian
Department of Pediatrics
The Hospital for Sick Children
The University of Toronto School of Medicine
Toronto, Ontario, Canada

Sa'ar Minha
MedStar Washington Hospital Center
Washington, DC

Marhisham Che Mood
Paediatric and Congenital Heart Centre
Institut Jantung Negara (National Heart Institute)
Kuala Lumpur, Malaysia

Jose Pablo Morales
Division of Cardiovascular Devices
U.S. Food and Drug Administration
Silver Spring, Maryland

Mamoo Nakamura
Heart Institute
Cedars-Sinai Medical Center
Los Angeles, California

Georg Nickenig
Department of Medicine II
University Hospital Bonn
Bonn, Germany

C. A. Nienaber
Department of Cardiology
University Hospital Rostock
Rostock, Germany

Fabian Nietlispach
University Heart Center
University Hospital Zurich
Zurich, Switzerland

Stéphane Noble
Department of Medical Specialties
University Hospital of Geneva
Geneva, Switzerland

Anthony Nobles
Westsachsen Hochschule
Zwickau, Germany

Eustaquio M. Onorato
Dipartimento Cardiovascolare
Humanitas Gavazzeni
Bergamo, Italy

Igor F. Palacios
Department of Medicine
Massachusetts General Hospital
Boston, Massachusetts

John L. Parks
Division of Cardiology
Medical University of South Carolina
Charleston, South Carolina

Carlos A. C. Pedra
Catheterization Laboratory for Congenital Heart Disease
Instituto Dante Pazzanese de Cardiologia
and
Hospital do Coração
São Paulo, Brazil

Simone R. F. Fontes Pedra
Echocardiography Laboratory for Congenital Heart
    Disease
Instituto Dante Pazzanese de Cardiologia
and
Hospital do Coração
São Paulo, Brazil

Alejandro Peirone
Pediatric Cardiology Section
Hospital Privado de Córdoba,
Córdoba, Argentina

C. Fábio A. Peralta
Hospital do Coração
and
Universidade de Campinas (UNICAMP)
São Paulo, Brazil

Augusto D. Pichard
MedStar Washington Hospital Center
Washington, DC

Fabien Praz
Department of Cardiology
Bern University Hospital
Bern, Switzerland

Worakan Promphan
Queen Sirikit National Institute of Child Health
Rangsit University
Bangkok, Thailand

Shakeel A. Qureshi
Department of Congenital Heart Disease
Evelina London Children's Hospital
London, United Kingdom

P. Syamasundar Rao
Department of Pediatrics and Medicine
The University of Texas/Houston Medical School
Memorial Hermann Children's Hospital
Houston, Texas

Oleg Reich
Children's Heart Center
University Hospital Motol
Prague, Czech Republic

John Reidy
Department of Radiology
Guy's Hospital
London, United Kingdom

Kristina Renkhoff
Cardiovascular Center Frankfurt
Sankt Katharinen Hospital
Frankfurt, Germany

Marcelo S. Ribeiro
Catheterization Laboratory for Congenital Heart
    Disease
Instituto Dante Pazzanese de Cardiologia
and
Hospital do Coração
São Paulo, Brazil

Phillip Roberts
The Heart Centre for Children
Childrens Hospital at Westmead
Westmead, Australia

Carlos E. Ruiz
Department of Cardiology in Pediatrics and Medicine
North Shore-LIJ School of Medicine
Hofstra University
New York, New York

Monique Sandhu
Division of Cardiology
Medical University of South Carolina
Charleston, South Carolina

Ulrich Schäfer
Division of Cardiology
Asklepios Klinik St. Georg
Hamburg, Germany

Martin B. E. Schneider
Department of Pediatric Cardiology
German Pediatric Heart Centre
Sankt Augustin, Germany

Gerhard C. Schuler
Department of Internal Medicine/Cardiology
University of Leipzig Heart Center
Leipzig, Germany

Peter Sick
Hopsital Barmherzige Brüder Regensburg
Regensburg, Germany

Horst Sievert
Cardiovascular Center Frankfurt
and
Sankt Katharinen Hospital
Frankfurt, Germany

Ulrich Sigwart
Department of Cardiology
University of Geneva
Geneva, Switzerland

Guilherme V. Silva
Texas Heart Institute
Houston, Texas

Jan-Malte Sinning
Department of Medicine II
University Hospital Bonn
Bonn, Germany

Daniel H. Steinberg
Division of Cardiology
Medical University of South Carolina
Charleston, South Carolina

Petr Tax
Children's Heart Center
University Hospital Motol
Prague, Czech Republic

Alejandro J. Torres
Pediatric Catheterization Laboratory
New York-Presbyterian Morgan Stanley Children's
    Hospital
New York, New York

Luis Trentacoste
Catheterization Laboratory for Congenital Heart
    Disease
Hospital de Niños Ricardo Gutiérrez
Buenos Aires, Argentina

R. Goekmen Turan
Department of Cardiology
University Hospital Rostock
Rostock, Germany

Laura Vaskelyte
Cardiovascular Center Frankfurt
Frankfurt, Germany

Joseph John Vettukattil
Congenital Cardiac Center
Helen DeVos Children's Hospital
Grand Rapids, Michigan

Ron Waksman
MedStar Washington Hospital Center
Washington, DC

Kevin P. Walsh
Mater Misericordiae Hospital
Dublin, Ireland

Nikos Werner
Department of Medicine II
University Hospital Bonn
Bonn, Germany

Brian Whisenant
Intermountain Heart Institute
Salt Lake City, Utah

Johannes Wilde
Department of Internal Medicine/Cardiology
University of Leipzig Heart Center
Leipzig, Germany

Neil Wilson
Department of Paediatric Cardiology
John Radcliffe Hospital
Oxford, United Kingdom

Stephan Windecker
Department of Cardiology
Bern University Hospital
Bern, Switzerland

Wen-Loong Yeow
Heart Institute
Cedars-Sinai Medical Center
Los Angeles, California

Evan M. Zahn
Congenital Heart Institute
Miami Children's Hospital
and
Arnold Palmer Women and Children's Hospital
Miami, Florida

Mario Zanchetta
Dipartimento Malattie Cardiovascolari
Azienda U.L.S.S.
Cittadella, Padova, Italy

1

How to design and operate a congenital-structural catheterization laboratory

John P. Cheatham

Introduction

What would Werner Forsmann say about what has happened since that fateful day, so long ago, when he performed the first cardiac catheterization on himself? Of course, he never actually reached his heart with the catheter the first time AND he was banished from his promising career as a young surgeon. However, his spirit exemplifies what has now become the modern-day interventional cardiologist. Since there is a distinction between the cardiologist trained to treat adults with predominant coronary artery and acquired cardiac disease and those cardiologists specially trained to manage congenital heart disease, the same can be said for the cardiac catheterization laboratories in which these patients are treated. For the purpose of this chapter, the design, equipment required, necessary inventory, and personnel requirements for the modern-day lab dedicated to advanced transcatheter therapy for the smallest newborn to the largest adult with complex congenital heart disease, will be discussed. The author readily acknowledges the biases instilled in him by his mentor and idol, Charles E. (Chuck) Mullins, MD, who has taught many of the congenital heart interventionalists across the globe (Figure 1.1a and b).

A new era

Historically, cardiothoracic surgeons and interventional cardiologists have had a somewhat competitive relationship. This is especially true with physicians treating coronary and acquired cardiac disease in adults. However, a "team concept" has always been important when establishing a center of excellence for the treatment of complex congenital heart disease. The collaborative spirit between the cardiac surgeon and the entire cardiology team has advanced therapies offered to patients. More recently, the unique relationship between the interventionalist and

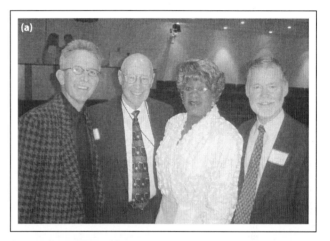

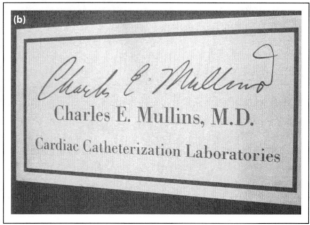

Figure 1.1 Charles E. (Chuck) Mullins, MD has taught and inspired many interventionalists specializing in congenital heart disease all over the world. (a) During the dedication ceremony at Texas Children's Hospital, Dr. Mullins gathers with some of his "aging" pupils and his longtime cath lab assistant. (b) The new cath labs were named in Chuck's honor ... an honor well deserved.

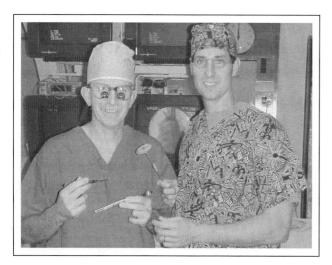

Figure 1.2 The unique and collegial relationship between the interventional cardiologist and cardiothoracic surgeon has fostered new Hybrid treatment strategies for complex congenital heart disease. However, sometimes the members of the team get confused and want each other's job!

surgeon has fostered combined transcatheter and surgical therapeutic options ... so-called Hybrid treatment[1–3] (Figure 1.2). This innovative spirit mandates a fresh and open mind to create the "ideal" venue, or Hybrid Suite, to expand the capabilities of the traditional cath lab and operating room.[4] Now, our colleagues in structural heart disease (SHD) have also learned the value in collaborating with their cardiac surgeon colleagues. Transcatheter aortic valve replacement (TAVR) has been the "lightning rod" to encourage this teamwork, and new Hybrid Suites are being designed in this field as well.

Hybrid Suite design

In planning an ideal Hybrid Suite, there are five major considerations: (1) personnel who will be participating in the procedure, (2) adequate space for the equipment and personnel, (3) equipment that is necessary, (4) informational management and video display, and (5) necessary inventory and consideration of costs.

Personnel

Traditionally, the team responsible for performing both diagnostic and interventional cardiac catheterizations in children and adults with congenital heart disease consists of the interventional cardiologist, an assisting fellow or cath lab nurse, and technicians and nurses who are responsible for monitoring the physiologic recorder and the x-ray imaging equipment, and for "circulating" in the room to assist with the procedure. These team members

were former ICU nurses, radiologic technicians, respiratory therapists, and paramedics who receive "on-the-job training." Specially trained registered cardiovascular invasive specialists (RCIS) are quite valuable in today's lab, as they are trained in all aspects of cath lab procedures and frequently have adult interventional experience. They are particularly helpful in treating adults with CHD and in the use of coronary stents, vascular closure devices, and small-diameter guidewires. All staff are "cross trained" to be able to run the imaging and hemodynamic equipment and rotate into any job necessary during the procedure. However, as the complexity of transcatheter procedures has evolved, many changes have been necessary to ensure safety and success.[5] A highly trained and competent assistant to the primary operator is imperative. A general pediatric cardiology fellow is usually inadequate to serve in this role today with the higher risk and complicated interventional procedures now performed. Therefore, it is becoming more common to have an advanced-level interventional cardiology fellow in the lab. However, many institutions do not have a general or advanced-level cardiology fellowship program, therefore, the role of a specially trained Interventional Nurse Practitioner has evolved and offers many advantages.

In addition to the team members mentioned above, dedicated cardiac anesthesia and cardiac ultrasound imaging is mandatory. This requires a staff anesthesiologist with assisting trainee or nurse anesthetist. A staff echocardiographer is also in attendance along with a fellow or technician. One gets the sense that the room is rapidly becoming crowded. By the way, dedicated anesthesia and echo equipment must find a home as well. With the new Hybrid procedures, the cardiothoracic surgeon and team will be present, which may include an assisting surgeon or resident, a scrub nurse, as well as the perfusionists and accompanying cardiopulmonary bypass machine. Now the suite really is shrinking! (Figure 1.3). The electrophysiologist and equipment when electrical therapy or a pacemaker is required can add up to 18 people, all with their specialized equipment, during a single Hybrid cardiac catheterization intervention for CHD!!! So, we have to design the suite to accommodate all of the personnel and the equipment.

Design: Space and ergonomics

The space required for a modern day Hybrid Cardiac Catheterization Suite is significantly more than a single-plane, adult coronary cath lab, or for that matter, the traditional biplane CHD cath lab built 10–20 years ago.[6–9] The suite design must account for the actual working space or procedure room, the control room, a computer "cold" room, an adjacent inventory supply room, and a new space very important to the modern suite ... the induction room, where all of the "team" can assess the

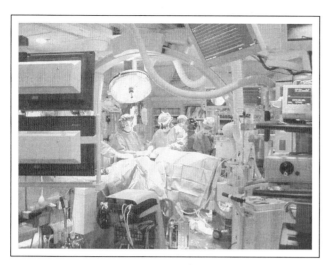

Figure 1.3 During a Hybrid cardiac procedure involving the surgical and interventional teams, as well as the perfusionist for cardiopulmonary bypass, the Hybrid Suite gets crowded very quickly. Space and proper ergonomics in design will overcome many obstacles in a traditional cath lab or operative suite.

patient and discuss the procedure, as well as administer sedative/anesthetic agents. With dedicated personnel now being assigned to the suites, it is desirable to also plan for administrative office space, personnel offices and work-space, a conference and editing room, a "break" area, and dressing rooms with bathroom and shower facilities. For the purpose of this chapter, we will confine our remarks to the essential space dedicated to the actual procedure being performed.

Ideally, the Hybrid Suite should be a minimum of 800 square feet (sq. ft), and preferably 900–1000 sq. ft (Figure 1.4). A square room, rather than the conventional

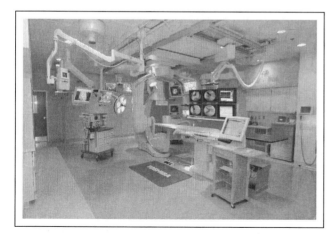

Figure 1.4 The appropriate space, design, and equipment are shown here in one of the Hybrid Suites at Columbus Children's Hospital. Note the flat-screen monitors, ceiling-mounted equipment, and video and equipment booms to allow easy access to the patient and informational imaging for all personnel.

rectangular suite, allows equal space around the catheter-ization table for complete patient accessibility ... 30" × 30" or 33′ × 33′ would be "ideal." This is especially important when interventional procedures may be performed from either femoral, jugular, or subclavian sites, and let us also not forget about transhepatic access. In the majority of Hybrid procedures, access is required through a median sternotomy and personnel will be on both sides of the table. There must be room for the anesthesiology team and anesthesia equipment at the head of the patient and to either side, while space must also be available for the echocardiography personnel and echo machine at the head of the patient during transesophageal echo (TEE), and at the end of the table for intracardiac echo (ICE) or intravascular ultrasound (IVUS) (Figure 1.5a and b). The

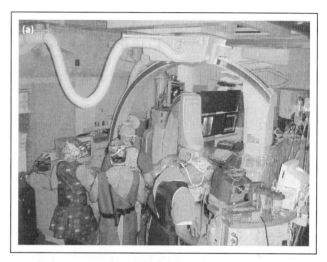

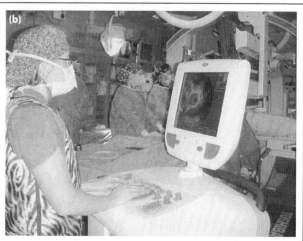

Figure 1.5 It is important to design appropriate space for the echo and anesthesia teams to be involved in transcatheter or Hybrid therapy for congenital heart disease. (a) The echo and anesthesia teams have a completely free space at the head of the table during TEE guidance of device closure. (b) In addition, dur-ing IVUS or ICE examination, the space at the foot of the table must also allow the team to do their job.

perfusionist and cardiopulmonary bypass machine will usually be positioned on the side opposite the surgeon and/or interventionalist, making the width of the room extremely important and different from a traditional cath lab … hence, a square room.

The control room should be as wide as the Hybrid Suite (25–33 ft) and approximately 10 ft in depth. This will allow all of the personnel, along with the physiologic and digital x-ray imaging equipment and monitors to be strategically placed. In addition, the digital review station and archiving system should be located in this room. In the combined interventional/electrophysiology suite, appropriate EP recording, pacing, radiofrequency ablation, and 3D mapping equipment must also be placed in the control room. This room should be designed in order for the personnel to view the procedure directly by looking down the table from the foot to the head of the patient (Figure 1.6). This ensures an unobstructed view of the procedure, regardless of the position of the biplane equipment or the team. Therefore, the patient table should be perpendicular to the control room. The adjacent computer or "cold room" size will be dependent on the manufacturer's specifications, but should allow easy access for maintenance or repair work to be performed. When building multiple suites, this room can be shared to conserve space.

The suite should also have an adjacent and ample supply room to store the extra inventory and consumable equipment that is not located in the cabinet storage within the procedure room. A blanket warmer is placed here, as well as other nonconsumable equipment. If possible, the adjacent supply room should be approximately 100–120 sq. ft and should be directly accessible from the procedure room

for maximum efficiency. If there are multiple suites, then a larger central supply room could be used that is accessible to both suites.

A relatively new concept in both surgery and interventional cardiology is the use of an "induction room" adjacent to the Hybrid Suite (Figure 1.7). This room becomes very important, since it allows the interventional, anesthesia, and surgical teams direct access to the patient and family, while maintaining a quiet and comforting environment to explain the procedures, perform history and physical examinations, and administer sedation. By installing small, space-efficient anesthesia machines that can be mounted on the wall, induction can be performed here as needed. In addition, this room may serve as a separate TEE room while an interventional catheterization is being performed, allowing maximum efficiency of the anesthesiology team. Ideally, this room should be approximately 12 ft × 17 ft, which will allow the appropriate family members and personnel to interact in a comfortable environment.

Not mentioned is the mandatory soil or "dirty" room where reusable equipment is washed; this must be separate from the "clean" scrub room, as per OSCHA standards. Also, when building two Hybrid Suites, it becomes apparent that a centrally located scrub area with two separate sinks be located immediately outside the procedure rooms with open access from both control rooms, but appropriate barriers for infection control. This allows maximum efficiency and entry into both suites, while maintaining safety and a sterile environment.

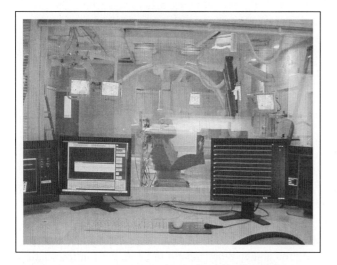

Figure 1.6 The control room should be designed to allow personnel to view the catheterization procedure without obstruction. Note the clear line of view down the table during the final phase of Hybrid Suite construction.

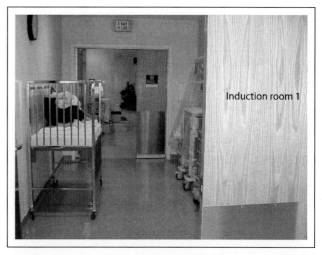

Figure 1.7 A relatively new concept is the use of an "induction room," which allows access to the patient and family by all team members in a quiet environment. Wall-mounted anesthesia equipment conserves space and allows sedation or induction of anesthesia as needed. The room should be directly connected to the Hybrid Suite, as shown here.

Equipment

What used to be a pretty simple list of equipment needs 15 years ago, has mushroomed into a huge cloud of needs, wants, and money! Biplane x-ray imaging equipment and a physiologic monitoring system with recording and reporting capabilities occupied most of the capital expense requirements of the traditional lab. However, the new Hybrid Suite's capital equipment list has grown proportionally, incorporating many services within a Heart Center.

Beginning with x-ray equipment, we certainly live in a new age of imaging. While some might argue the merits of biplane versus single-plane fluoroscopic and angiographic units, no one would dispute the clear advantages of displaying complex spatial anatomy using biplane cameras. This is especially true when performing transcatheter procedures in the tiniest preterm neonate to the 200 kg adult with complex CHD. So in a perfect world and without consideration of costs or space requirements, a modern biplane, digital cath lab is mandatory to achieve optimal imaging for the complicated interventional procedures of today.

Today, no one would argue the merits of digital (film-free) radiographic systems. The obvious advantages of digital technology are real-time access and viewing; no deterioration of images; ease of storage, management, and retrieval of image data; and labor savings. The digital images are easily accessible both inside and outside the hospital using a web server, as well as by remote satellite transmission. Yet, just as the "digital age" in cardiac catheterization began over two decades ago, we now live in the world of PC-based digital platforms and flat-panel detectors (FPD). This began with General Electric Medical's introduction of a single-plane FPD, then the PC-based digital platform for hemodynamic monitoring systems arrived in 2004, and culminated with the introduction of biplane FPD technology in 2005 by Siemens Medical and Toshiba Medical Systems Corporation. The targeted specialties for this new equipment are centers specializing in CHD cardiac catheterizations, advanced electrophysiology laboratories, and neuroradiology treatment centers.

We must ask, what are the advantages of FPD technology?[10,11] The definition of FPD is a compressed or flat detector that uses semiconductors or thin-film transistors (TFT), converts x-ray energy into electrical signals, and creates x-ray images. Currently, indirect-conversion FPD technology is used for biplane systems. Eventually, direct conversion technology may be used, once the "blanking" and frame rate limitations are overcome in the biplane configuration. Direct conversion will improve resolution, as the image is never converted into light. The FPD will likely replace all existing x-ray detectors, such as image intensifier (I.I.)-TV cameras and spot film cameras, as well as film screen systems. For cardiovascular work, the small profile of the detector size will allow a more compact design and

facilitate improved patient access. In addition, high image quality with improved blood vessel detectability by high modulation transfer function (MTF) and no distortion will be an advantage.

Finally, 3D digital tomography and interventions are now possible. A new imaging armamentarium that is proving extremely useful is 3D rotational angiography (3DRA). A single FPD is utilized and is rotated around the patient in ~4 s in a 200° arc while a continuous injection of contrast is being delivered. This image can be immediately displayed on the video monitor. More importantly, the data can be reconstructed by an image processor into a virtual 3D volume rendered image that can be viewed within 45–60 s. This 3D image has no limitations in demonstrating the complex anatomy in patients with CHD. One can view a structure from the patient's head, feet, back, front, and incorporating any angle of interrogation. One can also assess adjacent structures to evaluate their impact on the cardiac lesion. This greatly increases the interventionalists' understanding of spatial anatomy and defects … similar to a 3D CT scan. However, a great advantage is that transcatheter therapy can be performed with immediate 3DRA confirmation of the results (Figure 1.8). In the not too distant future 4DRA will become available. Some believe that the new technology of 3DRA and 4DRA may render biplane imaging equipment obsolete.

In the dedicated CHD Hybrid Suite, patient accessibility is equally important to high-quality imaging. Therefore, since the 3D gantry positioner was introduced by General Electric Medical nearly two decades ago, other companies now have realized the importance of patient access in a biplane lab. Since a three-dimensional gantry allows rotation of the C-arm in an X, Y, and Z axis, this allows additional space at the head of the table to accommodate the anesthesia and interventional teams. However, with the original design by GE and later Siemens Medical, the space was still crowded. The most recent and innovative design has come from Toshiba Medical Systems Corporation with a 5 axis C-arm positioner with biplane FPD (Infinix CF-i/BP), which allows movement in 5 axes around the patient, with rotation of the C-arm base to −135° or +135° which actually places the C-arm on the "foot" side of the lateral camera (Figure 1.9). This allows a completely "head-free zone" of 180° while in a biplane configuration, allowing easy access to the patient by the anesthesia, echo, and interventional teams (Figure 1.10). It is also highly beneficial to the electrophysiology service during complex studies with transvenous pacemaker implantation.

All teams must have not only free access to the patient, but also a clear line of sight to the image display monitors. Speaking of monitors, the days of the CRT monitors over. Flat-screen monitors have achieved comparable black-white, grayscale, and line resolution, and are ergonomically more versatile in a biplane laboratory. They take up less space, are lighter, and can be mounted on a

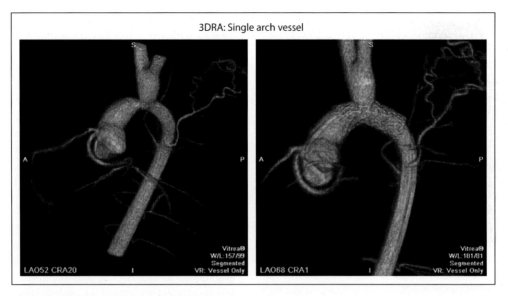

Figure 1.8 (**See color insert.**) A 3-dimensional rotational angiogram (3DRA) nicely demonstrates a complex postoperative aortic arch obstruction before and after stent therapy.

six-monitor gantry that can be strategically placed around the procedure table to allow optimal viewing by all personnel participating in the procedure, regardless of location (Figure 1.11). This gantry should be able to be placed on either side of the table, as well as over the table at the head or foot of the patient. Newer and larger, single multi-imaging monitors are becoming popular while allowing multiple sources of images to be displayed directly in front of the operator. In the Hybrid Suite, it is also important to install a surgical light mounted strategically on the ceiling. We also prefer to mount all other accessory equipment from the ceiling, that is, contrast injector with wall-mounted controls, local spotlight, and radiation shield.

The other components of x-ray imaging equipment found in the Hybrid Suite are fairly standard by today's standards. TV cameras using the charged-coupled device (CCD) technology, developed by Toshiba Medical Corporation, to improve brightness and resolution; x-ray tubes using spiral-grooved and liquid metal bearing technology, introduced by Phillips Medical to eliminate noise and reduce the delay in fluoro/digital acquisition; and high-frequency generators are now uniformly offered by all manufacturers. Furthermore, while using different technology, radiation dose management is a priority with all manufacturers to protect the patient and all those participating in the longer interventional catheterization procedures being performed today.[12] Advanced imaging processing (AIP) has been introduced by Toshiba Medical Systems to improve fluoroscopic images by reducing noise artifacts and eliminate frame averaging, which in turn allows "fluoro record" to be used instead of digital acquisition ... significantly reducing x-ray exposure (Figure 1.12). New innovations,

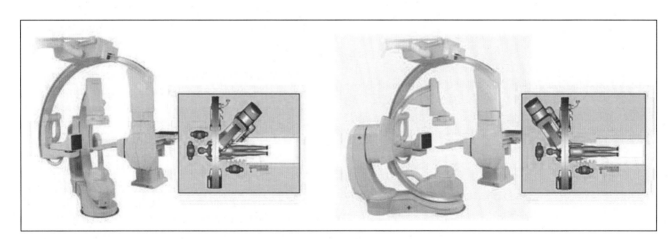

Figure 1.9 The new design of the Toshiba Infinix CF-i/BP positioners allows rotation of the C-arm base from −135° to +135°. This schematic drawing demonstrates the 180° of "head-free zone" afforded by this new design.

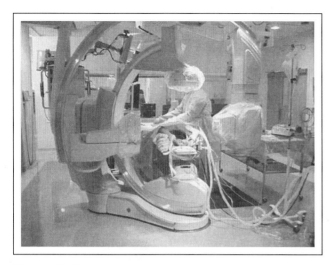

Figure 1.10 During a cardiac catheterization procedure, the open space at the head of the table is nicely demonstrated here. There is plenty of room for the interventional, echo, and anesthesia teams to perform their jobs.

such as "spot fluoroscopy" and "dose-tracking technology," are being introduced by the same manufacturer, which will further improve radiation safety for patients and personal in the Hybrid Suite.

An important, but forgotten, component of the new Hybrid Suite is the procedure table. Traditional cath lab tables have certain features that are well suited for x-ray imaging, patient positioning, quick and easy "free float" movement, and are electronically integrated into the manufacturer's x-ray imaging equipment. In addition, some tables have the ability to be placed in the Trendelenburg position. In comparison, the traditional operating room table is narrower, shorter, less "fluoro friendly," and does not provide

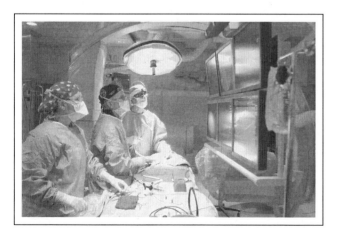

Figure 1.11 Flat-screen monitors have now approximated CRT monitors in terms of resolution. The lighter, more compact configuration of the flat-screen monitors allows a gantry holding six monitors to be easily positioned at any location for the Hybrid team to view the images, as depicted here during a Stage I Hybrid palliation for HLHS.

"free float" capabilities. Additionally, the table has the very important feature of 15–30° lateral tilt, which provides the cardiothoracic surgeon with exposure to the desired operative field ergonomically, while the Trendelenburg position is also possible. So, currently, either the surgeon or the interventionalist must make sacrifices while performing Hybrid procedures in the traditional operative or catheterization suite. A new Hybrid table is essential to facilitate new Hybrid management strategies for complex CHD. The table must be manufactured by the x-ray equipment companies in order to provide "connectivity" to the imaging equipment and possess tableside controls. This table must possess all of the above-mentioned specifications, so will require input from both cardiothoracic surgeons and interventional cardiologists as they are designed. Phillips Medical initially designed the first integrated Hybrid table, then Toshiba Medical Systems (Figure 1.13). Stay tuned for more in the future!

Informational management, video display, and transport

Staggering amounts of information are generated in today's healthcare environment and these data need to be readily available during the procedures. In our Heart Center, we attempted to provide access for angiography, echocardiography (including TTE, TEE, ICE, and IVUS), and the PACS system (CT, MRI, and chest x-ray) from any computer inside or outside the hospital with a dedicated web server and VPN access. This same information must be readily available in the new Hybrid Suites where complex procedures and decision making are being performed by the multidisciplinary team. The information needs to be accessible to all participants in the suite and must be specific to their assigned tasks. If the staff moves around the room, so must the displayed images. Furthermore, all of this information should be able to be transmitted to other sites within the hospital, that is, operative room, teleconference center, or research lab, as well as to sites anywhere in the world, that is, educational conferences, outside referring physicians for patient care, and teaching workshops. A dedicated and expansive archiving system is imperative for the digital technology of today. The data must be sent "seamlessly" between the archived source to the active procedure and/or educational site.

In an ideal world, money, space, and hospital administrative support would be unlimited. So, let us begin with the video display within the Hybrid Suite. Flat-screen monitors are strategically placed around the room, mounted to ceiling booms with a rotational axis that provides viewing from any location (Figure 1.14). We chose to enlist the expertise of Stryker Communications to fulfill these needs. Two monitors are mounted on three video booms, while one of the booms also serves as an equipment boom.

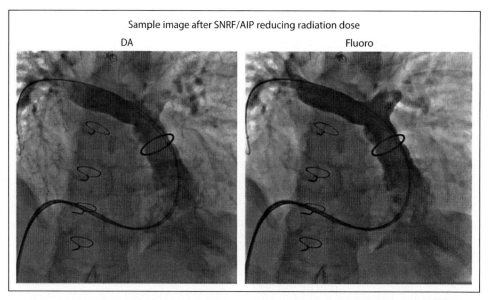

Figure 1.12 Advanced image processing (AIP) using signal noise reduction filter (SNRF) technology allows comparable diagnostic image quality compared with digital acquisition (DA) with significantly lower radiation dose, as seen in this patient before Melody TPV implant.

Mounted on the equipment boom is a defibrillator, fiber-optic surgeon's headlight, electrocautery, and a pan/tilt/zoom video camera. A second camera is mounted on the wall above the control room, providing expansive views of the suite and the procedures being performed. A video router is located within each suite and allows any image to be displayed on any video monitor, allowing each staff member optimal viewing of the information pertinent to their job. In turn, the video router in the Hybrid Suite is connected to a larger management and routing unit within the Teleconference Center, serving as the "mother ship" (Figure 1.15). All information can be transmitted anywhere in the world from this location. We believe this "video network topology" to be the framework of the future.

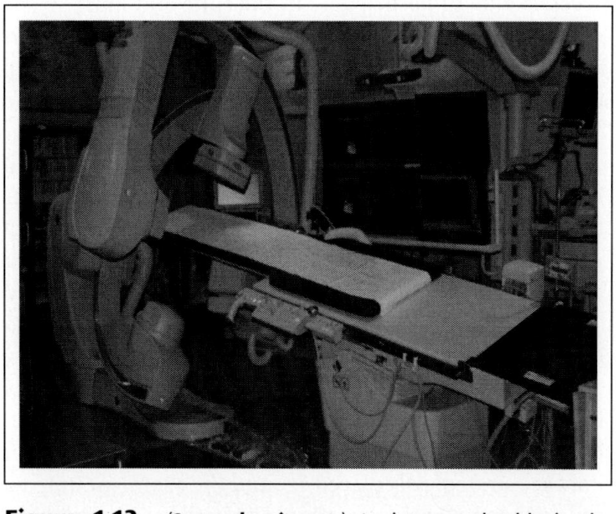

Inventory

Every cardiac catheterization procedure in patients with CHD requires a large inventory of "routine" consumable items. In addition, each interventional procedure requires an additional inventory of special and very expensive consumable materials. Words from my mentor, Dr. Mullins, are etched in my mind. "In a congenital heart laboratory, all consumable items must be available in a very wide range of sizes in order to accommodate every patient's size, from the tiniest premature neonate to the largest adult patient. A cardiac catheterization procedure NEVER should be compromised or terminated because of the lack of a necessary piece of consumable equipment." However, these special consumables will vary with the individual operator's experience and credentials, as well as with the availability of a particular device or material in any particular part of the world. Equally important in determining inventory is the individual hospital administrator's "budget" control. We are very fortunate to have tremendous hospital support, which seemingly allows unlimited access to all available consumables, that is, balloon catheters, devices, and delivery systems, stents, guidewires, RF perforating systems, all imaging

Figure 1.13 (**See color insert.**) An integrated table in the cardiac catheterization suite with x-ray equipment is mandatory. The ability of the table to "cradle or roll" and be placed in the Trendelenburg and reverse Trendelenburg positions is very important to the cardiac surgeon … as demonstrated in this photograph.

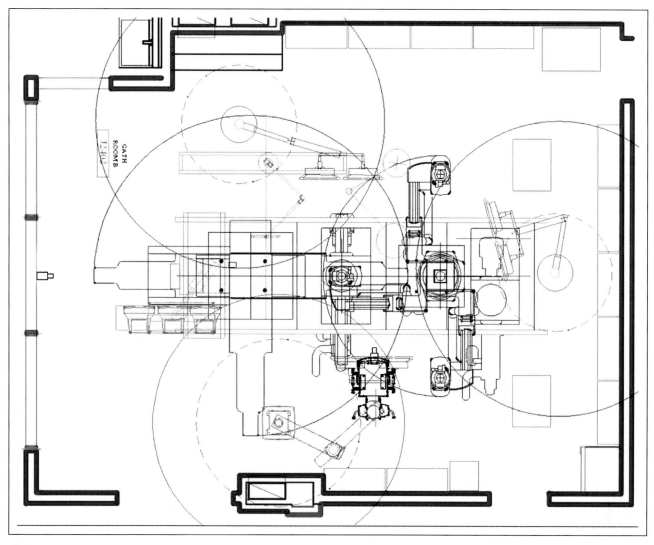

Figure 1.14   The schematic drawing of our Hybrid Suite demonstrates the importance of careful planning, input from multiple members of the Heart Center, and collaboration with several industry representatives. Note the video monitor and equipment boom design to ensure all personnel can view the appropriate images during the procedure, regardless of their location in the suite.

equipment (TTE, TEE, ICE, IVUS), and so on … which are justified and "reasonable." Now, we have to contend with stocking the extraordinarily expensive transcatheter heart valves! Accordingly, our inventory consumable costs are nearly US$2 million, so it is incumbent upon the cath lab manager and medical director to maintain strict inventory control and management. New "bar coders" can be used to scan all consumables used during the procedure to maintain an accurate accounting for billing purposes, as well as maintaining a computerized inventory and order management system. We have incorporated RFID technology (Mobile Aspects) in our suites that has proven to be extremely cost effective. The system tracts the inventory used for each patient, maintains par levels by reordering supplies, and bills the costs of the materials. Most new hemodynamic systems have an inventory management

program that can be used for this purpose. Unfortunately, economics, rather than necessity, will continue to dictate the practice of medicine.

Hybrid Cardiac Operating Suite

As the Hybrid procedures may be heavily weighted to a surgical component, it became clear that we needed to also design a Hybrid Cardiac Operating Suite to meet these needs (Figure 1.16a). The room design and equipment needs are a bit different from the Hybrid Cath Suite. The room space is similar, but a single-plane, ceiling-mounted FPD is more desirable in order to maintain the ergonomics of the surgical, anesthesia, and perfusion teams. A floor-mounted imaging system would be in the way, while the

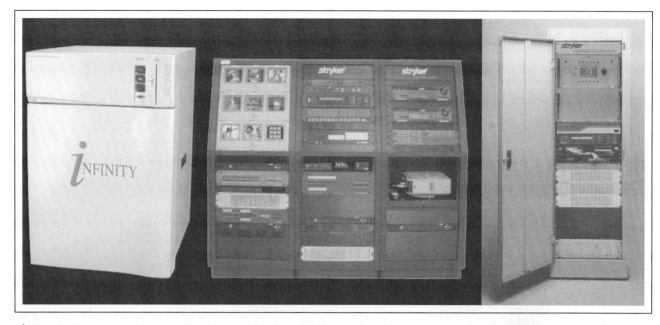

Figure 1.15   A large video router and informational management unit is located in our Teleconference Center and provides interconnectivity to the Hybrid Suites through the smaller video router and cameras within each suite. In turn, the operative suite and research laboratory can also be connected through the Teleconference Center, providing a "video network topology" for worldwide education and patient care.

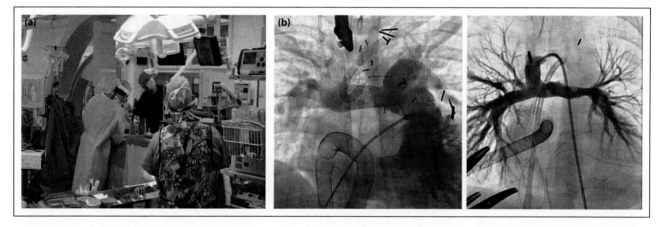

Figure 1.16   (**See color insert.**) The Hybrid Cardiac Operating Suite was the next evolution in Hybrid therapies and is used in both CHD and SHD. This will accommodate all members of the Hybrid team (a). Exit angiography can now be easily performed to assess the operative procedure before the patient returns to the ICU, as seen in these two patients: after pulmonary valve replacement and intraoperative stents and after Comprehensive Stage II repair for HLHS (b).

ceiling-mounted system can be parked and easily positioned at the table when needed. The video monitors and imaging equipment are similar to the Hybrid Cath Suite. The control and equipment rooms can be smaller.

We have introduced "exit angiography" in this suite to better understand the results of complex surgical treatment of CHD (Figure 1.16b). We may then elect to treat any residual anatomic abnormalities by either surgical or transcatheter techniques before the patient leaves the Operating Suite and minimize a "stormy" CTICU course. More recently, we have introduced 3DRA into the Hybrid

Cardiac Operative Suite to allow a more comprehensive evaluation in a single-plane environment (Figure 1.17).

Summary

In conclusion, collaboration between the interventional cardiologist and cardiothoracic surgeon continues to increase as the Hybrid strategies for complex CHD evolve. Making informational resources available when and where they are needed can have a dramatic impact on patient care.

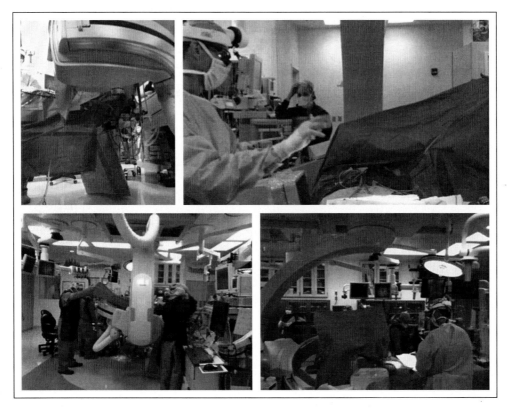

Figure 1.17   **(See color insert.)** The newest technology that has been added to the Hybrid Cardiac Operating Suite is 3DRA, as shown here in the meticulous setup in our suite.

The implementation of Hybrid Cardiac Catheterization and Operative Suites are a result of careful planning involving multiple disciplines, including Heart Center medical staff, equipment manufacturers, architects, contractors, and information technology specialists. Specially designed equipment and trained personnel are paramount to success. A huge inventory of consumables is required and must be judiciously managed. However, there is no substitute for a collegial and professional relationship and understanding among the Heart Center staff of the ultimate goals of success. Finally, it must be recognized that a progressive and forward-thinking hospital administrative staff is a prerequisite for the planning, building, and financial support necessary for the ideal Hybrid Cardiac Suites to become a reality.

References

1. Diab KA, Hijazi ZM, Cao QL, Bacha EA. A truly hybrid approach to perventricular closure of multiple muscular ventricular septal defects. *J Thorac Cardiovasc Surg* 2005;130(3):892–3.
2. Galantowicz M, Cheatham JP. Lessons learned from the development of a new hybrid strategy for the management of hypoplastic left heart syndrome. *Pediatr Cardiol* 2005;26(2):190–9.
3. Holzer R, Hijazi ZM. Interventional approach to congenital heart disease. *Curr Opin Cardiol* 2004;19(2):84–90.
4. Melvin DA, Chisolm JL, Lents JD, Chucta SD, Kish EC, Hardin J et al. A first generation hybrid catheterization laboratory: Ready for "prime time." *Catheter Cardiovasc Interv* 2004;63(1):123 (abst).
5. Mullins CE. History of pediatric interventional catheterization: Pediatric therapeutic cardiac catheterizations. *Pediatr Cardiol* 1998;19(1):3–7.
6. Mathewson JW. Building a pediatric cardiac catheterization laboratory and conference room: Design considerations and filmless imaging. *Pediatr Cardiol* 1996;17(5):279–94.
7. Verna E. Evolution of the catheterization laboratory: New instruments and imaging techniques. *Ital Heart J* 2001;2(2)116–7.
8. Section on Cardiology and Cardiac Surgery: American Academy of Pediatrics. Guidelines for pediatric cardiovascular centers. *Pediatrics* 2002; 109(3):544–9.
9. American College of Cardiology/Society for Cardiac Angiography and Interventions Clinical Expert Consensus Document on cardiac catheterization laboratory standards. A report of the American College of Cardiology Task Force on Clinical Expert Consensus Documents. *J Am Coll Cardiol* 2001;37(8):2170–214.
10. Holmes DR Jr, Laskey WK, Wondrow MA, Cusma JT. Flat-panel detectors in the cardiac catheterization laboratory: Revolution or evolution—What are the issues? *Catheter Cardiovasc Interv* 2004;63(3):324–30.
11. Chotas HG, Dobbins JT, Ravin CE. Principles of digital radiography with large-area, electronically readable detectors: A review of the basics. *Radiology* 1999;210:595–9.
12. Ross RD, Joshi V, Carravallah DJ, Morrow WR. Reduced radiation during cardiac catheterization of infants using acquisition zoom technology. *Am J Cardiol* 1997;79(5):691–3.

2

Operators' credentials and institutional requirements for congenital and structural heart disease

Ziyad M. Hijazi and Ted Feldman

Introduction

The category of congenital and structural (noncoronary) heart disease is large and growing. Congenital heart disease is the most common birth defect, with an incidence of approximately 1%. Most patients born with a cardiac defect live into adulthood. As of a few years ago in the United States, the number of adult patients with congenital cardiac defects (repaired, palliated, or unoperated) has exceeded those in the pediatric age group. Further, there are hundreds of thousands of patients who have valvular heart disease, including aortic valve stenosis, mitral regurgitation, and other valvular heart diseases. As the population ages, the number of patients with valvular heart disease is increasing.

The field of transcatheter treatment for congenital and structural/valvular heart disease has grown explosively over the past several years. Advances in new percutaneous devices and valves has enabled us to treat patients who only few years ago were thought to be either high-surgical-risk candidates or inoperable. The interest level in less invasive treatment options from patients and the medical community alike has increased significantly. Further, the recent regulatory approval of percutaneous valves and other devices to treat congenital and "structural" heart disease sparked the interest of many physicians and hospitals wanting to offer such treatment modalities to their patients.

While training program content, standards, credentialing, and board certifications for percutaneous coronary intervention have become well-developed, no such structure exists in the field of congenital, structural, or valvular heart disease therapies. In the absence of formalized criteria for training, some general principles are clear. Therefore, we believe that individuals and institutions that are interested in offering such therapies have to meet certain minimum criteria that will be discussed below.

Establishing a program in structural heart disease interventional therapies requires several key components (Table 2.1).

Operator knowledge base and training

Adequate knowledge in congenital and structural heart disease is essential for one individual to be able to care for and manage patients with various forms of congenital and structural heart disease. Currently, most interventional cardiovascular (CV) disease fellowship programs in the United States do not adequately train the individual to be able to perform or even care for such complex patients. We believe a minimum training of one year in a busy program that handles congenital and structural heart disease patients may be adequate to prepare such physicians on basic principles and to acquire core knowledge of the disease processes and treatment. The SCAI (Society for Cardiovascular Angiography and Interventions) has published a paper in which the core curriculum has been identified for pediatric invasive cardiologists who are to care for complex forms of congenital heart disease.[1] Also, the SCAI Structural Heart Disease Council has published

Table 2.1 Considerations for training
Knowledge base
Training
Simulation
Proctorship
Research trials
Multidisciplinary team
Institutional resources
Physical plant
Equipment/supplies
Personnel

another paper dealing specifically with the knowledge base for physicians who are to perform interventional procedures in adults with congenital and structural heart disease.[2]

Often, you may find a program that may be busy in one discipline or category of procedures but not in another. Therefore, the individual may seek further help/training from more than one program. The SCAI launched a survey in the United States of all programs that train physicians in congenital/structural heart disease.[3] In that survey, it was clear that not all institutions offer the entire spectrum in training. Further, the number of procedures performed in most institutions may not be large enough to train more than one individual. A similar survey is being arranged for European centers and perhaps other parts of the world.

Simulation/proctorship

The role of simulation in acquiring basic skills has seen dramatic increase in the last few years. Any new device that gets approval from the United States FDA includes in the regulatory process definition of a training program on how to use these devices once approved. Manufacturers and the FDA work together in setting the tone and process of device dissemination. For example, for atrial septal defect closure devices, prior to actually doing the case, the manufacturer requires the individual operator to attend a course. In that course, in addition to didactic lectures, there is a simulator where the operator gets trained on the device mechanics/techniques prior to doing any patient. Although, the simulators never exactly portray reality, they are the closest things to reality. The use of simulation in aviation training is well known.[4] There has been extensive experience with simulators in medicine, including anesthesiology for intubation and surgery for laparoscopic procedure training. For ASD closure, once the individual passes the training course, then the second phase moves to proctorship, where a certified proctor from the manufacturer visits and works with the individual on few cases. At the end of these training sessions, the proctor decides if the individual is ready to be an independent operator or he/she may require further training. This paradigm applies to the physician who is already out in practice, but does not provide a structure for training programs.

In contrast to coronary interventions, there are no published numbers to go by for certifying individuals in congenital/structural heart disease interventions. However, the American College of Cardiology/American Association for Thoracic Surgery (AATS)/Society of Thoracic Surgeons (STS)/SCAI have published a paper regarding transcatheter aortic valve implantation[5] in which a certain minimum number of procedures had to be acquired by the operators to be certified for the use of said valves. In that paper, the decision on certain numbers was not based on published evidence, but rather it was a consensus opinion. The published standards for coronary training create a paradox. The "magic number" for procedure volume for percutaneous coronary intervention (PCI) is 250 during an interventional fellowship. Congenital and structural procedure volumes are much lower than coronary, but many of the procedures are more complex. It is not possible to require even 100 cases during fellowship for most structural interventions.

Clinical research and clinical trials

One of the best avenues for training is participation in clinical trials. Many of the congenital and structural devices are new, and trials are ongoing to define their roles in practice, or to develop next-generation devices. Trial participation includes formal device training and also continued interaction with other operators regarding improvements in techniques and problem solving.

Institutional requirements

Any institution interested in offering patients transcatheter treatment for congenital and structural heart disease has to meet certain criteria. Obviously, the availability of cardiac surgery on the premises is essential. For congenital heart disease interventions, the presence of a program in congenital cardiac surgery is essential. This program should be performing all types of congenital cardiac surgery, from the simple to the most complex. Operations should be performed by at least one certified congenital cardiac surgeon. The need for a surgical program has less to do with surgery itself, and more to do with having an environment where decisions are made collaboratively. The institution should have a dedicated cardiac catheterization laboratory where cardiac catheterization (diagnostic/interventional) can be performed safely on such patients. For valvular heart transcatheter therapy, the presence of a hybrid suite is recommended with all the regulations that come with hybrid suites.[6] Detailed requirements have been determined by CMS (Centers for Medicare and Medicaid Services) for TAVR (transcatheter aortic valve replacement) procedures (Table 2.2).[7]

The cardiac catheterization/hybrid suite should be equipped with large inventory, including but not limited to:

Biplane fluoroscopy is preferable, but not essential; vascular closure devices and sheaths of varying sizes (from 6 to 24 Fr), length, and types, including Mullins sheaths; a wide variety of catheters (end holes, side holes, etc.); a variety of guide wires (hydrophilic, steerable, soft, stiff, extra stiff, and supra- and ultra-stiff), in regular length and exchange lengths; coronary and peripheral balloon dilation catheters of various sizes (balloon diameter and length), semi-compliant and noncompliant, low-pressure and high-pressure; stents of various sizes and design (open cell

Table 2.2   CMS operator and institutional requirement for TAVR

The patient (preoperatively and postoperatively) is under the care of a heart team: a cohesive, multidisciplinary team of medical professionals. The heart team concept embodies collaboration and dedication across medical specialties to offer optimal patient-centered care.

TAVR must be furnished in a hospital with the appropriate infrastructure that includes but is not limited to

1. On-site heart valve surgery program
2. Cardiac catheterization lab or hybrid operating room/catheterization lab equipped with a fixed radiographic imaging system with flat-panel fluoroscopy, offering quality imaging
3. Noninvasive imaging such as echocardiography, vascular ultrasound, computed tomography (CT), and magnetic resonance (MR)
4. Sufficient space, in a sterile environment, to accommodate necessary equipment for cases with and without complications
5. Post-procedure intensive care facility with personnel experienced in managing patients who have undergone open-heart valve procedures
6. Appropriate volume requirements per the applicable qualifications below

There are two sets of qualifications; the first set outlined below is for hospital programs and heart teams without previous TAVR experience and the second set is for those with TAVR experience.

Qualifications to begin a TAVR program for hospitals without TAVR experience:
The hospital program must have the following:

1. ≥50 total AVRs in the year prior to TAVR, including ≥10 high-risk patients
2. ≥2 physicians with cardiac surgery privileges
3. ≥1000 catheterizations per year, including ≥400 PCIs per year

Qualifications to begin a TAVR program for heart teams without TAVR experience:
The heart team must include:

1. Cardiovascular surgeon with:
   a. ≥100 career AVRs including 10 high-risk patients; or
   b. ≥25 AVRs in one year; or
   c. ≥50 AVRs in 2 years; and which include at least 20 AVRs in the last year prior to TAVR initiation
2. Interventional cardiologist with:
   a. Professional experience with 100 structural heart disease procedures lifetime; or
   b. 30 left-sided structural procedures per year of which 60% should be balloon aortic valvuloplasty (BAV). Atrial septal defect and patent foramen ovale closure are not considered left-sided procedures
3. Additional members of the heart team such as echocardiographers, imaging specialists, heart failure specialists, cardiac anesthesiologists, intensivists, nurses, and social workers
4. Device-specific training as required by the manufacturer

Qualifications for hospital programs with TAVR experience:
The hospital program must maintain the following:

1. ≥20 AVRs per year or ≥40 AVRs every 2 years
2. ≥2 physicians with cardiac surgery privileges
3. ≥1000 catheterizations per year, including ≥400 PCIs per year

Qualifications for heart teams with TAVR experience:
The heart team must include:

1. A cardiovascular surgeon and an interventional cardiologist whose combined experience maintains the following:
   a. ≥20 TAVR procedures in the prior year, or
   b. ≥40 TAVR procedures in the prior 2 years
2. Additional members of the heart team such as echocardiographers, imaging specialists, heart failure specialists, cardiac anesthesiologists, intensivists, nurses, and social workers

design vs. closed cell), short or long, bare and covered, and stent grafts for bail out dissections; snares of various sizes to retrieve foreign objects or to snare wires. Availability of valves of various sizes is a must if transcatheter valve replacement (aortic/pulmonic) is to be performed. The inventory is costly, and there are items that may not be used every 2 years, but their presence is essential. The cost of replacing expired inventory is part of "the cost of doing business," and this requires an institutional commitment. A failed procedure due to lack of proper equipment is no excuse!

Multidisciplinary team

The institution must have what is called a "heart team" on the premises. This concept has been adopted now by the major medical and surgical cardiovascular societies and is an integral part of the CMS requirements for institutions performing TAVR.[7] As stated in the CMS document, "The heart team concept embodies collaboration and dedication across medical specialties to offer optimal patient-centered care." The heart team should include interventional cardiologists who are trained and meet the procedure volume criteria for certification, cardiac and vascular surgeons who are also trained/certified, echocardiographers, CV anesthesiologists, perfusionists, nurse practitioners, and so on. The presence of other noncardiac services in the hospital is essential to manage these complex and often co-moribund patients, including pulmonologists, nephrologists, ID specialists, and others. The cardiology specialist has to develop considerable cross-specialty expertise as well, particulary with ultrasound and CT imaging.

Conclusion

Requirements for operator and institutional credentialing for congenital and structural interventions are largely undefined. The recent approval of TAVR has included criteria for this one procedure, and we will see more as other new devices are approved. In the meantime, some appreciation for a basic core curriculum[1] is essential, and each

operator has a responsibility to pursue his or her training in the spirit of becoming competent for a given procedure with the welfare of the patient as the guide, rather than simply complying with some arbitrary numerical procedure requirement. The experience we gain in training programs is usually just the beginning of a program of lifelong learning, and it takes many years to become proficient in the wide array of congenital and structural interventions. Structural intervention should be a full-time job for those who practice it!

References

1. Ruiz CE, Mullins CE, Rochini AP, Radtke WAK, Hijazi ZM, O'Laughlin MP et al. Core curriculum for the training of pediatric invasive/interventional cardiologists: Report of the Society for Cardiac Angiography and Interventions Committee on Pediatric Cardiology Training Standards. *Cath Cardiovasc Diag* 1996; 37:409–24.
2. Ruiz CE, Feldman TE, Hijazi ZM, Holmes DR, Webb JG, Tuzcu EM et al. Interventional fellowship in structural and congenital heart disease for adults. *Catheter Cardiovasc Interv* 2010;76:E90–105.
3. Marmagkiolis K, Hakeem A, Cilingiroglu M, Bailey SR, Ruiz C, Hijazi ZM et al. The Society for Cardiovascular Angiography and Interventions Structural Heart Disease Early Career Task Force Survey Results: Endorsed by the Society for Cardiovascular Angiography and Interventions. *Catheter Cardiovasc Interv* 2012; 80:706–11.
4. Gallagher AG, Cates CU. Virtual reality training for the operating room and cardiac catheterisation laboratory. *Lancet* 2004 Oct 23–29;364(9444):1538–40.
5. Tommaso CL, Bolman III RM, Feldman T, Bavaria J, Acker MA, Aldea G et al. Multisociety (AATS, ACCF, SCAI, and STS) Expert Consensus Statement: Operator and institutional requirements for transcatheter valve repair and replacement, Part 1: Transcatheter aortic valve replacement. *J Am Coll Cardiol* 2012;59:2028–42; originally published online Mar 1, 2012.
6. Bashore TM, Balter S, Barac A, Byrne JG, Cavendish JJ, Chambers CE et al. 2012 American College of Cardiology Foundation/Society for Cardiovascular Angiography and Interventions Expert Consensus Document on Cardiac Catheterization Laboratory Standards Update. *Cathet Cardiovasc Interven* 2012;80:E37–49.
7. National Coverage Analysis (NCA) for Transcatheter Aortic Valve Replacement (TAVR) (CAG-00430N). http://www.cms.gov/medicare-coverage-database/details/nca-details.aspx?NCAId=-257&NcaName=Transcatheter+Aortic+Valve+Replacement+%28TAVR%29&DocID=CAG-00430N&bc=gAAAAgAAAAA&.

3

Angiography

Lee Benson and Haverj Mikailian

Introduction

Accurate anatomical and physiological diagnosis is the foundation of a successful catheter-based therapeutic procedure. As such, a number of complementary imaging modalities have been developed to define, in real time, specific aspects of the heart and circulation for interventional applications. In the evolution of our understanding of the cardiovascular system, angiography and fluoroscopy were the first to be developed, and the angiography suite remains the cornerstone around which the interventional suite is built.

This chapter will include a discussion of standard angiographic approaches and how to achieve them. Emphasis will be placed on the application of these projections as applied to interventional procedures. A detailed description of the physical principles of image formation is beyond the scope of this chapter and the interested reader is referred to other sources for more detailed information.[1]

Angiographic projections

In the therapeutic management of the child with a congenital heart lesion, the spatial orientation and detailed morphology of the heart and great vessels are of critical importance. As the operator enters the laboratory, an overall understanding of the anatomy should have been synthesized, based on information from other imaging modalities such as chest roentgenography echocardiography, and computed tomographic, and magnetic resonance imaging. As such, the angiographic projections used in the procedure will be "tailored" to outline the lesion to allow appropriate measurements and guide the intervention.

In most children, the heart is oriented obliquely, with the left ventricular apex being leftward, anterior and inferior, and then the heart base (Figure 3.1). The interventricular septum is a complex geometric three-dimensional structure that takes an "S" curve from the apex to base (Figure 3.2), the so-called sigmoid septum. From

caudal to cranial, the interventricular septum curves through an arc of 100–120°. The right ventricle appears as an appliqué to the left. To address this unique topology, today's angiographic equipment allows a wide range of projections, incorporating caudocranial or craniocaudal angulations to outline or profile specific structures. The up-to-date laboratory of today consists of independent biplane-imaging chains, with which the proper selection of views minimizes overlapping and foreshortening of structures.[2]

Terminology

Angiographic projections are designated according to either the position of the recording detector (image intensifier or flat-panel detector) or the direction of the x-ray beam toward the recording device. Generally speaking, in cardiology the convention is the former, and all terminology discussed henceforth will use that convention. For example, when the detector is directly above a supine patient, the x-ray beam travels from posterior to anterior and the *angiographic projection* is designated posteroanterior (PA), but based on the detector *position*, it is called frontal, and the position of the detector by convention is at 0°. Similarly, when the detector is moved through 90°, to a position beside and to the left of the patient, a lateral (LAT) projection results. Between 0° and 90°, there are a multitude of projections termed left anterior oblique (LAO), and when the detector is moved to the right of the patient, a right anterior oblique projection (RAO) is achieved. As in the LAO projection, there are numerous RAO projections depending on the final angle from the midline. When the detector is posterior to the patient (the x-ray tube anterior), then a right (RPO) or left (LPO) posterior oblique projection occurs (Figure 3.3).

Standard detectors mounted on a C-arm or parallelogram, not only allow the above positions, but the detectors can be rotated around the transverse axis, toward the feet or head, expressed as caudal or cranial, respectively (Figure 3.4).

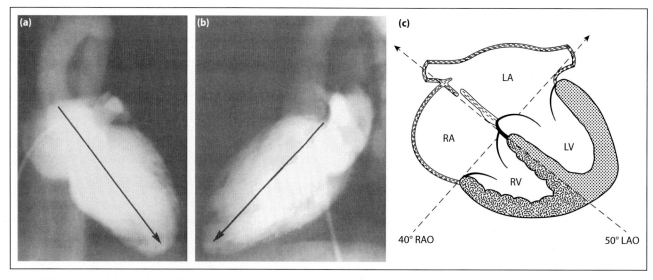

Figure 3.1 The typical lie of the heart in the chest. Panel (a)—frontal and (b)—LAT, projections of a left ventriculogram demonstrate the axis of the heart. The apex points anteriorly, inferiorly, and leftward. Panel (c) is a diagram of how standard mid-RAO and mid-LAO profile images of the axes of the heart. The RAO profiles the atrioventricular groove, and presents the ventricular septum en face. The mid-LAO view profiles the intraventricular septum, and separates the left and right ventricular and atrial chambers. (Modified from Culham JAG. Physical principles of image formation and projections in angiocardiography. In: Freedom RM, Mawson JB, Yoo SJ, Benson LN, Eds. *Congenital Heart Disease Textbook of Angiocardiography*. Chapter 2, figure 2-13. Armonk: Futura Publishing; 1997, pp. 39–93. With permission.)

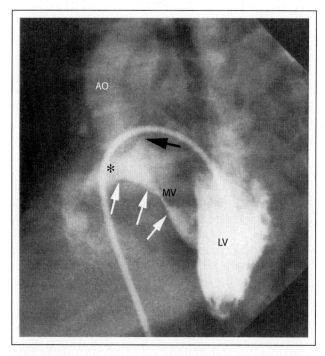

Figure 3.2 The sigmoid septum. A venous catheter is in the apex of the left ventricle through the mitral valve, in the long axis oblique projection. The sigmoid configuration of the septum is well seen (white arrows). Aortic–mitral continuity is noted (black arrow). Contrast is seen mixing across a ventricular defect (asterisk). (Modified from Culham JAG. Physical principles of image formation and projections in angiocardiography. In: Freedom RM, Mawson JB, Yoo SJ, Benson LN, Eds. *Congenital Heart Disease Textbook of Angiocardiography*. Chapter 2, figure 2-14. Armonk: Futura Publishing; 1997, pp. 39–93. With permission.)

In summary, the conventional terms RAO, LAO, PA, and left-LAT designate the position of the recording detector. The LAT position usually will have the detector to the left of the patient by convention, and will be so implied throughout this chapter. Finally, for clarification, while the term "projection" refers to the path of the x-ray beam, to be consistent with cardiological practice, projection or view will refer to the position of the detector.

Biplane angiography

As outlined in an earlier chapter discussing the ideal catheterization suite, dedicated interventional catheterization laboratories addressing congenital heart defects require biplane facilities.[3,4] Biplane angiography has the advantage of limiting contrast exposure and the assessment of evaluating the cardiac structures in real time in two projections simultaneously. However, this is at a cost, as these facilities are expensive, and with large flat-panel detectors, extreme simultaneous angulations can be compromised. The choice of a set of projections will depend on the information required, equipment capabilities, and the physical constraints to patient access. Standard biplane configurations include RAO/LAO, and frontal or LAT projections, with additional cranial or caudal tilt. The possible combinations are endless (Table 3.1 and Figure 3.5).

The cranial–LAO projections

A clear working understanding of these projections is of critical importance in developing a flexible approach to

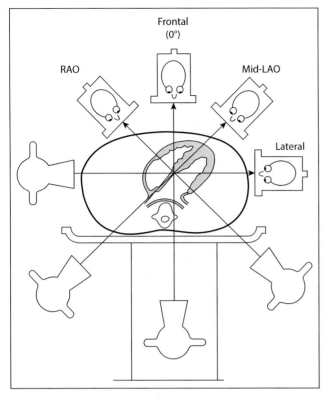

Figure 3.3 Naming the standard projections with the x-ray tube under the table. This diagrams the various positions of the detector/x-ray tube. The patient is supine, and the view is from the patient's feet, looking toward the head. (Modified from Culham JAG. Physical principles of image formation and projections in angiocardiography. In: Freedom RM, Mawson JB, Yoo SJ, Benson LN, Eds. *Congenital Heart Disease Textbook of Angiocardiography.* Chapter 2, figure 2-15. Armonk: Futura Publishing; 1997, pp. 39–93. With permission.)

congenital heart defect angiography and intervention. The practice of using "cookbook" projections for each case *may* allow acceptable diagnostic studies, but will fall short of the detail required to accomplish an interventional procedure. However, a comprehensive understanding of the normal cardiac anatomy, especially the interventricular septum, allows the operator to adjust the projection to optimize profiling the region of interest.

There are a number of "rules of thumb" that allow the operator to judge the steepness or shallowness of an LAO projection. Of importance is the relationship of the cardiac silhouette to the spine, the ventricular catheter, and the ventricular apex.

To optimize the profile of the midpoint of the *membranous ventricular septum*, (and thus the majority of perimembranous defects), two-thirds of the cardiac silhouette should be to the right of the vertebral bodies (Figures 3.6 and 3.7). This will result in a cranially tilted-left ventriculogram showing the left ventricular septal wall, the apex (denoted by the ventricular catheter) pointing toward the bottom of the image. A shallower projection will have more of the cardiac silhouette toward the left of the spine and profiles more of the inferobasal component of the septum, which is ideal for *inlet-type ventricular defects*. This projection allows for evaluation of atrioventricular valve relationships, inlet extension of perimembranous defects, and posterior muscular defects. A steeper LAO projection can be used to profile the *outlet extension of a perimembranous defect, and anterior muscular and apical defects*. As noted in Figure 3.6, the ventricular catheter in the cardiac apex can be used to help guide the projection, but only if it enters the chamber through the mitral valve. If catheter entry is through the ventricular defect or retrograde it tends to be more basal and left LAT.

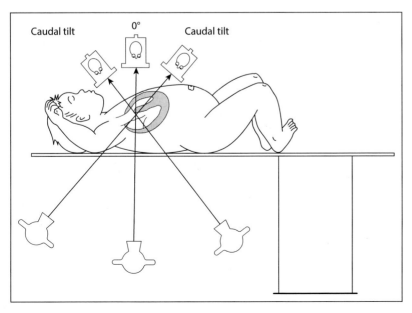

Figure 3.4 Naming the standard projections with the x-ray tube under the table. Cardiological convention is such that cranial and caudal tilt refers to the detector position. (Modified from Culham JAG. Physical principles of image formation and projections in angiocardiography. In: Freedom RM, Mawson JB, Yoo SJ, Benson LN, Eds. *Congenital Heart Disease Textbook of Angiocardiography.* Chapter 2, figure 2-16. Armonk: Futura Publishing; 1997, pp. 39–93. With permission.)

Table 3.1 Summary of projections

Projection	Angles	
Single-plane projections		
Conventional RAO	40° RAO	
Frontal	0°s	
Shallow LAO	1–30°	
Straight LAO	31–60°	
Steep LAO	61–89°	
Left-LAT	90° left	
Cranially tilted RAO	30° RAO + 30° cranial	
Cranially tilted frontal (sitting-up view)	30° or 45° cranial	
Cranially tilted shallow LAO	25° LAO + 30° cranial	
Cranially tilted mid-LAO (long-axis oblique)	60° LAO + 20° or 30° cranial	
Cranially tilted steep LAO (hepatoclavicular view)	45–70° LAO + 30° cranial	
Caudally tilted frontal	45° caudal	
Biplane combinations	**A plane**	**B plane**
AP and LAT	0°	Left-LAT
Long axial oblique (LXO)	30° RAO	*60° LAO + 20–30° cranial*
Hepatoclavicular view	*45° LAO + 30° cranial*	120° LAO + 15° cranial
Specific lesions		
RVOT-MPA (sitting up)	*10° LAO + 40° cranial*	Left- LAT
Long axial for LPA (biplane)	30° RAO	60° LAO + 30° cranial
LPA long axis (single plane)		60° LAO + 20° cranial
ASD	*30° LAO + 30° cranial*	
PA bifurcation and branches	*30° caudal + 10° RAO*	*20° caudal*

Note: Primary projections are in italics.
RAO = right anterior oblique, LAO = left anterior oblique, AP = anteroposterior, LAT = lateral, RVOT = right ventricular outflow tract, MPA = main pulmonary artery, LXO = long axis oblique, LPA = left pulmonary artery, ASD = atria septal defect, PA = pulmonary artery.

Modification of the cranial LAO projection will have to be made if there is a discrepancy in chamber sizes, and the septum rotated, such that a steeper or shallower projection may be required. Also, it is assumed that the patient is laying flat on the examining table, but if the head is turned to the right or a pad under the buttocks, it will rotate the thorax such that the LAO projection is steeper and the detector is caudal. This has to be compensated for during the setup for the angiogram. The clue in the former case is that more of the heart silhouette is over the spine.

The first step in setting up a cranial–LAO projection is to achieve the correct degree of steepness or shallowness. After that, the degree of cranial tilt has to be confirmed, so that the basal–apical septum is elongated. This can be estimated by seeing how much of the hemidiaphragm is superimposed over the cardiac silhouette; the more superimposition, the greater the cranial tilt. Additionally, the degree of cranial tilt can be determined by looking at the course of the ventricular catheter; it appears to be foreshortened or coming directly at the viewer as the degree of cranial angulation is decreased (Figure 3.8).

Three-dimensional rotational angiography

Digital imaging using flat-panel detectors allows the acquisition of cross-sectional images by rotating the detector on a C-arm around the object. The acquired volume data set can be manipulated on a workstation to generate a three-dimensional angiographic image and/or computerized tomography (CT)-quality soft-tissue imaging that can be used in real time during the procedure (Figure 3.9). The technology was first designed and applied for interventional neurovascular procedures.[5-7] However, its utility

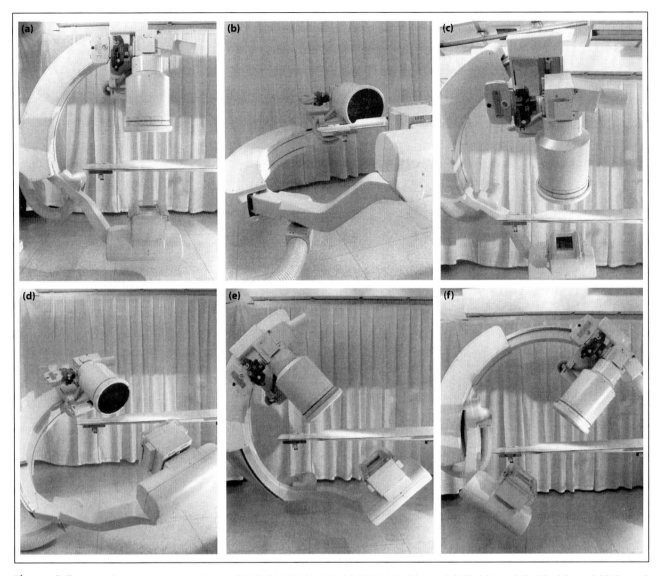

Figure 3.5 Standard projections. (a) Frontal (PA). (b) LAT. (c) RAO. (d) Mid-LAO with cranial tilt. (e) Cranially tilted frontal (sitting up). (f) Caudally tilted frontal. (Modified from Culham JAG. Physical principles of image formation and projections in angiocardiography. In: Freedom RM, Mawson JB, Yoo SJ, Benson LN, Eds. *Congenital Heart Disease Textbook of Angiocardiography*. Chapter 2, figure 2-17. Armonk: Futura Publishing; 1997, pp. 39–93. With permission.)

in obtaining a unique intraprocedural evaluation of the three-dimensional anatomy resulted in a rapid diffusion of the technology to other areas of interventional radiology. Until recently, its application outside interventional radiology was limited. In 2008, Noelker et al.[8] reported the use of 3-DRA for left atrial mapping during ablation procedures and Biasi et al.[9] reported its use in thoracic vascular interventions. In 2011, Glatz et al.[10] were the first to describe its application in children with congenital heart disease. In their study, 3-DRA was used for evaluation of the right ventricular outflow tract/central pulmonary arteries, cavopulmonary connection, pulmonary

veins, and distal pulmonary arteries. A number of subsequent publications[11-15] have demonstrated the usefulness of 3-DRA in defining the three-dimensional relationship between structures poorly defined by two-dimensional angiography, and in guiding pediatric interventional procedures (Figure 3.10).[16] The acquisition programs will vary among vendors. However, the essential components consist of a 5–7 s rotation of the C-arm at which time dilute contrast is injected for 1 or 2 s before the rotation begins. The location of the injection and whether pacing is used depends on the chambers or vessels to be visualized.[17] For example, for an arch obstruction, right ventricular pacing

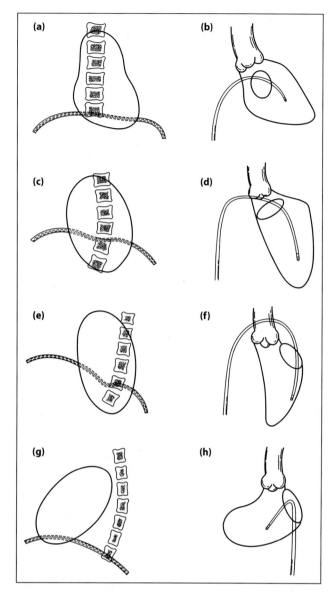

Figure 3.6 Setting up a standard LAO projection. To achieve the LAO projection, attempt to adjust the detector angle such that 2/3 of the cardiac silhouette is to the left of the spine as in (e). If a catheter is through the mitral valve in the left ventricular apex, it will point to the floor, as in (f). In this view, the intraventricular septal margin points toward the floor. The so-called four-chamber or hepatoclavicular view is achieved by having 1/2 the cardiac silhouette over the spine, as in (c). A catheter across the mitral valve will appear as in (d). A steep LAO projection will have the cardiac silhouette as in (g), and a transmitral catheter in the left ventricle will appear as in (h). (a) and (b) show the frontal projection. (Modified from Culham JAG. Physical principles of image formation and projections in angiocardiography. In: Freedom RM, Mawson JB, Yoo SJ, Benson LN, Eds. *Congenital Heart Disease Textbook of Angiocardiography.* Chapter 2, figure 2-19. Armonk: Futura Publishing; 1997, pp. 39–93. With permission.)

is typically used to reduce the stroke volume to allow the contrast to fill the vessel (Figure 3.11), while a nonpaced injection is used in the superior caval vein to examine a bidirectional cavopulmonary anastomosis (Figure 3.11). Diluted contrast is used (1:1 or 1:2) with 1–1.5 cm³/kg contrast used for an injection, and if the patient anesthetized, it is used with a breath hold. Several acquisition programs are available that can be used to optimize three-dimensional (volume rendered) or soft-tissue images. Once the acquisition is acquired, it can be rapidly (>5 min) reconstructed on a workstation in the laboratory. As such, it can be a valuable tool in planning and accomplishing an interventional procedure. Details of the technology are beyond the scope of this section, and the reader is referred to other works.[18–20] With newer acquisition programs, lower radiation doses are possible compared with the traditional digital biplane cine acquisitions.[10]

Cardiac catheterization and radiation exposure

Cardiac catheterization in children has evolved from a purely diagnostic test to a critical component of therapy. As such, the principles of radiation safety must take a central role in the planning and execution of these procedures due to the possible repeated exposures over a lifetime, the known increased radiosensitivity of children, and a longer time for side effects to manifest. Radiation exposure can be very high in the pediatric patient due to complexity of interventions, small body size, higher heart rates (requiring faster frame rates), and wide anatomical variations. The precautions recommended for adult patients equally apply to children, and should include low fluoroscopy frame rates during catheter manipulation, grid-free magnification in smaller children, single-frame acquisition for position documentation, and application of the ALARA (as low as reasonably achievable) principle (see below). As children born with congenital heart disease frequently undergo numerous diagnostic and therapeutic catheterizations, there is an ever-present, potentially harmful occurrence of cumulative long-term effects of radiation exposure.[21,22] This is problematic as the complex three-dimensional anatomy of congenital structural lesions frequently necessitates multiple acquisitions, which increases the radiation exposure. Imaging equipment employed for pediatric procedures should be designed and configured for image acquisition modified to accommodate variable procedural requirements with a wide age and weight range as seen in the pediatric laboratory.[23] Strategies for radiation exposure reduction and image quality in the pediatric population are well described[24] and the importance of exposure reduction is emphasized in the Image Gently and Step Lightly campaigns.[25]

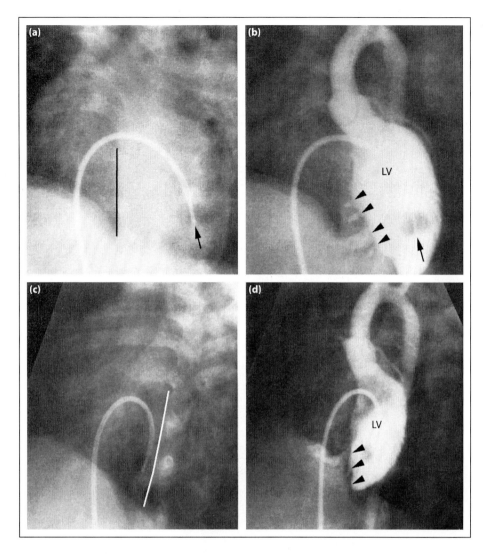

Figure 3.7   Achieving an LAO projection. (a): For a hepatoclavicular view, 1/2 of the cardiac silhouette is over or just left of the spine, with the catheter pointing toward the left of the image. During the injection, the apex and catheter (arrow) will point toward the bottom and left of the image. In this example, the basal (inlet) portion of the septum is intact. Multiple mid-muscular septal defects are not well profiled (arrowheads). In panel (c), the LAO projection is achieved with the catheter pointing toward the bottom of the frame, and the cardiac silhouette well over the spine. During the contrast injection (d), the mid-muscular defects are now better profiled. (Modified from Culham JAG. Physical principles of image formation and projections in angiocardiography. In: Freedom RM, Mawson JB, Yoo SJ, Benson LN, Eds. *Congenital Heart Disease Textbook of Angiocardiography.* Chapter 2, figure 2-20. Armonk: Futura Publishing; 1997, pp. 39–93. With permission.)

Specific lesions

Ventricular septal defect

The imaging of specific ventricular defects is beyond the scope of this chapter, but is commented upon in detail by various authors (Figure 3.12).[26] The injections to outline the septum and the lost margins, which circumscribe the defect(s), are best performed in the left ventricle using a power injector. Two orthogonal (right-angle) projections will give the best chance of profiling the lesion. However,

in precatheterization, the location of the defect should be well characterized by other imaging modalities, such that the projections chosen would give the optimal profile, with little modification. Table 3.1 lists single and biplane angulations for the various projections. For the perimembranous defect, the mid-cranial LAO projection, at about 50–60° LAO, and as much cranial tilt as the equipment and patient position will allow (Figure 3.13) should be attempted. Additional projections can include a shallow LAO with cranial tilt (the so-called four-chamber or hepatoclavicular view) to outline the basal septum or inlet

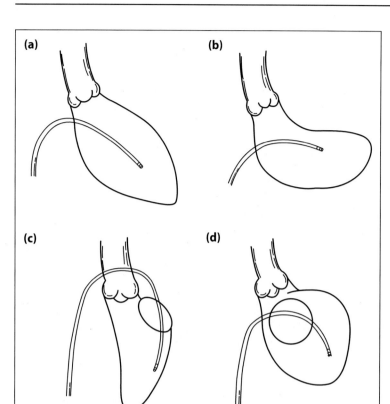

Figure 3.8 Obtaining the cranial tilt. In the standard RAO view, (a), the left ventricular apex points caudally and to the left. The LAO view will open the outflow from apex to base, as in diagram (c). If there is an upturned apex as in Fallot's tetralogy, the RAO view will appear as in (b). Adding cranial tilt to a mid-LAO projection will not effectively open the apex-to-base projection, and the appearance will be as looking down the barrel of the ventricles as in (d). (Modified from Culham JAG. Physical principles of image formation and projections in angiocardiography. In: Freedom RM, Mawson JB, Yoo SJ, Benson LN, Eds. *Congenital Heart Disease Textbook of Angiocardiography.* Chapter 2, figure 2-21. Armonk: Futura Publishing; 1997, pp. 39–93. With permission.)

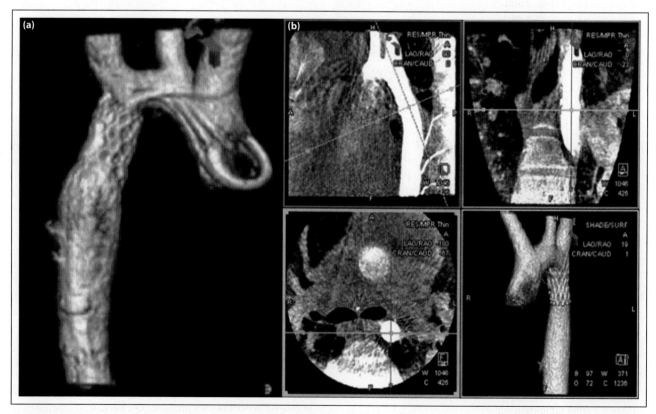

Figure 3.9 **(See color insert.)** Left panel (a), a volume-rendered image of a stented arch coarctation obtained from a rotational angiogram. In panel (b), from the same acquisition, the CT soft tissue images in the axial, coronal, and sagittal planes.

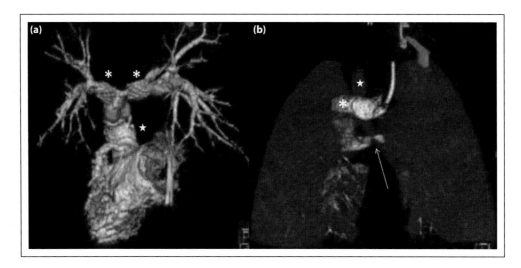

Figure 3.10 **(See color insert.)** Panel (a) A three-dimensional rotational angiogram from an injection in the right ventricle, viewed from the back (a projection not available in standard two-dimensional angiography), showing two endovascular stents (*) and the right ventricle to pulmonary artery conduit (star). Panel (b) shows a volume-rendered image from a cavopulmonary vein injection (*), reconstructed to show the relationship of the trachea (star) and a stenosis in the left pulmonary artery (arrow).

extension of a perimembranous defect. The RAO view will outline the high anterior and infundibular (outlet) defects.[27]

Coarctation of the aorta

Biplane angiography should be used to outline the arch lesion. Projections that can be used include LAO/RAO, PA and LAT, or a shallow or steep LAO (Figure 3.14). Our preference is a 30° LAO and left LAT, with 10–15° caudal tilt to minimize any overlapping structures, such as a ductal bump or diverticulum. Modifications to accommodate a right arch are generally mirror-image projections (i.e., 30° RAO and left LAT). The operator must be cautious to examine the transverse arch for associated hypoplasia, which may be foreshortened in the straight left-LAT projection. In such an instance, for a left arch, an LPO projection may elongate the arch. This is particularly important if an endovascular stent is to be implanted near the head and neck vessels.

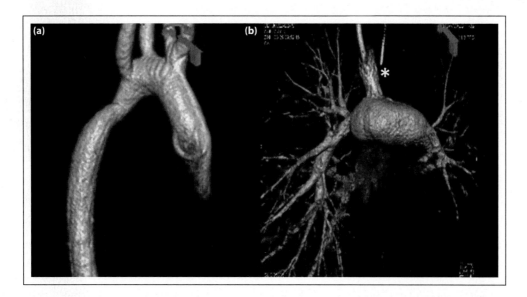

Figure 3.11 **(See color insert.)** Panel (a) is an image from a rotational angiogram from prior to stenting the arch obstruction. It was obtained during rapid right ventricular pacing to allow the diluted contrast time to fill the vessel throughout the time of acquisition. In panel (b), a cavopulmonary injection (*) is made without pacing, as the blood flow is slow, allowing filling of the anastomosis, and the proximal and distal pulmonary arteries during acquisition.

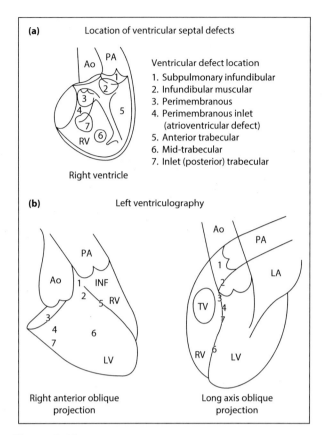

(a) Location of ventricular septal defects

Ventricular defect location
1. Subpulmonary infundibular
2. Infundibular muscular
3. Perimembranous
4. Perimembranous inlet
   (atrioventricular defect)
5. Anterior trabecular
6. Mid-trabecular
7. Inlet (posterior) trabecular

Right ventricle

(b) Left ventriculography

Right anterior oblique projection

Long axis oblique projection

Figure 3.12 The locations of various ventricular defects are diagrammed in panel (a) viewed from the right ventricle. In panel (b), the locations of these defects are noted as seen in an RAO or LAO projection.

Aortic valve angiography

Assessment of the diameter of the aortic valve in the setting of normally related great arteries with ventricular arterial concordance for balloon dilation is best performed using biplane in the long axis and RAO projections (Figure 3.15) (Table 3.1). Our preference is to obtain the diameter of the aortic valve from a ventriculogram, which profiles the hinge points of the leaflets. Caution must be observed when using an ascending aortogram, as one of the leaflets of the valve may obscure the margins of attachment.

The Mustard baffle

Children who have had a Mustard operation may develop over time obstruction to one or both limbs of the venous baffle (Figure 3.16). As atrial arrhythmias are not uncommon in this population, particularly as adults, pacing systems are frequently required for management. In this regard, enlargement of a stenotic, although at times asymptomatic, superior baffle is frequently required. The optimum projection to outline superior baffle obstruction for potential stent implantation is a cranial-angulated LAO projection (30° LAO and 30° cranial). This view will elongate the baffle pathway, allowing accurate measurement prior to stenting. For inferior baffle lesions, a frontal projection will allow adequate localization of the lesion. Leaks along the baffle are more problematic and require modification of the projection. The initial approach

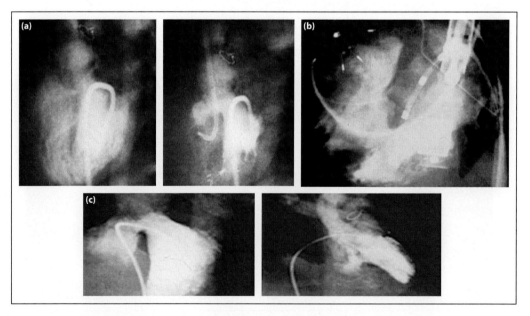

Figure 3.13 Panel (a) shows a left ventriculogram taken in the cranial–LAO projection. Note the apical, mid-muscular, and perimembranous septal defects. In panel (b), a modified hepatoclavicular view profiles a mid-muscular defect. Panel (c), left pane, is a left ventriculogram taken in the cranial–LAO view, with the catheter entering the ventricle through a perimembranous defect. Right pane, taken in the hepatoclavicular view with the catheter through the mitral valve, defines an inlet muscular defect in a child with a pulmonary artery band.

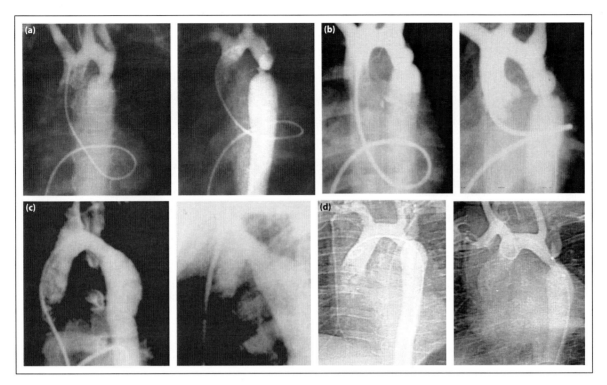

Figure 3.14   Panel (a), left pane, shows an ascending aortogram taken with a shallow-LAO projection without caudal angulation. The catheter was placed through a transeptal entry to the left heart. While the area of the coarctation can be seen, it is the caudal angulation that identifies the details of the lesion, including a small ductal ampulla, right pane. In panel (b), similar information is obtained, by employing caudal angulation to the frontal detector, right pane, while in the shallow-LAO projection in contrast to that information obtained without caudal angulation, left pane. In panel (c), left pane, hypoplasia of the transverse arch can be identified. However, in contrast, in the right pane, the degree of foreshortening is obvious. Panel (d), right pane, shows the standard LAO projection, of an ascending aortogram. In this case, there is overlap of the area of obstruction, transverse arch hypoplasia, and stenosis of the left subclavian artery, not defined until cranial angulation is employed, right pane.

should be a PA projection, with modifications in angulation made thereafter to best profile the lesion for device implantation, not too dissimilar to that of Fontan fenestration closure.

The secundum atrial septal defect and the fenestrated Fontan

Secundum atrial septal defects are best profiled in the 30° LAO with 30° cranial tilt (Figures 3.17 and 3.18). With the injection made in the right upper pulmonary vein, the sinus venous portion of the septum can be visualized, and anomalous pulmonary venous return can be ruled out. Additionally, any associated septal aneurysm can be outlined. With the application of transesophageal or intracardiac echocardiography, there is less fluoroscopic reliance on device positioning. When balloon sizing is performed, this projection will elongate the axis of the balloon for proper measurements.

The interventional management of the child with a fenestrated Fontan, whether an LAT tunnel or extracardiac connection, generally requires selective studies of the superior

and inferior caval vein and pulmonary circulations to determine the presence or absence of obstructive or hypoplastic pathways and whether venous collaterals have developed. As such, they must be addressed by angioplasty, stenting, or embolization techniques before consideration of fenestration closure. The development of venous collaterals after an extracardiac Fontan will generally develop either from the innominate vein, or from the right upper hepatic/phrenic vein, toward the neo-left atrium, less frequently from the right hepatic veins to the pulmonary veins. The optimum projection to outline these lesions is in the AP and LAT projections, with selective power injections in the appropriate vessel. The location and dimensions of the fenestration may also be defined in these views, but for ideal profiling, some degree of right or LAO may be required.

The bidirectional cavopulmonary connection

Second-stage palliation for a number of congenital defects consists of a bidirectional cavopulmonary connection (aka, the bidirectional Glenn anastomosis) (Figure 3.19). Since

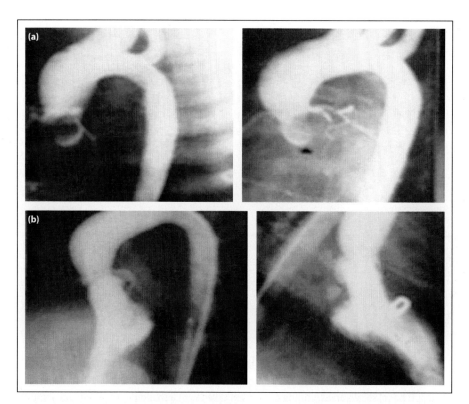

Figure 3.15   Intervention on the aortic valve requires accurate definition of the hinge points of the leaflets. In panel (a), long axis oblique views from an ascending aortogram, do not define the margins of the leaflets due to overlap of the cusps (bicuspid in these examples). In panel (b), long axis oblique (left) and RAO views, the left ventriculogram allows easier identification of the leaflet hinge points, where measurements can be made.

the caval to the pulmonary artery connection is toward the anterior surface of the right pulmonary artery (rather than on the upper surface), an AP projection will result in overlapping of the anastomotic site with the pulmonary artery. Therefore, to determine whether the anastomosis is obstructed, a 30° caudal with 10° LAO projection will generally open that region for better definition. Furthermore, this projection will outline the full extent of the right and left pulmonary arteries. The left-LAT projection with or without 10° caudal angulation will profile the anastomosis for its anterior–posterior dimension. Contrast injection must be made in the lower portion of the superior caval vein. The examination of venous collaterals can be performed from the AP and LAT projections in the innominate vein.

Pulmonary valve stenosis, Fallot's tetralogy, and pulmonary valve atresia with intact ventricular septum

Percutaneous intervention on isolated pulmonary valve stenosis is the assured procedure in the current era of catheter-based therapies (Figures 3.20 and 3.21). While

angiographic definition of the right ventricular outflow tract and valve is not complicated, several features must be kept in mind when approaching the angiography for an interventional procedure. In the case of isolated pulmonary valve stenosis and other right ventricular outflow tract lesions, because the outflow tract can take a horizontal curve, a simple AP projection will foreshorten the structure. Therefore, a 30° cranial with 15° LAO will open up the infundibulum, allowing visualization of the valve and the main and branch pulmonary arteries. The best definition of the hinge points of the valve, to choose the correct balloon size, is from the left-LAT projection. Occasionally, 10° or 15° caudal angulation of the LAT detector can be used to separate the overlap of the branch vessels seen on a straight left-LAT projection. However, this is not recommended, as it will also foreshorten the outflow tract, and the valve will appear off-plane, giving incorrect valve diameters.

Branch pulmonary artery stenosis

Pulmonary artery interventions are most common, and represent the most difficult angiographic projections to separate out individual vessels for assessment and

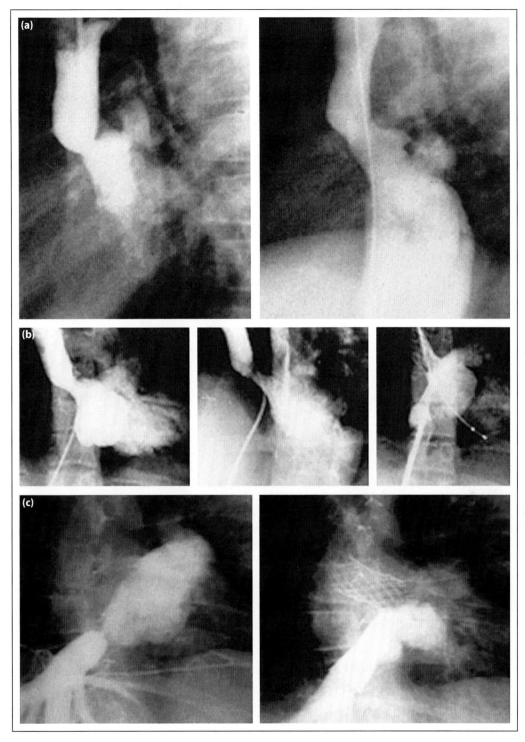

Figure 3.16   Baffle obstruction after a Mustard operation is, as the population ages, an increasingly common event. This is particularly so with the need to manage such patients with transvenous pacing devices. In panel (a), left pane, the presence of a superior baffle obstruction can be identified from the left-LAT projection. However, only with cranial angulation (cranial–LAO view), right pane, will the full extent of the lesion be detailed. This is particularly critical, as shown in panel (b), where the frontal view, left pane, does not show the full extent of the obstruction, and only from the angulated view will the length and diameter of the lesion be outlined (middle pane). A stent is placed, followed by a transvenous pacing system shown in the right pane from a frontal projection. For inferior baffle lesion, the frontal (PA) projection is optimal, panel (c), before (left) and after a stent is placed.

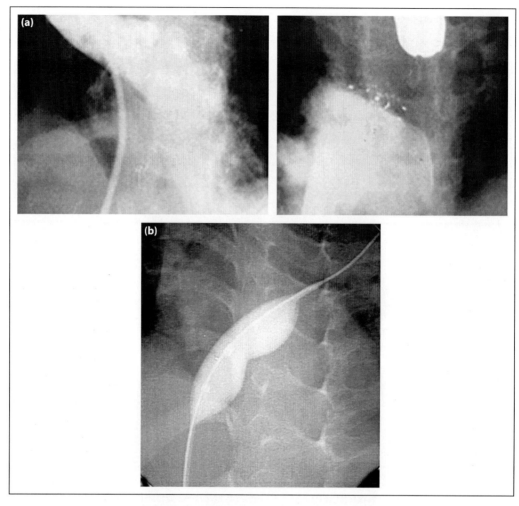

Figure 3.17 Use of angiography for septal defect definition and device placement in the setting of a secundum atrial septal defect has been supplanted by intracardiac and transesophageal techniques (panel a). However, fluoroscopy is still required for initial device localization, and in many laboratories, a short cine run is required to record the diameter of the static balloon to choose device size. In this case, we find the 30° LAO with 30° cranial tilt to best elongate the balloon to avoid foreshortening, panel (b).

potential intervention (Figures 3.22 through 3.24). A cranially tilted frontal projection with a left-LAT or RAO/LAO projection is frequently the first series of views that can be performed, as scout studies to map the proximal and hilar regions of the pulmonary circulation. The injection may be performed in either the ventricle or main pulmonary artery. Since there is frequent overlap to be seen in viewing the right ventricular outflow tract (see above), these standard views can be modified by increasing or decreasing the degree of RAO or LAO, and adding caudal or cranial tilt. Selective branch artery injections are best for detailed visualization, to plan the intervention. For the right pulmonary artery, a shallow-RAO projection with 10° or 15° cranial tilt will separate the upper- and middle-lobe branches, while a left-LAT with 15° caudal tilt will open up all the anterior vessels. Similarly, to maximize the elongated and posterior leftward-directed left pulmonary artery, a 60° LAO with 20° cranial is very effective, with

a caudal tilt on the LAT detector. Occasionally, in small babies after surgical reconstruction of the branch pulmonary arteries, the main pulmonary artery is aneurysmal and obscures the confluence. In this case, a steep 30° caudal projection with the frontal detector with 10–20° RAO will open up the bifurcation.

Summary

This short introduction to interventional angiography will allow the reader a point of departure to visualize the most common lesions. However, many cases occur that do not fall into a standard categorization and the operator must be prepared to alter the imaging projection to optimally define the lesion. Successful outcomes require patience, perseverance, and the learned experience of others.

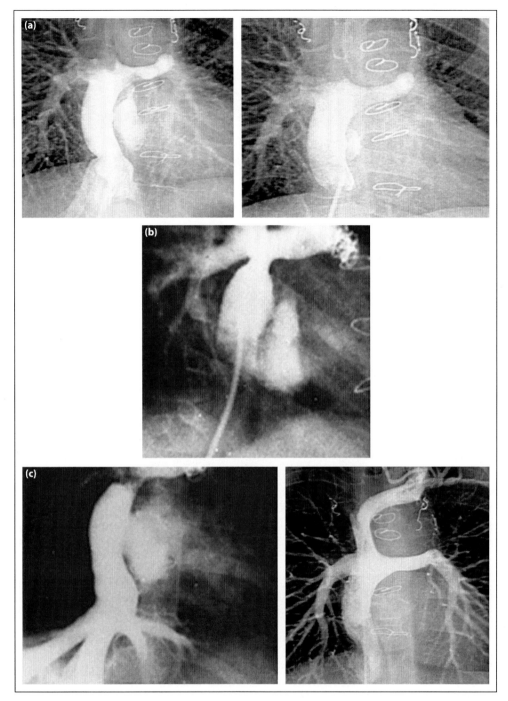

Figure 3.18   Panel (a) shows the appearance of a fenestrated extracardiac Fontan in the frontal projection, and its appearance after device closure. Generally, a frontal projection profiles the defect adequately, but at times, some angulation is required as seen in panel (b), where the defect is best profiled in a shallow-RAO view. Also note coils in the left superior caval vein, which developed after the Fontan procedure and required embolization. Occasionally, collateral vessels develop from the hepatic/phrenic vein (panel (c), left) or innominate vein (panel (c), right), where coils have been placed. The primary view is frontal (PA) and left-LAT.

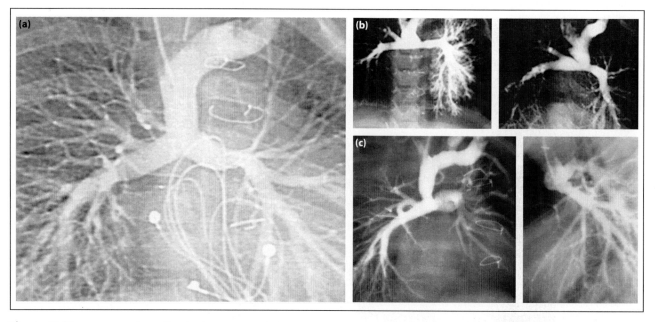

Figure 3.19 Because of an offset in the anastomosis between the superior caval vein and right pulmonary artery, the optimal view to see the anastomosis without overlap is shallow—with caudal tilt as seen in panel (a). Panel (b), left pane, is in the frontal projection, where overlap of the anastomosis obscures a potential lesion, as seen in the angulated view, right pane. The combination of an angulated frontal detector and caudal angulation of the LAT tube will allow definition of the anastomosis (left pane), and the pulmonary artery confluence (right pane), panel (c).

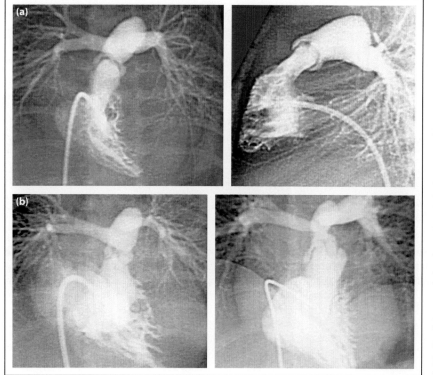

Figure 3.20 Panel (a) depicts the case of a typical isolated pulmonary valve stenosis in a neonate. The outflow tract is profiled in the cranially angulated frontal projection, with a slight degree of LAO angulation (left pane). The right ventriculogram outlines the form of the ventricle, the main pulmonary artery (and ductal bump) and the pulmonary artery confluence and branch dimensions. The LAT view (right pane) outlines the valve leaflets (thickened and doming) and allows accurate delineation of the valve structures for balloon diameter determination. In panel (b), two right ventriculograms in the cranially angulated slight LAO view depict the size of the annulus and main and branch pulmonary arteries (typical valve stenosis with left pulmonary hypoplasia, left pane; dysplastic valve stenosis, small nondilated main pulmonary artery, and proximal left branch pulmonary artery stenosis with poststenotic dilation, right pane).

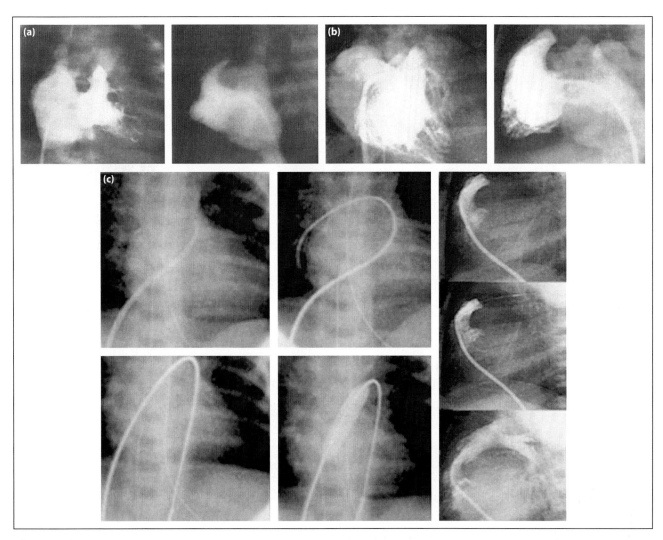

Figure 3.21   Angiographic projections for intervention in pulmonary atresia with intact septum are similar to that of isolated pulmonary valve stenosis. In panels (a) and (b), cranial angulation is critical to image the valve plate (left panes); while a left LAT will suffice for imaging the anterior–posterior aspects of the outflow tract. In valve perforation, it is critical to have visual control in two orthogonal planes, to avoid inadvertent infundibular perforation. A series of images during valve perforation is seen in panel (c). The left upper pane shows the catheter position; right upper pane, perforation and wire in the right pulmonary artery; left lower pane, the wire guide across the duct for stability; and in the right lower pane, balloon dilation of the valve. In the accompanying panel, viewed from the left-LAT projection, a series of images taken during perforation in the main pulmonary artery; top pane, position confirmation; middle pane, radio-frequency perforation; lower pane, angiography.

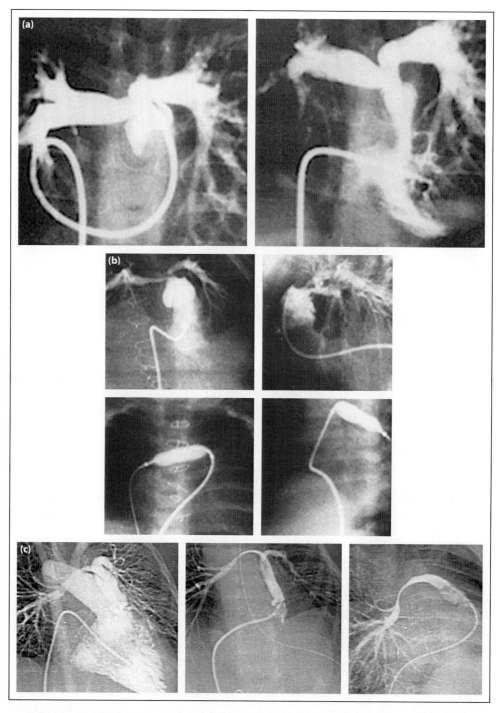

Figure 3.22   Angiography for selective intervention on the branch pulmonary arteries can be most difficult due to overlapping of structures. No single projection is totally representative and multiple views are frequently required. In panel (a), left pane, a scout film is taken in the main pulmonary artery; in the right pane, the right ventricle. Both images are taken in the cranial–LAO projection and in these examples clearly outline the outflow tracts and branch confluences. In panel (b), the dilated main pulmonary artery would have obscured the branch pulmonary artery confluence, and this cranial–LAO (left upper pane) and caudal left LAT (right upper pane) nicely details the anatomy for subsequent intervention (lower panes). In panel (c), an LAO-cranial projection outlines the crossed pulmonary arteries (left pane), as does a main pulmonary artery injection in the cranial projection (middle pane). The right pane identifies a stenotic lesion in the vessel from an RAO-cranial projection.

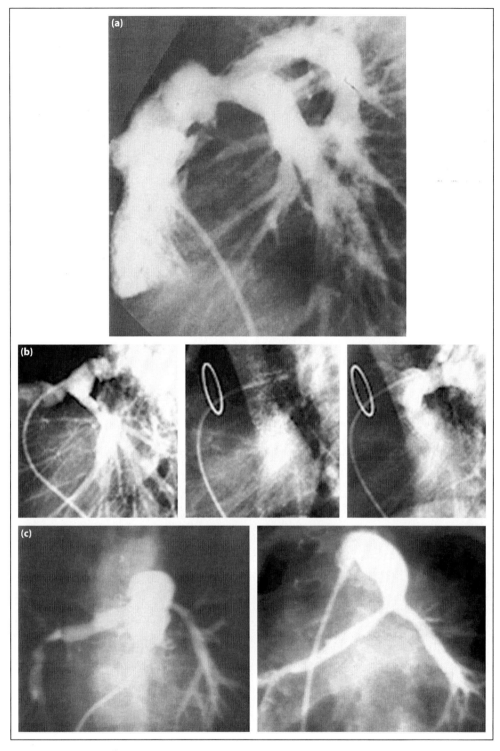

Figure 3.23   In panel (a), the image is taken from a left-LAT projection with caudal tilt. These will separate the proximal right and left pulmonary artery branches, and detail the main pulmonary artery. The outflow tract is foreshortened, and this view will mislead the operator when examining the diameter of the valve, and infundibulum. If such detail is required, a straight left LAT should be performed. In the caudal–LAT projection, the left pulmonary branch will sweep superiorly and toward the upper right corner of the image, while the left pulmonary artery will appear more medial and in the center of the image. In panel (b), the child had severe bilateral branch stenosis, (left pane), which persisted after surgical repair and valve insertion. Using the left-LAT view, stents could be placed in each branch (middle and right panes). In panel (c), severe main pulmonary artery dilation has obscured the confluence and very hypoplastic pulmonary arteries (left pane) in this child shortly after surgery. In this case, steep caudal angulation of the frontal tube with 10° or 15° LAO has detailed the lesion for the intervention (right pane).

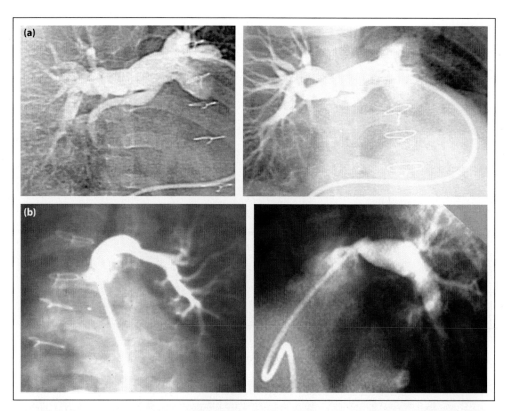

Figure 3.24 Selective injection into a branch pulmonary vessel will give the best-detailed image. However, overlapping the intrahilar branching vessels will interfere with interpretation if the lesion, as seen in panel (a), left pane, is taken in the RAO projection. By adding caudal tilt, as in this example, the tortuous path of the intrahilar vessel can be seen. In panel (b), left and right panes, cranial–LAO projection details the length of the left pulmonary artery and proximal areas of potential stenosis.

References

1. Culham JAG. Physical principles of image formation and projections in angiocardiography. In: Freedom RM, Mawson JB, Yoo SJ, Benson LN, Eds. *Congenital Heart Disease Textbook of Angiocardiography.* Armonk: Futura Publishing; 1997. pp. 39–93.
2. Freedom RM, Culham JAG, Moes CAF. *Angiocardiography of Congenital Heart Disease.* New York: Macmillan; 1984. pp. 10–16.
3. Beekman RH 3rd, Hellenbrand WE, Lloyd TR, Lock JE, Mullins CE, Rome JJ et al. ACCF/AHA/AAP recommendations for training in pediatric cardiology. Task force 3: Training guidelines for pediatric cardiac catheterization and interventional cardiology endorsed by the Society for Cardiovascular Angiography and Interventions. *J Am Coll Cardiol* 2005;46(7):1388–90.
4. Qureshi SA, Redington AN, Wren C, Ostman-Smith I, Patel R, Gibbs JL et al. Recommendations of the British Paediatric Cardiac Association for therapeutic cardiac catheterisation in congenital cardiac disease. *Cardiol Young* 2000;10(6):649–6.
5. Fahrig R, Fox AJ, Lownie S, Holdsworth DW. Use of a C-arm system to generate true three-dimensional computed rotational angiograms: Preliminary *in vitro* and *in vivo* results. *AJNR Am J Neuroradiol* 1997;18:1507–14.
6. Heran NS, Song JK, Mamba K, Smith W, Niimi Y, Berenstein A. The utility of DynaCT in neuroendovascular procedures. *AJNR Am J Neuroradiol* 2006;27:330–2.
7. Richter G, Engelhorn T, Struffert T et al. Flat panel detector angiographic CT for stent-assisted coil embolization of broad-based cerebral aneurysms. *AJNR Am J Neuroradiol* 2007;28:1902–8.
8. Noelker G, Gutleben KJ, Marschang H et al. Three-dimensional left atrial and esophagus reconstruction using cardiac C-arm computed tomography with image integration into fluoroscopic views for ablation of atrial fibrillation: Accuracy of a novel modality in comparison with multislice computed tomography. *Heart Rhythm* 2008;5:1651–7.
9. Biasi L, Ali T, Thompson M. Intraoperative DynaCT in visceral–hybrid repair of an extensive thoracoabdominal aortic aneurysm. *Eur J Cardiothorac Surg* 2008;34:1251–2.
10. Glatz AC, Zhu X, Gillespie J, Hanna BD, Rome JJ. Use of angiographic CT imaging in the cardiac catheterization laboratory for congenital heart disease. *J Am Coll Cardiol Img* 2010;3:1149–57.
11. Berman DP, Khan DM, Gutierrez Y, Zahn EM. The use of three-dimensional rotational angiography to assess the pulmonary circulation following cavo-pulmonary connection in patients with single ventricle. *Cath Cardiovas Interv* 2012;80:922–30.
12. Schwartz JG, Neubauer AM, Fagan TE, Noordhoek NJ, Grass M, Carroll JD. Potential role of three-dimensional rotational angiography and C-arm CT for valvular repair and implantation. *Int J Cardiovasc Imaging* 2011;27:1205–22.
13. Glockler M, Halbfab J, Koch A, Achenbach S, Dittrich S. Multimodality 3D-roadmap for cardiovascular interventions in congenital heart disease—A single-center, retrospective analysis of 78 cases. *Catheter Cardiovasc Interv* 2013;82:436–42 [Epub ahead of print].
14. Glöckler M, Koch A, Halbfaß J, Greim V, Rüffer A, Cesnjevar R, et al.. Assessment of cavopulmonary connections by advanced imaging: Value of flat-detector computed tomography. *Cardiol Young* 2013;23:18–26.

15. Glöckler M, Koch A, Greim V, Shabaiek A, Rüffer A, Cesnjevar R et al. The value of flat-detector computed tomography during catheterisation of congenital heart disease. *Eur Radiol* 2011;21:2511–20.

16. Fagan T, Kay J, Carroll J, Neubauer A. 3-D guidance of complex pulmonary artery stent placement using reconstructed rotational angiography with live overlay. *Catheter Cardiovasc Interv* 2012;79:414–21.

17. Noble S, Miro J, Yong G, Bonan R, Tardif JC, Ibrahim R. Rapid pacing rotational angiography with three-dimensional reconstruction: Use and benefits in structural heart disease interventions. *EuroIntervention* 2009;5:244–9.

18. Gupta R, Cheung AC, Bartling SH, et al. Flat-panel volume CT: Fundamental principles, technology, and applications. *Radiographics* 2008;28:2009–22.

19. Kalender WA, Kyriakou Y. Flat-detector computed tomography (FD-CT). *Eur Radiol* 2007;17:2767–79.

20. Kyriakou Y, Struffert T, Dorfler A, Kalender WA. Basic principles of flat detector computed tomography (FD-CT). *Radiologe* 2009;49:811–9.

21. Andreassi MG, Ait-Ali L, Botto N, Manfredi S, Mottola G, Picano E. Cardiac catheterization and long-term chromosomal damage in children with congenital heart disease. *Eur Heart J* 2006;27:2703–8.

22. de Gonzalez AB, Mahesh M, Kim K, et al. Projected cancer risks from computed tomographic scans performed in the United States in 2007. *Arch Intern Med* 2009;169:2071–7.

23. Strauss KJ. Pediatric interventional radiography equipment: Safety considerations. *Pediatr Radiol* 2006;36(Suppl 2):126–35.

24. Justino H. The ALARA concept in pediatric cardiac catheterization: Techniques and tactics for managing radiation exposure. *Pediatr Radiol* 2006;36(Suppl 2):146–53.

25. Sidhu MK, Goske MJ, Coley BJ, et al. Image Gently, Step Lightly: Increasing radiation exposure awareness in pediatric interventions through an international social marketing campaign. *J Vasc Interv Radiol* 2009;20:1115–9.

26. Ventricular septal defect. In: Freedom RM, Mawson JB, Yoo SJ, Benson LN, Eds. *Congenital Heart Disease Textbook of Angiocardiography*. Armonk: Futura Publishing; 1997. pp. 189–218.

27. Brandt PW. Axially angled angiocardiography. *Cardiovasc Intervent Radiol* 1984;7(3–4):166–9.

4

Hemodynamics

Mustafa Al-Qbandi and Ziyad M. Hijazi

Introduction

Hemodynamics, by definition, is the study of the motion of blood through the vascular system. In simple clinical application, this may include the assessment of a patient's heart rate, pulse quality, blood pressure, capillary refill, skin color, skin temperature, and other parameters.[1] As the complexity of the patient's status increases, invasive hemodynamic monitoring may be utilized to provide a more advanced assessment and to guide therapeutic interventions.

Invasive hemodynamic monitoring is now used routinely in many critical-care and intermediate-care units to assist in the assessment of single and multisystem disorders and their treatment. Hemodynamic monitoring might include waveform and numeric data derived from the central veins, right atrium (RA), right ventricle (RV), pulmonary artery, left atrium (LA), left ventricle (LV), aorta, and peripheral arteries.

Pressure itself is defined as force per area. This can be expressed in a variety of ways, such as pounds per square inch or kilograms per square centimeters. The standard international unit (SI) is the pascal (Pa). One pascal equals one newton per square meter. In practice, millimeters of mercury (mmHg) is the most commonly used unit of measure of blood pressure. One mmHg is the pressure exerted by a column of mercury that is 1 mm high at zero celsius at standard atmospheric pressure and equals 133.3 Pa.

$$1 \text{ mmHg} = 133.3 \text{ Pa} \quad \text{at zero Celsius}$$

Intra-arterial or direct arterial pressure measurement

The three components or characteristics of intravascular pressures measured through a fluid-filled catheter are

- Residual or static pressure inside the fluid-filled vessel.
- Dynamic pressure, which is caused by the imparted kinetic energy of the moving fluid (similar to the encountered fluid in arterial pressures when the catheter tip is directly facing the flow of fluid).

- Hydrostatic pressure, which results from the difference between the ends of the fluid-filled tubes (the tip of the catheter and the air-reference port of the transducer).

The most desired measurement during hemodynamic monitoring is residual or static pressure within the vessel or chamber being assessed. To achieve this goal, both dynamic and hydrostatic pressure components need to be eliminated. As stated above, dynamic pressures are encountered only in high or frequent flow rates or when the catheter tip is directed into the flow. This component is greatly reduced when assessing arterial blood pressure by the use of dampening services.

The hydrostatic pressure is the component to most consistently interfere with the accuracy of pressure measurements obtained through fluid-filled systems. Placement of the air-reference port at the level of the RA eliminates the effects of hydrostatic pressure within the fluid-filled column and provides accurate measurement within the peripheral artery.

All biomedical devices consist of three basic components:[1]

1. A transducer or device that detects the physiological event.
2. An amplifier that increases the magnitude of the signal from the transducer.
3. A recorder, meter, oscilloscope, or monitor to display the signal.

Right-sided pressure waveforms
Right-sided pressures

Hemodynamic data require examination of not only individual pressure waves, but also their timing to events on the electrocardiogram (ECG), particularly the QRS complex.[2] Correct interpretation of normal right heart pressure waveforms and careful examination of the unusual right heart hemodynamics and their timing in the cardiac cycle may reveal unanticipated pathophysiologic mechanisms.

Abnormalities of the waveforms can occur in the presence of arrhythmia or ventricular pacing. This must be considered when interpreting hemodynamic data. Therefore, ECG correlation is required for correct identification of these events.

Right atrium

In the RA, there is an 80–100 ms delay in the detection of mechanical events from their appearance on the ECG due to the length of tubing in the system.[1,3] During inhalation, the right atrial pressure falls, while in exhalation, the right atrial pressure increases (Table 4.1).

The right atrial pressure waveform consists of two major positive deflections, the "a" and "v" waves (Figure 4.1 and Tables 4.2 and 4.3).

The "a" wave results from right atrial contraction and immediately follows the P wave on the surface of ECG. Following the "a" wave and right atrial contraction, the pressure declines, defining the "x" descent. A small positive deflection, known as the "c" wave, may be seen reflecting closure of the tricuspid valve. Thereafter, the "x" descent continues as right atrial pressure declines due to right atrial relaxation. After full atrial relaxation and the nadir of the

Table 4.1 Normal physiologic respiratory effect on right atrial pressure

Inhalation: Intrathoracic pressure falls → RA pressure falls

Exhalation: Intrathoracic pressure increases → RA pressure increases

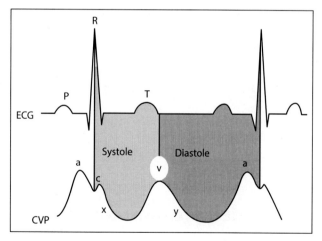

Figure 4.1 RA pressure tracing in a normal person. The "a" wave occurs simultaneously with atrial contraction; the "v" wave occurs during atrial filling; the "c" wave is coincident with the onset of ventricular contraction; the "x" descent corresponds to the fall in pressure after atrial contraction and the continued fall during early systole ("x"); and the "y" descent occurs after the opening of the tricuspid valve and with early diastolic filling. (From Internet: University of Iowa Children's Hospital. Home page section of arterial blood and central venous pressure monitoring devices. With permission.)

Table 4.2 Normal right atrial pressure waves

a Wave	1—Rise in pressure due to atrial contraction. 2—a Waves are larger in the presence of any resistance to RV filling (TS, RV failure, and cardiac tamponade), because resistance will increase pressure as the atrium attempts to contract and eject blood.
x Descent	Fall in pressure due to atrial relaxation.
c Wave	Rise in pressure due to ventricular contraction and bulging of the closed tricuspid valve.
v Wave	Rise in pressure during atrial filling.
y Descent	Fall in pressure due to the opening of the tricuspid valve and the beginning of ventricular filling.

Table 4.3 Abnormalities in right atrial tracings

Low mean atrial pressure	Hypovolemia Improper zeroing of the transducer
Elevated mean atrial pressure	Right ventricular failure Valvular disease (TS, TR, PS, and PR) Myocardial disease (RV ischemia, cardiomyopathy) Left heart failure (MS, MR, AS, AI, and cardiomyopathy) Increased PVR (PE, COPD, and primary pulmonary HTN) Pericardial effusion with tamponade physiology Atrial myxoma
Elevated a wave	Tricuspid atresia/stenosis Decreased RV compliance due to RV failure
Cannon a wave	A–V asynchrony (3rd degree AVB, VT, and V-pacer)
Absent a wave	Atrial flutter or fibrillation
Elevated v wave	TR RV failure Reduced atrial compliance (restrictive myopathy)
Equal a and v waves	Tamponade Constrictive physiology
Prominent x descent	Tamponade Subacute/chronic constriction RV ischemia
Prominent y descent	TR Constrictive pericarditis Restrictive myopathy
Blunted x descent	Atrial fibrillation RA ischemia
Blunted y descent	TS RV ischemia Tamponade
M or W waves	Diagnostic for RV ischemia, pericardial constriction, or CHF

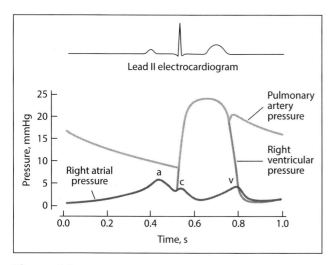

Figure 4.2 **(See color insert.)** The right ventricular pressure tracing is similar to that generated by the left ventricle except that the pressures are lower. (Courtesy of McGraw Hill.)

"x" descent, right atrial pressure rises due to increased volume from peripheral venous return. With right ventricular systole and the rapid increase in the right ventricular pressure, the tricuspid valve closes. The increasing right atrial pressure during right ventricular systole is the "v" wave; it reaches maximal amplitude just prior to the opening of the tricuspid valve. When the pressure in the RV falls below that of the RA, the tricuspid valve opens.

After the tricuspid valve opens, at the beginning of right ventricular diastole, the pressure in the RA rapidly falls, defining the "y" descent. After the "y" descent, the pressure in the RA equals the right ventricular end-diastolic

pressure (RVEDP) since the tricuspid valve is opened; it slowly increases as the RV fills.

The normal mean right atrial pressure is between 1 and 8 mmHg.

Jugular venous pulsations

The jugular venous pulse closely reflects changes in right atrial pressure, and also parallels changes observed in the vena cavae.[4,5] The variations in pressure within the RA are principally reflected by a change in volume for the venous system.

The venous pulse "a" and "c" waves have an average delay from the RA of approximately 60 ms, while the "v" wave delay is 80 ms; by comparison, the "y" trough delay is 90 ms, and the "x" trough is 110 ms. It also requires 60 ms for the right atrial "a" wave to reach the RV and cause a positive deflection in this chamber. These delays should be considered when examining the jugular venous pulse, as well as inferior vena caval pressure waves as a reflection of the right atrial pressure.[6]

Right ventricle

The RV pressure tracing (Figures 4.2 and 4.3) normally exhibits a peak systolic pressure equal to the one in the main pulmonary artery (PA) and is ≤30 mmHg. Generally, the RA and RV diastolic pressures are equal. The RV pressure during the first one-third of the diastole rises rapidly during the period of early diastolic filling. At the beginning of diastasis (this is the third phase of diastole) in which the RA and RV pressures are almost equal, filling is mainly the result of venous flow with the RA acting as a passive conduit. Also termed as the slow-filling period, the resistance to filling significantly increases, and the pressure

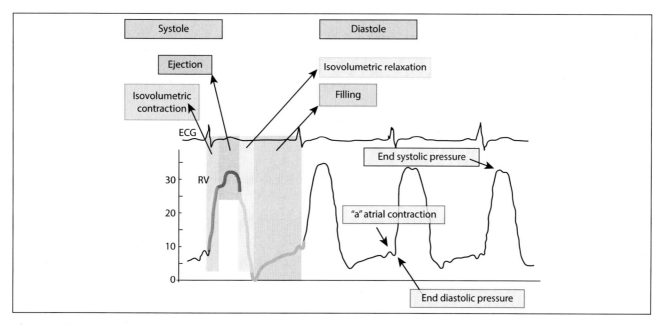

Figure 4.3 Example of RV pressure tracing in a normal person. The "a" wave represents atrial contraction. The shaded areas represent the contraction, ejection, relaxation, and filling periods.

then rises much more slowly until the onset of atrial systole "a" (Figure 4.2). This diastasis period is much shorter with rapid heart rates and the rapid-filling phase is immediately followed by atrial contraction.

The right ventricular waveform consists of the systole, a result of right ventricular contraction, and diastole occurring with right ventricular relaxation (Figure 4.3). During right ventricular systole, the pressure rapidly rises; when it is higher than that of the RA, the tricuspid valve closes. When the pressure exceeds that of the pulmonary artery, the pulmonic valve opens. The systolic waveform is rapid in upstroke and rounded in morphology; it occurs simultaneously with or immediately after the QRS complex on the surface ECG. The peak or maximal amplitude of this waveform is the right ventricular systole pressure. At the end of the systole, there is right ventricular relaxation and a rapid fall in pressure back to the baseline. This is the initiation of right ventricular diastole. When the pressure in the RV is lower than that of the pulmonary artery, the pulmonic valve closes. As the right ventricular pressure falls further, it becomes lower than that of the RA and the tricuspid valve opens.

Diastole consists of three periods generating three waveforms (Tables 4.4 and 4.5):

The first period, occurring at the onset of the tricuspid valve opening, produces an early rapid-filling wave during which approximately 60% of ventricular filling occurs.

Following this is a slow-filling period, accounting for approximately 15% of ventricular filling. Right atrial systole, which accounts for approximately 25% of right ventricular diastolic filling, produces an "a" wave that is simultaneous with and identical in morphology and amplitude to the "a" wave on the right atrial pressure tracing, since the tricuspid valve is opened and creates essentially one chamber. The pressure at the end of the "a" wave is termed the RVEDP.

The right ventricular pressure tracing is similar to that generated by the left ventricle, except that the pressures are lower.

The normal right ventricular diastolic pressure is 1–8 mmHg and the peak systolic pressure is 15–30 mmHg.

Pulmonary artery

The pulmonary artery waveform reflects systolic pressure resulting from rapid flow of blood into the pulmonary

Table 4.4 Right ventricular waves in systole and diastole

Systole
1. Isovolumetric contraction from TV closure to PV opening
2. Ejection from PV opening to PV closure
Diastole
1. Isovolumetric relaxation from PV closure to TV opening
2. Filling from TV opening to TV closure
   - Early rapid phase
   - Slow phase
   - Atrial contraction ("a" wave)

Table 4.5 Causes of right ventricular pressure changes

RV systolic pressure overload	RV systolic pressure reduced
Pulmonary HTN	Hypovolemia
Pulmonary valve stenosis	Cardiogenic shock
Right ventricular outflow obstruction	Tamponade
Supravalvular obstruction	
Significant shunt, ASD or VSD, TAPVC, and so on	
Increased PVR	

End-diastolic pressure overload	End-diastolic pressure reduced
Hypervolemia	Hypovolemia
CHF	TS
Diminished compliance	
Hypertrophy	
Tamponade	
TR	
Pericardial constriction	

artery from the RV during right ventricular systole. Since the pulmonic valve is opened, the waveform in the systole is identical in morphology and amplitude to that of right ventricular systole (Figure 4.4).

As right ventricular ejection ends, the pressure in the pulmonary artery falls in a similar manner to that in the RV. However, as right ventricular pressure falls below that of the pulmonary artery, the pulmonic valve closes, resulting in an incisura, or dicrotic notch, on the downslope of the pressure tracing. Pressure in the pulmonary artery continues to fall gradually as blood flows through the pulmonary arteries and veins into the left side of the heart, reaching a nadir or the end-diastolic pulmonary artery pressure.

Thereafter, the pressure falls during diastole to the level that is nearly equivalent to the mean LA pressure (or PCWP). Exceptions to the equivalency of PA diastolic pressure and mean LA pressure are

1. Rapid heart rate (the PA pressure does not have time to fall to the level of LA pressure during diastole)
2. Elevated pulmonary vascular resistance (PVR) with vasoconstriction

The mean PA pressure or diastolic PA pressure is elevated in response to any condition that (Table 4.6)

1. Increases LA or PCWP (e.g., LV diastolic dysfunction, MS, and mitral valve regurgitation [MR])
2. Increases PVR at the arterial level
3. Selectively obliterates a significant portion of pulmonary vascular bed upstream to the arteriolar level (e.g., multiple or large thromboemboli)

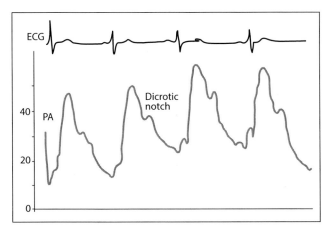

Figure 4.4 (**See color insert.**) Example of a PA pressure tracing in a normal person. Note the variation in peak systolic and diastolic pressures with respiration. The dicrotic notch appears shortly after the end of ejection and the closure of the pulmonic valve.

Table 4.6	Causes of change in pulmonary artery pressure
Elevated systolic PA pressure	**Reduced systolic PA pressure**
Primary pulmonary hypertension	Hypotension
Mitral stenosis	Pulmonary artery stenosis
Mitral regurgitation	Pulmonary valve stenosis/atresia
Congestive heart failure	Supra- or subvalvular pulmonary stenosis
Restrictive cardiomyopathy	Ebstein anomaly
Left-to-right shunt	Tricuspid valve stenosis/atresia
Pulmonary disease	
Reduced pulse pressure	**PA diastolic pressure > PCW pressure**
Right heart ischemia	Pulmonary disease
Tamponade	Pulmonary embolus
RV infarction	Tachycardia
Pulmonary embolism	

The waveform of the pulmonary artery is similar in morphology to that of the aorta. It is biphasic, but the pressure is lower.

The normal pulmonary artery systolic pressure is 15–30 mmHg and the normal pulmonary artery diastolic pressure is 4–12 mmHg.

Pulmonary artery capillary wedge pressure and left atrium

The pulmonary artery capillary wedge pressure (PCWP) (Figure 4.5) is an occluded pressure reflecting downstream

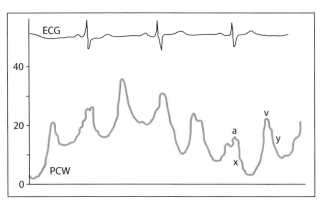

Figure 4.5 (**See color insert.**) Example of PCWP tracing, reflecting the LA pressure, in a normal person.

LA pressure provided there is proper positioning and there are no intervening anatomic obstructions (e.g., pulmonary venous obstruction, cor triatriatum). There is a time delay between the PCWP and the LA tracings of about 140–200 ms (Figure 4.6). The normal waveform consists of an "a" wave due to atrial contraction, a "v" wave reflecting left atrial filling during left ventricular contraction, a "c" wave (which may not be apparent on the PCWP tracing) due to mitral valve closure, and an "x" and "y" descent due to left atrial relaxation and left ventricular diastole, respectively. In the normal situation, the mean PCWP and end-diastolic PA pressure are approximately equal.

The normal mean left atrial pressure (and pulmonary capillary wedge pressure) is between 4 and 15 mmHg. When compared with the RA pressure tracing, LA pressure is always higher than RA pressure and the LA pressure pulse exhibits a normally dominant "v" wave (<15 mmHg) and a subordinate "a" wave (<12 mmHg). Tables 4.7 and 4.8 show the PCWP waves and the causes of change in PCWP waves.

Left ventricle

The pressure pulse (Figure 4.7) is characterized by a peak systolic pressure nearly equal to the peak aortic pressure (there may be a small mid-systolic or late-systolic pressure

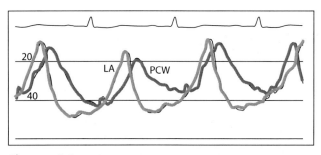

Figure 4.6 (**See color insert.**) PCW tracing (red tracing) "approximates" actual LA tracing (blue tracing) but is slightly delayed since pressure wave is transmitted retrograde through pulmonary veins.

Table 4.7 Causes of change in pulmonary artery pressure changes

PACWP Waves

"a" Wave: Atrial systole

High in MS, decreased LV compliance due to LV failure/valve disease

Cannon a waves: AV asynchrony (3rd degree AN block, V-pacer, and VT)

Absent a: Atrial flutter or fibrillation

Equal a and v: Tamponade and constrictive pericarditis

"c" Wave: Protrusion of MV into LA

"x" Descent: Relaxation of LA, downward pulling of mitral annulus by LV contraction

Prominent: Tamponade and constrictive pericaritis

Blunted: Atrial fibrillation and LA ischemia

"v" Wave

LV contraction

Height related to atrial compliance and amount of blood return and higher than a wave

High in VSD/MR/left or right ventricular failure

"y" Descent MV opening and LA emptying into LV

Prominent: MR, constrictive pericarditis, and restrictive cardiomyopathy

Blunted: MS, LV ischemia, and tamponade

Table 4.8 PCWP and LVEDP

PCWP not equal to LV end-diastolic pressure

- Mitral stenosis
- Atrial myxoma
- Cor triatriatum
- Pulmonary venous obstruction
- Decreased ventricular compliance
- Increased pleural pressure

gradient). In the absence of any obstruction to LV outflow, this peak pressure occurs at the end of the first third of systole. The peak-positive rate of rise of LV pressure (*dP/dt*) occurs before the opening of the aortic valve (AV); the peak-negative *dP/dt* occurs simultaneously with closure of the AV and marks the beginning of isovolumetric relaxation in the LV. Following AV closure, the LV pressure declines until decreasing the pressure differential between LV and LA causes the opening of mitral valve (MV). At end diastole, the pressure rises quickly in response to atrial systole. The LVEDP immediately precedes the beginning of isovolumetric contraction in the LV pressure pulse. In general, the mean PCWP, mean LAP, and LVEDP are all nearly equivalent in magnitude.

Comparing left-sided to right-sided pressures

- Diastolic amplitude similar between RV and LV tracings
- Systolic amplitude higher for LV than RV
- Duration of systole, isovolumetric contraction, and isovolumetric relaxation are longer for LV compared with RV
- Duration of ejection is shorter for LV than RV

Important abnormalities of left ventricular tracings

- Systolic pressure overload
  - Systemic hypertension
  - Aortic valve stenosis
  - Left ventricular outflow obstruction
  - Supravalvular obstruction
  - Coarctation of aorta
  - Significant atrial (ASD) or ventricular septal defect (VSD)
- Systolic pressure reduced
  - Hypovolemia
  - Cardiogenic shock
  - Tamponade

The LVEDP is elevated (>12 mmHg) in

1. LV diastolic volume overload (e.g., MR, aortic valve regurgitation [AR], and a large left-to-right shunt)
2. Concentric hypertrophy (decreased compliance), for example, aortic valve stenosis (AS) or long-standing HTN
3. Decreased myocardial contractility (dilated LV)
4. Restrictive or infiltrative cardiomyopathy
5. Constrictive pericardial disease (or a high-pressure pericardial effusion)
6. Ischemic heart disease (acute or chronic secondary-to-noncompliance, scar)

However, LVEDP is low in

1. MS
2. Hypovolemia

Ascending aorta

During ejection, normal pressure in the ascending aorta parallels LV pressure (Figure 4.7). Once the AV closes, the aortic pressure declines somewhat more slowly than the LV pressure. This reflects the accumulated pressure waves from the thoracic aorta and its tributaries as well as the capacitance of the aorta. Following the dicrotic notch, there is a brief increase in pressure due to some retrograde flow from the periphery into the ascending the aorta and the elastic recoil of the ascending aorta. Then as the blood runs off into the periphery, there is a gradual decline in the systolic arterial pressure until the next cardiac cycle. The rate and

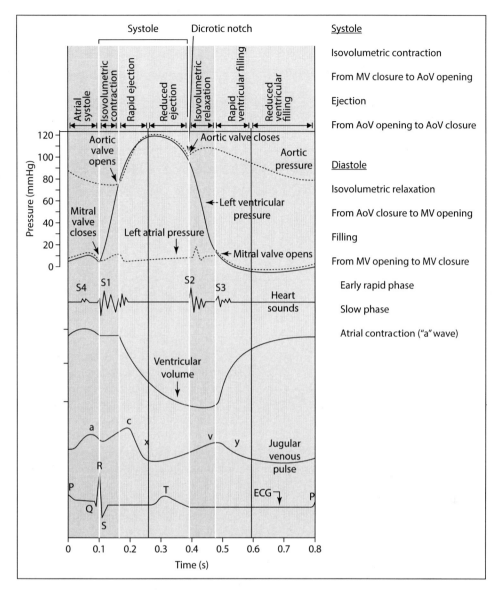

Figure 4.7 (**See color insert.**) Normal left and right pressure waves in correlation to ECG. The isovolumetric contraction and relaxation times are shaded in pink.

magnitude of decline of aortic pressure during diastole are dependent on

1. Aortic valve integrity (aortic insufficiency)
2. Capacitance and resistance of the peripheral circuit
3. Presence or absence of abnormal connection of aorta and the pulmonary circulation or the right heart (e.g., PDA)
4. Presence or absence of a large arteriovenous fistula

Pulse pressure (PP) is defined as the systolic minus the diastolic pressure

$$PP = \text{Systolic BP} - \text{Diastolic BP}$$

There are many causes of change in pulse pressure (Table 4.9).

Femoral or peripheral arterial pressure is not, and usually should not be equal to central aortic pressure. The overshoot of femoral artery pressure is due to summation of the pressure wave reflections generated by the expansion and recoil characteristics of the central aortic and large-artery elasticity. The peripheral or femoral artery pressure is almost always higher than the central aortic pressure (Figure 4.8).[7]

Pulsus bisferiens

The normal carotid arterial pulse tracing and the central aortic pulse waveform consist of an early component, the percussion wave, which results from rapid left ventricular ejection, and a second smaller peak, the tidal wave,

Table 4.9 Causes of change in aortic pressure	
Widened pulse pressure	**Reduced pulse pressure**
Systemic hypertension	Tamponade
Aortic insufficiency	Heart failure
Significant patent ductus arteriosus	Cardiogenic shock
	Aortic stenosis
Ruptured sinus of Valsalva aneurysm	
Systolic pressure elevated	**Systemic pressure reduced**
Systemic hypertension	Hypovolemia
Atherosclerosis	Aortic stenosis
Aortic insufficiency	Heart failure
Coarctation of aorta	

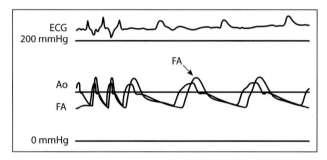

Figure 4.8 Simultaneously recorded pressures from the aortic root (Ao) and femoral artery (FA) demonstrating delayed transmission and a higher systolic pressure in the femoral artery. There is smoothing of the waveform and loss of the dicrotic notch.

presumed to represent a reflected wave from the periphery. The tidal wave may increase in amplitude in hypertensive patients or in those with elevated systemic vascular resistance. Radial and femoral pulse tracings demonstrate a single sharp peak in normal circumstances. Pulsus bisferiens is characterized by two systolic peaks of the aortic pulse during left ventricular ejection separated by a mid-systolic dip (Figure 4.9). Both percussion and tidal waves are accentuated. It is difficult to establish with certainty that the two peaks are occurring in the systole with simple palpation (pulsus bisferiens) versus one peak in the systole and the other in the diastole (dicrotic pulse).[8-10]

Pulsus bisferiens (Figure 4.9) is frequently observed in patients with hemodynamically significant (but not mild) aortic regurgitation. In patients with mixed aortic stenosis and aortic regurgitation, bisferiens pulse occurs when regurgitation is the predominant lesion. The absence of pulsus bisferiens does not exclude significant aortic regurgitation.

In most patients with hypertrophic cardiomyopathy, the carotid pulse upstroke is sharp and the amplitude is normal; pulsus bisferiens is rarely palpable but often recorded. The rapid upstroke and prominent percussion wave result from

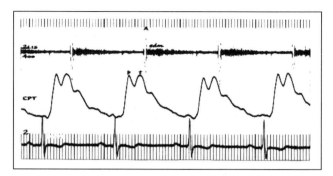

Figure 4.9 Pulsus bisferiens.

rapid left ventricular ejection into the aorta during early systole. This is followed by a rapid decline as left ventricular outflow tract obstruction ensues, a result of midsystolic obstruction and partial closure of the aortic valve. The second peak is related to the tidal wave. Occasionally, a bisferiens pulse is not present in the basal state but can be precipitated by the Valsalva maneuver or by inhalation of amyl nitrate.

Pulsus bisferiens is occasionally felt in patients with a large patent ductus arteriosus or arteriovenous fistula. A bisferiens quality of the arterial pulse is also rarely noted in patients with significant mitral valve prolapse and very rarely in normal individuals, particularly when there is a hyperdynamic circulatory state.

The mechanism of pulsus bisferiens is not clear. It appears to be related to a large, rapidly ejected left ventricular stroke volume associated with increased left ventricular and aortic *dp/dt*.

It is mainly seen in hypertrophic obstructive cardiomyopathy and aortic insufficiency.[8]

Pulsus alternans

Pulsus alternans (also termed mechanical alternans) is a variation in pulse amplitude occurring with alternate beats due to changing systolic pressure (Figure 4.10). The precise mechanism for pulsus alternans remains unclear; alternating preload (Frank–Starling mechanism) and incomplete relaxation have been proposed. Changes in afterload, which is lower before the strong beat because of the lower output during the weak beat, may also contribute. Pulsus alternans should not be diagnosed when the cardiac rhythm

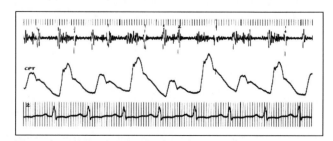

Figure 4.10 Pulsus alternans.

is irregular. Pulsus alternans is more common with faster heart rate.

It has also been suggested that a change in ventricular contractility is the primary mechanism. Changes in sarcoplasmic calcium pumps with alternate strong and weak beats appear to be the mechanism for changes in contractility. Thus, pulsus alternans may primarily result from an alternating contractile state of the ventricle. The magnitude of the alteration of pressure and stroke volume during pulsus alternans, indices of pump function, reflects the interaction of an alternating contractile state with changes in preload and afterload.[11,12]

Some of the causes of pulsus alternans are pericardial effusion, cardiomyopathy, congestive heart failure, and severe aortic regurgitation with left ventricular dysfunction.

Pulsus paradoxus

Systolic arterial pressure normally falls during inspiration, although the magnitude of decrease usually does not exceed 8–12 mmHg. These changes in pulse amplitude are not usually appreciated by palpation but can be established with the sphygmomanometer.

A more marked inspiratory decrease in arterial pressure exceeding 20 mmHg is termed pulsus paradoxus (Figure 4.11).[13] In contrast to the normal situation, this is easily detectable by palpation, although it should be evaluated with a sphygmomanometer. When the cuff pressure is slowly released, the systolic pressure at expiration is first noted. With further slow deflation of the cuff, the systolic pressure during inspiration can also be detected. The difference between the pressures during expiration and inspiration is the magnitude of pulsus paradoxus. The inspiratory decrease in systolic pressure is accentuated during very deep inspiration or Valsalva; thus, assessment of pulsus paradoxus should be made only during normal respiration.

In addition to tamponade, pulsus paradoxus can occur in chronic obstructive pulmonary disease, hypovolemic shock, and infrequently in constrictive pericarditis and restrictive cardiomyopathy. It is rarely observed in pulmonary embolism, pregnancy, marked obesity, and partial obstruction of the superior vena cava.

In hypertrophic obstructive cardiomyopathy, arterial pressure occasionally rises during inspiration (reversed pulsus paradoxus); the precise mechanism for this phenomenon is unclear.[13] In addition to changes in the amplitude, configurational changes of the carotid pulse may occur.

Cardiac output

In the cardiac catheterization laboratory, the cardiac output is usually determined by one of two methods: (1) measurement of oxygen consumption, or (2) the indicator-dilution method. Each of these techniques will be reviewed further.

Measurement of oxygen consumption (Fick method)

Adolph Fick initially described this technique in 1870.[14] The principle used is that the uptake of a substance by any organ system is the product of the arteriovenous concentration difference of that substance and the blood flow to that organ. Hence, if the lungs are used as the end organ, the pulmonary blood flow (which is equal to the systemic blood flow in the absence of an intracardiac shunt) can be determined by measuring the arteriovenous difference in the oxygen across the lungs and the uptake of oxygen by the lungs. Oxygen content is calculated by estimating the oxygen-carrying capacity of the patient's blood, as hemoglobin-bound oxygen. This is the volume of oxygen that could be carried on hemoglobin at 100% saturation. This is calculated by

$$Hb \text{ (g/L)} \times 1.36.$$

Usually, this is in the order of 200 mL/L, although it varies with Hb. The content of each sample is then computed by multiplying by the saturation. Thus, if Hb is 140 g/L and saturation in a sample is 70%, then oxygen-carrying capacity is

$$140 \times 1.36 = 190 \text{ mL/L}$$

and oxygen content will be

$$190 \times 70\% = 133 \text{ mL/L}.$$

The left ventricular oxygen content:

$$1.36 \times \text{Hemoglobin concentration} \times \text{LV oxygen saturation}.$$

The mixed venous (pulmonary artery) oxygen content:

$$1.36 \times \text{Hemoglobin concentration} \times \text{PA oxygen saturation}.$$

The value 1.36 is derived from the fact that 1 g of hemoglobin, when 100% saturated, combines with 1.36 mL of oxygen.
Therefore,

$$CO(L/min) = \frac{O_2 \text{ consumption (mL/min)}}{Ao - PA \, O_2 \text{ content (mL/L)}}$$

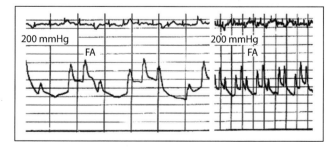

Figure 4.11   Pulsus paradoxus.

There are two techniques traditionally used for the determination of oxygen consumption:

1. Douglas bag method
2. Metabolic hood or the polarographic method

However, it is important to remember that no matter what method is used, the patient needs to be breathing comfortably at a steady state. The other source of error is the use of supplemental oxygen by the patient during the procedure; this makes it difficult to calculate the oxygen content of inspired air. To minimize this error, it is suggested that supplemental oxygen therapy must be discontinued for at least 15 min prior to determination of cardiac output by the Fick method. Alternatively, VO_2 can be estimated as 3 mL O_2/kg/min or 125 mL/min/m^2.

Indicator-dilution method

This method uses the mean concentration and transit time of an artificial substance that is added to the bloodstream. The most commonly used method is cold saline (thermodilution) injected into the RA and the resulting temperature change is detected in the PA. Another indicator not commonly used these days is the indocyanin green dye. The dye is injected into the central circulation (preferably PA) and is then detected in a systemic artery.

Thermodilution

Room temperature (or iced) normal saline solution is injected into the SVC or RA through the proximal port of the Swan–Ganz catheter, the thermistor that is located at the tip of the catheter is inserted in the PA.[15,15-17] If room-temperature saline is used, there must be at least 10°C difference between the injectate and body temperature. A dilution curve is then constructed as cool saline passes the thermistor tip. The CO is then calculated by the computer using the area under the curve as done for the dye indicator technique (total of 3–5 outputs should be done). In a number of studies, this method has shown good correlation with the Fick method for calculation of cardiac output.

CO is calculated by the following formula:

CO (mL/s)

$$= \frac{\text{Volume injected (mL)} \times \text{Temperature difference (°C)}}{\text{Area under the curve (°C.s)}}$$

To get the CO in L/min, the above value is multiplied by 0.06. MR or AR does not directly influence the downslope of the indicator-dilution curve. However, severe TR results in poor mixing in the RA and subsequent loss of the indicator to the body tissue before it reaches the PA.

Important hemodynamic equations:

1. Mixed venous oxygen saturation:[18]

$$MV \text{ sat} = \text{Sat SVC} - \frac{\text{Sat SVC} - \text{Sat IVC}}{4}$$

Usually, it is in the range of 60–80%.

2. Cardiac output

$$CO = SV \times HR$$

$$CO = \frac{\text{Oxygen consumption (mL/min)}}{AVO_2 \text{ difference (mLO}_2\text{/L blood)}}$$

AVO_2 is the difference between arterial and mixed venous (pulmonary artery) O_2 content

$$O_2 \text{ content} = \text{Saturation} \times 1.36 \times \text{Hemoglobin concentration}$$

3. Simple shunt calculation Qp:Qs

$$Qp:Qs = \frac{\text{Sat Ao} - \text{Sat MV}}{\text{Sat PV} - \text{Sat PA}}$$

4. Cardiac index (L/min.m^2)

$$CI = \frac{CO \text{ (L/min)}}{BSA \text{ (m}^2\text{)}}$$

Normal 2.5–4.2 L/min.m^2.

5. Stroke volume (mL)

$$SV = \frac{CO \text{(mL/min)}}{HR}$$

6. Stroke index (mL/beat.m^2)

$$SI = \frac{SV \text{(mL/beat)}}{BSA \text{ (m}^2\text{)}}$$

7. Stroke work

$$SW = (\text{Mean LV systolic P} - \text{Mean LV diastolic P}) \times SV \times 0.0144$$

8. Pulmonary artery resistance (Wood units)

$$PAR = \frac{\text{Mean PAP} - \text{Mean LAP (or PCWP)}}{Qp}$$

You can use CO instead of Qp in the absence of intracardiac shunting. Multiply by 80 for results in metric units (dynes.s.cm^{-5}) (i.e., PVRI). Normal range for PVRI is 225–315 dynes.s.cm^{-5}

$$\text{Mean PAP} = \text{PAD} + \frac{\text{PAS} - \text{PAD}}{3}$$

The normal range of mean pulmonary artery pressure (PAP) is 11–18 mmHg.

9. Total pulmonary resistance (Wood units)

$$\text{TPR} = \frac{\text{Mean PAP}}{\text{CO}}$$

Multiply by 80 for results in metric units (dynes.s.cm^{-5}) (i.e., TPRI).

10. Systemic vascular resistance (Wood units)

$$\text{SVR} = \frac{\text{Mean systemic arterial BP} - \text{Mean RAP}}{\text{CO}}$$

Multiply by 80 for results in metric units (dynes.s.cm^{-5}) (i.e., obtain the SVRI). The normal range for SVRI is 1970–2390 dynes.s.cm^{-5}.

$$\text{Mean AP} = \text{DBP} + \frac{\text{SBP} - \text{DBP}}{3}$$

The normal range for mean atrial pressure (MAP) is 80–100 mmHg.

Vascular resistance

Vascular resistance is the impediment offered by the vascular bed to flow. The greatest resistance occurs at the site of the greatest drop in pressure (arterioles). Whether it is on the left or right side, it is a measurement of ventricular afterload.

The percentage of total vascular resistance estimated for each region of the systemic vascular is: aorta and larger arteries: 9%; small arteries and branches: 16%; arterioles: 41%; capillaries: 27%; venules: 4%; small veins: 1%; and large veins: 2%.

However, vascular resistance is dependent on the properties of the vessel and its contained fluid, with a pattern of unidirectional and constant blood flow (microcirculation). Vascular impedance is the impediment offered to flow at the input of a vascular bed where pulsatile flow is involved (aorta and arteries).

Estimation of vascular resistance

The hemodynamic expression of Ohms's law helps one to understand how the circulation is controlled. Similarly, the Poiseuille equation for flow of homogeneous fluids states

$$\text{Resistance} = \frac{P}{Q} = \frac{8\eta L}{r4}$$

where
  Q = volume flow
  P = change in pressure
  r = radius of tube
  L = length of tube
  η = viscosity of the fluid

In the vascular system, the key factor is the radius of the vessel. The smaller the vessel diameter, the greater the resistance. This can be simplified to

$$\text{Flow (Q)} = \frac{\text{Pressure}}{\text{Resistance}}$$

Arterial pressure = Cardiac output × Vascular resistance

The resistance is a ratio, relating pressure and flow, and reflects the vasomotor tone in arterioles, terminal arterioles, and precapillaries sphincter (Tables 4.10 and 4.11).

$$\text{Vascular resistance (mmHg/L/min)} = \frac{\text{Arterial pressure (mmHg)}}{\text{Cardiac output (L/min)}}$$

Data in these formulae are expressed in liters per minute (blood flow), and pressures are in millimeters of mercury. These equations yield resistance in arbitrary resistance units (R units). They may be converted into dyne.cm.s^{-5} by using the conversion factor 80. mmHg/L/min is termed as a hybrid unit or Wood unit. If multiplied by 80, then the unit will be in dyne.cm.s^{-5}.

Table 4.10 Normal values for systemic and pulmonary vascular resistance		
	Normal reference values Wood units	dyne.cm.s^{-5}
Systemic vascular resistance SVR = (Mean Ao − Mean RA)/Qs	10–20	770–1500
Pulmonary vascular resistance PVR PVR = (Mean PA − Mean LA)/Qp	0.25–1.5	30–180

Table 4.11   Causes of change in pulmonary and systemic vascular resistance

Increased systemic vascular resistance	Decreased systemic vascular resistance[19]	Increased PVR
Systemic HTN Cardiogenic shock with compensatory arteriolar constriction	Inappropriately high cardiac output Arteriovenous fistula Severe anemia High fever Sepsis Thyrotoxicosis	Primary lung disease Eisenmenger syndrome Elevated pulmonary venous pressure Left-sided myocardial dysfunction Mitral/aortic valve disease Left-sided obstructive chd

Systemic vascular resistance (SVR)

$$= \frac{(\text{Mean Ao} - \text{Mean RA})}{\text{Qs}}$$

Pulmonary vascular resistance (PVR)

$$= \frac{(\text{Mean PA} - \text{Mean LA})}{\text{Qp}}$$

Qs: systemic blood flow; Qp: pulmonary blood flow.

Shunt detection and measurements

Shunt detection

1. Indocyanine green method
   - Indocyanine green (1 cm³) is injected as a bolus into the right side of the circulation (pulmonary artery).
   - Concentration is measured from peripheral artery.
   - Appearance and washout of dye produces initial first-pass curve followed by recirculation in normal adults.
   - Nowadays, this method is not used in modern cardiac catheterization laboratories.
   - However, there is resurgence using this method to accurately detect right-to-left shunt in patients with patent foramen ovale.
2. Oximetric method
   - Obtain O_2 saturations in sequential chambers, identifying both step-up and drop-off in O_2 sat. It is important that the samples used for this calculation are acquired with the patient breathing air or an oxygen-enriched mixture not exceeding 30%. If higher concentrations of oxygen (50% or greater) are to be used (e.g., to test for pulmonary vascular reactivity), then the calculation of pulmonary blood flow (and Qp:Qs ratio) should involve measurement of pO_2 on at least the pulmonary vein sample (preferably also the pulmonary artery sample). This allows inclusion of dissolved oxygen in the calculation (a more complex calculation, which necessitates calculation of the oxygen content of the samples). The oximetric method is not very sensitive for small shunts (<1.3:1). As the RA receives blood from several sources, SVC, IVC, and coronary sinus:

   - SVC: Saturation most closely approximates true systemic venous saturation
   - IVC: Highly saturated because kidneys receive 25% of CO and extract minimal oxygen
   - Coronary sinus: Markedly desaturated because heart maximizes O_2 extraction

$$\text{MV sat} = \frac{3 \times \text{sat SVC} + \text{sat IVC}}{4}$$

   - Oxygen saturation samples should be taken from
   - IVC (at L4–5 and diaphragm levels)
   - SVC (at innominate vein level and RA level)
   - RA (high, mid, and low levels)
   - RV (mid, apex, and outflow tracts)
   - PA (MPA and left and right PAs)
   - LV (left ventricle)
   - AO (ascending, descending below ductus)

Shunt measurement

Pulmonary-to-systemic blood flow Qp:Qs

Estimation of oxygen content $= 1.36 \times \text{Hgb} \times O_2 \text{ saturation}$

$$\text{Systemic blood flow (SBF)} = \frac{O_2 \text{ consumption}}{\text{Ao } O_2 - \text{MVO}_2}$$

$$\text{Pulmonary blood flow (PBF)} = \frac{O_2 \text{ consumption}}{\text{Pv } O_2 - \text{Pa } O_2}$$

Oxygen consumption VO_2 measured either by

Resting oxygen uptake = Basal metabolic rate by Douglas bag method or

Formula $VO_2 = 2 \times 125 \text{ mL } O_2/\text{min} = 250 \text{ mL } O_2/\text{min}$

In children, the largest source of error is in the assessment of oxygen consumption.[19-23] Traditionally, this has been measured using a hood and gas pump that extracts all exhaled air and passes it through a mixing system before measuring the oxygen content. The difference between inhaled oxygen content and exhaled oxygen content, coupled with the flow maintained by the pump, allows estimation of oxygen consumption. This method involves several assumptions. First, it assumes that the pump caters for all exhaled air and that none is "lost." Second, it assumes effective mixing before the oxygen measurement. Third, it assumes (at least with some equipment) that the volume of exhaled air is the same as that of inhaled air, which is only true if carbon dioxide production is identical with oxygen uptake (in some labs, a respiratory quotient—respiratory exchange ratio [RER]—of 0.8 is assumed). It also requires very accurate measurements of flow through the pump. Additionally, it requires very precise measurements of the oxygen level in exhaled air, which has in the past required the use of large and cumbersome equipment (a mass spectrometer). Patients being catheterized under anesthesia may require a closed-circuit method, which is also laborious and time-consuming to perform. In either case, it is essential that the medical and technical personnel involved be very familiar with the equipment and the methodology, and that they perform such measurements on a regular basis.

Oxygen consumption is not measured routinely; when measurements are required, it is often difficult or impossible to obtain satisfactory measurements—for example, because the staff who are familiar with the apparatus are unavailable, and the personnel involved with the procedure are unfamiliar with the equipment and lack confidence/competence in obtaining the necessary data. Normal values for oxygen consumption obtained from children of varying age and sex and at different heart rates have allowed the use of "assumed oxygen consumption."[22]

Gradients and valve stenosis

Aortic valve stenosis

Stenosis of the aortic valve causes obstruction to blood flow from the left ventricle to the aorta. As a result, there is a systolic pressure gradient across the valve with a higher pressure in the left ventricle than the aorta.

Echocardiography has largely reduced the need for cardiac catheterization in the evaluation and monitoring of patients with aortic stenosis (Table 4.12). The 2006 American College of Cardiology/American Heart Association (ACC/AHA) guidelines on the management of valvular heart disease included recommendations for the diagnostic evaluation of adolescents and young adults with congenital aortic stenosis and the use of echocardiography for the evaluation and monitoring of older patients with aortic stenosis.[24,25]

Table 4.12 Severity of aortic stenosis in adults

	Aortic jet velocity (m/s)	Mean gradient (mmHg)	Valve area (cm²)
Normal	≤2.0	<5	3.0–4.0
Mild	<3.0	<25	>1.5
Moderate	3.0–4.0	25–40	1.0–1.5
Severe	>4.0	>40	<1.0[a]

Source: Adapted from Bonow RO. *Circulation* 2008;118:e523.
Note: Critical aortic stenosis has been hemodynamically defined as a valve area <0.75 cm² and/or an aortic jet velocity >5.0 m/s. However, the decision about valve replacement is not solely based on hemodynamics, as some patients who meet these criteria are asymptomatic, while others with less severe measurements are symptomatic. In patients with severe aortic stenosis who also have a low cardiac output state, the aortic jet velocity and mean gradient may be lower than that indicated above (low-gradient aortic stenosis)
[a] Severe aortic stenosis is also considered to be present if the valve area indexed by body surface area is <0.6 cm²/m².

The guidelines recommended cardiac catheterization for hemodynamic assessment in older adults in only one setting: in symptomatic patients in whom noninvasive tests are inconclusive or provide discrepant results from clinical findings regarding the severity of aortic stenosis. There may be a larger role in adolescents and young adults with congenital aortic stenosis. Also, with the emergence of percutaneous transcatheter aortic valve replacement, patients undergo full hemodynamic assessment of the gradient prior to and after valve implantation.

A precise assessment of the aortic valve gradient can be obtained by the simultaneous measurement of the aortic pressure (as assessed with a pigtail catheter above the aortic valve or a long 5 F or 6 F long sheath), and the left ventricular pressure (measured using the transseptal technique or longer 4 F pigtail catheter inserted into the long sheath). However, if the aortic pressure is obtained from the peripheral artery, realignment of the pressure tracing is necessary, since the peripheral arterial pressure is delayed temporarily compared with the central aortic pressure.

Determining the transvalvular gradient is done by simultaneous measurement of pressures obtained from a catheter in the aorta and one in the left ventricle positioned via a transseptal approach. However, it is more common for the left ventricular catheter to be placed retrogradely via the aorta. With this technique, after measurements are made in the left ventricle, the catheter is quickly pulled back to a level just above the aortic valve and the aortic pressure is measured. However, the transvalvular gradient may increase by the presence of a catheter across the stenotic aortic valve, thereby reducing the effective antegrade orifice area.[3] This effect is proportional to the severity of the underlying aortic stenosis.

The time-honored method of evaluating the severity of aortic stenosis (Figure 4.12) is a calculation of the

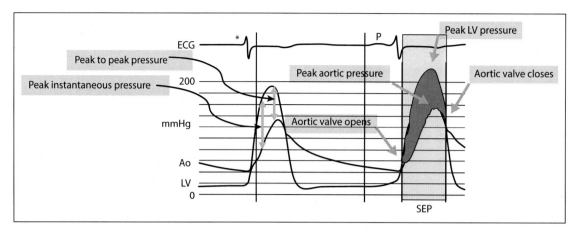

Figure 4.12 **(See color insert.)** Simultaneously recorded pressures from the left ventricle (LV) and aorta (Ao) in a patient with aortic stenosis. There is a systolic pressure gradient (red shaded area) in which the LV systolic pressure is greater than that in the aorta. The pressure gradient and systolic ejection period (SEP, in s/beat) are used in the Gorlin formula to calculate the aortic valve area (aortic valve area = cardiac output ÷ [44.3 x SEP x HR x square root mean gradient]). The peak instantaneous gradient is the maximal pressure difference between Aorta and LV when the pressures are measured at the same moment. The peak-to-peak gradient is the difference between the maximal pressure in the aorta and the maximal pressure in LV. (Redrawn from Kern MJ (ed). *Cardiac Catheterization Handbook*, 2nd ed. St. Louis: Mosby-Year Book; 1995. With permission.)

aortic valve area (AVA in cm²) based on the formulations described by Cannon and Gorlin[26,27] and Hakki et al.:[28]

AVA by Gorlin

$$= \frac{\dfrac{\text{CO in cc/min}}{\text{SEP} \times \text{HR}}}{\text{K} \times 44.3 \times \sqrt{\text{Mean aortic valve gradient in mmHg}}}$$

where CO = cardiac output (mL per beat), SEP = systolic ejection period (s per beat), and it is measured from the time the semilunar valves open, and ventricular contraction propels blood into the great arteries, to the point of when the semilunar valves close. SEP is calculated by measuring at 100 mm/s paper speed. K is the combined constant and is 1.0 for aortic, pulmonic, and tricuspid valves, and 0.85 for the mitral valve.

For example: CO = 4.3 L/min, HR = 95 beats/min, SEP = 0.22 s/beat, and mean gradient = 40 mmHg

$$\text{AVA} = \frac{(4.3 \times 1000/0.22 \times 95)}{44.3 \times \sqrt{40}} = \frac{205.7}{279.1} = 0.7 \text{ cm}^2$$

A more simplified formula is

AVA by Hakki[29] formula

$$= \frac{\text{CO}}{44.3 \times \sqrt{\text{Peak-to-peak gradient}}} = \frac{\text{CO in mL/min}}{44.3 \times \sqrt{P1 - P2}}$$

$P1$ = peak LV pressure, $P2$ = peak Ao pressure.

A reduced aortic pressure and the existence of a pressure gradient between the left ventricle and the aorta are the principal findings relating to the aortic pressure among

patients with aortic valvular stenosis. In addition, the rise in aortic pressure is slow and delayed compared with the pressure rise in the left ventricle.

In addition to an increased systolic pressure, abnormalities of diastolic pressure may be observed because of left ventricular hypertrophy with reduced compliance. Although the mean left ventricular diastolic pressure may be normal or elevated, the left ventricular end-diastolic pressure is most commonly elevated, a result of atrial contraction and filling of the noncompliant left ventricle. Thus, there is usually a prominent "a" wave with increased amplitude.

The left atrial pressure tracing shows large "a" waves because of the combination of a hypertrophied left atrium and a stiff or noncompliant left ventricle; this reflects the increased pressure generated during atrial contraction and filling of the left ventricle.

Low-gradient valvular aortic stenosis

An important group of patients with aortic stenosis consists of symptomatic patients who have low-gradient aortic stenosis, defined as a small transvalvular gradient (<30 mmHg), and a low cardiac output, with a calculated AVA of ≤0.7 cm².[29] In these patients, there is often doubt about whether the aortic valve is sufficiently stenotic to account for the symptoms or the patient has only mild aortic valvular disease and the symptoms are resulting from a significant reduction in left ventricular function due to a myopathic problem.

The concern about low-gradient aortic stenosis is justified, since the Gorlin formula is flow dependent and tends to underestimate the valve area when the cardiac output is low, that is, <3 L/min.[26,30,31] Since cardiac output measured at the time of cardiac catheterization greatly influences the clinical evaluation and subsequent management decisions, a pharmacologic stimulation of cardiac output (such as Dobutamine)[32] is often required for further evaluation to facilitate the decision regarding surgery in these patients. Maneuvers that increase cardiac output will almost always increase the calculated valve area, except in truly severe aortic stenosis. Aortic valve resistance calculations are rarely used for clinical decision making.

Common maneuvers that have been employed in the cardiac catheterization laboratory to induce left ventricular outflow tract (LVOT) gradients include:

- Valsalva maneuver—Valsalva lowers preload due to reductions in venous return.
- Administration of nitroglycerin that lowers preload through venodilation.
- Postextrasystolic potentiation—Postextrasystolic potentiation produces an increase in left ventricular inotropy and contractility, which may result in an increase in systolic anterior motion (SAM) and outflow obstruction, and a decrease in aortic pulse pressure (Brockenbrough effect).
- Isoproterenol infusion—Isoproterenol infused at an initial rate of 1 μg/min and then increased by 1 μg every minute until a heart rate of 120–150 beats/min is reached or the LV outflow pressure gradient reaches 55 mmHg. Isoproterenol is no longer used in the catheter lab.

Acute aortic valve regurgitation

Acute AR does not allow sufficient time for myocardial adaptation, and LV moves quickly up its diastolic pressure–volume curve, causing a marked elevation of LVEDP and early closure of the mitral valve. The left ventricular pressure tracing reveals a steep rise in diastolic pressure and a markedly elevated left ventricular end-diastolic pressure (which is equivalent to the aortic end-diastolic pressure). There is minimal increase in LVED volume or fiber length, and the total stroke volume cannot increase sufficiently to compensate for the regurgitant volume; thus, forward SV and CO fall. The high LVEDP also serves to minimize the runoff into LV; therefore, the diastolic pressure in the aorta may remain near normal and the arterial pulse pressure increases very little, if at all.[3]

Chronic aortic valve regurgitation

In this case, the LV has time to adapt to the volume overload by using the Frank–Starling mechanism (increased fiber stretch). The hemodynamic and afterload conditions in chronic AR resemble those of chronic MR with two important differences: (1) the total SV is ejected into a high-impedance circuit (the aorta and systemic arteries), and because the total forward SV is augmented, the LV and

aortic systolic pressures are elevated (>160 mmHg); and (2) because the AV is incompetent, the diastolic pressure in the aorta falls to subnormal levels during diastole, thereby reducing the diastolic perfusion pressure across the coronary arterial bed. The pulse pressure, which is defined as the systolic minus the diastolic pressure, is therefore widened. Since eccentric myocardial hypertrophy is associated with a sizable increase in total myocardial oxygen demand, patients with AR are particularly prone to develop angina in the absence of coronary artery disease (CAD).

In aortic regurgitation, the left ventricular stroke volume (A) (measured angiographically) is greater than the forward stroke volume (F) (determined by the Fick cardiac output); the difference is the regurgitant fraction (RF) that leaks back into the left ventricle during each cardiac cycle.

$$RF = \frac{[\text{Stroke volume (A)} - \text{Stroke volume (F)}]}{\text{Stroke volume (A)}}$$

The ACC/AHA guidelines[24,25] for the management of patients with valvular heart disease recommended cardiac catheterization in patients with aortic regurgitation in only one setting: when noninvasive tests are inconclusive or provide discrepant results from clinical findings. Cardiac catheterization should be performed with aortic root angiography and measurement of left ventricular pressure to assess the severity of the regurgitation, aortic root size, and left ventricular function.

Mitral valve stenosis

Regardless of the cause, there is impairment of blood flow from the left atrium into the left ventricle, resulting in a pressure gradient between the two chambers during diastole.

The ACC/AHA guidelines on the management[24,25] of valvular heart disease included recommendations for the use of cardiac catheterization for hemodynamic evaluation in patients with mitral stenosis (Table 4.13).

The severity of mitral stenosis as reflected by the mean mitral valve gradient (MVG) is measured during diastole by the simultaneous comparison of the left ventricular pressure (obtained with a left ventricular catheter positioned retrogradely from the aorta), and the left atrial pressure directly measured using a transseptal catheter or indirectly with a pulmonary artery catheter measuring the capillary wedge pressure. In most cases, a gradient is present, although it decreases during diastole because of slow but continuous left atrial emptying. With atrial systole, however, the gradient increases and is markedly higher than the left ventricular end-diastolic pressure. The volume of blood in the left atrium and the mean left atrial pressure are both increased during this period. After mitral valve opening, the pressure only gradually decreases and the "y" descent is gradual. The "a" wave, which is due to left atrial contraction, is markedly increased because of the stenosis.[3,7]

Table 4.13   ACC/AHA guideline summary: cardiac catheterization in mitral stenosis

Class I—There is evidence and/or general agreement that cardiac catheterization for hemodynamic evaluation is useful in patients with MS in the following settings:

• To assess the severity of MS if noninvasive tests are not conclusive or there is a discrepancy between the results of noninvasive tests and clinical findings related to the severity of MS.
• When there is a discrepancy between MVA and the Doppler-derived mean gradient, catheterization should include left ventriculography to evaluate the severity of mitral regurgitation.

Class IIa—The weight of evidence or opinion is in favor of usefulness of cardiac catheterization for hemodynamic evaluation in patients with MS in the following settings:

• To assess the exercise-induced hemodynamic response of the pulmonary artery and left atrial pressures when there is a discrepancy between clinical symptoms and hemodynamics at rest.
• To assess the cause of severe pulmonary arterial hypertension if it is out of proportion to the severity of MS determined by noninvasive testing.

Class III—There is evidence and/or general agreement that cardiac catheterization for hemodynamic evaluation in patients with MS is not useful in the following settings:

• To assess mitral valve hemodynamics when two-dimensional and Doppler echocardiographic findings are consistent with clinical findings.

Source: Data from Bonow RO. *J Am Coll Cardiol* 2006; 48:e1.

Since the diastolic filling period is important in the assessment of MVGs (Figure 4.13), the heart rate's effect upon the MVG is important. The gradient is higher with a faster heart rate since less time is available for left atrial emptying with a reduced diastolic period. By comparison, the gradient is lower with a slower heart rate.

A simplified method for estimating the mean MVG has been developed in which mean left ventricular diastolic pressure is estimated as LVEDP/2,[33] thus

$$MVG = \text{Mean LAp} - \frac{LVEDP}{2}$$

The calculation of mitral valve area (MVA in cm²) based on the formulations described by Gorlin and Gorlin is [27]

Mitral VA by Gorlin

$$= \frac{\dfrac{CO \text{ in cc/min}}{DFP \times HR}}{K \times 44.3 \times \sqrt{\text{Mean mitral valve gradient in mmHg}}}$$

where CO = cardiac output (mL per min), DFP = diastolic filling period (s per beat), and K is the constant factor for the mitral valve 0.85 (for aortic, pulmonary, or tricuspid valves, K = 1). The Gorlin formula is best applied to patients in sinus rhythm without mitral regurgitation, normal left ventricular function, and no other concomitant valve lesions.

Acute mitral regurgitation

With acute mitral regurgitation, the left ventricle and (more importantly) the left atrium have not had time to adapt to the regurgitant volume overload, resulting in low compliance chambers. As a result, with the onset of systole and the large volume of regurgitant blood flow, the left atrial pressure rises abruptly, causing a very tall "v" wave. Because of this "v" wave, the pressure gradient between the left atrium and left ventricle declines by the end of the systole; the amplitude of the "v" wave and that of the left ventricular systole are nearly equivalent. The diastolic pressure of the left ventricle is increased because of an increase in the end-diastolic volume within an undilated and noncompliant chamber.[7]

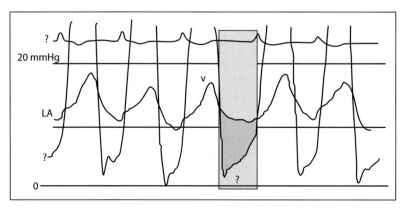

Figure 4.13   **(See color insert.)** LA and LV pressure tracings in a patient with MS. Shaded area represents the mitral valve gradient. DFP = diastolic filling period. The planimetered area (green shaded) is used to calculate mean valve gradient (MVG).

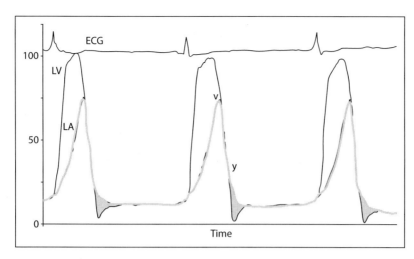

Figure 4.14 (**See color insert**.) LV and LA pressure tracings in isolated, severe MR and atrial fibrillation. The "a" and "c" waves in the LA tracing (blue pressure tracing) are not evident and the "v" wave is accentuated.

Chronic mitral regurgitation

Normal MV closure, which prevents the systolic backflow of blood into the LA, depends on the complex interaction of each of the components of the valve apparatus (LA wall, the annulus, the MV leaflets, the chordae, the papillary muscles, and the LV wall). Abnormalities in the anatomy and function of any of these components lead to valvular regurgitation. The regurgitant flow produces a large left atrial pressure wave immediately with the onset of ventricular systole. During the initial part of diastole, the left atrium rapidly decompresses with a large antegrade flow to the left ventricle.

Pressure measurements (Figure 4.14) either in the PCW or LA positions usually reveal an elevated "v" wave (>20 mmHg peak value), followed by a relatively rapid "y" descent as the MV opens and an excessive inflow of blood traverses the MV.[34] There is commonly a small pressure gradient across the MV during early diastole, reflecting functional MS in the presence of increased flow. If the MR is relatively acute and severe, a very large "v" wave is generated owing to the fact that the LA remains relatively normal sized and noncompliant and LV shortening remains normal to supranormal. Conversely, in long-standing severe MR, the "v" wave may be extremely small owing to massive dilatation of the LA and a significant increase in its capacitance. When myocardial contractility becomes severely diminished, depression of the total stroke volume may also contribute to the lack of generation of a significantly elevated "v" wave.

The left ventricle is volume overloaded due to the excess blood volume (generated during the prior systolic regurgitant beat) flowing during diastole from the left atrium. However, since the compliancy of the left ventricle increases, the left ventricular systolic and diastolic pressures are normal or only slightly increased. Although the left ventricular stroke volume is increased, the forward stroke volume is normal because a part of the stroke volume regurgitates back into the left atrium. The left ventricular pressure waveforms in systole and diastole are therefore normal.

The effective CO depends on the severity of the regurgitation, the acuteness versus chronicity of the process, the adaptation of the LV to the volume overload, and the maintenance of normal myocardial contractility.

In combined MS/MR, significant dilatation of the LA is seen owing to the combined pressure and volume overload of the chamber. In this setting, the pressure recordings from the left heart reveal an early and mid-diastolic pressure gradient across the MV, but if the DFP is sufficiently long, the LA and LV pressures equilibrate during the period of slow ventricular filling. The "v" wave is often dominant, reflecting the augmented systolic expansion and dilatation of the LA. The amount of regurgitation is calculated as the difference between total LV stroke volume (measured on contrast LV angiogram) and the stroke volume calculated from a Fick or indicator-dilution CO and the resting HR.

The left ventricular stroke volume (A) (measured angiographically) is greater than the forward stroke volume (F) (determined by the Fick cardiac output); the difference is the RF that leaks back into the left atrium during each cardiac cycle:

$$RF = \frac{[\text{Stroke volume (A)} - \text{Stroke volume (F)}]}{\text{Stroke volume (A)}}$$

Pulmonary valve stenosis

Diagnostic cardiac catheterization is rarely required in patients with pulmonic stenosis (PS) due to the extensive characterization of valvular structure, severity of stenosis, and right ventricular size and function derived from echocardiography. Invasive hemodynamic measurements and ventriculography may be useful when the severity of

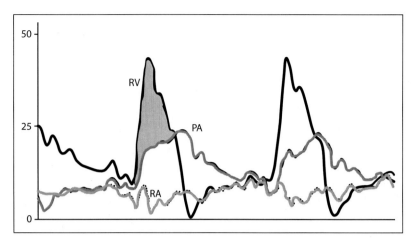

Figure 4.15 **(See color insert.)** Simultaneous pressure recordings from RV, PA (red tracing), and RA (blue tracing) in a patient with pulmonic valve stenosis. The shaded area is the pulmonic valve stenosis gradient.

stenosis is unclear or a significant secondary infundibular stenosis is suspected in addition to the valvular stenosis (Figure 4.15).

The ACC/AHA guidelines recommended cardiac catheterization for evaluation of the severity of PS in only one condition (Table 4.14): if the peak jet velocity on the Doppler echocardiography is >3 m/s (estimated peak systolic gradient >36 mmHg).[24,25] Balloon valvotomy is usually performed during the same procedure, if clinically indicated (Table 4.13).

PS is congenital in 95% of cases; rare causes include carcinoid syndrome and rheumatic valve disease. Although PS can be a feature of other types of congenital heart disease (e.g., tetralogy of Fallot), 80% of cases are isolated as PS. The abnormal valve is classified as unicommissural (with prominent systolic doming of leaflets and eccentric orifice),

bicuspid (with fused commissures), or dysplastic (severely thickened and deformed leaflets). Rarely, PS can be associated with the aneurysm of the PA.

Cardiac catheterization in a moderate-to-severe obstruction of the PV places a pressure overload on the RV that, in turn, leads to significant right ventricular hypertrophy (RVH). The pressure tracings from RV and PA (Figure 4.15) can be used to calculate the mean gradient similar to the method used for AS. Pulmonic valve area can also be calculated by the Gorlin[27] formula as follows:

Pulmonary valve area by Gorlin

$$= \frac{\dfrac{CO\ in\ cc/min}{SEP \times HR}}{K \times 44.3 \times \sqrt{Mean\ RV\ to\ PA\ gradient\ in\ mmHg}}$$

Pulmonary valve regurgitation

The basic cardiac defect in pulmonary regurgitation (PR) is retrograde leakage of blood from the main PA into the RV during diastole. Unless the pulmonary artery diastolic pressure (PADP) is severely elevated, the driving force between the PA and RV is not large, and the RF of the stroke volume remains relatively small. Moreover, the RV can tolerate a relatively large volume overload, and thus, the patient with PR commonly exhibits no impairment of CO either at rest or during exercise. Also, the RVEDP and RAP are not elevated unless there is an associated pressure overload on RV, or PR is long-standing.

Tricuspid valve stenosis

Tricuspid stenosis (TS) is a rare clinical condition, with rheumatic disease accounting for more than 90% of cases. In patients with rheumatic MV disease, only 3–5% have concurrent TS.

Table 4.14 ACC/AHA guideline summary: balloon valvotomy for pulmonic stenosis in adolescents and young adults

Class I—There is evidence and/or general agreement that balloon valvotomy should be performed in adolescents and young adults with PS in the following settings:

• Symptoms of angina, syncope, or dyspnea on exertion with an RV-to-pulmonary artery peak-to-peak gradient >30 mmHg at cardiac catheterization.
• Asymptomatic patients with an RV-to-pulmonary artery peak-to-peak gradient >40 mmHg at cardiac catheterization.

Class IIb—The weight of evidence or opinion is less well established for the usefulness of balloon valvotomy in adolescents and young adults with PS in the following setting:

• Asymptomatic patients with an RV-to-pulmonary artery peak-to-peak gradient of 30–39 mmHg at cardiac catheterization.

Source: Data from Bonow RO. *J Am Coll Cardiol* 2006; 48:e1.

Tricuspid valve regurgitation

Secondary tricuspid regurgitation (TR) is much more common than primary TR. Functional TR resulting from pulmonary HTN is seen in patients with significant left-sided heart disease, those with primary pulmonary HTN, and those with pulmonary disease leading to cor pulmonale. Functional TR also occurs in patients with RV dilatation as seen with RV infarction or an ASD. TR occurs in as many as 30–50% of patients with rheumatic mitral valve disease.

The normal tricuspid valve (TV) orifice area is 8–12 cm²; significant symptoms and signs of TS may be seen when the valve area is compromised to ≤2 cm². As with MS, the gradient across the valve is dependent on the diastolic filling period and cardiac output. Thus, exercise is associated with a significant increase in the gradient across the valve. The RA pressure pulse in TS is characterized by an exaggerated "a" wave (if in sinus rhythm). As with MS, there is slowing of the "y" descent and the absence of diastasis between the RA and RV pressure pulses (Figure 4.15). HR influences the pressure gradient as it does in MS. These effects are subtle though, since in most cases the valve gradient is not more than 5–8 mmHg.

Cardiac Tamponade

The pericardial space normally contains 5–10 mL of fluid that may be detected by echocardiography. This fluid serves as a lubricating material to allow normal rotation and translation of the heart during the cardiac cycle. A wide variety of disorders can result in pericardial effusion. When the intrapericardial (IP) pressures exceed the pressures in the cardiac chambers, impaired cardiac filling occurs; this is known as tamponade physiology. As the pericardial pressures increase, filling of each cardiac chamber is affected sequentially, starting with lower-pressure chambers (atria). The compressive effect of the fluid is seen best in the phase of cardiac cycle when pressure is lowest in that chamber (diastole for the ventricle and systole for atrium). In severe tamponade, diastolic pressures in all cardiac chambers are equal and elevated.

Diastolic equilibration or pressures are the hallmark of cardiac tamponade. Hence, accurate measurement of pressures in right- and left-sided chambers is mandatory when tamponade is suspected, although this is rarely necessary these days with the advent of echocardiography. The pressure tracings should be recorded simultaneously, along with the respiratory cycle. Ideally, both right and left heart catheterization should be done to show the equalization of diastolic pressures in these chambers. However, if PCWP tracings are of good quality, and if clinical, noninvasive, and hemodynamic data are consistent with tamponade, left heart catheterization may be omitted. When the IP pressure has increased to equal RA pressure, cardiac tamponade begins.

With the rise in IP pressure, the venous pressure rises to maintain intracardiac volume. In early cardiac tamponade without preexisting heart disease, the IP and RA pressures are equal but only slightly elevated. Furthermore, PCWP (or LA pressure) remains higher than the RA pressure. When cardiac tamponade becomes more severe, the RA and IP pressures remain equal and rise progressively as the tamponade gets more severe. The point at which the RA, and PCWP (or LA pressure) become equal defines classic cardiac tamponade (this finding is not pathognomonic; other conditions can cause this equalization such as constrictive pericarditis). RA and PCWP should be recorded simultaneously rather than sequentially. The height to which the venous pressure is elevated depends on the severity of tamponade. In milder cases, these pressures range from 7 to 10 mmHg. In moderate cases, pressures are 10–15 mmHg and are often accompanied by reduction in cardiac output and arterial BP.

Severe tamponade is characterized by pressures in the range of 15–30 mmHg usually accompanied by profound reduction in CO and arterial BP, which at this stage will demonstrate pulsus paradoxus (Figure 4.11). Often, there is a narrow pulse pressure before the drop in peak systolic pressure. In establishing the diagnosis of cardiac tamponade, special attention should be paid to the waveform of RA and PCWP tracings. Inspiratory decrease in RA pressure should be observed. Cardiac tamponade exerts its abnormal pressure on heart chambers throughout the cardiac cycle. However, ventricular ejection is faster than venous return, causing cardiac volume to decrease. With this event, there is a slight decline in IP pressure. For this reason, venous return is confined to the period of ventricular systole that translates to prominence of "x" descent and absence of "y" descent of venous pressure. Thus, in typical tamponade, RA pressure is elevated and equal to PCWP and shows an inspiratory drop and absence of "y" descent. This is in contrast to constrictive pericarditis that demonstrates a sharp "x" and "y" descents.

References

1. Baim DS, Grossman W. *Cardiac Catheterization, Angiography, and Intervention.* 5th ed. Baltimore: Williams & Wilkins; 2005.
2. Kern MJ. Hemodynamic rounds series II: Pitfalls of right-heart hemodynamics. *Cathet Cardiovasc Diagn* 1998;43:90–4.
3. Kern MJ, Feldman T, Bitar S. Hemodynamic data. In: *The Cardiac Catheterization Handbook.* 5th ed. St. Louis: Mosby-Year Book; 2011. pp. 126–7.
4. Morgan BC, Abel FL, Mullins GL, Guntheroth WG. Flow patterns in cavae, pulmonary artery, pulmonary vein, and aorta in intact dogs. *Am J Physiol* 1966;210:903–9.
5. Brecher GA, Hubay CA. Pulmonary blood flow and venous return during spontaneous respiration. *Circ Res* 1955;3:210–14.
6. Tavel ME. Normal sounds and pulses: Relationships and intervals between the various events. In: *Clinical Phonocardiography and External Pulse Recording.* 2nd ed. Chicago: Year Book Medical Publishers; 1972. p. 35.

7. Kern MJ, Lim MJ, Goldstein JA. *Hemodynamic Rounds: Interpretation of Cardiac Pathophysiology from Pressure Waves Analysis*. 3rd ed. Philadelphia: Wiley-Blackwell; 2009. pp. 86–7.
8. Fleming PR. The mechanism of the pulsus bisferiens. *Brit Heart J* 1957;19:519–24.
9. Lewis T. The pulsus bisferiens. *Brit Med J* 1907;1:918–20.
10. Talley JD. Recognition, etiology, and clinical implications of pulsus bisferiens. *Heart Dis Stroke* 1994;3:309–11.
11. Lab MJ, Seed WA. Pulsus alternans. *Cardiovasc Res* 1993;27:1407–12.
12. Lablanche JM, Thieuleux FA, Bertrand ME. Pulsus alternans: Alternation of relaxation parameters. *Arch Mal Coeur Vaiss* 1984;77:1540–6.
13. Massumi RA, Mason DT, Vera Z, Zelis R, Otero J, Amsterdam EA. Reversed pulsus paradoxus. *N Engl J Med* 1973;289:1272–5.
14. Acierno LJ. Adolph Fick: Mathematician, physicist, physiologist. *Clin Cardiol* 2000;23:390–1.
15. Wood EH. Diagnostic applications of indicator-dilution technics in congenital heart disease. *Circ Res* 1962;10:531–68.
16. Freed MD, Keane JF. Cardiac output measured by thermodilution in infants and children. *J Pediatr* 1978;92:39–42.
17. Sibille L, Prasquier R, Vallois JM, Gaudebout C, Pocidalo JJ. Cardiac output measurement with a simplified thermodilution technique. Comparison with the Fick method. *Biomedicine* 1975;23:64–7.
18. Miller HC, Brown DJ, Miller GA. Comparison of formulae used to estimate oxygen saturation of mixed venous blood from caval samples. *Brit Heart J* 1974;36:446–51.
19. Lindahl SG. Oxygen consumption and carbon dioxide elimination in infants and children during anaesthesia and surgery. *Brit J Anaesth* 1989;62:70–6.
20. Lundell BP, Casas ML, Wallgren CG. Oxygen consumption in infants and children during heart catheterization. *Pediatr Cardiol* 1996;17:207–13.
21. Kappagoda CT, Greenwood P, Macartney FJ, Linden RJ. Oxygen consumption in children with congenital diseases of the heart. *Clin Sci* 1973;45:107–14.
22. LaFarge CG, Miettinen OS. The estimation of oxygen consumption. *Cardiovasc Res* 1970;4:23–30.
23. Wilkinson JL. Haemodynamic calculations in the catheter laboratory. *Heart* 2001;85:113–20.
24. Bonow RO, Carabello BA, Chatterjee K et al. Focused update incorporated into the ACC/AHA 2006 guidelines for the management of patients with valvular heart disease: A report of the American College of Cardiology/American Heart Association Task Force on Practice Guidelines (Writing Committee to Revise the 1998 Guidelines for the Management of Patients with Valvular Heart Disease): Endorsed by the Society of Cardiovascular Anesthesiologists, Society for Cardiovascular Angiography and Interventions, and Society of Thoracic Surgeons. *Circulation* 2008;118:e523–661.
25. Patel MR, Bailey SR, Bonow RO et al. ACCF/SCAI/AATS/AHA/ASE/ASNC/HFSA/HRS/SCCM/SCCT/SCMR/STS 2012 appropriate use criteria for diagnostic catheterization: A report of the American College of Cardiology Foundation Appropriate Use Criteria Task Force, Society for Cardiovascular Angiography and Interventions, American Association for Thoracic Surgery, American Heart Association, American Society of Echocardiography, American Society of Nuclear Cardiology, Heart Failure Society of America, Heart Rhythm Society, Society of Critical Care Medicine, Society of Cardiovascular Computed Tomography, Society for Cardiovascular Magnetic Resonance, Society of Thoracic Surgeons. *J Thorac Cardiovasc Surg* 2012;144:39–71.
26. Cannon SR, Richards KL, Crawford M. Hydraulic estimation of stenotic orifice area: A correction of the Gorlin formula. *Circulation* 1985; 71:1170–8.
27. Gorlin R, Gorlin SG. Hydraulic formula for calculation of the area of the stenotic mitral valve, other cardiac valves, and central circulatory shunts. I. *Am Heart J* 1951;41:1–29.
28. Hakki AH, Iskandrian AS, Bemis CE et al. A simplified valve formula for the calculation of stenotic cardiac valve areas. *Circulation* 1981;63:1050–5.
29. Carabello BA. Advances in the hemodynamic assessment of stenotic cardiac valves. *J Am Coll Cardiol* 1987;10:912–9.
30. Cannon JD Jr., Zile MR, Crawford FA Jr., Carabello BA. Aortic valve resistance as an adjunct to the Gorlin formula in assessing the severity of aortic stenosis in symptomatic patients. *J Am Coll Cardiol* 1992;20:1517–23.
31. Cannon SR, Richards KL, Crawford MH et al. Inadequacy of the Gorlin formula for predicting prosthetic valve area. *Am J Cardiol* 1988;62:113–6.
32. deFilippi CR, Willett DL, Brickner ME et al. Usefulness of dobutamine echocardiography in distinguishing severe from nonsevere valvular aortic stenosis in patients with depressed left ventricular function and low transvalvular gradients. *Am J Cardiol* 1995;75:191–4.
33. Cui W, Dai R, Zhang G. A new simplified method for calculating mean mitral pressure gradient. *Catheter Cardiovasc Interv* 2007;70:754–7.
34. Freihage JH, Joyal D, Arab D et al. Invasive assessment of mitral regurgitation: Comparison of hemodynamic parameters. *Catheter Cardiovasc Interv* 2007;69:303–12.

5

Transesophageal 2D and 3D echocardiographic guidance

Joseph John Vettukattil

The technique of transcatheter intervention has evolved into highly complex and time-consuming mini-robotic device implantations that require careful preoperative assessment and intraprocedural guidance. Imaging techniques, too, have advanced to facilitate these procedures and assist the interventionist. Often, the echocardiologist and interventionist have developed an interdependency to achieve the best procedural outcome, reducing time, complication rate, and radiation dose. With the advance of real-time three-dimensional transesophageal imaging (3DTEE), 2DTEE has become almost redundant due to the limited spatial dimensions it can provide. Currently, TEE is used for most transcatheter interventions enhanced with 3D imaging. This includes accurate measurements of the aortic valve hinge points for valvoplasty and transcatheter valve implantation;[1] closure of aortic, mitral, and tricuspid paravalvar leaks (PVLs); transseptal puncture; left atrial appendage (LAA) closure; mitral valve annuloplasty; application of mitra-clip and similar devices; Fontan and Mustard baffle fenestrations; atrial septal defect (ASD) and patent foramen ovale (PFO) closure; and for congenital and acquired ventricular septal defect (VSD) closures. An extensive discussion of all these aspects is beyond the scope of this chapter, but some important aspects will be highlighted.

Preparation

The patient typically fasts for 6 hours before the introduction of the TEE probe. Under deep sedation with local anesthetic aerosol spray or preferably under general anesthetic, the probe is gently introduced while the patient does the swallowing movements lying in a lateral decubitus position. A mouth guard is applied to protect the patient as well as the probe. Ideally, the output from the echo monitor should be displayed by the side of the angiography display system with the operator positioned at the same side as the

interventionist, allowing easy observation of the procedure and direct interactions.

Before imaging begins, all related information, including previous imaging and hemodynamics, must be reviewed to plan the procedure. Depending on the nature of the intervention, 2D and 3D data sets are collated and analyzed. Appropriate measurements are made and quantification of the severity of the lesion, nature, location, morphology, and the best approach for intervention are identified and discussed with the interventionist.

With the advances in miniaturization and computing technology, 2DTEE is possible almost at any age. 3D probes are currently available only for children weighing 28 kg or above. However, in critical lesions where the 3D information is likely to significantly change the management plan, patients as small as 18 kg have had 3DTEE performed safely.

Image acquisition, analysis, and display

Depending on the diagnostic system available, it is important to have presets to optimize the quality of images and to achieve the best frame rates possible. Focusing on the anatomy of interest, gain, depth, and number of cardiac cycles to be synchronized must be determined before starting the image acquisition.

Live 3D catheter guidance

Live 3D zoom is the best setting for continuous monitoring of the device and catheter position during an intervention. The probe is positioned perpendicular to the area of interest whenever possible, so that the best echo signals captured attain optimum resolution for immediate display. Both lateral and vertical sector widths are set to include the whole of the structure of interest to be captured within the 3D frame. Details of the settings for individual lesions will be dealt with in the discussion of specific interventions.

Imaging for structural interventions

Mitral paravalvar leak

PVL is most commonly encountered with mitral prostheses. However, it is also seen with any prosthetic valve implantation. While assessing PVL in mitral prostheses, the actual area of dehiscence can be detected as an area of echo drop-out outside the sewing ring with appropriate adjustment of the gain settings. This must be confirmed by the presence of regurgitant jet on color-flow imaging.[3] In order to facilitate communication between the echocardiologist/cardiographer and the interventionist, the location of the dehiscence is best described in a standardized way, although it may be described in relation to internal landmarks such as the LAA, aortic valve, or the crux of the heart. The anatomic location of mitral PVL is best displayed in a clockface view with the aorta at the 12 o'clock position and the LAA between 9 and 10 o'clock positions (Figure 5.1). Various factors such as the anatomic location, size, shape, extent, course, severity, dimensions, proximity to the valve struts, nature of the adjoining tissue, mechanism of the lesion, exit and entrance points (especially in the para-aortic lesions), stability of the valve, the possible impact of device placement and suitability for interventions, and the best device for the specific intervention should be clearly defined before the intervention is attempted. Often, the

PVL in the lateral aspect of the mechanical valve can be better accessed through the transseptal approach, whereas the transapical approach or a high septal puncture is necessary to gain access to the medially placed defects (Figure 5.2). A retrograde approach through the aortic valve may be suitable for some lesions in the anterolateral position (8–11 o'clock) and transseptal puncture from the superior vena cava (SVC) is favored by some for the more medially located lesions.

The echocardiologist should guide the interventionist throughout the procedure by describing the position of the tip of the sheath and the delivery system in relation to the anatomy of interest and neighboring structures, while carefully evaluating for any potential complication. It is preferable for the echocardiologist to interrupt the procedure to obtain accurate assessment when in doubt rather than provide inaccurate guidance.

Mitral PVLs may be multiple and the adjoining tissue is often friable. The suture lines may be tense, which has caused the lesion in the first instance; hence, further tension through the placement of an oversized device may increase the defect size. The medial defects are best approached through transapical or a hybrid approach (Figure 5.3). However, a high transseptal approach may also be appropriate to access a medial defect (between the 1 and 5 o'clock position).

Tricuspid PVL is less common, as the tricuspid valve is easily accessible and visible for the surgeon during the valve replacement. Even when present, the leaks are well tolerated except when there are associated lesions causing pulmonary or right ventricular hypertension. When present, it is best approached via the superior caval route. It is also possible to achieve a stable catheter and guide wire position by placing the guide wire in the branch pulmonary arteries (PAs).

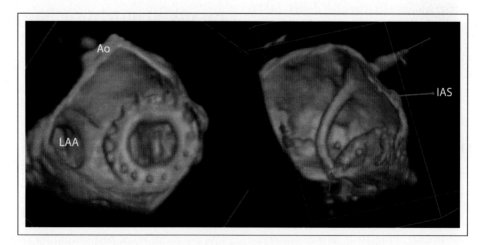

Figure 5.1   **(See color insert.)** The standard clockface display of a paravalvar leak with aorta at 12 o'clock position and LAA at 9 o'clock position (on the right). Here, the intervention is performed through the transseptal approach. The sheath comes out through the transseptal puncture being guided to the regurgitant orifice (arrow on the left).

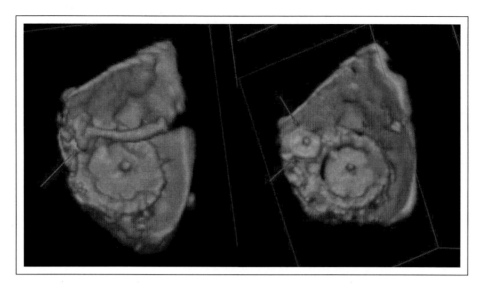

Figure 5.2   (**See color insert.**) The LA disk of the PVL device being positioned under 3D guidance (left arrow) and postdevice deployment on the right (red arrows).

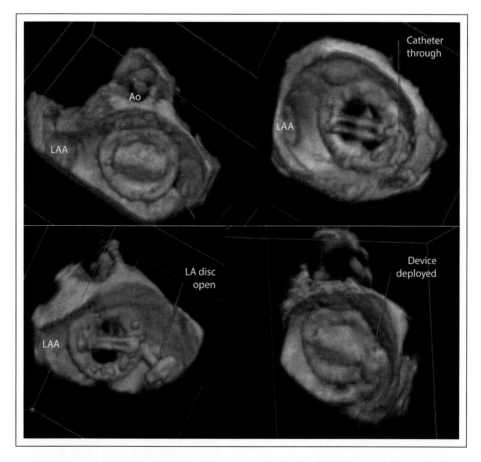

Figure 5.3   (**See color insert.**) Mitral PVL medial lesion at 3 o'clock position shown in these 3DTEE images. The approach here was through the transapical route. Catheter positioning and device manipulation is shown through serial images from left to right. Left upper image shows the defect. Upper right image shows the catheter passing through the defect. The lower two images illustrate the device placement and release in final position.

Aortic PVL

When aortic PVL is present, often 3D assessment can be best obtained preoperatively through trans thoracic echocardiography (TTE). The course and nature of the defect is easily demonstrable with TTE prior to TEE. Specific aspects to be considered when assessing the aortic PVL are the length and course of the tract, proximity to the coronaries, and relationship to the conduction system. It is also important to differentiate aortic PVLs from aorta to LV tunnels or fistulas.

Quantifying the severity of PVL is very similar to assessing mitral regurgitation. If 3DTEE is not available, multiplane 2D color-flow Doppler imaging is necessary to obtain a better understanding of the defect. On real time 3-Dimensional echocardiography (RT3DE), the flow through a significant lesion may be visible as an echogenic 3D shadow. When this is present, it always signifies a hemodynamically important lesion (Video 5.1) and live-color 3D images should always be obtained for assessing the dimensions and shape of the regurgitant orifice. Color 3D multiplanar reformatting or MPR is the best method for assessing these lesions. Ideally, the size of the defect should be expressed in relation to the circumference of the valve.

2DTEE is very sensitive in accurately identifying the leak (88%) and pointing out the exact location can be challenging, as the regurgitant jet may be overshadowed by the prosthetic valve. Transducer position behind the left atrium in TEE enables the visualization of mitral PVL unobscured by the prosthesis.

3DTEE

Mitral PVL is best visualized by the live zoom mode. To assess the position of the leak in relation to the rest of the cardiac structures, the display is standardized by positioning the anatomic structures in a clockface manner. Thus, the aorta is displayed anteriorly at 12 o'clock position and the LAA laterally at the 9 o'clock position, rendering the interatrial septum medially and the posterior wall of the left atrium at 6 o'clock position. Live-color 3D may be used to compare and visually quantify the leak. To derive the regurgitant orifice area, the most accurate method in experienced hands is the 3D MPR using color 3D full-volume loops. When aligned in anatomically appropriate planes, and frozen in peak systolic frame, vena contracta measured in three orthogonal planes gives the nearest possible data pertaining to the regurgitant orifice. A majority of the PVLs in mitral position are seen between 3 and 9 o'clock positions. For procedural guidance, 3D zoom function is most reliable and so is visualization of the catheter tip. The larger area of the cardiac anatomy is visible in this mode compared with live 3D. The echocardiologist/echocardiographer should be able to guide the interventionalist to the

area of the leak with accurate visualization of the regurgitant orifice in relation to the catheter tip.

Trans catheter aortic valve implantation (TAVI)

The aortic valve does not have a true fibrous ring supporting the valve leaflets and, hence, it is not symmetric or circular (Figure 5.4). The geometry of the valve is further altered by the degree of thickening, calcification, and its morphology (number of leaflets and the degree and plane of fusion). The relative tension in neighboring chambers and the aortic wall itself also influences the morphology and shape of the "annulus," raising concerns about the accuracy of the measurement in one plane using 2DTEE. The assumed circularity of the aortic annulus leads to erroneous estimates resulting in discrepancy of measurements between different imaging techniques and modalities. TEE-measured aortic annular size is 1.36 mm more than the TTE. One cannot overemphasize the role of 3D MPR in accurately measuring the distances between the hinge points of the aortic valve leaflets in peak systole.

The 2DTEE-based measurements have been shown to be comparable to CT measurements. Using short-axis views, the opening of the aortic valve should be classified as central or eccentric and the severity, location, and symmetry of the aortic valve calcification accurately described.

During TAVI, the prosthesis anchors according to the resistance of the tissues behind the aortic leaflets. During implantation, the native aortic valve leaflets are crushed against the aortic wall and the differences in the tension across the valve may cause asymmetric deployment of the prosthesis and contribute to the risk of compression of the coronary arteries. In order to minimize the risk of coronary occlusion, it is advisable to measure the distance from the

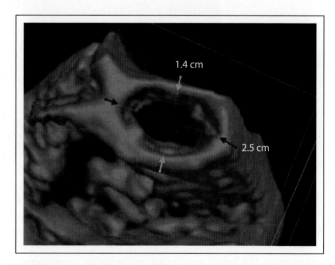

Figure 5.4 **(See color insert.)** Asymmetry of the aortic valve "annulus" seen on 3DTEE imaging.

aortic annulus to the ostia of the coronary arteries and to compare this with the length of the leaflets measured in a long-axis view. This measurement is best achieved with 3D MPR as the accurate visualization of the hinge points of the valve leaflets is possible, which may be in a different plane to that of the coronary ostia. Although the leaflets are typically shorter than the annular–ostial distances, those patients in whom the leaflet length exceeds the annular-ostial distances are at risk of ostial occlusion when the valve is deployed and the native leaflets are crushed to the side.

Although balloon inflation is normally performed during rapid right ventricular pacing to reduce stroke volume, the balloon may still migrate during inflation, particularly in those patients with severe septal hypertrophy or with a smaller sino-tubular junction. The loss of right ventricular capture or ventricular extra systole may also result in balloon migration. TEE may be used to confirm a stable position during inflation and to monitor the behavior of the calcified aortic leaflets during inflation.

During the deployment of the prosthesis, TEE is very helpful in confirming accurate positioning of the valve and is generally used in conjunction with fluoroscopy. The optimal position for the Edwards SAPIEN™ valve is with the ventricular side of the prosthesis positioned 2–4 mm below the annulus in the left ventricular outflow tract immediately following deployment; TEE is used to confirm satisfactory positioning and function of the prosthesis. When the prosthesis is positioned too low, it may impinge on the mitral valve apparatus or it may be difficult to stabilize in patients with marked septal hypertrophy. The native valve leaflets may also fold over the prosthesis and compromise the prosthetic valve function. If the prosthesis is implanted too high, it may migrate up the aorta and obstruct the coronary ostia, or cause significant PVL.[2]

It is important to confirm that all the prosthetic leaflets are moving well, that the valve stent has assumed a circular configuration (using 2D or 3D views), and that there is no significant valvar or PVL. Some regurgitation through the prosthesis will be common, while the delivery apparatus and/or guide wire remain across the valve and may persist, to a lesser degree, after their removal, as it may take a few minutes postimplant for the leaflets to completely recover from being crimped for deployment. Until this occurs, the leaflets may not coapt completely and mild transient regurgitation may be observed at the coaptation point. TEE views with continuous-wave, pulsed-wave, and color Doppler should be used to confirm satisfactory prosthetic valve position and function. To aid this, transgastric views may be obtained.

Aortic regurgitation has also been reported as a consequence of residual native aortic valve leaflet tissue prolapsing into the prosthesis, interfering with leaflet motion and coaptation. This may result from deficient containment of residual native aortic tissue by the prosthesis and/or positioning the valve too low. Monitoring complications such as perforation, clot formation, and tamponade is crucial

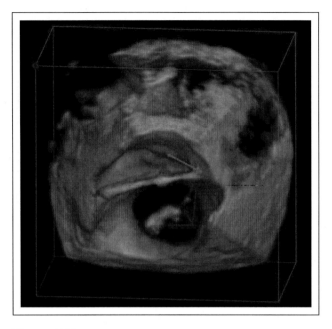

Figure 5.5 **(See color insert.)** 3D image of clot formation at the septal puncture site during LAA closure. Guide wire is through the transseptal puncture site (green arrow) and clot is attached to the interatrial septum (red arrow).

during deployment. Device embolization and atrioventricular (AV) block are more common with Corevalve. Damage or distortion of the subvalvar mitral apparatus by the delivery system, although uncommon, is possible. Asymmetric left ventricular wall motion abnormalities may indicate acute coronary occlusion. Cardiac tamponade, or right ventricular or septal perforation are other complications that need to be watched for during the procedure. Rarely does dissection or rupture of the aortic root occur.

Left atrial appendage closure

Achieving a low septal puncture and accurate measurement of the landing zone for LAA closure devices are very important aspects for successful closure. With 3DTEE, better visualization of the morphology and dimensions of the landing zone can be made from a full-volume loop with MPR. It is equally important to watch for complications during the procedure, as thromboembolism or pericardial tamponade can be detrimental if not identified promptly (Figure 5.5).

Congenital interventions

ASD and PFO closure

Assessment of deficiency in the interatrial septum to determine the feasibility of device closure has been mostly performed using the multiplane 2DTEE imaging. More recently, 3DTEE has significantly improved the visualization of these defects, so that accurate sizing may be

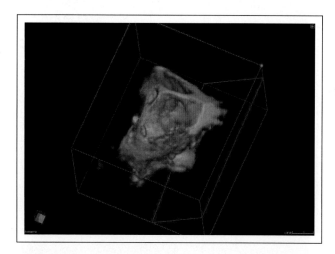

Figure 5.6 (**See color insert.**) Small secundum ASD at the region of the oval fossa viewed from the LA.

achieved, avoiding the need for balloon sizing. 2D imaging can often determine the hemodynamic significance and morphology of the defect. It also helps to identify the secundum defects from others, such as the sinus venosus or primum defects, which may be unsuitable for device closure. It is very important to ascertain the anatomic type of the defect, morphologic variations relating to size, shape, consistency, and adequacy of the margins, plane of the defects, and spatial orientation of the defect in 4D.[4]

During 2DTEE assessment, the viewing angle is rotated throughout the visible planes noting the relative position of the defect with regard to anatomic landmarks. It is important to identify the pulmonary veins as they open into the left atrium, the mouth of the coronary sinus, and opening of the systemic veins. At 0°, the crux of the heart with AV junction identifying the rim of the defect from the AV valves is made. Then the probe is rotated to visualize the coronary sinus at about 25–30 degrees with angulation. Following this, the aortic rim is best seen between 30 and 50 degrees, and at 90 degrees, the bicaval view is obtained. During device deployment, the best view is at 40–45 degrees, where the plane of the defect in relation to the aortic margin and the course of the delivery system is best visualized.

For 3D imaging, live 3D zoom is the most appropriate mode to visualize the plane and the morphologic characteristics of the defect, while adjusting the gain settings to define the margins well (Figures 5.6 through 5.9). 3D MPR must be used for accurate identification of the size of the defect(s) in atrial diastole. 3D assessment also helps to avoid oversizing and the need for balloon sizing. It reduces the potential for residual defects, and helps to detect and define associated malformations.

In addition to reducing the procedure time and radiation, in experienced hands, the information obtained by 3DTEE is superior to other imaging techniques, including intra cardiac echocardiography (ICE).

Transseptal puncture

TEE guidance is very helpful in transseptal procedures and baffle fenestrations. In this regard, left atrial appendage

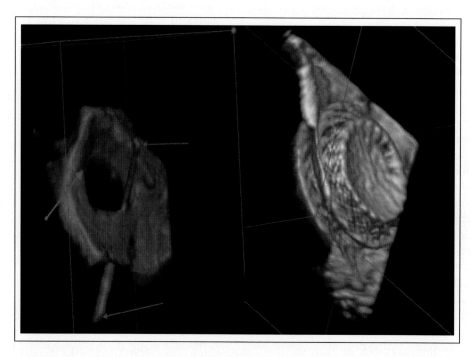

Figure 5.7 (**See color insert.**) A large ASD with adequate margins (except deficient aortic rim) closed with an Occlutech™ device. The defect with catheter passing from the IVC to the LA on the left and the device in position on the right.

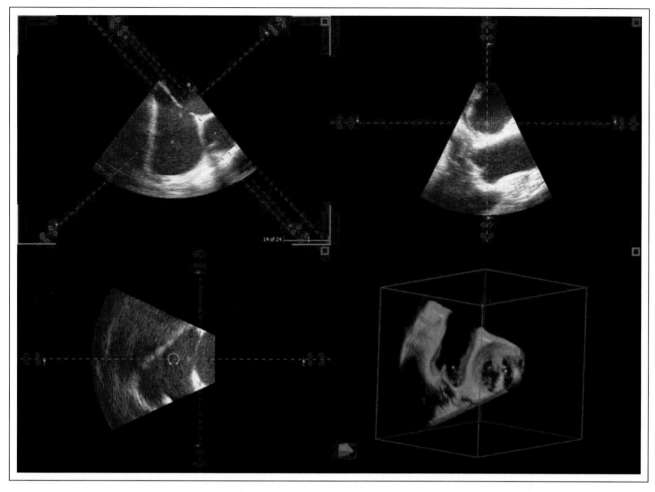

Figure 5.8   (**See color insert.**) Two ASDs in parallel identified as single defect on 2DTEE but visualized as two separate defects in 3DTEE.

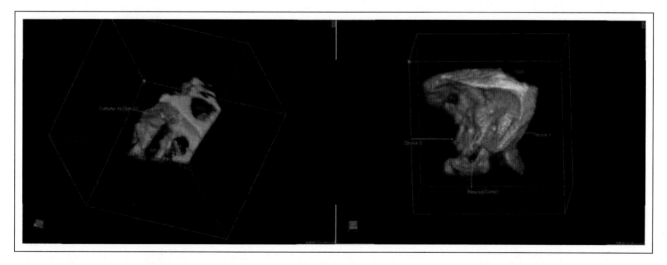

Figure 5.9   (**See color insert.**) 3DTEE showing two ASDs separated by a firm septum closed using two devices sitting comfortably, adjacent to each other with a small residual defect.

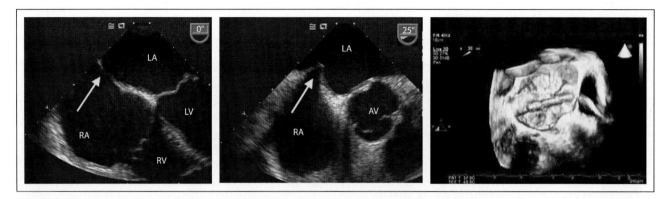

Figure 5.10 (See color insert.) Transseptal puncture under 2DTEE and 3DTEE guidance.

closure and relief of pulmonary vein stenosis and associated procedures benefit from TEE guidance (Figure 5.10).

Summary

Advanced cardiac imaging techniques through miniaturization and computing power have revolutionized visualization of the cardiac morphology and function leading to better bedside assessment and percutaneous catheter interventional therapy. Mastering these techniques provides new challenges. With the advent of high-speed Internet access, training and learning with collaborative research has become a reality. This is expected to further assist in the interactions and improved management of structural and congenital heart defects.[5]

References

1. Black D, Ahmad Z, Lim Z, Salmon A, Veltdman G, Vettukattil J. The accuracy of three-dimensional echocardiography with multiplanar reformatting in the assessment of the aortic valve annulus prior to percutaneous balloon aortic valvuloplasty in congenital heart disease. *J Invasive Cardiol* 2012;24(11):594–8.
2. Zamorano JL, Badano LP, Bruce C, Chan K-L, Gonçalves A, Hahn RT et al. EAE/ASE recommendations for the use of echocardiography in new transcatheter interventions for valvular heart disease. *Eur J Echocardiogr* 2011;12:557–84.
3. Wunderlich N, Franke J, Wilson N, Sievert H. 3D Echo guidance for structural heart interventions. *Interv Cardiol Rev* 2009;4(1):16–32.
4. Vettukattil JJ, Ahmed Z, Salmon AP, Mohun T, Anderson RH. Defects in the oval fossa: Morphologic variations and impact on transcatheter closure. *J Am Soc Echocardiogr* 2013;26(2):192–9.
5. www.3dechocardiography.com.

6

Intracardiac echocardiography (ICE)

Damien Kenny, Qi-Ling Cao, and Ziyad M. Hijazi

Introduction

The ideal multimodality intraprocedural imaging system to facilitate and guide the ever-increasingly complex array of congenital and structural heart interventions is one of the "holy grails" of interventional cardiology. The ideal system would provide detailed (real-time 3-D) near- and far-field images with minimal invasiveness, low cost, minimal interventional interference, and easy interface with the user, which ideally would be the interventionalist performing the procedure. Many of the intraprocedural imaging modalities available to the interventionalist (including CT, MRI, transthoracic echocardiography [TTE], and transesophageal echocardiography [TEE]) provide some of these functions but each has its own limitations. Intracardiac echocardiography [ICE] is attractive in that it provides excellent near-field and reasonable far-field imaging without the need for anesthesia and with minimal interference with the intervention, and it is manipulated entirely by the interventionalist performing the procedure. Radiation exposure through fluoroscopy may also be minimized. Consequently, it has become one of the most widely used ultrasound-based imaging adjuvants in the catheterization laboratory, obviating the need for support for anesthesiologists and echocardiographers, providing a potential procedural cost savings.[1] This chapter evaluates the historical development of ICE and the available systems, and provides examples of the congenital and structural interventions in which it has proved itself invaluable.

Historical perspectives and currently available systems

Ultrasound-tipped catheters were described in the 1970s, and later evolved into high-frequency intravascular ultrasound imaging probes to evaluate coronary artery disease in the 1980s.[2,3] It has only been over the past two decades that intracardiac transducers have been developed to evaluate intracardiac anatomy.[4,5] This has involved an evolution from high-frequency low-power catheters with 360° axial imaging capabilities for intravascular imaging to the development of lower-frequency transducers with greater depth penetration and more focused evaluation of segmental anatomical structures. Initial systems maintained radial imaging capabilities, and reports that assessed ventricular size and function soon followed.[6,7] However, it was with the realization of intracardiac imaging to guide interventional procedures, particularly initially in the field of electrophysiology, with need for access to the left atrium,[8,9] that significant developments were made in respect to maneuverability and advanced imaging support techniques.[10] Linear-array transducers gave way to phased-array catheters with lower frequencies and Doppler imaging capabilities.[11,12] Since this time and in line with the resurgence in transseptal puncture to access the left heart for structural interventions, ICE has evolved into one of the most widely used imaging modalities for noncoronary interventional cardiac procedures.[13] A list of cardiac interventional procedures for which ICE has been utilized is provided (Table 6.1).

Currently, there are five commercially available intracardiac imaging systems (Table 6.2).[14] The Ultra ICE™ system (Boston Scientific, San Jose, California) is a mechanical single-element system that is covered fully in another chapter and will not be discussed further here. The other systems are side-looking 64-element catheters without integrative functionality for 3-D electrophysiological mapping systems. The systems designed specifically for 3-D mapping integration are beyond the scope of this chapter and reference will be limited to Table 6.2. The AcuNav system (Biosense Webster, Diamond Bar, California) (Figure 6.1) is a side-looking 64-element phased-array transducer with four-way (anterior/posterior/left/right) handle steerability and a locking knob available as 8 and 10 F single-use catheters. The transducer has a frequency that varies from 5.5 to 10 MHz and scans in the longitudinal monoplane providing a 90° sector image with tissue penetration of 12 cm for the 10 F system and 16 cm for the 8 F system. The entire catheter system is freely torquable, providing the potential for imaging through multiple planes of the

Table 6.1 Interventions utilizing ICE imaging

Intervention	Advantages	Disadvantages
ASD closure	Good profiling of the entire interatrial septum, including the inferior portion Obviates the need for heavy sedation or general anesthesia	May be more difficult to interpret multiple or complex ASDs
PFO closure	As above with clear imaging of variants in PFO anatomy and tunnel morphology Limits the need for fluoroscopy	Catheter stability may be an issue during device deployment
VSD closure	Excellent profiling of the membranous septum in a number of different achievable views	May not be optimal for midmuscular or more apical defects
Aortic valvuloplasty/TAVR	Provides excellent accurate imaging of the aortic valve annulus May fit the workflow pattern of TAVR better than TEE as the procedure evolves	Limited experience to date, although this is likely to evolve
Pulmonary valvuloplasty/tPVR	Provides excellent imaging of the pulmonary valve, including assessment of residual stenosis or new regurgitation following intervention Limits the requirement for repeated angiography	May be perceived as expensive and unnecessary in this setting
Mitral valvuloplasty	Used to guide transseptal puncture and mitral interventions with full operator control	Left heart structures, particularly the left atrial appendage, may be a challenge to image from the right heart
Transseptal puncture	Provides detailed imaging of the atrial septum with its inherent anatomical variations No need to move the probe when using fluoroscopy	Lack of multiplanar imaging may limit the immediate view of the needle position following puncture
Left atrial appendage occlusion	Operator dependence	May require imaging from the left atrium to obtain detailed views, which may require a second transseptal access

Table 6.2 Commercially available ICE systems

Device name	Company	Features
UltraICE	Boston Scientific	9 F nonsteerable rotational motor-driven gray scale-only system (see Chapter 7)
AcuNav	Siemens, Biosense Webster	Side-looking 64-element phased-array four-way steerability, 8 F and 10 F; gray scale, color Doppler, tissue Doppler, 3-D localization with Cartosound
EP Med View Flex Catheter	St Jude Medical	Runs side-looking 64-element catheter on the Viewmate scanner, 10 F introducer, two-way flex color Doppler, gray scale, tissue Doppler 8–2 MHz
ClearICE	St Jude Medical	Derived from the hockey stick, 64-element side-looking highly steerable four-way side-looking array with two sets of electrodes for integration of 3-D localization with NavX; runs on the GE Vivid *i* scanner; gray scale, tissue Doppler, synchronization mapping, 2-D speckle tracking
SoundStar Catheter	Biosense Webster	This is a new catheter, just now marketed as a 10 F (3.33-mm) device with integrated ultrasound array (like AcuNav) but with the CARTO magnetic sensor in the tip.
AcuNav V	Siemens	Provides real-time volume imaging, but limited clinical experience to date

Source: Taken (with additions) from Hijazi ZM, Shivkumar K, Sahn DJ. *Circulation* 2009;119:587–96.

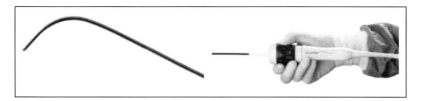

Figure 6.1 The AcuNav catheter. Left: The tip of the catheter can be manipulated in four different directions. Right: The control handle has three knobs: one to move the tip in posterior/anterior directions; one to move the tip right/left; and the last knob is a locking one that will fix the tip in the desired orientation.

heart, and with the locking system, allowing maintenance of a stable, fixed-tip orientation that gives the interventionalist freedom to provide "hands-free" imaging during the desired intervention. The system can provide full Doppler capabilities, including spectral, color, and tissue imaging.

Imaging protocols

The catheter is introduced through an appropriately sized sheath (8 or 10 F) in the femoral vein. The connection to the echocardiographic machine must be kept dry and a sterile cover is required for the cable. A longer 30 cm sheath may be used to ensure that the rigid ICE catheter clears some of the curves of the pelvis. Either way, fluoroscopic guidance should be used to screen catheter advancement into the mid-right atrium to ensure there is no trauma to the venous conduits to the heart. In adult patients, the AcuNav catheter can be introduced in the same (femoral) vein used for the septal device delivery. However, for patients weighing less than 35 kg (i.e., children), the contralateral femoral vein is used. When ICE is being used for mitral valve interventions requiring large venous sheaths, again the contralateral femoral vein is preferred.

Standard views

With the ICE catheter in the mid-right atrium aligned parallel to the spine, this is referred to as the neutral or "home" view. With the transducer rotated so that it is facing the tricuspid valve, the inflow, apical, and outflow portions of the right ventricle should be clearly seen. Further clockwise rotation will demonstrate the left ventricular outflow tract with the aortic valve and the ascending aorta with further rotation demonstrating the mitral valve and the left atrial appendage (LAA). Counterclockwise rotation is used to reestablish the home view and from here various maneuvers can be used to image the area of interest.

Atrial septum

The use of ICE during atrial septal defect (ASD) and patent foramen ovale (PFO) closure is well reported and has become the imaging modality of choice in adults,[15–17] often facilitating early hospital discharge.[18] At the start of the

case, a complete evaluation of the defect(s) and surrounding anatomy is performed. The intensity of this interrogation will in part depend on the adequacy and completeness of imaging prior to the procedure. For patients with an ASD, the size of the defect via 2-D imaging (with and without being stretched by a balloon) as well as the measurement of surrounding rims is obtained. Contrast injection via agitated saline microbubbles is performed for patients with a PFO to confirm the presence of a right-to-left shunt.

Stepwise protocol for ICE imaging to guide ASD or PFO closure

Step 1: From the "home view," the ICE catheter is flexed posteriorly using the knob so that the transducer faces the interatrial septum. Fluoroscopy showing the position of the catheter as well as a corresponding anatomic diagram is shown in Figure 6.2. The ICE image obtained shows the interatrial septum as well as the coronary sinus and pulmonary veins, depending on the exact location of the transducer. This can be referred to as the "septal view" (Figure 6.2b). One can obtain further views by locking the tip in this position and rotating the entire handle or by fine adjustments of the posterior/anterior or right/left knobs.

Step 2: The ICE catheter itself is then advanced in a cephalad direction toward the superior vena cava (SVC). This can be referred to as the SVC or "long-axis view." A fluoroscopic image showing the position of the catheter, as well as a corresponding anatomic diagram, is shown in Figure 6.2c. The ICE image obtained is also shown. In this plane, the transducer faces the interatrial septum and the SVC can be seen as it relates to the right atrium. The interatrial septum is shown in a superior/inferior plane and corresponds to the TEE long-axis view. Greater portions of the SVC can be seen by continued advancement of the ICE catheter in this flexed position toward the SVC. Greater portions of the inferior septum can be similarly imaged by withdrawing the ICE catheter toward the inferior vena cava in the flexed position. A defect of the interatrial septum can be well profiled, and the superior and inferior rims as well

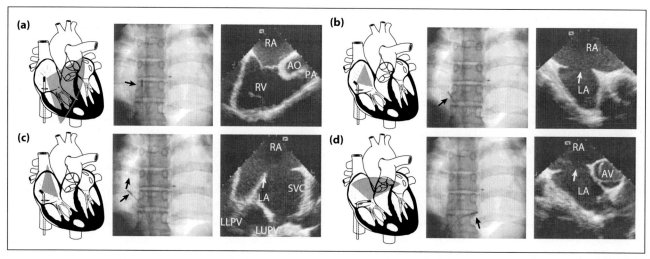

Figure 6.2 (a) Images in the home view. Left: Sketch representing the heart with the position of the intracardiac catheter inside the heart with the ultrasonic array box in the neutral "home view" position. The shaded area represents structures seen in this view. Middle: A cine fluoroscopy image showing the position of the ICE catheter (arrow) in the mid-right atrium with the transducer facing the tricuspid valve and parallel to the spine. Right: An actual intracardiac echocardiographic image with the ultrasonic box in the neutral home view position. The tricuspid valve and right ventricle outflow and inflow are well seen in this position. The aortic valve and pulmonic valve can also be seen. AO: aortic valve; RA: right atrium; PA: pulmonary artery; RV: right ventricle. (b) Images in the septal view. Left: Sketch representing the heart with the position of the intracardiac catheter inside the heart with the ultrasonic array box in the posterior flexed position looking at the atrial septum "septal view." The shaded area represents structures seen in this view. Middle: A cine fluoroscopy image showing the position of the ICE catheter (arrow) in the right atrium with the transducer flexed posterior looking at the septum. Right: An actual intracardiac echocardiographic image with the ultrasonic box in the septal view. The atrial septal defect (arrow) and the left and right atria are well seen. (c) Images in the long-axis "caval view." Left: Sketch representing the heart with the position of the intracardiac catheter inside the heart with the ultrasonic array box in the posterior flexed position with a cephalad advancement looking at the atrial septum and the superior vena cava caval view. The shaded area represents structures seen in this view. Middle: A cine fluoroscopy image showing the position of the ICE catheter (black arrow) in the right atrium with the transducer flexed posterior looking at the superior vena cava (white arrow). Right: An actual intracardiac echocardiographic image with the ultrasonic box in the caval view. The atrial septal defect (arrow), the left and right atria, the left pulmonary veins, and superior vena cava are all well seen. SVC: superior vena cava; LLPV: left lower pulmonary vein; LUPV: left upper pulmonary vein. (d) Images in the "short-axis view." Left: Sketch representing the heart with the position of the intracardiac catheter inside the heart with the ultrasonic array box in the flexed position and the entire handle rotated clockwise until the imaging transducer is above the tricuspid valve looking at the aorta from below. In this position, fine rotation of the knobs can demonstrate different parts of the atrial septum. The shaded area represents structures seen in this view. Middle: A cine fluoroscopy image showing the position of the ICE catheter (black arrow) in the right atrium with the transducer above the tricuspid valve. Right: An actual intracardiac echocardiographic image with the ultrasonic box in the short-axis view. The atrial septal defect (arrow), the left and right atria, and the aortic valve are all well seen. This view is similar to a TEE short-axis view with the left atrium in the far field (opposite to the TEE).

as the diameter of the defect can be measured. In this view, both the right and left pulmonary veins may also be imaged, depending on the exact angle of the imaging plane.

Step 3: The catheter (in its locked position) is then rotated clockwise until it sits in a position with the transducer near the tricuspid valve annulus, and inferior to the aorta. A fluoroscopic image showing the catheter position and a corresponding anatomic diagram is shown in Figure 6.2d. The ICE image obtained is also shown. In this view, the aortic valve can be seen in short axis as well as the interatrial septum. This corresponds to the basal short-axis view obtained with TEE and is known as the "short-axis view." However, the right atrium is in

the near field and the left atrium is in the far field, which is opposite of what is seen with TEE.

Prior to the actual device-deployment procedure, the above views are obtained in order to image the ASD or PFO. Additional views can be obtained by advancing the catheter through the ASD or PFO into the left atrium (see below). From this position, an equivalent of the transthoracic four-chamber view can be obtained with views of the mitral valve, LV, and RV. The catheter can be further manipulated to view the LAA, which may be helpful in procedures to occlude the LAA. The catheter is then withdrawn back to the right atrium. During the exchange wire and delivery sheath positioning, the long-axis view is felt to best delineate

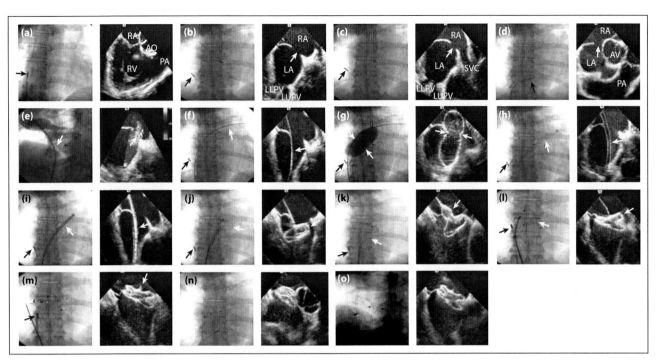

Figure 6.3 Cine fluoroscopic and ICE images in a 54-year-old female patient with a large secundum ASD who underwent closure using a 28 mm Amplatzer septal defect. (a) Left: Cine of the ICE catheter in the home view (arrow). Right: Image obtained showing the tricuspid valve, right ventricle, aorta, and pulmonary artery. (b) Septal view images. Left: ICE transducer (arrow) facing the septum. Right: ICE image obtained demonstrating the defect (arrow), pulmonary veins, and left and right atria. (c) Caval view images. Left: ICE transducer (arrow) facing the upper septum and looking at the superior vena cava. Right: ICE image obtained demonstrating the defect (arrow), SVC, pulmonary veins, and left and right atria. (d) Short-axis view images. Left: ICE transducer (arrow) above the tricuspid valve. Right: ICE image obtained demonstrating the defect (arrow), aortic valve, pulmonary artery, and left and right atria. (e) Left: Angiogram in the right upper pulmonary vein demonstrating the defect (arrow). Right: ICE image with color in septal view demonstrating the defect and shunt (arrow). (f) Left: Cine fluoroscopy image demonstrating the ICE catheter (black arrow) in the septal view position during passage of the exchange guide wire (white arrow) through the defect into the left upper pulmonary vein. Right: Corresponding ICE image showing the guide wire (arrow) through the defect. (g) Left: Cine fluoroscopy image demonstrating the ICE catheter (black arrow) in the septal view position during balloon sizing of the defect to obtain the stretched diameter (white arrows). Right: Corresponding ICE image showing the indentations on the balloon (arrows). (h) Left: Cine fluoroscopy image demonstrating the ICE catheter (black arrow) in the septal view position during passage of the delivery sheath (arrow) into the left atrium. Right: Corresponding ICE image showing the delivery sheath (arrow) inside the left atrium. (i) Left: Cine fluoroscopy image demonstrating the ICE catheter (black arrow) in the septal view position during passage of a 28-mm Amplatzer Septal Occluder within the sheath (arrow). Right: Corresponding ICE image showing the device inside the sheath (arrow). (j) Left: Cine fluoroscopy image demonstrating the ICE catheter (black arrow) in the septal view position during deployment of the left atrial disk (arrow) of a 28-mm Amplatzer Septal Occluder in the left atrium. Right: Corresponding ICE image showing the left disk in the left atrium (arrow). (k) Left: Cine fluoroscopy image demonstrating the ICE catheter (black arrow) in the septal view position during deployment of the connecting waist (arrow). Right: Corresponding ICE image showing the connecting waist (arrow). (l) Left: Cine fluoroscopy image demonstrating the ICE catheter (black arrow) in a modified septal short-axis view position during deployment of the right atrial disk (arrow). Right: Corresponding ICE image showing the right atrial disk (arrow). (m) Left: Cine fluoroscopy image demonstrating the ICE catheter (black arrow) in a modified septal short-axis view position after the device has been released from the cable (white arrow). Right: Corresponding ICE image showing the device after it has been released (arrow). (n) Left: Cine fluoroscopy image demonstrating the ICE catheter in a modified short-axis view position. Right: Corresponding ICE image showing the aortic valve and both disks of the device. (o) Left: Cine fluoroscopy image in the four-chamber view demonstrating the position of the device. Right: ICE image with color Doppler showing good device position and no residual shunt.

intracardiac relations. Device deployment is monitored in the long-axis view as well to demonstrate the relation of the disks to the interatrial septum. Figure 6.3a–o demonstrates a case of a patient with a large secundum ASD who underwent device closure. This figure demonstrates all the steps involved in device closure using the Amplatzer Septal

Occluder. Color Doppler imaging as well as contrast echocardiography is used to assess for the presence or absence of any residual shunts. For assessment of residual right-to-left shunting following PFO closure, a Valsalva maneuver may be performed with greater efficacy than in patients who have undergone TEE-guided closure (Figure 6.4).

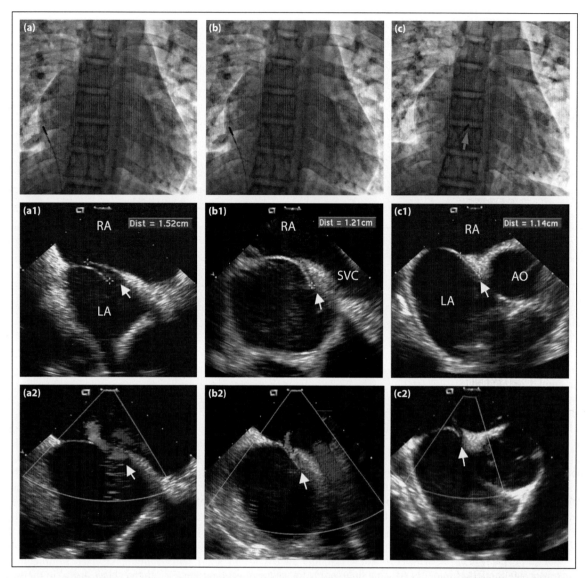

Figure 6.4 **(See color insert.)** A series of images outlining PFO closure with the Gore Septal Occluder. (a–c) Initial diagnostic assessment of the PFO. (a–a2) The septal view of the atrial septum with and without color Doppler (demonstrating L–R shunt) with corresponding position of the ICE catheter on fluoroscopy outlined by the red arrow. (b–b2) The long-axis view (c–c2) demonstrating the short-axis view with the tunnel length measuring between 11 and 15 mm (a1, b1, c1). (d–f) Fluoroscopy images with ICE catheter position (red arrow) with the corresponding ICE image below. (d) R–L shunt of bubble contrast across the PFO with (e) clearly showing the wire crossing the defect and (f) balloon sizing of the defect, which is optional outside of most clinical trails. (g–i) Delivery of the HELEX device with corresponding fluoroscopy and ICE images in various views. (i) The left atrial component of the device deployed with (j, k) demonstrating the device pulled back to the septum and further deployment of the right atrial component of the device with it fully deployed in the long-axis (k) and short-axis views (l). (m, n) Release of the device on fluoroscopy with corresponding postdeployment ICE assessment with short-axis views and long-axis views with and without color (o1, o2, p1, p2).

Stepwise protocol using ICE to guide VSD

The use of ICE to guide transcatheter ventricular septal defect (VSD) closure has been described.[19]

Step 1: ICE imaging is initiated in the RA with the "home-view" similar to ASD and PFO closure as described above. From this position, the RA, the RV inflow, and the membranous/perimembranous portion of the interventricular septum (IVS) are seen. The defect within the IVS is noted and its relationship to the tricuspid valve is shown in Figure 6.5a.

Step 2: The short-axis view is similar to that obtained during ASD and PFO closure. The catheter is flexed posteriorly and locked. The entire handle is rotated clockwise and advanced slightly just above the tricuspid valve until the short-axis view is achieved, with the transducer in

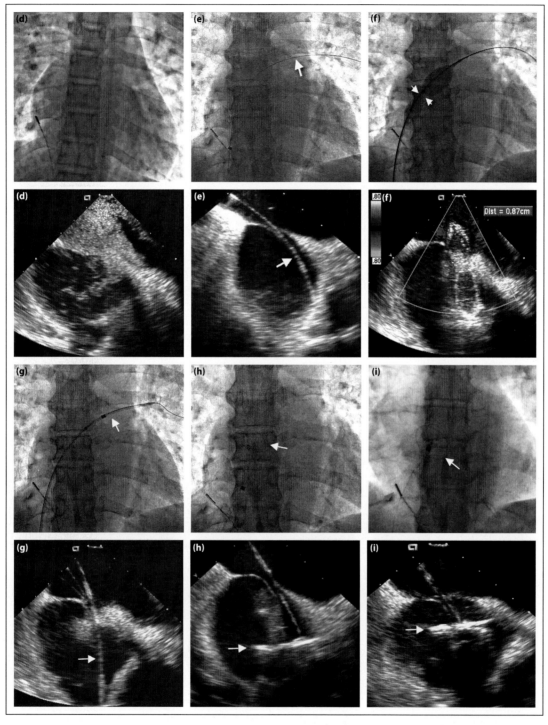

Figure 6.4 (continued) A series of images outlining PFO closure with the Gore Septal Occluder. (a–c) Initial diagnostic assessment of the PFO. (a–a2) The septal view of the atrial septum with and without color Doppler (demonstrating L–R shunt) with corresponding position of the ICE catheter on fluoroscopy outlined by the red arrow. (b–b2) The long-axis view (c–c2) demonstrating the short-axis view with the tunnel length measuring between 11 and 15 mm (a1, b1, c1). (d–f) Fluoroscopy images with ICE catheter position (red arrow) with the corresponding ICE image below. (d) R–L shunt of bubble contrast across the PFO with (e) clearly showing the wire crossing the defect and (f) balloon sizing of the defect, which is optional outside of most clinical trails. (g–i) Delivery of the HELEX device with corresponding fluoroscopy and ICE images in various views. (i) The left atrial component of the device deployed with (j, k) demonstrating the device pulled back to the septum and further deployment of the right atrial component of the device with it fully deployed in the long-axis (k) and short-axis views (l). (m, n) Release of the device on fluoroscopy with corresponding postdeployment ICE assessment with short-axis views and long-axis views with and without color (o1, o2, p1, p2).

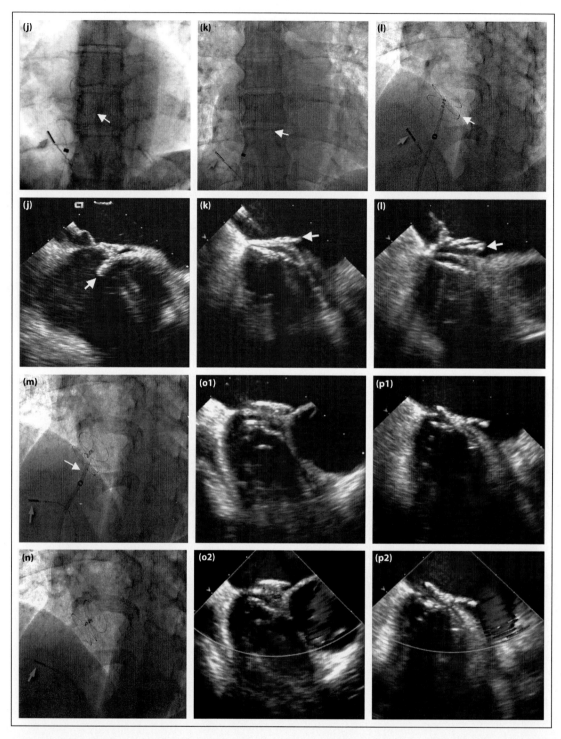

Figure 6.4 (continued) A series of images outlining PFO closure with the Gore Septal Occluder. (a–c) Initial diagnostic assessment of the PFO. (a–a2) The septal view of the atrial septum with and without color Doppler (demonstrating L–R shunt) with corresponding position of the ICE catheter on fluoroscopy outlined by the red arrow. (b–b2) The long-axis view (c–c2) demonstrating the short-axis view with the tunnel length measuring between 11 and 15 mm (a1, b1, c1). (d–f) Fluoroscopy images with ICE catheter position (red arrow) with the corresponding ICE image below. (d) R–L shunt of bubble contrast across the PFO with (e) clearly showing the wire crossing the defect and (f) balloon sizing of the defect, which is optional outside of most clinical trails. (g–i) Delivery of the HELEX device with corresponding fluoroscopy and ICE images in various views. (i) The left atrial component of the device deployed with (j, k) demonstrating the device pulled back to the septum and further deployment of the right atrial component of the device with it fully deployed in the long-axis (k) and short-axis views (l). (m, n) Release of the device on fluoroscopy with corresponding postdeployment ICE assessment with short-axis views and long-axis views with and without color (o1, o2, p1, p2).

an anterior–superior plane as shown in Figure 6.5b. A fluoroscopic image of the catheter and the corresponding ICE image are shown. This view demonstrates the location and size of the defect, the aortic valve, and the pulmonic valve.

Step 3: A four-chamber view is obtained by maneuvering the ICE catheter into the mid-RA with the tip positioned slightly anterior (close to the interatrial septum), and rotation such that the orientation of the imaging transducer faces the LV as shown in Figure 6.5c with the accompanying fluoroscopic and ICE images. In this view, the entire left atrium and ventricle can be seen, as well as part of the right atrium and ventricle. This view is important to show disk deployment and the position of the disk in relation to the IVS.

In patients with an associated atrial communication (ASD or PFO), the ICE catheter can be advanced across the atrial defect from the RA into the LA under fluoroscopic guidance.

Full reassessment following device deployment both pre- and postrelease is essential to ensure that the device is well positioned, without significant residual leak or impingement on surrounding structures.

ICE to guide aortic valve interventions

Balloon aortic valvuloplasty for calcific aortic stenosis has enjoyed a revival with the evolution of transcatheter aortic valve replacement (TAVR). Experience using ICE imaging during TAVR has been published with the suggestion that ICE will fit the workflow with TAVR better than TEE as the procedure becomes more established.[20] A stepwise approach to balloon aortic valvuloplasty using ICE is outlined in Figure 6.6. ICE also provides excellent imaging of the aortic root and has been used to guide the closure of complex aortic-atrial fistulae (personal experience).

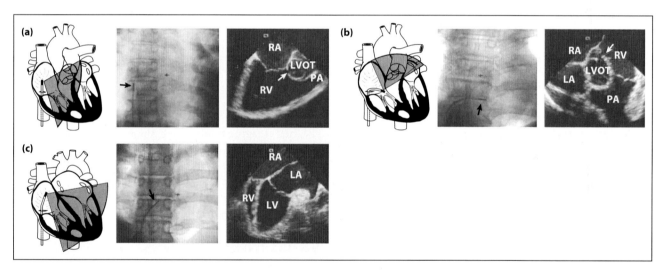

Figure 6.5 Transcatheter closure of perimembranous VSD. (a) Images in the home view. Left: Sketch representing the heart with the position of the intracardiac catheter inside the heart with the ultrasonic array box in the neutral home view position. The shaded area represents structures seen in this view. Middle: A cine fluoroscopy image showing the position of the ICE catheter (arrow) in the mid-right atrium with the transducer facing the tricuspid valve and parallel to the spine. Right: An actual intracardiac echocardiographic image with the ultrasonic box in the neutral home view position. The tricuspid valve, right ventricle outflow and inflow are well seen in this position. The aortic valve and pulmonic valve can also be seen. A perimembranous VSD can also be seen in this view (arrow). LVOT: left ventricle outflow tract; RA: right atrium; PA: pulmonary artery; RV: right ventricle. (b) Images in the short-axis view with more posterior flexion. Left: Sketch representing the heart with the position of the intracardiac catheter inside the heart with the ultrasonic array box in the flexed position and the entire handle rotated clockwise until the imaging transducer is above the tricuspid valve looking at the aorta and left ventricle outflow tract from below. In this position, fine rotation of the knobs can demonstrate different parts of the membranous ventricular septum. The shaded area represents structures seen in this view. Middle: A cine fluoroscopy image showing the position of the ICE catheter (arrow) in the right atrium with the transducer above the tricuspid valve. Right: An actual intracardiac echocardiographic image with the ultrasonic box in the short-axis view. The defect (arrow), the left ventricle outflow tract, right ventricle, and relation of the defect to the aortic valve are well seen. (c) Images in the four-chamber view. Left: A sketch representing the heart with the position of the intracardiac catheter inside the heart with the ultrasonic array box in the anterior flexed position close to the atrial septum looking at the four chambers of the heart. In this position, fine rotation of the knobs can demonstrate different parts of the membranous ventricular septum. The shaded area represents structures seen in this view. Middle: A cine fluoroscopy image showing the position of the ICE catheter (arrow) in the right atrium with the transducer near the septum in the anterior flexed position. Right: An actual intracardiac echocardiographic image with the ultrasonic box in the four-chamber view. All four chambers are seen.

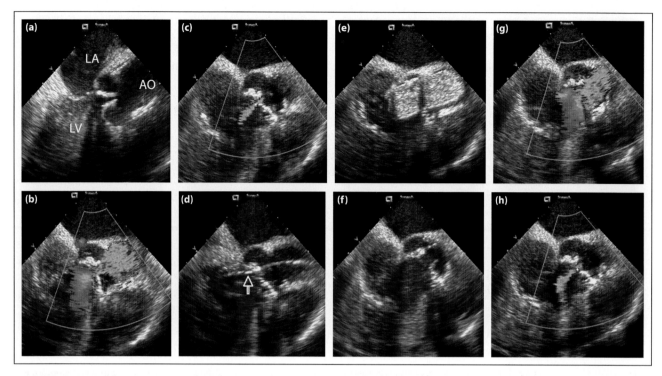

Figure 6.6 A series of ICE images outlining balloon aortic valvuloplasty. (a) The thickened stenotic aortic valve with significant systolic flow turbulence (b) and trace aortic incompetence (c) seen on color Doppler. (d) The wire across the aortic valve with balloon inflation clearly seen on (e). Improved valve opening is seen on 2-D imaging (f) with a wider systolic color Doppler jet across the valve (g) and minimal increase in aortic regurgitation (h).

ICE to guide mitral valve interventions

The use of ICE to guide balloon mitral valvuloplasty is well reported.[21,22] The mitral valve can be well profiled from the right heart, as indicated in Figure 6.7. An initial assessment of the inflow portion of the mitral valve can be carried out with clockwise rotation from the home view. Additionally, with appropriate maneuvers, the LAA may be interrogated for thrombus in this view. Then, with posterior deflection and rotation of the handle, the catheter tip can be advanced into the right ventricle, and following removal of the flexion, the catheter tip will move into the low right ventricular outflow tract. Gradual clockwise rotation of the catheter is subsequently performed and provides sequential images of the left ventricle, the mitral subvalvular apparatus, and the mitral valve leaflets.

Following full assessment, ICE imaging can then be used to guide transseptal puncture to access the mitral valve with the balloon. The use of ICE for transseptal puncture is routine in patients undergoing electrophysiology interventions within the left atrium,[23] and potential anatomical variants of the septum, including atrial septal aneurysm that may complicate transseptal puncture, are clearly outlined with ICE. The process is outlined in Figure 6.7.

Usual imaging planes for balloon positioning are from within the RA; however, imaging from the RV as outlined above may also be used and is preferable to get the entire left ventricle in the long-axis view.

ICE to guide pulmonary valve interventions

The use of ICE for percutaneous pulmonary valvuloplasty has been reported.[24] Accurate intracardiac assessment of residual pulmonary gradients and development of pulmonary regurgitation pre and post each ballooning may help to gauge how aggressive an approach is indicated. Accessing the RV as indicated above from the home view with posterior flexion and careful advancement across the tricuspid valve under fluoroscopy is relatively straightforward. Once across the tricuspid valve, release of the flexion will open up the pulmonary valve. This approach to guide percutaneous pulmonary valve replacement is outlined in Figure 6.8.

Established and evolving applications of ICE

ICE imaging has been reported in a range of other interventions, including LAA occlusion[25] and interatrial baffle

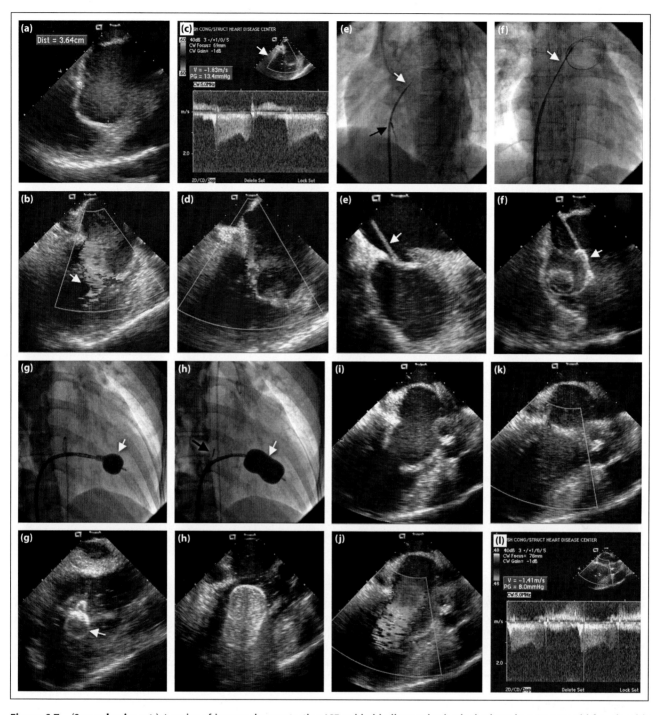

Figure 6.7 (**See color insert.**) A series of images demonstrating ICE-guided balloon mitral valvuloplasty in a 36-year-old female with previous rheumatic heart disease. (a–d) Evaluation of the mitral annulus (a), stenosis (b), Doppler gradient (c), and degree of mitral regurgitation (d). (e) A fluoroscopy image outlining the transseptal needle position (white arrow) with the ICE catheter position outlined by the black arrow and corresponding ICE image below demonstrating tenting of the atrial septum in the long-axis view. (f) The wire across the atrial septum in the left atrium on fluoroscopy and ICE. (g, h) Fluoroscopy images of the various stages of inflation of the Inoue balloon (white arrows) with the ICE catheter position (black arrow (h)) and the corresponding ICE images. (i–l) Further ICE assessment of the mitral valve with significant improvement in valve opening both on 2-D (i) and color Doppler (j) imaging with trivial mitral regurgitation (k) and satisfactory reduction in mean transmitral Doppler gradient (l).

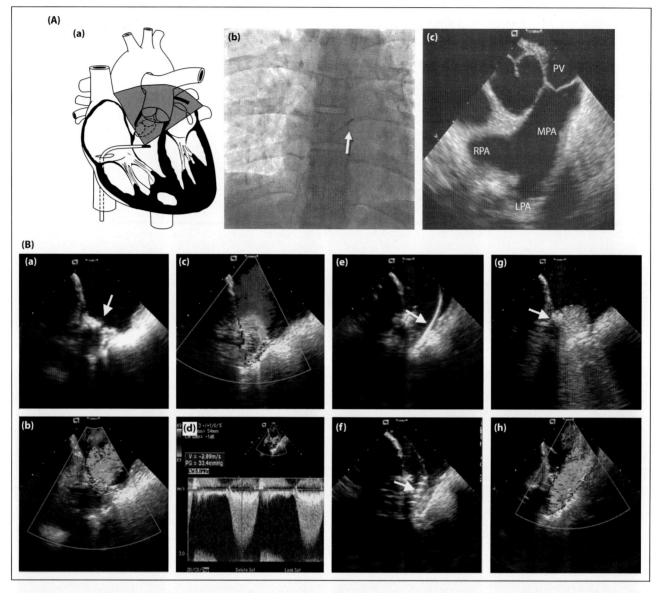

Figure 6.8 (**See color insert**.) (A) (a, b) A diagrammatic representation with corresponding fluoroscopy image of the ICE catheter position within the RV with the transducer directed up toward the pulmonary valve. (c) The ICE image. (B) Series of images demonstrating transcatheter pulmonary valve replacement with the Edwards SAPIEN valve. (a) The thickened stenotic homograft valve (white arrow) with prominent pulmonary regurgitation (b). Color (c) and spectral Doppler (d) assessment confirm significant obstruction. (e) The wire across the valve (white arrow) with the predilated bare metal stent in position (white arrow (f)). Stent inflation (g) leads to free pulmonary regurgitation (h). (i) Clear demonstration of the SAPIEN valve within the prestented RVOT, and following inflation (j), the functioning valve is clearly seen (k, m, n) with minimal pulmonary regurgitation (l). Repeat spectral Doppler confirms minimal estimated residual transvalvar Doppler gradient (o, p).

occlusion following an atrial switch procedure.[26] The range of applications for ICE within the field of electrophysiology are beyond the scope of this textbook, but evolving approaches are investigating the potential for integration of ultrasound imaging with electroanatomical mapping, fusion, and overlay images to guide atrial ablation.[13,14] Novel imaging approaches have also been reported from within the pericardium (percutaneous intrapericardial cardiac echocardiography—PICE), which may help to improve some of the imaging limitations that exist from within the heart.[14,27]

The most exciting development in regard to congenital and structural interventions is the development of 3-D imaging properties within an intracardiac echocardiographic catheter (Figure 6.9). The Siemens Acunav V system is a real-time volume ICE (VICE) catheter that is deliverable through a 10 F sheath, and is 90 cm long providing 22° × 90° volume. The system requires the Siemens

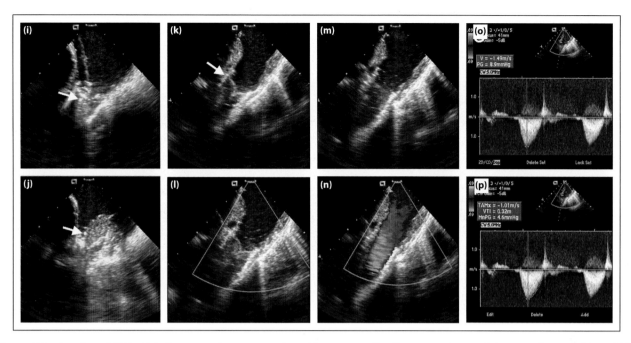

Figure 6.8 (continued) (A) (a, b) A diagrammatic representation with corresponding fluoroscopy image of the ICE catheter position within the RV with the transducer directed up toward the pulmonary valve. (c) The ICE image. (B) Series of images demonstrating transcatheter pulmonary valve replacement with the Edwards SAPIEN valve. (a) The thickened stenotic homograft valve (white arrow) with prominent pulmonary regurgitation (b). Color (c) and spectral Doppler (d) assessment confirm significant obstruction. (e) The wire across the valve (white arrow) with the predilated bare metal stent in position (white arrow (f)). Stent inflation (g) leads to free pulmonary regurgitation (h). (i) Clear demonstration of the SAPIEN valve within the prestented RVOT, and following inflation (j), the functioning valve is clearly seen (k, m, n) with minimal pulmonary regurgitation (l). Repeat spectral Doppler confirms minimal estimated residual transvalvar Doppler gradient (o, p).

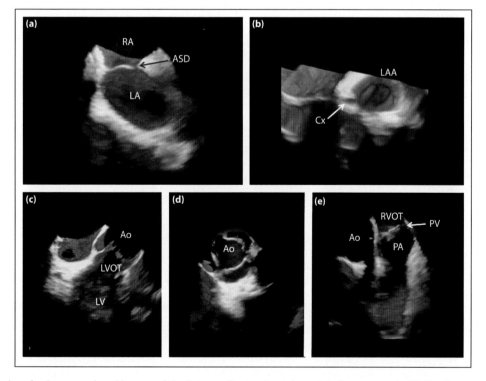

Figure 6.9 A series of volume-rendered images of the intracardiac anatomy (annotated) as assessed with the Siemens Acunav V system real-time volume ICE (VICE) catheter. RA: right atrium; LA: left atrium; ASD: atrial septal defect; LAA: left atrial appendage; Cx: circumflex artery; LV: Left ventricle; LVOT: left ventricular outflow tract; Ao: aorta; PA: pulmonary artery; RVOT: right ventricular outflow tract; PV: pulmonary valve.

SC2000TM volume-imaging ultrasound system. The system provides nonstitched, instantaneous full-volume imaging of the heart in one single heart cycle. If images comparable to 3-D TEE are possible with a straightforward interface, this will provide a significant imaging advance for assessing complexities within the atrial septum and other intracardiac structures amenable to transcatheter interventions.

Conclusions

ICE has evolved into the imaging modality of choice in an evolving number of congenital and structural interventions. It provides excellent imaging, without the need for general anesthesia, that is operator driven, obviating the need for support from echocardiographers. It is likely that evolving technologies will continue to develop to support 3-D imaging, reduction in catheter sizes, and improvement in far-field imaging capabilities so that the need for fluoroscopic imaging with its associated risks will continue to decline.

References

1. Alboliras ET, Hijazi ZM. Comparison of costs of intracardiac echocardiography and transesophageal echocardiography in monitoring percutaneous device closure of atrial septal defect in children and adults. *Am J Cardiol* 2004;94:690–2.
2. Bom N, Lancee CT, Van Egmond FC. An ultrasonic intracardiac scanner. *Ultrasonics* 1972;10:72–6.
3. Glassman E, Kronzon I. Transvenous intracardiac echocardiography. *Am J Cardiol* 1981;46:1255–9.
4. Seward JB, Khandheria BK, McGregor CG, Locke TJ, Tajik AJ. Transvascular and intracardiac two-dimensional echocardiography. *Echocardiography* 1990;7:457–64.
5. Valdes-Cruz LM, Sideris E, Sahn DJ et al. Transvascular intracardiac applications of a miniaturized phased-array ultrasonic endoscope: Initial experience with intracardiac imaging in piglets. *Circulation* 1991;83:1023–7.
6. Fisher JP, Wolfberg CA, Mikan JS et al. Intracardiac ultrasound determination of left ventricular volumes: *In vitro* and *in vivo* validation. *J Am Coll Cardiol* 1994;24:247–53.
7. Vazquez de Prada JA, Chen MH, Guerrero JL et al. Intracardiac echocardiography: *In vitro* and *in vivo* validation for right ventricular volume and function. *Am Heart J* 1996;131;320–8.
8. Tardif JC, Vannan MA, Miller DS et al. Potential applications of intracardiac echocardiography in interventional electrophysiology. *Am Heart J* 1994;127:1090–4.
9. Mitchel JF, Gillam LD, Sanzobrono BW et al. Intracardiac ultrasound imaging during transseptal catheterization. *Chest* 1995;108:104–8.
10. Tardiff JC, Cao QL, Schwartz SL, Pandian NG. Intracardiac echocardiography with a steerable low-frequency linear-array probe for left sided heart imaging from the right side: Experimental studies. *J Am Soc Echocardiogr* 1995;8:132–8.
11. Bruce CJ, Nishimura RA, Rihal CS et al. Intracardiac echocardiography in the interventional catheterization laboratory: Preliminary experience with a novel phased-array transducer. *Am J Cardiol* 2002;89:635–40.
12. Li P, Dairywala IT, Liu Z et al. Anatomic and hemodynamic imaging using a new vector phased-array intracardiac catheter. *J Am Soc Echocardiogr* 2002;15:349–55.
13. Kim SS, Hijazi ZM, Lang RM, Knight BP. The use of intracardiac echocardiography and other intracardiac imaging tools to guide noncoronary cardiac interventions. *J Am Coll Cardiol* 2009;53:2117–28.
14. Hijazi ZM, Shivkumar K, Sahn DJ. Intracardiac echocardiography during interventional and electrophysiological cardiac catheterization. *Circulation* 2009;119:587–96.
15. Mullen MJ, Dias BF, Walker F, Siu SC et al. Intracardiac echocardiography guided device closure of atrial septal defects. *J Am Coll Cardiol* 2003;41:285–92.
16. Hijazi Z, Wang Z, Cao Q et al. Transcatheter closure of atrial septal defects and patent foramen ovale under intracardiac echocardiographic guidance: Feasibility and comparison with transesophageal echocardiography. *Catheter Cardiovasc Interv* 2001;52:194–9.
17. Bartel T, Konorza T, Arjumand J et al. Intracardiac echocardiography is superior to conventional monitoring for guiding device closure of interatrial communications. *Circulation* 2003;107:795–7.
18. Ponnuthurai FA, van Gaal WJ, Burchell A et al. Safety and feasibility of day case patent foramen ovale (PFO) closure facilitated by intracardiac echocardiography. *Int J Cardiol* 2009;131:438–40.
19. Cao QL, Zabal C, Koenig P, Sandhu S, Hijazi ZM. Initial clinical experience with intracardiac echocardiography in guiding transcatheter closure of perimembranous ventricular septal defects: Feasibility and comparison with transesophageal echocardiography. *Catheter Cardiovasc Interv* 2005;66:258–67.
20. Bartel T, Bonaros N, Müller L et al. Intracardiac echocardiography: A new guiding tool for transcatheter aortic valve replacement. *J Am Soc Echocardiogr* 2011;24:966–75.
21. Salem MI, Makaryus AN, Kort S et al. Intracardiac echocardiography using the AcuNav ultrasound catheter during percutaneous balloon mitral valvuloplasty. *J Am Soc Echocardiogr* 2002;15:1533–7.
22. Green NE, Hansgen AR, Carroll JD. Initial clinical experience with intracardiac echocardiography in guiding balloon mitral valvuloplasty: Technique, safety, utility, and limitations. *Catheter Cardiovasc Interv* 2004;63:385–94.
23. Daoud EG, Kalbfleisch SJ, Hummel JD. Intracardiac echocardiography to guide transseptal left heart catheterization for radio frequency catheter ablation. *J Cardiovasc Electrophysiol* 1999;10:358–63.
24. Vaina S, Ligthart J, Vijayakumar M et al. Intracardiac echocardiography during interventional procedures. *Euro Intervention* 2006;1:454–64.
25. Ho IC, Neuzil P, Mraz T et al. Use of intracardiac echocardiography to guide implantation of a left atrial appendage occlusion device (PLAATO). *Heart Rhythm* 2007;4:567–71.
26. Kuppahally SS, Litwin SE, Green LS et al. Utility of intracardiac echocardiography for a trial baffle leak closure in repaired transposition of the great arteries. *Echocardiography* 2010;27:E90–3.
27. Horowitz BN, Vaseghi M, Mahajan A et al. Percutaneous intrapericardial echocardiography during catheter ablation: A feasibility study. *Heart Rhythm* 2006;3:1275–82.

7

Intracardiac echocardiography by Ultra ICE

Eustaquio M. Onorato, Francesco Casilli, and Mario Zanchetta

Introduction

With the rapid development of percutaneous interventional procedures for diseases that were once approached surgically, there has been a concomitant increased interest of intracardiac echocardiography (ICE™) in clinical settings, specifically to assist transseptal left heart catheterization[1,2] or transseptal catheter placement,[3–5] radio-frequency catheter ablation of cardiac arrhythmias,[6–8] and transcatheter closure of atrial septal defect (ASD)[9–11] or patent foramen ovale (PFO).[9,12]

This chapter aims to provide interventional cardiologists with an overview of the use of the mechanical single-element system intracardiac echocardiography by Ultra ICE (IntraCardiac Ultrasound imaging catheter, EP Technologies, Boston Scientific Corporation, San Jose, California) (Table 7.1).

The mechanical single-element system provides rotational images in two orthogonal views similar to magnetic resonance imaging (MRI).

Table 7.1 Main characteristics of the Ultra ICE ultrasound intracardiac probe

FDA approval: June 20, 1997
- Mechanical scanning system
- Unique siliceous piezoelectric crystal
- 8.5 Fe "over-the-wire" catheter
- 9 MHz frequency
- Radial scanning at 360°
- Images on a plane perpendicular to the long axis of the catheter
- Imaging field: 10 cm
- Platforms: ClearView Ultra System, Galaxy System, iLab System (EP Technologies, Boston Scientific Corporation)
- Single-operator use
- Three-dimensional reconstruction

FDA, Food and Drug Administration.

Rotational intracardiac ultrasound system

The Ultra ICE catheter, model 9900, consists of a central inner core and a catheter body (8.5 Fr) that has, at its distal end a sonolucent window, which incorporates a unique siliceous piezoelectric crystal at a frequency of 9 MHz (Figure 7.1). At its proximal end, it has a connector for the motor drive unit, which allows the rotation of the transducer and the transmission and reception of ultrasound waves. The central inner core consists of a flexible wire with a high torsion and rotation capacity that transfers to the transducer a circular movement with a speed ranging from 1600 to 1800 rpm. The resulting wave is propagated on a transverse plane, perpendicular to the long axis of the catheter, to create a two-dimensional image presented as a video tomographic section (radial at 360°) in real time on a dedicated review station compatible with Boston Scientific Ultrasound Imaging Systems (ClearView® Ultra™ and Galaxy® Systems) (Figure 7.2), including the most recent iLab® System (Figure 7.3). This represents the user interface and allows modification of the image magnification, gray scale, luminosity, and contrast as well as the storage of the images in a digital format. In particular, iLab System has a new intuitive user interface, a large high-definition monitor, a good touchpad interface, automatic enhancement of ICE images, and a modular hardware design that is easy to upgrade. The radio-opaque tip of the Ultra ICE catheter is designed to allow easy placement and to serve as a fluoroscopic marker during the procedure. The area of interest is then the central point in the ultrasound image, providing a clear view of what needs to be visualized along with the surrounding structures. Moreover, the catheter may be automatically withdrawn up to a maximum distance of 15 cm by a pullback device at a constant speed of 0.2–0.5 to 1.0–2.0 mm/s. The data so obtained may be stored in a personal computer (TomTec Imaging System, Unterschleinheim, Germany) (Video 7.1), which, in turn, provides accurate measurements and a three-dimensional

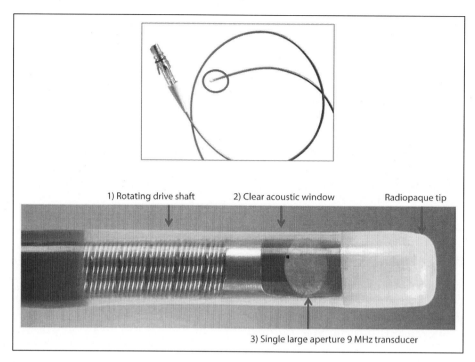

1) Rotating drive shaft 2) Clear acoustic window Radiopaque tip

3) Single large aperture 9 MHz transducer

Figure 7.1 (**See color insert.**) The distal end of the Ultra ICE catheter. (1) Flexible wire with high torsion and rotation capacity; (2) sono-lucent window; (3) unique siliceous piezoelectric crystal with a frequency of 9 MHz.

reconstruction of the examined structures. In addition, it is possible to obtain a high reproducibility in spatial terms with less operator dependency, finding the same plane at successive studies with an error of only a few millimeters or even less. With the Ultra ICE catheter, the penetration depth is about 5.0 cm, but because the scanning is radial, the useful imaging field is actually about 10 cm, with axial and lateral resolutions of 0.27 and 0.26 mm, respectively.

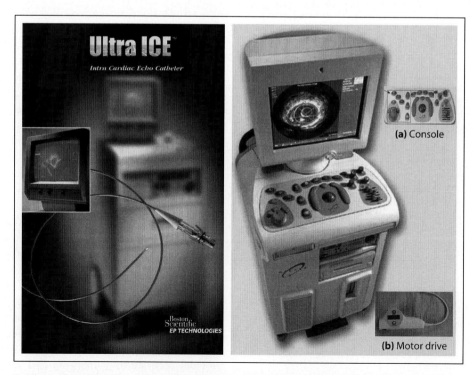

(a) Console

(b) Motor drive

Figure 7.2 (**See color insert.**) Dedicated review stations: ClearView Ultra System (left) and Galaxy System (right) with console (a) and motor drive unit (b). (From EP Technologies, Boston Scientific Corporation. With permission.)

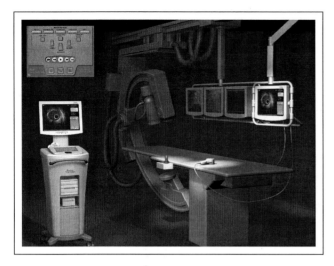

Figure 7.3   (See color insert.) The Boston Scientific iLab System allows the option of fully integrating the hardware into the cardiac catheterization and electrophysiology laboratories, providing the integration of real-time fluoroscopic and echocardiographic images according to a modality immediately usable by operators; details of iLab System review station (top). (From EP Technologies, Boston Scientific Corporation. With permission.)

The Ultra ICE catheter, a single-use disposable device, is introduced through the femoral vein and advanced toward the right heart with an "over-the-wire" 8.5 Fr precurved introducer, available in several lengths and curves (distal curvature angle ranging from 0° to 140°) (Figure 7.4). This allows the operator to navigate the catheter in the right heart chambers and to manipulate the distal portion of the catheter containing the transducer in various directions. Before insertion, the Ultra ICE catheter requires an exhaustive

preparation, including sterile apyrogenic water rinsing of the sonolucent camera by a dedicated preparation needle (Fluid Dock™) to eliminate any air, which otherwise could lead to decreased imaging quality.

Rotational intracardiac echocardiography by Ultra ICE is designed to provide the combination of real-time imaging and soft tissue visualization, which cannot be duplicated by fluoroscopy, preoperative imaging (CT or MRI), or electroanatomic mapping. Thus, it can bring valuable clinical information, either when used by itself or in conjunction with these other imaging modalities.

Image presentation and examination technique

Although an innumerable series of planes can be displayed by Ultra ICE, four views of the axial plane and only one view of the longitudinal long-axis plane have to be commonly utilized for an exhaustive evaluation of the structures from the inner confines of the right atrium and great veins (Table 7.2). Because the majority of these various planes bears little similarity to routine angiographic images or commonly utilized transthoracic (TT) and transesophageal echocardiography (TEE) sections, the Ultra ICE images obtained are not readily understood by physicians, so there is the need to describe in detail these new unique views. The Ultra ICE uses two tomographic views, that is the *axial* and the *parasagittal long-axis* planes, with results that are appropriate for a comparative study of the morphology and relationships of the cardiac structures. Keeping in mind that the radiological standard format of an imaging presentation gives a view on the scan plane from below, looking at the heart from the inferior vena cava upward to the cardiac base, physicians no longer need to reorient the images mentally in order to figure out the relative position of structures displayed by Ultra ICE, because the imaging orientation is displayed with similar right–left and anterior–posterior MRI orientation, consistent with familiar recommendations of any standard radiological format.

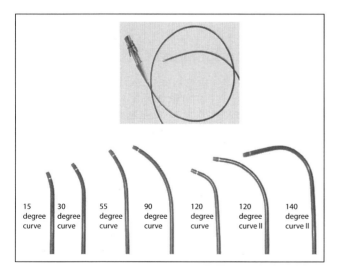

15 degree curve | 30 degree curve | 55 degree curve | 90 degree curve | 120 degree curve | 120 degree curve II | 140 degree curve II

Figure 7.4   (See color insert.) The Ultra ICE catheter is introduced through the femoral vein and advanced toward the right heart with an over-the-wire 8.5 Fr precurved introducer available in several lengths and curves.

Table 7.2 Standard scan planes during mechanical interrogation by Ultra ICE	
Scan	**Transducer position**
Axial	
Great vessels	T 5°–6°
SVC–RA junction	T 6°
Aortic valve	T 6°–7°
Cavo-tricuspid isthmus	T 8°
Parasagittal long axis	
Four chamber	Central on FO

T, thoracic intervertebral disk; RA, right atrium; SVC, superior vena cava; FO, fossa ovalis.

Intracardiac echocardiographic axial views

An examination is begun by navigating the Ultra ICE catheter and neutrally placing the transducer into the superior vena cava, then subsequently withdrawing it as a unit through the body of the right atrium toward the inferior vena cava. The axial transducer orientation will be in the horizontal plane of the body and in the short axis of the right atrium. In order to appropriately display the image in an MRI orientation, two specific anatomic landmarks have to be used. The first one is the crista terminalis, which appears as a bright and thick structure, located at the junction between the posterior smooth wall and the anterolateral trabeculated portion of the right atrium. The second one is the right atrial appendage, which is defined as a large Snoopy nose-like structure.

During the intracardiac ultrasound interrogation, the scan sections have to be rotated electronically in order to display the right atrial appendage at 12 o'clock and the crista terminalis at 10 o'clock position on the screen (Table 7.3). This is an essential step when interrogating the cardiac structure by ICE: so, the left-sided structures will be displayed to the viewer's right and right-sided structures to the viewer's left, whereas the anterior structures will be to the top of the screen and the posterior structures to the bottom of the screen. This orientation of the image is familiar to MRI views of the cardiac morphology and, in the history of echocardiography, has not been used until now.

Great vessels axial plane

The axial view of the great vessels is recorded with the catheter neutrally placed in the center of the superior vena cava and parallel to its long axis, with the transducer positioned between the 5th and 6th intervertebral disks of the thoracic spine, in order to achieve an ideal perpendicular angle of incidence of the ultrasound beam to the vessel wall (Figure 7.5a). Note that even though the technique and image magnification of near and far fields differ, MRI and Ultra ICE images are shown with the same orientation: left-sided

structures at the operator's right, anterior structures at the top of the image, and so on. The Ultra ICE axial view of the plane of the great vessels allows visualization of the superior vena cava, ascending aorta, and right upper pulmonary vein in the short axis, whereas the right pulmonary artery is cut in its long axis. The right ventricular outflow tract, the pulmonary trunk, and the left pulmonary artery are not clearly imaged due to poor lateral resolution in the far field, and they pass anterior and leftward of the aorta (Table 7.4). On the great vessels view, it is possible to evaluate the spatial orientation of the great arteries as well as to visualize the ascending aorta (to assess its enlargement, or the presence of a dissection) and the proximal right pulmonary branch (to view the thrombus) pathologies. Moreover, the high location of partial anomalous pulmonary venous drainage may be easily identified by Ultra ICE.

Superior vena cava–right atrium junction axial plane

The axial view of the superior vena cava–right atrium junction plane is recorded by minimal withdrawal of the catheter, with the transducer neutrally positioned at the body of the 6th intervertebral disk of the thoracic spine (Figure 7.5b). On the superior vena cava–right atrium junction plane, the Ultra ICE allows visualization of the right atrial appendage, crista terminalis, left atrium with right upper pulmonary vein entry, and ascending aorta (Table 7.5). The usefulness of the superior vena cava–right atrium junction axial plane is in evaluating the motion characteristics of the right atrial appendage, in determining the presence of intra-atrial masses, and in identifying the crista terminalis. Moreover, the lower entry of partial anomalous pulmonary venous drainage is easy to identify in this plane.

Aortic valve axial plane

A further caudal pullback of the catheter into the right atrium with the transducer positioned between the 6th and the 7th intervertebral disk of the thoracic spine allows the axial view of the aortic valve plane to be obtained (Figure 7.5c). The aortic valve is viewed in its short axis astride the right and left atria; the atrial septum is transversely scanned in its entirety and the fossa ovalis with its antero-superior and postero-inferior rims may be well appreciated (Table 7.6). The aortic valve view is crucial in determining aortic valve abnormalities, in evaluating the origin of the right and left coronary ostia, and in providing qualitative and quantitative assessments of the atrial septum and its abnormalities, such as secundum ASD, PFO, and atrial septal aneurysm (ASA). In the area of the atrial septum, the fossa ovalis is qualitatively identifiable as a distinct component of the atrial septum, characterized

Table 7.3 Anatomic landmarks and their spatial orientation

Structures	Scan plan	Orientation (hour)
Aortic root	Great vessels	2:00
SVC	Great vessels	9:00
Right PA	Great vessels	6:00
Crista terminalis	SVC–RA junction	10:00
Right auricle	SVC–RA junction	12:00

SVC, superior vena cava; RA, right atrium; PA, pulmonary artery.

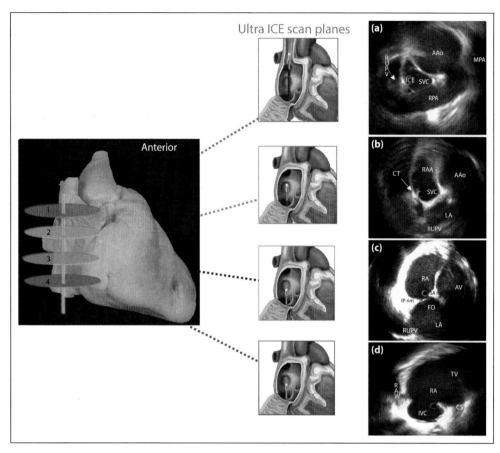

Figure 7.5   (See color insert.) Intracardiac echochograophic axial views: (a) *Great vessels axial plane*, SVC, superior vena cava; RUPV, right upper pulmonary vein; RPA, right pulmonary artery; AAo, ascending aorta; MPA, mean pulmonary artery; (b) *Superior vena cava–right atrium junction axial plane*, SVC, superior vena cava; RAA, right atrial auricle; CT, crista terminalis; RUPV, right upper pulmonary vein; Aao, ascending aorta; (c) *Aortic valve axial plane*: the aortic valve is viewed in its short axis astride the right and left atria, whereas the atrial septum is transversally scanned in its entirety and the fossa ovalis with its superior–anterior and inferior–posterior rims may be well appreciated, RA, right atrium; AV, aortic valve; LA, left atrium; RUPV, right upper pulmonary vein; FO, fossa ovalis; SA rim, superior–anterior rim; IP rim, inferior–posterior rim; (d) *Cavotricuspid isthmus axial plane*, RA, right atrium; TV, tricuspid valve; RAW, right atrial wall; CS, coronary sinus; IVC, inferior vena cava.

by a thin membranous region within a thicker muscular septum. Moreover, the same useful parameters may be quantitatively measured, such as the systolic and diastolic transverse atrial septal diameters, the dimensions of the ASD and fossa ovalis, and the fossa ovalis distances to the inlet of the inferior vena cava (postero-inferior rim) or to the outer aortic wall (antero-superior rim).

Cavotricuspid isthmus axial plane

The inferior vena cava–right atrial junction plane is obtained by further caudal withdrawal of the catheter with the transducer positioned at the level of the body at the 8th intervertebral disk of the thoracic spine (Figure 7.5d). In this plane, it is possible to visualize the right lateral wall,

Table 7.4   Great vessels axial plane: Interrogated structures

Right superior pulmonary vein
Superior vena cava
Ascending aorta
Right pulmonary artery branch
Pulmonary trunk
Transverse pericardial sinus

Table 7.5   Superior vena cava–right atrium junction axial plane: Interrogated structures

Right appendage
Superior vena cava
Crista terminalis
Ascending aorta
Left atrium
Pulmonary trunk
Right superior pulmonary vein drainage in left atrium

Table 7.6 Aortic valve axial plane: Interrogated structures

Right atrium
Aortic valve
Left atrium
Interatrial septum:
  Fossa ovalis
  Antero-superior rim
  Postero-inferior rim

Table 7.7 Cavo-tricuspid isthmus axial plane: Interrogated structures

Right atrium
Antero-lateral right atrium parietal wall
Inferior vena cava
Eustachian valve
Cavo-tricuspid isthmus
Coronary sinus
Tricuspid annulus
Kock's triangle

inferior vena cava, Eustachian valve, ostium of the coronary sinus with Thebesian valve, tricuspid annulus, and tricuspid valve (Table 7.7).

The cavotricuspid isthmus plane is frequently used during radio-frequency ablation procedures in order to perform catheterization of the coronary sinus and to identify the location and the boundaries of the Kock's triangle with its apex pointing upwards. Moreover, the Ultra ICE is able to clearly elucidate the morphologic developmental deficiency that underlies the inferior vena cava types of sinus venosus defects.

Intracardiac echocardiographic parasagittal view

Long-axis four-chamber plane

The long-axis view is obtained with a 55° precurved introducer sheath advanced up to the end of the catheter and turned posterior and leftward, to longitudinally scan the atrial septum (Figure 7.6). The transducer orientation will be in the long axis of the body and oblique to the long axis of the heart. The resulting image replicates a truncated apex-up four-chamber view, without the need of image reorientation. Thus, the examiner can potentially make a transition from a transverse to a longitudinal plane, without needing to change the image orientation. Two precautions will help to avoid this problem: first, strict attention should be paid not to modify the position of the motor drive unit that interfaces between the imaging console and the Ultra ICE catheter; second, the precurved long sheath is used to rotate the Ultra ICE catheter in order to maintain an optimal performance between the transducer and the drive-shaft. On

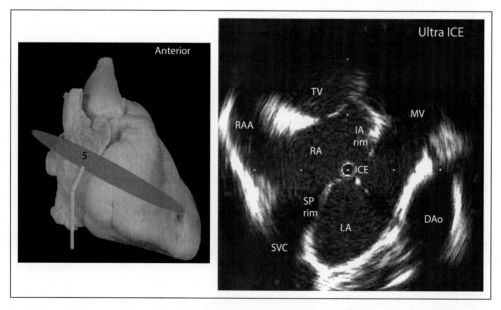

Figure 7.6 (**See color insert.**) *Long-axis four-chamber plane*: The long-axis view is obtained with a 55° precurved introducer sheath advanced up to the end of the catheter and turned posterior and leftward, to longitudinally scan the atrial septum. On this plane, it is possible to visualize the right and left atria, right and left atrial auricles, tricuspid and mitral valves, and the descending aorta. Moreover, the atrial septum is longitudinally scanned and the fossa ovalis with its inferior–anterior and superior–posterior rims can be well appreciated. SVC, superior vena cava; RA, right atrium; RAA, right atrial auricle; FO, fossa ovalis; TV, tricuspid valve; MV, mitral valve; LA, left atrium; DAo, descending aorta; SP rim, superior–posterior rim; IA rim, inferior–anterior rim.

Table 7.8   Long-axis four-chamber parasagittal plane: interrogated structures

Right and left atria
Tricuspid and mitral valves
Atrioventricular junction
Interatrial septum:
 Fossa ovalis
 Antero-inferior rim
 Postero-superior rim

this plane, it is possible to visualize the right and left atria, right and left atrial appendages, tricuspid and mitral valves, and the descending aorta. Moreover, the atrial septum is scanned longitudinally and the fossa ovalis with its antero-inferior and postero-superior rims can be well appreciated (Table 7.8). Ostium primum and ostium secundum ASDs may be predictably appreciated with an optimized long-axis four-chamber view. The systolic and diastolic longitudinal atrial septal diameters, the dimensions of the ASD and the fossa ovalis, and the fossa ovalis distances to the inlet of the inferior vena cava (postero-inferior rim) as well as the coronary sinus or atrioventricular junction (antero-inferior rim) may be measured accurately. Finally, abnormalities such as ASA, or lipomatous hypertrophy of the atrial septum may be readily detected on this section by Ultra ICE.

Current uses of ultra ice in the cardiac catheterization laboratory

The applications of Ultra ICE in the cardiac catheterization laboratory include monitoring and guiding catheter-based closure of ASD and PFO with or without ASA as well as in diagnosing associated atrial septal abnormalities (Table 7.9).

Table 7.9   Main applications of Ultra ICE consist of (a) monitoring and guiding catheter-based interventional procedures and (b) diagnosing associated atrial septal abnormalities

a. Catheter-based interventional procedures:
• Ostium secundum atrial septal defect
• Patent foramen ovale with/without atrial septal aneurysm

b. Associated atrial septal abnormalities:
• Ostium primum atrial septal defect
• Sinus venosus defects
• Right-sided partial anomalous pulmonary venous drainage
• Lipomatous hypertrophy of the atrial septum
• Eustachian valve and Chiari's network

Anatomical features of the interatrial septum, the morphology of the valve-like opening of the PFO, the degree of mobility of the septum primum, and the size of the ASD/PFO defects are all variable and require careful evaluation by the operator prior to implantation of the closure device. The relationship of the ASD/PFO to the surrounding structures has to be considered when choosing the correct closure device.[13]

The pivotal roles of Ultra ICE during catheter-based procedures are the following:

1. Ultra ICE can distinguish between the septum primum (low echo signal intensity) and the septum secundum (high signal intensity) (Figure 7.7), whereas on transesophageal ultrasound these structures are of similar echogenicity.
2. It can be helpful to confirm the presence of additional structural anomalies such as partial anomalous drainage of pulmonary veins.
3. It can be used to evaluate the spatial relationship of the ASD with other structures such as the aorta, superior and inferior caval veins, coronary sinus, mitral, and tricuspid valves (Figures 7.5 and 7.6).
4. It allows morphometric evaluation of the ASD directly rather than using indirect measurements of a balloon catheter.

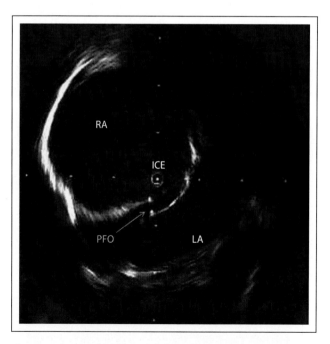

Figure 7.7 Rotational intracardiac echocardiography (Ultra ICE intracardiac echo catheter, EP Technologies, Boston Scientific Corporation) showing the usual tunnel-like shape of the PFO. Long-axis four-chamber parasagittal view. RA, right atrium; LA, left atrium; ICE, intracardiac echocardiographic catheter; PFO, patent foramen ovale.

The most frequently used method for the selection of the ASD occluder and its deployment are the balloon-sizing maneuver[14,15] and TEE monitoring.[16] Although both TEE and balloon sizing are considered as important requirements for a successful procedure, their positive predictive accuracy and specificity are low.[17–19] Moreover, both these methods have drawbacks: in particular, balloon sizing can give inaccurate measurements, causing possible over- or underestimation of the selected occluder size. Selection of an inappropriate-sized device may result in multiple attempts at deployment, which in turn may cause septum primum membrane damage, eventually enlarging the defect.[20] TEE usually requires general anesthesia with or without endotracheal intubation. Furthermore, aspiration, airway obstruction, esophageal perforation, and vocal cord dysfunction have been infrequently reported.[21,22] Finally, the esophageal probe is usually not well tolerated by the conscious patient. On the other hand, Ultra ICE facilitates the monitoring and guiding of catheter closure of ASD and PFO (Figure 7.8), thus eliminating the cumbersome balloon-sizing maneuver and the need for general anesthesia or deep sedation during transesophageal echocardiographic monitoring. Indeed, in the cardiac catheterization laboratory Ultra ICE permits a proper measurement of the size of the ASD (major and minor axis of the fossa ovalis, rim length) and the selection of an appropriately sized device by simply using two standardized orthogonal views (the axial view on the aortic valve plane and the parasagittal view on the four-chamber plane) (Tables 7.7 and 7.8, Figure 7.9). Finally, selection of the appropriate size of the atrial septal occluder device can be easily achieved using a mathematical formula available in a simple software program.[23]

In all 135 ASD patients of our preliminary series, high-quality images of the atrial septum were obtained, which allowed measurement of the size of the defect and to

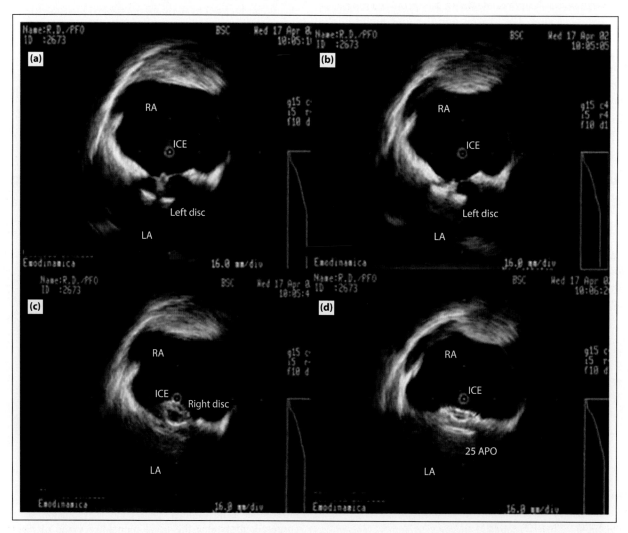

Figure 7.8   PFO closure monitoring by rotational intracardiac echocardiography (Ultra ICE). In the long-axis four-chamber parasagittal view: (a) left disk opening of the Amplatzer PFO occluder 25 mm (APO 25); (b) APO 25 left disk toward the atrial septum; (c) APO 25 right disk opening; (d) device correctly implanted (personal data). RA, right atrium; LA, left atrium; ICE, intracardiac.

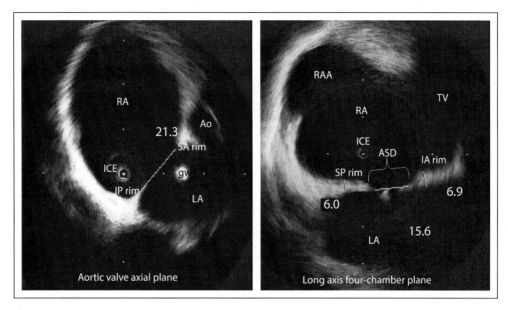

Figure 7.9 Two standardized orthogonal views: the *axial* view on the aortic valve plane (left) and the *parasagittal long-axis* view on the four-chamber plane (right) are used during catheter atrial septal defect (ASD) closure to provide quantitative and qualitative information for proper occluder device size selection. RA, right atrium; LA, left atrium; RUPV, right upper pulmonary vein; FO, fossa ovalis; SA rim, superior–anterior rim; IP rim, inferior–posterior rim; SVC, superior vena cava; RAA, right atrial auricle; TV, tricuspid valve; MV, mitral valve; Ao, aorta; SP rim, superior–posterior rim; IA rim, inferior–anterior rim; ICE, intracardiac echocardiographic catheter.

visualize more clearly the occluder during the different stages of its deployment[24] (Figure 7.10). All the patients underwent transcatheter ASD closure under local anesthesia alone without Ultra ICE-related complications. The cumulative rates of complete occlusion were 97.7% at 24 hours and 98% at 3 years.[24]

PFO may have a large variety of associated anatomical features: mild–moderate ASA, large ASA, multiperforated fossa ovalis (Video 7.2), hypertrophic or lipomatous rims, and long-tunnel PFO (Video 7.3 and Video 7.4). These different anatomical characteristics, often combined with each other, may impact on immediate procedural results

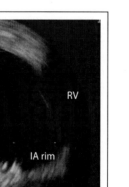

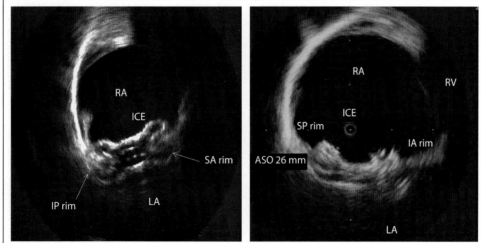

Figure 7.10 Ultra ICE is able to clearly visualize an implanted Amplatzer septal occluder (ASO) device. The occluder device is seen in both orthogonal views, on the left, the *axial* view on the aortic valve plane, and on the right, the *parasagittal long-axis* view on the four-chamber plane. RA, right atrium; LA, left atrium; RV, right ventricle; SA rim, superior–anterior rim; IP rim, inferior–posterior rim; SP rim, superior–posterior rim; IA rim, inferior–anterior rim; ICE, intracardiac echocardiographic catheter.

and outcomes. The ability to assess the different features by Ultra ICE has been suggested as the key to lowering the incidence of potential failures or complications and increasing the long-term occlusion rates. The goal of PFO closure is to eliminate the interatrial shunt, thus abolishing the risk of recurrent paradoxical thrombo-embolism. In patients with long-tunnel PFO, ASA, or anatomical features requiring large occluder devices, the risk of residual shunting is higher and, therefore, the use of echocardiography during the procedure may be useful to measure the defect accurately, to select the most appropriate device size, and to help in the positioning and delivering of the occluder device (Figure 7.11). In 2012, Vigna and colleagues described intraobserver and interobserver variability for fossa ovalis dimensions to be greater with TEE than with rotational Ultra ICE in patients undergoing percutaneous PFO closure. A significant disagreement may be observed between TEE and ICE measurements in terms of fossa ovalis dimensions and the subsequent device selection, particularly in the presence of ASA.[25]

To summarize, the main advantages of Ultra ICE during catheter-based procedures are

1. Appropriate selection of the type and the size of the device, avoiding balloon sizing
2. Optimal monitoring of device deployment, mainly because of its ability to provide images at 360° reconstruction

3. Good tolerance by the patient for a relatively prolonged time period
4. Ease of performance (single operator)
5. Limited fluoroscopic exposure time

The major drawbacks are

1. No color-Doppler capability
2. Additional costs (dedicated review stations and disposable catheter)

Associated atrial septal abnormalities

Mechanical interrogation of intracardiac structures may be useful in diagnosing other atrial septal abnormalities that may represent contraindications to interventional procedures.

ASA refers to a redundancy of the septum primum tissue bulging into the right and/or the left atrium. ASA is rarely present as an isolated lesion ("lone" ASA),[26] whereas it is usually associated with congenital or acquired heart disease.[27] The prevalence of ASA in the general population ranges from 1% in autopsy studies[28] to 2.2–4.9% in TEE series.[29] ASA is frequently associated with a PFO in 50–89% of patients; this association has emerged as potentially increasing the risk of stroke occurrence or relapse.[30] Furthermore, PFOs seen in the presence of ASA tend to be larger compared with those seen without ASA.[31] The ICE

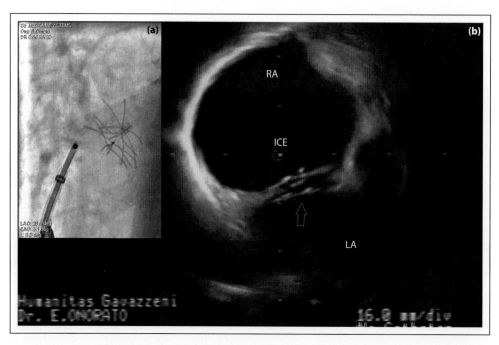

Figure 7.11   PFO closure using CARDIA PFO occluder (CARDIA, Inc., Burnsville, Minnesota) under fluoroscopic (a) and Ultra ICE (b) control and monitoring. Rotational intracardiac echocardiography (Ultra ICE) (b) shows the septum primum sandwiched between two umbrellas of the device. RA, right atrium; LA, left atrium; ICE, intracardiac echocardiographic catheter; intrasept device (orange arrow).

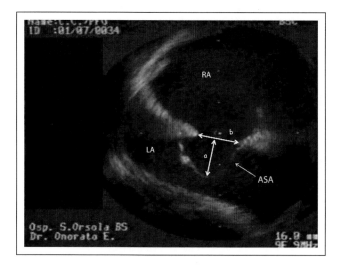

Figure 7.12 Rotational intracardiac echocardiography (Ultra ICE) showing PFO with ASA according to criteria published by Hanley: protrusion of interatrial septum, or part of it, > or = to 15 mm beyond plane of interatrial septum (a > or = to 15 mm) or phasic excursion of interatrial septum during cardiorespiratory cycle; diameter of the base of the aneurysmal portion of the atrial septum measuring ≥15 mm (b). Long-axis four-chamber parasagittal view (personal experience). RA, right atrium; LA, left atrium; ICE, intracardiac echocardiographic catheter; PFO, patent foramen ovale; ASA, atrial septal aneurysm.

definition of ASA agrees entirely with TT and TEE criteria, previously published by Hanley et al.:[32] The diameter of the base of the aneurysmal portion of the atrial septum measuring ≥15 mm, bulging of the atrial septum or fossa ovalis ≥15 mm, and phasic excursion of the atrial septum or fossa ovalis during the cardiorespiratory cycle ≥15 mm in total amplitude (Figure 7.12). The major advantages of ICE over TEE are the larger field views and the superior soft tissue contrast, allowing for an easy and precise evaluation of ASA. The presence of ASA is not associated with an increased rate of complications or decreased success rate of PFO closure;[33] however, a very large ASA may be problematic and needs to be individually considered when selecting the type or size of the device for closure.

The *ostium primum ASD* can be clearly identified in the presence of developmental deficiency of the antero-inferior rim on the long-axis four-chamber plane, underlining the fact that this malformation involves the atrioventricular canal (Figure 7.13).

The superior and inferior vena cava types of *sinus venosus defect* are shown unequivocally by Ultra ICE; in fact, mechanical ultrasound interrogation may clearly show that these interatrial communications are outside the confines of the fossa ovalis, with the mouths of the superior or inferior vena cava having biatrial connection and overriding the intact antero-superior or postero-inferior muscular borders of the fossa ovalis, respectively (Figure 7.14).

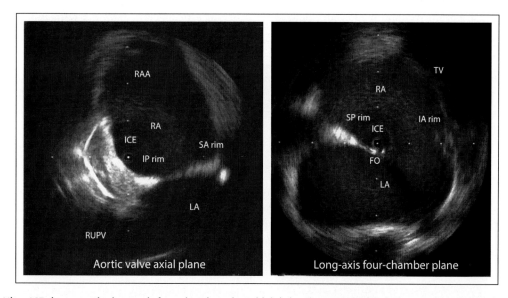

Figure 7.13 Ultra ICE shows on the long-axis four-chamber plane (right) the absence of the inferior–anterior rim (*ostium primum atrial septal defect*) while on the aortic valve axial plane (left) the integrity of interatrial septum with well-represented superior–anterior and inferior–posterior rims. RA, right atrium; RAA, right atrial auricle; FO, fossa ovalis; TV, tricuspid valve; LA, left atrium; RUPV, right upper pulmonary vein; SP rim, superior–posterior rim; IA rim, inferior–anterior rim; SA rim, superior–anterior rim; IP rim, inferior–posterior rim; ICE, intracardiac echocardiography probe.

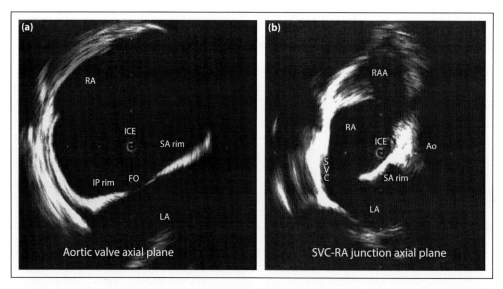

Figure 7.14   (a) Aortic valve axial plane showing an intact fossa ovalis with well-represented rims. (b) Ultra ICE shows a *superior vena cava type of sinus venosus defect* characterized by interatrial communication outside the confines of the fossa ovalis, with the mouths of the superior vena cava having biatrial connection and overriding the intact inferior–posterior muscular borders of the fossa ovalis. RA, right atrium; RAA, right atrial auricle; FO, fossa ovalis; Ao, ascending aorta; LA, left atrium; SVC, superior vena cava; SA rim, superior–anterior rim; IP rim, inferior–posterior rim; ICE, intracardiac echocardiography probe.

Moreover, the *right-sided partial anomalous pulmonary venous drainage* can be diagnosed as a "drop-out" (high connection pattern) or a "tear-drop" (low connection pattern) appearance of the superior vena cava on the great vessels plane or on the superior vena cava–right atrial junction plane, respectively.

Finally, the *lipomatous hypertrophy of the atrial septum*, characterized by massive fatty deposits in the secundum atrial septum and a septum secundum ≥15 mm thick, can

be differentiated from myxoma, thrombus, or tumors[34] (Figure 7.15).

When this condition is associated with ASD, it could be considered as a contraindication to all catheter-based closure procedures due to the impossibility of achieving a correct device deployment, independent of the closure systems. Lesser degrees of atrial septal hypertrophy, between 6 and 14 mm, represent a more common condition, especially in patients with high blood pressure

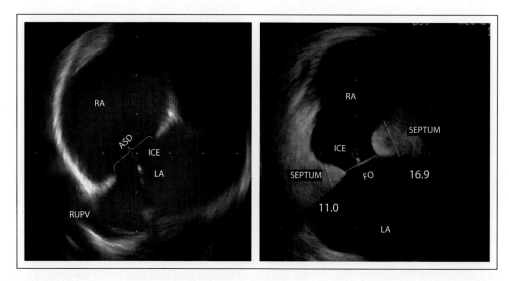

Figure 7.15   Ultra ICE can identify massive fatty deposits in the secundum atrial septum with a septal thickness ≥15 mm. On the left, an atrial septal defect (ASD) with normal septum secundum thickness; on the right, a case of *lipomatous hypertrophy of the atrial septum*. RA, right atrium; LA, left atrium; ASD, atrial septal defect; RUPV, right upper pulmonary vein; FO, fossa ovalis; ICE, intracardiac echocardiography probe.

and in obese and elderly female patients, and are relative contraindications.

Other applications of Ultra ICE

Other current applications of Ultra ICE involve interventional electrophysiologic procedures, cardiac biopsy, assessment of procedural complications, transseptal puncture, and monitoring of endovascular thoracic and abdominal aortic aneurysm repair (Table 7.10).

The following *electrophysiologic procedures* are monitored easily by Ultra ICE:

- Radio-frequency catheter ablation of the superior portion of the sinus junction in inappropriate sinus tachycardia[6]
- Radio-frequency catheter ablation of the slow posterior pathway in atrioventricular nodal reentrant tachycardia[35]
- Radio-frequency catheter ablation of the crista terminalis in ectopic right atrial tachycardia[36]

Table 7.10   Other current applications of Ultra ICE

- Interventional electrophysiology
- Transseptal puncture
- Assessment of procedural complications
- Cardiac biopsy
- Thoracic and abdominal aortic endoprosthetic procedure monitoring
- Left atrial appendage percutaneous closure, percutaneous mitral valvuloplasty, transcatheter mitral valve repair, transcatheter aortic valve implantation (TAVI)

- Radio-frequency catheter ablation of the cavo-tricuspid isthmus in atrial flutter

The most useful Ultra ICE plane during radio-frequency ablation procedures is the axial cavo-tricuspid isthmus plane, because it allows anatomic details to be obtained in order to perform catheterization of the coronary sinus and to identify the location and the boundaries of the Koch's triangle.

Another useful application of Ultra ICE is in safely and effectively assisting *transseptal puncture* of the septum primum during mitral valvuloplasty, ablation of left-sided arrhythmias (atrial fibrillation or left-sided accessory pathways ablation),[37] or in the presence of a previously implanted atrial septal occluder device.[38]

Ultra ICE may show the tip of Mullins transseptal sheath and the Brockenbrough needle seated against the middle of the fossa ovalis, causing a slight "tenting effect" (Figure 7.16). Performing a successful transseptal puncture involves not only making sure the needle passes through the fossa, but also assuring the needle avoids structures such as the aorta and the left atrial free wall. Being able to visualize those structures by Ultra ICE can provide an added measure of confidence, particularly in cases of associated anatomical abnormalities (lipomatous hypertrophy of the septum, ASA, double-layer septum), complex congenital heart disease, or when using radio-frequency to perforate the septum.

An emerging application for the Ultra ICE involves crossing the septum and then monitoring and helping to guide *left-sided procedures* (*electrophysiologic procedures*). In this setting, ICE is designed to allow the user to

- Visualize the left atrial anatomy
- Confirm catheter location relative to the anatomy

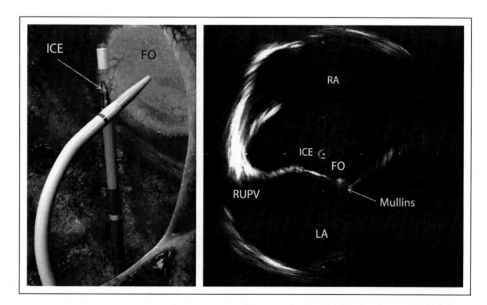

Figure 7.16   (See color insert.) Ultra ICE permits continuous monitoring of the transseptal puncture showing the tip of Mullins transseptal sheath and the Brockenbrough needle seated against the middle of the fossa ovalis, causing a slight "tenting effect." RA, right atrium; LA, left atrium; ICE, intracardiac echocardiography probe; RUPV, right upper pulmonary vein; FO, fossa ovalis.

- Verify tip-to-tissue contact
- Identify location of the esophagus relative to the ablation catheter
- Characterize acute lesion morphology: swelling, dimpling, and crater formation
- Monitor any early signs of thrombus formation, stenosis, or pericardial effusion

Moreover, Ultra ICE permits early recognition of *procedural complications* such as device embolization, device thrombosis, cardiac perforation, and tamponade. Pericardial effusion may be detected as an echo-free space outside the right atrial free wall, whereas the bright parietal echo signal may be seen intermittently, depending on the size of the effusion.

Cardiac biopsy can be facilitated using Ultra ICE guidance, particularly in high-risk cases in which abnormal tissue is adjacent to thin walls or delicate structures. It allows exact delineation of tumor tissue, enabling the operator to guide the bioptome and avoid inadvertent damage to the thin atrial or ventricular walls or valve apparatus.

Finally, during *vascular endoprosthesis implantation at the thoracic or subrenal aortic level*, the mechanical probe may be used to provide an exact evaluation of the lesion and to ensure that the expansion of the endograft is complete and symmetric. The echocardiographic examination with a mechanical transducer is particularly useful for two main reasons: first, to confirm the aortic pathology and the previous morphometric evaluation obtained by computed tomography or MRI, and second, to determine the complete and symmetric expansion of the endoprosthesis struts, in order to reduce the risk of acute and subacute graft occlusion.[39]

Potential future applications of this innovative ultrasound monitoring could be *left atrial appendage percutaneous closure* and, when Doppler capabilities will be available, *percutaneous mitral valvuloplasty, transcatheter mitral valve repair*, and *TAVI*.

Conclusions

The major advantages of Ultra ICE technology are

1. A 100% duty cycle combining imaging of cardiac anatomy and interventional systems, in the sense that images are continuously available during all the stages of catheter-based procedures, allowing not only immediate pre- and postprocedure imaging but also vision-guided and sophisticated monitoring of the interventions
2. A high spatial resolution, no acoustic barriers, or interference from irregular cardiac and respiratory cycle
3. Excellent soft tissue-contrasting capabilities and the ability to image cardiac structures deep within the heart

4. Obtaining specific tomographic views with ease, generally less operator dependence, and considerably less operator dexterity than TT or TEE
5. An effective manipulation of the Ultra ICE catheter by means of a precurved long sheath and to rotate the transducer to critically optimize an image-specific orientation

These advantages are determined by a short distance of interrogated tissue from the transducer and a relatively homogeneous fluid path due to the only uniform omnidirectional backscatter of the red cells. This image quality and wealth of information dramatically reduce examination time and renders Ultra ICE a valuable tool not only for diagnosis but also for *in vivo* morphometry. However, a thorough understanding of the tomographic imaging from the inner confines of the right atrium and great veins requires anatomic and radiological identification and validation for a rapid feedback and a reliable study.

Limitations that still exist and features that may limit the optimal use of a mechanical array technology include

1. Relatively large Ultra ICE delivery catheter
2. Potentially overall increased cost of interventional procedures due to the need of a dedicated system and disposable catheter
3. Abrupt transitions from the transverse to the longitudinal plane
4. Lack of Doppler hemodynamic and parametric capabilities
5. Inadequate depth penetration for imaging the pulmonary artery trunk and the ventricles with the catheter positioned in the right atrium

The major clinical application of the Ultra ICE is facilitating the catheter-based interventional procedures. It should contribute to the pediatric and adult cardiology armamentarium for both diagnostic and therapeutic procedures, because the imaging catheter can remain in place for the entire procedure with excellent patient tolerance, discovering a new route to sophisticated interventions.

Disclosure: The authors have nothing to disclose regarding the content of this manuscript.

References

1. Mitchel JF, Gillam LD, Sanzobrino BW et al. Intracardiac ultrasound imaging during transseptal catheterization. *Chest* 1995;108:104–8.
2. Epstein LM, Smith I, Tenhoff H. Nonfluoroscopic transseptal catheterization: Safety and efficacy of intracardiac echocardiographic guidance. *J Cardiovasc Electrophysiol* 1998;9:625–30.
3. Mangrum JM, Mounsey JP, Kok LC et al. Intracardiac echocardiography-guided, anatomically based radiofrequency ablation of focal atrial fibrillation originating from pulmonary veins. *J Am Coll Cardiol* 2002;39:1964–72.

4. Johnson SB, Seward JB, Packer DL. Phased-array intracardiac echo-cardiography for guiding transseptal catheter placement: Utility and learning curve. *Pacing Clin Electrophysiol* 2002;25:402–7.

5. Hung JS, Fu M, Yeh KH et al. Usefulness of intracardiac echocardiography in complex trans-septal catheterization during percutaneous transvenous mitral commissurotomy. *Mayo Clin Proc* 1996;71:134–40.

6. Chu E, Kalman JM, Kwasman MA et al. Intracardiac echocardiography during radiofrequency catheter ablation of cardiac arrythmias in humans. *J Am Coll Cardiol* 1994;24:1351–7.

7. Kalman JM, Olgin JE, Karch MR et al. Use of intracardiac echocardiography in interventional electrophysiology. *Pacing Clin Electrophysiol* 1997;20:2248–62.

8. Olgin JE, Kalman JM, Chin M et al. Electrophysiological effects of long, linear atrial lesions placed under intracardiac ultrasound guidance. *Circulation* 1997;96:2715–21.

9. Hijazi ZM, Wang Z, Cao Q et al. Transcatheter closure of atrial septal defects and patent foramen ovale under intracardiac echocardiographic guidance: Feasibility and comparison with transesophageal echocardiography. *Catheter Cardiovasc Interv* 2001;52:194–9.

10. Jan SL, Hwang B, Lee PC et al. Intracardiac ultrasound assessment of atrial septal defect: Comparison with transthoracic echocardiographic, angiocardiographic, and balloon-sizing measurements. *Cardiovasc Interv Radiol* 2001;24:84–9.

11. Zanchetta M, Pedon L, Rigatelli G et al. Intracardiac echocardiography evaluation in secundum atrial septal defect transcatheter closure. *Cardiovasc Interv Radiol* 2003;26:52–7.

12. Zanchetta M, Rigatelli G, Onorato E. Intracardiac echocardiography and transcranial Doppler ultrasound to guide closure of patent foramen ovale. *J Invasive Cardiol* 2003;15:93–6.

13. Delgado V, van der Kley F, Schalij MJ et al. Optimal imaging for planning and guiding interventions in structural heart disease: A multi-modality imaging approach. *Eur Heart J* 2010;12(Supplement E):E10–23.

14. King TD, Thompson SL, Mills NL. Measurements of the atrial septal defect during cardiac catheterization. Experimental and clinical results. *Am J Cardiol* 1978;41:41–2.

15. Hijazi ZM, Cao Q, Patel HT et al. Transesophageal echocardiographic results of catheter closure of atrial septal defect in children and adults using the Amplatzer devices. *Am J Cardiol* 2000;85:1387–90.

16. Masura J, Gavora P, Formanek A et al. Transcatheter closure of secundum atrial septal defects using the new self-centering Amplazter septal occluder. *Cathet Cardiovasc Diagn* 1997;42:388–93.

17. Hellenbrand WE, Fahey JT, McGowan FX et al. Transesophageal echocardiographic guidance of transcatheter closure of atrial septal defect. *Am J Cardiol* 1990;66:207–13.

18. Metha RH, Helmcke F, Nanda NC et al. Uses and limitations of transthoracic echocardiography in the assessment of atrial septal defect in the adult. *Am J Cardiol* 1991;67:288–94

19. Godart F, Rey C, Francart C et al. Two-dimensional echocardiographic and color Doppler measurements of atrial septal defect, and comparison with the balloon-stretched diameter. *Am J Cardiol* 1993;72:1095–7.

20. Lee CH, Kwok OH, Chow WH. Pitfalls of atrial septal defect using meditech sizing balloon. *Cathet Cardiovasc Interv* 2001;53:94–5.

21. Daniel WG, Erbel R, Kasper QW et al. Safety of transesophageal echocardiography. A multicenter survey of 10,419 examinations. *Circulation* 1991;83:817–21.

22. Urbanowicz JH, Kernoff RS, Oppenheim G et al. Transesophageal echocardiography and its potential for esophageal damage. *Anesthesiology* 1990;72:40–3.

23. Zanchetta M, Onorato E, Rigatelli G et al. Intracardiac echocardiography-guided transcatheter closure of secundum atrial septal defect. A new efficient device selection method. *J Am Coll Cardiol* 2003;42:1677–82.

24. Zanchetta M, Rigatelli G, Pedon L et al. Transcatheter atrial septal defect closure assisted by intracardiac echocardiography: 3-year follow-up. *J Interv Cardiol* 2004;17(2):95–8.

25. Vigna C, Marchese N, Zanchetta M et al. Echocardiographic guidance of percutaneous patent foramen ovale closure: Head-to-head comparison of transesophageal versus rotational intracardiac echocardiography. *Echocardiography* 2012;29:1103–10.

26. Lazar AV, Pechacek LW, Mihalick MJ et al. Aneurysm of the interatrial septum occurring as an isolated anomaly. *Cathet Cardiovasc Diagn* 1983;9:167–73.

27. Mugge A, Daniel WG, Angermann C et al. Atrial septal aneurysm in adult patients. A multicenter study using transthoracic and transesophageal echocardiography. *Circulation* 1995;91:2785–92.

28. Silver MD, Dorsey JS. Aneurysms of septum primum in adults. *Arch Pathol Lab Med* 1978;102:62–5.

29. Pearson AC, Nagelhout D, Castello R et al. Atrial septal aneurysm and stroke: A transesophageal echocardiographic study. *J Am Coll Cardiol* 1991;18:1223–29.

30. Mas JL, Arquizan C, Lamy C et al. Recurrent cerebrovascular events associated with patent foramen ovale, atrial septal aneurysm, or both. *N Engl J Med* 2001;345:1740–6.

31. Marazano M, Roudaut R, Cohen A et al. Atrial septal aneurysm. Morphological characteristics in a large population: Pathological associations. A French multicenter study on 259 patients investigated by transoesophageal echocardiography. *Int J Cardiol* 1995;52:59–65.

32. Hanley PC, Tajik AJ, Hynes JK et al. Diagnosis and classification of atrial septal aneurysm by two-dimensional echocardiography: Report of 80 consecutive cases. *J Am Coll Cardiol* 1985;6:1370–82.

33. Krumsdorf U, Keppeler P, Horvath K et al. Catheter closure of atrial septal defects and patent foramen ovale in patients with an atrial septal aneurysm using different devices. *J Interv Cardiol* 2001;14:49–55.

34. Levine RA, Weyman AE, Dinsmore RE et al. Non-invasive tissue characterization: Diagnosis of lipomatous hypertrophy of the atrial septum by nuclear magnetic resonance imaging. *J Am Coll Cardiol* 1986;7:688–92.

35. Fisher WG, Pelini MA, Bacon ME. Adjunctive intracardiac echocardiography to guide slow pathway ablation in human atrioventricular nodal reentrant tachycardia: Anatomic insights. *Circulation* 1997;96:3021–9.

36. Kalman JM, Olgin JE, Karch MR et al. Crystal tachycardias: Origin of right atrial tachycardias from the crista terminalis identified by intracardiac echocardiography. *J Am Coll Cardiol* 1998;31:451–9.

37. Citro R, Ducceschi V, Salustri A et al. Intracardiac echocardiography to guide transseptal catheterization for radiofrequency catheter ablation of left-sided accessory pathways: Two case reports. *Cardiovasc Ultrasound* 2004;2:20.

38. Santangeli P, Di Biase L, Burkhardt JD et al. Transseptal access and atrial fibrillation ablation guided by intracardiac echocardiography in patients with atrial septal closure devices. *Heart Rhythm* 2011;8(11):1669–75.

39. Zanchetta M, Rigatelli GL, Pedon L et al. IVUS guidance of thoracic and complex abdominal aortic aneurysm stent-graft repairs using an intracardiac echocardiography probe: Preliminary report. *J Endovasc Ther* 2003;10:218–26.

8

Cardiac computed tomography and magnetic resonance imaging in the cath-lab

Robert Kumar, Vladimir Jelnin, Chad Kliger, and Carlos E. Ruiz

Introduction

The mathematical basis of x-ray image reconstruction dates back to 1917 when Radon,[1] an Austrian mathematician, published an analytical solution to the problem of reconstructing an object from multiple projections. The actual application of mathematical image reconstruction techniques of radiographic medical imaging was first reported in 1961 by Oldendorf,[2] and the first clinical computerized tomography was developed by the Nobel laureate Sir Godfrey N. Hounsfield. He applied the early mathematical theories to reconstruct the internal structure of the body from a number of different x-ray measurements, using a translate/rotate process that was repeated until the entire circumference of the body was scanned.[3-5] Since then, computed tomography (CT) has become one of the most important x-ray-based imaging technologies.

The use of CT as a cardiac diagnostic modality in the past was hindered primarily by the limitations of temporal resolution. This was improved with the introduction of electron beam CT (EBCT) in the mid-1980s. The main technological advantage of EBCT was the absence of a mechanically rotating x-ray source, resulting in higher temporal resolution.[6] With EBCT, electrons are fired from a generator and electromagnetically deflected to sweep across four tungsten target rings located in the gantry beneath the patient. EBCT reduced acquisition time to 100 ms/image or less, thereby being able to "freeze" cardiac motion and produce clear cross-sectional images of the heart. This technology resulted in the birth of cardiac CT.

Conventional CT has evolved with the introduction of spiral, or helical, CT technology. Since the early 1990s, the use of multidetector CT (MDCT) has stimulated a renewed interest in cardiac CT imaging, and has essentially replaced EBCT. Further advances in technology and the development of fusion-imaging techniques have allowed new applications of CT imaging for improved preprocedural planning and guidance within the cardiac catheterization laboratory.

Principles of cardiac computed tomography

CT technology has advanced rapidly over the last several years, and many of the technical principles are beyond the scope of this chapter. However, certain aspects of CT image acquisition are important to understand for obtaining the high-quality CT images necessary for preprocedural planning and guidance during interventional procedures. The majority of cardiac CT studies today are performed using helical CT. Helical CT scanning utilizes a spiral or helical path of the x-ray tube around the body, while the table moves continuously through the gantry. Collected volumetric data are then reconstructed into single transaxial planes using an interpolation algorithm,[7-9] as opposed to obtaining transaxial images using an x-ray tube rotating around the body in a stepwise fashion (step-and-shoot).

In the early 1990s, helical CT started using multirow detectors (MDCT) currently capable of generating 256 slices or more of varying thickness with each gantry rotation. Instead of one detector row, multiple parallel detector rows acquire data, allowing for much faster scan times. MDCT scanners can produce submillimeter resolution with commonly used 64-slice systems demonstrating a spatial resolution as low as 0.5 mm. To produce high-quality cardiac images needed for procedural guidance, a minimal imaging artifact must be present. Attention to proper ECG gating, minimizing patient motion during the scan, and ensuring adequate contrast enhancement are important details to consider during the acquisition. In addition, the scan should be tailored to the specific patient and procedure, such that sufficient coverage of relevant anatomy is obtained. Specific cardiac acquisition protocols should be used.[10,11]

Image postprocessing techniques

Two techniques for postprocessing of CT data have helped expand the role of CT in guiding structural heart disease interventions: 3-D volume-rendering (VR) and curved multiplanar reconstruction (CMPR). These computer reconstruction techniques allow the visualization of human organs in three dimensions, and the ability to manipulate the image to obtain precise 2-D and 3-D measurements. All major CT manufacturing companies can deliver their own dedicated 3-D workstation with each scanner, and most of them have similar functionality and tools. All existing techniques use the original cross-sectional CT images as the source. The quality of final 3-D reconstructed images is directly related to the spatial resolution of the source image (voxel size). Combining all voxels of the data set and using specified reconstruction techniques (i.e., postprocessing) allows the visualization of the anatomy in 3-D views (Figure 8.1).

Volume-rendering techniques are based on assigning specific colors and opacities to voxels, depending on their densities.[12,13] Standard color and opacity presets are usually available in the majority of 3-D workstations. By changing the opacities of the voxel values corresponding to specific tissues, it is possible to make various tissues appear transparent or opaque depending on the anatomical structure being examined (Figure 8.2). Flexibility in changing a variety of parameters, including the color scheme and opacity, allows adjustment of the images to the needs of the individual procedure. Volume-rendered

images are useful for obtaining measurements of cardiac defects and structures of interest, such as paravalvar leaks (PVLs), ventricular pseudoaneurysms, and prosthetic valve frames (Figure 8.3). Manipulation of volume-rendered images prior to a procedure can be useful for planning access approach and determining the appropriate device and delivery equipment.

Multiplanar reconstruction (MPR) allows the observer to change the plane of view from axial to sagittal, coronal, or oblique views, a standard method used for basic CT imaging. The CMPR method is widely used for vessel visualization and analysis.[12] With CMPR, the cut plane is not linear, but curved and defined by a centerline created by the operator to follow the vessel curvature. The resulting image is a flattened representation (reformation) of the curved plane. CMPR may be used for planning access routes in procedures requiring large delivery sheaths, which may be occlusive to smaller vessels and pose a significant risk of vascular injury.

Rationale of CT guidance in structural heart disease interventions

Fluoroscopy has long been the dominant imaging modality used to guide interventional procedures in the catheterization laboratory. However, fluoroscopy has several limitations as a sole imaging modality for complex structural

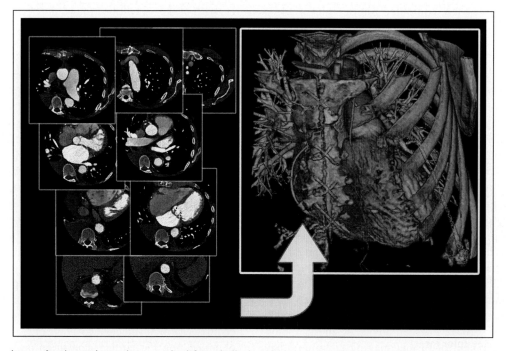

Figure 8.1 **(See color insert.)** 2-D data acquired from helical multidetector CT (MDCT) scanning can be reconstructed into 3-D volume-rendered images using postprocessing techniques.

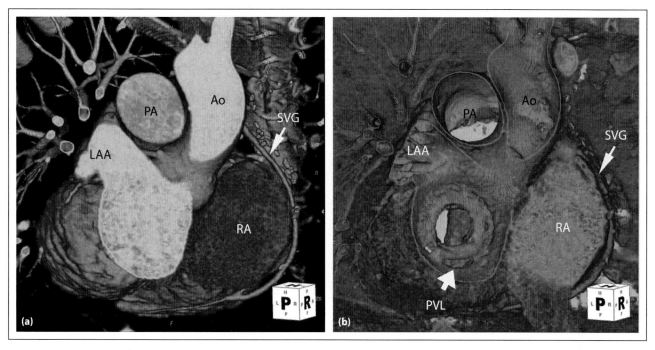

Figure 8.2   **(See color insert.)** 3-D reconstruction of a cardiac CTA study. The image can be manipulated to examine different cardiac structures by selectively changing the opacities of voxels with different densities. (a) The course of a patent saphenous vein graft (SVG, arrow) is clearly seen. (b) The same image in (a) after making high-density voxels more transparent. The SVG (thin arrow) is not seen as well as in (a), but a prosthetic mitral valve with a paravalvar leak (PVL, thick arrow) is now identified.

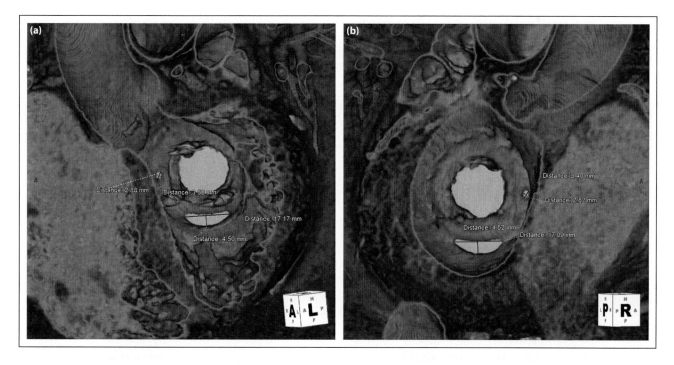

Figure 8.3   **(See color insert.)** Volume-rendered CT images are useful for making accurate measurements of cardiac structures. In this case, the dimensions of two mitral paravalvar leaks are measured from the ventricular side (a) and the atrial side (b) prior to consideration of percutaneous PVL closure.

heart disease interventions. 3-D anatomic interrelationships are difficult to accurately assess with 2-D fluoroscopy alone. Accurate measurements in 3-D space are difficult to assess; the position of catheters and therapeutic devices within the heart may be misinterpreted and radiolucent soft-tissue structures are poorly visualized under fluoroscopy, often requiring frequent contrast injections to identify the target location.

Computed tomography angiography (CTA) represents a modality from which accurate 2-D and 3-D measurements can be made and 3-D anatomy can be seen in multiple angulations for procedural planning and guidance. Recent technological advances have allowed for complementary imaging modalities to be used in conjunction with fluoroscopy to guide structural cardiac interventions.[14] The integration of multimodality imaging with fluoroscopy in the catheterization laboratory, also known as fusion imaging, now provides an alternative to traditional fluoroscopically guided catheterization. For example, the fusion of CT and MRI data with 2-D fluoroscopy has been described to be feasible and accurate for coronary sinus lead implantation during cardiac resynchronization therapy device placement.[15,16] Similar techniques of imaging fusion are now being incorporated into a variety of structural heart disease interventions. Continuous display of relevant 3-D structures while manipulating catheters under fluoroscopy is valuable to the interventionalist and may lead to reduced procedural times, radiation dose, and contrast administration. The fusion of 3-D CT or MRI data with fluoroscopic imaging now represents a new paradigm of imaging guidance that may expand the potential for procedural success and safety in structural heart disease interventions.

Overview of CT–fluoroscopy fusion

Merging preacquired CT data with live fluoroscopic images, or CT–fluoroscopy fusion, has a variety of applications for intraprocedural imaging guidance. CT–fluoroscopy fusion involves the process of 3-D data reconstruction, segmentation of cardiac and thoracic structures, and accurate registration of the 3-D data to fluoroscopy. First, axial CTA data obtained prior to the procedure must be reconstructed into 3-D images using volume-rendering techniques. Segmentation is then performed, a postprocessing technique, in which the 3-D images are either automatically or manually "segmented" to identify important structures such as the aorta, cardiac chambers and valves, coronary arteries, trachea, lungs, and ribs (Figure 8.4). These structures can then be added or subtracted from the image for guidance depending on the procedural component of interest.

Next, the 3-D images are registered to live fluoroscopy. At the beginning of the procedure, fluoroscopy for registration is performed in two orthogonal planes, such as left anterior oblique (LAO) and right anterior oblique (RAO) projections, at least 20° apart. Radiopaque structures, such as prosthetic heart valves, dense vascular calcification, and

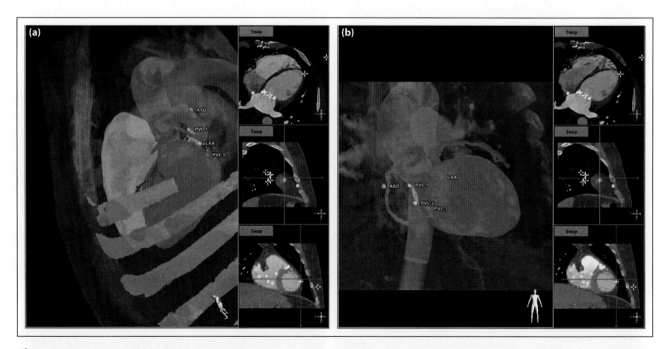

Figure 8.4 **(See color insert.)** Segmentation of 3-D volume-rendered CT images for preprocedural planning. (a) The aorta and coronary arteries (red), right ventricle (green), left ventricle (purple), and ribs (tan) are segmented. The locations of an atrial septal defect (blue dot), three paravalvar leaks (PVL 1–3), and left atrial appendage (LAA) are marked (yellow dots). (b) The image in (a) is rotated to show the same structures in a different orientation. Segmented structures can be added or removed. In this case, the ribs were removed to better visualize the left ventricle.

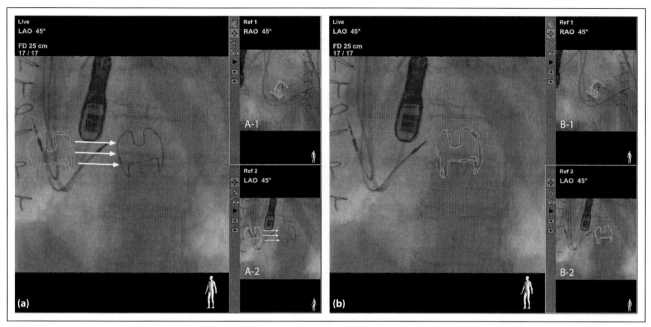

Figure 8.5 **(See color insert.)** Registration of 3-D CTA data to live fluoroscopy. (a) The outline of a prosthetic mitral valve frame (orange) is overlaid onto the fluoroscopy screen. It is then adjusted to correspond to the same size, location, and orientation as the radiopaque frame seen on fluoroscopy using specialized software (Philips HeartNavigator, Best, Netherlands). (b) Once the CTA data are properly registered, the movement of the C-arm will be tracked, and the CT overlay images will automatically move and rotate accordingly (B-1 and B-2). Additional structures and landmarks from the CTA data can be added or removed as needed for procedural guidance.

vertebrae are typically used for registration. When internal markers are not present, contrast opacification of the aorta can be performed during cineangiography to provide a radiopaque structure for CT registration. Using registration software, such as HeartNavigator (Philips Healthcare, Best, Netherlands) or Innova 3-D (GE Healthcare, Chalfont St. Giles, UK), the reconstructed 3-D CT images are adjusted to correspond to the same size, location, and orientation as seen on fluoroscopy using radiopaque structures in orthogonal views (Figure 8.5).

For the subsequent duration of the procedure, the previously segmented structures can be overlaid onto the fluoroscopy screen as needed, and specific landmarks can be placed. As the C-arm rotates and the fluoroscopic view changes, the movement is tracked, and the overlaid CT images are automatically adjusted accordingly. The use of CT–fluoroscopy fusion imaging for guidance in several structural heart disease interventions will be discussed in the examples below.

Transcatheter valve replacement

Transcatheter aortic valve replacement

Over the past few years, the rapid worldwide increase in transcatheter aortic valve replacement (TAVR) procedures has fueled a growing interest in multimodality imaging for procedural planning and guidance, and MDCT has emerged to play a vital role in the procedural

planning for TAVR.[14,17,18] Currently, two devices are in widespread use for TAVR: the balloon-expandable SAPIEN valve (Edwards Lifesciences, Irvine, CA, USA) and the self-expanding CoreValve (Medtronic, Minneapolis, MN, USA).

In cases using a femoral or subclavian artery approach for the insertion of the delivery sheath, a detailed knowledge of the peripheral vasculature is important due to the risk of vascular complications related to the large sheath sizes for these devices (18–24 Fr). 3-D volume-rendered reconstruction of the peripheral vasculature can help assess the tortuosity and atherosclerotic disease that may increase the risk of complications during vascular access (Figure 8.6a). Measurements of the iliac, femoral, and subclavian arteries can be accurately performed using CMPR to assess the ability of these arteries to accommodate the delivery sheath (Figure 8.6b).

After an access route has been identified, CT imaging provides detailed information regarding the aortic annulus, aortic root, and coronary arteries (Figure 8.7a–e). Accurate measurements of the aortic valve annulus are important to minimize the risk of paravalvar regurgitation, and 3-D modalities such as MDCT may provide more accurate measurements than 2-D TTE or TEE.[18] With MDCT, the aortic valve annular diameter, perimeter, and area can be measured for optimal sizing of the prosthesis, leaflet and annular calcification can be assessed, and the distance from the annulus to the coronary ostia can be measured to assess the potential for coronary artery obstruction from the prosthesis or densely calcified aortic valve leaflets. The dimensions of the sinus

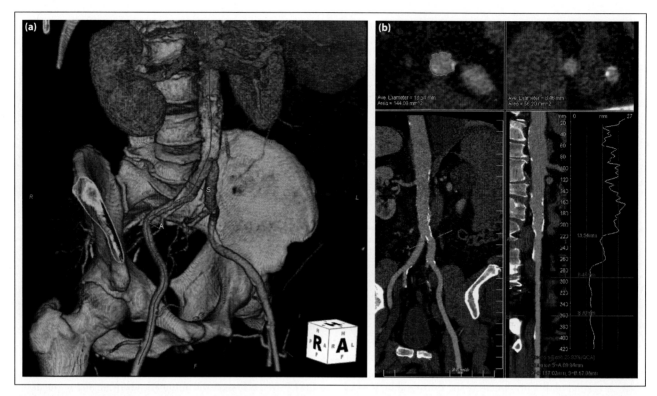

Figure 8.6   **(See color insert.)** CTA images of the peripheral vasculature in a patient prior to transcatheter aortic valve replacement (TAVR). (a) 3-D volume-rendered CTA images can identify tortuosity and atherosclerotic disease that increase the risk of vascular complications. In this case, the iliofemoral vessels are mildly tortuous, and calcification of the descending aorta is present. (b) Curved multiplanar reconstruction (CMPR) in the same patient allows accurate measurements of the iliofemoral vessels. In this patient, TAVR was successfully performed using femoral artery access.

of Valsalva, sinotubular junction, and ascending aorta can also be assessed by MDCT, and the angulation and spatial orientation of the aortic root structures can be determined. Manipulation of the 3-D volume-rendered CT images can identify the optimal fluoroscopic views to be used during device deployment, in which the three leaflets of the aortic valve lie in a single plane, such that the prosthetic valve may be deployed at an optimal depth below all the leaflets to avoid a supra-annular or low implantation (Figure 8.8a and b).

After preprocedural assessment, CT–fluoroscopy fusion can be a valuable tool for successful TAVR implantation. If femoral artery access is to be used, CT registration of the iliofemoral system can be performed using the pelvis and femoral bones for registration. An outline of the iliofemoral system can be overlaid onto fluoroscopy to identify the optimal femoral artery puncture location (Figure 8.9a–c). During positioning and deployment of the prosthetic valve, the C-arm is rotated into the optimal fluoroscopic angulation previously identified by CT, in which the aortic valve leaflets lie in a single plane. Using the registration process outlined previously, an outline of the aorta and coronary arteries can be overlaid onto the fluoroscopy screen to aid in device positioning (Figure 8.9c). Additionally, an outline of the prosthesis at an optimal implant depth can be utilized to minimize the number of contrast injections needed for deployment. The

use of preprocedural CT imaging and CT–fluoroscopy fusion guidance can be used to minimize complications associated with vascular access and malpositioning of the prosthesis.

Transcatheter pulmonary valve implantation

Transcatheter pulmonary valve implantation with the Melody valve (Medtronic, Minneapolis, MN, USA) has demonstrated encouraging results in patients with right ventricular outflow tract (RVOT) conduit dysfunction, either obstruction or pulmonary insufficiency.[19] Preprocedural CTA examination can provide detailed assessment of the RVOT and pulmonary valve annulus dimensions; identify the course of the left coronary artery, which may potentially be compressed during valve deployment; and identify additional stenosis of the pulmonary arteries or branches. CT guidance during valve deployment can be used to optimize the sizing and positioning of the Melody valve (Figure 8.10a–d).

Transcatheter mitral valve-in-valve implantation

Patients with degenerated bioprosthetic mitral prostheses, who are considered inoperable based on estimated surgical risk, have been successfully treated with transcatheter

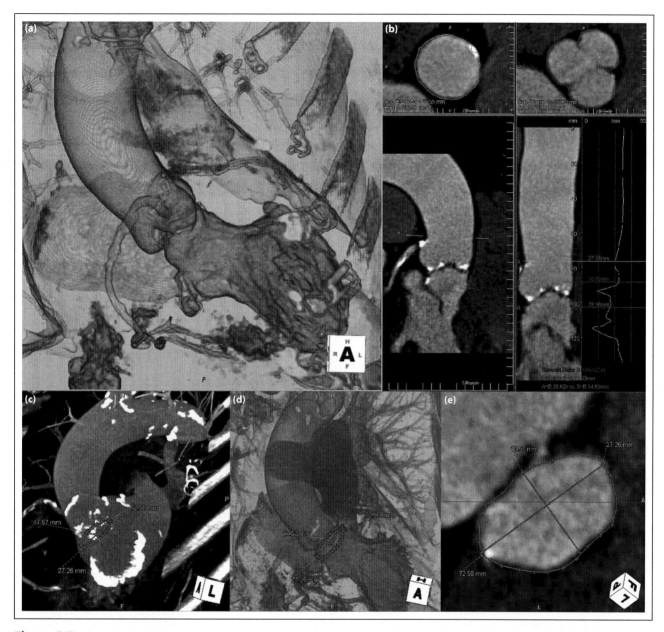

Figure 8.7 **(See color insert.)** CTA assessment of the aortic valve and adjacent structures prior to transcatheter aortic valve replacement (TAVR). (a) 3-D volume-rendered CTA images provide an overview of the size and angulation of the ascending aorta during preprocedural planning for TAVR. (b) Curved multiplanar reconstruction (CMPR) of the ascending aorta is used to measure the aorta at the sinotubular junction (green outline, top left panel) and the sinus of Valsalva (red outline, top right panel). (c–e) Multiple images are used for the assessment of the aortic valve annulus. (c) Demonstrates surrounding calcium (white) in relationship to the aortic annular plane (green outline) using a maximum-intensity projection (MIP). (d) Demonstrates the spatial orientation of the aortic annular plane (green outline) in a volume-rendered image. (e) Shows a cross section of the annulus using CMPR to make accurate measurements of the aortic annulus perimeter and maximum and minimum diameters.

valve-in-valve implantation. Mitral valve-in-valve implantation may be performed using a retrograde transapical approach or an antegrade transseptal approach. Preprocedural CTA imaging can be used to obtain precise measurements of the mitral bioprosthesis prior to choosing a transcatheter valve and to select the optimal route of access for the procedure (Figure 8.11a–d).

CT guidance for site-specific puncture

Structural heart disease interventions may involve peripheral arterial or venous access, transseptal access, or percutaneous transapical access. Needle puncture for these

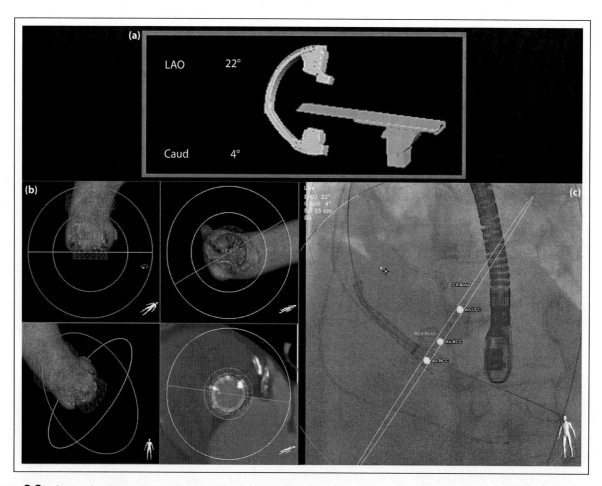

Figure 8.8 **(See color insert.)** 3-D volume-rendered CTA images are used to identify the optimal plane for device deployment during transcatheter aortic valve implantation (TAVR), in which all three aortic valve leaflets lie in a single plane. (a, b) The predicted C-arm angulation to achieve the desired orientation can be identified by CTA prior to the procedure. A volume-rendered CTA image of the aorta can be rotated to align the aortic valve leaflets, with the plane containing all three represented by the yellow circle (b). In this case, a model of a CoreValve is placed in the CTA image to identify the optimal device position. (c) A fluoroscopic view in the predetermined C-arm angulation during CoreValve deployment. The preacquired CTA images have been registered to the fluoroscopic images, and the outline of the aorta (red) and the base of each aortic valve leaflet (yellow dots) are overlaid onto the fluoroscopy screen. The plane of the leaflets is represented by the yellow circle.

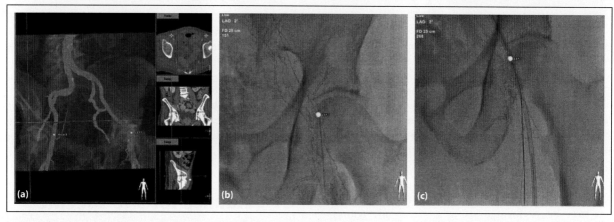

Figure 8.9 **(See color insert.)** (a) The iliofemoral system is segmented after 3-D reconstruction of CTA data in a patient undergoing transcatheter aortic valve replacement (TAVR). The planned puncture sites of both femoral arteries are marked with yellow dots. (b) After the CTA data have been registered to the fluoroscopic images, CT overlay imaging is used to guide femoral artery access. The needle is guided toward the planned puncture site in the left femoral artery (yellow dot). (c) After accessing the femoral artery, the vessel is pre-closed (Prostar XL, Abbott Vascular, Abbott Park, IL, USA) prior to insertion of the delivery sheath.

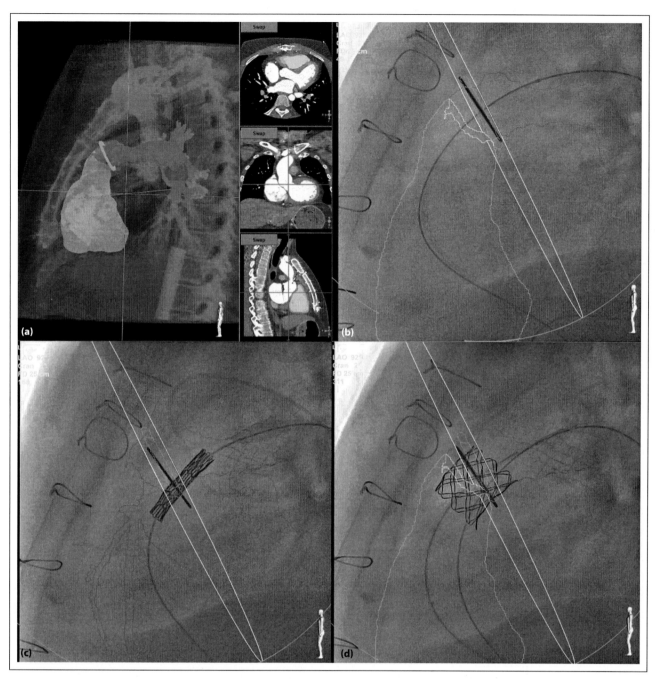

Figure 8.10   (See color insert.) CT guidance during implantation of a transcatheter Melody valve (Medtronic, Minneapolis, MN, USA) in a patient with tetralogy of Fallot and severe pulmonary insufficiency of a right ventricular outflow tract conduit. The patient also had severe stenosis of the left main pulmonary artery. (a) 3-D volume-rendered CTA images identify the right ventricle (green) and proximal pulmonary vasculature (magenta). The pulmonary valve prosthesis in the RVOT conduit is also identified (orange). The CT data are then registered to fluoroscopy for CT overlay guidance. (b) A fluoroscopic image with CT–fluoroscopy fusion imaging used to mark the outline of the right ventricle (green) and pulmonary arteries (magenta). The plane of the pulmonary valve is identified with a yellow circle. (c) A fluoroscopic image with the Melody valve being positioned prior to deployment. CT–fluoroscopy fusion imaging is used to identify the left ventricle and left coronary artery (red outline) to assess for potential coronary compression during valve deployment. A stent is visible in the left pulmonary artery that was placed prior to deploying the Melody valve. (d) A fluoroscopic image showing the Melody valve in the final position.

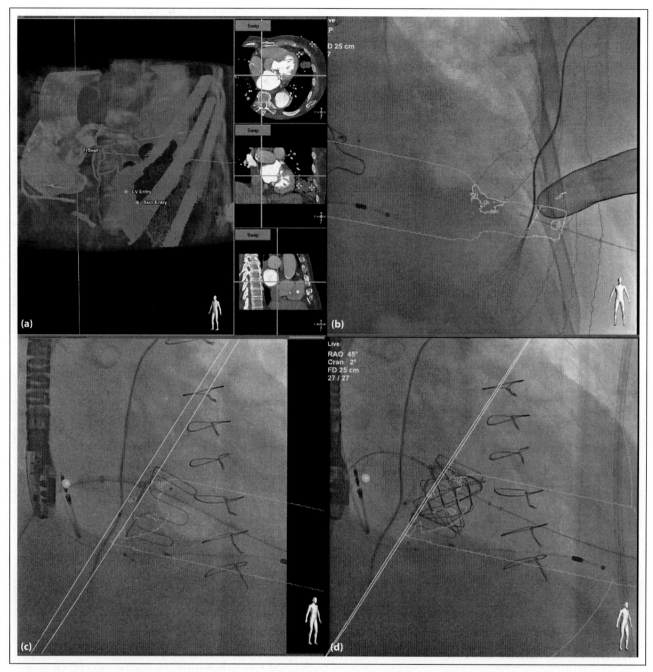

Figure 8.11 **(See color insert.)** CT guidance for mitral valve-in-valve implantation in a patient with a degenerated bioprosthetic mitral valve using a Melody transcatheter valve. An antegrade transseptal approach was used to deliver the Melody valve, with transapical access used to snare and exteriorize the guide wire to create a "rail-wire" for secure device delivery. (a) 3-D volume-rendered CTA images are segmented to identify the aorta and coronary arteries (red), left atrium (orange), and ribs (magenta). The transapical skin and left ventricle entry points (green dots) and planned transseptal puncture site (gray dot) are marked. (b) A fluoroscopic image showing transapical access using CT overlay guidance. After the CTA data have been registered to fluoroscopy, the skin entry point (green dot) is placed on the fluoroscopic image for access guidance. A manually constructed cylinder coaxial to the mitral valve is overlaid onto the fluoroscopic image to guide the angle of needle entry. (c) The transseptal guide wire has been exteriorized through the transapical access site to create a rail-wire, and a catheter is advanced over the wire. The transseptal puncture site was marked for guidance (blue dot). (d) The Melody valve is deployed within the degenerated mitral bioprosthesis over the rail-wire.

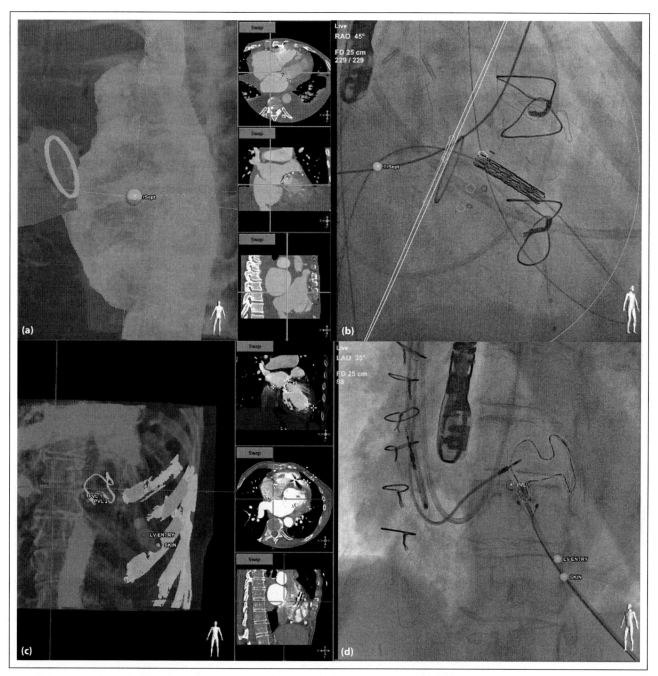

Figure 8.12   **(See color insert.)** CT guidance for site-specific transseptal and transapical access. (a, b) CT guidance for transseptal access during a mitral valve-in-valve implantation procedure using a Melody transcatheter pulmonary valve (Medtronic, Minneapolis, MN, USA). The patient has a degenerated mitral bioprosthetic valve and was deemed to be inoperable. (a) Shows segmentation of the left atrium (orange) and the left ventricle (purple) from 3-D volume-rendered CTA images. The mitral valve prosthesis is marked (green circle). The ideal transseptal puncture site for delivery of the Melody valve is marked (blue dot). (b) Shows a fluoroscopic image during delivery of the Melody valve. Transseptal access was obtained and a rail-wire was snared in the aorta and exteriorized through the femoral artery to deliver the Melody valve. CT data were registered to fluoroscopic images, and CT overlay guidance was used for site-specific transseptal puncture (blue dot). (c, d) CT guidance for an aortic paravalvar leak (PVL) closure. (c) Shows segmentation of the prosthetic aortic valve (orange) and ribs (green). The PVL is marked (red dots) and the skin and left ventricular entry points are identified (green dots) at a safe distance from the lung, coronary arteries, and ribs. A manually constructed cylinder is placed between the skin and ventricular entry points to identify the angle of needle entry. (d) Shows a fluoroscopic image during the procedure, with a catheter extending through the left ventricular apex to the aortic valve, and two Amplatzer Vascular Plug II devices (St. Jude Medical, St. Paul, MN, USA) being deployed across the PVL (red dot).

procedures must be accurate to minimize complications and provide optimal access to the target lesion. CT guidance for obtaining accurate femoral artery access was described above. Using similar techniques of 3-D volume rendering, segmentation, and registration to fluoroscopy, CT guidance can also be used for obtaining accurate and safe transseptal and transapical access (Figure 8.12a–d).

Left atrial appendage exclusion

Left atrial appendage (LAA) exclusion has been shown to be a promising treatment option for reducing stroke risk in atrial fibrillation in patients who are poor candidates for anticoagulation.[20-22] Currently available devices for LAA exclusion include the Amplatzer Cardiac Plug (ACP) (St. Jude Medical, Plymouth, MN, USA), The WATCHMAN device (Atritech, Plymouth, MN, USA), and the Lariat Suture Delivery System (SentreHeart, Palo Alto, CA, USA).

Detailed knowledge of the LAA anatomy is imperative for the device choice and sizing, and can be challenging to assess by 2-D echo due to the complex anatomical configuration of the LAA and the wide variation in LAA morphologies. Improper sizing and positioning of the ACP or WATCHMAN device may lead to perforation of the LAA, incomplete exclusion of the appendage, or device embolization. CT imaging can provide detailed anatomic assessment of the LAA prior to the procedure (Figure 8.13a

and b), and CT–fluoroscopy fusion during the procedure can be used to guide device delivery and positioning.

Paravalvar leak closure

PVLs of aortic and mitral prosthetic valves have been successfully closed percutaneously with a variety of devices.[23] Preprocedural planning using CT imaging can identify the leak location and size, assess for significant calcification within the tract or adjacent annular tissue, and assist in choosing the appropriate access route. Identification of the leak location by fluoroscopy alone can be challenging, and CT–fluoroscopy fusion can be a valuable tool for guidance during percutaneous PVL closure. By allowing markers to be placed in the location of PVL on the fluoroscopy screen, CT–fluoroscopy fusion can facilitate access, wire crossing, and device deployment (Figure 8.14a–e).

Alcohol septal ablation

Patients with hypertrophic obstructive cardiomyopathy (HOCM) may benefit from alcohol ablation of the septal artery when septal hypertrophy results in left ventricular outflow tract (LVOT) obstruction.[24] However, arterial supply to the septum varies widely between patients. CTA may help identify optimal candidates for septal ablation.

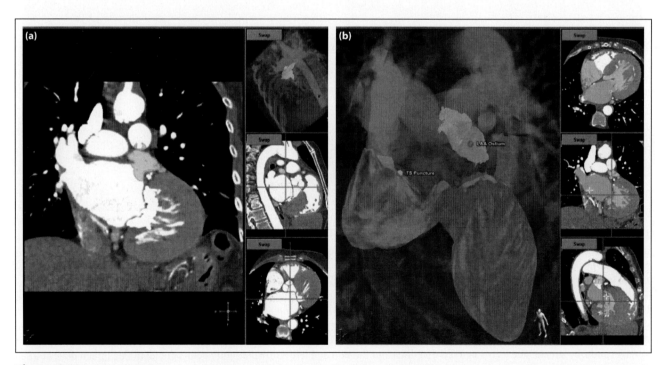

Figure 8.13 **(See color insert.)** (a) The size, morphology, and orientation of the left atrial appendage (LAA, yellow shading) can be assessed by CTA prior to LAA exclusion. Improper sizing of an exclusion device may lead to perforation, incomplete exclusion, or device embolization. (b) For procedural guidance, the cardiac chambers and LAA are segmented on volume-rendered CT images. The planned transseptal (TS) puncture site is identified and marked with a blue dot. The images can then be registered to fluoroscopy and used for CT overlay guidance during the procedure.

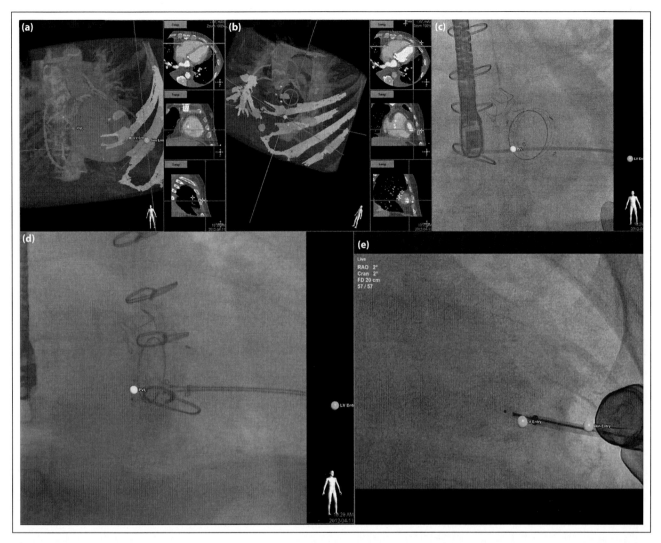

Figure 8.14 **(See color insert.)** CT guidance for paravalvar leak (PVL) closure using transapical access. (a, b) Segmentation of volume-rendered CT images is used to identify the 3-D location of the PVL (yellow dot), as well as the skin and left ventricular puncture sites (blue dots), in relationship to surrounding structures. (c) After registering the CT data to fluoroscopic images, CT overlay guidance is used for crossing the PVL (yellow dot) with a guide wire and advancing a delivery sheath. The radiopaque portion of the mitral bioprosthesis used for registration is identified by the green circle. (d) Two Amplatzer Vascular Plug II devices (St. Jude Medical, St. Paul, MN, USA) are deployed across the PVL using CT overlay guidance. (e) An Amplatzer duct occluder device (St. Jude Medical, St. Paul, MN, USA) is used to close the left ventricular access site (blue dot).

CT–fluorosocopy fusion imaging can be used to guide catheter delivery during percutaneous alcohol septal ablation (Figure 8.15).

Ventricular pseudoaneurysm closure

Ventricular pseudoaneurysms may form after trauma, myocardial infarction, or endocarditis. Larger pseudoaneurysms may cause heart failure and pose a risk of sudden death from spontaneous rupture.[25] Percutaneous closure has been reported in several cases. CT imaging can help identify optimal candidates for percutaneous closure based on the defect size and location, and CT–fluoroscopy fusion may provide intraprocedural guidance for device sizing and deployment (Figure 8.16a–c).

Percutaneous treatment of aortic coarctation

Coarcation of the aorta in adult patients is a rare disorder that can be successfully treated by surgery, or balloon angioplasty with or without stent placement.[26–28] CTA imaging of the aorta is useful prior to catheter-based

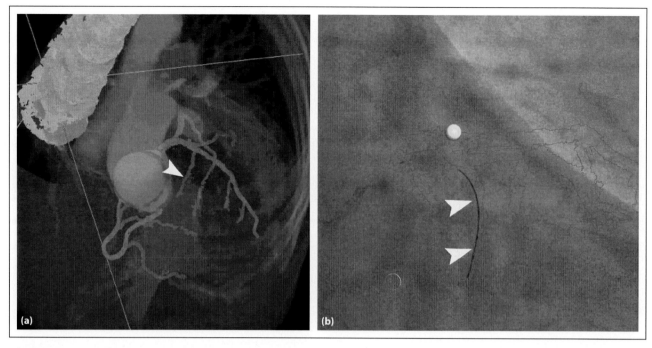

Figure 8.15   **(See color insert.)** CT guidance for alcohol septal ablation in a patient with hypertrophic obstructive cardiomyopathy (HOCM). (a) Prior to performing an alcohol septal ablation procedure for HOCM, 3-D volume-rendered CTA images are used to segment the coronary arteries (red). The first septal perforator artery is identified (arrowhead). (b) CT overlay guidance for alcohol septal ablation. After registration of the CT data to fluoroscopic images, the coronary arteries are identified (red outline). The ostium of the first septal perforator is marked (yellow dot). A guide wire (white arrowheads) is advanced into the first septal perforator (arrowheads) using CT guidance and the position is confirmed by contrast angiography prior to injection of ethanol.

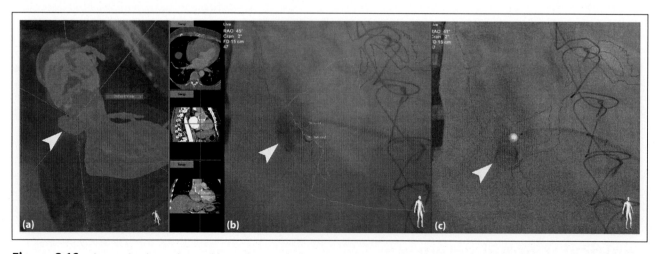

Figure 8.16   **(See color insert.)** CT guidance for ventricular pseudoaneurysm closure. This patient developed a pseudoaneurysm in the left ventricular outflow tract (LVOT) after aortic valve replacement for endocarditis. (a) 3-D volume-rendered CTA images are segmented to identify the aorta and coronary arteries (red), left ventricle (purple), and a pseudoaneurysm in the LVOT (magenta). (b) A catheter is advanced into the pseudoaneurysm from a transapical approach, and contrast is injected into the pseudoaneurysm to confirm the catheter location. The pseudoaneurysm had two ostia communicating with the LVOT, identified as ostium 1 (purple circle) and ostium 2 (red dot). (c) Embolization coils (Cook Medical, Bloomington, IN, USA) are successfully deployed into the pseudoaneurysm using CT overlay guidance.

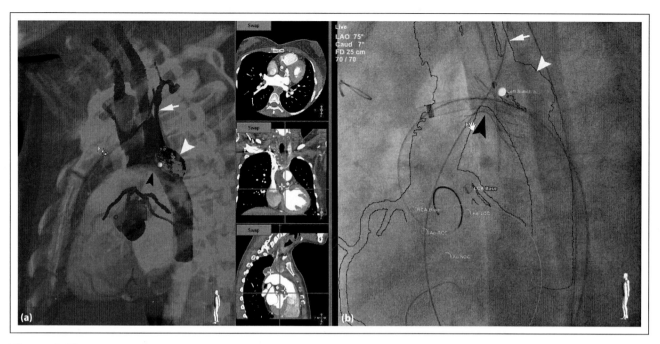

Figure 8.17   **(See color insert.)** CT imaging guidance for aortic stent placement in a patient with coarctation of the aorta. This patient had coarctation repair in childhood and later had a left carotid artery to descending aorta graft placed. She developed symptomatic recurrent coarctation with a high gradient across the coarctation. CTA identified a severe ostial subclavian stenosis in addition. (a) Volume-rendered 3-D CTA images are segmented to show the aorta and location of the coarctation (black arrow), coronary arteries, left subclavian artery (white arrow) with ostial stenosis (yellow dot), and left carotid artery to descending aorta graft (white arrowhead). The length and diameter of the coarctation, distance from aortic arch branch vessels, and diameter of the proximal and distal aortic segments were measured on CTA images prior to the procedure. (b) A Palmaz XL 3110 stent (Johnson and Johnson, New Brunswick, NJ) was placed across the coarctation using fluoroscopy with CT overlay guidance. After registration of the CT data to fluoroscopic images, the outline of the aorta, coronary arteries, and left carotid artery to descending aorta graft are placed on the fluoroscopy screen for guidance (red outlines). The ostium of the stenotic left subclavian artery is identified (yellow dot). A subclavian artery stent was placed after implantation of the aortic stent.

treatment to obtain detailed information regarding the size of the aorta, the length of coarctation, and the size and location of major vessels arising from the aortic arch. CT–fluoroscopy fusion can be used to guide stent implantation (Figure 8.17).

Conclusion

CT imaging is a powerful tool for planning and guidance of structural heart disease interventions due to its high-resolution images and 3-D visualization of cardiac structures. The software for CT–fluoroscopy fusion, such as HeartNavigator (Philips Healthcare, Best, Netherlands) or Innova 3D (GE Healthcare, Chalfont St. Giles, UK), represents a major advance in the guidance for structural heart disease interventions by combining 3-D data with 2-D fluoroscopy. We have provided a few examples of procedures utilizing CT–fluoroscopy fusion guidance, but fusion-imaging guidance may be used during almost any structural heart disease intervention. In addition to CTA, fusion imaging using MRI or echocardiography is also possible. Though there is limited clinical experience with CT–fluoroscopy fusion

imaging at this time, this technology has great potential to increase procedural success and safety as fusion-imaging techniques become more widely adopted.

References

1. Radon J. Uber die bestimmung von funktionen durch ihre integralwerte langs gewisser manningfaltigkeiten. *Bu Succss Akad Wiss* 1917;69:262.
2. Oldendorf WH. Isolated flying spot detection of radio-density discontinuities displaying the internal structural pattern of a complex object. *IRE Trans Bio-Med Elect BME* 1961;8:68.
3. Hounsfield GN. Computed medical imaging: Nobel Lecture, December 8, 1979. *J Comput Assist Tomogr* 1980;4:665.
4. Hounsfield GN. Computerized transverse axial scanning (tomography): I. Description of system. *Br J Radiol* 1973;46:1016.
5. Hounsfield GN. Picture quality of computed tomography. *Am J Radiol* 1976;127:3.
6. Boyd D. Computerized transmission tomography of the heart using scanning electron beams. In Higgins CB, Ed. *CT of Heart and the Great Vessels: Experimental Evaluation in the Clinical Application.* New York: Futura; 1983.
7. Kalender WA, Seissler W, Klotz E, et al. Spiral volumetric CT with single-breath-hold technique, continuous transport, and continuous scanner rotation. *Radiology* 1990;176:181.

8. Kalender WA, Polacin A. Physical performance characteristics of spiral CT scanning. *Med Phys* 1991;18:910.

9. Crawford CR, King KF. Computed tomography scanning with simultaneous patient translation. *Med Phys* 1990;17:967.

10. Bae KT. Optimization of contrast enhancement in thoracic MDCT. *Radiol Clin North Am* 2010;48:9–29.

11. Lu JG, LV B, Chen XB et al. What is the best contrast injection protocol for 64-row multi-detector cardiac computed tomography? *Eur J Radiol* 2010;75:159–65.

12. Calhoun PS, Kuszyk BS, Health DG et al. Three-dimensional volume rendering of spiral CT data: Theory and method. *Radiographics* 1999;19:745–64.

13. Johnson PT, Fishman EK. Postprocessing techniques for cardiac computed tomographic angiography. *Radiol Clin North Am* 2010;48:687–700.

14. Delgado V, van der Kley F, Schalij MJ et al. Optimal imaging for planning and guiding interventions in structural heart disease: A multimodality imaging approach. *Eur Heart J Suppl* 2010;12:E10–E23.

15. Auricchio A, Sorgente A, Soubelet E et al. Accuracy and usefulness of fusion imaging between three-dimensional coronary sinus and coronary veins computed tomographic images with projection images obtained using fluoroscopy. *Europace* 2009;11:1483–90.

16. Duckett SG, Ginks MR, Knowles BR. Advanced image fusion to overlay coronary sinus anatomy with real-time fluoroscopy to facilitate left ventricular lead implantation in CRT. *Pacing Clin Electrophysiol* 2011;34:226–34.

17. Leipsic J, Gurvitch R, Labounty TM et al. Multidetector computed tomography in transcatheter aortic valve implantation. *JACC Cardiovasc Imaging* 2011;4:416–29.

18. Gurvitch R, Webb JG, Yuan R et al. Aortic annulus diameter determination by multidetector computed tomography: Reproducibility, applicability, and implications for transcatheter aortic valve implantation. *JACC Cardiovasc Interv* 2011;4:1235–45.

19. McElhinney DB, Hellenbrand WE, Zahn EM et al. Short- and medium-term outcomes after trancatheter pulmonary valve placement in the expanded multicenter US melody valve trial. *Circulation* 2010;122:507–16.

20. Fountain RB, Holmes DR, Chandrasekaran K et al. The PROTECT AF (WATCHMAN left atrial appendage system for embolic protection in patients with atrial fibrillation) Trial. *Am Heart J* 2006;151:956–96.

21. Holmes DR, Reddy VY, Turi ZG et al. Percutaneous closure of the left atrial appendage versus warfarin therapy for prevention of stroke in patients with atrial fibrillation: A randomised non-inferiority trial. *Lancet* 2009;374:534–42.

22. Bartus K, Han FT, BednarekJ et al. Percutaneous left atrial appendage suture ligation using the LARIAT device in patients with atrial fibrillation: Initial clinical experience. *J Am Coll Cardiol* 2012;62(2):108–18.

23. Kliger C, Eiros R, Isasti G et al. Review of surgical prosthetic paravalvular leaks: Diagnosis and catheter-based closure. *Eur Heart J* 2012;34(9):638–49.

24. Ball W, Ivanov J, Rakowski H et al. Long-term survival in patients with resting obstructive hypertrophic cardiomyopathy: Comparison of conservative versus invasive treatment. *J Am Coll Cardiol* 2011;22:2313–21.

25. Vlodaver Z, Coe JI, Edwards JE. True and false left ventricular aneurysms. Propensity for the latter to rupture. *Circulation* 1975;3:567–72.

26. Forbes TJ, Kim DW, Du W et al. Comparison of surgical, stent, and balloon angioplasty treatment of native coarctation of the aorta: An observational study by the CCISC. *J Am Coll Cardiol* 2011;58:2664–74.

27. Warnes CA, Williams RG, Bashore TM et al. ACC/AHA 2008 Guidelines for the Management of Adults with Congenital Heart Disease: A report of the American College of Cardiology/American Heart Association Task Force on Practice Guidelines. *Circulation* 2008;118:714–833.

28. Baumgartner H, Bonhoeffer P, De Groot NM et al. Task Force on the Management of Grown-up Congenital Heart Disease of the European Society of Cardiology (ESC). Guidelines for the management of grown-up congenital heart disease. The Task Force on the Management of Grown-up Congenital Heart Disease of the European Society of Cardiology (ESC) endorsed by the European Pediatric Cardiology (AEPC). *Eur Heart J* 2010;31:2915–7.

9

Ultrasound guidance

Jamie Bentham and Neil Wilson

Introduction

Increased access to portable high-resolution ultrasound will not convince a congenital and structural interventionist to change his or her practice and join the ever-increasing number of anesthetists, interventional radiologists, intensivists, and emergency room physicians who now use real-time ultrasound-guided vascular access as their first-line technique. What will prove convincing, however, is if it can be demonstrated that the technique is superior in certain circumstances and affords advantages over conventional techniques by providing additional information and reducing the risk of complications. This is the sole objective of this chapter.

Background

Complication rates for vascular access reach appreciable proportions (5–19%).[1–3] As interventional cardiologists, our confidence in our own abilities to obtain vascular access in a safe manner may be misplaced. What is unarguable is that any potential means of reducing complications of vascular access should be explored.[3]

From the literature it is evident that for some vessels at least a higher success rate for vascular access is achieved with real-time ultrasound guidance. For the purposes of this chapter, success needs to be carefully defined as the ability to secure an appropriately sized sheath into the correct position in the chosen vessel such that the intervention can be undertaken with the least amount of trauma or risk to the vessel. Complication rates increase with the number of attempts at vessel access, the vessel chosen, the size of the patient, and the size of the sheath. Some of these factors may be mitigated by technique while some are an inherent part of a given procedure. Ultrasound guidance serves only to offer a potential reduction in risks associated with vessel entry. While including ultrasound as part of an access technique will not remove much of the overall risk to vessels, its very real advantages nonetheless merit exploration. Important consideration must be given to the very real concept of training:

with the best teacher in the world, there will be a learning curve for junior operators that will carry the potential for multiple attempts, vessel perforation, and complications. We all acknowledge that trainees must be trained and anything to streamline and facilitate their achieving competence at vascular access can only be encouraged.

Technique

Like all techniques, ultrasound-guided access takes time to learn, has distinct advantages and disadvantages, and has its own particular pitfalls.

Many different ultrasound machines are available and some are inexpensive. Higher processing power undoubtedly offers improved image quality and is a worthwhile investment, although the costs are substantially greater. Higher-resolution linear probes (>7 MHz) with a small footprint are easiest to handle and provide the best-quality superficial imaging (<8 cm). Lower-frequency probes are rarely required even with femoral vessels in large adult patients. The preset functions for vascular access on the machine provide a useful starting point, but image optimization always improves the quality of the image obtained, even if only by adjusting gain and depth. Orientation of the probe is critical in understanding the relationship of the vessels viewed on the screen, but will vary depending on the position of the operator in relation to the patient. For example, for head and neck vessels, where the operator is usually superior to the patient, in short axis, the left side of the screen displays structures toward the patient's left side, whereas for femoral vessels, it is preferable to orientate the left side of the screen to display structures to the patient's right. Keeping structures beneath the left aspect of the probe on the left of the screen is an important rule to remember. Before placing the probe into position, it is essential to locate the expected position of the vessel based on surface landmarks (SLMs).

The short-axis view is the most informative for vessel interrogation and then subsequently for needle-guided vessel entry. The vessels appear as an echolucent structure

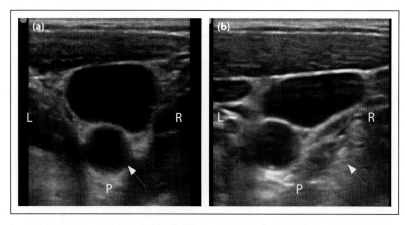

Figure 9.1   Preparation for right internal jugular vein ultrasound-guided access. The patient's head is turned to the left in (a) but is in a midline position in (b). The RIJV and right common carotid artery (arrow) are in an anterio-posterior orientation in (a), but in (b) the RIJV is brought lateral to the RCCA. This is a useful maneuver to reduce the risk of inadvertent RCCA puncture through the posterior wall of the RIJV. The RIJV size in (a) is accentuated with a Valsalva. The vein is compressible in (b). The arterial wall is thicker than the vein and pulsation would be evident on a moving image. Left, L; right, R; posterior, P.

and confirmation of the vessels' identity can be swiftly performed by combining anatomical appearance and location, compressibility, injection of agitated saline, or duplex scanning (color Doppler and 2D ultrasound combined, Figure 9.1). According to published studies, misidentification of the vessel is a common cause of unintentional arterial access. It is important to distinguish between arterial and venous pulsatility due to transmission from the adjacent artery or from respiratory variation. Overreliance on vessel pulsatility is unwise in cardiac patients given the potential absence of such in cases of coarctation of aorta, aortic stenosis, and in patients on ventricular assist or cardiopulmonary bypass. Likewise, venous pulsation in patients with serious right heart compromise with tricuspid regurgitation can be confounding.

One pitfall for ultrasound-guided vascular access is the potential for inadvertent entry into a vessel at a point either too distal or too proximal. Strict adherence to SLMs alongside ultrasound-guided access affords the best approach by combining the safety of established SLM-based techniques developed to avoid vital structures with the added advantage of real-time imaging of the needle as it enters the vessel with ultrasound. If the needle tip is not followed with ultrasound, there is potential for inadvertent vessel entry or damage to surrounding structures as the needle enters spaces not intended to be accessed with an increased risk of harm. The technique is thus strictly complementary and the usual principles of central venous and arterial access need to be stringently adhered to.

The usual preparation of the patient for catheterization is followed by asking an assistant to help sheath the ultrasound probe inside a sterile cover containing sterile ultrasound gel. The operator then applies additional sterile ultrasound gel to the outside of the sheathed probe for acoustic contact with the skin. Having located the vessel

for entry and confirmed the SLM, align the target vessel in the center of the screen in short axis (Figure 9.1). The distance of the vessel from the skin as well as the size of the vessel can be measured if required and is occasionally of use if large sheaths are to be introduced through small vessels, for example, in stenting coarctation of the aorta. Long-axis orientation is useful for visualizing vessel entry and with practice it becomes second nature to manipulate the probe between the different axes. The advantage of using long-axis imaging is that short axis, although easier to use initially, fails to give information about the needle trajectory, including the depth of insertion of the needle. It is important that the needle is advanced only as the tip is visualized (Figure 9.2). This often requires moving the probe over the needle closer to the site of skin entry and is facilitated by changing from a short axis to a long axis. On approaching the vessel, the needle is initially seen to indent the vessel before the vessel is entered (Figure 9.2). Learning the feel of the needle entering the vessel, aspirating as one advances, and using a bare needle with an arterial puncture are all useful methods of avoiding puncturing the posterior wall of the vessel (Figure 9.1). Although occasionally difficult to avoid in small pediatric patients, transfixing vessels in this manner is likely to be associated with a higher rate of vascular complications as the posterior puncture site undoubtedly continues to bleed and form a hematoma. Correct position of the wire advanced through the introduced needle should be confirmed in the usual way before placing a sheath.

Ultrasound affords additional advantage when difficult vascular access is likely. These situations are frequently encountered in congenital practice and include occluded vessels (Figure 9.3), multiple previous catheters or cardiac surgery, prolonged intensive care stay, body habitus, coagulopathy, hypovolemia or hemodynamic instability, and poor tolerance of the supine position.

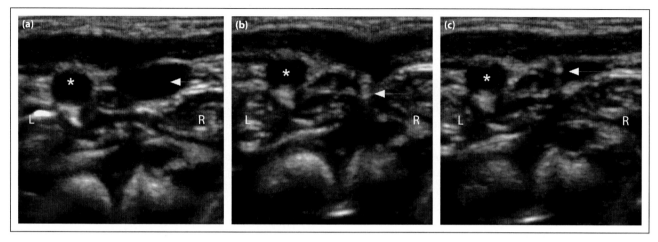

Figure 9.2   Right internal jugular vein ultrasound-guided access in a neonate. (a) The RCCA (*) is well separated from the RIJV (arrow). (b) The needle (arrow) s seen to compress the vein such that the anterior wall almost meets the posterior wall. It is clearly evident how the vessel is easily transfixed and the artery entered should the relationship of the vessels be similar to Figure 9.1a. (c) The needle can be facilitated to enter the vessel by approaching the vessel wall at a steep angle. The end of the needle is seen in the vessel before the guide wire is introduced (arrow). Left, L; right, R.

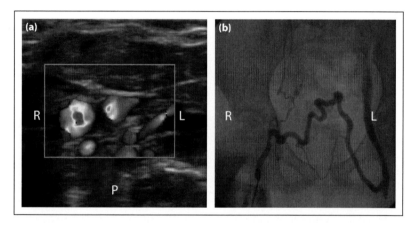

Figure 9.3   (**See color insert.**) Right femoral vein cannulation. (a) Color Doppler is useful for confirming arterial and venous flow and can facilitate access. (b) Ultrasound-guided access often allows access to smaller vessels, although these may not be useful in securing a sheath for intervention as demonstrated here, where an angiogram through the access needle demonstrates right femoral vein occlusion. The left femoral vein appears patent.

Before any complex interventional procedure, consideration should be given to the approaches available to improve the likelihood of success.

Vascular access

Internal jugular vein, subclavian vein, and common carotid arterial access

The internal jugular (IJ) vein usually runs lateral to the carotid artery within the carotid sheath with the vagus nerve and deep to the sternocleidomastoid muscle (SCM). In almost one quarter of patients, however, the IJ vein lies anterior or medial to the carotid artery (5%).[4] This proportion increases markedly with the rotation of the head

and neck toward the contralateral side (Figure 9.1). Using SLMs, IJ vessel entry is at the point of Sedillot's triangle (made of the sternal and clavicular heads of the SCM medially and laterally and the clavicle inferiorly) with the needle directed toward the ipsilateral nipple. It will not be surprising to find reported central line placement failure rates and complications with an SLM approach to be similar to the rates of the variation in the anatomy (around 5% failure to enter the IJ and 5% for inadvertent arterial puncture). The superiority of ultrasound in locating the vessel arrangement in the neck and the demonstration of a reduction in complication rates has resulted in European and American expert guidance in favor of the technique.[5,6] The studies on which this guidance is based demonstrate a small improvement in overall success of real-time ultrasound-guided access versus SLM approach, but more importantly there was a significant reduction, both in time to cannulation and in the number of attempts required.[2,7]

Ultrasound is occasionally used for entering the subclavian vein by a supraclavicular approach, but is used infrequently for an infraclavicular approach because of the intense reflection of ultrasound from the clavicle generating an acoustic shadow beneath. The subclavian vein follows a more consistent route than the IJ vein with the most common approach being the point of needle insertion just inferior to the junction of the middle and medial third of the clavicle at the deltopectoral groove. Inadvertent ultrasound-guided, steep needle-angle approaches may cause an inexperienced operator to puncture the pleura. The needle should be directed toward the sternal notch in the coronal plane with the needle entering the skin at a very low angle to the chest wall if ultrasound is used. This is difficult to visualize with ultrasound and probably does not assist with the technique.

Common carotid artery access is infrequently performed, but remains an important option for neonatal aortic valvuloplasty as it affords the most direct approach to the aortic valve. Although some perform an arterial cutdown, we access the carotid artery using ultrasound guidance similar to the approach to access the IJ vein. The difficulties encountered relate to the mobility of the vessel in the neck and the angle of approach is often disconcertingly steep as a consequence. In view of the small distance to the aortic valve using this approach, great care needs to be made when placing the arterial sheath as the dilator will typically advance too far and need withdrawing in a small neonate. For this reason, we recommend the use of the shortest available sheath/dilator configuration. The ease this approach affords to what can occasionally be a difficult procedure offsets, to some extent as yet unrealized, concerns about the integrity of the carotid artery following the procedure.

Femoral venous and arterial access

The common femoral artery and vein lie within the femoral triangle bordered superiorly by the inguinal ligament, medially by the adductor longus muscle, and laterally by the sartorius muscle. The vein usually lies medial to the artery although it may lie posterior to the artery, particularly in children (36–45% depending on leg posture). When attempting cannulation further distal to the inguinal ligament, this relationship is less consistent (Figure 9.3). The artery lies at the midpoint of the inguinal ligament (between the anterior superior iliac spine and the pubic tubercle). SLM femoral access for cardiac catheterization is the most frequently adopted approach for the congenital interventional cardiologist and arguably there is little to be gained from introducing a new procedure into a time-pressured laboratory schedule. When compared with ultrasound-guided IJ venous access, the evidence

is less well documented, but this may simply reflect the infrequent practice of this technique. Evidence in favor of reduction in the number of attempts, reduced time for vessel access, and reduced inadvertent vessel access can be found.[8] An increased overall vessel access rate is unlikely to be realized in experienced hands.[9] There is a suggestion of an associated reduction in vascular complication rates.[9] For femoral access requiring a large sheath, such as placement of a stent for coarctation of aorta, ultrasound-guided access allows targeting of the common femoral artery above its bifurcation, accessing the largest vessel possible while staying below the inguinal ligament.

Transhepatic venous access

Increasing familiarity with transhepatic venous access in interventional practice has opened up another avenue for vascular access in circumstances where an inferior approach to the atria is preferred (e.g., atrial septal defect closure and patent ductus arteriosus closure) and conventional approaches are not an option, as in patients with bilateral femoral vein or inferior caval vein occlusion, or those with an anatomically interrupted inferior caval vein ascending above the diaphragm as an azygos continuation. Fluoroscopic guidance and ultrasound guidance are used together to facilitate access to a hepatic rather than a portal vein (Figure 9.4). Our preference is to adopt an approach midway between the xiphisternum and the right midaxillary line, directing the needle toward the right atrium beginning immediately underneath the costal margin. Some prefer a more lateral approach using a longer needle. Using a combination of duplex ultrasound to facilitate needle guidance toward a vein ascending in the direction of the right atrium, we also have fluoroscopy in place and a syringe with contrast attached to the needle (Figure 9.4). Once a vessel is entered, it is straightforward to put down the ultrasound probe, gently aspirate, and then inject to ensure that the hepatic vein is of sufficient caliber and a straight enough course to accommodate a sheath and catheter.

Ultrasound-guided pericardiocentesis

Once the technique of ultrasound guidance of vascular access has been mastered, it becomes second nature to employ ultrasound to facilitate pericardial access in a similar way to transhepatic access as discussed above. For large collections, particularly in adults, this will be largely redundant and urgency may necessitate more immediate action. However, for pediatric cases, pericardiocentesis can occasionally prove more difficult and ultrasound guidance here has its uses. From a subxiphoid approach angling toward the tip of the left scapula, an apical collection is easily accessed. Collections behind the left ventricle will require a more left lateral approach and collections in front of the right ventricle while beginning subxiphoid will

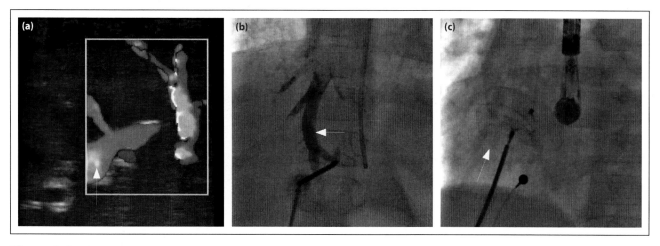

Figure 9.4   **(See color insert.)** Transhepatic access for atrial septal defect closure in a patient with left atrial isomerism and interrupted inferior caval vein with azygous continuation. (a) Ultrasound is useful for identifying large hepatic venous vessels with a direct path toward the right atrium. (b) A hand angiogram through the needle is still performed to confirm flow toward the right atrium and that the vein is of sufficient caliber for the final sheath size intended (arrow). (c) Here, access has been secured and an 8 French sheath used to close a large atrial septal defect (arrow, Amplatz septal occluder). This procedure would have been difficult from either an internal jugular or subclavian vein approach.

require a deceptively anterior approach. The needle can be directly targeted at the largest pocket of fluid and the tip of the needle visualized to enter the pericardial collection.

Conclusions

Introduction of ultrasound-guided vascular access into interventional practice is gaining in popularity. It affords advantages that are likely to result in reduced vascular complications. Understanding the technique and the common pitfalls and following this with an investment of time in perfecting the technique will improve the accuracy and speed of vascular access in many different situations as well as give useful additional information to guide large sheath placement and choice of vascular approach in complex procedures.

References

1.   McGee DC, Gould MK. Preventing complications of central venous catheterization. *New Engl J Med* 2003;348:1123–33.

2.   Hind D, Calvert N, McWilliams R et al. Ultrasonic locating devices for central venous cannulation: Meta-analysis. *BMJ* 2003;327:361.

3.   Bergersen L, Marshall A, Gauvreau K et al. Adverse event rates in congenital cardiac catheterization—A multi-center experience. *Catheter Cardiovasc Interv* 2010;75:389–400.

4.   Denys BG, Uretsky BF. Anatomical variations of internal jugular vein location: Impact on central venous access. *Crit Care Med* 1991;19:1516–9.

5.   Troianos CA, Hartman GS, Glas KE et al. Guidelines for performing ultrasound guided vascular cannulation: Recommendations of the American Society of Echocardiography and the Society of Cardiovascular Anesthesiologists. *J Am Soc Echocardiogr* 2011;24:1291–318.

6.   Grebenik CR, Boyce A, Sinclair ME, Evans RD, Mason DG, Martin B. NICE guidelines for central venous catheterization in children. Is the evidence base sufficient? *Br J Anaesth* 2004;92:827–30.

7.   Troianos CA, Jobes DR, Ellison N. Ultrasound-guided cannulation of the internal jugular vein. A prospective, randomized study. *Anesth Analg* 1991;72:823–6.

8.   Seto AH, Abu-Fadel MS, Sparling JM et al. Real-time ultrasound guidance facilitates femoral arterial access and reduces vascular complications: FAUST (Femoral Arterial Access with Ultrasound Trial). *JACC Cardiovasc Interv* 2010;3:751–8.

9.   Iwashima S, Ishikawa T, Ohzeki T. Ultrasound-guided versus landmark-guided femoral vein access in pediatric cardiac catheterization. *Pediatr Cardiol* 2008;29:339–42.

10

Percutaneous transfemoral access with big sheaths

Noa Holoshitz and Ziyad M. Hijazi

Introduction

Cardiac catheterization is based on the notion that the heart can be accessed through the peripheral vasculature without the need for a "surgical" incision. This, however, means that vascular puncture and closure are performed without direct visualization of the blood vessel and this can lead to complications. The most common complications of any type of cardiac catheterization procedure are access site related.[1,2] Nowhere is this more important than when considering vascular access with large sheaths. In today's age of transcatheter valve implantation, percutaneous access with large sheaths in both the femoral artery and femoral vein has become common practice.[3–7] It is the standard in some institutions to continue to perform a surgical "cutdown" to access the femoral arteries for large sheath insertion for certain procedures such as transcatheter aortic valve replacement (TAVR). However, the authors' experience along with multiple clinical reports have shown that in most patients, large sheaths may be inserted into either the femoral vessels for TAVR or other procedures through a percutaneous approach safely, if a few precautions are taken.[8–14] In this chapter, we will briefly review the procedures that require large sheath insertion as well as techniques for obtaining access and percutaneous closure for large sheaths.

Historical perspective

Cardiac catheterization was initially performed in humans in 1929[15] and was adapted as a diagnostic tool in the 1940s and the 1950s in all types of cardiac physiology. Initially, all procedures were done through a surgical cutdown approach to the brachial vessels as pioneered by Sones and Shiley.[16] However, in 1953, Seldinger proposed a novel percutaneous approach to access the femoral vessels without the need of a surgical incision.[17] The Seldinger technique, which is how it has become widely known, was adopted in the cardiac

catheterization lab in the 1970s and is now used for essentially every diagnostic and interventional catheterization procedure. Historically, diagnostic and interventional cardiac catheterizations were performed using a 6–8 Fr sheath. With the development of interventional procedures in structural and congenital heart disease, larger sheaths were required for device implantation. As sheath size requirements have increased, so has the potential for vascular complications. Therefore, much focus has been placed on developing methods for smooth insertion of large-bore femoral sheaths and obtaining adequate closure postprocedure.

Procedures requiring large sheaths

Venous

To this day, many procedures in structural and congenital interventions require a large femoral venous sheath. In fact, the major limitation of the original congenital cardiac intervention, the atrial septal defect (ASD) closure performed by King and Mills in 1976,[18] was the very large delivery system it required (22–24 Fr). Therefore, structural and congenital interventionalists have become very comfortable obtaining large femoral venous access, even in young children. Luckily, the femoral veins are very forgiving and have the ability to be stretched and therefore the potential for complication is less than in the arterial system. In current practice, ASD closure using an Amplatzer Septal Occluder (St. Jude Medical, St. Paul, MN) can be performed using anywhere from a 6 Fr venous sheath for the smallest device (4 mm) to a 12 Fr sheath for the largest device (38 mm). Other procedures that may require a large venous sheath include left atrial appendage occlusion using the WATCHMAN (Boston Scientific, Natick, MA) or Amplatzer Cardiac Plug (St. Jude Medical) (12–14 Fr). Perhaps some of the most exciting procedures in structural and congenital interventions are the ones that require the largest sheaths. Transcatheter pulmonic valve replacement (TPVR) has been performed since 2000 with the Melody valve (Medtronic, Minneapolis, MN) or, more recently, the SAPIEN valve (Edwards Lifesciences, Irvine, CA). The Melody Ensemble Delivery System (Medtronic) is available in 18, 20, and 22 mm diameter sizes, and is implanted through a 22 Fr venous sheath. The Edwards SAPIEN valve is available for use in the pulmonic position through the COMPASSION trial[19] in 23 or 26 mm size and is implanted through a 22 or 24 Fr sheath, respectively, in the femoral vein. The MitraClip (Abbott Laboratories, Abbott Park, IL) system for the reduction of mitral regurgitation continues to undergo clinical trials in the United States; however, it is approved for use in Europe. It requires an initial transseptal puncture with the appropriately sized sheath followed by delivery of the clip through a 24 Fr venous sheath. In both the US Melody valve trial and the COMPASSION trial, there were no reports of vascular complications.[19,20]

Arterial

Large percutaneous arterial access is more complicated than venous access because of the potential for serious complications. Again, as with large venous sheaths, structural and congenital interventionalists have been at the forefront of procedures requiring large arterial sheaths. The first ballooning of the aortic valve and aortic coarctation occurred in the mid-1980s and required 12–14 Fr arterial sheaths. This was followed by stenting of aortic coarctation in 1989, which required up to a 12 Fr sheath. Of course, the procedure that has gained the most attention for its large arterial sheath requirement is TAVR, which was first performed in 2002. As TAVR has become more widely used, a lot of work has gone into making the large femoral artery access and hemostasis safer. Although some centers still use surgical cutdown to obtain arterial access for TAVR, we believe that it can be performed safely percutaneously and we will review our techniques in the next section. The current TAVR valve systems include the SAPIEN valve, which is available commercially in the 23 and 26 mm sizes (which require a 22 Fr and 24 Fr arterial sheath, respectively), the SAPIEN XT valve, which is available commercially in Europe and through the PARTNER II trial in the United States in 23, 26, and 29 mm sizes (requiring a 18, 19, and 20 Fr Sheath, respectively), and the Medtronic CoreValve, which is available in the United States through the clinical trial and is available in 23, 26, and 29 mm sizes and requires an 18 Fr arterial sheath. In the PARTNER trial, the rate of major vascular complications was 16.2% in the inoperable arm of the trial and 11% in the high-risk arm.[21,22] There have been a lot of advances in new valve technology with one of the main emphasis points being miniaturization of the valve delivery system in an effort to reduce vascular complications.

Obtaining access with large sheaths

Finding the "landing zone"

The most important step in obtaining arterial access with a large-caliber sheath is to ensure that the puncture site is in the common femoral artery (CFA). The ideal level of access is the mid-CFA, approximately 1–2 cm below the inguinal ligament (Figure 10.1). If the puncture is too low, the profunda femoris artery (PFA) or the superficial femoral artery (SFA) may be entered, which can lead to local complications such as vessel laceration, pseudoaneurysm, arteriovenous fistula, thrombosis, or excessive bleeding.[23–30] In addition, the larger the sheath-to-artery size ratio, the greater the risk of vascular obstruction and failure of closure. The SFA and PFA both taper as they branch from the CFA and therefore are not ideal for placement of larger sheaths. However, if the arterial puncture is too high, the external iliac artery (EIA) may be entered, which may significantly increase the risk of a retroperitoneal bleed (RPB). Even in routine percutaneous coronary interventions, which typically utilize sheaths in the 6 Fr range, there may be an 18-fold increase of RPB in the setting of high arterial puncture.[30]

We routinely use a combination of fluoroscopy and angiography using a 5 Fr sheath from the contralateral vessel to ensure that our large-caliber sheath access is in the desirable location; above the CFA bifurcation and below the inferior epigastric artery, approximately at the middle third of the common femoral head (Figure 10.1). Although trials conducted have not shown any evidence to support the routine use of fluoroscopy to reduce femoral artery access site complications,[31–33] the studies did not utilize concomitant angiography and used a traditional 18-gauge needle as opposed to a micropuncture needle to obtain access.

Prior to performing a procedure that requires a large-caliber arterial sheath such as TAVR, we fully evaluate the femoral vessels by both angiography and CT angiogram to make sure that the vessels will accommodate the large sheath. We typically look for approximately 7 mm vessels for a 22 Fr sheath and approximately 8 mm vessels for a 24 Fr sheath. It is also important to evaluate the amount of tortuosity and calcification of the ileo-femoral arteries, which is best done by CT angiogram (Figure 10.2).[34,35] A vessel with very little calcification may accommodate a large sheath even if the diameter is borderline, while a heavily calcified vessel will not.

Contralateral access

After assessing the femoral vessels, we typically start our procedures obtaining access on the contralateral side using a 5 Fr sheath. We use a micropuncture needle for all of our access and use fluoroscopy to direct the needle to the middle third of the femoral head. Once we have arterial blood return from the needle, we advance a 0.018" wire through

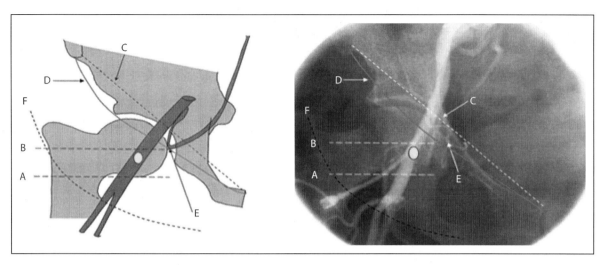

Figure 10.1   (**See color insert.**) "Landing zone" for the placement of percutaneous femoral sheaths. (a) Lower margin of the femoral head. (b) Center point of the femoral head. (c) Line connecting the anterior superior iliac crest and symphysis pubis for approximation of inguinal ligament location. (d) Actual inguinal ligament location. (e) Point where the inferior epigastric artery descends below the inguinal ligament before turning cranial. (f) Inguinal crease. Yellow circle is the target for needle entry into common femoral artery. (Courtesy of Dr. Zultan Turi. With permission.)

the needle and insert a 4 Fr micropuncture dilator and sheath over the wire. At this point it is possible to perform an angiogram through the small sheath to ensure proper sheath position prior to insertion of a 5 or 6 Fr sheath. This contralateral sheath will then be used as a guide in obtaining access on the opposite side as well as for closure using the "crossover" technique,[36–38] which will be discussed later in the chapter.

Placement of large sheath

Once the contralateral sheath is in place and correct placement has been verified by angiogram, a pigtail catheter is advanced into the abdominal aorta, just above the level of the iliac bifurcation. Using 20–30 mL of dye, an aorta angiogram is performed with focus on the common femoral artery on the side where the large sheath will be placed (Figure 10.3a). This angiogram will show the operator exactly where the femoral artery bifurcation is and where the inferior epigastric artery takes off, so that the appropriate landing zone can be defined. If the camera is not moved, it is possible to do an image overlay at this point in order to perform fluoroscopy directed access with a micropuncture needle. The same technique described above is used to obtain access with the micropuncture needle and like with the initial sheath insertion, once the 4 Fr micropuncture

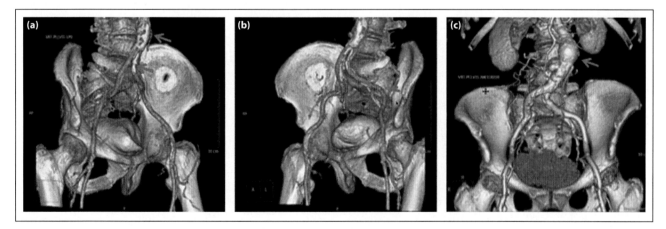

Figure 10.2   (**See color insert.**) Three-dimensional reconstruction of CT angiogram for the evaluation of ileo-femoral arteries. (a) RAO projection demonstrating moderate calcification of the abdominal aorta and iliac bifurcation (large arrows) as well as mild calcification and narrowing of the left common femoral artery (small arrow). (b) LAO projection of the same patient demonstrating moderate tortuousity (arrowheads), which was not as well appreciated on the RAO view. (c) An AP projection of a patient with moderate abdominal aorta calcification and aneurysm (arrow).

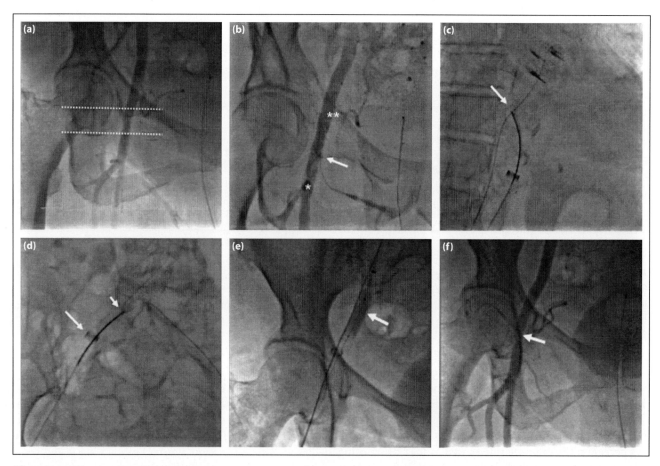

Figure 10.3 Stepwise approach for crossover technique by fluoroscopy. (a) Angiogram of the right common femoral artery being performed through the contralateral side demonstrating the ideal landing zone (between dashed lines). (b) Angiogram through the micropuncture sheath (arrow) demonstrating good position above the femoral bifurcation (*) and below the interior epigastric artery (**). (c) A snare inserted through the large sheath in the right groin is used to capture a wire that was inserted through the left groin (arrow). (d) The large sheath is retracted (large arrow) and the snare pulls the wire from the left groin into the right common iliac artery (small arrow), thereby creating an arterial bridge. The wire will be externalized through the large sheath. (e) A small balloon is inflated to low atmospheres in the right external iliac artery in order to occlude blood flow while the sheath is removed and the ProGlide sutures are tightened. A final angiogram (f) shows no evidence of dye extravasation or dissection. There is a slight narrowing (arrow) at the location of the ProGlide sutures.

sheath is in place, we confirm correct placement with an angiogram (Figure 10.3b).

After the location of the sheath has been verified by angiography, we turn our attention to "preclosure" of the vessel. The preclosure technique has been described extensively for use with large arterial and venous sheaths.[9–12,39] Two ProGlide sutures are preloaded over an 0.035″ wire through the margins of the arteriotomy before predilatation and access-site sheath insertion. They are deployed in the 10 o'clock and 2 o'clock positions and are left outside the body for closure at the end of the procedure (Figure 10.4). Then, over the same 0.035″ wire, the large arterial sheath can now be inserted with serial dilations under fluoroscopic guidance to ensure a smooth insertion.

Another approach for obtaining large-caliber arterial access is by the use of ultrasound guidance,[40–43] which has been shown to have results that are comparable or perhaps

superior to the technique we described. The technique visualizes the femoral bifurcation as well as the needle entry into the vessel for accurate placement. Ultrasound is commonly used by interventional radiologists; however, cardiologists typically feel more comfortable using fluoroscopy. Although several ultrasound systems have been developed for the purpose of obtaining femoral access, most catheterization laboratories do not have dedicated ultrasound vascular access guidance systems, whereas fluoroscopy utilizes technology and methods that are uniformly available.

It is important to note that especially in the world of congenital interventional cardiology, large sheaths may be used in the venous circulation as opposed to arterial circulation. As previously mentioned, the procedures that require the largest venous sheaths are the TPVRs. Because the risk of serious bleeding is so much less with venous access, we do not usually use the contralateral side to guide

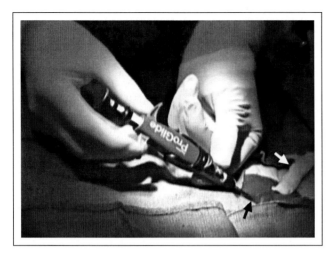

Figure 10.4   Preclosure of femoral artery with two ProGlide sutures. ProGlide sutures being deployed in the 2 o'clock position (black arrow). The first set of sutures have already been deployed in the 10 o'clock position and are wrapped in gauze (white arrow).

us. However, it is important to use fluoroscopic landmarks and slowly advance the large sheath under fluoroscopy to prevent any damage to the vessel. It is also important to periodically ensure that the wire over which the sheath and dilators are being inserted is free, in order to prevent kinking of the wire.

Hemostasis

For arterial access, "preclosure" with two ProGlide sutures is probably the most commonly used method to achieve hemostasis when a large sheath is involved. We routinely use this for our TAVR procedures as well as for smaller "large" sheaths such as for coarctation stenting. In conjunction to preclosure, we use the crossover technique to achieve proximal balloon tamponade of the vessel during sheath removal.[36,37]

The first step in the crossover technique involves retraction of the large-caliber sheath from the aorta into the common iliac artery with injection of contrast to ensure ostial iliac patency with no dissection. A soft wire such a 0.035" Terumo exchange length GlideWire (Terumo Corporation, Somerset, NJ) then needs to be passed from the contralateral vessel into the main vessel and externalized through the large sheath creating an "arterial bridge." Some operators propose using an angled catheter such as an internal mammary or Judkins right to direct the soft wire from the contralateral side. We have found that passing a Goose Neck snare through the large sheath to capture the soft wire is an easy way to create this bridge (Figure 10.3c,d). Once the wire is externalized through the large sheath, a compliant balloon such as a 10–12 mm TYSHAK (NuMED, Hopkinton, NY) is

passed from the contralateral vessel and positioned in the ostial to proximal common iliac artery on the side of the large sheath (Figure 10.3e). The balloon is inflated gently to low atmosphere and the large sheath is withdrawn to the ileo-femoral junction. Contrast injection through the large sheath at this point will identify any perforation and demonstrate occlusion of blood flow by the balloon. When proximal hemostasis is achieved with the balloon, the large sheath is removed and the two ProGlide sutures are tightened. If there is still some oozing at this point, manual pressure may be applied. A final angiogram (Figure 10.3f) will confirm complete hemostasis and the absence of perforation or dissection. At this point if a perforation is suspected, a covered stent may be placed from the contralateral side since the sheath and wire are already in place. It is also important to work closely with a vascular surgeon who may perform a surgical cutdown as a bailout when hemostasis is not achieved. With the balloon inflated proximally to tamponade flow, the surgeon has the leisure of not rushing through the procedure, as there is less of a concern that the patient will become hemodynamically unstable from bleeding.

Alternate methods

Although the crossover technique with double preclosure is commonly used, there are other alternatives for obtaining hemostasis in the femoral artery. For example, the ProStarXL (Abbott Vascular) suture-mediated closure device is approved for closure up to 24 Fr sheaths and multiple studies have shown it to be safe and effective for closure of large arterial sheaths for TAVR and infrarenal and thoracic endovascular aneurysm repair (EVAR and TEVAR).[44] There have also been reports of using a single ProGlide suture to obtain hemostasis with "smaller" arterial sheaths used for the SAPIEN XT aortic valve (18 or 19 Fr sheaths).[45] The data seem to indicate that in this patient population, a single ProGlide suture placed at the beginning of the case is an effective and safe way for obtaining hemostasis. While it is usually the suture-mediated closure device that is used for obtaining hemostasis in large arterial sheaths, there was a small case study published from the University of Pennsylvania using one or two 8 Fr AngioSeal collagen-mediated closure device (St. Jude Medical) for closure of arteriotomies in the 9–12 Fr range for balloon aortic valvuloplasty.[46]

Venous hemostasis

When large sheaths are placed in the femoral veins, there may still be significant access site complications. However, given the nature of the venous circulation, bleeding is seldom as serious. Other complications that may occur include dissection or occlusion of the vein, as well as a deep venous thrombosis. There have been reports of using preclosure

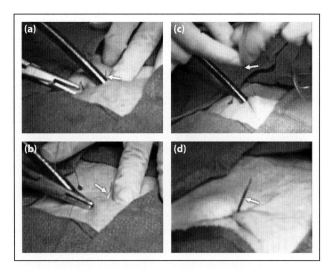

Figure 10.5   (**See color insert.**) Figure-of-eight suture. (a) The first stitch is placed distal to the sheath deep in the subcutaneous tissue (arrow). (b) The second stitch is placed just above the sheath, more superficially than the first one (arrow), thereby creating a figure-of-eight. (c) The fisherman's knot is tied (arrow) and the suture is tightened as the sheath is removed. (d) The final appearance of the stitch, which compresses the femoral vein underneath to achieve hemostasis.

with two Perclose ProGlide sutures in venous procedures requiring large sheaths such as transcatheter pulmonic valve implantation.[39] Suture-mediated closure devices have also been shown to be safe and effective in children requiring venous closure after large sheath implantation.[47] We, however, typically chose to use the figure-of-eight suture for hemostasis on the venous side. We have used the figure-of-eight suture successfully in venous sheaths up to 24 Fr. The details of this method of hemostasis have been described in multiple publications.[48,49] A 0-Vycril suture on a needle is used to make one deep stitch just distal to the sheath and one superficial stitch just proximal to the sheath, thereby creating a figure-of-eight (Figure 10.5a,b). A fisherman's knot is then tied (Figure 10.5c) and the knot is pushed down while the sheath is removed. The knot compresses the soft tissue and holds the pressure on the venous site (Figure 10.5d). We typically leave these sutures in overnight and remove them the next morning; however, some groups advocate leaving them in only for the 4 h duration of bed rest.[49]

Summary

In today's age of structural and congenital interventions, it is imperative that the interventionalist be comfortable in obtaining large-caliber access in both the femoral artery and vein. This may be performed safely by using a combination of angiography and fluoroscopy guided technique. Hemostasis is obtained using preclosure with a suture-mediated closure device for the artery and a figure-of-eight suture for the femoral vein. Studies have shown that these methods are comparable to surgical cutdown in the rates of vascular complications. Although there is much work on "miniaturization" of transcatheter valves, these procedures will most likely be more widespread in the future and therefore the skills described here will continue to be in use.

References

1. Tavakol M, Ashraf S, Brener SJ. Risks and complications of coronary angiography: A comprehensive review. *Glob J Health Sci* 2012;4(1):65–93.
2. Phillips BL Cabalka AK, Hagler DJ et al. Procedural complications during congenital cardiac catheterization. *Congenit Heart Dis* 2010;5:118–23.
3. Webb JG, Pasupati S, Humphries K et al. Percutaneous transarterial aortic valve replacement in selected high-risk patients with aortic stenosis. *Circulation* 2007;116:755–63.
4. Grube E, Schuler G, Buellesfeld L et al. Percutaneous aortic valve replacement for severe aortic stenosis in high-risk patients using the second- and current third-generation self-expanding CoreValve prosthesis: Device success and 30-day clinical outcome. *J Am Coll Cardiol* 2007;50:69–76.
5. Cribier A, Eltchaninoff H, Tron C et al. Treatment of calcific aortic stenosis with the percutaneous heart valve: Mid-term follow-up from the initial feasibility studies: The French experience. *J Am Coll Cardiol* 2006;47:1214–23.
6. Webb JG, Chandavimol M, Thompson CR et al. Percutaneous aortic valve implantation retrograde from the femoral artery. *Circulation* 2006;113:842–50.
7. Bonhoeffer P, Boudjemline Y, Saliba Z et al. Percutaneous replacement of pulmonary valve in a right-ventricle to pulmonary-artery prosthetic conduit with valve dysfunction. *Lancet* 2000;356:1403–5.
8. Solomon LW, Fusman B, Jolly N et al. Percutaneous suture closure for management of large French size arterial puncture in aortic valvuloplasty. *J Invasive Cardiol* 2001;13:592–6.
9. Feldman T. Femoral artery preclosure: Finishing a procedure before it begins. *Catheter Cardiovasc Interv* 2001;53:448.
10. Lee WA, Brown MP, Nelson PR et al. Total percutaneous access for endovascular aortic aneurysm repair ("Preclose" technique). *J Vasc Surg* 2007;45:1095–101.
11. Sharp, A, Michev, I, Maisano F et al. A new technique for vascular access management in transcatheter aortic valve implantation. *Catheter Cardiovasc Interv* 2010;75:784–93.
12. Badawi RA. Technique for hemostasis and closure after percutaneous aortic valve replacement. *Catheter Cardiovasc Interv* 2010 Mar 26. [Epub ahead of print].
13. Nakamura M, Chakravarty T, Jilaihawi H et al. Complete percutaneous approach for arterial access in transfemoral transcatheter aortic valve replacement—A comparison with surgical cutdown and closure. *Catheter Cardiovasc Interv* 2013 Jul 19 [Epub ahead of print].
14. Holper EM, Kim R, Mack M et al. Randomized trial of surgical cutdown versus percutaneous access in transfemoral TAVR. *Catheter Cardiovasc Interv* 2014;83(3):457–64.
15. Forssmann W. Die Sondierung des rechten Herzens. *Klin Wochenschr* 1929;8:2085.
16. Sones FM JR, Shiley EK, Proudfit WL, Westcott RM. Cinecoronary arteriograph. (abstr) *Circulation* 1959;20:773.
17. Seldinger SI. Catheter replacement of the needle in percutaneous arteriography: A new technique. *Acta Radiol* 1953;39:368.
18. King TD, Mills NL. Nonoperative closure of atrial septal defects. *Surgery* 1974;75:383–8.

19. Kenny D, Hijazi ZM, Kar S et al. Percutaneous implantation of the Edwards SAPIEN transcatheter heart valve for conduit failure in the pulmonary position: early phase 1 results from an international multicenter clinical trial. *J Am Coll Cardiol* 2011;58:2248–56.

20. Zahn EM, Hellenbrand WE, Lock JE, McElhinney DB. Implantation of the Melody transcatheter pulmonary valve in patients with a dysfunctional right ventricular outflow tract conduit. *J Am Coll Cardiol* 2009;54(18):1722–9.

21. Leon MD, Smith CR, Mack K et al. for the PARTNER Trial Investigators. Transcatheter aortic valve implantation for aortic stenosis in patients who cannot undergo surgery. *N Engl J Med* 2010;367:1957.

22. Smith CR, Leon MD, Mack MJ et al. For the PARTNER Trial Investigators. Transcatheter versus surgical aortic-valve replacement in high-risk patients. *N Engl J Med* 2011;364:2187.

23. Kahlert P, Al-Rashid F, Weber M et al. Vascular access site complications after percutaneous transfemoral aortic valve implantation. *Herz* 2009;34:398–408.

24. Bleiziffer S, Ruge H, Mazzitelli D et al. Survival after transapical and transfemoral aortic valve implantation: Talking about two different patient populations. *J Thorac Cardiovasc Surg* 2009;138:1073–80.

25. Belli AM, Cumberland DC, Knox AM et al. The complication rate of percutaneous peripheral balloon angioplasty. *Clin Radiol* 1990;41:380–3.

26. Kim D, Orron DE, Skillman JJ et al. Role of superficial femoral artery puncture in the development of pseudoanuerysm and arterio-venous fistula complicating percutaneous transfemoral cardiac catheterization. *Catheter Cardiovasc Diagn* 1992;25:91–7.

27. Noto TJ Jr, Vetrovec GW. Cardiac catheterization 1990: A report of the Registry of the Society for Cardiac Angiography and Interventions (SCAI). *Catheter Cardiovasc Diagn* 1991;24:75–83.

28. Rapoport S, Sniderman KW, Morse SS et al. Pseudoanuerysm: A complication of faulty technique in femoral arterial puncture. *Radiology* 1985;154:529–30.

29. Altin RS, Flicker S, Naidech HJ. Pseudoanuerysm and arterio-venous fistula after femoral artery catheterization: Association with low femoral punctures. *Am J Roentgenol* 1989;152:629–31.

30. Sherev DA, Shaw RE, Brent BN. Angiographic predictors of femoral access site complications: Implications for planned coronary percutaneous interventions. *Catheter Cardiovasc Interv* 2005;65:196–202.

31. Abu-Fadel MS, Sparling JM, Zacharias SJ et al. Fluoroscopy vs. traditional guided femoral arterial access and the use of closure devices: A randomized controlled trial. *Catheter Cardiovasc Interv* 2009;74:533–9.

32. Turi ZG. Fluoroscopy guided vascular access: Asking the right question, but getting the wrong answer? *Catheter Cardiovasc Interv* 2009;74:540–2.

33. Turi ZG. Optimizing vascular access: Routine femoral angiography keeps the vascular complication away. *Catheter Cardiovasc Interv* 2005;65(2):203–4.

34. Leipsic J, Gurvitch R, Labounty TM et al. Multidetector computed tomography in transcatheter aortic valve implantation. *J Am Coll Cardiol Cardiovasc Imaging* 2011;4(4):416–29.

35. Apfaltrer P, Henzler T, Blanke P, Krazinski AW, Silverman JR, Schoepf UJ. Computed tomography for planning transcatheter aortic valve replacement. *J Thorac Imaging* 2013;28(4):231–9.

36. Sharp ASP, Michev I, Maisano F et al. A new technique for vascular access management in transcatheter aortic valve implantation. *Catheter Cardiovasc Interv* 2010; 75:784–93.

37. Genereux P, Webb J, Svenson L et al. Vascular complications after transcatheter aortic valve replacement. Insights from the PARTNER trial. *J Am Coll Cardiol* 2012;60:1043–52.

38. Buchanan GL, Chieffo A, Montorfano M et al. A "modified crossover technique" for vascular access management in high-risk patients undergoing transfemoral transcatheter aortic valve implantation. *Catheter Cardiovasc Interv* 2013;81:579–83.

39. Hamid T, Rajagopal R, Pius C et al. Preclosure of large-sized venous access sites in adults undergoing transcatheter structural interventions. *Catheter Cardiovasc Interv* 2013;81:586–90.

40. Arthurs ZM, Starnes BW, Sohn VY et al. Ultrasound-guided access improves rate of access-related complications for totally percutaneous aortic aneurysm repair. *Ann Vasc Surg* 2009;22:736–41.

41. Pitta S, Prasad A, Rihal C et al. Feasibility and efficacy of ultrasound-guided femoral artery access. *Catheter Cardiovasc Interv* 2010;75:S47–162.

42. Seto AH, Abu-Fadel MS, Sparling JM et al. Real-time ultrasound guidance facilitates femoral arterial access and reduces vascular complications: FAUST (Femoral arterial Access with UltraSound Trial). *J Am Coll Cardiol Cardiovasc Interv* 2010;3:751–8.

43. Gedikoglu M, Oguzkurt L, Gur S, Andic C, Sariturk C, Ozkan U. Comparison of ultrasound guidance with the traditional palpation and fluoroscopy method for the common femoral artery puncture. *Catheter Cardiovasc Interv* 2013;82(7):1187–92.

44. Thomas C, Steger V, Heller S et al. Safety and efficacy of the Prostar XL vascular closure device for percutaneous closure of large arterial access sites. *Radiol Res Practice* 2013;2013:875484.

45. Kahlert P, Al-Rashid F, Plicht B et al. Suture mediated arterial access site closure after transfemoral aortic valve implantation. *Catheter Cardiovasc Interv* 2013;81:E139–50.

46. Bui QT, Kolansky DM, Bannan A et al. "Double wire" angio-seal closure technique after balloon aortic valvuloplasty. *Catheter Cardiovasc Interv* 2010;75:488–92.

47. Ozawa A, Chaturvedi R, Lee KJ, Benson L. Femoral vein hemostasis in children using a suture-mediated closure device. *J Interv Cardiol* 2007;20:164–7.

48. Cilingiroglu M, Salinger M, Zhao D, Feldman T. Technique of temporary subcutaneous "figure-of-eight" sutures to achieve hemostasis after removal of large-caliber femoral venous sheaths. *Catheter Cardiovasc Interv* 2011;78(1):155–60.

49. Morgan GJ, Waragai T, Eastaugh L, Chaturvedi RC, Lee KJ, Benson L. The Fellows stitch: Large caliber venous hemostasis in pediatric practice. *Catheter Cardiovasc Interv* 2012;80:79–82.

11

Percutaneous subclavian access

Christian Frerker, Ulrich Schäfer, and Karl-Heinz Kuck

Introduction

In 2002, transcatheter aortic valve implantation (TAVI) was successfully introduced as a new treatment option for aortic valvular stenosis.[1] Since then, rapidly rising implantation numbers have proven the feasibility and safety of this promising technology.[2-4] When percutaneous aortic valve implantation was in its infancy, it was still necessary to expose the arterial access vessel surgically under general anesthesia. Today, it is usually a truly percutaneous procedure for femoral access with the use of preclosure systems, meaning that the interventions can be carried out under sedation or only local anesthesia. Nevertheless, vascular complications remain a significant cause of mortality and morbidity with an incidence of 7–15%.[5,6] Despite the increasing experience with different access-site techniques and preclosure devices, failure to close the percutaneously created arteriotomy remains a dangerous problem with transfemoral TAVI. These facts require a detailed preprocedural assessment of the access paths, as well as precise management and experience if complications occur. In addition to the transfemoral access site, several other access sites have been proposed. Safety and feasibility of a transsubclavian approach, using a surgical cutdown with subsequent surgical repair after TAVI, have been demonstrated.[7,8] With increasing experience, a truly percutaneous technique for the axillary access was developed—"the Hamburg Sankt Georg Approach."[9]

Anatomy

Owing to the widespread confusion about the correct anatomic terminology, it should be mentioned that even with a surgical cutdown to the artery, the implantation is always done via the axillary artery and not via the subclavian artery. By definition, the axillary artery begins at the lateral border of the first rib as a continuation of the subclavian artery. It changes its name to brachial artery at the lower (inferior) border of the teres major muscle. On its way, the axillary artery is divided into three segments according to its relation to the pectoralis minor muscle.

Technique

The ipsilateral double-puncture technique for femoral access has shown good results.[6] Building on these good results, this special technique should also be used for axillary access for safety reasons and complication management. Emphasis should be given to the fact that compression treatment is rather difficult if not impossible (especially in obese patients) in this particular anatomical region (as opposed to the common femoral artery).

The first step of the procedure is a puncture of the ipsilateral brachial artery with subsequent insertion of a 6 Fr sheath. Over this distal brachial spot, retrograde dye injection (5–10 cc) is applied to visualize the diameter of the axillary artery with its branches to the shoulder joint. In addition, a second puncture of the femoral artery with the insertion of a 6 Fr sheath needs to be performed. Following these two punctures, a small wire (e.g., a 0.018″ Plywire 400 cm, GlobalMed) is advanced over a regular diagnostic JR4 catheter (previously placed over the brachial artery into the descending aorta) and snared down into the femoral artery, thereby establishing an arterio-arterial monorail access path. The wire serves as a safety net and can be used for balloon blockade or for endovascular stent graft implantation from two access sites if needed. The length of 400 cm allows sufficient length of wire at both arterial sites (brachial and femoral). For safety reasons, an appropriate balloon (regular PTA [percutaneous transluminal angioplasty] balloons 6–10 mm, 20–40 mm length) should always be inserted over the femoral monorail access path into the descending aorta. This balloon is kept in place during the complete procedure for immediate vessel occlusion if needed. With the use of fluoroscopy and the arterio-arterial wire as a landmark, the axillary artery should be punctured significantly lateral to the rib cage and below the clavicle. Care has to be taken to puncture very lateral to avoid the pneumothorax and to have the opportunity to compress the very distal axillary artery if needed. In addition, puncturing the side branches of the axillary artery, that is, the superior thoracic artery, thoracoacromial artery, and lateral thoracic artery should be avoided. After successful puncture of the axillary artery, a 6 Fr can be introduced and heparin should be given to achieve an activated clotting time (ACT) >250 ms. The wire should be left in place (distal aorta) and preclosure devices (i.e., ProStar® XL 10 Fr or two ProGlide® 6 Fr; Abbott Vascular Devices, Redwood City, California, USA) should to be inserted over a regular J-wire into the direct puncture site. Care has to be taken to prevent the ProStar from going into the ascending aorta due to the excess length of the ProStar and the short distance from the puncture site to the aortic valve. Our own experience demonstrated that the use of a ProStar displayed more complications than two ProGlide systems (*n* = 24, closure success: ProStar 37% vs. two ProGlide 100%, *p* < 0.01).[9] Nevertheless, it has to be mentioned that usage of either ProStar or ProGlide is considered as "off-label usage" for that specific indication. After the insertion of a preclosure device, a device sheath can be carefully introduced (usually over a stiff intervention wire).

At the end of the procedure, the device sheath has to be carefully pulled back and a balloon catheter (regular PTA balloons 6–10 mm, 20–40 mm length) should be advanced into the axillary artery and inflated with 4–8 atmospheres to provide hemostasis for closure of the access site. The device sheath can then be removed under "dry conditions" and the sutures provided by the ProStar XL or the two ProGlide systems tied down to obtain successful hemostasis. Finally, a control angiogram of the axillary artery should be performed over the sheath placed in the brachial artery using a small amount of contrast. Closure of the brachial artery should be effected by manual compression followed by a pressure bandage. The femoral artery puncture site can be closed either by manual compression or by using a closure device.

Basic steps of percutaneous axillary access:

1. Puncture of the ipsilateral brachial artery, insertion of a 6 Fr sheath, and dye injection (5–10 cc) to visualize the diameter of the axillary artery.
2. Puncture of the femoral artery, insertion of a 6 Fr sheath and a wire (400 cm) via the brachial artery with down-snaring into the femoral artery, thereby establishing an arterio-arterial monorail access path.
3. For safety reasons, an appropriate balloon (regular PTA balloons 6–10 mm, 20–40 mm length) has to be inserted over this monorail access path from the femoral artery into the descending aorta (kept in place) for immediate vessel blockade if needed.
4. Direct puncture of the axillary artery (significantly lateral of the rib cage and below the clavicula) with the use of fluoroscopy and the arterio-arterial wire as a landmark and insertion of a 6 Fr sheath.
5. Heparin should be given to achieve an ACT >250 ms.
6. Insertion of preclosure devices (i.e., ProStar XL 10 Fr or two ProGlide 6 Fr) over a second wire into the direct puncture site.

7. Careful introduction of a device sheath.
8. Do the procedure.
9. Removal of the device sheath with the blocking balloon (regular PTA balloons 6–10 mm, 20–40 mm length) inflated proximal to the puncture site (4–8 atmospheres).
10. After the removal of the device sheath, the sutures of the preclosure system have to be tied down to obtain successful hemostasis.
11. Control angiography of the axillary artery via the side port of the sheath in the brachial artery.

Complications

The biggest concern for direct puncture of the axillary artery is the risk of major bleeding and dissection. In case of a complication such as a flow-limiting dissection or persistent bleeding, retrograde or antegrade treatment of the injured axillary vessel segment can be performed using balloon dilation and/or stent implantation (covered stent graft for significant bleeding/perforation, fenestrated stent for dissection). In addition, retrograde angiography via the side port of the brachial sheath can always be performed. In general, endovascular treatment of the subclavian and axillary artery with stents has been proven to be feasible and safe in numerous studies with an immediate success rate of 93–100%.[10,11] Owing to the histological differences between the axillary artery and the femoral artery, different approaches and closure devices could be anticipated. The subclavian and axillary arteries have layers of elastic fibers in the media. In contrast, the media layer of the femoral artery between the internal and external elastic laminae contains mainly smooth muscle cells with few strands of elastic fibers. Furthermore, the fibrous adventitia of the femoral artery is usually thicker than that of the axillary artery.[9] Thus, the use of self-expanding stents is recommended in the subclavian and axillary artery. The greater elasticity of the subclavian artery challenges the appropriate stent size for the prevention of endoleaks with subsequent persistent bleeding. The major disadvantage of self-expandable stent grafts is the relatively large sheath size that has to be used (usually 8–10 Fr compared with 6–7 Fr for balloon-expandable stentgrafts).

In case of complications that cannot be managed percutaneously, a balloon can be positioned and inflated within a more proximal segment of the axillary artery in order to achieve temporary hemostasis until subsequent surgical reconstruction is possible. The long arterio-arterial circuit wire remains *in situ* as a safety guard to secure re-access into the vessel at all times.

The incidence of major bleeding according to Valve Academic Research Consortium (VARC) was 0% in a series of 24 patients, indicating the feasibility and safety of this approach.[9] The percutaneous access serves to minimize vascular trauma and to enhance the clinical benefit.

The risk of stroke is published in a range of 0–4% even in vessels with severe calcification or chronic total occlusion.[10,11]

The risk of injury to the internal thoracic artery remains an issue that may exclude patients from a trans-axillary approach, especially if the internal mammary artery (IMA) is grafted to the coronary arteries (relative contraindication).

Summary

This new technique allows a completely percutaneous axillary approach with the use of a preclosure device. The key factor is to assure access at all times for the treatment of life-threatening vessel injuries. With the establishment of a long "safety-net" wire with two access points (i.e., brachial and femoral artery) to the axillary artery, this criterion is nicely met. The wire should always be placed before direct puncture, preclosure, and device sheath insertion into the axillary artery. Last but not least, with this wire in hand, vessel closure can be performed without haste under controlled conditions.

References

1. Cribier A, Eltchaninoff H, Bash A et al. Percutaneous transcatheter implantation of an aortic valve prosthesis for calcific aortic stenosis: First human case description. *Circulation* 2002;106:3006–8.

2. Smith CR, Leon MB, Mack MJ et al. Transcatheter vs. surgical aortic valve replacement in high risk patients. *N Engl J Med* 2011;364:2187–98.

3. Grube E, Laborde JC, Gerckens U et al. Percutaneous implantation of the CoreValve self-expanding valve prosthesis in high-risk patients with aortic valve disease: The Siegburg first-in-man study. *Circulation* 2006;114(15):1616–24.

4. Gurvitch R, Toggweiler S, Willson AB et al. Outcomes and complications of transcatheter aortic valve replacement using a balloon expandable valve according to the Valve Academic Research Consortium (VARC) guidelines. *EuroIntervention* 2011;7:41–8.

5. Rodes-Cabau J, Webb JG, Cheung A et al. Transcatheter aortic valve implantation for the treatment of severe symptomatic aortic stenosis in patients at very high or prohibitive surgical risk: Acute and late outcomes of the multicenter Canadian experience. *J Am Coll Cardiol* 2010;55(11):1080–90.

6. Frerker C, Schewel D, Kuck KH et al. Ipsilateral arterial access for management of vascular complication in transcatheter aortic valve implantation. *Catheter Cardiovasc Interv.* 2013;4:592–602.

7. Petronio AS, De Carlo M, Bedogni F et al. Safety and efficacy of the subclavian approach for transcatheter aortic valve implantation with the CoreValve revalving system. *Circ Cardiovasc Interv* 2010;3:359–66.

8. Modine T, Obadia JF, Choukroun E et al. Transcutaneous aortic valve implantation using the axillary/subclavian access: Feasibility and early clinical outcomes. *J Thorac Cardiovasc Surg* 2011;141:487–91, 491.e1

9. Schäfer U, Ho Y, Frerker C et al. Direct percutaneous access technique for transaxillary transcatheter aortic valve implantation: "The Hamburg Sankt Georg Approach." *J Am Coll Cardiol Cardiovasc Interv* 2012;5(5):477–86.

10. Sixt S, Rastan A, Schwarzwalder U et al. Results after balloon angioplasty or stenting of atherosclerotic subclavian artery obstruction. *Catheter Cardiovasc Interv* 2009;73:395–403.

11. AbuRahma AF, Bates MC, Stone PA et al. Angioplasty and stenting versus carotid-subclavian bypass for the treatment of isolated subclavian artery disease. *J Endovasc Ther* 2007;14:698–704.

12

Access from the common carotid artery

Grazyna Brzezinska-Rajszys

It is rare for access from the carotid artery to be required for the purposes of cardiac catheterization. Nowadays, this approach is reserved mostly for balloon valvuloplasty in newborns with aortic valve stenosis. It may also be used for access to stenting of the arterial duct and, in rarer cases, stenting coarctation of the aorta. In experienced hands, it is a safe approach and simplifies crossing the stenosed aortic valve and reduces vascular complications associated with the femoral arterial approach in very small patients.[1–7] It also shortens the time of the procedure, which is especially important in sick neonates.[7] The carotid artery approach is also very useful for interventions in which relatively large sheaths are required.[8] With some technical modifications, it can be useful for aortic valve implantation.[9] The choice of access via the right or left common carotid artery depends on the planned interventional procedure and the anatomy of the aortic arch and its branches.

Ultrasound assessment of the morphology and the flow through the carotid artery after neonatal surgical cutdown has shown that the carotid artery is well preserved in more than 95% of the patients,[4,6] although an asymptomatic obstruction may occasionally be present.[10]

The common carotid artery cutdown should be performed by a surgeon or a cardiologist trained in this technique.

Technique

The carotid artery takes its course in the triangle formed by the clavicle and the sternal and clavicular bellies of the sternocleidomastoid muscle insertions entering the chest under the head of the clavicle.

The patient is placed in a supine position with a wedge placed under the back to elevate the shoulders, with the head slightly turned to the opposite side to expose the neck and keep the chin away from the operating field. Forceful neck extension or serious leftward rotation of the head should be avoided as it may change the cervical vascular anatomy. Careful positioning of the patient is important as it improves identification of surface landmarks.

Anatomic landmarks, including the sternal notch, the clavicle, and the sternocleidomastoid muscle, should be assessed before preparation and draping for the procedure. The carotid artery should be palpated and its course determined. The common carotid artery lies lateral to the trachea, usually under the medial sternal head of the sternocleidomastoid muscle. General anesthesia and controlled ventilation is important.

Percutaneous access is performed by many and may include the use of high-frequency ultrasound guidance; see Chapter 9 for vascular access.

The carotid artery cutdown should be a sterile procedure. A transverse skin incision (parallel to the clavicle) is made above the sternocleidomastoid muscle halfway between the jugular notch and the thyroid cartilage. After the skin incision, the platysma should be blunt dissected and the medial border of the sternocleidomastoid muscle exposed. The common carotid artery takes its course together with the internal jugular vein and the vagus nerve as a neurovascular bundle medial to the sternocleidomastoid muscle.

The common carotid artery is identified, located medially and deeper than the jugular vein. The artery is exposed with blunt dissection and an adequate length of artery is mobilized to allow proximal and distal control with vascular loops of rubber or silk. A purse-string suture of 7-0 or 6-0 monofilament (Prolene) is placed between the vascular loops. Arterial puncture is performed in the center of the purse-string. Gentle traction on both vascular loops helps to control the bleeding. The artery is entered with the needle and a guide wire is introduced through it (Figure 12.1). An appropriate-sized sheath is introduced over the guide wire. It is important to check carefully the position of the end of the sheath under fluoroscopy, as in neonates it can reach the aortic valve. If the balloon is then kept partially in the sheath during its inflation, it can cause serious damage to the sheath and may cause difficulties in its removal. The patient should be heparinized with 100 units/kg. In neonates, cerebral ultrasonography should be performed before the procedure to

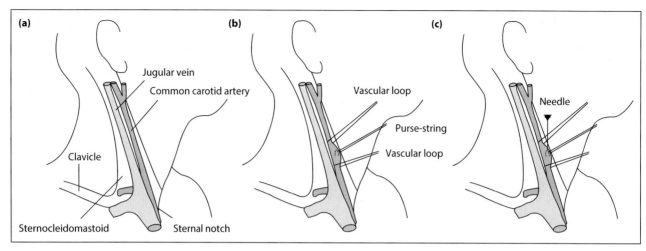

Figure 12.1 The technique for right carotid artery approach. (a) Anatomic landmarks and carotid anatomy. (b) Preparation of the carotid artery with vascular loops and purse-string. (c) Arterial puncture in the middle of the purse-string.

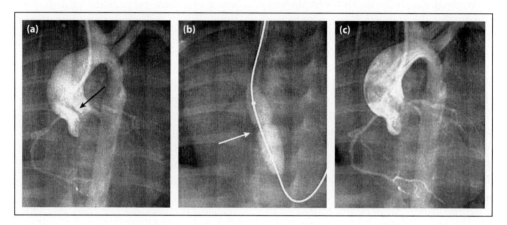

Figure 12.2 Right carotid artery access for aortic balloon valvuloplasty in a neonate. (a) Aortography before valvuloplasty with the jet of unopacified blood (arrow). (b) Balloon valvuloplasty catheter placed across the valve; the indentation on the balloon reflects the level of the stenotic valve (arrow). (c) Aortography after successful balloon valvuloplasty.

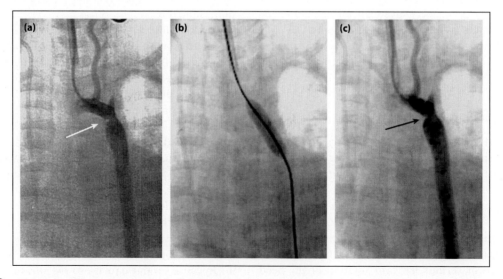

Figure 12.3 Right carotid artery access for balloon angioplasty of coarctation of the aorta in a neonate. Procedure performed after aortic valvuloplasty during the same session. (a) Aortography before angioplasty shows native coarctation of the aorta (arrow). (b) Balloon angioplasty catheter placed in the isthmus. (c) Aortography after successful balloon angioplasty.

exclude cerebral hemorrhage because this may influence heparinization.

Once the sheath is in place, intervention such as balloon dilation or stent implantation can be performed. After the procedure, while traction is maintained on both vascular loops, the sheath is removed, and the purse-string is tied to produce hemostasis. The vascular loops are then removed. The flow through the artery is checked by palpation and the wound is closed by a subcutaneous suture. The wound should be covered with a sterile dressing.

An ultrasound scan with visualization of the carotid artery and Doppler examination with measurements of the blood velocity should be repeated before discharge from the hospital.

Complications

With a careful surgical technique, complications related to carotid access are very rare. Periprocedural complications such as arterial thrombosis or arterial damage treated with its ligation were reported in earlier series and should be treated individually.[6,10] Carotid artery stenosis is a potential complication of this approach, but seems to be exceptional.[6] In an angiography performed 3 months after balloon aortic valvuloplasty, a normal right carotid artery was demonstrated.[3] At midterm follow-up, in some patients with ultrasound examination, the site of surgical incision could be identified without flow disturbances.[10]

One of the main limitations of this procedure is the need for specialized training in the technique or the need for a surgeon to perform carotid arteriorotomy.

Examples of applications

The carotid artery approach can be used for balloon valvuloplasty in neonates with isolated critical aortic valve stenosis (Figure 12.2). In patients with associated coarctation of the aorta, balloon angioplasty of coarctation can be performed through the carotid approach during the same session (Figure 12.3).[2,7] The carotid artery approach can be used for stent implantation into the aorta in small children (Figure 12.4),[8] for stent implantation into the pulmonary artery via Blalock–Taussig shunt in patients with complex congenital heart defects with pulmonary trunk atresia and pulmonary artery stenosis (Figure 12.5), and for occlusion

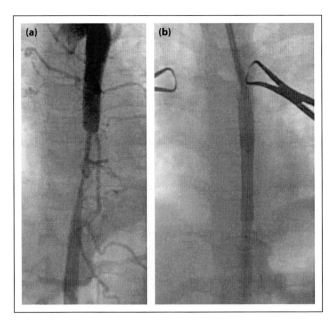

Figure 12.4   A stent implantation into the thoracic aorta for middle aortic syndrome by right carotid artery access. (a) Angiogram shows severe narrowing of lower thoracic aorta. (b) Stent implantation into the aorta.

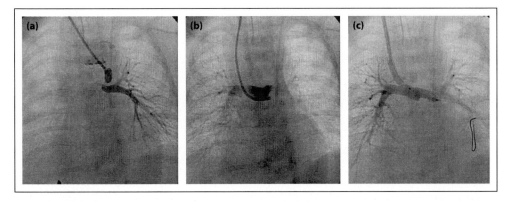

Figure 12.5   Right carotid artery access for stent implantation into the left pulmonary artery via right-modified Blalock–Taussig shunt. (a) Angiography in the arterial duct shows severe stenosis of the pulmonary artery end of the duct. (b) Arteriography of pulmonary arteries with catheter placed through the Blalock–Taussig shunt shows severe stenosis of the left pulmonary artery. (c) Arteriography through the sheath after stent implantation in the left pulmonary artery. Note that catheter and guide wire are still in the pulmonary artery.

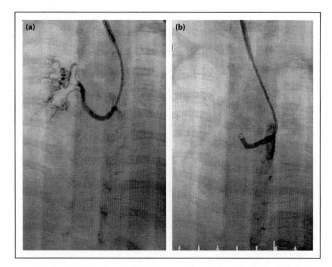

Figure 12.6 Right carotid artery access for embolization of major aorto-pulmonary collateral after a switch operation for transposition of the great arteries in a neonate. Selective angiography in collateral before (a) and after the procedure (b).

of important aorto-pulmonary collaterals, mostly in neonates after surgery (e.g., after an arterial switch operation) (Figure 12.6).

Conclusion

Access from the common carotid artery performed carefully is safe and very helpful. The indications for this technique should be analyzed in detail before planning an interventional procedure, taking into consideration also the vascular anatomy. Nowadays, with modern low-profile balloon catheters, the role of common carotid artery access is diminishing, but in special circumstances, it should still be considered. In low-weight patients with critical aortic stenosis, this easy access seems to be very important, reducing the time of the procedure and complications related to damage of the femoral artery.

The carotid access should be a technique available in pediatric catheter laboratories. In centers familiar with this approach, it is used more frequently than aortic balloon valvuloplasty for different occasions.

References

1. Fischer DR, Ettedgui JA, Park SC, Siewers RD, del Nido PJ. Carotid artery approach for balloon dilation of aortic valve stenosis in the neonate: A preliminary report. *J Am Coll Cardiol* 1990;15:1633–6.
2. Carminati M, Giusti S, Spadoni I et al. Balloon aortic valvuloplasty in the first year of life. *J Interv Cardiol* 1995;8(6 Suppl):759–66.
3. Maeno Y, Akagi T, Hashino K et al. Carotid artery approach to balloon aortic valvuloplasty in infants with critical aortic valve stenosis. *Pediatr Cardiol* 1997;18:288–91.
4. Weber HS, Mart CR, Kupferschmid J, Myers JL, Cyran SE. Transcarotid balloon valvuloplasty with continuous transesophageal echocardiographic guidance for neonatal critical aortic valve stenosis: An alternative to surgical palliation. *Pediatr Cardiol* 1998;19:212–7.
5. Fagan TE, Ing FF, Edens RE, Caldarone CA, Scholz TD. Balloon aortic valvuloplasty in a 1,600-gram infant. *Catheter Cardiovasc Interv* 2000;50:322–5.
6. Robinson BV, Brzezinska-Rajszys G, Weber HS et al. Balloon aortic valvotomy through a carotid cutdown in infants with severe aortic stenosis: Results of the multi-centric registry. *Cardiol Young* 2000;10:225–32.
7. Pedra CA, Pedra SR, Braga SL et al. Short- and midterm follow-up results of valvuloplasty with balloon catheter for congenital aortic stenosis. *Arq Bras Cardiol* 2003;81:120–8.
8. Brzezinska-Rajszys G, Qureshi SA, Ksiazyk J et al. Middle aortic syndrome treated by stent implantation. *Heart* 1999;81:166–70.
9. Modine T, Sudre A, Delhaye C et al. Transcutaneous aortic valve implantation using the left carotid access: Feasibility and early clinical outcomes. *Ann Thorac Surg* 2012;93:1489–94.
10. Borghi A, Agnoletti G, Poggiani C. Surgical cutdown of the right carotid artery for aortic balloon valvuloplasty in infancy: Midterm follow-up. *Pediatr Cardiol* 2001;22:194–7.

13

Transhepatic access

Makram R. Ebeid

Introduction

With the advances in catheter techniques, alternative access routes have been sought to overcome anatomical limitations. One of the obstacles encountered by catheter operator is the inability to use the traditional femoral vein approach to perform cardiac catheterization and/or intervention. This may be due to anatomical constraints such as interruption of the inferior vena cava or occlusion of the femoral veins as a result of previous line placement (Figure 13.1). In the presence of occluded femoral vessels, alternate routes are sought to perform cardiac catheterization and/or interventions. The internal jugular or subclavian vein approach may be appropriate in some instances. In other instances where the patient has undergone cavopulmonary anastomosis, it may be impossible to reach the area of interest using this approach. Additionally, manipulating the catheters from that approach may be difficult in certain areas of the heart.

History

In the mid-1990s, the transhepatic approach emerged as an alternative to the traditional femoral venous approach for cardiac catheterization and/or intervention.[1-2] A number of catheter operators subsequently reported favorable experiences with varying degrees of success and applicability.[3-8] Some (including the author) felt that it is the preferred approach to be utilized in certain instances even when alternative venous routes are available.[5,9] The knowledge and skills to perform this approach should be acquired by the experienced pediatric interventionist to be used when deemed appropriate. This approach is more favorable than neck approaches for some interventions (personal experience) and for catheter manipulations and may be even more attractive than the traditional femoral approach in some cases, as will be discussed.

Physiological anatomy

The liver contributes about 2% of the total body weight. It contains 50,000–100,000 lobules, constructed around the central vein connecting to the hepatic vein and into the inferior vena cava.[10] Surrounding the hepatic lobule is the portal triad, formed from the tributaries of the bile duct, the portal vein, and the hepatic artery.[11] It receives blood supply from two sources: the portal vein (75%) and the

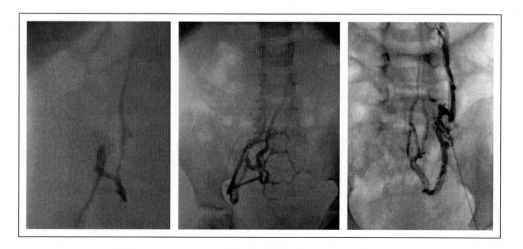

Figure 13.1 Angiograms outlining occluded femoral veins in three patients.

hepatic artery (25%). Most of the liver is covered by the peritoneum.[10] Approximately 10% of the total blood volume is stored in the liver at any given time.[10] This volume can increase two- to threefold in cases of elevated right atrial pressure. The liver lies close to the abdominal wall on its right and lateral anterior surface.[12] Its diaphragmatic aspect (superior, right, and anterior borders) forms the convex surface of the liver lying beneath the diaphragm and is separated from its visceral (inferior) border by a sharp narrow inferior border. The gall bladder is located in the inferior surface approximately 4–5 cm to the right of the midline.[12] The projections of the liver on the body surface have acquired added significance in the performance of a transhepatic approach. The projections vary depending upon the position of the individual as well as the body build, especially the configuration of the thorax. In the erect position, the liver extends downward to the 10th or 11th rib in the right midaxillary line. Here, the pleura projects downward to the 10th rib and the lung to the 8th. The inferior margin of the liver crosses the costal arch in the right lateral body line, approximately at the level of the pylorus (transpyloric line). In the horizontal position, the projection of the liver moves a little upward.[11]

Precatheter planning

A careful history review is necessary to exclude underlying liver disease and to elicit a history of anticoagulation and antiplatelet regimen as well as a history of abdominal surgery, which are all very important in the planning. We generally like to avoid antithrombin, but not necessarily antiplatelet medications prior to the transhepatic catheterization. The latter would usually favor closing the tract postprocedure (see later). When indicated, lab work to evaluate the bleeding and liver function should be considered. The knowledge of the liver location in patients with complex congenital heart disease and suspected heterotaxy to evaluate the liver location is mandatory prior to the procedure. Ultrasound should be obtained if not previously done in such cases. A history indicative of elevated central venous pressure (as in Fontan patients or patients with right-sided lesions) is important in order to plan for pre- and postmanagement of the patients, though in itself is not a contraindication to this approach. History of previous abdominal surgery is very important. The presence of scar tissue makes placement of the sheath more difficult. It also favors closure of the tract postprocedure.

Technique

The procedure can be performed under conscious sedation or general anesthesia. In cases of conscious sedation, the area of entry should be well anesthetized and that includes the subcutaneous tissue as well as deep into the

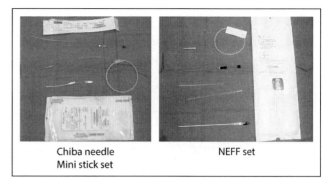

Figure 13.2   Transhepatic set. Left: Chiba needle with Mini-Stick kit. Right: Neff set.

subcapsular area and the hepatic parenchyma, since the needle entry and sheath placement can be painful. It is important to monitor the blood pressure during the procedure which is usually done using an indwelling arterial catheter. A long needle (21- or 22-gauge needle) with or without an obturator, as the Chiba needle or the Neff set (Cook, Bloomington, IN), is usually used (Figure 13.2). Alternative needles can be used such as the Mini-Stick needle (Mini-Stick™ kit, Boston Scientific, Natick, MA), which is a 21-gauge needle and shorter than the Chiba needle. The appropriate needle length is chosen by examining the length under fluoroscopy and the distance it needs to cross. We generally prefer the Mini-Stick needle in the younger patients. An 0.018 inch wire with a floppy end is needed to be introduced through the needle. A transitional/coaxial sheath that allows upsizing the wire size will facilitate placing the required dilator and sheath to perform the procedure; it is part of the Neff set or can be obtained in separate kits such as the Mini-Stick kit or commercially available transradial kits provided by Merit (Merit Medical Systems, South Jordan, UT). The procedure can be done in single- or biplane laboratories. The image intensifier is set at 0° antero-posterior projection and 90° lateral projections (when biplane fluoroscopy is utilized). The needle is introduced under fluoroscopy in the mid- to anterior axillary line below the costal margin angled superiorly, posteriorly, and medially toward the patient's left shoulder (Figure 13.3 and Video 13.1). Alternative approaches include introducing the needle midway between the xiphoid sternum and right mid-axillary line, directing the needle to the right atrium at 20–30° angle[6] or the mid-liver in the intercostal spaces, below the diaphragm, as guided by fluoroscopy (Hijazi Z, MD, personal communication).

The needle commonly used is 15 cm long. The needle/obturator is introduced until it is 1/2" from the midline. A "pop" may be felt when the needle is in a large vein. The obturator is removed and a contrast-filled syringe is applied to the needle. Gentle aspiration is performed while withdrawing the needle until blood is obtained. Once blood is obtained, the needle is held steady and a small

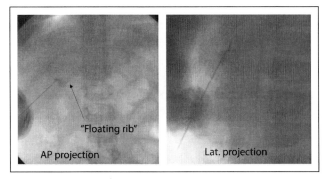

Figure 13.3   Needle orientation in the antero-posterior and lateral projections.

contrast injection is performed while acquiring the image on antero-posterior and lateral projections to outline the hepatic vein (Video 13.2). Distinction between hepatic and portal veins is done by noticing the direction of the flow of the blood (Figure 13.4a and Video 13.3). Occasionally, despite outlining a hepatic vein, the vein is seen to be very tortuous with sharp curves, which makes it more difficult to use for the catheterization (Figure 13.4b). The needle may have to be readjusted slightly or pulled further while small injections are performed to outline a useful hepatic vein. A small amount of contrast in the liver parenchyma can outline the target hepatic vein for subsequent attempts. The needle can be manipulated while injecting contrast toward the desired vein (Video 13.4). However, too much

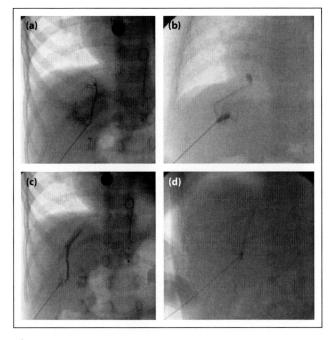

Figure 13.4   (a) Angiogram outlines a portal vein. Note the direction of blood flow. (b) A tortuous hepatic vein is seen. Its course would make it difficult to introduce the wire/sheath. (c, d) Two favorable hepatic veins useful for placing the sheath and performing the cardiac catheterization.

contrast in the hepatic parenchyma can interfere with visualizing the hepatic vein at subsequent attempts. Hand injection can outline unexpected issues such as thrombosis of hepatic portion of the inferior vena cava (IVC), thus precluding that route (Video 13.5). Once a suitable hepatic vein is identified (Figure 13.4c and d), the syringe is removed and the wire is inserted under fluoroscopy guidance. The wire should advance smoothly and easily along the tract to the heart. As long as no resistance is met, the wire can be manipulated along the hepatic veins to the atrium (Video 13.6). The easy advancement of the wire is one of the most pleasant feelings for the catheterizer during the procedure. We attempt to maintain the stiffer part of the wire along the transhepatic tract. Thus, the wire is advanced to the right atrium and preferably positioned in the superior vena cava or in the pulmonary veins if there is an atrial septal defect. Alternatively, the wire is maintained in the right atrium or the right ventricle. When the wire course is straight, the sheath advancement is usually easy (Video 13.7). Depending on the sheath size, multiple dilators may be used to dilate the hepatic tract and allow for insertion of the required sheath. Frequently, a transitional sheath such as the Mini-Stick kit or Neff set is used. By the use of this sheath, the 0.018 inch wire can be upsized to a larger and stiffer wire (0.035–0.038 inch). Alternatively, a second 0.018 inch wire can be placed alongside, especially if there is concern about premature removal of the initially placed wire. This will provide a larger, more effective wire caliber, which can be used to advance stiffer dilators/sheaths (Figure 13.5). Rarely, despite placing the wire, it may be difficult or impossible to advance the required sheaths and dilators. This may happen because of the sharp angle the floppy wire may take when it curves in the capsular space/liver parenchyma while entering the hepatic vein. In these rare instances when the sheath and the dilator would not follow, the procedure may have to be repeated by entering a higher intercostal space (Figure 13.6). Preferably, the entry point should be the subcostal area, though by depending on the hepatic position, one or two intercostal spaces above can also be used, allowing a straighter wire/sheath course. In small infants, the sheath may need to be advanced while holding and stabilizing the dilator under fluoroscopy to avoid potential dilator trauma to the heart (Video 13.7). Ultrasound has been used as an adjunct or instead of fluoroscopy to identify a suitable hepatic vein and obtain transhepatic access.[8,13,14] Johnston et al.[13] used ultrasound to access the hepatic vein in eight patients. This identified the central hepatic vein with the straightest course, which facilitated placing the sheath with less tenting. The ultrasound transducer was covered with a sterile sleeve allowing imaging within the sterile field. Imaging of the vein is performed in multiple planes along the subcostal area until the best location for puncture is identified. Also, imaging can measure the depth of the vein and the distance the needle would need to be advanced. Additionally, the

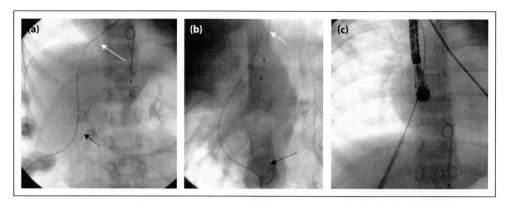

Figure 13.5   Antero-posterior (a) and lateral projections (b) of transhepatically placed wire making a sharp angle (black arrow). Notice that two 0.018″ caliber wires (white arrow) are placed side by side, which facilitated placing a large-caliber dilator. (c) Subsequently, a super-stiff wire was positioned in the innominate vein allowing placing an 11 French sheath for ASD closure.

ultrasound is used to identify the gall bladder position and the needle course as it enters the hepatic parenchyma, guiding the needle tip toward the hepatic vein. Once the needle tip is identified in the hepatic vein, the trocar, if used, can be removed and the wire advanced under ultrasound and/or fluoroscopy guidance. Mcleod et al.[8] used ultrasound

in five of six procedures to identify a large hepatic vein. Post (or during the procedure if necessary) ultrasound can assess for the presence of retro- or intraperitoneal bleeding. The use of heparin is based on the planned procedure, arterial line placement, and operator preference. If heparin is used, it is administered after obtaining access. The decision

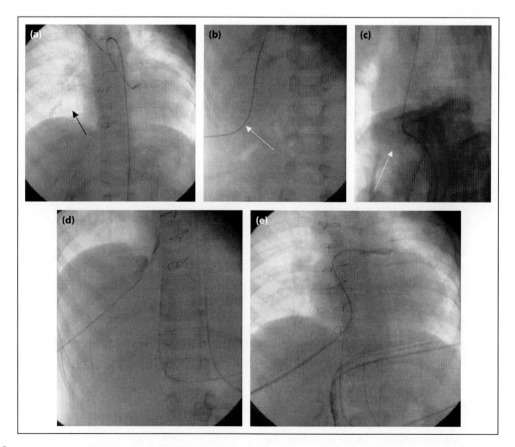

Figure 13.6   (a) A floppy wire was successfully placed in the right pulmonary vein using the subcostal approach. Antero-posterior (b) and lateral (c) projections of the wire show a sharp tight curve. Despite using multiple dilators, it was not possible to place the required sheath. (d) A repeat hepatic puncture slightly higher avoided the sharp tight curve of the wire and allowed easy placement of the required sheath (e).

to reverse heparin before removal of the sheath is guided by the activated clotting time, heparin dose, time elapsed from administering heparin, and the procedure performed. We prefer to avoid heparin reversal, if possible, in cases of atrial septal device placement. The presence of postoperative adhesions can make hepatic entry more difficult and requires multiple transitional and stiff dilators and wires. The stainless-steel hollow wire available in the Neff set can be used to stiffen the transitional sheath and allow advancing it. Special care should be exercised to avoid shearing the 0.018 inch wire while advancing the hollow wire with the transitional sheath. Once the transitional sheath is in place, the wire can be upsized to a stiffer and larger-caliber wire.

Catheter manipulations

After obtaining the transhepatic access and placing the appropriate sheath, catheter manipulations using that route can differ from catheter manipulations using other approaches. Most of the approaches from the transhepatic route need preshaped catheters with reasonably good torque, as the Judkins right-type catheters, Judkins left (with the tip cutoff), and occasionally some with tight curves, such as the Shepherd hook or Simmons-type curved catheters (Merit Medical Systems).

Right heart

Right and left superior vena cava

Entry to the superior vena cava is relatively simple with the aid of guide wire and preshaped catheters. Entry to the coronary sinus and left superior vena cava is generally easier than other approaches since the transhepatic route directs the catheter posteriorly toward the coronary sinus (Figure 13.7).

Inferior vena cava

Usually, the entry to the inferior vena cava is straightforward. Occasionally, the wire needs to be directed from the right atrium to the inferior vena cava by a preshaped catheter such as Simmons or Cobra-type curved catheter (Merit Medical Systems).

Right ventricle

Entry into the right ventricle involves more manipulation since the transhepatic route carries the catheter posteriorly and leftward. The wire should be directed with the aid of a preshaped catheter anteriorly to the right ventricle. This is carried out relatively simply by Judkins right-type catheters (Figure 13.8). Alternatively, balloon-directed catheters or custom-made, specially angulated transhepatic sheaths can be used (Cook), which may facilitate transhepatic catheter manipulations.

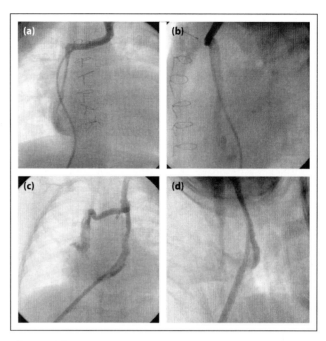

Figure 13.7 Entry to the right superior vena cava (a, b) and left superior vena cava (c, d). Note the straight entry to the coronary sinus and left superior vena cava.

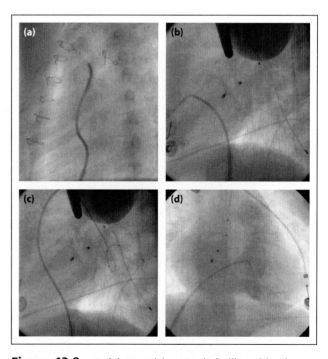

Figure 13.8 A right-ventricle entry is facilitated by the use of preshaped curved catheters to allow redirecting the wire/catheter from the posterior leftward transhepatic orientation to anterior/rightward direction toward the right ventricle. Shown is the catheter in a left anterior oblique projection (a), lateral (b, c), and antero-posterior projections (d).

Pulmonary artery and branches

The entry from the right ventricle to the main pulmonary artery is relatively simple and similar to the entry from the femoral vessels (Figure 13.9a–c) (Video 13.8). The entry is facilitated by using preshaped catheters (or sheaths) and floppy wires. Directing the catheter/wire to the left pulmonary artery guides it into a relatively smooth curve (Figure 13.9f) when compared with the right pulmonary artery (Figure 13.9d and e). This lends itself well to interventions on the left pulmonary artery, whether to perform balloon angioplasty or stent placement. Intervention on the right pulmonary artery is also feasible, though it involves more curvature.[15]

In the absence of femoral vein access, other routes for closure of the *patent ductus arteriosus* have been sought. Using the transhepatic approach lends itself to easily closing the persistent patent ductus arteriosus.[16]

Atrial septum and left heart structures

Atrial septum

The transhepatic approach directs the catheter leftward and posteriorly. It lends itself to direct access to the atrial septum and the left atrium. This feature is very helpful in interventions on the atrial septum, whether performing balloon atrial septostomy (Video 13.9) or closing atrial

septal defects. In cases of placing devices, especially in cases of large atrial septal defects, the delivery sheath is almost perpendicular to the atrial septum, which aligns the device in a plane parallel to the atrial septum (Figure 13.10).[17] Even when the femoral vein is not occluded, this approach will avoid other maneuvers described to align the atrial septal device parallel to the septum (Figure 13.11), avoiding prolapse of any part of the device through the deficient rim.[18,19] This approach will also avoid the difficulties encountered if the device were to be deployed using the internal jugular approach when the femoral vein is not accessible.[20] In cases of intact atrial septum where access to the left heart is needed, transseptal entry can be safely performed. The needle curve may need to be manually adjusted to have less curvature since the entry is more perpendicular (personal experience, Figure 13.12).

Left atrium: Entry to the left atrium is facilitated by the transhepatic route. This route directs the catheter posteriorly and leftward toward the left atrium and to the pulmonary veins (Figure 13.13). Though this route directs the catheter toward the left pulmonary veins, right and left pulmonary veins can be easily accessed through intra-atrial communications, especially in single ventricles with large intra-atrial communications. This allows easy assessment of the pulmonary veins as well as the ability to obtain wedge angiograms and pressures to assess the pulmonary artery tree, including the main pulmonary arteries and conduits (Videos 13.10 and 13.11). This approach would

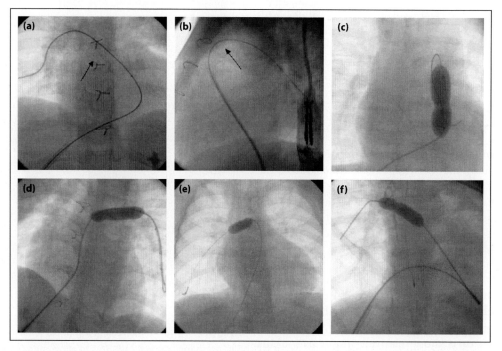

Figure 13.9 Transhepatic interventions in the pulmonary artery system. Antero-posterior (a) and lateral projections (b) of transhepatic stent placement (arrow) in a stenosed homograft. (c) Pulmonary balloon valvuloplasty. (d) Balloon angioplasty of the left and right pulmonary arteries (e, f). Notice the relatively smooth curve of the left pulmonary artery catheter as contrasted with the somewhat sharper curve of the right pulmonary artery catheter.

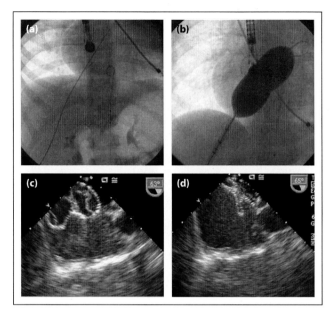

Figure 13.10 Crossing the atrial septal defect using this approach is simple (a). Note the straight catheter course. (b) Balloon sizing shows the orientation of the atrial septum almost perpendicular to the transhepatic approach, which renders itself for ease of placement of occluder devices (c, d) Transesophageal imaging planes with (c) and without (d) tension on the cable. Note that even with tension applied, the device is oriented parallel to the septum and does not change with release of the tension.

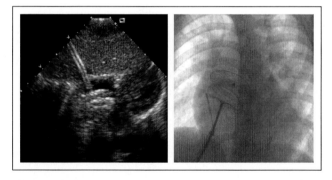

Figure 13.11 The delivery sheath and cable are seen to be perpendicular to the atrial septum echo, facilitating closure of a large ASD.

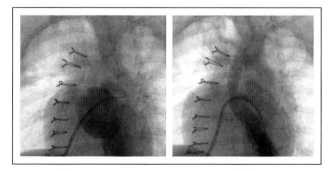

Figure 13.12 Transhepatic entry to the LA and the LV using a transseptal needle in a patient with Williams syndrome. Note the supra-aortic stenosis.

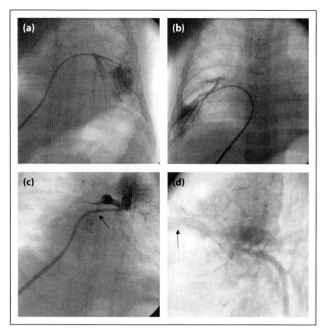

Figure 13.13 A left atrial entry is facilitated by this approach. Shown are two patients with occluded femoral vessels and hypoplastic left heart syndrome. Obtaining these angiograms using the internal jugular approach would have been more difficult. (a, b) Left and right pulmonary vein wedge angiograms outlining the distal pulmonary arteries in a patient with Norwood stage I. (c, d) Antero-posterior and lateral left pulmonary vein wedge angiograms outlining a Sano modification (arrow).

allow easier assessment of the pulmonary artery tree than the internal jugular especially in small infants with single ventricles.

Left ventricle: Entry to the left ventricle will require turning the catheter anteriorly from its straight posterior approach. It can sometimes be accomplished with balloon-directed catheters with or without the use of a tip deflector or preshaped wires (Figure 13.14). It may also be facilitated by the use of precurved catheters with sharp curves, such as a Judkins left catheter with the tip cutoff, allowing the placement of a wire in the left ventricle, and exchanging the catheter for a more flexible one with a smoother curve.

Single ventricle: The transhepatic approach lends itself well to patients with single ventricles. The elevation in the central venous pressures in these patients, which results in dilated hepatic veins, frequently facilitates obtaining access (Video 13.12). Actually, in this subset of patients, if access is difficult, unusual anatomical issues should be considered, such as thrombosis of the IVC (video) or hepatic veins stenosis (congenital or acquired). Prior to completion of the total cavopulmonary anastomosis, the transhepatic approach allows the use of sheaths larger than those which otherwise may be safely placed in the artery for intervention on the aortic side when indicated (Figure 13.15 and Video 13.13). Stenting of branch pulmonary

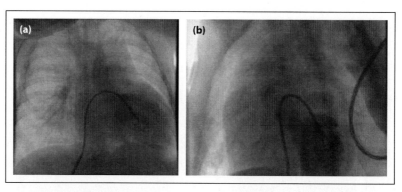

Figure 13.14 Right anterior oblique (a) and left anterior oblique (b) of a left ventriculogram using the transhepatic approach.

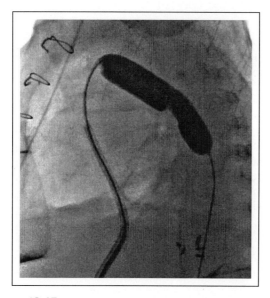

Figure 13.15 Transhepatic balloon angioplasty of coarctation in a patient with a palliated single ventricle allowed use of a relatively large sheath sparing the artery.

arteries in patients with complex single ventricles is quite feasible using this approach (Video 13.14).

Central line placement

After establishing the transhepatic access, a peel-away sheath is positioned in place. A sufficient amount of local anesthetic is infiltrated and a tunnel measuring a few centimeters is formed by the use of a hemostat extending from the entry site. A Broviac catheter (CR Bard, Salt Lake City, UT) is cut to the required length and introduced along the tunnel and into the peel-away sheath. Once the catheter is in place, the sheath is removed. The catheter and the entry sites are sutured. Alternatively, an antibiotic-treated catheter can be used, which may not require tunneling (Cook). The latter may be inserted through the peel-away sheath or

over a wire or both after being cut to the required length and then sutured in place.

Closure of the tract

Closure of the transhepatic tract using coils[1] or Gelfoam (Upjohn, Kalamazoo, MI)[5] has been suggested[1,2] to avoid retroperitoneal bleeding and liver hematoma. Others have felt that this is not necessary.[8] Conservative management has been demonstrated successfully in two cases with significant retroperitoneal bleeding.[19] The decision to close the tract continues to be debatable. Our practice has been to consider closure in patients who require relatively large sheaths or those who had prior abdominal surgery. In these patients, the presence of postoperative adhesions interferes with the hemostasis process and can result in prolonged bleeding.

Many occlusion devices can be used for the purpose of closing the intrahepatic access tract. If a coil or a plug is to be used, the tract can be outlined by placing a catheter smaller than the sheath size proximal to the hepatic vein. The sidearm of the sheath is used to inject dye while the catheter (4 or 5 French) is used to deliver the occlusion coil or plug. The sheath is slowly withdrawn while small hand injections are performed using the sidearm. This identifies the tract well (Figure 13.16) and avoids premature sheath withdrawal from the tract, especially in instances where the liver may have shifted because of unrecognized intraperitoneal or capsular bleeding.[2,21] Controlled-release devices are preferred for closure, such as detachable coils or one of the Amplatzer vascular plug family (St Jude Medical, Plymouth, MN) (Figure 13.17), which allows accurate placement and avoids the potential of device or coil embolization. This is especially important since, in the event of embolization, venous access would have been lost. Gelfoam has been used,[6] though its radiolucency makes it less attractive.

Postremoval of the sheath, extra attention to the entry site while obtaining hemostasis is necessary, especially if

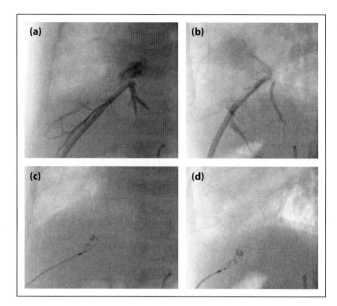

Figure 13.16 (a, b) Antero-posterior and lateral angiograms using the sheath sidearm while slowly withdrawing the sheath outlines the position of the tract. (c, d) A flipper coil is shown placed in the transhepatic tract.

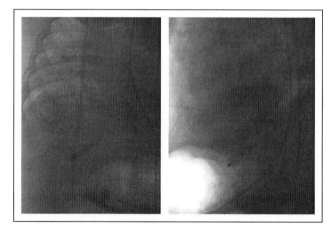

Figure 13.17 Transhepatic tract closed using a second-generation Amplatzer vascular plug.

the tract is not closed. The absence of blood oozing from the skin site does not mean that hemostasis has been achieved inside the liver parenchyma. The entry site should be held firmly against the liver parenchyma for at least 10 min even if visible skin hemostasis has been achieved prior to that. This is achieved by applying upward pressure on the subcostal area, pushing the liver parenchyma upward against the rib cage along the entry site.

Postcatheterization care

Postcatheterization care is similar to the regular cardiac catheterization care. We have not routinely performed an

ultrasound, blood count, or liver profile. Need and impact on management should be assessed on a case-by-case basis. Most patients are transferred to the regular floor and discharged the following day except if indicated otherwise. If an ultrasound is performed, there is almost always some degree of intraperitoneal fluid seen. Its significance is judged based on the clinical findings.

Complications

Potential complications may include intra/retroperitoneal bleeding, hemobilia, pneumothorax, pleural effusions, perforation of the gall bladder, portal vein thrombosis, and liver abscess/peritonitis. Fortunately, serious complications are infrequent and account for <5% with the majority being managed conservatively. The complication rate can be minimized by careful attention to details, administering antibiotics when necessary, and coil closure when indicated. The most common reported complication is retroperitoneal bleeding with an estimated incidence of clinically detected bleeding of <5%.[21,22] It is likely that in all these patients, some degree of self-limiting intra/retroperitoneal bleeding occurs. Serious retroperitoneal bleeding is rare but can be fatal. Careful attention to the details of the catheterization should minimize this risk. Most of these patients, even with clinically detectable intraperitoneal bleeding, can be managed with a conservative approach.[21] The latter approach has been advocated for managing even some traumatic liver injuries,[23-26] which has been traditionally addressed surgically. Transient elevation in liver function tests was also reported[19] and responded to removal of an indwelling central line.

Conclusion

The transhepatic cardiac approach has lent itself to the arena of cardiac catheterizations and interventions. In the absence of other venous routes, it may be the only available approach. In other instances, it may be the preferred approach for accessing certain areas of the heart and for the successful performance of the planned catheterization or intervention.[27]

References

1. Shim D, Lloyd TR, Cho KJ, Moorehead CP, Beekman RH III. Transhepatic cardiac catheterization in children: Evaluation of efficacy and safety. *Circulation* 1995;92:1526–30.
2. Sommer RJ. New approaches for catheterization and vascular access: The transhepatic technique. *Progr Pediatr Cardiol* 1996;6:95–104.
3. Sommer RJ, Golinko RJ, Mitty HA. Initial experience with percutaneous transhepatic cardiac catheterization in infants and children. *Am J Cardiol* 1995;75:1289–91.
4. Johnson JL, Fellows KE, Murphy JD. Transhepatic central venous access for cardiac catheterization and radiologic intervention. *Catheter Cardiovasc Diagn* 1995;35:168–71.

5. Wallace MJ, Hovsepian DM, Balzer DT. Transhepatic venous access for diagnostic and interventional cardiovascular procedures. *Vasc Interv Radiol* 1996;7:579–82.

6. Book WM, Raviele AA, Vincent RN. Repetitive percutaneous transhepatic access for myocardial biopsy in pediatric cardiac transplant recipients. *Catheter Cardiovasc Diagn* 1998;45(2):167–9

7. Fischbach P, Campbell RM, Hulse E et al. Transhepatic access to the atrioventricular ring for delivery of radiofrequency energy. *J Cardiovasc Electrophysiol* 1997;8(5):512–6.

8. McLeod KA, Houston AB, Richens T, Wilson N. Transhepatic approach for cardiac catheterization in children: Initial experience. *Heart (British Cardiac Society)* 1999;82(6):694–6.

9. Shim D, Lloyd TR, Beekman RH. Transhepatic therapeutic cardiac catheterization: A new option for the pediatric interventionalist. *Catheter Cardiovasc Interv* 1999;47:41–5.

10. Guyton AC, Hall JE. The liver as an organ. In: *Textbook of Medical Physiology*. 11th ed. Philadelphia: Elsevier Saunders; 2006. pp. 859–60.

11. Netter FH. Part III liver, biliary tract and pancreas. In: Oppenheimer E. Ed. *The Ciba Collection of Medical Illustrations, Volume 3, A Compilation of Paintings on The Normal and Pathological Anatomy of the Digestive System*. 2nd ed. Summit, NJ: Ciba; 1967. pp. 4–6.

12. Healy JC, Borley NR. Abdomen and pelvis. In: Standring S. Ed. *Gray's Anatomy. The Anatomical Basis of Clinical Practice*. 39th ed. Churchill Livingstone, Philadelphia: Elsevier; 2005. p. 1214.

13. Johnston TA, Donnelly LF, Frush DP, O'Laughlin MP. Transhepatic catheterization using ultrasound-guided access. *Pediatr Cardiol* 2003;24(4):393–6.

14. Gazzera C, Fonio P, Gallesio C, Camerano F, Doriguzzi Breatta A, Righi D et al. Ultrasound-guided transhepatic puncture of the hepatic veins for TIPS placement. *Radiol Med* 2013;118(3):379–85. doi: 10.1007/s11547-012-0853-3. Epub 2012 June 28.

15. Ebeid MR. Transhepatic approach for rehabilitation of stenosed pulmonary arteries. *Ann Pediatr Cardiol* 2010;3(1):25–30.

16. Ebeid, M, Kosek MA, Aggarwal A, Gaymes C. Transhepatic closure of the persistently patent ductus arteriosus (PDA). *Catheter Cardiovasc Interv* 79(5):S17 (Abs).

17. Ebeid MR, Joransen JA, Gaymes CH. Transhepatic closure of atrial septal defect and assisted closure of modified Blalock/Taussig shunt. *Catheter Cardiovasc Interv* 2006;67:674–8.

18. Wahab H, Bairam AR, Cao Q, Hijazi ZM. Novel technique to prevent prolapse of the Amplatzer septal occluder through large atrial septal defect. *Catheter Cardiovasc Interv* 2003;60:543–5.

19. Varma C, Benson LN, Silversides C, Yip J, Warr MR, Webb G et al. Outcomes and alternative techniques for device closure of the large secundum atrial septal defect. *Catheter Cardiovasc Interv* 2004;61:131–9.

20. Sullebarger JT, Sayad D, Gerber L, Ettedgui J, Jimmo-Waumans S, Alcebol PC. Percutaneous closure of atrial septal defect via transjugular approach with the Amplatzer septal occluder after unsuccessful attempt using the cardioSEAL device. *Catheter Cardiovasc Interv* 2004;62:262–5.

21. Erenberg FG, Shim D, Beekman RH, III. Intraperitoneal hemorrhage associated with transhepatic cardiac catheterization: A report of two cases. [see comment]. *Catheter Cardiovasc Diagn* 1998;43(2):177–8.

22. Kadir S. Transhepatic cholangiography and biliary drainage. In: Kadir S. Ed. *Current Practice of Interventional Radiology*, Philadelphia: Decker; 1991. pp. 497–511.

23. Andersson R, Bengemanrk S. Conservative treatment of liver trauma. *World J Surg* 1990;14:483–6.

24. McConnel DB, Trunkey DD. Nonoperative management of abdominal trauma. *Surg Clin N Am* 1990;70:677–88.

25. Uranus S, Mischinger HJ, Pfeifer J, Kronberger L, Rabl H, Werkgartner G et al. Hemostatic methods for the management of spleen and liver injuries. *World J Surg* 1996;20:1107–12.

26. Demetriades D, Rabinowitz B, Sofianos C. Non-operative management of penetrating liver injuries: A prospective study. *Br J Surg* 1986;73:736–7.

27. Ebeid MR. Transhepatic vascular access for diagnostic and interventional procedures: Techniques, outcome and complications. *Catheter Cardiovasc Interv* 2007;69:594–606.

14

Transseptal left heart catheterization

Guilherme V. Silva and Igor F. Palacios

Transseptal catheterization, which allows access to the left atrium, is the first step of the percutaneous mitral valvuloplasty procedure and one of the most crucial. Transseptal left heart catheterization was introduced independently in 1959 by Ross and Cope, and later modified by Brockenbrough and Mullins.[1-4] The procedure was introduced as an alternative to the methods available at that time, such as directly measuring left atrial and left ventricular pressures using either the transbronchial or transthoracic approaches.[5] The developments of the flotation pulmonary artery catheter in 1970 by Swan and Ganz[6] and retrograde cardiac catheterization of the left ventricle led to a significant decline in the utilization of the transseptal technique. Furthermore, with fewer patients with valvular disease and improved echocardiography, a smaller number of cardiologists were trained to perform the procedure.[7,8] With fewer procedures came fewer qualified personnel, and, because of concern over potentially grave complications and associated mortality, the procedure attained an "aura of danger and intrigue."[9] With the introduction of interventional procedures such as percutaneous mitral valvuloplasty, antegrade percutaneous aortic valvuloplasty, and now radio-frequency ablation of left-sided bypass tracts, there has been an increased demand for, and rekindled interest in, transseptal catheterization.[10,11] We will describe the technique, indications, and complications of transseptal left heart catheterization in this chapter.

Traditional technique

The physician performing a transseptal catheterization must be aware of the indications and contraindications of this technique and should be very familiar with the anatomy of the interatrial septum. Transseptal catheterization is performed using the percutaneous technique only from the right femoral vein. Although the right subclavian and the right jugular veins have been used occasionally, these are not standard techniques. Transseptal catheterization is also possible from the left femoral vein, but it is more painful to

the patient due to the sharp angulation between the left iliac vein and the inferior vena cava. Biplane fluoroscopy, if available, is the ideal imaging system. However, a single-plane C-arm fluoroscope, which can be rotated from the anteroposterior (AP) to lateral position, may also be used.

There are two different transseptal needles: the Ross needle and the Brockenbrough needle. The Ross needle is a 17-gauge needle, has a more pronounced curve, and is typically used with the Brockenbrough catheter. The Brockenbrough needle is more frequently utilized. It is an 18-gauge needle, which tapers at the distal tips to a 21 gauge, and is typically used with the Mullins sheath.

Prior to attempted puncture of the interatrial septum, full familiarity with the transseptal apparatus (Mullins sheath and dilator, Brockenbrough needle and stylet, and the Palacios transseptal kit [Cook]) is essential. The Mullins transseptal introducer (Cook) is composed of a 59-cm sheath and a 67-cm dilator. The distance the dilator protrudes from the sheath should be noted prior to the procedure. The Brockenbrough needle is 71 cm in length. The flange of the needle has an arrow that points to the position of the tip of the needle. Before use, the operator should be sure that the needle is straight and that the arrow of the flange is perfectly aligned with the needle tip. This arrow will allow the operator to know exactly where the distal tip of the needle is pointing. When the needle tip lies just within the dilator, there is approximately 1.5–2 cm distance between the dilator hub and the needle flange. This measurement should also be noted.

Once satisfied with the spatial relationship of the components of the transseptal system, a 0.032–0.035 inch J wire is positioned at the junction of the superior vena cava and left innominate vein from the right femoral vein. Venipuncture must be as horizontal as possible to facilitate manipulation of the transseptal system and permit maximal transmission of pulsations. Tactile as well as visual clues are important in properly identifying the puncture site. To ease insertion of the Mullins sheath, predilatation with an 8 F dilator is recommended. A pigtail catheter is positioned retrogradely in the right coronary sinus. To correctly identify the aorta with the use of the pigtail catheter and biplane fluoroscopy, the spatial relationship of the ascending aorta and its surrounding structures should be known. The pigtail catheter must be flushed with heparinized saline every 3 min to prevent clot formation and embolic complications.

Before proceeding, the right and left heart borders and apical pulsations are surveyed under fluoroscopy. Under fluoroscopic guidance, the Mullins sheath and dilator are advanced over the J wire into the superior vena cava/left innominate vein junction. The sheath must never be advanced without the wire, as the stiff dilator can readily perforate the inferior vena cava, superior vena cava, or right atrium. Once the Mullins sheath is properly placed, the wire is removed. The Brockenbrough needle is then advanced to lie just inside the dilator, using the predetermined distance between the needle flange and dilator as a guide. When advancing the needle to this position, it must rotate freely within the dilator and not be forcibly turned to prevent damage to the needle tip or dilator. Occasionally, there is some resistance to the advance of the transseptal needle through the iliac vein or the inferior vena cava, particularly at the pelvic brim. Under these circumstances, the needle should not be forcibly advanced; instead, the needle with its stylet inside and the Mullins sheath should be advanced as a unit through the areas of resistance.

Once properly advanced to the tip of the Mullins dilator, the Brockenbrough needle is double-flushed, and the manometer line connected. To avoid confusion, we recommend displaying only this single pressure tracing, and on a 40–50 mmHg scale. At this point, proper orientation of the

assembly is critical. The side arm of the sheath and needle flange should always have the same orientation. Initially, they point horizontally and to the patient's left. This directs the tip of the apparatus medially in the anteroposterior fluoroscopic view. The entire system is then rotated clockwise until the needle flange arrow and sheath sidearm is positioned at 4 o'clock (with the patient's forehead representing 12 o'clock and the patient's occipital 6 o'clock). This directs the assembly to the left and slightly posterior.

Under anteroposterior fluoroscopy, the entire system is then withdrawn across three sequential landmark "bumps," or leftward movements of the needle. These landmark "bumps" represent the movement of the apparatus (1) as it enters the right atrium/superior vena cava junction, (2) as it moves over the ascending aorta where the tactile sensation of aortic pulsations aids in localization, and (3) as it passes over the limbus to intrude into the fossa ovalis. On a lateral view, the correct position for puncture of the apparatus is posterior and inferior to the aorta (marked by the pigtail catheter) (Figure 14.1).

The system is advanced (needle within the dilator) until further movement is limited by the limbus. In approximately 10% of cases, the foramen ovale is patent and the apparatus directly enters the left atrium. In the remainder, the tip of the Brockenbrough needle is advanced into the left atrium under continuous fluoroscopic and pressure monitoring. Care should be taken to advance only the tip of the needle and not the entire apparatus. Successful penetration of the septum is heralded by a change from right atrial to left atrial pressure waveform, accompanied by a small but definite lateral

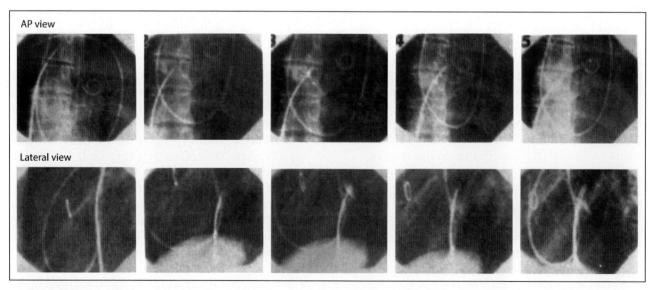

Figure 14.1 Simultaneous AP and lateral views during transseptal left heart catheterization. A pigtail catheter is positioned retrogradely in the right coronary sinus to correctly identify the aorta with the use of biplane fluoroscopy. Under anteroposterior fluoroscopy, the entire system is then withdrawn across three sequential landmark "bumps," or leftward movements of the needle. These landmark "bumps" represent movement of the apparatus (1) as it enters the right atrium/superior vena cava junction, (2) as it moves over the ascending aorta where the tactile sensation of aortic pulsations aids in localization, and (3) as it passes over the limbus to intrude into the fossa ovalis. On a lateral view, the correct position for puncture of the apparatus is posterior and inferior to the aorta.

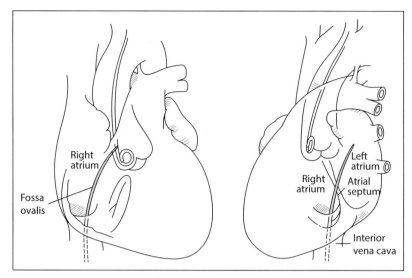

Figure 14.2 Under anteroposterior fluoroscopy, the entire system is then withdrawn across three sequential landmark "bumps," or leftward movements of the needle (right-side panel). On a lateral view, the correct position for puncture of the apparatus is posterior and inferior to the aorta (left-side panel). The proper orientation of the Mullins sheath/dilator in the left atrium after successful puncture of the interatrial septum: In the anteroposterior view (left), the sheath lies at the midportion of the right atrial silhouette. In the lateral view (right), it is located posterior and inferior to the aortic valve plane (demarcated by the pigtail catheter).

movement of the needle tip on fluoroscopy. A palpable "pop" may occur with septal penetration, confirmed by injecting contrast, which should flow freely into the left atrium. If the pressure tracing is damped, injection of contrast will aid in localizing the puncture site. If there is staining of the interatrial septum, the needle must be advanced farther. A stained septum must not be interpreted as failure and, in fact, the tattooed septum may indeed be used as a guide for future attempts. If the left atrium cannot be entered, the entire system must be withdrawn to the inferior vena cava/right atrial junction, the needle removed, and the J wire advanced through the Mullins system and repositioned in the superior vena cava for a second attempt. If there is aortic or pericardial staining, or the presence of an aortic pressure tracing, the tip of the needle must be removed and the patient reevaluated prior to a second attempt. If the procedure is being performed in preparation for percutaneous mitral balloon valvuloplasty or antegrade aortic balloon valvuloplasty, we generally postpone a second attempt for another day because the patient would need systemic anticoagulation. If the aorta is entered only with the needle (not the dilator) in a diagnostic transseptal puncture, where prolonged anticoagulation is not needed, the puncture may be attempted again.

The proper positioning of the needle after successful puncture is at the midportion of the right atrial silhouette in the anteroposterior view. In the lateral view, it lies posterior and inferior to the aortic valve plane, as demarcated by the pigtail catheter (Figure 14.2). Slight variations in the technique may be required in the presence of abnormal atrial or aortic anatomy and with different interventional procedures. In patients with left atrial enlargement, the septum lies more horizontally. The site of puncture is more posterior and inferior. In aortic valve disease accompanied by a dilated aorta, the septum is more vertical. The fossa ovalis and the puncture site are, therefore, more superior and slightly anterior. With right atrial enlargement, the transseptal apparatus may not reach to the septum. A gentle curve placed on the needle 10–15 cm

from the distal tip may allow engagement of the fossa ovalis. During double-balloon percutaneous mitral balloon valvuloplasty (PMV) or with antegrade percutaneous aortic balloon valvuloplasty (PAV), a low puncture site in the middle posterior third of the septum provides a straight pathway to the mitral orifice and apex of the left ventricle to facilitate manipulation of guide wires and catheters. A slightly higher puncture is preferred when using a single Inoue balloon to allow the straightest course for the flow-directed distal balloon through the mitral valve (Figure 14.3).

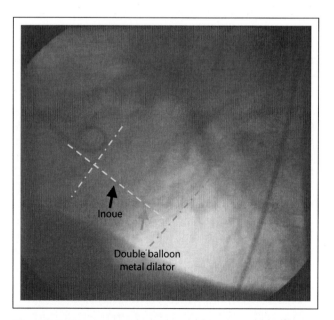

Figure 14.3 A transseptal puncture site according to planed procedure. The interatrial septum below the aortic knob identified by the pigtail in the right coronary cusp is divided into three thirds. The upper third is preferentially used for the Inoue technique, the middle third for the double-balloon technique of PMV and for antegrade aortic balloon valvuloplasty, while the lower third is preferentially used for the Cribier metallic dilator technique of PMV.

After successful septal puncture, the entire system is rotated counterclockwise to 3 o'clock and carefully advanced under fluoroscopic and hemodynamic guidance until it is certain the dilator lies within the left atrium. The needle is withdrawn into the dilator. The sheath is then advanced into the left atrium, keeping the needle within the sheath to avoid puncturing the left atrium. The needle and dilator are then removed and the sheath double-flushed prior to being connected to the manometer line. If the sheath has entered an inferior pulmonary vein, it must be withdrawn slightly with counterclockwise rotation to position it in the left atrium. Care should be taken after entering the left atrium with the needle. Perforation of the left atrial wall could occur if the system is advanced without careful pressure and fluoroscopic monitoring. If the left atrial pressure becomes damped, the apparatus may be against the left atrial wall and further advancement of the system could result in perforation and tamponade. Immediately after the completion of transseptal left heart catheterization, heparin, 5000 units, is administered intravenously.

Echocardiographic-assisted transseptal puncture

Traditionally (as described above), the location of the fossa ovalis, as the ideal transseptal puncture site, has been done by fluoroscopy. More recently, transesophageal (TEE) and intracardiac echocardiography (ICE) have been utilized to guide transseptal puncture.[12] TEE is particularly useful in locating and guiding the transseptal operator in site-specific interatrial septal puncture. Superior/inferior orientation of the transseptal puncture is best accomplished in the bicaval view (90°) and anterior/posterior orientation is seen best in the four-chamber view (0°). Immediately after septal puncture with the Brockenbrough needle, the left atrium entry can be confirmed by injecting agitated saline through the needle and visualizing bubbles in the left atrium. This offers added safety to the procedure, as the operator can confirm left atrial access prior to advancing the dilator and sheath. TEE is particularly helpful in procedures where site-specific interatrial septum puncture is mandatory, such as for the deployment of the MitraClip™ device (Abbott Vascular, Illinois, USA). When using the MitraClip device, the operator needs a superior-posterior transseptal approach in order to have "room" to manipulate the device in the left atrium and position the clip perfectly so as to "grab" the A2 and P2 portions of the mitral valve.

An echocardiographic-assisted transseptal can also be done using the ICE (AcuNavICE, Siemens Medical Systems, Mountain View, California, USA). During atrial septal puncture, ICE is able to locate the needle tip position precisely and provide a clear visualization of the "tenting effect" on the fossa ovalis. From the "home view" (where the tricuspid valve is visualized) posterior tilt and slight clockwise rotation of the catheter will commonly offer the operator an interatrial septal view that is comparable to the bicaval view for TEE (superior/inferior orientation). If further clockwise rotation of the catheter is performed, the short-axis view of the aorta will be displayed offering anterior/posterior orientation for transseptal puncture. In addition, ICE can also confirm successful entering of the left atrium by the injection of agitated saline solution through the transseptal needle.

Modified technique: Using an angioplasty guide wire for enhanced safety

This modified technique was described to address the issue of left atrial entry with a dilator and sheath after successful transseptal needle puncture.[13] Using the traditional technique described above, after successful puncture of the interatrial septum, the operator should turn the needle/sheath/dilator apparatus to a 3 o'clock orientation to safely enter the left atrium without damaging the left atrial appendage. In addition to entrance into the aorta (which can be avoided by confirming left atrial pressure tracing prior to advancing sheath and dilator), one of the most feared complications of transseptal puncture is posterior or free left atrial wall perforation/damage. This usually occurs when advancing the sheath/dilator unit after successful left atrial puncture by the needle. In theory, this can be avoided by assessing the heart shadow under fluoroscopy or pressure-tracing "dampening" while advancing the sheath/dilator unit. The proposed modified technique involves advancing a 0.014 inch angioplasty guide wire through the Brockenbrough needle immediately after the left atrial pressure confirms correct needle positioning in the LA. The angioplasty guide wire is then advanced into the left upper pulmonary vein in the anteroposterior x-ray projection (Figure 14.4). Using the angioplasty guide wire as a rail, the needle/sheath and dilator unit are advanced without significant concern into the body of the left atrium. This technique might be particularly useful in patients with smaller left atrial sizes (such as young patients with recurrent atrial fibrillation undergoing ablation), or in patients with a very redundant/"floppy" septum primum, or in patients with a scarred interatrial septum (status: post-multiple transseptals or post-cardiac surgery), where either small atrial volume or extensive manipulation of the transseptal apparatus is needed, respectively; thus, increasing the risk of left atrial perforation when advancing sheath/dilator unit.

Indications

In the past, in the majority of cases, transseptal catheterization was performed for diagnostic purposes. However,

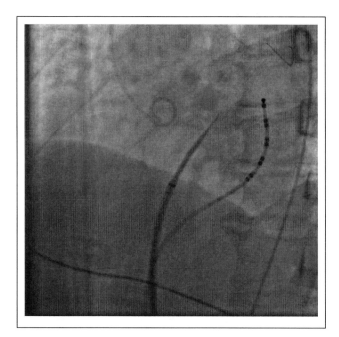

Figure 14.4 A lateral x-ray view showing advancement of the 0.014″ angioplasty guide wire through the transseptal needle into the left upper pulmonary vein.

today interventional procedures requiring access to the left atrium comprise a large group of patients in need for the transseptal technique.[10,11]

Transseptal left heart catheterization should be performed whenever direct measurement of left atrial pressure is needed (when accuracy of pulmonary capillary wedge pressure is questionable) or retrograde access to the left ventricle is unobtainable or dangerous. In patients with mitral stenosis and pulmonary artery hypertension, the true capillary wedge may be unobtainable or inaccurate[5,10,11,14] and there is a slightly higher incidence of pulmonary artery perforation with balloon floatation in the pulmonary arteries. In patients with prosthetic mitral valves, the pulmonary capillary wedge pressure may overestimate the diastolic gradient across the valve. A false mitral gradient could be the result of either the presence of pulmonary hypertension and/or a phase delay in the pulmonary wedge "v" waves, resulting in a higher mean diastolic gradient compared with the left atrial pressure obtained by transseptal catheterization (Figure 14.5). This may lead to the calculation of an erroneously small prosthetic mitral valve area and unnecessary repeated mitral valve surgery.[15] In mitral regurgitation, the regurgitant fraction can be quantified by injecting indocyanine green dye into the left ventricle and obtaining dye curves by sampling the left atrium and femoral artery.[14]

Aortic valvular disease or aortic valve replacement may preclude safe retrograde left ventricular catheterization. In patients with mechanical aortic valves, retrograde catheterization is not possible. Many cardiologists prefer

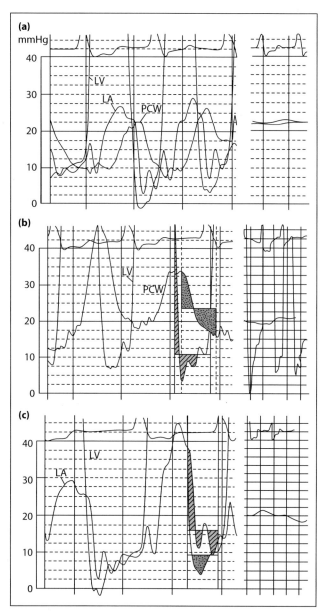

Figure 14.5 In patients with prosthetic mitral valves, the pulmonary capillary wedge pressure may overestimate the diastolic gradient across the valve. A false mitral gradient could be the result of either the presence of pulmonary hypertension and/or a phase delay in the pulmonary wedge "v" waves resulting in a higher mean diastolic gradient compared with the left atrial pressure obtained by transseptal catheterization. This may lead to the calculation of an erroneously small prosthetic mitral valve area and unnecessary repeat mitral valve surgery.

the transseptal technique in patients with bioprosthetic aortic valves or native aortic stenosis to avoid damaging the valve during catheterization. In critical aortic stenosis, the transaortic gradient is more reliable when left ventricular and ascending aortic pressures are measured simultaneously via transseptal puncture. When the valve area is 0.6 cm² or less, the catheter itself may significantly

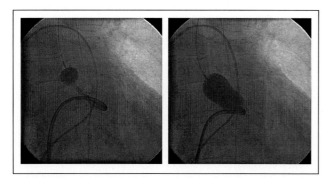

Figure 14.6   Antegrade aortic balloon valvuloplasty using the Inoue balloon catheter.

obstruct the orifice and falsely increase the recorded gradient[16] or result in transient hemodynamic deterioration. In heavily calcified valves, transseptal catheterization may avert possible dislodgement and embolization of calcium.[7] Transseptal left heart catheterization should be performed in patients with aortic valve replacements in whom evaluation of the aortic gradient or ventriculography is needed.

Other diagnostic uses for transseptal catheterization include aortic valve endocarditis where crossing the valve could be deleterious and the evaluation of dynamic left ventricular outflow obstruction, both allowing simultaneous recording of left ventricular and aortic pressures, and in distinguishing dynamic outflow obstruction from catheter entrapment. Transseptal catheterization allows direct measurement of left atrial pressure in mitral regurgitation, cor triatriatum, and pulmonary hypertension, and provides access for pulmonary vein angiography in evaluating pulmonary atresia and pulmonary veno-occlusive disease.[14]

The resurgence of interest in transseptal catheterization is a direct result of its role in interventional procedures. Transseptal catheterization is a prerequisite in percutaneous mitral valvuloplasty[17] and antegrade percutaneous aortic valvuloplasty[18] (Figure 14.6). Likewise, in the pediatric population, balloon atrial septostomy in the treatment of transposition of the great arteries, pulmonary atresia with intact ventricular septum, total anomalous pulmonary venous return, and tricuspid atresia each may require transseptal catheterization.[19]

Currently, the vast majority of radio-frequency ablations of left-sided bypass tracts are performed via retrograde left ventricular catheterization. However, successful ablation of left free wall, posteroseptal, and septal bypass tracts have been reported using a transseptal approach.[20] A transseptal approach may allow for the ablation of otherwise inaccessible pathways and, perhaps, may facilitate the procedure in some patients, reducing both their discomfort and radiation exposure.

Contraindications

Contraindications to transseptal catheterization include

1. Obstruction of the inferior vena cava (e.g., by tumor, thrombus, therapeutic ligation, or filter placement).
2. Systemic anticoagulation.
3. Bleeding diathesis.
4. Anatomic deformity such as severe kyphoscoliosis or patients with previous pneumonectomy resulting in severe rotation of the heart.
5. Congenital deformities resulting in obscured landmarks of the atrial septum.
6. Thrombus in the right or the left atrium documented by echocardiography. Patients with previous clinical emboli can have transseptal catheterization if they have been adequately anticoagulated with coumadin and the left atrium is free of thrombus by TEE.
7. Presence of atrial myxoma.
8. Patients with large right atrium represent a particular problem because of the flattening of the septum and sometimes the inability of the needle to touch the interatrial septum.

Complications

In part, the decline in the frequency of transseptal catheterization can be ascribed to concern over potentially lethal complications. Penetration of the inferior vena cava, atria, or aorta can occur and may lead to tamponade and/or death.[1,2,21,22] Earlier studies utilized a single anteroposterior fluoroscopic view and, in some series, used larger-gauge needles than today. Lateral fluoroscopy allows the visualization of the needle to place it posterior and inferior to the aortic valve plane, thus avoiding penetration of the aorta and an extreme posterior needle position, which risks left atrial perforation. Today, transseptal catheterization can be performed safely with low incidence of complications[5,7,10,11,14] that reflects operator experience and perhaps the addition of biplane fluoroscopy. Others, however, have reported low complication rates utilizing single-plane fluoroscopy.[3,4] The transseptal "needle tip only" can inadvertently puncture the atria or the aorta. However, adverse sequelae do not develop provided that this inadvertent puncture is immediately recognized before the apparatus is advanced further. In a series utilizing biplane fluoroscopy, inadvertent pericardial punctures occurred in 3/217 patients (1.4%) and none resulted in tamponade.[23] Several series have noted that in operations following uneventful transseptal catheterizations, blood-stained pericardial fluid is not infrequently present, implying unnoticed atrial puncture during the procedure.[22,24] Cardiac tamponade occurs with advancement of the larger dilator and not with inadvertent needle puncture. Cardiac tamponade occurs less frequently in patients with prior cardiac surgery, making transseptal catheterization safer in postoperative patients. Tamponade is less likely to occur because of the obliteration of the pericardial space by adhesions.[25]

Two-dimensional transthoracic, transesophageal, and intravascular echocardiography have been used as adjuncts to fluoroscopy to avoid such complications. The interatrial septum and aorta are best visualized in the apical four-chamber view and saline contrast allows localization of the needle before and after septal puncture.[26] Needle tip punctures are not eliminated, and occurred in 1 of 13 transseptal catheterizations (with no adverse sequelae).[24]

Systemic embolization is another grave complication of transseptal catheterization. Cerebral emboli are most frequently reported, but emboli to coronary, splanchnic, renal, and femoral arteries have occurred.[1-4,21-28] We do not routinely order echocardiograms prior to diagnostic transseptal catheterization unless the patient is at high risk for an atrial thrombus (e.g., atrial fibrillation, mitral stenosis). As part of the evaluation for percutaneous mitral valvuloplasty, patients obtain an echocardiogram to visualize the atrial appendage and the presence of thrombus, as well as to be ranked by echo score.[1] Transseptal catheterization in the presence of a nonechogenic atrial myoxoma has resulted in tamponade.[29] It is also conceivable that not all thrombi are visible by echo. In addition to thrombus, embolization of air to the coronary and cerebral vessels has occurred,[29] as well as embolization of a perforated guide catheter, later discovered in the left popliteal artery.[21] Bleeding and vasovagal reactions occur more frequently, but are more easily managed.

Early studies utilized a single anteroposterior view, accounting for higher morbidity and mortality than occurs today. Lateral fluoroscopy allows orientation of the catheter posterior and inferior to the aorta and reduces inadvertent penetration of the aorta and left atrium. A high success rate has been reported using modified single-plane fluoroscopy. A right anterior oblique (40–50°) view provides an end-face view of the atrial septum and defines the inferior, posterior, and superior borders of the right atrium. A pigtail in the aorta demarcates its posterior wall and the level of the aortic valve. The recommended point of puncture lies midway between the posterior borders of the right atrium and aorta, and 1–3 cm below the aortic valve.[3] Using this technique, atrial puncture occurred in 2/118 (1.7%) and cardiac tamponade in 1/106 (0.9%), for an overall inadvertent puncture rate of 1.3%.[6,7] This suggests a marked improvement over previous series relying solely on anteroposterior fluoroscopy, but higher numbers are needed before definite conclusions can be drawn. The modified technique offers no advantage over biplane fluoroscopy, although it has been suggested that it may be more appropriate for less-experienced, "low-volume" operators because it provides a greater margin of safety in terms of locating the area of septal puncture.[3]

Several authors have suggested that there is a "learning curve" for transseptal catheterization, and that the majority of complications occur in the first 25–50 procedures.[14,29,30] Even at a leading academic catheterization laboratory, the technique had to be "relearned" for percutaneous mitral valvuloplasty, resulting in 2/61 (3.3%) incidence of tamponade resulting from transseptal catheterization.[31] A higher rate of complications has been noted when the procedure is not regularly performed.[32]

The rate of unsuccessful attempts at transseptal catheterizations also varies with operator experience. Inability to engage the septum in up to 1.4–7% of attempts has been reported, varying with different patient populations.[23,24,33,34]

In conclusion, transseptal left heart catheterization remains an important skill of the interventional cardiologist. Although for diagnostic purposes the technique is less requested than in the past, it remains a necessity in percutaneous mitral valvuloplasty, antegrade percutaneous aortic valvuloplasty, and atrioseptostomy, and may offer advantages in radio-frequency ablation of left-sided pathways. In the proper hands, and with the proper equipment, there is little additional risk over routine left heart catheterization. Experienced operators are essential in assuring low morbidity and mortality.

References

1. Braunwald E. Transseptal left heart catheterization. *Circulation* 1968;37(Suppl III):74–9.
2. Nixon PGF, Ikram H. Left heart catheterization with special reference of the transeptal method. *Br Heart J* 1965;28:835–41.
3. Croft CH, Lipscomb K. Modified technique of transseptal left heart catheterization. *J Am Coll Cardiol* 1985;5:904–10.
4. Doorey AJ, Goldenberg EM. Transseptal catheterization in adults: Enhanced efficiency and safety by low-volume operators using a "non-standard" technique. *Catheter Cardiovasc Diag* 1991;8:535–42.
5. Dunn M. Is transseptal catheterization necessary? *J Am Coll Cardiol* 1985;6:1393–4.
6. Swan HJC, Ganz W, Forrester J, Marcus H, Diamond G, Chonette D. Catheterization of the heart in man with use of a flow directed balloon-tipped catheter. *N Engl J Med* 1970;283:447–51.
7. Schoonmaker FW, Vijay NK, Jantz RD. Left atrial and ventricular transseptal catheterization review: Losing skills? *Catheter Cardiovasc Diag* 1987;13:233–8.
8. Lundovist CB, Olsson SB, Varnauskas E. Transseptal left heart catheterization: A review of 278 studies. *Clin Cardiol* 1986;9:21–6.
9. Baim DS, Grossman W. Percutaneous approach, including transseptal catheterization and apical left ventricular puncture in cardiac catheterization, angiography and intervention, 1991.
10. Clugston R, Lau FYK, Ruiz C. Transseptal catheterization update 1992. *Catheter Cardiovasc Diag* 1992;26:266–74.
11. Roelke M, Smith AJC, Palacios IF. The technique and safety of transseptal left heart catheterization. The Massachusetts General Hospital experience with 1,279 procedures. *Catheter Cardiovasc Diag* 1994;32:332–9.
12. Babaliaros VC, Green JT, Lerakis S, Lloyd M, Block PC. Emerging applications for transseptal left heart catheterization old techniques for new procedures. *J Am Coll Cardiol* 2008;51(22):2116–22.

13. Hildick-Smith D, McCready J, de Giovanni J. Transseptal puncture: Use of an angioplasty guidewire for enhanced safety catheterization and cardiovascular interventions. 2007;69:519–21.

14. O'Keefe JH, Vlietstra MB, Hanley PC, Seward JB. Revival of the transseptal approach for catheterization of the left atrium and ventricle. *Mayo Clin Proc* 1985;60:790–5.

15. Schoenfield MH, Palacios IF, Jutter AM, Jacoby SS, Block PC. Underestimation of prosthetic mitral valve areas: Role of transseptal catheterization in avoiding unnecessary repeat mitral valve surgery. *J Am Coll Cardiol* 1985;5:1387–92.

16. Carabello BA, Barry WH, Grossman W. Changes in arterial pressure during left heart pullback in patients with aortic stenosis: A sign of severe aortic stenosis. *Am J Cardiol* 1979;44:424–7.

17. Palacios IF. Techniques of balloon valvotomy for mitral stenosis. In: Robicsek F. Ed. *Cardiac Surgery: State of the Art Reviews.* Philadelphia, PA: Hanley R Belfus; 1991. pp. 229–38.

18. Block PC, Palacios I. Comparison of hemodynamic results of antegrade versus retrograde percutaneous balloon aortic valvuloplasty. *Am J Cardiol* 1987;60:659–62.

19. Rashkind WJ. Transcatheter treatment of congenital heart disease. *Circulation* 1983;67:711–6.

20. Saul JP, Hulse JE, Hulse E et al. Catheter ablation of accessory atrioventricular pathways in young patients: Use of long vascular sheaths, the transseptal approach, and a retrograde left posterior parallel approach. *J Am Coll Cardiol* 1993;21:571–83.

21. Lindeneg O, Hansen AT. Complication in transseptal left heart catheterization. *Acta Med Scand* 1966;180:395–9.

22. Adrouny AZ, Sutherland DW, Griswold HE, Ritzman LW. Complications with transseptal left heart catheterization. *Am Heart J* 1963;65:327–33.

23. Ali Khan MA, Mulins CE, Bash SE, Al Yousef S, Nihill MR, Sawyer W. Transseptal left heart catheterisation in infants, children, and young adults. *Catheter Cardiovasc Diag* 1989;17:198–201.

24. Singleton RT, Scherlis L. Transseptal catheterization of the left heart: Observations in 56 patients. *Am Heart J* 1960;60(6):879–85.

25. Folland ED, Oprian C, Giancomini J et al. Complications of cardiac catheterization and angiography in patients with valvular heart disease. *Catheter Cardiovasc Diag* 1989;17:15–21.

26. Kronzon I, Glassman E, Cohen M, Winer H. Use of two-dimensional echocardiography during transseptal cardiac catheterization. *J Am Coll Cardiol* 1984;4(2):425–8.

27. Libanoff AJ, Silver AW. Complications of transseptal left heart catheterization. *Am J Cardiol* 1965;16:390–3.

28. Peckham GB, Chrysohou A, Aldridge H, Wigle ED. Combined percutaneous retrograde aortic and transseptal left heart catheterization. *Br Heart J* 1964;26:460–8.

29. Henderson MA. Transseptal left atrial catheterization (letter). *Catheter Cardiovasc Diag* 1990;21:63.

30. Laskey WK, Kusiak V, Unkreter WJ, Hirshfield JW Jr. Transseptal left heart catheterization: Utility of a sheath technique. *Catheter Cardiovasc Diag* 1982;8:535–42.

31. Wyman RM, Safian RD, Portway V, Skillman JJ, Mckay RG, Baim DS. Current complications of diagnostic and therapeutic cardiac catheterization. *J Am Coll Cardiol* 1988;12:1400–6.

32. Lew AS, Harper RW, Federman J, Anderson ST, Pitt A. Recent experience with transseptal catheterization. *Catheter Cardiovasc Diag* 1983;9:601.

33. Gordon JB, Folland ED. Analysis of aortic valve gradients by transseptal technique: Implications for noninvasive evaluation. *Catheter Cardiovasc Diag* 1989;17:144–51.

34. Weiner RI, Maranhao V. Development and application of transseptal left heart catheterization. *Catheter Cardiovasc Diag* 1988;15:112–120.

15

Percutaneous transapical access

Robert Kumar, Chad Kliger, Vladimir Jelnin, and Carlos E. Ruiz

Good people often reinvent a procedure that has already been invented, when there is a need for it and when the times are ripe for it.

WJ Kolff[1]

Introduction

Percutaneous entry into the left ventricle (LV) from a transapical approach through the intact chest wall provides a simple, direct route of access to many cardiac structures, and can be successfully utilized for a variety of diagnostic and interventional procedures for patients with structural heart disease (SHD). Transapical ventricular access methods can be divided into surgical access and closure via a lateral thoracotomy, percutaneous entry with surgical closure, and entirely percutaneous entry and closure. Successful percutaneous transapical access has been described for delivery of sheaths up to 12 Fr,[2] and will be described here in detail.

The feasibility of percutaneous transapical access for hemodynamic assessment in patients with aortic stenosis was described as early as the 1950s.[3] In 1964, Levy and Lillehei reported their results of transapical LV puncture in 122 patients with aortic stenosis using a 17–21 gauge Teflon catheter, with one procedural death related to contrast injection into the myocardium.[4] In the 1980s, transapical access was described as a means to obtain intraventricular pressures in patients with mechanical mitral prosthetic valves and aortic stenosis, in whom the LV was difficult to enter from a retrograde aortic approach, and a transseptal approach posed a risk of catheter entrapment within the mechanical prosthesis.[5] These authors reported a complication rate similar to that of using a transseptal approach.

Transapical access for purely hemodynamic assessment has become infrequent due to improved noninvasive hemodynamic assessment with Doppler echocardiography and newer invasive methods of hemodynamic assessment such as high-fidelity pressure wires that can be used to cross mechanical prosthetic valves.[6,7] Recently, there has been increasing interest in the use of transapical access for

cardiac structural interventions, with advances in imaging and device technology expanding the applicability of this approach. A thorough understanding of the access technique and the management of potential complications are necessary prior to adopting transapical access into clinical practice.

To date, percutaneous transapical access has been utilized for numerous interventional procedures, including paravalvular leak closure, pseudoaneurysm closure, and ventricular septal defect closure. Additionally, transapical access can be used for the creation of a "rail-wire" to facilitate sheath and device delivery, a technique potentially helpful for transcatheter mitral valve therapies. With future advancements in technology, in particular dedicated transapical closure devices, and new techniques for multimodality imaging fusion, the applicability of percutaneous transapical access may continue to expand.

Case selection

Transapical access can provide entry into the left ventricle with favorable characteristics for successful SHD intervention. Many SHD defects are located within the left ventricle at locations that make guide-wire crossing or device delivery difficult from an antegrade transseptal or retrograde transaortic approach due to unfavorable angles for entry (Figure 15.1). In addition, the direction and tortuosity of a defect tract, dense calcification surrounding the target lesion, or the presence of prosthetic heart valves may introduce additional challenges. In other cases, severe peripheral atherosclerotic disease may limit safe access through a peripheral artery approach, and transapical access may offer a safe alternative route of ventricular entry. Overall, any SHD defect in communication with the LV can be approached using transapical access. In appropriately selected cases, a transapical approach may provide superior equipment deliverability and control and result in reduced fluoroscopy time and increased procedural success rates.

All cases being considered for a transapical procedure should be discussed with a multidisciplinary team

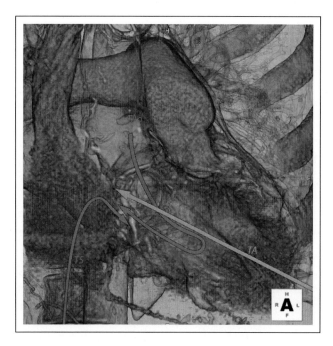

Figure 15.1 (**See color insert.**) In this example, a 3-D volume-rendered CTA image depicts a target lesion near the mitral valve with unfavorable angles for wire crossing and device delivery through a retrograde aortic (TAo) or transseptal approach (TS) (red arrows). Alternatively, transapical access (TA) offers a more direct approach to the target lesion (green arrow).

that includes interventional cardiologists, cardiothoracic surgeons, imaging specialists, and an anesthesiologist. Patients should be deemed high risk for surgical intervention and all potential approaches thoroughly considered prior to undergoing a transapical intervention.

Contraindications

Transapical access is associated with a small but significant risk of serious complications and should be chosen in carefully selected patients.[2,4] Prior to undergoing a transapical procedure, the patient should undergo a complete history and physical examination. A detailed history should be obtained that includes prior cardiothoracic surgery and time since the last surgery, prior chest radiation, presence of a bleeding diathesis, and degree of pulmonary hypertension. The chest wall should be examined by thorough inspection and palpation, with any deformity impeding entry identified.

The majority of our experiences with percutaneous transapical access is in patients with prior cardiothoracic surgery. Patients with prior thoracic surgery may have disrupted pericardium, which may reduce the potential for tamponade. Even in cases with surgical preservation of the pericardium, the presence of adhesions may reduce the risk of bleeding at or around the transapical puncture site. CT surgery less than 3 months prior to planned transapical

puncture may place the patient at higher bleeding risk, and alternative access routes or surgical closure should be considered.

The presence of a bleeding diathesis, or hypocoaguable state, also places the patient at increased risk of bleeding and procedural-related complications. Whether congenital or acquired, alternative access should be considered in the presence of a hypocoaguable state. Thrombocytopenia, with a platelet count less than 50,000/mm³ is a contraindication due to bleeding risk. Low-molecular-weight heparins and oral anticoagulants should be discontinued prior to the procedure, with a goal International Normalized Ratio (INR) less than 1.5. When an anticoagulant lacks reliable laboratory assessment, the anticoagulant must be discontinued with sufficient time for drug elimination and unfractionated heparin can be utilized as a bridge when necessary. Several patients undergoing transapical access have been treated with aspirin and clopidogrel, but safety with the use of alternative antiplatelet agents remains unclear.

Pulmonary hypertension with pulmonary artery pressures greater than two-thirds systemic pressure is an additional contraindication for the transapical approach. In our experience, the only procedural mortality occurred in a patient with suprasystemic pulmonary hypertension who developed electromechanical dissociation.

The use of chronic steroid therapy or immunosuppressants may result in reduced tissue integrity and impaired wound healing, making safe percutaneous transapical closure a challenge in these patients.

Preprocedural imaging

Multimodality imaging assessment must be performed to obtain the necessary information for procedural planning of transapical access. 2-D and 3-D transthoracic and transesophageal echocardiography (TTE/TEE), utilizing real-time 3-D zoom and full-volume acquisition with color flow provides assessment of ventricular chamber size, myocardial wall thickness, and the presence of wall motion abnormalities. Areas of thinned, scarred myocardium and focal wall motion abnormalities near the site of transapical access should be avoided during directed puncture. In addition, the presence of apical thrombus is a contraindication to a transapical procedure and can be assessed for by TTE/TEE, with the additional use of an echo contrast agent for improved visualization of thrombus when suspected.

Baseline pleural and pericardial effusions are also important to identify when present. Consideration should be made for the placement of preprocedure drains with planned maintenance during the short term for postprocedural management. Furthermore, echocardiography provides detailed information regarding the intended structural heart defect, including size, location, and its relationship to surrounding structures (Figure 15.2a).

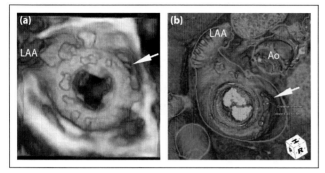

Figure 15.2 (**See color insert.**) (a) 3-D TEE demonstrates the presence of a prosthetic mitral valve with a paravalvular leak (white arrow). Defect size, location in relation to the prosthetic valve, and relationship to surrounding structures are identified. The left atrial appendage (LAA) can be used as a reference point for identifying the location of the leak. (b) A 3-D volume-rendered CTA image in a similar projection as the TEE image in (a), showing the mitral paravalvular leak (white arrow) and surrounding structures. Measurements can be made for device selection and sizing. Based on the location of the defect, an access route can be chosen.

Cardiac-computed tomographic angiography (CTA) has evolved to be a useful tool for procedural planning in SHD interventions. Helical CTA with retrospective ECG gating and multiphase reconstruction can generate 3-D and 4-D volume-rendered images from which the spatial orientation of the target lesion and surrounding structures can be identified, and measurements can be accurately performed (Figure 15.2b). A thorough understanding of the anatomic relationships of the cardiac apex, papillary muscles, coronary arteries, lung, and ribs is necessary prior to obtaining transapical access and can easily be assessed by CTA (Figure 15.3b). The distance from the skin surface to the left ventricular apex can be accurately measured by CTA, and the intercostal space with the optimal location and angle of entry from the chest wall to the apex can be determined. A puncture site should be chosen at a safe distance from the lung and coronary arteries while remaining coaxial to the target lesion. The sternum may be used as a reference point, and the distance from the sternum to the planned puncture site can be measured and used for access guidance (Figure 15.3a). From our experience, CTA imaging is essential for safe planning and guidance and should be utilized for all transapical procedures.

Percutaneous ventricular access technique

Patient preparation

Percutaneous left ventricular access can be performed in a standard cardiac catheterization lab or in a hybrid operating room equipped with C-arm fluoroscopy. The procedure

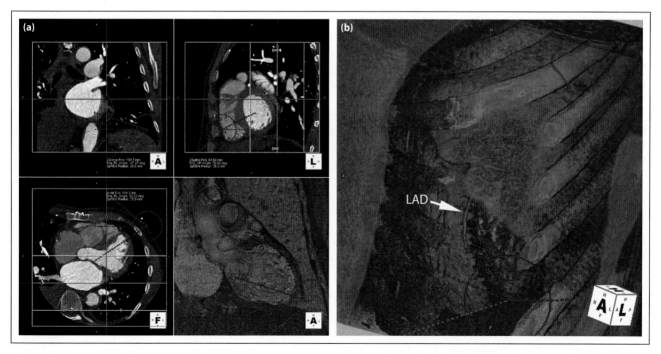

Figure 15.3 (**See color insert.**) (a) Helical CTA images can be viewed in multiple planes and with 3-D reconstruction to identify an optimal puncture site and angle of entry that is coaxial to the target lesion. The distance from the skin surface to the left ventricle can be measured by CTA. The distance from the sternum to the planned puncture site can be measured as a reference for guiding access. (b) 3-D volume-rendered CTA images are used to assess the location of coronary arteries (left anterior descending artery, white arrow) and lung tissue to avoid inadvertent puncture during transapical access. The rib interspace through which the ventricle will be accessed can be identified.

is performed with the patient intubated and sedated under general anesthesia. Equipment for management of complications and surgical bailout should be readily available in the laboratory prior to starting the procedure. A full TEE assessment should be performed in the intubated patient prior to obtaining transapical access to obtain baseline hemodynamics, document the presence and size of pleural and pericardial effusions, and confirm the characteristics of the structural defect. All aspects of the procedure thereafter should be performed under real-time TEE guidance in addition to live fluoroscopy.

After the patient is sedated, an arterial line should be placed for hemodynamic monitoring. In cases of significant pulmonary hypertension, a pulmonary artery catheter may be inserted for additional monitoring. Radiolucent defibrillator pads should be placed on the chest and back. The patient should then be prepped in sterile fashion from the clavicles to the groin, and the chest wall should be thoroughly cleansed with clorhexidine and covered with an antimicrobial incise drape (Ioban, 3M, St. Paul, MN, USA). It is often helpful to position the patient with the arms elevated, perpendicular to the table, and the elbows bent at 90°, with careful attention to positioning to avoid nerve injury. This position provides excellent exposure of the chest wall, but limits cranial angulation of the image intensifier. Alternatively, the patient may be placed with the arms down alongside the patient if the arms do not obscure the skin entry point, usually anterior to the anterior axillary line. Placing the arms at the side of the patient, however, may cause a slight change in the position of thoracic structures in relation to the ribs and decrease the accuracy of measurements obtained from a preprocedural CTA. After the patient is properly positioned and prepped, the exact location of skin entry for apical access should be identified. The distance from the sternum to the ventricular apex on the skin surface can be measured from the preprocedure CTA and confirmed with manual palpation of the point of maximal impulse. The skin can be marked accordingly.

Fusion imaging guidance

If the catheterization laboratory is sufficiently equipped, CTA imaging obtained prior to the procedure can be used for CT-fluoroscopy fusion guidance using specialized software. Details of CT-fluoroscopy fusion guidance are discussed in detail in Chapter 8.

Briefly, CT-fluoroscopy fusion involves 3-D reconstruction of preprocedural CTA data. The cardiac structures are 3-D volume rendered and automatically segmented to identify the left atrium, left ventricle, and aorta. Segmentation of the coronary arteries (specifically, the left anterior descending artery with diagonal branches), lungs, and ribs is performed manually. Subsequently, the images are analyzed and the transapical puncture site is determined with

the skin and left ventricle entry aligned to the SHD defect, away from lung parenchyma, coronary arteries, and papillary muscles. Key transapical access landmarks are placed to identify three points: skin entry, left ventricle epicardial entry, and the SHD defect that requires intervention.

The CTA images are then registered to contrast-enhanced fluoroscopy of the aorta or fixed internal radiopaque markers in the chest, such as a prosthetic heart valve, and overlaid onto live fluoroscopy (Figure 15.4a–c).[8]

If CT-fluoroscopy fusion-imaging software is unavailable, CTA images in equivalent angulations can be projected on a monitor adjacent to the fluoroscopic image to help guide ventricular access. TTE imaging at the apex with the probe in a sterile sleeve can also provide imaging guidance during transapical access. If there is concern for coronary artery puncture, a left coronary angiogram can be performed to identify the course of the left anterior descending (LAD) and diagonal branches (Figure 15.5). When concern for lung trauma exists, the anesthesiologist may choose to intubate the patient with a double-lumen endotracheal tube that allows selective deflation of the left lung to avoid lung puncture during ventricular access.

Technique

After the puncture site has been determined, the skin is then entered at the predetermined location using a 21-gauge micropuncture needle (7 cm), which is guided toward the site of LV epicardial entry. Larger needles (e.g., Chiba 16 cm, St. Jude Medical, St Paul, MN, USA) may be necessary with an LV myocardial depth of greater than 5 cm from the skin surface. A 3-cc syringe filled with contrast attached to the needle can be used to confirm intraventricular location of the needle. A 0.018 inch guide wire is then advanced into the left ventricle, then into the left atrium or aorta, with the position of the wire confirmed by fluoroscopy and TEE. A 5 or 6 Fr radial sheath (Cook Medical, Bloomington, IN, USA) is then advanced into the left ventricle directly over the 0.018 inch guide wire, and upsized to a 7–12 Fr sheath as needed for the procedure (Figure 15.4d). Alternatively, the 0.018 inch guide wire can be upsized to a 0.035 inch guide wire using a micropuncture kit, and a braided sheath of appropriate size such as a Raabe sheath (Cook Medical) can be directly used. Multiple sheath exchanges increase the risk of access site-related bleeding and should be minimized. 6–8 Fr sheaths are used routinely for device delivery, and sheaths up to 12 Fr have been used successfully without surgical exposure.[2] After the sheath is placed, intravenous heparin is administered at a dose of 70–100 units per kilogram. An activated clotting time of greater than 250 s is maintained for the duration of the procedure until all devices have been deployed in the target lesion.

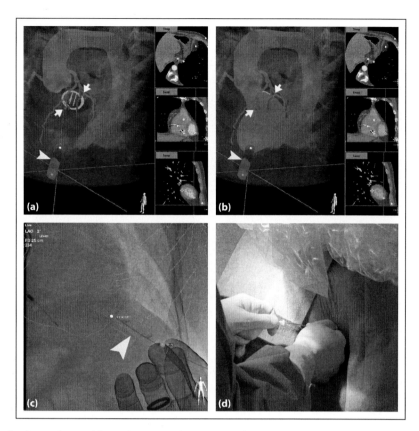

Figure 15.4 (**See color insert.**) CT guidance for transapical access. (a) 3-D volume-rendered CT images are segmented to identify relevant structures: aorta and coronary arteries (red) and mitral valve prosthesis (orange). Two mitral paravalvular leaks (PVL) are marked (red dots). The skin and ventricular planned puncture sites are marked (skin—green dot, left ventricle—white dot). A cylinder is manually constructed to connect the skin and ventricular entry points (yellow arrow). (b) The left ventricle (purple) is added to the image to show the relationship of the ventricle to the skin and ventricular puncture sites. (c) After the CT data have been registered to the fluoroscopic images, an outline of the left ventricle and the cylinder containing the skin and ventricular puncture sites (skin—green dot, left ventricle—white dot) are overlaid onto the fluoroscopy screen and used for access guidance. (d) After a 0.018 inch guide wire has been advanced into the left ventricle, a sheath is advanced over the wire. In this case, a 4 Fr micropuncture sheath is being used to exchange the guide wire for a 0.035 inch guide wire, and a larger sheath will then be advanced over the 0.035 inch guide wire.

Access closure

Traditional surgical technique

Access to the left ventricular apex is gained through a left anterolateral mini-thoracotomy, typically between the 5th and 6th intercostals space. Two purse-string pledgeted sutures placed within the apical myocardium, away from the coronary vasculature, are used to close the site of TA entry. The pericardium, if present, can be partially closed over the apex and a left lateral chest tube inserted. The intercostal incision is closed in a standard fashion.

Percutaneous technique

The proper closure of the apical access site is instrumental to minimizing bleeding complications. Sheath sizes smaller than 5 Fr may not require a closure device, though our current practice is to routinely use a closure

device regardless of sheath size. While there is currently no FDA-approved device for apical closure, several devices have been successfully used "off-label" to close the apex percutaneously. These devices have included embolization coils (Cook Medical) and several of the Amplatzer family of closure devices (St. Jude Medical)—muscular ventricular septal defect (mVSD), Amplatzer vascular plug II (AVP), and Amplatzer ductal occluder (ADO) devices. The largest reported experience is with the 6-4 ADO, which is most commonly used in our laboratory.[2] After all devices for treatment of the target lesion have been deployed, anticoagulation is reversed with intravenous protamine. The transapical access site should be closed when the activated clotting time is less than 170 s. If using an ADO for closure, the device is advanced through the sheath into the left ventricle, and the disk configured just distal to the sheath. The sheath and ADO are then withdrawn carefully, and a contrast injection through the sheath will identify when the sheath is in the pericardial space with

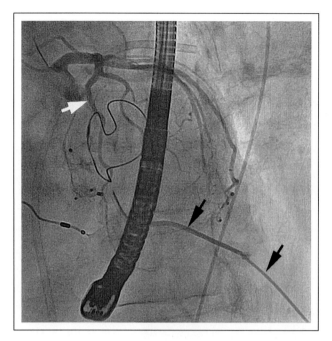

Figure 15.5 A left coronary angiogram can be performed to identify the course of the coronary arteries during transapical access. A catheter is advanced into the ventricle (black arrows) avoiding the LAD (white arrow) or its branches.

the device secured against the inner wall of the myocardium (Figure 15.6a–c). Elongation of the device body within the myocardium and systolic compression should be noted. The device is then released with the stem of the device secure within the myocardium. Next, the sheath and delivery cable are removed and the soft tissue track is quickly sealed with injection of a foam hemostatic matrix

(SurgiFlo, Johnson & Johnson, New Brunswick, NJ, USA). Finally, TEE and fluoroscopy should be used to confirm the stable position of all devices.

Multiple transapical access

Repeat SHD interventions using transapical access can be performed. In addition, double transapical access for simultaneous deployment of devices can be performed if necessary. It is important, however, to maintain a safe distance between transapical entry points, such that two distinct punctures are available for closure without interference between closure devices. While our experience has not resulted in any adverse events due to multiple LV access sites (up to three transapical accesses in a single patient have been performed), avoiding multiple LV accesses is reasonable when possible due to limited long-term data.

Structural heart disease procedures using percutaneous transapical access

The largest experience of SHD interventions using fully percutaneous transapical access is with paravalvular leak repairs. Several other procedure types have been successfully performed with percutaneous transapical access, including ventricular septal defect closure, pseudoaneurysm closure, and externalizing guide wires from the left ventricle to create a "rail-wire" for device delivery from an antegrade transseptal or retrograde transaortic approach. In general, procedures performed from a transapical

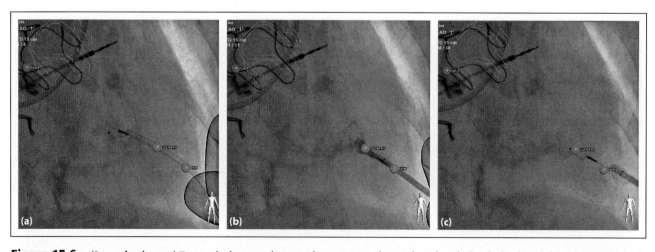

Figure 15.6 (**See color insert.**) Transapical access closure using a 6-4 Amplazter ductal occluder device (ADO). (a) The ADO device is advanced through the sheath into the left ventricle. The skin and left ventricular entry points (green dots) are identified using CT overlay imaging, as are the mitral prosthetic valve frame (orange) and the mitral paravalvular leak with closure devices in place (red dot). (b) The sheath and ADO are withdrawn until the sheath is in the pericardial space and the disk of the ADO device is secure against the inner wall of the myocardium. The position of the sheath is confirmed by contrast injection. (c) After the device is properly positioned, the sheath is withdrawn and the ADO is released.

approach are performed in a similar fashion to a transseptal or transaortic approach, though shorter catheters and guide wires may be used. Often, a stiff wire such as the Inoue wire (Toray Industries, New York, NY, USA) is placed in the left atrium after obtaining transapical access and left in place as a "safety wire" until device deployment to prevent loss of the transapical access site during device and wire manipulation. If transapical access is used for the creation of a rail-wire, a guide wire from a peripheral access site is placed in the left atrium or aorta, and snared using an endovascular snare advanced through a JR4 catheter from the transapical access site, or vice versa. The snared wire is then externalized through the secondary access site and used as a "rail" to secure delivery of a closure device or transcatheter valve (Figure 15.7a–d). Delivery of the therapeutic device, especially large-diameter devices, is usually done through the peripheral access site to avoid larger transapical sheath sizes.

Complications

Intraprocedural complications from interventions using transapical access have been reported as high as 25%,[9] and may include coronary artery laceration, lung trauma, right ventricular puncture, pericardial effusion or tamponade, hemothorax, and death. Coronary laceration can be avoided with CT-imaging guidance and coronary angiography when obtaining transapical access, but if laceration occurs, the patient may require placement of a covered stent or coil embolization. Emergent surgery for coronary repair may be necessary if the laceration is too distal for percutaneous treatment. Hemothorax is the most frequent reported complication[9] and may be due to bleeding from the LV puncture site or arterial laceration. TEE will identify the presence of hemothorax during the procedure, which can then be treated with emergent chest tube insertion under fluoroscopic guidance. Hemothorax

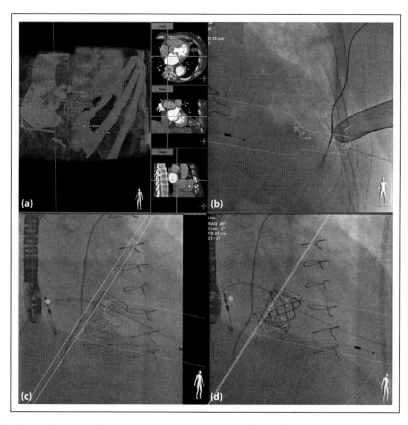

Figure 15.7 (**See color insert.**) Transapical access for a mitral valve-in-valve implantation in a patient with a degenerated mitral valve prosthesis. (a) 3-D volume-rendered CTA images are segmented to identify the aorta and coronary arteries (red), left atrium (orange), ribs (magenta), and partial left lung (blue). The planned transseptal puncture location (gray dot) and LV and skin entry points (green dots) are marked. The frame of the mitral valve prosthesis is identified (green outline). (b) After the CTA images are registered to fluoroscopy, transapical access is obtained with a micropuncture needle at the previously identified skin entry site (green dot), at an angle coaxial to the mitral valve. A manually constructed cylinder from the CTA data (green outline) connecting the skin entry to the mitral valve is overlaid onto the fluoroscopy screen and used to guide LV puncture. (c) After obtaining transseptal and transapical access (blue dot—transseptal puncture site), a guide wire is snared and exteriorized. A catheter is advanced over the rail-wire across the mitral valve. (d) A Melody transcatheter valve (Medtronic, Minneapolis, MN, USA) is successfully deployed within the frame of the degenerated mitral valve prosthesis over the rail-wire.

may also develop postprocedure and can be identified by chest x-ray. Thoracentesis, chest tube placement, or thoracotomy may be required. Pericardial effusion can occur from bleeding at the LV puncture site and can be quickly recognized by TEE or hemodynamic instability if tamponade develops. In this situation, emergent pericardiocentesis should be performed. As previously mentioned, it is important to note that all patients undergoing transapical interventions at our institution had prior cardiac surgery, and postsurgical adhesions and disrupted pericardium may decrease the chance for tamponade to develop. The presence of intact pericardium on preprocedural CTA may be determined prior to transapical interventions. In the event of unsuccessful closure device deployment and loss of the transapical access route, emergent surgical closure via a lateral thoracotomy should be performed. In our experience, the single procedural death was due to electromechanical dissociation in a patient with severe pulmonary hypertension, though the exact mechanism of electrical instability remains undetermined. Finally, it should be noted that there is no data on complication rates for transapical SHD interventions in patients without prior cardiac surgery, and reported outcomes for transapical interventions cannot be extrapolated to a nonsurgical population.

Conclusions and future directions

With proper preprocedural planning and careful access and closure technique, percutaneous transapical access offers a safe access route for performing complex structural interventions. The advantages of using a transapical access route may include reduced fluoroscopy time,[2] superior device control and positioning, and increased procedural success rates. As device technology improves, a greater number of procedures may be able to be performed using a fully percutaneous transapical approach, including

transcatheter aortic and mitral valve therapies, and even right-sided interventions for tricuspid and pulmonic valve disease. Dedicated access closure devices are currently being tested that may simplify transapical procedures and reduce complication rates. Advances in device technology and new imaging technologies, such as multimodality imaging fusion, will allow a greater number of operators to successfully adopt percutaneous transapical access for structural heart disease interventions, and the ventricular apex may well become the "optimal gateway" to the heart.

References

1. Kolff WJ, Norman JC. Transapical left ventricular bypass. *Chest* 1971;60:110–1.
2. Jelnin V, Dudiy Y, Einhorn BN et al. Clinical experience with percutaneous left ventricular transapical access for interventions in structural heart defects: A safe access and secure exit. *J Am Coll Cardiol* 2011;4:868–74.
3. Brock R, Milstein BB, Ross DN. Percutaneous left ventricular puncture in the assessment of aortic stenosis. *Thorax* 1956;11:163–71.
4. Levy MJ, Lillehei CW. Percutaneous direct cardiac catheterization—A new method, with results in 122 patients. *N Engl J Med* 1964;271:273–80.
5. Morgan JM, Gray HH, Gelder C et al. Left heart catheterization by direct ventricular puncture: Withstanding the test of time. *Catheter Cardiovasc Diagn* 1989;16:87–90.
6. Parham W, Shafei A, Rajjoub H et al. Retrograde left ventricular hemodynamic assessment across bileaflet prosthetic aortic valves: The use of a high-fidelity pressure sensor angioplasty guidewire. *Catheter Cardiovasc Interv* 2003;59:509–13.
7. Jang-Ho B., Lerman A, Yang E et al. Feasibility of pressure wire and single arterial puncture for assessing aortic valve area in patients with aortic stenosis. *J Invasive Cardiol* 2006;18:359–62.
8. Li JH, Haim M, Movassaghi B et al. Segmentation and registration of three-dimensional rotational angiogram on live fluoroscopy to guide atrial fibrillation ablation: A new online imaging tool. *Heart Rhythm* 2009;6:231–7.
9. Pitta SR, Cabalka AK, Rihal CS. Complications associated with left ventricular puncture. *Catheter Cardiovasc Interv* 2010;7:998–9.

16

Recanalization methods for postcatheter vessel occlusion

Frank F. Ing

Background

It is not an uncommon experience for a cardiologist to take a patient with congenital heart disease (CHD) to the catheterization laboratory and spend excessive time to gain vascular access for a diagnostic or interventional procedure. A typical scenario is for the operator to encounter difficulty threading a wire into the femoral vein in spite of excellent blood return from the percutaneous needle. After many attempts, the operator may give up and assume the femoral vein to be occluded. Alternatively, some may inject a small amount of contrast into the needle to evaluate the vein and if occlusion is discovered, the contralateral femoral vein is attempted. If both veins are occluded or multiple venous access is necessary for a complicated intervention, alternative venous access (jugular, transhepatic, etc.) is used. While alternative venous access is helpful, the direct femoral venous access is best for a majority of cardiac catheterization procedures. Unfortunately, CHD patients who have had multiple cardiac catheterizations or multiple surgeries, especially in infancy, or have had chronic indwelling lines placed in the femoral vein are the most susceptible to femoral vein occlusions. These same patients are also the ones who require femoral vein access the most. Similarly, chronic indwelling lines in the upper body or transvenous pacing wires can also cause obstruction of various large upper body veins, including the subclavian, jugular, and innominate veins, and the superior vena cava (SVC), especially in small patients. The current chapter will review some techniques to evaluate the occluded veins and recanalize these vessels.

Clinical presentation, anatomy, and pathophysiology

For the most part, CHD patients who develop femoral vein occlusions remain asymptomatic. Most likely, the occlusion developed at a very young age and venous collaterals to the paravertebral venous system develop and, together with the deep femoral venous system, maintain adequate venous return from the leg. Occasionally, the occlusion is a long segment and involves the iliac vein and even the distal inferior vena cava (IVC). In that case, the paravertebral venous system will channel blood to the contralateral iliofemoral venous system and eventually back to the IVC, usually at the level of the renal veins. The pathophysiology of this type of venous obstruction is different from the adult who presents with IVC obstruction due to abdominal and pelvic malignancies and/or various thrombophilic syndromes. IVC syndrome (leg pain, edema, venous ulcerations) from the latter cause is most likely due to acute obstruction and inadequate development of collateral venous channels. In the upper body, the subclavian vein, innominate vein, or SVC may become obstructed, leading to upper arm edema and various degrees of SVC syndrome. This is commonly found in patients who have had a Mustard or Senning repair for d-transposition of the great arteries or have had chronic indwelling lines or transvenous pacing wires. If there is adequate venous collateralization, the patient may be asymptomatic. In the latter group, it is often discovered at the time of pacing-wire replacement.

History of the procedure

While there are many reports of stenting the obstructed IVC and iliofemoral vein in adults,[1-6] there is only scant literature on stenting of obstructed veins in children or patients with CHD.[7,8] Ing et al. first reported a series in which stents were used to recanalize severely stenotic or occluded iliofemoral veins or IVC in CHD patients for the purpose of reestablishing vascular access for future repetitive cardiac catheterizations or surgeries.[7] In that series, 24 patients received 85 stents in 22 iliofemoral

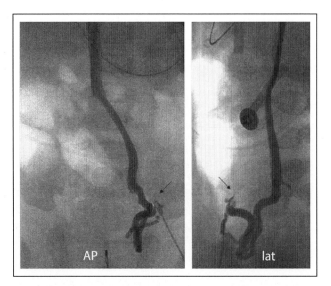

Figure 16.1   "Beak" (arrows) of occluded left superficial femoral vein shown in AP and lateral projection.

veins and 6 IVCs. Thirteen of the 28 vessels were completely occluded and various techniques were used to cross the occlusion for stent implantation. The fact that 85 stents were necessary suggested that most of these occlusions were long segments and multiple overlapping stents were used. Descriptions of recanalizing obstructed innominate veins and SVC baffles for postoperative Mustard or Senning patients and/or during pacing-wire replacements have also been reported.[9–11]

Technique of recanalization
Iliofemoral veins and IVC

Owing to the lack of signs or symptoms of an occluded iliofemoral venous system in CHD patients undergoing cardiac catheterization, the operator must have a high index of suspicion and be prepared to handle an occlusion, especially if the patient has a history of multiple vascular access as an infant. When excellent blood return from a needle is not met with successful passage of a guide wire into the femoral vein, one should make a small hand injection into the needle to evaluate the vessel rather than simply remove the needle to start again. If the femoral vein is occluded, contrast will enter into venous collaterals that commonly circulate into the paravertebral venous system and eventually exit into a more proximal patent iliac system or IVC or contralateral iliofemoral venous system. An angiogram should be performed in both anteroposterior (AP) and lateral projections to evaluate these vessels. Special attention should be paid at the beginning of the injection to look for the "beak" of the remnant superficial femoral vein (Figure 16.1) before superimposition by contrast in the venous collaterals. Even when the angiogram is taken at 30–60 frames per second, only 1–2 frames may show this "beak." Sometimes the "beak" is obvious, and at other times it can be very subtle, as shown in two patients in Figures 16.2 and 16.3. The lateral projection is particularly helpful because of the anterior course of the superficial femoral vein remnant in contrast to the venous collateral flow, which takes a more posterior course

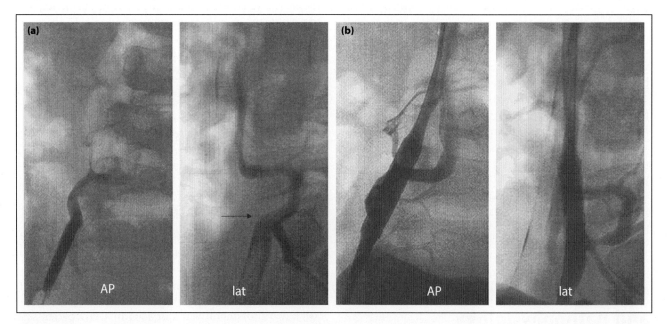

Figure 16.2   (a) In this patient, the "beak" of the occluded right femoral vein is superimposed by the posterior paravertebral venous collateral and not seen in the AP projection. It is very subtle (arrow) in the lateral projection and could be easily missed. (b) Wide patency of vessel after stent implantation.

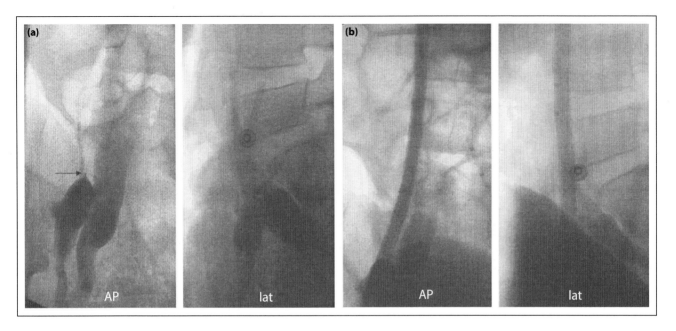

Figure 16.3   (a) In this patient, the remnant "beak" (arrow) of the occluded right femoral vein is only subtly visible in the AP projection and obscured by the venous collateral vessel on the lateral projection. (b) Femoral vein access is reestablished after implantation of three overlapping stents.

into the paravertebral venous system. When this "beak" is identified, there is high likelihood for a successful recanalization. First, a small (0.014–0.018″) guide wire is passed into the tip of the "beak" under fluoroscopic guidance. The needle is replaced with a cannula to secure the initial access. Occasionally, an angled guide wire is all that is needed to push past the "beak" and up the occluded vessel. More commonly, the wire will simply buckle. The cannula should be exchanged for a 4–5 Fr dilator, which prevents the wire from buckling during its advancement. With support from the dilator, which is pushed up to the tip of the "beak," the angle guide wire is advanced. If the front end of the wire is too soft, then the stiffer back end of the wire can be used. The wire is advanced in small increments (mm), followed by advancement of the dilator. The wire is removed and repeated small hand injections are made to evaluate the course (Figure 16.4a and b). Contrast may stain the lumen of the thrombosed vessel. This sequence is repeated until contrast is seen flowing freely in the proximal patent vessel, which could be the iliac vein if the occluded segment is short or even as far as the IVC if there is a long segment occlusion (Figure 16.4c and d). It is important to note the anterior course of this vessel and to assess for extravasation (Figure 16.5a–c). Once the wire is passed into the patent segment, the occluded segment can be serially dilated with either progressively larger dilators or dilation balloons until it is large enough to accommodate a sheath. It is advisable to use a long sheath (such as a Mullins sheath) to secure a long-segment occlusion for the cardiac catheterization. The planned procedure should be performed first and the vessel should be stented

at the end of the planned procedure. An angiogram of the entire length of the iliofemoral venous system and IVC should be performed in order to assess the diameters for proper stent and balloon size selection. When a single stent is inadequate to cover the entire length of the occluded segment, multiple overlapping stents should be used starting from the most cranial end (Figure 16.6a and b). When the occlusion involves the IVC, patency is often seen at the level of the renal veins, most likely due to the high flow of these veins back into the IVC. Presently, only balloon-expandable stents are used in growing children to accommodate future further dilation as the child grows. The Genesis stent is a good choice for these vessels. Balloon size selection should be based on the normal caliber of the adjacent patent vessel. During stent implantation, a clamp is placed on the inguinal ligament to define the caudal limit for stent positioning. A needle is usually placed on the groin, parallel to the femoral vein course, to help determine the level at which the tip of the needle can enter the stent. By positioning the stent such that the most caudal edge can be entered by the percutaneous needle, future access into the stent is ensured even if the stent becomes reoccluded. However, keep in mind that on the lateral projection, the stent should not be positioned too anteriorly so that flexion of the hips will distort the stent. In general, if the stent is positioned such that its most caudal edge is in the mid-portion of the bladder, it is safe from hip flexion. At the end of the procedure, the hips can be flexed under lateral fluoroscopy to ensure stent positioning. Follow-up angiogram should be taken to evaluate inflow (Figure 16.7a–c). If the distal femoral vein is small or

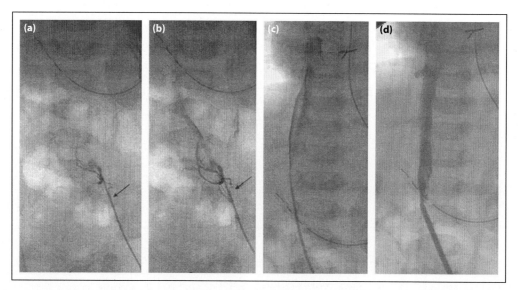

Figure 16.4 (a, b) An angled guide wire or the stiff end of a 0.014–0.018" wire through a 4–5 Fr dilator is advanced in small increments through the occluded vein. Small hand injections are taken through the dilator (arrows) to evaluate the occluded vessel course. Contrast stains the occluded segment or enters into the smaller collateral. (c) When the patent IVC is entered, contrast flows freely into the right atrium. (d) The dilator is exchanged out for a long sheath.

the inflow into the stent appears inadequate, there is a possibility of stent reocclusion. This should not pose a hemodynamic problem since the vein was occluded in the first place prior to recanalization. However, by having the stent in place, future catheterizations can still be performed even if the stent occludes. By using biplane fluoroscopic guidance, a needle can be directed into the lumen of the radiopaque

stent and advanced further into the patent vessel distally. As long as the needle remains inside the stent, extravasation is avoided. As shown in the Figures 16.8 and 16.9, multiple catheterizations were performed for cardiac biopsies in a transplant patient in whom an occluded femoral vein was stented and became reoccluded due to poor inflow. As the child grew, longer (Chiba) needles were needed to reach

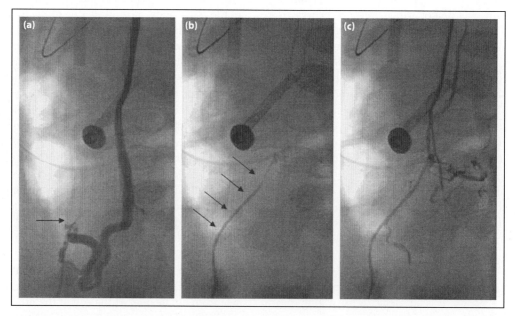

Figure 16.5 (a–c) The anterior course of the femoral and iliac veins (arrows) is noted during advancement of the wire and dilator in the lateral projection.

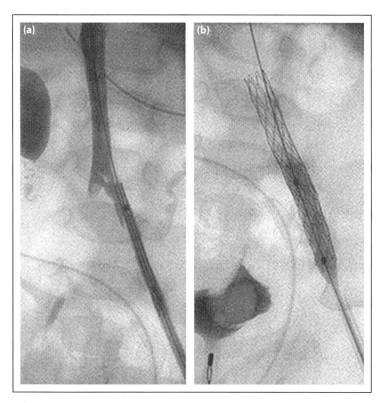

Figure 16.6   (a) Stent and balloon are positioned across the most proximal segment of the occluded left iliac vein. (b) A second stent is implanted more distally in the occluded superficial femoral vein segment and telescoped into the first stent.

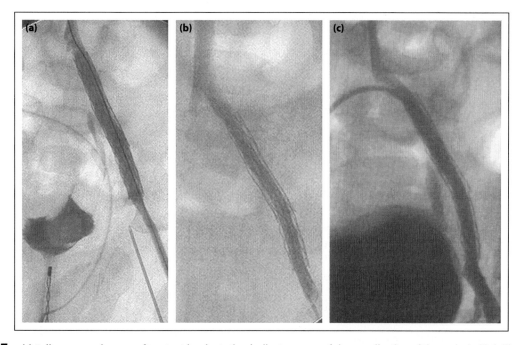

Figure 16.7   (a) Follow-up angiogram after stent implantation indicates successful recanalization of the occluded left iliac and femoral vein. (b, c) Follow-up cardiac catheterization (for other interventions) 4 months (b) and 18 months (c) later show patency of the stented segment. A thin layer of intima is noted within the stents.

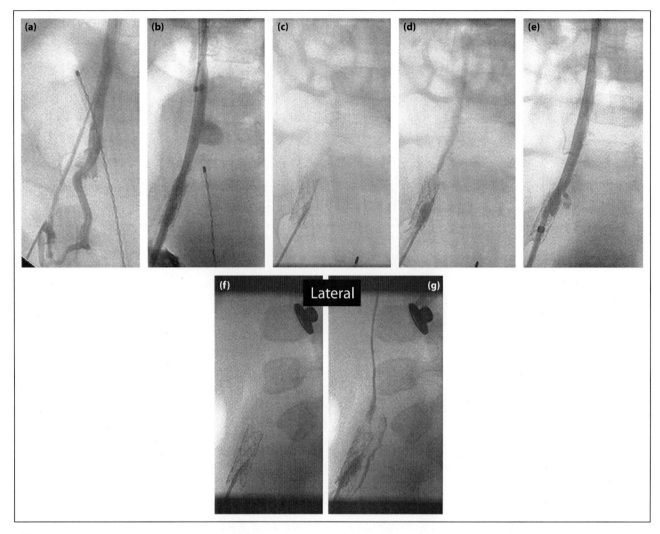

Figure 16.8 (a) Right femoral vein occlusion was found in this 3-month-old infant after orthotopic heart transplant rendering cardiac biopsy difficult due to vascular access. (b) A stent was implanted initially. (c) Owing to poor distal venous inflow, the stent was found to be reoccluded during a follow-up cardiac catheterization. (d) However, using the radiopaque stent as a target, a needle can be introduced back into the stent. (e) The occluded stent and vessel can be recannulated. (e–g) Lateral projection of the same patient. Using both AP and lateral views, the needle can be easily guided back into the occluded stent to regain vascular access of the femoral vein.

the stent edge, but once there, a wire was easily advanced through the thrombosed stent and finally into the more cranial patent segment of the femoral vein. Following stent implantation in a systemic vein, lifetime antiplatelet therapy with low-dose aspirin is prescribed. Occasionally, the occluded venous segments can be quite extensive, requiring multiple stents involving bilateral femoral and iliac veins as well as the IVC as shown in Figures 16.10 through 16.13.

Innominate veins and SVC

Techniques of recanalization are similar to those used for occluded iliofemoral vessels. In those patients with a pacing wire, following removal, an angiogram often can locate the potential intraluminal space permitting a wire to be passed followed by initial angioplasty. A long sheath

is then passed over the same wire for stent implantation before reinsertion of a pacing wire (Figure 16.14a–c). When complete occlusion of the SVC is encountered (SVC baffle of Mustard), access is obtained from both the internal jugular (IJ) and femoral veins. Angiograms above and below the occluded site are taken. With a target well defined in both the AP and lateral projections, a transseptal needle can be used to traverse the occluded segment followed by angioplasty and stent implantation (Figure 16.15a–f).

Follow-up data

There are few data on the long-term results of stented peripheral systemic veins in patients with CHD. Midterm

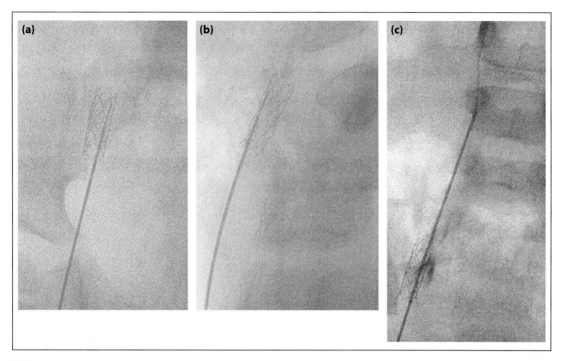

Figure 16.9   (a–c) This transplanted patient has had multiple follow-up catheterizations over 5 years. As the child grew, the stent shifted further cranially. A longer (Chiba) needle is needed to gain access into the occluded stent using the AP (a) and lateral (b) views. Free flow of contrast into the IVC is noted in (c).

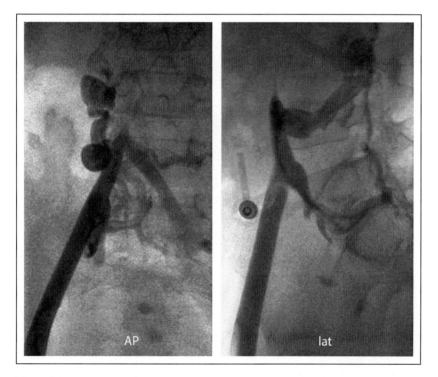

Figure 16.10   This patient with complex congenital heart disease was found to have significant distal IVC occlusion at the level of the iliac bifurcation. Bifurcating stents will be needed to recanalize the distal IVC without jailing either iliac vein. Note the extension venous collaterization into the paravertebral venous system.

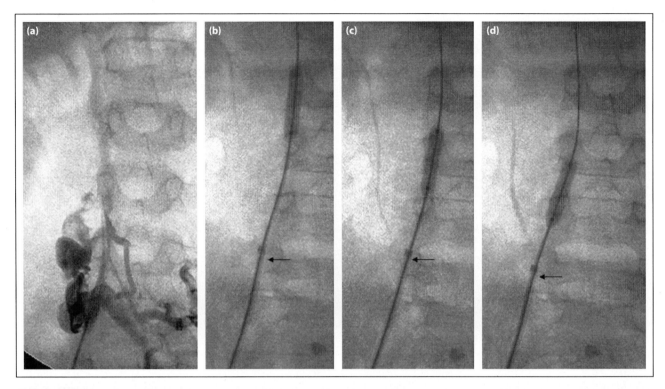

Figure 16.11 (a) Angiogram after the wire and dilator were advanced past the IVC occlusion. (b–d) Initial balloon dilation of the occluded distal IVC and right iliac vein was performed to permit passage of sheath (arrow) into the IVC.

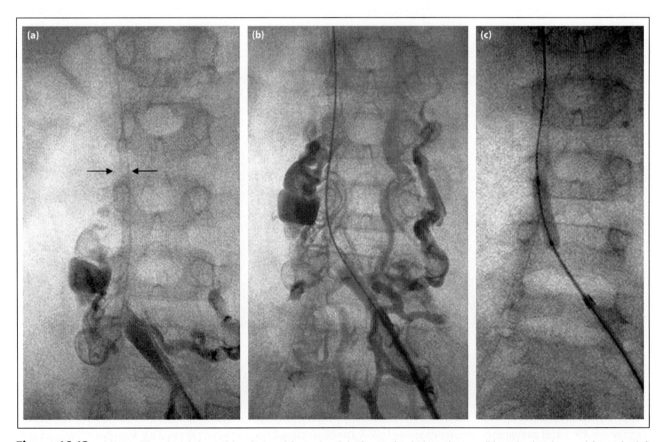

Figure 16.12 (a) A Mullins sheath (arrow) is advanced from the right femoral vein into the IVC. (b) A wire is advanced from the left femoral vein to cross the occluded IVC segment. (c) Balloon dilation is carried out at the junction of the distal IVC and left iliac bifurcation.

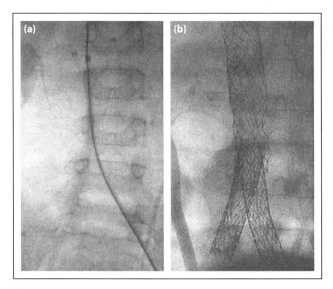

Figure 16.13   (a) Bilateral sheaths are placed from the femoral veins into the IVC for stent implantation. (b) Two overlapping stents are implanted in the distal IVC and two bifurcating stents in the bilateral iliac veins.

follow-up data were available in the paper by Ing et al., which reported a patency rate of 87% for 12 patients (15 vessels). Two stented veins were found to be occluded due to poor inflow, but were easily recannulated and redilated for successful cardiac catheterization. In another (unpublished) series of 27 patients in whom 53 stents were implanted, follow-up catheterization was performed in 12 patients at mean 2.2 years showing a stent patency rate of 83% (10/12

vessels) while intimal hyperplasia was found in 25% (3/12 vessels).[12] Two occluded stents were easily recanalized. A longer-term follow-up is warranted.

Summary

In summary, patients with CHD who have undergone multiple cardiac catheterizations or surgeries during infancy may develop occlusions of the iliofemoral venous system in spite of the lack of signs or symptoms. In addition, large upper-body systemic veins, including the innominate vein and SVC, can become obstructed as a result of certain surgical repairs performed for CHD or due to chronic indwelling lines or even transvenous pacing wires. Again, symptoms vary depending on the development of adequate venous pop-off collaterals.

Recanalization and stenting of these occluded vessels can be achieved. For the femoral veins, if the remnant superficial femoral vein "beak" can be identified during angiography, the attempt is likely to be successful. Preservation of femoral vein access with this technique may avoid more complicated alternative venous access routes and simplify future diagnostic or interventional cardiac catheterizations. For innominate vein obstructions found during pacing-wire replacement, angiograms showing the pathway of a transvenous pacing wire can help to identify the potential pathway across the obstruction. For SVC occlusion, having a target on the other side of the obstruction allows the safe use of a transseptal needle to gain access through the occluded segment.

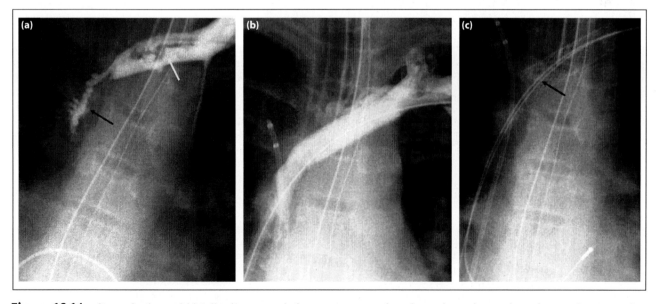

Figure 16.14   **(See color insert.)** (a) Following removal of a transvenous pacing wire, an innominate vein angiogram shows complete occlusion of the vessel as it enters into the SVC (red arrow). Proximally, thrombus is noted along the vessel (yellow arrow). (b) Angiogram taken following stent implantation showing wide patency of the innominate vein into the SVC. (c) New pacing wires (black arrow) are passed across the stented innominate vein.

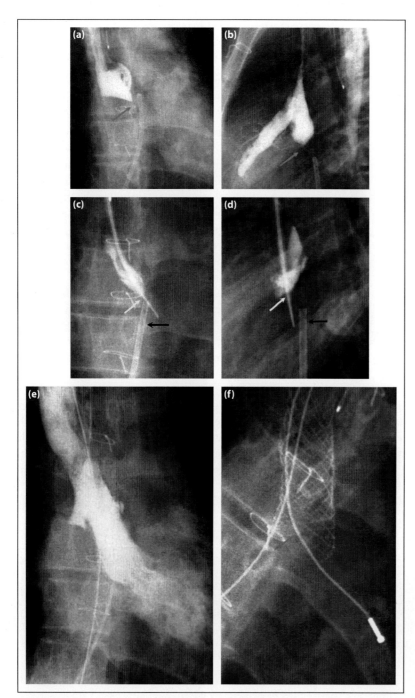

Figure 16.15 (**See color insert.**) AP (a) and lateral (b) projection of complete SVC occlusion (red arrows) in a patient with d-transposition of the great arteries s/p Mustard repair. AP (c) and lateral (d) projection of successful transseptal needle puncture across the occluded segment (yellow arrows). A catheter was inserted from the femoral vein and positioned below the occluded site in the right atrium to act as a target (black arrows) for the transseptal needle. (e) Angiogram post-SVC baffle stent showing wide patency of flow into the "neo-right atrium." (f) New transvenous pacing wires placed through the stented SVC baffle.

References

1. Charnsangavej C, Carrasco CH, Wallace S et al. Stenosis of the vena cava: Preliminary assessment of treatment with expandable metallic stents. *Radiology* 1986;161:295–8.
2. Nazarian GK, Bjarnason H, Dietz CA, Bernadas CA, Hunter DW. Iliofemoral venous stenosis: Effectiveness of treatment with metallic endovascular stents. *Radiology* 1996;200:193–9.
3. Fletcher WS, Lakin PC, Pommier RF, Wilmarth T. Results of treatment of inferior vena cava syndrome with expandable metallic stents. *Arch Surg* 1998;133:935–8.
4. Change TC, Zaleski GX, Funaki B, Leaf J. Treatment of inferior vena cava obstruction in hemodialysis patient using Wallstents: Early and intermediate results. *Am J Radiol* 1998;171:125–8.
5. Funagi B, Szymski GX, Leef JA et al. Treatment of venous outflow stenoses in thigh grafts with Wallstents. *Am J Roentgenol* 1999;172:1591–6.
6. Raju S, Neglén P. Percutaneous recanalization of total occlusions of the iliac vein. *J Vasc Surg* 2009;50:360–8.
7. Ing FF, Fagan TE, Grifka RG et al. Reconstruction of stenotic or occluded iliofemoral veins and inferior vena cava using intravascular stents: Re-establishing access for future cardiac catheterization and cardiac surgery. *JACC* 2001;37:251–7.

8. Ward CJB, Mullins CE, Nihill MR et al. Use of intravascular stents in systemic venous and systemic venous baffle obstructions: Short-term follow-up results. *Circulation* 1995;91:2948–54.

9. Ing FF, Mullins CE, Grifka RG et al. Stent dilation of superior vena cava/innominate vein obstructions permits transvenous pacing lead implantation. *Pacing Clin Electrophysiol* 1998;21:1517–30.

10. Hill KD, Fleming G, Curt Fudge J, Albers EL, Doyle TP, Rhodes JF. Percutaneous interventions in high-risk patients following Mustard repair of transposition of the great arteries. *Catheter Cardiovasc Interv* 2012;80(6):905–14.

11. Sadagopan SN, Veldtman GR, Roberts PR. Extraction of chronic pacing lead and angioplasty for complete superior baffle obstruction in complex congenital heart disease. *Pacing Clin Electrophysiol* 2008;31(12):1661–3.

12. Ing FF. Unpublished series from Children's Hospital of San Diego.

17

Transpericardial access

Randall J. Lee, Krzysztof Bartus, and Nitish Badhwar

Introduction

Percutaneous pericardiocentesis was initially described in 1840 by Frank Schuh. Since the twentieth century, percutaneous access to the pericardial space has been widely accepted as the preferred procedure for the treatment of cardiac tamponade and/or the diagnosis of pericardial effusions. Clinical diagnosis of cardiac tamponade was described by Claude Beck and referred to as "Beck's triad," consisting of hypotension, an increased venous pressure, and a quiet heart.[1]

Echocardiography has become the standard method for confirmation of the existence of a pericardial effusion, localization of the effusion, size determination, and hemodynamic consequences. Echocardiography diagnosis of cardiac tamponade is determined by abnormal septal motion, collapse of the right atrium and/or right ventricle, and decreased respiratory variation of the inferior vena cava.[2] Various techniques for pericardial access have been described that include the apical, subxiphoid, transatrial, and transbronchial approaches.

A commonly taught method for performing a pericardiocentesis has been the subxiphoid approach, which uses a spinal needle inserted in the midline inferior to the subxiphoid with the needle directed at a 45° angle from the abdominal wall and 45° from the midline directed toward the left shoulder. Ancillary technologies such as echocardiography (ECG) recordings have been used to assist in pericardiocentesis. An alligator clip can be attached to the end of the spinal needle and to a lead of an ECG machine. The spinal needle is advanced until either a premature ventricular contraction (PVC) is seen or ST segment elevation occurs. Commonly, cardiac pulsations are felt prior to the ECG evidence of myocardial irritation (PVC) or myocardial injury (ST elevation). Echocardiography can be used to localize the pericardial effusion, visualize the myocardium, and identify adjacent organs while guiding the needle toward the pericardial effusion. The use of echocardiography has minimized the risk of performing a pericardiocentesis.

Loculated pericardial effusions may require echocardiographic- and fluoroscopic-guided pericardiocentesis using nonstandard entry sites where effusions are identified at the point closest to the skin.[3] More recently, pericardial access has been adapted for epicardial interventions. This chapter will describe how to perform a "dry" pericardial access approach for epicardial therapeutic interventions.

Anatomy of the pericardium

The pericardium is a closed fibroserous sac surrounding the heart and roots of the great vessels. The pericardium is composed of an outermost layer, the fibrous pericardium, and an inner layer, the serous pericardium. The inner layer is divided into the parietal pericardium and visceral pericardium. The parietal pericardium is fused to the fibrous layer, while the visceral pericardium composes part of the epicardium. The potential space between the parietal pericardium and visceral pericardium is the pericardial cavity that contains pericardial fluid, which lubricates the heart.

The fibrous pericardium is contiguous with the external coats of the great vessels and the pretracheal layer of the deep cervical fascia. The fibrous pericardium is also connected superiorly to the sternum by the sternopericardial ligaments and inferiorly to the central tendon of the diaphragm. Via these connections, the pericardium minimizes the motion of the heart within the mediastinum.

The roots of the aorta, the superior vena cava, the right and left pulmonary arteries, and the four pulmonary veins are connected with the fibrous pericardium. The inferior vena cava does not receive any covering from the fibrous pericardium. The serous pericardial reflections form two tubes around the roots of the great vessel and define the boundaries constituting the transverse and oblique sinus. One set of reflections forms a tube that surrounds the aorta and pulmonary trunk, while the second set of reflections form a tube that engulfs the superior vena cava, the inferior vena cava, and the four pulmonary veins. The transverse sinus is the passage between the two tubes formed anteriorly by the serous pericardium surrounding the aorta and pulmonary trunk and inferiorly by the serous pericardium surrounding the four pulmonary veins, superior vena cava, and inferior vena cava. The oblique sinus is the recess in the most posterior aspect of the pericardial cavity formed by the serous pericardial reflections surrounding the pulmonary veins and the inferior vena cava; and posteriorly by the pericardium that lies anterior to the esophagus.

The anterior surface of the pericardium is partially covered by the lungs and pleura, but the lower aspect of the anterior surface of the pericardium forms the posterior aspect of the anterior mediastinal space. The anterior mediastinum is a virtual space bounded anteriorly by the sternum and posteriorly by the anterior surface of the heart (Figure 17.1b). This virtual space contains mediastinal fat on the surface of the heart and the thymus that is at the most superior aspect of the anterior mediastinal space. The posterior pericardium is in contact with the bronchi, the esophagus, the descending thoracic aorta, and the posterior part of the mediastinal surface of each lung. The posterior pericardium forms the anterior aspect of the posterior mediastinum. The heart is considered to be the middle mediastinum. Laterally, the pericardium

is surrounded by pleurae with the phrenic nerve and the esophageal plexus innervating the parietal pericardium.[4]

In addition to providing lubrication to the heart, functional roles of the pericardium include minimizing the motion of the heart within the mediastinum, preventing infections and restricting excessive dilatation of the heart in the setting of acute volume overload. However, increased fluid within the pericardial cavity can lead to increased pressure within the pericardial cavity limiting filling of the heart, creating cardiac tamponade, and necessitating therapeutic pericardiocentesis.

Conventional approach for epicardial therapeutic interventions

A "dry" pericardial access approach has been described by Sosa and colleagues during their description of catheter ablation of epicardial ventricular tachycardias in patients with Chagas disease and cardiomyopathy.[5] The technique described used a subxiphoid approach that generally

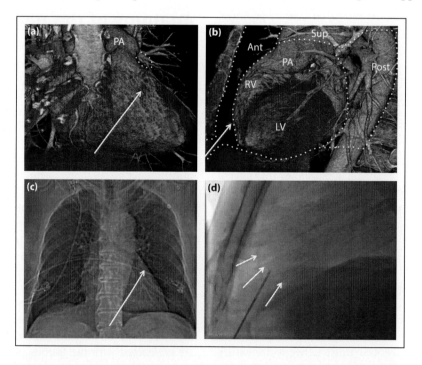

Figure 17.1 (**See color insert.**) The orientation of the pericardial access for LAA ligation utilizing the LARIAT™ suture delivery device. Pericardial access for LAA ligation utilizing the LARIAT suture delivery device requires an anterior access approach into the pericardial space. As seen in the anteroposterior view (AP) of the 3D reconstruction of the CT angiogram (a), the LAA (delineated by the dashed line) is lateral to the pulmonary artery (PA) and appears to be in front of the hilum. The needle is directed (direction of the arrow) just lateral to the LAA, which is generally toward the left shoulder. In the fluoroscopic image, the needle (arrow) would be directed just lateral to the hilum (c). The lateral view of the 3D reconstruction of the CT angiogram (b) demonstrates the virtual space of the anterior mediastinal space (Ant). The needle (arrow) is directed through the sternocostal triangle that allows for the needle to pass under the xiphoid process and above the diaphragm into the anterior mediastinal space, thus avoiding damage to the diaphragm and avoiding abdominal organs. The 90° left lateral fluoroscopic view allows for the needle to be advanced to the myocardial border (d). Ant: anterior mediastinal space, Sup: superior mediastinal space, Post: posterior mediastinal space. RV: right ventricle, PA: pulmonary artery, LV: left ventricle.

resulted in a posterior pericardial access to target the left ventricle. The technique has been adapted and generally is taught as a subxiphoid approach. Spinal needles have been used for "dry" pericardiocentesis. However, needles such as the Pajunk needle (Pajunk, Norcross, GA, USA) that have a curved bevel and an asymmetrical opening with the advantage of directing the guide wire away from the myocardium if the curved portion of the needle is toward the myocardium and the needle opening is directed away from the myocardium (Figure 17.2). After infiltration of the skin and subcutaneous tissue with local anesthesia, the needle is inserted just below the subxiphoid process at a 45° angle from the abdominal cavity and 45° from the midline, directed toward the left shoulder. Guidance of the needle in the anterior-posterior fluoroscopic view allows for visualization of the inferior aspect of the heart border. After the needle has been advanced past the subcutaneous tissue and approaches the inferior aspect of the heart border, the stylet is removed and a 5- to 10-cc syringe with a 50:50 solution of contrast and saline is connected to the needle. Upon advancement of the needle toward the heart, a small amount of contrast is injected to delineate the fibrous pericardium. Commonly, cardiac pulsations can be felt through the needle as it comes into contact with the pericardium. The contrast injection will demonstrate a "tenting" of the fibrosis pericardium before entry into the pericardial cavity. The tenting is best seen in the 90° left lateral fluoroscopic view (Figure 17.3d). Entry into the pericardial cavity will generally be associated with a "popping" sensation as the needle passes through the outer layer of the pericardium. Additionally, passing of the needle through the outer layer of the pericardium can be seen fluoroscopically by the release of the "tenting" of the pericardium and the

needle tip beyond the contrast staining of the pericardium (Figure 17.3e). Once the needle is through the outer layer of the pericardium, the injection of contrast into the pericardial cavity is noted by the pooling of the contrast inferiorly around the cardiac border (Figure 17.3f). A 0.035 J guide wire is passed through the needle into the pericardial space to allow for dilators and sheaths to be inserted into the pericardial cavity.

Anterior pericardial access approach

Recently, an anterior pericardial access approach has been used for LAA ligation with the LARIAT™ suture delivery device.[6] Procedural success of the LAA ligation is predicated on successfully obtaining an anterior pericardial access to allow the LARIAT suture delivery device to travel anteriorly over the right ventricular surface to approach the LAA at its most anterior aspect to allow the LARIAT snare to be passed over the entire LAA.

An 18 G Touhy or Pajunk epidural needle is recommended for the anterior pericardial access approach. The unique feature of the Pajunk needle is its spoon-like curvature at the end of the needle with an asymmetrical opening (Figure 17.2). When the opening is directed superiorly, the needle will slide up the anterior surface of RV when entering the pericardial cavity and directing the J wire up the anterior surface of the RV (Figure 17.4a).

Pericardial access for LAA ligation with the LARIAT suture delivery device needs to be directed lateral to the LAA in the AP fluoroscopic view (Figure 17.1a). The pericardial puncture is initiated 2–3 cm inferior to the xiphoid process. After infiltration of the skin and subcutaneous tissue with local anesthesia, the needle is passed superficially in the subcutaneous tissue toward the xiphoid process and parallel to the sternum. A shallow angle with respect to the abdomen assures that the needle does not enter the abdominal cavity. The needle is passed just below the xiphoid process through the sternocostal triangle (Larrey's triangle) to enter the anterior mediastinal space. To assure an anterior pericardial access approach, a 90° left lateral fluoroscopic view is used to clearly allow for the visualization of the cardiac silhouette and the apex of the heart (Figures 17.1 and 17.3). The needle is directed 1–2 cm above the acute margin of the heart. Entering the pericardial space 1–2 cm above the acute margin of the heart prevents the J wire from slipping posteriorly. Once the pericardial needle has entered the pericardial space, a 0.035 J guide wire is inserted through the needle. The guide wire advances superiorly over the anterior surface of the RV (Figure 17.3a). The importance of using the 90° left lateral view to gain anterior access to the pericardial space was demonstrated in our initial experience of 183 patients undergoing LAA ligation with the

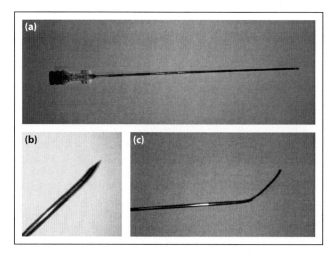

Figure 17.2 Pajunk needle. The Pajunk needle (a) has a curved bevel at the end of the needle with an asymmetrical opening (b) that facilitates the needle sliding along the surface of the heart. The asymmetric opening of the needle directs the guide wire along the heart surface rather than straight out into the myocardial wall (c).

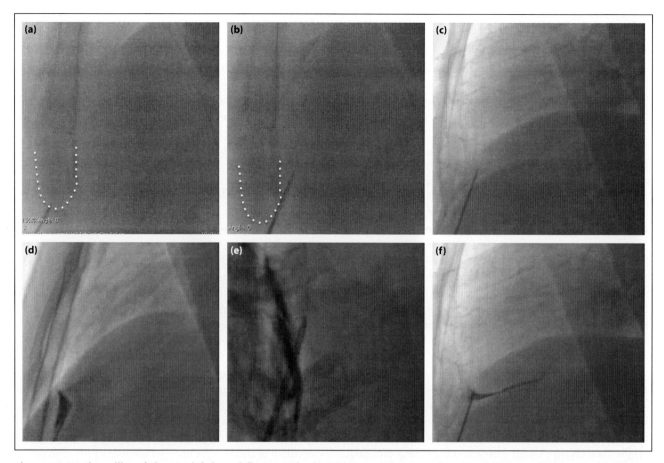

Figure 17.3 The utility of the 90° left lateral fluoroscopic view. The 90° left lateral fluoroscopic view allows for visualization of the needle in relationship to the sternum (highlighted by the dashed line) and the myocardial border. In (a), the needle approach is too superficial. Visualization of the sternum allows the operator to direct the needle just under the sternum passing through the sternocostal triangle (b), above the diaphragm and toward the myocardial border (c). A small injection of 50:50 contrast:saline allows for the visualization of the needle against the fibrous pericardium creating "tenting" of the pericardium (d). Passing the needle through the fibrous pericardium and parietal pericardium is generally associated with the tactile feeling of a "pop" and release of the tenting with visualization of the needle past the contrast dye front (e). Correct entry into the pericardial space is delineated by contrast pooling on the inferior surface (f).

LARIAT device, 32 of 140 patients (23%) required two or more pericardial access attempts to gain an anterior pericardial access when using an anteroposterior or shallow left anterior oblique fluoroscopic view. In contrast, only 1 of 39 patients required a second pericardial access attempt when utilizing the 90° left lateral fluoroscopic view.[7]

Helpful suggestions

One of the most common concerns of a "dry" pericardiocentesis is perforation and/or laceration of the RV. Avoidance of a perforation of the RV includes the use of contrast to delineate the pericardium and advancing the needle in 1 mm increments either when "tenting" occurs or when myocardial pulsations are palpated via the needle. If the needle tip moves past the dye front, additional contrast should be injected to determine if the pericardial space has been entered. Additionally, the needle should not be perpendicular to the surface of the heart at the pericardial entry point. The sudden release of pressure as the needle punctures through the pericardium may result in the advancement of the needle by up to 1 cm relative to the pericardium, thus perforating the RV. A needle angle of 30–45° to the surface of the heart allows the needle to slide up the anterior surface of the heart, thus minimizing perforation of the RV. If the patient is intubated, having the anesthesiologist hold respiration will decrease the cardiac movement, helping to avoid sudden changes in the heart's position.

If myocardial staining occurs or PVCs are observed, the needle should be withdrawn 1–2 mm before inserting the J guide wire. The J guide wire should pass easily within the pericardial space without resistance. Any buckling or resistance of the wire as it exits the needle tip infers that either the wire is in myocardial tissue or the needle has slipped out of the pericardial space. If the needle tip is in the myocardium,

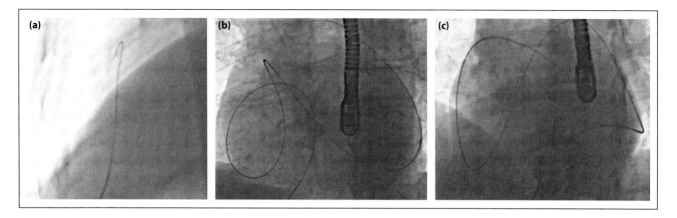

Figure 17.4 Verification of correct entry into the pericardial space. The initial entry for an anterior pericardial approach is directing the needle 1–2 cm above the apex of the heart on the anterior surface of the heart. The bevel is directed upward and away from myocardial surface encouraging the guide wire to travel superiorly along the anterior surface of the heart (a). Verification of the guide wire within the pericardial space is performed in a 30–40° LAO fluoroscopic view and AP fluoroscopic view. The LAO fluoroscopic view is used as the wire is being advanced within the pericardial cavity to assure that the guide wire passes the spine and outlines the left cardiac border (b). This assures that the guide wire is not in the RV. A second fluoroscopic view such as an AP fluoroscopic view (c) is used to assure that the guide wire is not in the mediastinal space and that adhesions are not present.

advancing the guide wire against resistance could lead to passing the guide wire through the myocardium into the RV, laceration of the myocardium, or "stitching" the myocardium where the guide wire traverses the myocardium and exits back into the pericardial space, thus appearing be in the proper position. Dilation over a guide wire that has been "stitched" through the myocardial wall will result in myocardial laceration or perforation. Passing the guide wire into the RV is generally associated with PVCs. If the RV is perforated, removal of the needle from the RV generally has little clinical consequence unless the needle is moved sideways, potentially resulting in abrasion or laceration of the myocardium. Perforation of the RV with the needle generally leads to 30- to 50-cc pericardial fluid. In our initial 183 patients undergoing pericardiocentesis for LAA ligation, RV puncture occurred in 32 patients with only two patients having greater than 100 cc of hemopericardium.[7] Both patients were treated conservatively with no clinical consequences.

A micropuncture needle has been used for "dry" pericardial access. The advantage of a micropuncture needle is that any perforation of the heart should lead to decreased bleeding and less laceration of the heart. The disadvantage of the micropuncture needle is a loss of tactile sensation and it is easier to pass the needle through tissue with an increased likelihood of perforating the heart. The needle is also flimsy and bends easily; thus, redirecting the needle is virtually impossible.

A shallow left anterior oblique (LAO) fluoroscopic view (30°) is used to confirm that the J wire outlines the left cardiac silhouette, which ensures that the J wire is not in the right ventricle (RV) (Figure 17.4b). In the LAO fluoroscopic view, the RV cavity does not go beyond the spine. Therefore,

if the J guide wire is outlining the left cardiac silhouette, the J guide wire cannot be in the RV. A second fluoroscopic view, generally the AP fluoroscopic view, is used to assure that the J guide wire is in the cardiac silhouette and not in the pleural space (Figure 17.4c).

Complications

Complications associated with pericardiocentesis are due to the needle penetrating the heart and surrounding structures such as coronary arteries, lungs, stomach, colon, and liver.[8] Complication rates vary between 4% and 40%.[9–14] Complications include coronary artery puncture or aneurysm, left internal mammary artery puncture or aneurysm, arrhythmias, pneumothorax, hemothorax, pneumopericardium, infections, arterial bleeding, hepatic injury, or injury to other vital abdominal organs.

Anterior versus conventional posterior pericardial access approach

The technique of directing the needle parallel to the sternum and entering the anterior mediastinal space via the sternocostal triangle would seem to be a safer approach versus the more conventionally taught approach of angulating the needle at 45°.

The use of the 90° lateral fluoroscopic view helps to direct the needle just below the xiphoid process to enter through the sternocostal triangle into the anterior mediastinal space (Figures 17.1 and 17.3), thus entering the virtual space and avoiding organs within the abdomen. Once the anterior mediastinal space has been entered via the sternocostal triangle, the pericardial cavity can be entered either anteriorly or posteriorly. This approach minimizes perforation of vital organs within the abdomen and avoids injuring the diaphragm.

References

1. Sternbach G. Claude Beck: Cardiac compression triads. *J Emerg Med* 1988;6(5):417–9.
2. Fagan SM, Chan KL. Pericardiocentesis: Blind no more!. *Chest* 1999;116(2):275–6.
3. Molkara D, Tejman-Yarden S, El-Said H, Moore JW. Pericardiocentesis of noncircumferential effusions using nonstandard catheter entry sites guided by echocardiography and fluoroscopy. *Congenit Heart Dis* 2011;6(5):461–5.
4. 13. Lachman N, Syed FF, Habib A et al. Correlative anatomy for the electrophysiologist, part II: Cardiac ganglia, phrenic nerve, coronary venous system. *J Cardiovasc Electrophysiol* 2011;22:104–10.
5. Sosa E, Scanavacca M, d'Avila A, Pilleggi F. A new technique to perform epicardial mapping in the electrophysiology laboratory. *J Cardiovasc Electrophysiol* 1996;7:531–6.
6. Bartus K, Han F, Bednarek J, Myc J et al. Percutaneous left atrial appendage suture ligation using the LARIAT in patients with atrial fibrillation: Initial clinical experience. *J Am Coll Cardiol* 2013;62:108–18.
7. Bartus K, Lee RJ, Morelli R, Badhwar N. Anterior pericardial access for left atrial appendage ligation. (Submitted for publication).
8. Loukas M, Walters A, Boon JM, Welch TP, Meiring JH, Abrahams PH. Pericardiocentesis: A clinical anatomy review. *Clin Anat* 2012;25(7):872–81.
9. Vayre F, Lardoux H, Pezzano M et al. Subxiphoid pericardiocentesis guided by contrast two-dimensional echocardiography in cardiac tamponade: Experience of 110 consecutive patients. *Eur J Echocardiogr* 2000;1(1):66–71.
10. Salem K, Mulji A, Lonn E. Echocardiographically guided pericardiocentesis—The gold standard for the management of pericardial effusion and cardiac tamponade. *Can J Cardiol* 1999;15(11):1251–5.
11. Tsang TS, Freeman WK, Barnes ME et al. Rescue echocardiographically guided pericardiocentesis for cardiac perforation complicating catheter-based procedures. The Mayo Clinic experience. *J Am Coll Cardiol* 1998;32(5):1345–50.
12. Sacher F, Roberts-Thomson K, Maury P et al. Epicardial ventricular tachycardia ablation a multicenter safety study. *J Am Coll Cardiol* 2010;55:2366–72.
13. Schmidt B, Chun KR, Baensch D et al. Catheter ablation for ventricular tachycardia after failed endocardial ablation: Epicardial substrate or inappropriate endocardial ablation? *Heart Rhythm* 2010;7:1746–52.
14. Koruth JS, Aryana A, Dukkipati SR et al. Unusual complications of percutaneous epicardial access and epicardial mapping and ablation of cardiac arrhythmias. *Circ Arrhythm Electrophysiol* 2011;4:882–8.

18

Surgical access (transapical, transatrial, transaortic, femoral, subclavian)

Mirko Doss

There are several modes of delivery of transcatheter aortic valve replacement (TAVR) devices. The first delivery route was the antegrade transvenous route, initially described and used by Cribier, to implant the first aortic transcatheter valve.[1] After an initial series of patients, this route was abandoned for the retrograde transfemoral approach, which proved to be technically easier to perform.

Apart from the percutaneous transfemoral route, there are several other access routes that require a surgical cutdown. These are the transapical access, direct aortic, subclavian, and carotid access modes.

Direct transaortic access

Direct access to the aortic valve is obtained through a partial upper sternotomy or minithoracotomy in the second right intercostal space. Patients require intubation and general anesthesia. Patients with prior coronary artery bypass surgery with proximal anastomoses on the ascending aorta, horizontal aorta, short ascending aorta (<5 cm), radiation of the chest, and porcelain aorta are not good candidates for this access (Figure 18.1).

Prior to skin incision, the chest computerized tomogram (CT) is evaluated to identify the location of the aorta (lateralization, calcification, length of ascending aorta >5 cm, and depth from sternum).

Partial upper sternotomy

The right second intercostal space is identified and marked. A 5 cm skin incision is performed from the fossa juglaris to the second intercostal space along the centerline of the sternum. The subcutaneous tissue is then dissected down to the sternum and the muscles of the right intercostal space, adjacent to the sternum, are incised. Care is taken not to injure the right-sided internal thoracic artery. A J-type sternotomy is then performed, from the manubrium of the sternum to the second intercostal space. The right side of the divided sternum is then

elevated and the substernal tissues are dissected, including the internal thoracic artery. Then, a miniretractor is inserted and the sternum is spread. Mediastinal tissue is dissected away and the pericardium, with the ascending aorta beneath it, is identified. The pericardium is incised in a longitudinal fashion along the path of the ascending aorta. Stay sutures are placed in such a way that the ascending aorta is pulled into an optimal position for access. Now, a spot on the distal part of the ascending aorta is chosen, keeping in mind that at least 5 cm is needed for valve system insertion. In a noncalcified portion of the ascending aorta, a double purse-string suture, using 4-0 Prolene™, is placed and secured with tourniquets.

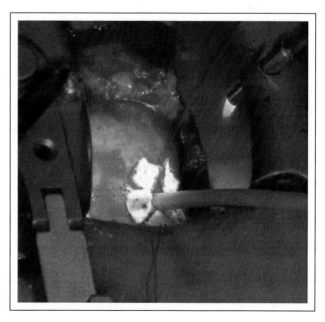

Figure 18.1 **(See color insert.)** Surgical access to the ascending aorta as used in the transaortic approach. An incision in the right 2nd intercostal space is made, the aorta exposed, and a pledgeted purse-string suture placed. The sheath for valve deployment is introduced from the cranial aspect of the patient and directed toward the aortic valve.

Heparin is administered after making sure that there is no bleeding from the suture sites. The ascending aorta is then punctured by the Seldinger technique in the middle of the purse-string suture. A 6 F sheath is inserted and a guiding catheter advanced through the aortic valve, into the left ventricular cavity. The guide wire is exchanged for a stiff wire, using a pigtail catheter. A 24 F sheath is then advanced over the stiff wire, into the ascending aorta. The procedure now is the same as a regular transfemoral arterial procedure.

After successful valve deployment, the sheath is removed and the purse-string sutures tied.
Additional sutures might be necessary if there is bleeding from the puncture site.
Heparin is reversed. The sternotomy is closed in the regular fashion.

Minithoracotomy in the right second intercostal space

The minithoracotomy in the second intercostal space provides a means of accessing the aorta from a more lateral angle and avoiding a sternotomy. This might be advantageous in patients with an elongated ascending aorta that is displaced into the right mediastinum. The second intercostal space on the right is identified and marked. A 5 cm skin incision is performed, starting at the lateral end of the sternum. The subcutaneous tissues and intercostal muscles are divided. Care is taken not to injure the right internal thoracic artery. A miniretractor is inserted and the ribs spread. Access to the ascending aorta is gained through the pleura and pericardium, which is incised in a longitudinal fashion along the path of the aorta.

Stay sutures are placed in such a way that the ascending aorta is pulled into an optimal position for access. Now, a spot on the distal part of the ascending aorta is chosen, keeping in mind that at least 5 cm is needed for valve system insertion. In a noncalcified portion of the ascending aorta, a double purse-string suture, using 4-0 Prolene, is placed and secured with tourniquets.

Heparin is administered after making sure that there is no bleeding from the suture sites. The ascending aorta is then punctured by the Seldinger technique in the middle of the purse-string suture. A 6 F sheath is inserted and a guiding catheter advanced through the aortic valve, into the left ventricular cavity. The guide wire is exchanged for a stiff wire, using a pigtail catheter. A 24 F sheath is then advanced over the stiff wire, into the ascending aorta. The procedure now is the same as a regular transfemoral procedure.

After successful valve deployment, the sheath is removed and the purse-string sutures tied.
Additional sutures might be necessary if there is bleeding from the puncture site.

Heparin is reversed. The thoracotomy is closed in the regular fashion.

Transapical aortic valve implantation

After preoperative screening and sizing of the native aortic annulus by transesophageal echocardiography and CT angiography, patients are taken to the hybrid angiography suite (Figure 18.2).

Patients with extreme deformities of the chest, right pneumonectomy with displacement of the heart below the sternum, and severe chronic obstructive pulmonary disease (COPD) might not be ideal candidates for the transapical approach. Patients are placed in a supine position.

The procedure is performed under general anesthesia. As a safety net, femoral vessels are either exposed or an arterial and venous 6 F sheath placed.

The position of the apex of the heart is determined by transthoracic echocardiography or fluoroscopy and marked. Preoperative evaluation of the CT scan is also helpful in determining lateralization of the apex.

A 5 cm minithoracotomy, usually in the 5th intercostal space, is performed. The intercostal muscles are divided and a miniretractor inserted. The ribs are spread. The apex is palpated through the pericardium and the right position thus confirmed.

Pericardial fatty tissue is resected and the pericardium incised laterally. Four stay sutures are placed and the apex exposed. Care is taken to identify the bare spot of muscle

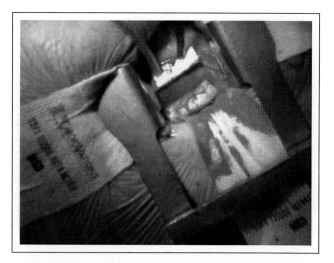

Figure 18.2 (See color insert.) Surgical access to the apex of the left ventricle as used in the transapical approach. An incision in the left 5th intercostal space is made, the apex and left anterior descending artery exposed, and a purse-string suture placed. A soft tissue retractor facilitates access and exposure to the apex. In this figure, a parallel U-stitch technique is used as a purse-string, secured with two pledgets and tourniquets.

on the anterior surface of the left ventricle as well as the left anterior descending artery.

A pledgeted double purse-string suture or double U-stitch suture (3-0 Prolene) is placed on the apical aspect of the left ventricle, taking care to include the bare spot of muscle, taking large bites preferably with a medium half (MH) tapered needle and double armed Prolene suture (polypropylene suture is indicated for use in general soft tissue approximating and/or ligation, especially for use in cardiovascular procedures), thus ensuring transmurality and sparing the left anterior descending artery.

A bipolar epicardial or transvenous pacing wire is placed and tested. The left ventricular apex is punctured and a soft guide wire passed antegradely across the stenotic aortic valve under fluoroscopic and echocardiographic guidance. A 14 F soft sheath is introduced and positioned across the aortic valve. A 0.0035" superstiff guide wire (Amplatz superstiff; 260 cm, Boston Scientific) is then positioned across the aortic arch and "anchored" into the descending aorta. The sheath is partially withdrawn and a 20 mm balloon valvuloplasty catheter positioned under fluoroscopic and echocardiographic guidance. Balloon valvuloplasty is performed once during a brief episode of rapid ventricular pacing (180–220/min). The balloon catheter and apical sheath are withdrawn and a 26 F transapical delivery sheath inserted. The valve is then pushed into position across the native annulus. Fluoroscopic and echocardiographic imaging is used to position the valve and single-shot aortic root angiography is used to confirm the intra-annular position below the coronary ostia. During a second brief episode of rapid ventricular pacing, the valve is deployed. Repeat dilatation is indicated in the presence of moderate paravalvular leakage. Valve function is immediately assessed by using angiographic and echocardiographic visualization. The transapical sheath is removed and the apex securely closed with the purse-string sutures. To avoid tearing of the ventricle, this is done under a brief period of rapid pacing to decompress the left ventricle. Intercostal blockade is performed using a local anesthetic. The pericardium is partially closed over the apex and a left lateral chest tube is inserted.

The minithoracotomy is closed in the standard fashion.

Transfemoral access

The common femoral artery is the preferred access site (Figure 18.3). If not of adequate size, the external iliac or even common iliac artery can be used. Patients are often treated with mild sedation only, when treated percutaneously. However, if a surgical cutdown is indicated, general anesthesia becomes necessary. Indications for a surgical cutdown can be severe calcifications at the access site, borderline vessel size, a need for accessing the common iliac artery, or a wish to suture a graft onto the vessel for sheath insertion.

For a surgical cutdown, patients are intubated and placed under general anesthesia. The left or right groin is draped.

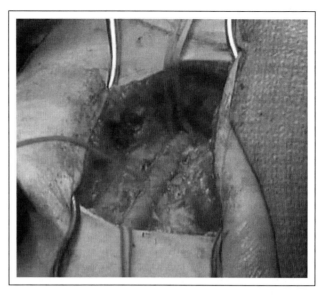

Figure 18.3   (See color insert.) Surgical access to the common femoral artery as used in the transfemoral approach. The vessel and its side branches are snared with vessel loops.

The incision is made along the line of the inguinal band. This ensures that the common femoral artery is accessed at its largest caliber. After the subcutaneous tissue is divided, the inguinal band is identified by palpation. Along its lower border, the common femoral artery is found. It is dissected and secured with vessel loops, proximal and distal to the planned puncture site. Care is taken not to injure the femoral nerve and lymphatic vessels. Medial to the femoral artery, the femoral vein is identified and dissected. It can be used for pacemaker insertion.

A purse-string suture using the 5-0 Prolene suture is then placed on a soft spot on the femoral artery. Heparin is administered and the center of the purse-string is punctured. A 6 F sheath is inserted and a guiding catheter is advanced through the aortic valve into the left ventricular cavity. The guiding wire is exchanged for a stiff wire, using a pigtail catheter. An 18 F sheath is then advanced over the stiff wire, through the common iliac artery, and into the descending aorta. Deployment of the transcatheter valve is then performed in the usual way.

After valve implantation, the sheath is removed and the purse-string on the femoral artery tied.

Heparin is reversed and a Redon drain inserted in the wound. The groin is then closed in the usual fashion.

Subclavian access

The subclavian artery, if of adequate size, can be used with all transfemoral systems (Figure 18.4).

Patients should be intubated and placed under general anesthesia for the procedure. Some centers have performed this procedure with local anesthesia only, in selected cases.

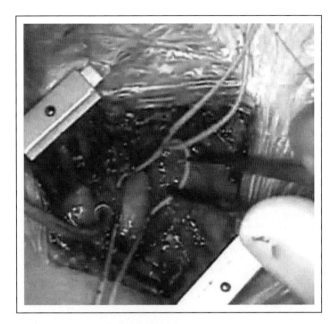

Figure 18.4 **(See color insert.)** Surgical access to the axillary artery as used in the subclavian approach. The incision is made in the lateral portion of the clavicle. The pectoral muscle above the artery is split and the vessel and its side branches are snared with vessel loops.

Patients with stenoses or inadequate artery size, severe calcifications of the subclavian artery or aortic arch, horizontal aorta, or previous use of the internal thoracic artery as an *in situ* bypass graft are not ideal candidates for this access.

The left subclavian artery is used more often than the right one, as it allows for a better orientation of the delivery system, across the aortic arch and the aortic annulus, in a similar fashion as the transfemoral approach. Access to the subclavian artery is gained via an incision below the right clavicle. The incision can be made in the midportion or the lateral portion of the clavicle. The minor and major pectoral muscles are exposed and split if necessary. Then the subclavian vein is identified. Using scissors, the subclavian artery is then dissected, taking care not to disrupt the nervous fibers of the brachiocephalic plexus. Control of the subclavian artery is then gained by applying vessel loops proximal and distal to the desired entry point. Heparin is administered. A purse-string suture using a 5-0 Prolene suture is placed. The artery is then punctured by the Seldinger technique in the middle of the purse-string suture. A 6 F sheath is inserted and a guiding catheter advanced through the aortic valve, into the left ventricular cavity. The guiding wire is exchanged for a stiff wire, using a pigtail catheter. An 18 F sheath is then advanced over the stiff wire, through the subclavian artery, into the aortic arch and ascending aorta. The procedure now is the same as a regular transfemoral procedure.

When removing the system, care has to be taken to cause local dissection. Pulse pressure should be checked distal to the tied purse-string after vessel closure.

Transatrial access

The aortic valve can also be accessed via the right and left atrium (Figure 18.5).

A minithoracotomy in the 4th intercostal space provides a means of accessing the left and right atrium from a lateral angle and avoiding a sternotomy. This might be advantageous in patients who have contraindications for transapical and transfemoral access. Furthermore, entanglement of the mitral apparatus and a transseptal puncture pose additional challenges for this access. The 4th intercostal space on the right is identified and marked. A 5 cm skin incision is performed, starting at the midclavicular line and extending to the anterior axillary line. The subcutaneous tissues and intercostal muscles are divided. Care is taken not to injure the right lung. A miniretractor is inserted and the ribs are spread. Access to the atrium is gained through the pleura and pericardium, which is incised in a longitudinal fashion along the path of the superior and inferior vena cava.

Stay sutures are placed in such a way that the left or right atrium is pulled into an optimal position for access. Now,

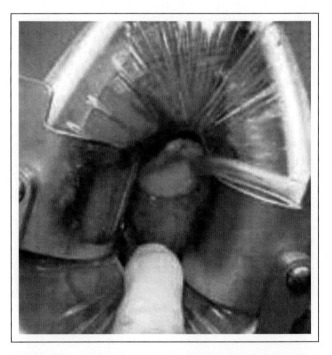

Figure 18.5 **(See color insert.)** Surgical access to the right atrium as used in the transatrial approach. An incision in the right 4th intercostal space is made, the aorta exposed, and a purse-string suture placed. The sheath for valve deployment is introduced from the cranial aspect of the patient and directed toward the aortic valve.

basically any spot can be chosen on the atrium and a purse-string suture, using 4-0 Prolene, is placed and secured with tourniquets.

Heparin is administered after making sure that there is no bleeding from the suture sites. The atrium is then punctured by the Seldinger technique in the middle of the purse-string suture and a guide wire advanced through the aortic valve.

If coming via the right atrium, additional transseptal negotiation is needed to access the aortic valve, by passing through the left atrium and mitral valve.

If accessed through the left atrium only, the mitral valve needs to be passed. An 18 F sheath is then inserted and transcatheter valve implantation performed in the usual way. After valve deployment, Heparin is reversed, the sheath removed, and the purse-string tied. An intercostal blockade is performed using a local anesthetic. The pericardium is closed and the intercostal space readapted. A left lateral chest tube is inserted. The minithoracotomy is closed in the standard fashion.

Comment

The most common access for the implantation of transcatheter aortic valves is the transfemoral approach. Significant advancements in delivery techniques and devices, especially lower profile and expandable sheaths, have increased the number of patients qualifying for this approach and thus more than half of all transcatheter procedures are performed via this access.

Originally performed by a surgical cutdown, most procedures are now done percutaneously.[2] Vascular complications, once associated with an increased mortality rate, are now being treated by endovascular means. Patients who are identified to have an increased risk for vascular complications, such as dissections and rupture, are now being treated by alternative access routes. The key advantage of the transfemoral approach is its less-invasive nature, when compared with all other access options. The main disadvantages remain its dependability on vessels size and the unpredictable endoluminal damage caused by the passage of the delivery system through a potentially diseased aortic arch.[3]

Alternatively, the transaortic approach has been used. It was originally developed for the use of the Medtronic CoreValve (Medtronic, Minneapolis, MN, USA) because the longer device profile precluded its use via the transapical way in patients unsuited for transfemoral implantations. However, it is now being used with the Edwards SAPIEN device (Edwards Lifesciences, Irvine, CA, USA) as well.[4] The advantage of the transaortic approach is its user-friendliness, which includes direct delivery at a short distance and access through a purse-string suture in the ascending aorta with which all cardiac surgeons are proficient. Its main disadvantage is the need for a surgical incision, especially the ministernotomy and the necessity

of accessing the ascending aorta, which if diseased might put the patient at an increased risk of stroke. In recent publications, however, it was demonstrated that almost all patients are candidates for this approach, even with calcifications present on the ascending aorta.[5] In patients with bypass grafts in the proximal ascending aorta, its use is questionable.

Another widely used access for transcatheter implantation is the transapical approach. It was introduced with the Edwards SAPIEN device and has proven its versatility by not being size dependant. Early learning-curve issues with bleeding and hemodynamic compromise have been addressed by standardization of purse-string suture technique and anesthesiological management. Therefore, transapical access has been established as the second most commonly used approach and now provides excellent short- and long-term outcomes.[6] Some view the need for a minithoracotomy as a disadvantage. Currently, there are several automated apical closure devices being developed that promise a percutaneous trocar-based transapical approach. The major advantages of this approach are its straight-line antegrade passage through the aortic valve, steerability within the aortic root, and short delivery distance, allowing for the most precise valve deployment of all available access forms.[7]

If the above-mentioned access routes fail, subclavian and transatrial approaches remain as alternatives. The subclavian approach was first used for the CoreValve device, when transfemoral access was not possible.[8] Subclavian artery exposure is well known to surgeons for arterial cannulation for cardiopulmonary bypass. Although the artery is not often diseased distally, it can be relatively small in caliber and is subject to dissection and disruption on manipulation. Additionally, its use is of concern in patients with previous bypass grafts using the left internal thoracic artery.[9]

In rare cases, a transatrial approach can be chosen. Patients with small peripheral vessels, porcelain aorta, subclavian stenoses, post-left-sided pneumonectomy, and thorax deformities fall into this category. However, I would recommend that, owing to the broader experience, low complication rates, and operator friendliness of the alternate access routes described, this technique should remain in reserve until there are no other good alternatives.

References

1. Cribier A, Eltchaninoff HA, Bash A. Percutaneous transcatheter implantation of an aortic valve prosthesis for calcific aortic stenosis: First human case description. *Circulation* 2002;106:3006–8.
2. Toggweiler S, Gurvitch R, Leipsic J. Percutaneous aortic valve replacement: Vascular outcomes with a fully percutaneous procedure. *J Am Coll Cardiol* 2012;59:113–8.
3. Eggebrecht H, Schmermund A, Voigtländer T, Kahlert, P, Erbel R, Mehta RH. Risk of stroke after transcatheter aortic valve implantation (TAVI): A meta-analysis of 10,037 published patients. *Eurointervention* 2012;8(1):129–38.

4. Bapat VN, Thomas M, Hancock J, Wilson K. First successful trans-catheter aortic valve implantation through the ascending aorta using the Edwards SAPIEN THV system. *Eur J Cardiothorac Surg* 2010;38:811–3.

5. Bapat VN, Attia RQ, Thomas M. Distribution of calcium in the ascending aorta in patients undergoing transcatheter aortic valve implantation and its relevance to the transaortic approach. *J Am Coll Cardiol Interv* 2012;5:470–6.

6. Doss M, Buhr EB, Martens S, Moritz A, Zierer A. Transcatheter-based aortic valve implantations at midterm: What happened to our initial patients? *Ann Thorac Surg* 2012;94(5):1400–6.

7. Walther T, Simon P, Dewey T, Wimmer-Greinecker G, Falk V, Kasimir MT et al. Transapical minimally invasive aortic valve implantation: Multicenter experience. *Circulation* 2007;116(11 Suppl):I240–5.

8. Bruschi G, Fratto P, De Marco F. The trans-subclavian retrograde approach for transcatheter aortic valve replacement: single-center experience. *J Thorac Cardiovasc Surg* 2010:140:911–5.

9. Leon MB, Piazza N, Nikolsky E. Standardized endpoint definitions for transcatheter aortic valve implantation clinical trials: A consensus report from the Valve Academic Research Consortium. *J Am Coll Cardiol* 2011;57:253–69.

19

Fetal cardiac interventions

Carlos A. C. Pedra, Simone R. F. Fontes Pedra, and C. Fábio A. Peralta

Introduction

Maxwell, Allan, and Tynan from the United Kingdom were the first to report a fetal aortic valvoplasty in 1990.[1] Since then, fetal cardiac interventions have been performed for some complex congenital heart diseases (CHD) such as aortic stenosis (AS), hypoplastic left heart syndrome (HLHS) with intact or highly restrictive interatrial septum (IAS), and pulmonary atresia (PA) or critical pulmonary stenosis (CPS) with intact ventricular septum (IVS). Considerable technical difficulties encountered in the early experiences were mainly due to limitations of imaging, equipment, and fetal lie unsuitability. Optimal patient selection was also challenging. However, with evolving and improving imaging and catheter/balloon technology, and the capability of changing fetal position *in utero* or performing the procedure through a limited uterine exposure, such procedures were revitalized by the Boston group from 2000 onward and became an integral part of the treatment algorithm for such complex CHD. The hypothesis behind these procedures has been that a prenatal intervention may remodel cardiac morphology and function to such an extent that they may favorably alter the *in utero* natural history, resulting in improved pre- and postnatal outcomes, including an increased likelihood of achieving a biventricular (BV) circulation. The technique has been standardized and reproduced with few variations among centers.[2] In this chapter, we review the indications, techniques, and current results of fetal cardiac interventions.

Indications

In general, fetal cardiac procedures are undertaken only after ruling out major extracardiac malformations and signs of chromosomal abnormalities by ultrasonographic examination.

Critical AS and evolving HLHS[2-7]: AS should be the dominant lesion with echocardiographic visualization of a thickened, immobile aortic valve with turbulent or decreased color Doppler flow. The Doppler-derived gradient should not be used to select patients, because of frequently associated left ventricular (LV) dysfunction and endocardial fibroelastosis (EFE). The LV diastolic length should be above the lower limit of normal (Z score >−2) at the time of diagnosis. Occasionally, our group may also consider performing aortic valvoplasty in smaller LVs (LV diastolic length Z score between −2 and −3) not only with the hope of preventing LV hypoplasia but also to improve LV function and promote antegrade flow across the aortic valve to theoretically improve cerebral and myocardial perfusion in pre- and postnatal periods, respectively. Evolving HLHS is diagnosed based on functional parameters such as reversed blood flow in the transverse aortic arch (TAA), left-to-right flow across the IAS, monophasic mitral valve (MV) inflow, and moderate-to-severe LV dysfunction in midgestation. Fetal aortic valvoplasty should be performed under 30 weeks' gestational age.

HLHS and intact or highly restrictive IAS[8]: Unequivocal prenatal echocardiographic diagnosis of established HLHS with either an intact IAS or a tiny (≤1 mm) atrial septal defect (ASD) or patent foramen ovale (PFO) and prominent flow reversal in the pulmonary veins should be made. Fetal atrial septoplasty and ASD creation is ideally performed between 29 and 32 weeks' gestation in order to promote survival until term.

PA/IVS or CPS/IVS and evolving HRHS[9,10]: Patients should have a prenatal echocardiographic diagnosis of PA/IVS or CPS/IVS with the following features: membranous PA, with identifiable pulmonary valve (PV) leaflets or membrane, no or minimal systolic opening, and no or minimal color Doppler ultrasound flow across the PV; an IVS; left-to-right shunting across a patent ductus arteriosus (PDA); and right heart hypoplasia, with a tricuspid valve (TV) annulus Z score below ≤2 and an identifiable but qualitatively small right ventricle (RV) with no evidence of RV growth after 2–4 weeks of serial echocardiographic evaluation. Cases with fetal diagnosis of major RV to coronary artery connections should be excluded. Pulmonary valvoplasty is performed between 24 and 30 weeks' gestation.

Critical AS, severe mitral regurgitation (MR), giant left atrium (LA), and hydrops[11]: These fetuses have normal-sized LV and reversed flow in the TAA. They form a unique and challenging subgroup of patients that have been described as such only recently.[11] Aortic valvoplasty and atrial septostomy should be considered between 30 and 34 weeks' gestation as a "salvage" procedure, to diminish the risk of fetal loss due to conspicuous hydrops, associated with pulmonary veins and right ventricular compression.

Technique

Fetal cardiac interventions should be performed in centers with obstetrics backup.[2] Although special units have been designed and used for these procedures, they are usually conducted in the operating room (OR) by a multidisciplinary team, which includes a fetal medicine specialist, a fetal/pediatric cardiologist, and an interventionist. In our experience, the fetal cardiologist is responsible for the patient selection, and pre- and postprocedural echocardiographic assessment. The fetal medicine specialist conducts fetal positioning and anesthesia, and simultaneously

controls the puncture needle and the ultrasound probe. The interventionists (usually two) handle the catheters and guide wires, while the fetal medicine specialist holds onto the needle to keep its position during the procedure.[2]

We prefer to perform such interventions under maternal conscious sedation and regional spinal blockade conducted by an anesthesiologist.[2] This approach is crucial to attain an appropriate fetal lie by external manipulation, if needed (Figure 19.1). Maternal positioning is maintained with left uterine displacement. Maternal hypotension is avoided by fluid and vasopressor (ephedrine) administration. To promote uterine relaxation and avoid contractions after procedural manipulations, mothers are given nifedipine 20 mg TID for 48–72 h, starting 12–24 h before the procedure. When a large polyhydramnios is present and may impair appropriate needle access to the target structure, it is evacuated using a 15-cm-long 21G Chiba needle (Cook, Bloomington, IN, USA). If ideal fetal positioning cannot be attained by external manipulation, the procedure should be abandoned and attempted at another time. In our experience, we do not perform any interventions through a maternal abdominal wall incision and uterine exposure. After optimal fetal position is achieved, the fetus is anesthetized using a mixture of fentanyl (5–10 µg/kg), pavulon

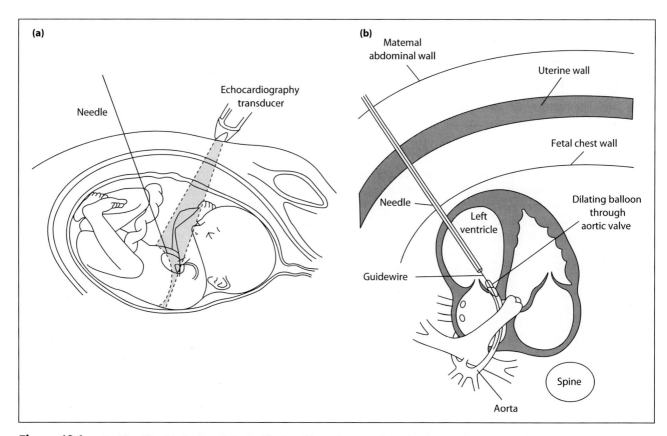

Figure 19.1 Ideal fetal lie. (a) The fetus is in the ideal position. The cannula and stylet are shown traversing the maternal abdomen, the uterus, and the anterior aspect of the fetal chest under ultrasound guidance. (b) The positions of the cannula in the left ventricle and the dilating balloon are shown.

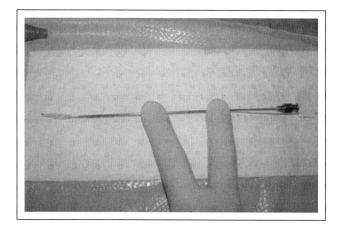

Figure 19.2 Catheter and needle setup. Premarked system used to perform the fetal cardiac interventional procedures. The wire is secured with a tape with its tip advancing 1–2 cm beyond the tip of the catheter balloon. The balloon catheter shaft is marked with a tape that abuts the hub of the needle when the system is advanced through it.

(10 μg/kg), and atropine (20 μg/kg) given intramuscularly or in the umbilical cord using a 21–22G Chiba needle.

Cardiac access is obtained through direct needle puncture of the fetal heart via the uterus and the fetal chest wall (Figure 19.1). Under continuous two-dimensional ultrasound guidance, a 15-cm-long 17–19 gauge Chiba needle (with a stylet) is advanced to the target fetal cardiac chamber (LV, RV, or right atrium [RA]). The imaging plane is carefully adjusted to yield a picture in which both the entire needle length and the target cardiac chamber are included in the field of view. A premarked system (a rapid-exchange 6- to 10-mm-long coronary balloon premounted over a cut-off 0.014 inch floppy-tip guide wire) is advanced to the

desired location (Figure 19.2). The needle, guide wire, and balloon shafts are premeasured and marked, so that positioning within the fetal heart is known from external measurements rather than the ultrasound imaging alone. The balloon shaft is marked with sterile tapes, so that no more than the full length of the balloon is extruded out of the Chiba needle tip, when fully advanced. The guide wire is also fixed with sterile tapes, so that no more than 3–4 cm of the distal flexible guide wire straight tip extrudes out from the balloon tip (Figure 19.2).

The LV or the RV is entered at the apex, with the needle course parallel to the outflow tract, directed at the stenotic/atretic semilunar valves (Figure 19.1). In this way, the valves can be crossed almost blindly, with minimal guide wire and catheter manipulation. For PV perforation, the same needle that was used for apex entry is advanced through the atretic PV. Occasionally, a transplacental and/or subcostal transhepatic needle course is required to reach the desired location, depending on the placenta and fetal positions. After stylet removal, the catheter system is introduced and advanced until the shaft mark reaches the proximal hub of the needle. Balloon positioning for inflation is based on the external aforementioned measurements and ultrasound imaging, with emphasis on the visualization of the guide wire in the ascending aorta (for critical AS), or in the right pulmonary artery or descending aorta through the PDA (for PA/IVS) or in the LA or one of the dilated pulmonary veins (for atrial septoplasty). Balloons are inflated with pressure gauges to allow precise estimates of inflation diameters. Balloon diameters 10–30% larger than the aortic or pulmonary valve annulus are selected for valve dilation (Figure 19.3). Two to four inflations are performed depending on the fetal clinical status. For atrial septoplasty, a 17G Chiba needle with a

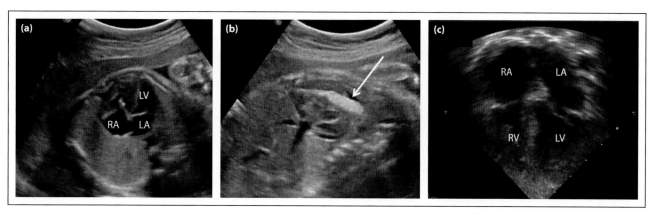

Figure 19.3 Outcomes after fetal pulmonary valvoplasty for critical pulmonary valve stenosis and a hypoplastic right ventricle. (a) Four-chamber view in fetal life. The right ventricle is hypertrophied and does not reach the apex of the heart. The tricuspid valve is smaller than the mitral valve. The Z value of the RV length was –2.5. (b) The balloon is inflated across the pulmonary valve (arrow) in the fetus. The RV was entered at its apex. (c) Four-chamber view of the heart at the age of 1 year. This patient underwent neonatal pulmonary valvoplasty and ductal stenting. Significant RV growth can be observed. The Z value of the RV length increased to 0. LA: left atrium; RA: right atrium; LV: left ventricle; RV: right ventricle.

greater internal lumen diameter is used in order to accommodate the profile of larger dilating balloons. The largest possible balloon is usually 4 mm, expandable to 4.7 mm. Although we have not attempted to implant stents in the IAS, this may be achieved using special catheters specifically designed by the Boston Children's Hospital group for fetal interventions. The 17G Chiba needle is advanced through the thin-walled RA in a perpendicular course toward the IAS. The same needle is used to perforate the IAS to gain access to the LA. Once the tip of the needle is seen in the body of the dilated LA, the premarked system is advanced, until the tape mark on the catheter balloon shaft reaches the proximal hub of the Chiba needle. At this point, the whole system is brought back as a unit until the balloon straddles the IAS. The balloon is inflated with enough pressure to achieve the maximum balloon diameter but the pressure is kept below the burst pressure limit. A second puncture within the IAS is performed using similar techniques, if the newly created ASD is judged to be too small to relieve the left atrial hypertension. After the valves or the IAS is dilated, the whole system (needle + balloon + wire) is withdrawn as a unit through the fetal cardiac wall and out of the fetal and maternal bodies. In order to avoid shearing off of the balloon from the catheter shaft, no attempt is made to bring the balloon back into the needle lumen. Small-volume unit doses of epinephrine (1–10 μg/kg) and atropine should be available for immediate fetal intracardiac injection to treat hemodynamic instability due to significant and persistent fetal bradycardia (<80–100 bpm for 3–5 min). Also, a new 21–22G Chiba needle should be readily available for pericardial drainage in case of tamponade.

After the procedure, mothers are hospitalized overnight. The fetuses are assessed by ultrasound later on the same day and/or the following day before planned maternal discharge. Echocardiography is performed at intervals determined by the primary fetal cardiologist.

Results

A technically successful aortic or pulmonary valvoplasty is defined as one in which a balloon is inflated across the valve, with unequivocal evidence of antegrade flow and/or new aortic/pulmonary regurgitation (AR or PR), depending on the valve being dilated, as assessed by color Doppler echocardiography.[2–7,9,10] We have considered postprocedural AR as a marker of effective dilatation.[2] Interestingly, it improves significantly or disappears until birth due to unknown reasons. It is well tolerated in the fetal life due to the low systemic vascular resistance, determined by the placental circulation and high end-diastolic left ventricular pressure secondary to severe LV dysfunction.

A technically successful atrial septoplasty is defined as one in which there is unequivocal echocardiographic

evidence of a newly created ASD at the conclusion of the intervention or on the following day, associated with a reduction in LA size and improvement in the pulmonary vein Doppler pattern.[8] The ASD size is determined by measuring the width of the color jet (vena contracta) (Figure 19.4).

Possible procedural complications

Significant morbidity to mothers is rarely encountered in the literature. On the other hand, fetal hemodynamic instability due to fetal bradycardia and significant hemopericardium is a common complication, especially in procedures that involve ventricular access.[12] Several mechanisms have been postulated to explain this, including a cholinergically mediated bradycardiac response triggered by a ventricular reflex and potentiated by sympathetic withdrawal, and reduced cardiac output resulting from ventricular distortion during ventricular puncture.[12] Given the high frequency of such complications, prophylactic atropine administration during fetal anesthesia, intracardiac therapeutic injection of epinephrine and atropine, and prompt pericardial drainage should be considered part of the standard of care in such interventions. Fetal loss may happen and although it is more commonly associated with hemodynamic instability and hemopericardium, other contributing factors, such as fetal and maternal anesthetic issues and mechanical stimuli, may also play a role. Premature labor may ensue as in any other fetal intervention. This highlights the importance of adequate uterine relaxation.

Outcomes in fetuses with AS and evolving HLHS

In general, a neonatal BV circulation is achieved in about a third of fetuses who had undergone *in utero* aortic valvoplasty.[2–7] Acknowledging that "fetal AS with evolving HLHS" is intrinsically a disease of the LV myocardium, it seems that only a subset of patients would eventually achieve a BV circulation. This can be best predicted by a multivariable threshold scoring system, which includes a LV long-axis Z score >0, a LV short-axis Z score >0, an aortic annulus Z score >3.5, an MV annulus Z score >2, a high-pressure LV defined by the presence of MR, or AS with a maximum systolic gradient of ≥20 mmHg and milder degrees of EFE.[5,6]

Although appropriate patient selection is crucial for optimal outcomes, we still intervene in an occasional fetus who has morphologic and functional characteristics that do not completely meet the above-mentioned criteria. Fetuses that have smaller and borderline LVs may theoretically benefit from the procedure due to improved coronary flow and

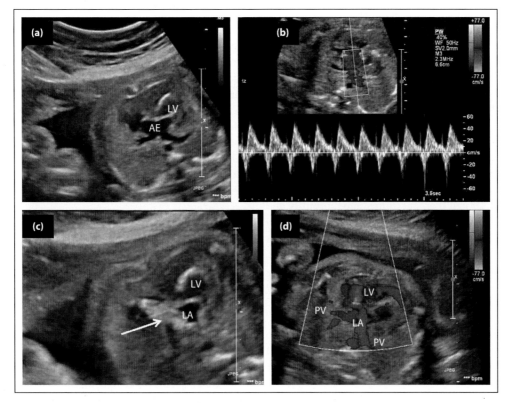

Figure 19.4 **(See color insert.)** Fetal atrial septostomy in a patient with hypoplastic left heart syndrome and restrictive atrial septal defect. Echocardiographic views. (a) The left atrium and the pulmonary veins are dilated. (b) Doppler pattern in the pulmonary vein showing bidirectional flow due to a prominent "a" wave. (c) Balloon (arrow) inflated across the interatrial septum after transseptal puncture. (d) Immediate result after fetal atrial septostomy showing reduction in left atrial size and an unobstructed flow across the interatrial septum on color flow mapping (red color). LA: left atrium; LV: left ventricle; PV: pulmonary vein.

preservation of myocardial function, which may have a positive impact on neonatal outcomes, regardless of the surgical strategy (Norwood vs. hybrid).[2] In addition, promoting forward flow across the aortic valve *in utero* may theoretically help to minimize the neurodevelopmental abnormalities secondary to retrograde TAA perfusion, observed in fetuses with established HLHS. Moreover, progressive growth of the left heart structures during fetal life and in infancy, resulting in an eventual BV repair, has been observed in two patients in our experience (Figure 19.5).

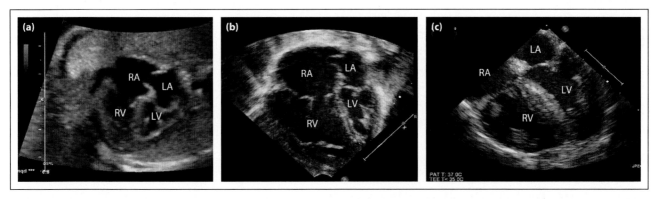

Figure 19.5 Outcomes after fetal aortic valvoplasty for critical aortic stenosis and evolving hypoplastic left heart syndrome. Four-chamber echocardiographic view in the fetus, neonate, and infant. (a) Before fetal aortic valvoplasty, the LV does not reach the apex and is severely dysfunctional and hypoplastic with a Z score of LV length of –2.5. There is significant and diffuse endocardial fibroelastosis. (b) After birth, the neonate underwent balloon aortic valvoplasty and a hybrid procedure. The LV is mildly dysfunctional and almost reaches the apex. The Z score of LV length is –2.0. (c) After LV overhaul and surgical aortic valvoplasty at the age of 9 months, the LV has attained normal size (Z score of LV length is –1.0) and function. LA: left atrium; RA: right atrium; LV: left ventricle; RV: right ventricle.

We have employed a staged strategy for such patients, with fetal aortic valvoplasty followed by a neonatal hybrid procedure ± balloon aortic valvoplasty. This approach works as a bridge to a possible BV repair later in infancy. The LV size and function are serially reassessed by echo, and a cardiac catheterization and an MRI study are performed before surgery. Left ventricular overhaul with BV conversion[13] is undertaken, if growth of the LV is deemed satisfactory (Figure 19.5).

Although postnatal LV diastolic dysfunction may be an issue in patients who have undergone fetal aortic valvoplasty and achieved a BV circulation,[14] in our experience, this is a lesser evil than the immediate morbidity and mortality and long-term complications of a univentricular pathway, such as inexorable deterioration in the cardiovascular function, arrhythmias, protein-losing enteropathy, and thromboembolic events.

In our own experience with fetal aortic valvoplasty (unpublished data), technical success was attained in 12/13 patients. Four of these had severe MR and gigantic LA. BV circulation was achieved in 50% of patients, including two with initially borderline LV and significant EFE (Figure 19.5). Figure 19.6 depicts a flowchart on the outcomes after fetal aortic valvoplasty at our center.

Outcomes in fetuses with AS, severe MR, and gigantic LA

A recently published series showed that this condition is commonly associated with either fetal loss or prematurity and carries a poor prognosis, no matter what procedure is performed in the pre- or postnatal periods.[11] Probably in utero ASD creation or enlargement should also be performed along with aortic valve dilation. Establishing a reliable decompressing pathway for the giant LA seems to be crucial to relieve pulmonary vein and RV compression, systemic venous congestion, and increased cardiac output. In our limited experience, two out of four patients with this condition died in the early neonatal period due to prematurity and hydrops, despite successful fetal aortic valve dilation. One patient died at the age of 5 months after complications arising from percutaneous and surgical aortic valvoplasties and MV replacement. One is still being followed after a successful hybrid procedure (Figure 19.6).

Outcomes in fetuses with HLHS and intact or highly restrictive IAS

In the Boston Children's Hospital experience, fetuses with HLHS who underwent in utero ASD creation or enlargement are born with higher saturations and a more stable clinical initial course.[8] However, surgical mortality after the Norwood operation remains higher than in those patients in whom no intervention was performed in utero. This may be due to the still limited number of patients, but it is unclear whether the procedure performed in late gestation is efficacious, in terms of preventing the development of secondary pulmonary vascular and parenchymal changes.

Our experience consists of five technically successful cases. One fetus died the following day due to unclear reasons. One is still in utero. In two patients, the IAS was highly restrictive at birth and the resultant systemic

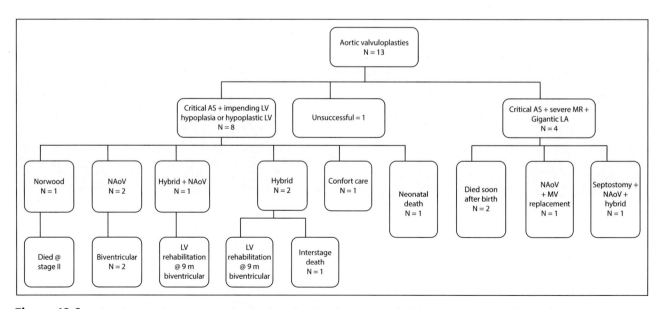

Figure 19.6 Flowchart on the outcomes after fetal aortic valvoplasty at Hospital do Coração, São Paulo, Brazil. AS: aortic stenosis; LV: left ventricle or left ventricular; MR: mitral regurgitation; LA: left atrium; NAoV: neonatal aortic valvoplasty; MV: mitral valve.

hypoxia prompted urgent atrial septostomy. Both died due to several complications after a hybrid approach and prolonged hospitalization. In the other patient, in whom a 3.5 mm ASD was created at 32 weeks' gestation, in spite of an initial favorable clinical course and stability in the neonatal period, she eventually died of pulmonary arterial hypertension due to pulmonary vein arterialization at the age of 6 months, after a Glenn/Norwood operation.

Outcomes in fetuses with PA/CPS and evolving HRHS

In utero pulmonary valvoplasty for PA/IVS or CPS/IVS is more challenging from the technical standpoint due to the heavily trabeculated RV and a smaller RV cavity, which may be associated with a significant failure rate, especially at the beginning of the learning curve.[10] Despite this, it seems that fetuses who undergo a successful intervention show a significant growth of the right ventricular structures from midgestation to late gestation, when compared with control fetuses, who did not undergo prenatal intervention and had univentricular outcomes after birth.[10] In our experience with five fetuses, technical failure was observed in one. One is still *in utero*. The remaining three patients had CPS/IVS and showed significant growth of the RV structures after fetal intervention. They achieved a BV circulation after initial neonatal palliation with pulmonary valvoplasty and ductal stenting (Figure 19.3).

Conclusions

Currently, available data in the literature justify expanding the availability of fetal catheter interventions as a treatment option to centers with the infrastructure and commitment to do these procedures. Nevertheless, they should still be restricted to referral centers, which can amass a critical volume of experience to ensure clinical competence. It is clear that some fetuses do benefit from these interventions, especially balloon aortic valvoplasty. In this regard, prenatal intervention on the aortic valve should be regarded only as a part of a process of overhaul of left heart structures, which will need to continue postnatally, irrespective of the type of eventual circulation. Clearly, more fetuses need to be studied both with and without fetal intervention, preferably in a multicenter registry or in a prospective randomized trial.

References

1. Maxwell D, Allan L, Tynan MJ. Balloon dilation of the aortic valve in the fetus: A report of two cases. *Br Heart J* 1991;65:256–8.
2. Pedra SF, Peralta CF, Pedra CAC. Future directions of fetal interventions in congenital heart disease. *Intervent Cardiol Clin* 2013;2:1–10.
3. Tworetzky W, Wilkins-Haug L, Jennings RW, van der Velde ME, Marshall AC, Marx GR et al. Balloon dilation of severe aortic stenosis in the fetus: Potential for prevention of hypoplastic left heart syndrome: Candidate selection, technique, and results of successful intervention. *Circulation* 2004;110:2125–31.
4. Mäkikallio K, McElhinney DB, Levine JC, Marx GR, Colan SD, Marshall AC et al. Fetal aortic valve stenosis and the evolution of hypoplastic left heart syndrome: Patient selection for fetal intervention. *Circulation* 2006;113:1401–5.
5. McElhinney DB, Marshall AC, Wilkins-Haug LE, Brown DW, Benson CB, Silva V et al. Predictors of technical success and postnatal biventricular outcome after in utero aortic valvuloplasty for aortic stenosis with evolving hypoplastic left heart syndrome. *Circulation* 2009;120(15):1482–90.
6. McElhinney DB, Vogel M, Benson CB, Marshall AC, Wilkins-Haug LE, Silva V et al. Assessment of left ventricular endocardial fibroelastosis in fetuses with aortic stenosis and evolving hypoplastic left heart syndrome. *Am J Cardiol* 2010;106:1792–7.
7. Arzt W, Werttaschnigg D, Veit I, Klement F, Gitter R, Tulzer G. Intrauterine aortic valvuloplasty in fetuses with critical aortic stenosis: Experience and results of 24 procedures. *Ultrasound Obstet Gynecol* 2011;37:689–95.
8. Marshall AC, Levine J, Morash D, Silva V, Lock JE, Benson CB et al. Results of in utero atrial septoplasty in fetuses with hypoplastic left heart syndrome. *Prenat Diagn* 2008;28(11):1023–8.
9. Tulzer G, Arzt W, Franklin RC, Loughna PV, Mair R, Gardiner HM. Fetal pulmonary valvuloplasty for critical pulmonary stenosis or atresia with intact septum. *Lancet* 2002;360(9345):1567–8.
10. Tworetzky W, McElhinney DB, Marx GR, Benson CB, Brusseau R, Morash D et al. In utero valvuloplasty for pulmonary atresia with hypoplastic right ventricle: Techniques and outcomes. *Pediatrics* 2009;124:e510–8.
11. Vogel M, McElhinney DB, Wilkins-Haug LE, Marshall AC, Benson CB, Juraszek AL et al. Aortic stenosis and severe mitral regurgitation in the fetus resulting in giant left atrium and hydrops. Pathophysiology, outcomes, and preliminary experience with prenatal cardiac intervention. *J Am Coll Cardiol* 2011;57:348–55.
12. Mizrahi-Arnaud A, Tworetzky W, Bulich LA, Wilkins-Haug LE, Marshall AC, Benson CB et al. Pathophysiology, management, and outcomes of fetal hemodynamic instability during prenatal cardiac intervention. *Pediatr Res* 2007;62(3):325–30.
13. Emani SM, Bacha EA, McElhinney DB, Marx GR, Tworetzky W, Pigula FA et al. Primary left ventricular rehabilitation is effective in maintaining two-ventricle physiology in the borderline left heart. *J Thorac Cardiovasc Surg* 2009;138:1276–82.
14. Friedman KG, Margossian R, Graham DA, Harrild DM, Emani SM, Wilkins-Haug LE et al. Postnatal left ventricular diastolic function after fetal aortic valvuloplasty. *Am J Cardiol* 2011;108:556–60.

20

Special considerations in small children and newborns

Martin B. E. Schneider

Introduction

Since balloon atrioseptostomy was introduced by Rashkind et al.[1] in the early 1960s, the number of transcatheter interventions in newborns and small infants has continuously increased. Today, a broad variety of interventional procedures can be performed safely in very small patients on a routine basis. These interventional procedures include preoperative palliations such as the Rashkind procedure, alternative treatment options to surgical procedures such as balloon dilatation in pulmonary valve stenosis and a wide spectrum of postoperative interventions to optimize surgical results.

The major limitation of transcatheter interventions in this age group is the size of the vessels in relation to the size of the catheter materials.

Different materials and techniques play a key role in successful interventional procedures in newborns, especially as many of these interventions are performed in emergency situations. Therefore, the first part of this chapter focuses on vascular access options and selected catheter materials.

The second part emphasizes the technical aspects of interventions in small patients, by presenting examples of emergency and elective procedures. This part can only provide a small overview of a wide spectrum of interventional procedures and will be continued by other authors in some of the following chapters.

Vascular access options in small patients

In order to minimize damage to arterial vessels and potential subsequent complications such as thrombosis and embolization, which threaten perfusion of distal tissues, venous access should be preferred, whenever possible.

The most common access site is the femoral vein, followed by the jugular vein.

In newborns, the umbilical vein can serve as an alternative site. As this vein enters the right atrium close to the foramen ovale, it is suitable for transseptal interventions such as the Rashkind procedure or antegrade balloon dilatation in critical aortic stenosis (Figure 20.1).[2–4]

Interventional procedures on the right side of the heart such as balloon dilatation in pulmonary valve stenosis are easier to perform via the femoral vein because the inferior vena cava drains into the right atrium close to the tricuspid valve.

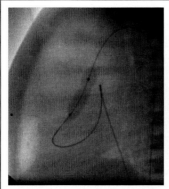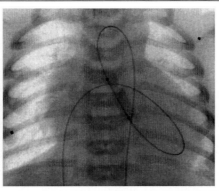

Figure 20.1 Antegrade balloon dilatation in critical aortic stenosis in a newborn.

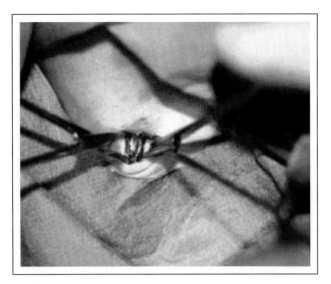

Figure 20.2 **(See color insert.)** Recommendations for axillary artery cutdown.

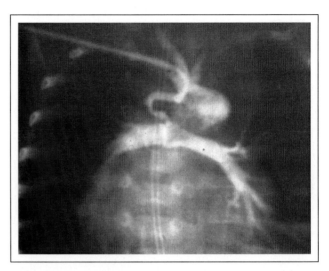

Figure 20.3 Vascular access from the right axillary artery is used for stent implantation into an arterial duct that originates from the aortic arch.

If arterial access is required, the femoral artery is commonly used. For specific interventions, a cutdown of the axillary or right carotid artery (Figure 20.2) may be necessary.

1. Use sharp instruments for the skin incision only.
2. Use two blunt curved clamps for tissue preparation.
3. There is a nerve bundle in this region that resembles the axillary artery. Check for pulsation to correctly identify the arterial vessel.
4. After preparation, the artery should be held and marked by two strings.
5. Puncture the artery with a Seldinger technique while tightening the distal string.

Such approaches may be needed for interventional occlusions of major aorto-pulmonary collateral arteries (MAPCAs), dilatation or stent implantation in renal artery stenosis, and stent implantation into modified Blalock–Taussig shunts or into the ductus arteriosus, if the duct originates from the aortic arch (Figure 20.3).[5–7]

Materials

Although many manufacturing companies offer a broad spectrum of various catheter materials for adult patients, the number of catheters that are specifically designed for very small infants is still limited. Therefore, pediatric interventionists may want to look at catalogs from companies that offer catheters to the adult cardiologists, urologists, radiologists, and especially neuroradiologists: they may find materials they can potentially use for interventional procedures in the very young children.

The following part of the chapter will provide an overview of materials often used in small patients at our center. While this is not exhaustive, it may give the reader a

glimpse of the difficulties encountered in performing procedures in this age group.

Sheaths

In patients with a bodyweight of less than 3 kg, anything larger than a 4 French sheath for the arterial site or a 7 French sheath for the venous site should be avoided. Bigger sheaths carry the risk of severe damage to the vessels. Terumo Radiofocus (Terumo, Leuven, Belgium) sheaths are preferred because of their smooth surface and their favorable ratio of a comparatively bigger inner lumen and a smaller outer diameter.

Sheaths of 3 French are available (e.g., by BALT Company, Montmorency, France); however, the 3 French catheter materials have some disadvantages. Most of these catheters such as the Pigtail or the Cobra are relatively rigid, which makes them prone to kinking during intravascular manipulations. Furthermore, the inner lumen of 3 French catheters appears to be too small for adequate contrast-medium injection for angiography.

Guide wires

For diagnostic catheterization, we use 0.018-, 0.025-, and 0.035-inch Teflon-coated guide wires THSF (Cook, Bloomington, IN, USA) almost exclusively. The advantage of these guide wires is their very soft tip at a stiff but flexible end. This stiff end can be preshaped easily by pulling it gently over the thumb before insertion. Depending on the individual anatomy, different guide wire shapes can be created for maneuvering a catheter into difficult positions. We use a preshaped stiff end of the guide wire for the majority of complex catheter maneuvers.

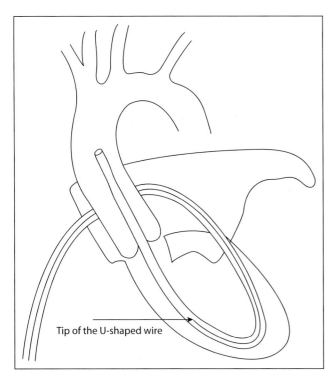

Figure 20.4   Antegrade positioning of a 4 French wedge catheter across the aortic valve (see also Figure 20.1). The cardiologist positions the U-shaped stiff end of a 0.018-inch Teflon-coated guide wire at the apex of the left ventricle and holds it there with the right hand, while the left hand pushes the catheter over the guide wire to the left ventricular outflow tract and across the aortic valve.

The following examples illustrate how individually shaped stiff ends of guide wires can facilitate procedures in specific anatomical positions.

A U-shape of the 0.018-inch guide wire helps position a 4 French wedge catheter across the aortic valve in an antegrade fashion (Figure 20.4).[2–4]

The same guide wire, but with an S-shaped stiff end, is used to maneuver the same catheter across the pulmonary valve (Figure 20.5).

Alternatively, a mild C-shape of a 0.035-inch guide wire can guide a Cobra catheter with its opposite C-shape into the same anatomical position (Figure 20.6).

The C-shaped guide wire supports the Cobra catheter at the tricuspid valve level. To enter the right ventricular outflow tract and then the pulmonary artery, the bent tip of this catheter can be used to hold the guide wire in position with its tip in the middle part of the right ventricle and pushing the catheter while twisting it counterclockwise.

The 0.018- and 0.025-inch guide wires are used for the 4 and 5 French Berman angiographic and the Berman wedge catheters (Arrow, Reading, PA, USA). With the 0.035-inch guide wire catheters such as the Cobra, the Pigtail, or the Judkins can be maneuvered.

Coronary guide wires can be helpful for some interventional procedures such as dilatations with coronary

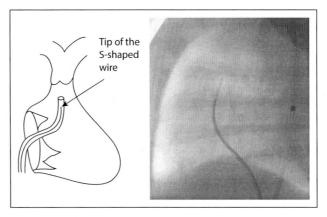

Figure 20.5   Entering the pulmonary artery using a 4 French wedge catheter and the stiff end of a 0.018-inch Teflon-coated guide wire (left: Schematic of the antero-posterior view; right: Lateral view).

angioplasty balloons, or recanalization of obstructed vessels, or perforation of the pulmonary valve in membranous pulmonary valve atresia.

For recanalization of vessels, a stiff and sharp guide wire such as the Cross-it 400 XT Hi Torque (Guidant Corporation, Indianapolis, IN, USA) is recommended.

Floppy and soft tips, for example, the Wizdom 3-cm soft tip (Cordis Corporation, Bridgewater, NJ, USA), or the Pilot 50 (Guidant), are suitable to access small distorted vessels. In this situation, the Terumo guide wires can be used as an alternative.

Stent implantation should always be performed with the support of stiff guide wires. The guide wire size depends on the inner lumen of the catheter of the stent/balloon assembly. If a 0.035-inch guide wire fits into the inner lumen of a balloon catheter, the 0.035-inch Teflon-coated THSF guide wire (Cook) can be recommended for procedures even in small patients. If the inner lumen of the balloon catheter varies from 0.018 to 0.025 inches, the 0.018 SV 5 straight guide wire (Cordis) with its short floppy tip provides excellent support for the stent once mounted onto the balloon.

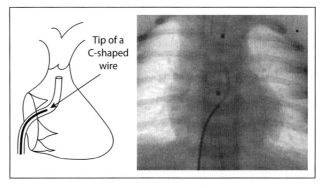

Figure 20.6   Entering the pulmonary artery using a 4 French Cobra catheter and the stiff end of a 0.035-inch Teflon-coated guide wire (left: schematic of an AP view; right: fluoroscopic AP view).

List of catheter materials often used in newborns and small patients

Diagnostic catheters

Angiographic catheters

- Berman angiographic catheter (Arrow) 4 and 5 French, 0.018-inch and 0.025-inch lumen
- Pigtail 4 French Terumo, 0.038-inch lumen
- Pigtail catheters 4 and 5 French, 0.035-inch lumen
- Pigtail 3 French catheter BALT, 0.021-inch lumen
- Cobra with side holes, 4 and 5 French, 0.035-inch lumen
- NIH catheter 4 and 5 French, 0.035-inch lumen

End-hole catheters

- Berman wedge catheter (Arrow) 4 and 5 French, 0.018- and 0.025-inch lumen
- Cobra 4 and 5 French (Cordis) 0.035-inch lumen
- Judkins R and L (Cordis), 4 and 5 French different curves, 0.035-inch lumen (Judkins catheters are quite long (>100 cm) for small patients)
- Terumo catheters 4 French (Terumo): Cobra, Non Taper Angle, and Straight Taper, 0.038-inch lumen

Interventional materials

Rashkind balloon catheters. For the standard Rashkind procedures in full-term babies, the Miller balloon (Edwards Lifesciences, Irvine, CA, USA) can be used. These catheters are labeled as 5 French, but at least a 6 French sheath is necessary to introduce the balloon with some effort. However, it passes easily through a 7 French sheath.

In preterm babies, the Z-5 atrioseptostomy catheter from NuMED (Hopkinton, NY, USA) with a 9.5-mm-diameter, noncompliant balloon and 1 mL maximum volume can be recommended (Figure 20.7). This catheter needs a 5 French introducer and a 0.014-inch guide wire. The use of a guide wire is highly recommended because the surface of the noninflated balloon is quite rough, offering potential damage to vessels and intracardiac structures. Therefore, the Rashkind procedure should be performed under fluoroscopy with the guiding wire securely positioned in the left upper pulmonary vein.

Balloon catheters. The NuMED company produces balloon catheters specifically designed for small patients. The Tyshak-Mini series with balloon diameters between 4 and 10 mm need relatively small introducer sizes of 3–4 French only. It is important to remember that these balloons have to be guided by 0.014-inch guide wires exclusively. Alternatively, the Tyshak II balloons from 4- to 8-mm diameter fit into 4 French introducer sheaths and can be guided by 0.018-inch (maximum 0.021 inch) guide wires.

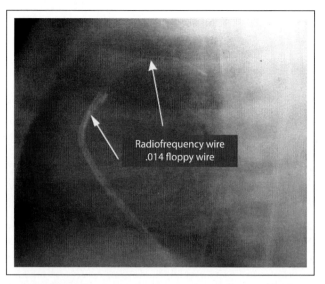

Figure 20.7 Perforation of an atretic pulmonary valve. The radio-frequency guide wire and a 0.014-inch floppy guide wire were positioned together with their ends at the tip of a 4 French Cobra catheter. After perforation, the radio-frequency guide wire must be pulled back, and the floppy guide wire must be advanced across the hole simultaneously.

These balloons are excellent for valvuloplasties, particularly for antegrade dilatation of aortic valve stenosis.

The SAVVY balloons from Cordis 2- to 6-mm diameter) are useful for dilatation of rigid stenoses. These balloons have a very low profile. The maximum inflation pressure is up to 10 atmospheres. With a guide wire lumen of 0.018 inch, they fit into a 4 French introducer.

Coronary angioplasty catheters are commonly used in newborns. Collaborating with adult cardiologists helps us select the most appropriate coronary balloon for our small patients from their wide spectrum of materials designed for the adult patient.

Stents. One of the greatest limitations from a device material point of view is the use of stents in newborns, as they are not designed to stay in the human body for life.[8] One of the few short peripheral stents, the Palmaz P128 (Cordis Corporation) with the potential for redilatation of up to 19-mm diameter, was removed from the market several years ago. That stent could be implanted easily into the vessels of small infants and redilated to adjust for patient growth. It was replaced by the Genesis PG 1910P stent[9] with a minimum length of 19 mm—a length that is too long for most small patients. Other companies have developed new stents of different sizes and lengths such as the EV3 stent (Ev3, Plymouth, MN, USA) and new-generation stents such as the Formula stent from Cook. Although they were able to miniaturize the introducer systems to 5 or 7 French, a 4 French system, which would be needed for a safe arterial access route in small babies, is not yet available.

Basically, there are three different indications for stent implantation in newborns and small infants:

1. *Short-term palliation for a time period of several weeks up to 6 months.*[10] Examples are palliative stenting of critical coarctation or stenting of the arterial duct. As these stents are only needed for a short period of time, redilatation to adjust for patient growth is very rarely necessary. Therefore, the stents used for such indications are mainly premounted coronary stent systems with a diameter of 3.5–4.5 mm and a length between 8 and 12 mm. The decision about which stent type will be used often depends on what the adult catheterization laboratory has in stock, for example, the coronary balloon catheters mentioned above.

   Arterial duct stents can usually stay in place for life because most of them will close spontaneously due to intimal hyperplasia after several months. Coronary stents in other anatomical locations, however, do need to be surgically removed. Thus, implantations of coronary stents in newborns and small infants warrant discussion with the surgical team and careful planning for future procedures as part of an interdisciplinary therapeutic concept.

2. *Midterm stent strategies*[11,12] *for a time period of 6 months up to 2 years, followed by surgical removal.* Balloon-expandable peripheral stents with the potential of redilation from 4 mm up to 10- to 12-mm diameter are required. These stents are premounted stent–balloon assemblies in general, which is their major advantage. We often use Cordis Genesis Palmaz Blue stents on Slalom balloons of the Medium series. The balloon diameters used in small patients range from 4 to 8 mm and the stent lengths from 12 to 18 mm. All of them have a 0.018-inch lumen and need 5 or 6 French introducers. For example, in patients with hypoplastic pulmonary arteries and MAPCAs, the stents can be implanted into the right ventricular outflow tract to increase antegrade flow into the pulmonary arteries to promote vessel growth. These stents can be redilated to adjust for patient growth during the first 1 or 2 years of life until the size of the pulmonary arteries has become adequate for complete surgical repair of tetralogy of Fallot (TOF), instead of unifocalization.

3. *Long-term stent treatment.* There are very few situations where stents with the potential for redilatation up to 19 or 20 mm can be used, even in small infants;[12] for example, implantation into the central part of a systemic vein. Today, one of the shortest stents available for small patients is the Genesis PG1910P (Cordis). It is 19-mm long and fits with a balloon into a 7 French introducer at minimum. Therefore, it can only be implanted in small patients

via a venous access route. The Intrastent LD Max from EV3 Company is shorter than 19 mm, but it is even more difficult to mount onto balloon catheters with a very low profile.

Miscellaneous

For transcatheter perforation of atretic valves[7,13] in this age group, stiff guide wires or laser catheters or radiofrequency wires can be used. We have experiences with the radio-frequency method only and use a 1 French ablation guide wire with a 0.25-mm tip from the Osypka Company (Rheinfelden, Germany). This guide wire fits along with a 0.014-inch floppy guide wire into an end-hole catheter with an inner lumen of 0.035 or 0.038 inch (Figure 20.7). After successful perforation of the atretic valve, the ablation guide wire can be removed carefully by simultaneously pushing the floppy guide wire across the newly created hole for further dilatation of the previously atretic valve.

Techniques

The second part of this chapter will demonstrate technical aspects of transcatheter interventions in newborns and small infants. The selected cases will exemplify how interventional procedures may replace or facilitate surgeries or optimize surgical results.

For each case, we will present the anatomical problem first, followed by the interventional solution. Finally, we will discuss the technical aspects required to achieve the interventional objectives.

Case 1: Pulmonary valvuloplasty and arterial duct stenting in duct-dependent pulmonary circulation

A newborn with a bodyweight of 2.9 kg was diagnosed with critical pulmonary valve stenosis and a hypoplastic right ventricle. Three interventional procedures were necessary to dilate the stenotic pulmonary valve and to perform staged arterial duct stenting at day 2, 3, and 6 of life (Figures 20.8 and 20.9).[7,13,14]

Technical aspects of case 1

Intervention on the second day of life: dilation of the pulmonary valve. A 4 French Cobra catheter was positioned in the right ventricular outflow tract with the aid of a C-shaped stiff end of a 0.035-inch Teflon-coated guide wire (see above). The guide wire was exchanged for a 0.014-inch floppy Wizdom guide wire. The floppy guide wire was easily advanced across the stenotic valve and distally into the

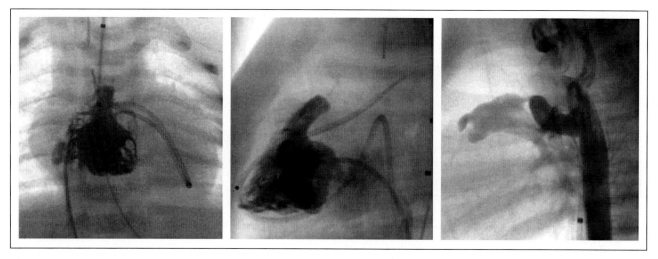

Figure 20.8 Case 1: Anatomy prior to interventional treatment.

peripheral pulmonary artery. Alternatively, one can try to push the guide wire across the duct into the descending aorta. It is important to position the stiff part of the floppy guide wire at the level of the valve, otherwise the guide wire position may be lost while changing the Cobra catheter with the balloon catheter.

Once the correct guide wire position is achieved, the end-hole catheter needs to be withdrawn while pushing the guide wire forward at the same time. Then the balloon catheter is advanced over the guide wire to the position of the valve. In this patient, we used a 6-mm-diameter 2-cm-long Tyshak-Mini balloon. Of note, a second catheter is placed in the ascending aorta from a retrograde approach. This catheter was used for a final angiogram to demonstrate the size and shape of the arterial duct after balloon dilatation of the pulmonary valve. The venous access route replaced an arterial puncture. The duct was shown to be wide open with a diameter of more than 5 mm. Therefore, implantation of a coronary stent was not possible at this time. The prostaglandin infusion was stopped to allow the arterial duct to constrict.

After 24 hours, the arterial oxygen saturation decreased and the patient was taken to the catheterization laboratory again.

Intervention on the third day of life: stent implantation in the arterial duct. For stent implantation, a 4 French Pigtail catheter was introduced via the femoral artery into the descending aorta. At the same time, a 4 French Cobra catheter was positioned in the pulmonary artery (see above), and a 0.018-inch SV-5 straight guide wire was pushed through the narrowed duct deep into the descending aorta. Subsequently, a premounted 12-mm-long Cordis Genesis stent, 1240 PPS, on a 4-mm-diameter Opta-PRO balloon was positioned in the duct via the femoral vein. The stent was inflated at the narrowed duct segment at the pulmonary artery end. The ampulla was shown to be too wide for the safe placement of a second stent.

Intervention at the sixth day of life: second stent into the arterial duct. At this time, the duct ampulla was narrow enough for the safe implantation of a second stent. A stent of the same type as the first was placed in a telescope

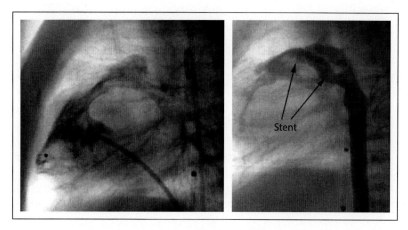

Figure 20.9 Case 1: Interventional result.

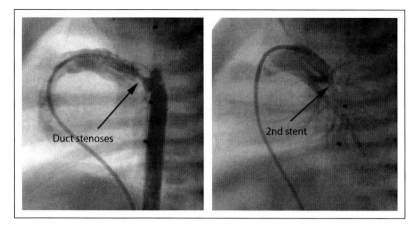

Figure 20.10 Stenting the arterial duct in telescope technique in order to cover the whole duct.

technique behind the first stent in order to cover the whole duct (Figure 20.10).

This case clearly illustrates the necessity of covering the whole length of the arterial duct, when stent implantation is performed.

Case 2: Stenting of the hypoplastic aortic arch in complex duct-dependent systemic circulation

A 4-week-old preterm baby with a body weight of 1.8 kg was diagnosed with a complex univentricular left heart lesion, consisting of a rudimentary subaortic right ventricle, a restrictive ventricular septal defect, and a hypoplastic aortic arch with coarctation. In addition to the complex cardiac defect, this patient had other medical problems related to prematurity.

At this time, he was not deemed to be a surgical candidate, so a combined interventional/surgical strategy was developed (Figure 20.11). The hypoplastic aortic arch and the coarctation were to be stented first to wean the patient off prostaglandins, to allow for patient's growth and weight gain, and finally to perform an elective Norwood

procedure, once the patient reached a body weight of 2500–3000 mg and was in a reasonable clinical condition.[10]

Technical aspects of case 2

Palliative stenting of the aortic arch and the coarctation. After puncture of the femoral artery, a 3 French introducer was placed. Contrast was injected through a 3 French Cobra catheter to visualize the aortic arch. A second 4 French Berman angiographic catheter was positioned in the ventricle for angiography during stent implantation but, due to the large size of the left ventricle and the pulmonary arteries, adequate visualization of the aortic arch could not be achieved, and so this catheter was removed.

Extracardiac structures such as the endotracheal tube or the trachea must be used as landmarks during implantation. Three premounted coronary Cordis Velocity stents each with a length of 8 mm and a balloon diameter of 4.5 mm were implanted by telescopic technique to allow the stents to conform to the slight curve of the aortic arch, instead of straightening the arch with a single stent. In order to avoid dislocation of the first stent while implanting the second, it is recommended to start with the most proximal stent. To minimize damage to the artery, the 3

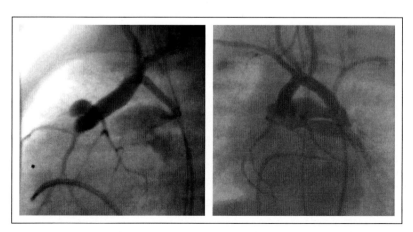

Figure 20.11 Case 2: Anatomy before (left) and after (right) intervention.

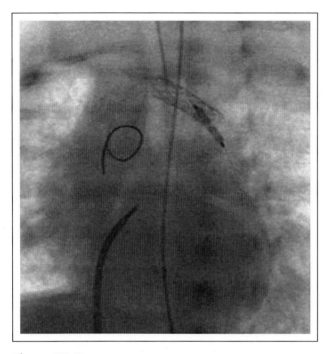

Figure 20.12   Stenting of hypoplastic arch and coarctation.

French sheath was removed and the premounted stents were carefully advanced over a 0.014-inch guide wire directly through the skin. The first stent was positioned at the origin of the right subclavian artery, partly covering the right carotid artery. About 30% of the length of the second stent was telescoped into the first stent. The second stent overlapped the origin of the left carotid artery. The last stent was partly placed into the second with its distal part at the duct level to treat the coarctation (Figure 20.12).

As we used coronary stents with no significant potential for future redilation, these stents had to be cut open surgically or even removed later on. During the Norwood operation 3 months later, one of the stents was removed and the other two stents were cut open in their entire length.

Case 3: Stenting of the right ventricular outflow tract in severe tetralogy of Fallot, complicated by major aorto-pulmonary collateral arteries

The third case is of a 3-day-old patient with a body weight of 2.7 kg and severe TOF with severe right ventricular outflow tract obstruction, pulmonary valve stenosis, hypoplastic pulmonary arteries, and MAPCAs (Figures 20.13 and 20.14).

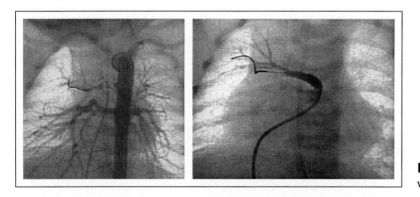

Figure 20.13   Case 3: Anatomy prior to interventional treatment.

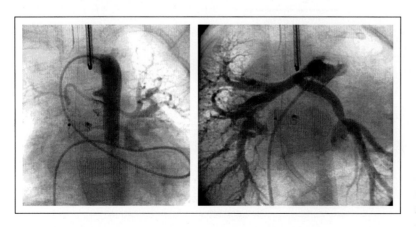

Figure 20.14   Case 3: Interventional result after 6 months.

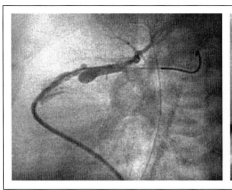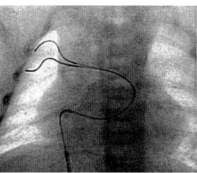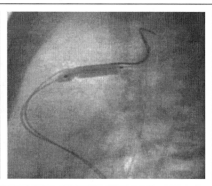

Figure 20.15   Critical pulmonary stenosis from the lateral aspect (left), entering the right upper lobe artery by a coronary guide wire and a second "body wire" (middle), balloon dilation of the critical pulmonary stenosis (right).

Technical aspects of case 3

First interventional catheterization at 3 days of age: balloon dilatation and stent implantation into the right ventricular outflow tract. The pulmonary artery was entered with a Cobra catheter. In order to have stable access to the pulmonary artery, two floppy 0.014-inch guide wires (so-called buddywire technique) instead of one should be inserted deep into the pulmonary artery of the right upper lobe. A 4.5-mm-diameter coronary balloon catheter (over-the-wire system) was used for predilatation of the valve (Figure 20.15).

After predilatation, a 4 French Cobra catheter was passed over the two guide wires into the right pulmonary artery and then the two guide wires were exchanged with the stiff end of a C-shaped 0.035-inch Teflon-coated guide wire (Figure 20.16).

A Palmaz Genesis stent of 12-mm length, premounted on a 6-mm-diameter Opta PRO balloon, was implanted between the right ventricular outflow tract and the main pulmonary artery. This stent–balloon assembly needs a 6 French introducer.

After stent placement, the left and right lower-lobe pulmonary artery could be identified.

Second interventional catheterization at 7 weeks of age: implantation of a second stent and MAPCA occlusion. The infant underwent repeat catheterizations for elective stent redilatation. At this time, a severe stenosis of the main pulmonary artery distal to the stent was noted and a second stent implanted using a telescope technique. The technique was identical to the first intervention, and the stent was of the same type.

After implantation of the second stent (Figure 20.17), the MAPCAs to the right lung were occluded in order to promote the growth of the right pulmonary artery by eliminating competitive blood flow from the aorta (Figure 20.18). The left-sided MAPCA remained open because of an absent left upper-lobe pulmonary artery.

After a further 4 months, the stents were redilated up to a diameter of 9 mm to allow for patient growth and thus promote further development of the pulmonary arteries. The patient underwent surgical repair of TOF instead of unifocalization at 9 months of age.

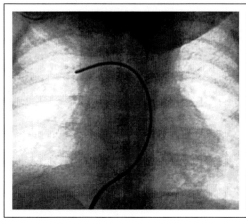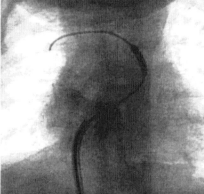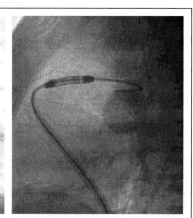

Figure 20.16   The two guide wires were exchanged with the stiff end of a C-shaped 0.035-inch Teflon-coated guide wire (left); position of the pre-mounted stent: AP view (middle), lateral view (right).

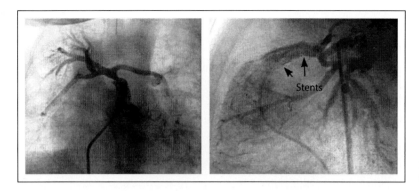

Figure 20.17   Stented right ventricular out-flow tract: AP view (right), lateral view (left).

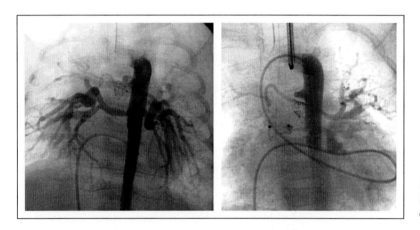

Figure 20.18   Mayor aorto-pulmonary collateral arteries before occlusion (left) and after occlusion (right).

Case 4: Revascularization of obstructed Blalock–Taussig shunt 2 days after surgery

A patient with TOF and hypoplastic pulmonary arteries developed severe cyanosis 2 days after surgical placement of a modified Blalock–Taussig shunt (from the right subclavian artery to the main pulmonary artery). The cause of the cyanosis was acute shunt thrombosis.[15] He underwent emergency cardiac catheterization at 12 days of age with a body weight of 3.4 kg (Figure 20.19).

Technical aspects of case 4

Interventional revascularization of an obstructed aorto-pulmonary shunt. In this situation, arterial access is required. A 4 French Cobra catheter was inserted via the femoral artery and a hand injection of contrast revealed complete obstruction of the Blalock–Taussig shunt. The shunt was recanalized with a 0.014-inch Cross-it 400 XT Hi Torque guide wire and dilated with a 2.5-mm SAVVY balloon. Alternatively, coronary balloon catheters with diameters between 1.5 and

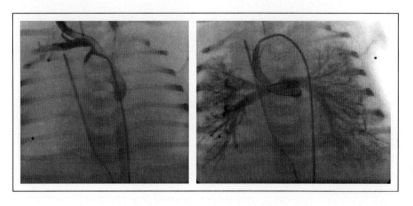

Figure 20.19   Case 4: Anatomy before (left) and after (right) intervention.

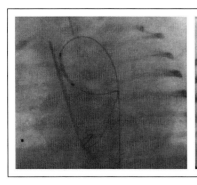
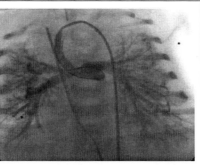

Figure 20.20 Stent implantation into the arterial duct: stent before (left) and after (right) balloon inflation.

2.5 mm can be used. The advantage of the SAVVY balloon is the over-the-wire technique. Most of the coronary balloons work on a monorail basis. This can cause problems in a severely curved route such as the connection between the arterial trunk and the proximal part of the shunt.

The initial dilatation was followed by another dilatation with a 4-mm Tyshak II balloon.

To provide the balloon catheters with sufficient support on their sharply angled route, the guide wire was pushed retrograde across the pulmonary valve and fortuitously across the tricuspid valve into the superior vena cava (SVC). A few minutes after dilatation, shunt thrombosis recurred and the oxygen saturation decreased. An angiogram demonstrated partial occlusion of the shunt.

At this point, the decision for stent implantation was made. Using a 4 French Terumo nontapered angled catheter, the 0.014-inch guide wire was exchanged with a 0.18 SV-5 straight guide wire, and the 4 French arterial introducer was exchanged with a 5 French sheath.

A premounted Palmaz Genesis stent (PG1540PPS, Cordis) was implanted in a retrograde fashion via a short sheath in the femoral artery (Figure 20.20), resulting in stable oxygen saturation of 80–83%. High-dosed heparin was administered at that time.

If stent implantation is necessary in a surgically placed shunt, any coronary stent system can be used. The balloon catheter should be approximately 10% bigger than the fixed diameter of the shunt to give the stent enough apposition to minimize the risk of migration. Redilation is not necessary in an artificial shunt.

Case 5: Recanalization of completely obstructed superior vena cava

This case describes a completely obstructed vein. The patient had a sinus venosus defect with an overriding SVC. He underwent neonatal surgical repair. During surgery, the SVC was reimplanted because of its overriding upon the defect. Five days after surgery, an echocardiogram showed complete obstruction of the SVC. Over time, these patients may develop pleural effusions and venous congestion of the upper half of the body.

The patient was taken to the catheterization laboratory 5 days after surgery at 4 weeks of age with a body weight of 2.8 kg (Figures 20.21 and 20.22).

Technical aspects of case 5

Interventional recanalization of complete SVC obstruction 5 days after surgery. The first angiogram was performed from the right internal jugular vein. A complete obstruction of the SVC was noted. As the thrombus was not organized yet, the SVC was passed with a 0.014-inch soft floppy guide wire (Wizdom). The tip of the guide wire was pushed deep into the IVC and snared through additional access in the right femoral vein by a 10-mm-diameter

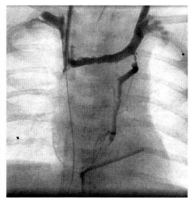
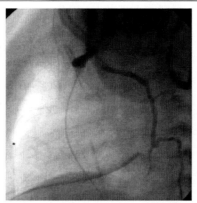

Figure 20.21 Case 5: Anatomy before interventional treatment.

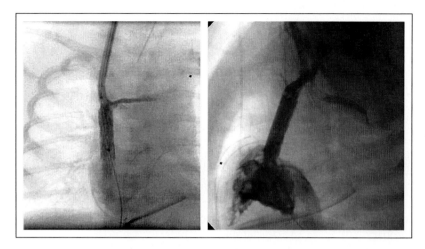

Figure 20.22 Stented SVC in a very small infant: AP view (left), lateral view (right).

snare. Then, two 4 French end-hole catheters (i.e., straight Terumo catheter) were inserted through both venous access sites. Holding the two catheters in a close kissing position, one of them was withdrawn from the sheath by pulling it while pushing the other catheter. This catheter connection between the femoral and the jugular access sites allows the operator to position a broad variety of guide wires. In this case, we changed the 0.014-inch guide wire with a stiff 0.18-inch SV 5 straight guide wire and removed the end-hole catheter.

Balloon dilation with a 5-mm-diameter Tyshak balloon (Figure 20.23) was unsuccessful because the vein collapsed immediately after deflation of the balloon. The primary cause of obstruction was not a thrombotic event, but more likely stretching of the surgically reinserted SVC, which led to the vessel collapse first. Subsequently, a thrombus developed at that site.

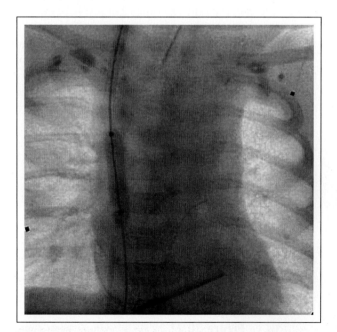

Figure 20.23 Balloon dilation of obstructed superior caval vein.

Stent implantation was considered the best solution for this problem. However, in this case, we had to choose a stent with the potential to stay in the SVC for life. Reoperation of a stented SVC carries significant surgical risks unrelated to patient size and age.

A Genesis PG 1910P stent[9] with the potential for redilation up to a diameter of 19 mm was manually mounted on a Tyshak II balloon catheter with a balloon length of 20 mm and diameter of 5 mm. Owing to the low profile of the balloon, it was not possible to achieve an adequate fixation to the catheter. Therefore, the same balloon, which was used during dilation, was used again. A previously inflated balloon has a rough surface compared with an unused balloon. We inflated the balloon very slightly while mounting the stent and we glued the stent onto the balloon with some contrast medium (Neil Wilson, personal communication).

This stent–balloon assembly was tested outside the patient's body by pushing it through a 7 French sheath to see whether it passed through. After this, a second 7 French short sheath was introduced from the jugular vein and positioned across the obstructed SVC to cover the stent during insertion.

Once the stent was positioned correctly, the sheath was withdrawn very slowly to expose the stent. Injection of contrast medium through this 7 French sheath showed an excellent angiogram of the SVC and the correct position of the stent.

Case 6: Interventional VSD closure in infants

An 11-month-old girl with a body weight of 7 kg suffered from multiple swiss cheese VSDs.[16] Surgical pulmonary artery banding, closure of two large and three small VSDs, and pulmonary artery debanding had already been performed.

Owing to additional muscular VSDs close to the apex, the right ventricular pressure after debanding was still near-systemic (Figure 20.24), and decision for interventional closure of the VSDs was made (Figure 20.25).

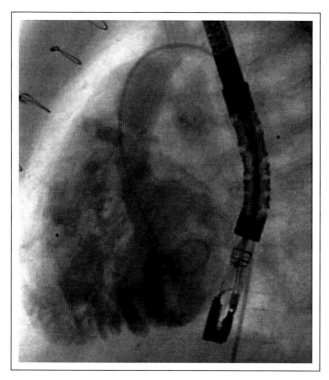

Figure 20.24   Lateral left ventricular angiogram demonstrating diffuse residual left-to-right shunts after surgery. The interventricular septum is not clearly visualized.

Technical aspects of case 6

Interventional closure of multiple VSDs using Amplatzer Duct Occluder II and an Amplatzer Vascular Plug IV. The first Amplatzer Duct Occluder II (ADO II) system was implanted from the right internal jugular vein. After identifying one of the larger VSDs with a 4 French right Judkins catheter under echocardiographic guidance, an 0.018-inch Terumo guide wire was advanced to the pulmonary artery and snared from the venous side (Figure 20.26) and pulled out of the sheath in the right internal jugular vein.

Over the guide wire, a 5 French long sheath was advanced through the VSD by pushing it from the venous side and pulling from the arterial side simultaneously. After crossing the

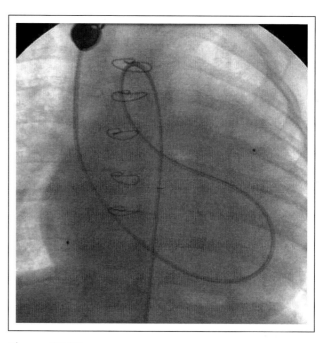

Figure 20.26   Venous–arterial loop from right internal jugular vein across one of the VSDs to the right femoral artery.

VSD, the guide wire and the arterial catheter were removed and replaced with a 4 French Pigtail catheter in the left ventricle for check angiography. Afterward, the 6 × 6 ADO II was introduced into the long sheath and positioned across the VSD in such a way that its distal part was located on the LV side and the proximal part on the RV side (Figure 20.27).

After confirming the correct position of the device by echocardiography and angiography, the device was released.

The second device, a 5-mm Amplatzer Vascular Plug IV (AVP IV) was implanted directly from the left side. As this device can be delivered easily through a 4 French diagnostic Judkins catheter, the snaring procedure for device implantation from the right side of the heart is not necessary. After identifying and marking an additional defect, the Judkins catheter was pushed deep into the right ventricle for a stable catheter position while the device was advanced. The AVP IV can be loaded into this catheter and

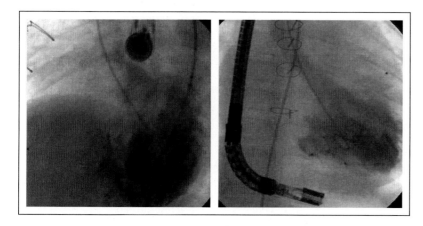

Figure 20.25   Interventional result: mild residual shunt at the level of the two devices (left: lateral view; right: frontal view).

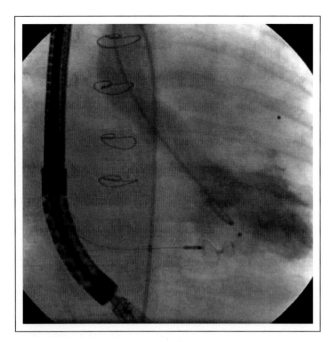

Figure 20.27   Positioning ADO II across a VSD under echocardiographic guidance.

its distal part opened in the right ventricular part of this tunnel-like VSD. By pulling the catheter back, the left disk opens on the LV side of the VSD (Figure 20.28). Like other Amplatzer devices, the AVP IV is delivered by unscrewing it from the wire.

The long shape of these devices fits well into swiss cheese VSDs in a typically thickened and spongy myocardium.

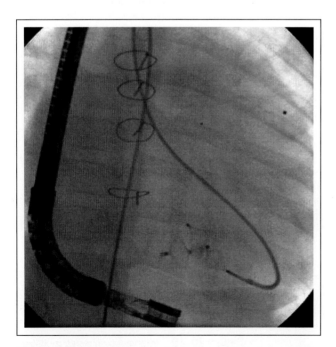

Figure 20.28   The AVP IV device is positioned close to the ADO II in a tunnel-like VSD.

Another advantage is the miniaturized delivery catheter that fits through a 4 or 5 French long sheath. Therefore, it can be used even in very young patients with body weights of less than 3 or 4 kg.

Case 7: Stenting of a restrictive persistent foramen ovale in preterm babies

A baby with prenatal diagnosis of hypoplastic left heart syndrome (HLHS) and a severely restrictive PFO was delivered at 36 weeks gestational age via cesarean section with a birth weight of 2.5 kg.[17] Her echocardiogram confirmed HLHS with mitral and aortic atresia and an almost completely obstructed, thickened interatrial septum. Immediately after birth, she was transferred to the catheterization laboratory. Under echocardiographic guidance, the small left atrium was accessed with a long sheath and the stiff end of a 0.035 guide wire (Figure 20.29).

Figure 20.30 demonstrates the interventional result after implantation of a 6 × 12 mm Palmaz Blue stent and redilatation to a diameter of 8 mm. Of note, the position of the stent is quite anterior due to a tiny (only 1.3 mm) ascending aorta.

Technical aspects of case 7

As newborns with HLHS and a severely restrictive PFO are in critical condition after delivery, the time for transport to the catheterization laboratory as well as the procedure time should be as short as possible. Three physicians are required for the procedure: one well-trained cardiologist performing the peri-interventional transthoracic echocardiogram (TTE), the other two physicians performing the stent procedure. It is crucial to realize that the restrictive or even obstructed PFO will be located far more anteriorly than usual because the ascending aorta is very small, thus giving the interatrial septum room to move more

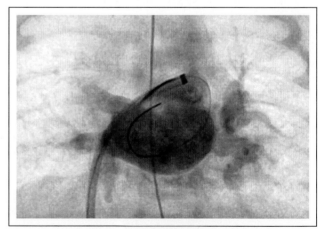

Figure 20.29   A 6 French long sheath is positioned in the left atrium. The coronary guide wire is used to minimize the risk of perforation of the left atrial wall. The pulmonary veins are distended and there is no shunt across the PFO.

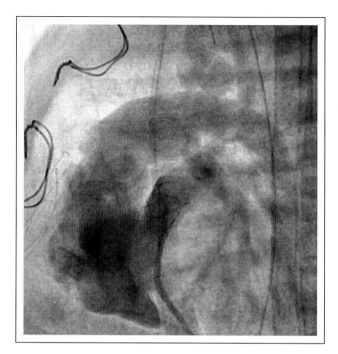

Figure 20.30 Angiography: stented interatrial septum from lateral view.

ventrally. The size of the required atrial communication in a newborn with HLHS is usually between 6 and 8 mm. We recommend a premounted stent as well as a long sheath so that the deflated balloon can be withdrawn into the sheath without risk of dislodging the stent, because the rough balloon surface may get caught in the struts of the stent. Positioning of the stent/balloon assembly should be performed under echocardiographic guidance (Figure 20.31).

Position of the stent after implantation: lateral angiographic view (Figure 20.30), echocardiographic view (Figure 20.31). This

case is only one example of the wide range of various complex interventional procedures in very small patients illustrated in this chapter. However, given the large number and variety of congenital heart lesions and their specific intricacies, it is impossible to cover or foresee all potential interventional treatment options.

The use of materials from medical specialties other than pediatric cardiology enables us today to perform many interventional procedures before or after surgery, or even instead of surgery.

New technologies need to be explored and developed to treat small patients with stent implantation in particular, but without the necessity for later surgical removal.

Bioabsorbable stents or breakable stents (Figure 20.32; see also Figure 20.33) may present a solution to this problem in the near future.[18–21]

A new stent concept: Breakable stent from Osypka Company in Germany

The new Osypka baby stent is a pre-mounted balloon-stent assembly with a stent length of 15 mm and a balloon diameter of 6 mm. The stent is made of stainless steel. Both balloon and stent fit through a 4 French sheath and run on a 0.018 inch guide wire.

This stent is supposed to support the vessel lesion for 1 to 2 years and will be destroyed by over dilation using a 10–12 mm diameter balloon. A row of hook and eyelet connections running longitudinally along the stent opens by over dilating and the circumference integrity will be destroyed. Therefore, this stent can be used in small babies or infants and can stay for a lifelong period without the need for surgical removal.

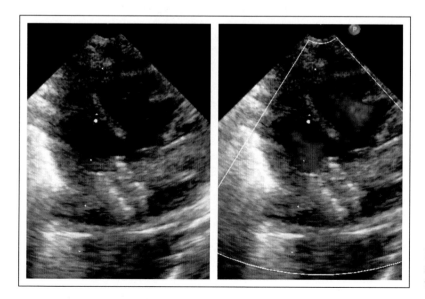

Figure 20.31 **(See color insert.)** TTE 2D (left) and color Doppler (right) images of the stent position after implantation.

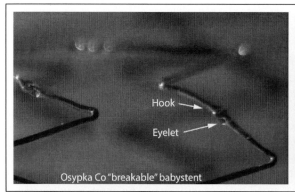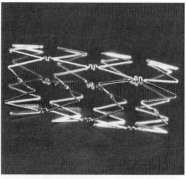

Figure 20.32   A 4 French stent/balloon assembly with a 6 mm diameter. The stent loses its hook-and-eyelet connection by overdilating it to 10–12 mm (see also Figure 20.33).

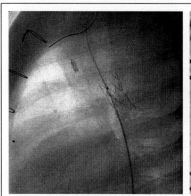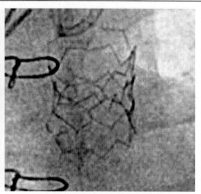

Figure 20.33   First-in-man. The new baby stent after implantation in a small infant with HLHS and aortic recoarctation (6-mm diameter) (right) and after 27 months and redilatation to 12 mm (left). Most of the hooks-and-eyelets are already disconnected.

References

1. Rashkind WJ, Miller WW. Creation of an atrial septal defect without thoracotomy. A palliative approach to complete transposition of the great arteries. *JAMA* 1966;196:991–2.
2. Pass RH, Hellenbrand WE. Catheter intervention for critical aortic stenosis in the neonate. *Catheter Cardiovasc Interv* 2002;55:88–92.
3. Peuster M, Fink C, Schoof S, Von Schnakenburg C, Hausdorf G. Anterograde balloon valvuloplasty for the treatment of neonatal critical valvar aortic stenosis. *Catheter Cardiovasc Interv* 2002;56:516–21.
4. Piechaud JF. Issues in transcatheter treatment of critical aortic stenosis in the newborn infant. *J Interv Cardiol* 2001;14:351–5.
5. Gewillig M, Boshoff DE, Dens J, Mertens L, Benson LN. Stenting the neonatal arterial duct in duct-dependent pulmonary circulation: New techniques, better results. *J Am Coll Cardiol* 2004;43:107–12.
6. Gibbs JL, Rothman MT, Rees MR, Parsons JM, Blackburn ME, Ruiz CE. Stenting of the arterial duct: A new approach to palliation for pulmonary atresia. *Br Heart J* 1992;67:240–5.
7. Schneider M, Zartner P, Sidiropoulos A, Konertz W, Hausdorf G. Stent implantation of the arterial duct in newborn with duct-dependent. *Circulation Eur Heart J* 1998;19:1401–9.
8. Qureshi SA, Sivasankaran S. Role of stents in congenital heart disease. *Expert Rev Cardiovasc Ther* 2005;3:261–9.
9. Forbes TJ, Rodriguez-Cruz E, Amin Z, Benson LN, Fagan TE, Hellenbrand WE et al. The Genesis stent: A new low-profile stent for use in infants, children, and adults with congenital heart disease, *Catheter Cardiovasc Interv* 2003;59:406–14.
10. Fink C, Peuster M, Hausdorf G. Endovascular stenting as an emergency treatment for neonatal coarctation. *Cardiol Young* 2000;10:644–6.
11. Gewillig M, Boshoff D, Mertens L. Creation with a stent of an unrestrictive lasting atrial communication. *Cardiol Young* 2002;12: 404–7.

12. Schneider MBE, Zartner P, Duveneck K, Lange PE. Various reasons for repeat dilation and of stented pulmonary arteries in paediatric patients, *Heart* 2002;88:510–4.
13. Ovaert C, Qureshi SA, Rosenthal E, Baker EJ, Tynan M. Growth of the right ventricle after successful transcatheter pulmonary valvotomy in neonates and infants with pulmonary atresia and intact ventricular septum. *J Thorac Cardiovasc Surg* 1998;115:1055–62.
14. Rosenthal E, Qureshi SA, Tynan M. Percutaneous pulmonary valvotomy and arterial duct stenting in neonates with right ventricular hypoplasia. *Am J Cardiol* 1994;74:304–6.
15. Chessa M, Piazza L, Butera G, Rana Y, Medda M, Carminati M. Images in cardiovascular medicine. Transcatheter balloon recanalization of an occluded modified Blalock–Taussig shunt. *Ital Heart J* 2003;4:285.
16. Knauth AL, Lock JE, Perry SB, Jenkins KJ. Transcatheter device closure of congenital and postoperative residual ventricular septal defects. *Circulation* 2004;110:501–7.
17. Vlahos AP, Lock JE, McElhinney DB, van der Velde ME. Hypoplastic left heart syndrome with intact or highly restrictive atrial septum. *Circulation* 2004;109:2326–30.
18. Ewert P, Riesenkampff E, Neuss M, Kretschmar O, Nagdyman N, Lange PE. Novel growth stent for the permanent treatment of vessel stenosis in growing children: An experimental study. *Catheter Cardiovasc Interv* 2004;62:506–10.
19. Peuster M, Wohlsein P, Brugmann M, Ehlerding M, Seidler K, Fink C et al. A novel approach to temporary stenting: Degradable cardiovascular stents produced from corrodible metal-results 6–18 months after implantation into New Zealand white rabbits. *Heart* 2001;86:563–9.
20. Schneider MBE, Fischer G, Lange PE. First human use of a new "PFM-Babystent." *Heart* 2003;89:83.
21. Sigler M, Schneider K, Meissler M, König K, Schneider MBE. Breakable stent for interventions in infants and neonates: An animal study and histopathological findings. *Heart* 2006;92(2):245.

21

Congenital aortic valve stenosis: Background and valvuloplasty in children and adults

Oleg Reich and Petr Tax

Anatomy

In congenital aortic valve stenosis, the aortic annulus may be hypoplastic to some extent, the leaflets may be thickened, and the commissures may be fused to varying degrees. Dysplastic or unicuspid valves (Figure 21.1a) often seen in newborns are present in about 10% of infants and 3% of older children in whom the treatment is indicated. Trileaflet valves (Figure 21.1b) are seen in 25% of infants and 40% of older patients who require treatment. The majority of the stenotic valves are bicuspid.[1] There are two forms of bicuspid aortic valves: balanced or "anatomically bicuspid" and unbalanced or "functionally bicuspid." The "anatomically bicuspid" valve is composed of two equal-sized cusps with two sinuses of Valsalva (Figure 21.1c). The "functionally bicuspid" valve also opens as bicuspid, but it has three sinuses, two of them adjacent to a fused cusp, which is actually formed by two unequal cusps conjoined by an unopened commissure. The fused cusp is larger than the opposite one, hence "unbalanced bicuspid valve" (Figure 21.1d). This anatomical concept is important in regard to the prognosis of the valvuloplasty.[1] In the balanced bicuspid valves as well as in trileaflet stenotic valves, the orifices are usually enlarged by splitting of the functioning commissures, whereas in the unbalanced bicuspid valves, the fused cusp is often torn aside from the rudimentary commissure (Figure 21.2),[2] presumably due to unequal rigidity of the different-sized cusps.

Pathophysiology

Aortic stenosis causes left ventricular pressure overload. Despite this pressure overload, the wall stress throughout systole is usually not higher than normal because of increased left ventricular wall thickness. Another compensatory mechanism is a lengthening of the ejection time at the expense of the diastole duration. Owing to adaptation, the systolic left ventricular function is usually well maintained over a long period of time. Diastolic function varies according to the severity of the left ventricular hypertrophy. In pronounced hypertrophy, the compliance of the left ventricular wall is markedly decreased and the left ventricular end-diastolic pressure is elevated. Elevated end-diastolic pressure and a shortened diastole duration contribute to a limitation of the subendocardial coronary flow. In severe stenosis, restriction of the coronary flow causes subendocardial ischemia during exercise or even at

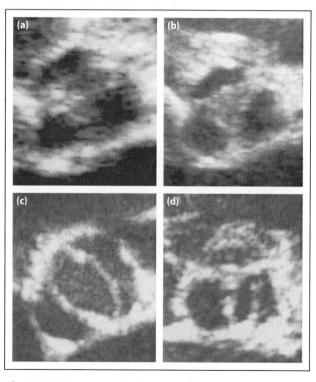

Figure 21.1 The anatomy of congenital aortic stenosis assessed by two-dimensional echocardiography in parasternal short-axis view. (a) Unicuspid valve, (b) trileaflet valve, (c) balanced bicuspid ("anatomically bicuspid") valve, and (d) unbalanced bicuspid ("functionally bicuspid") valve.

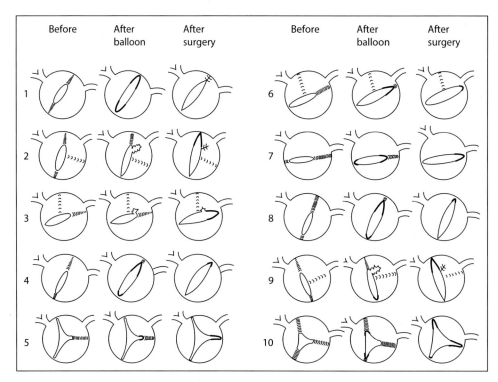

Figure 21.2   Schematic drawing of valves before intervention, after balloon dilation, and after surgical correction. Bold lines show change obtained with each intervention. (From Solymar L et al. *J Thorac Cardiovasc Surg* 1992;104(6):1709–13.)

rest. Acute myocardial ischemia during exercise may cause ventricular arrhythmias and syncope or sudden death. Another sign of severe stenosis is the inability of the left ventricle to increase the cardiac output adequately with exercise, which is reflected by an insufficient systolic pressure rise or even by a systolic pressure drop on exertion.

Clinical symptoms

Some infants present with congestive heart failure due to the left ventricular dysfunction. In some, subendocardial ischemia causes left ventricular endocardial fibroelastosis and fibrosis of the papillary muscles with mitral insufficiency. The majority of patients are asymptomatic and the disease is usually diagnosed because of the presence of a murmur. Other common signs are fatigue, exertional dyspnoea, angina pectoris, and syncope. More than 70% of the patients with severe aortic stenosis may die suddenly.[3]

Indications for treatment

The normal aortic valve area is approximately 2.0 cm²/m². Aortic stenosis is considered mild when the area is above 0.8 cm²/m², moderate with the area of 0.5–0.8 cm²/m², and severe with the area less than 0.5 cm²/m². With a normal cardiac output, severe stenosis causes a peak systolic gradient of over 75 mmHg and a mean gradient of over 40 mmHg. Necessary treatment is indicated based on the clinical and echocardiographic criteria:

- In all patients with Doppler peak systolic gradient ≥75 mmHg and/or mean gradient ≥40 mmHg
- In patients with left ventricular strain on the ECG and peak gradient of ≥60 mmHg
- Regardless of the gradient in patients presenting with syncope, low cardiac output, or severe left ventricular dysfunction

The gradient must be measured at rest and any factors that may increase the resting cardiac output, such as anemia, must be excluded. In borderline cases, an exercise test is performed and if subendocardial ischemia or a hypotensive reaction occurs, treatment is indicated. In patients with moderate to severe aortic regurgitation, surgical treatment is preferred to valvuloplasty.

Alternatives

Studies that compared valvuloplasty with surgical valvotomy have reported almost identical results.[4,5] Therefore, in patients with aortic stenosis and zero to mild aortic regurgitation, valvuloplasty is the method of choice. In patients with more than mild aortic regurgitation, the Ross procedure or valve replacement is indicated.

History of the procedure

Percutaneous balloon valvuloplasty was first described in 1983.[6] A year later, the effectiveness of the method in gradient reduction and the low incidence of restenosis shortly after the procedure was documented in children with congenital aortic stenosis.[7] In 1986, the first balloon valvuloplasty was performed in a newborn with critical aortic stenosis.[8]

Precatheter imaging

All the information needed for the indication for valvuloplasty is obtained by echocardiography. The aortic valve gradient is assessed by continuous-wave Doppler from a subcostal, apical, suprasternal, and right subclavicular approach, and the highest gradient measured is considered. The peak gradient is calculated from maximum flow velocity and the mean gradient using a time–velocity integral.

The morphology of the aortic valve is assessed by means of two-dimensional imaging from parasternal long- and short-axis views. The aortic annulus diameter is measured between the hinge points of the valve leaflets in the two-dimensional parasternal long-axis view (Figure 21.3). The annulus must be carefully scanned by transducer angulation so that the maximum possible diameter is obtained. With such a measurement, almost perfect agreement between the echocardiography and aortography is achieved in the annulus diameter measurements.[1] Aortic insufficiency is assessed by color-flow mapping and pulsed Doppler.

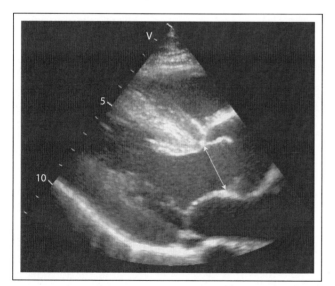

Figure 21.3 The aortic annulus diameter is measured between the hinge points of the valve leaflets in the two-dimensional parasternal long-axis view. The annulus must be carefully and thoroughly scanned by transducer angulation so that the maximum possible diameter is obtained.

Anesthesia

General anesthesia is used to avoid restlessness and agitation that can occur during valve dilation due to severely impaired cardiac output or chest pain. In patients in good clinical condition, endotracheal intubation is not necessary. Anesthetics are chosen and administered so that adequate spontaneous ventilation is preserved. The most common medications are

- Intravenous *ketamine* 1% 2.0–2.5 mg/kg and *midazolam* 0.2–0.3 mg/kg followed by a continuous infusion of *ketamine* in a 1 mg/kg/hour dosage
- In children older than 6 years—*propofol* 1.5–2.0 mg/kg along with a slow injection of *sufentanil* 1–2 µg/kg followed by a continuous infusion of *propofol* in a dose of 100–200 µg/kg/min.

Local anesthesia of the groin supplements the general anesthesia. Oxygen is administered by a face mask prior to and during the dilation.

Access

Catheters are usually inserted through the femoral arteries. With a reliable echocardiographic measurement of the aortic annulus (see the earlier section, "Precatheter Imaging"), a sheath of a diameter appropriate for the intended balloon catheter can be used from the beginning of the procedure. The largest contemporary balloons can be inserted through 9 to 11 F sheaths, therefore, the limb perfusion is usually not at risk even in a long procedure. If, however, any concern exists in this respect, a double-balloon technique (see the upcoming section, "Double-Balloon Technique") should be considered.

Occasionally, it may be impossible to pass the guide wire from the retrograde approach to the left ventricle. In such cases, the procedure can be completed from the femoral venous access. First, the foramen ovale patency is explored by a catheter inserted through a short sheath, which is then exchanged for an appropriate long sheath if a transseptal puncture is required.

Protocol of hemodynamic assessment

Pressure gradients

Crossing the stenotic aortic valve is often not easy and once the catheter is in the left ventricle it is not wise to pull it back. Therefore, the gradient is usually measured by a simultaneous recording of the pressures in the left ventricle and the aorta. Alternatively, the pullback gradient can be measured by a catheter capable of pressure transmission while maintaining the guide wire in place, such as Multi-Track™ by NuMED. Simultaneous measurement can readily be obtained with two catheters. Another option is to measure the distal pressure by a cannula in the femoral artery or by a sheath side port, provided that the diagnostic catheter is at least 1 F thinner than the sheath. However, with the use of a peripheral artery, the gradient is artificially reduced by the effect of pulse amplification.[9]

Catheter-measured gradients are usually lower than those measured by Doppler echocardiography. The reasons are numerous:

- Doppler measures instantaneous gradient whereas a catheter measures peak-to-peak gradient. The peak pressure in the aorta is somewhat delayed compared with the left ventricular pressure (Figure 21.4).[10]
- Doppler tends to overestimate the gradients due to the pressure recovery effect.[11,12]
- If a peripheral artery is used, the gradient is reduced by the pulse-amplification effect.
- During the catheterization, cardiac output is somewhat diminished due to anesthesia or sedation compared with the echocardiographic measurements performed in a completely awake state. With a given valve area, less flow results in lower gradient.

Because of the last point, Doppler gradients are usually used for valvuloplasty indication, whereas a comparison of the catheter-measured gradient prior to and after the valvuloplasty serves as an instant measure of its effectiveness.

Aortic valve area

The most accurate criterion as well as the assessment of valvuloplasty success is the calculation of the aortic valve area. This method requires correct simultaneous pressure recordings from the left ventricle and the ascending aorta along with correct measurement of the cardiac output. Using the *Gorlin formula*, the aortic valve area (A_{AOV}) in cm^2 is calculated from the systemic flow (Qs) in liters per minute, heart rate (HR) in beats per minute, systolic ejection time (SET) in seconds per heart cycle, and the mean systolic gradient (ΔP) in mmHg:

$$A_{AOV} = \frac{1000 \cdot Qs}{44.3 \cdot HR \cdot SET \cdot \sqrt{\Delta P}}$$

If the systemic flow is indexed per m^2 of body surface area, the valve area is obtained in cm^2/m^2. The actual routine is as follows:

1. In several consecutive heart cycles, the area between left ventricular and aortic pressure curves and the *SET* is measured (Figure 21.4).

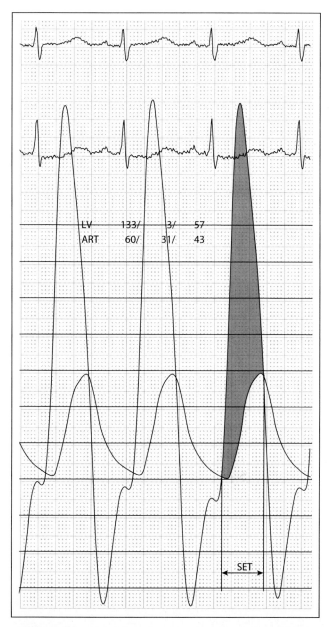

Figure 21.4 A simultaneous recording of pressures in the left ventricle (LV) and in the aorta (ART). The shaded area between the curves and the systolic ejection time (SET) are used for the calculation of the aortic valve area.

2. For each cycle, the area in mm^2 is divided by the *SET* in mm and the result is divided by the recorder excursion in mm per 1 mmHg. This way, the mean systolic pressure gradient in mmHg is obtained. The average mean systolic pressure gradient calculated from all the measured cycles is entered into the formula as the ΔP.

3. *SET* is converted from mm to seconds by dividing it by the recorder speed in mm/second and the average *SET* from all the measured cycles is entered into the formula.

Angiography

Biplane aortography with contrast injection into the aortic root is performed to measure the valve annulus, assess the position of aortic valve orifice, and exclude or document aortic valve incompetence. The aortic annulus diameter is measured between the leaflet hinge points in the frontal projection. Aortography is also used to choose a balloon of the proper length (Figure 21.5).

Balloon

An ideal balloon catheter should have a low profile and fast inflation and deflation times. There is no need for high-pressure balloons, but they should be noncompliant. Whereas in infants, slim catheter shafts and introducers are necessary, in older patients, thicker shafts capable of accommodating thicker guide wires are preferable as they can better support the balloon position during the left ventricular contraction. For proper balloon selection, it is essential to have a wide variety of balloon sizes with the smallest possible balloon diameter increments instantly available.

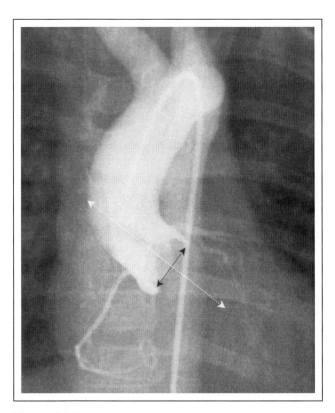

Figure 21.5 Aortography in the frontal projection. The aortic annulus diameter is measured between the leaflets, hinge points (black arrow) and the proper balloon length is assessed according to the measurement in the long axis of the left ventricular outflow tract and ascending aorta (white arrow).

Balloon diameter

The optimum valvuloplasty result would be maximum gradient relief with minimum valve incompetence. Such a result, however, is seldom obtained and a reasonable goal should be to decrease the gradient below the indication level and at the same time keep the valve incompetence to a minimum. Therefore, a more conservative balloon policy is employed:

- The balloon diameter should not exceed the diameter of the aortic annulus.[13,14]
- It is wise to start with a balloon diameter of about 90% of the aortic annulus and eventually increase its size by 1 mm, if the gradient was not reduced sufficiently and the aortic valve remained competent.

Double-balloon technique

The aortic valve dilation can be performed by simultaneous inflation of two balloons introduced into the valve from both the femoral arteries (Figure 21.6). Advantages of this double-balloon technique are as follows:

- Compared with one big balloon, two smaller balloons usually require smaller introducers and, accordingly, the risk of femoral artery injury is decreased.
- With two balloons, apposition is never complete and blood can vent between them; this reduces the forces expelling the balloons out of the valve during left ventricular systole and avoids a severe aortic pressure drop during the dilation.[15]
- It is believed that in bicuspid valves, the two balloons comply better with the valve anatomy and therefore are less likely to cause a cusp disruption than a single balloon.[16]
- The double arterial access enables the most accurate measurement of the gradient and the valve area by a simultaneous pressure recording in the left ventricle and the ascending aorta (see the earlier section, "Protocol of Hemodynamic Assessment").

A disadvantage of the double-balloon technique is the need for two guide wires to be passed through the aortic valve into the left ventricle, which may prolong the procedure. The *effective diameter* (D_{eff}) of a combination of two balloons with diameters D_1 and D_2 may be calculated from the following equation[17] (*arccos* is arcus cosinus):

$$D_{eff} = \frac{D_1 \times \left(\pi - \arccos\left(\dfrac{D_1 - D_2}{D_1 + D_2} \right) \right) + D_2 \times \arccos\left(\dfrac{D_1 - D_2}{D_1 + D_2} \right) + 4 \times \sqrt{\dfrac{D_1 \times D_2}{4}}}{\pi}$$

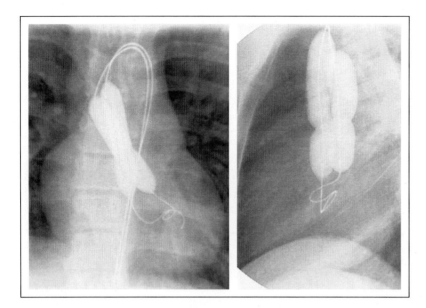

Figure 21.6 The double-balloon technique in frontal and lateral projections. The aortic valve dilation is performed by a simultaneous inflation of two balloons introduced into the valve from both the femoral arteries.

or roughly but simply:

$$D_{eff} = \frac{D_1 + D_2}{1.22}$$

Balloon length

A balloon of the optimum length should safely straddle the aortic valve without overlapping the mitral valve chordae. The optimum ratio of the balloon length to the balloon diameter is ≥3 and it should never be <2.

Balloon burst pressures

Rated burst pressures of valvuloplasty balloons range from 5 to 8 atm in the smallest diameters to 1.5 to 3 atm in the largest ones. The specified rated burst pressures should never be reached. The use of manometer-equipped inflation syringes for valvuloplasty is not always practical. Rather than watching the manometer dial, the operator should carefully observe the balloon position and the waist caused by the stenotic valve. Once the waist disappears, the inflating pressure should be released immediately. As a safety measure, syringes with different cylinder diameters (nominal volumes) can be used to reach different inflation pressures (Figure 21.7).

Brands available

A variety of PTV (percutaneous transluminal valvuloplasty) catheters are produced by NuMED (now available through B. Braun Medical, Inc.), such as Tyshak®, Tyshak II®, Tyshak Mini, Z-MED™, Z-MED II™, Coefficient™, and Nucleus™. They provide a wide range of balloon diameters from 4 to 30 mm with 1–2-mm increments. An adequate

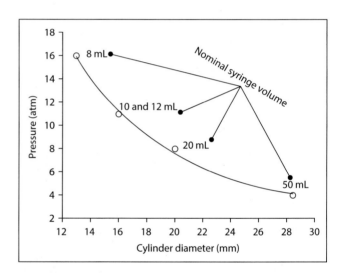

Figure 21.7 Maximum pressure attainable using different syringes.

range of balloon lengths is provided for each diameter. The Z-MED, Z-MED II, and Coefficient catheters provide higher-rated burst pressures than the Tyshak, Tyshak II, and Tyshak Mini catheters. The Tyshak and Z-MED catheters accommodate thicker guide wires, and have slightly higher-rated burst pressures than the Tyshak II, Tyshak Mini, Z-MED II, and Coefficient balloon catheters. With the combination of a thicker shaft and a thicker wire, Tyshak and Z-MED balloons can resist the left ventricular ejection power better and therefore are preferred in older children.

The Nucleus balloon catheter was specially designed with a waist in the middle portion to assure a stable position in the valve during inflation. It is therefore particularly suitable for aortic valvuloplasty. It is available in diameters from 10 to 30 mm with 2 mm increments and a variety of balloon length choices for each diameter.

X™Line catheters by NuMED (Tyshak-X™, Z-MED-X™, Z-MED II-X™, and Nucleus-X™) have a radiopaque braided inner tubing that provides better pushability and increased stiffness compared with the basic models. Small balloon diameters are not available in the X™Line. Tyshak-X, Z-MED-X, and Z-MED II-X start at 8 mm diameter. The smallest Nucleus-X balloon diameter is 18 mm.

VACS II and VACS III by Osypka are other low-profile balloons available in diameters 4–30 mm with 1 mm increments up to 18 mm with the exception of 11 and 13 mm, which are not available. Above 18 mm diameter, the increments are 2 mm. Two to four different lengths are available per diameter, except for the 4, 5, and 6 mm diameters, that come with the single length of 20 mm.

Another option is Cristal Balloon by Balt. The available balloon diameters range from 8 to 40 mm with increments of 2 to 3 mm up to 30 mm diameter, and 5 mm increments above that. There is only a single balloon length for each diameter, except for balloon diameters of 12 and 15 mm, which are available in different lengths. The semicompliant construction of these balloons enables predictable variation of diameters at a set pressure above or below the nominal level. The actual diameter for a given pressure is assumed from a compliance chart provided by the manufacturer. The semicompliance of the catheters may actually be a setback for the aortic valvuloplasty where a precise balloon sizing is essential and the use of balloon inflation devices equipped with a pressure gauge is impractical (see the sections "Balloon Diameter" and "Balloon Burst Pressures").

Valvuloplasty

Heparin in a dose of 100 IU per kg of body weight is administered immediately after vascular access is established. Hemodynamic measurements and aortography are performed. A systolic frame of the aortography in which the position of the effective orifice is documented by a jet of noncontrast blood is used as a road map (Figure 21.8a). Angulated catheters such as cobra, Judkins right coronary, or left coronary bypass catheters or a pigtail catheter are used to guide a hydrophilic polymer-coated guide wire (such as Radiofocus® by Terumo) through the valve orifice. The angle of interrogation is adjusted by two different kinds of movement: in the frontal plane by pushing or pulling the catheter and in the sagittal plane by catheter rotation. The guide wire is guided into the orifice by repeated gentle, yet sufficiently rapid, to-and-fro movements until it slides into the left ventricle. If the angle of attack is considered appropriate and the guide wire cannot cross the valve, straight-tip wire may be replaced for an angled-tip one and vice versa. If, however, the ideal angle of interrogation cannot be attained, the catheter is exchanged for one with a different angulation. In a difficult situation, the tip of a pigtail catheter may gradually be cut off to provide fine angle changes. Once the valve is crossed by the guide wire, the catheter is advanced to the left ventricle and the pressure gradient is measured. A J-shaped exchange wire is then inserted toward the left ventricular apex and an appropriate balloon catheter is advanced over the wire. The

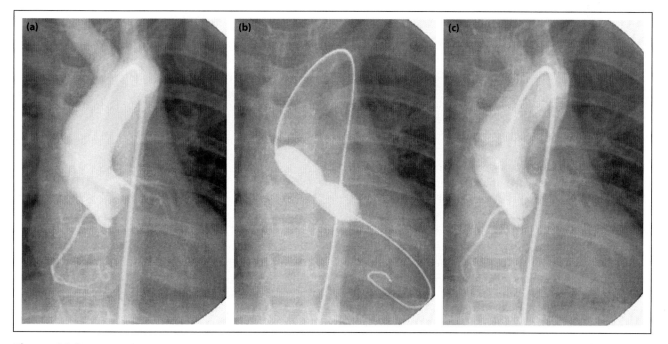

Figure 21.8 Aortic valvuloplasty from a retrograde approach. (a) On the aortogram prior to the procedure, doming of the aortic valve and severely narrowed effective orifice is depicted by noncontrast blood. (b) Waist on the balloon caused by the stenotic valve. (c) The effective orifice has been significantly enlarged by the valvuloplasty.

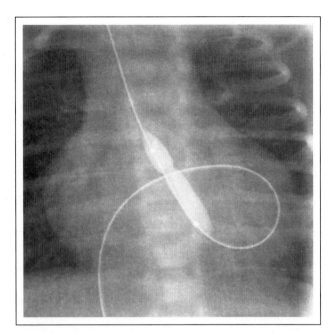

Figure 21.9 Antegrade aortic valvuloplasty in an infant.

exchange wire should be directed to the apex rather than to the inflow portion of the left ventricle so that the mitral valve is not exposed to risk by the balloon inflation.

In rare cases, it may be impossible to pass the guide wire from the retrograde approach to the left ventricle. In such patients, the procedure may be performed from an antegrade approach using patent foramen ovale or a transseptal puncture (Figure 21.9). This way the catheter is introduced into the left ventricular inflow; a J-shaped hydrophilic polymer-coated guide wire is turned upward from the left ventricular apex into the aortic valve and advanced to the descending aorta. The catheter is then pushed over the guide wire to the descending aorta, the guide wire is exchanged, and an appropriate balloon catheter is advanced into the valve. During the dilation, care is taken to protect the anterior mitral leaflet and its chordae by keeping the loop in the left ventricle wide open and extended as far as possible into the apex.

To prevent air embolism due to balloon rupture, the balloon is gently flushed with CO_2 before the insertion. It may be further purged and air removed after insertion by fluoroscopically controlled flushes with diluted contrast medium while the balloon is still in the descending thoracic aorta. Using the balloon radiopaque markers and the road map, the balloon is then positioned to straddle the aortic valve and gradually inflated. Before the full inflation is reached, tiny position adjustments can be made, if necessary. Once the waist caused by the stenotic valve (Figure 21.8b) has been abolished, the balloon is quickly deflated. During inflation, the balloon in the valve should remain as steady as possible. Displacement of the balloon prior to its full inflation prevents the effective valve dilation and

to-and-fro movement of the inflated balloon may cause injury to the valve leaflets or surrounding tissues. There are four measures to minimize or prevent the balloon movement during the dilation:

- *Rigid shaft-wire combination.* This can be achieved by using thicker shafts along with thicker guide wires (see the section "Brands Available") or by using stiff exchange guide wires, such as Amplatz Extra Stiff manufactured by Cook. The diameters of these guide wires start at 0.025 inch, which is thin enough to be used even with the low-profile balloon catheters (in Tyshak from 4 mm balloons and in Tyshak II and VACS II from 9 mm balloons).
- *Double-balloon technique.* During a simultaneous inflation of two balloons, the aortic orifice is never fully obstructed and, thus, presumably the forces responsible for the balloon displacement are weaker in comparison to the single-balloon technique.
- *Adenosine-induced transient ventricular asystole.*[18] A 0.3 mg/kg dose of adenosine is used to fill an intravenous line and rapidly flushed. The cannula and the vein used should be wide enough to withstand rapid injection. The femoral vein and the external jugular vein are good choices. The subsequent asystole usually lasts for 5–10 s, sufficient time to perform the dilation safely.
- *Rapid right ventricular pacing.*[19] A bipolar pacing catheter is introduced into the right ventricular apex. VVI pacing at a rate of 220–240 impulses per minute is started immediately before the balloon inflation and stopped immediately after its deflation. A standby defibrillator ready to terminate eventual sustained ventricular tachycardia or fibrillation must be within reach.

Unlike the adenosine administration that sometimes fails, rapid ventricular pacing is effective in all cases in the prevention of the balloon movement and the protocol should be always used to hold the balloon steady in the correct position. With the stable balloon position and the full obliteration of the balloon waist, a single balloon inflation usually will suffice to reduce the gradient, provided that the balloon diameter was chosen properly.

Postprocedure protocol

After valvuloplasty, the balloon catheter is replaced by a diagnostic catheter, the guide wire is removed, and the gradient is measured. If it is intended to calculate the aortic valve area after the dilation, the cardiac output must be measured again at this point. The aortography is then repeated to assess the widening of the effective orifice by a change in the jet diameter (Figure 21.8c) and to evaluate aortic insufficiency. A complete echocardiographic evaluation is performed on the following day.

Pitfalls and problems

Occasionally, left anterior hemi-block or even complete left bundle branch block is produced by compression of the conductive tissue caused by the balloon. This is always self-limiting and requires no treatment. Severe damage to the valve leaflets, myocardium, and the aortic wall can be prevented by avoiding oversized balloons and by keeping the inflated balloon stable in the aortic valve. A vessel injury may result from the balloon rupture. Therefore, care is taken to operate always below the balloon rated burst pressure (see the earlier section, "Balloon Burst Pressures"). The mitral valve may be injured by the balloon inflation, if the exchange wire is accidentally threaded through the anterior leaflet chordae. Therefore, a safe position of the wire tip in the ventricular apex and the wire course anterior to the mitral valve apparatus in the lateral view must be confirmed before each inflation. Proper access and hemostasis techniques along with the use of low-profile balloons help to prevent vascular damage.

Postcatheter management

In children and young adults, the sheaths are usually withdrawn in the catheterization laboratory at the end of the procedure. Before the removal, the activated clotting time should be less than 200 s. Thus, in very short procedures, circulating *heparin* must be at least partially neutralized by *protamine sulfate*. Hemostasis is achieved by manual compression of the catheter entry site. A pulse oximeter is attached onto a toe involved to measure the peripheral pulsation. The compression force should be balanced so that the distal pulses are still measurable while bleeding and hematoma formation are safely controlled. Only rarely, with the use of the largest sheaths, a vascular hemostatic device such as Angio-Seal® (Quinton), VasoSeal™ (Datascope), or Perclose ProGlide® (Abbott) is required to seal the artery. After hemostasis is achieved, the patient is transferred to an intensive care unit for further monitoring and subsequently discharged 24 hours after the procedure, if no complications have occurred.

Results

Good short-term results have been demonstrated in a large cohort of children in a multicentric study.[20] Midterm results, however, have shown a substantial incidence of restenosis, development of severe aortic insufficiency, and reinterventions.[21,22] In our 189 patients treated with valvuloplasty at the age of 5 weeks to 23 years with a median follow-up period of 7.5 years, the restenosis rate was 15% and severe aortic insufficiency developed in 20%. Similar rates have been observed by others.[23] While restenosis may be successfully treated by a repeated valvuloplasty in

the majority of cases,[24] aortic regurgitation is progressive in the long term,[1,25] and many patients require surgery during their childhood and early adulthood. The actuarial probability of survival 14 years after the valvuloplasty is 93% in infants and 98% in older patients, but the probability of surgery-free survival is only 52% in infants and 65% in older patients. The "functionally bicuspid" aortic valve has been documented to be an independent predictor of severe postvalvuloplasty aortic insufficiency and the need for surgery.[1]

References

1. Reich O, Tax P, Marek J, Rázek V, Gilík J, Tomek V et al. Long term results of percutaneous balloon valvoplasty of congenital aortic stenosis: Independent predictors of outcome. *Heart* 2004;90:70–6.
2. Solymar L, Sudow G, Berggren H, Eriksson B. Balloon dilation of stenotic aortic valve in children. An intraoperative study. *J Thorac Cardiovasc Surg* 1992;104:1709–13.
3. Campbell M. The natural history of congenital aortic stenosis. *Br Heart J* 1968;30:514–26.
4. Gatzoulis MA, Rigby ML, Shinebourne EA, Redington AN. Contemporary results of balloon valvuloplasty and surgical valvotomy for congenital aortic stenosis. *Arch Dis Child* 1995;73:66–9.
5. Justo RN, McCrindle BW, Benson LN, Williams WG, Freedom RM, Smallhorn JF. Aortic valve regurgitation after surgical versus percutaneous balloon valvotomy for congenital aortic valve stenosis. *Am J Cardiol* 1996;77:1332–8.
6. Lababidi Z. Aortic balloon valvuloplasty. *Am Heart J* 1983;106:751–2.
7. Lababidi Z, Wu JR, Walls JT. Percutaneous balloon aortic valvuloplasty: Results in 23 patients. *Am J Cardiol* 1984;53:194–7.
8. Lababidi Z, Weinhaus L. Successful balloon valvuloplasty for neonatal critical aortic stenosis. *Am Heart J* 1986;112:913–6.
9. Marshal HW. Physiologic consequences of congenital heart disease. In: Hamilton WF, Dow P. Eds. *Handbook of Physiology: Section 2. Circulation.* Washington DC: American Physiologic Society; 2005. p. 417.
10. Beekman RH, Rocchini AP, Gillon JH, Mancini GB. Hemodynamic determinants of the peak systolic left ventricular-aortic pressure gradient in children with valvar aortic stenosis. *Am J Cardiol* 1992;69:813–5.
11. Cape EG, Jones M, Yamada I, VanAuker MD, Valdes-Cruz LM. Turbulent/viscous interactions control Doppler/catheter pressure discrepancies in aortic stenosis. The role of the Reynolds number. *Circulation* 1996;94:2975–81.
12. Gjertsson P, Caidahl K, Svensson G, Wallentin I, Bech-Hanssen O. Important pressure recovery in patients with aortic stenosis and high Doppler gradients. *Am J Cardiol* 2001;88:139–44.
13. Helgason H, Keane JF, Fellows KE, Kulik TJ, Lock JE. Balloon dilation of the aortic valve: Studies in normal lambs and in children with aortic stenosis. *J Am Coll Cardiol* 1987;9:816–22.
14. Phillips RR, Gerlis LM, Wilson N, Walker DR. Aortic valve damage caused by operative balloon dilatation of critical aortic valve stenosis. *Br Heart J* 1987;57:168–70.
15. Mullins CE, Nihill MR, Vick GW, Ludomirsky A, O'Laughlin MP, Bricker JT et al. Double balloon technique for dilation of valvular or vessel stenosis in congenital and acquired heart disease. *J Am Coll Cardiol* 1987;10:107–14.
16. Beekman RH, Rocchini AP, Crowley DC, Snider AR, Serwer GA, Dick M et al. Comparison of single and double balloon valvuloplasty in children with aortic stenosis. *J Am Coll Cardiol* 1988;12:480–5.
17. Yeager SB. Balloon selection for double balloon valvotomy. *J Am Coll Cardiol* 1987;9:467–8.

18. De Giovanni JV, Edgar RA, Cranston A. Adenosine induced transient cardiac standstill in catheter interventional procedures for congenital heart disease. *Heart* 1998;80:330–3.

19. Daehnert I, Rotzsch C, Wiener M, Schneider P. Rapid right ventricular pacing is an alternative to adenosine in catheter interventional procedures for congenital heart disease. *Heart* 2004;90:1047–50.

20. Rocchini AP, Beekman RH, Ben Shachar G, Benson L, Schwartz D, Kan JS. Balloon aortic valvuloplasty: Results of the valvuloplasty and angioplasty of congenital anomalies registry. *Am J Cardiol* 1990;65:784–9.

21. Moore P, Egito E, Mowrey H, Perry SB, Lock JE, Keane JF. Midterm results of balloon dilation of congenital aortic stenosis: Predictors of success. *J Am Coll Cardiol* 1996;27:1257–63.

22. Galal O, Rao PS, Al Fadley F, Wilson AD. Follow-up results of balloon aortic valvuloplasty in children with special reference to causes of late aortic insufficiency. *Am Heart J* 1997;133:418–27.

23. Jindal RC, Saxena A, Juneja R, Kothari SS, Shrivastava S. Long-term results of balloon aortic valvulotomy for congenital aortic stenosis in children and adolescents. *J Heart Valve Dis* 2000;9:623–8.

24. Shim D, Lloyd TR, Beekman RH. Usefulness of repeat balloon aortic valvuloplasty in children. *Am J Cardiol* 1997;79:1141–3.

25. Balmer C, Beghetti M, Fasnacht M, Friedli B, Arbenz U. Balloon aortic valvoplasty in paediatric patients: Progressive aortic regurgitation is common. *Heart* 2004;90:77–81.

22

Congenital aortic valve stenosis: Special considerations in neonates

Alejandro J. Torres and William E. Hellenbrand

Aortic valve stenosis occurs in 3–6% of patients with congenital heart disease with males being affected 3–5 times as often as females. The anatomic types of aortic valve stenosis include unicuspid, bicuspid, tricuspid, quadricuspid, and undifferentiated aortic valves. Bicuspid aortic valve is the most common malformation of the aortic valve and is present in up to 1.3% of the general population and in 70–85% of pediatric patients with aortic stenosis. Most neonates requiring intervention have either a unicuspid or a severely stenotic bicuspid valve. Aortic stenosis sometimes occurs within single families but the pattern of occurrence appears to be multifactorial. The recurrence risk in the offspring of an affected father is approximately 3% whereas it is 15% if the mother is affected. Bicuspid aortic valve and coarctation of the aorta are the most common cardiac anomalies in patients with Turner's syndrome (monosomy XO).[1]

In the neonate, critical aortic stenosis is a complex disorder, frequently associated with varying degrees of left ventricular and annular hypoplasia, mitral valve anomalies, and endomyocardial fibroelastosis. Other cardiovascular anomalies such as aortic coarctation, patent ductus arteriosus, and ventricular septal defect occur in 20% of the patients. Numerous studies have described different methods of scoring in an attempt to define the lower limit of left ventricular hypoplasia that would be adequate to support the full systemic circulation. In severe cases, staged univentricular palliation or transplantation is indicated.[2–7] Neonates with critical aortic stenosis suffer from low cardiac output and shock secondary to poor left ventricular function, myocardial ischemia, and/or mitral insufficiency; therefore, prompt intervention is required. Percutaneous balloon valvoplasty and surgical valvotomy are comparable in terms of immediate gradient relief but both remain palliative procedures. A number of patients will eventually require aortic valve surgery for progressive valve insufficiency, refractory obstruction at multiple levels, or a mixed lesion. Open or closed surgical valvotomy was the only technique available until the mid-1980s. Percutaneous balloon aortic valvuloplasty was first introduced in 1984 and has since become the first-line treatment for aortic valve stenosis.[8–12]

Diagnosis, precatheterization assessment, and management

Transthoracic echocardiography is the imaging method of choice to establish the morphology and function of the aortic valve, assess left ventricular function, and rule out other congenital cardiac anomalies. The number and morphology of the aortic valve cusps are best determined from the parasternal short-axis view. In many cases, the leaflets are immobile and a systolic opening cannot be visualized. Although defining the details of the aortic valve anatomy is important, it does not modify the management plan for these patients. The annulus is usually 5–8 mm in diameter and poststenotic dilatation of the ascending aorta is commonly seen.

Several studies have shown a correlation of the size of various left-sided heart structures and hemodynamic relations with survival of biventricular repair in critical aortic stenosis (Figure 22.1).[3,4,11] All studies use scores based on echocardiographic measurements to predict the ability of the left ventricle to support systemic cardiac output. A multivariate equation and a risk factor analysis were first described by Rhodes et al. in 1991.[6] In this study, the equation for the discrimination score for survival included indexed aortic root diameter, indexed mitral valve area, and left ventricular long axis to heart long axis ratio. In 2006, Colan et al.[13] revised the previous score and included the Z score of the aortic valve annulus and the degree of endocardial fibroelastosis. A predictive scoring system for aortic stenosis was also devised by the Congenital Heart Surgeon Society.[14,15] Although the use of these scores has improved the selection among these patients, their

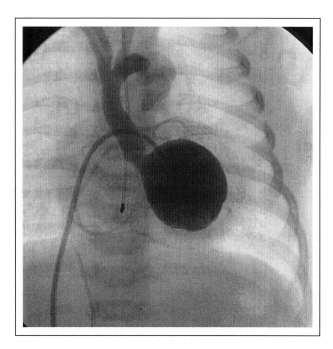

Figure 22.1 LV angiogram in a patient with critical aortic stenosis. Rhodes's scoring system based on threshold values for LV mass, mitral valve area, relative long-axis dimension, and aortic root diameter was used to predict outcome. Single ventricular palliation was recommended, as three risk factors were present.

predictive value remains imperfect. Therefore, they should be used to guide initial management but not as the definitive criteria.[16] Medical centers taking care of these patients should develop and become familiar with their own decision algorithms.

Quantitative assessment of flow velocities using Doppler recordings is routinely used to determine the severity of aortic stenosis. Caution should be exercised when interpreting Doppler measurements, as this technique is flow dependent. Thus, in patients with poor left ventricular systolic function and low cardiac output, a low transvalvular peak velocity may be obtained, even in the presence of severe stenosis. These patients should be distinguished from those with primary cardiomyopathy and severe left ventricular dysfunction in whom the normal aortic valve motion is limited in systole. In these cases, the transvalvular peak velocity is low but the aortic valve has a normal appearance, and there is no poststenotic dilatation of the ascending aorta. In conclusion, a low-pressure gradient measured with Doppler is of less significance in newborns with aortic stenosis than in older children and can mislead the diagnosis, if other echocardiographic and clinical findings are not considered. Indications for intervention in neonates are thus based on assessment of systemic perfusion, ventricular function, and valve morphology. Current guidelines for balloon valvoplasty in newborns include (1) patients with preserved left ventricular function and

a mean gradient across the aortic valve of ≥50 mmHg by Doppler interrogation and (2) patients with an abnormal aortic valve and systemic circulation dependent on right-to-left shunt across a patent arterial duct, by definition critical aortic stenosis and those with an abnormal valve who are able to maintain cardiac output without a duct but present with left ventricular dysfunction, regardless of the measured gradient across the aortic valve.[12,17]

Newborns with aortic stenosis often present with some degree of ventricular dysfunction and not infrequently in cardiogenic shock. Advances in prenatal diagnosis have allowed for proper procedural planning when the need of early intervention is suspected. Those patients who present in shock should be hemodynamically stabilized as much as possible but intervention should not be postponed for this reason. Mechanical ventilation and sedation should be initiated as soon as the diagnosis is made to decrease the oxygen demand. Acid–base status, blood count, coagulation times, and electrolytes should be evaluated and corrected if necessary.[12] Prostaglandin (PGE1) infusion is started to augment cardiac output in the setting of a failing and obstructed left ventricle. We recommend inserting both venous and arterial umbilical catheters since these catheters can later be used for vascular access during the catheterization. Inotropic support is commonly initiated to increase the cardiac output. Those agents with the least chronotropic effect, such as dopamine or dobutamine, are the most commonly used. Their effect on the heart rate should be carefully monitored because a decrease in the filling time of the left ventricle can further compromise the cardiac output.

Catheterization

General anesthesia with complete sedation and paralysis are preferable to decrease the cardiac output demands and facilitate the procedure. Warming lights, heating blankets, or other devices to avoid excessive thermal stress are important. Extracorporeal membrane oxygenation (ECMO) should be considered prior to the procedure in patients who present with cardiogenic shock. Resuscitation equipment and intravenous drugs, including external defibrillator, cross-matched blood, and inotropic and antiarrhythmic agents should be available in the catheterization laboratory.[12]

Technique

The crossing of the aortic valve with a guide wire can be achieved either from the aorta (retrograde approach) or from the left ventricle (antegrade approach). Each of these approaches has its limitations and disadvantages.

Retrograde approach

Catheters can be advanced into the ascending aorta using the femoral artery, umbilical artery,[10,12–18] or the surgically exposed right common carotid artery[19–21] or the right subscapular artery.[22] The umbilical artery is preferable when still patent. A 0.018"–0.021" J-Rosen guide wire is advanced into the aorta through either a 3 Fr or 5 Fr umbilical catheter, which is then exchanged for an imaging catheter. It is important to remember that both umbilical arteries travel from the umbilicus toward the groins and catheters should be advanced in that direction when introduced and not upward as with the umbilical vein. If the femoral artery is used instead, the procedure can be performed with a 3 Fr sheath and a 3 Fr thin-walled pigtail. The imaging catheter is placed in the ascending aorta and a 5 Fr Berman angiographic catheter is advanced from the inferior vena cava through the patent foramen ovale into the left ventricle. The gradient across the aortic valve can be measured by simultaneous recording of the aortic and left ventricular pressure. In hemodynamically unstable patients, we do not perform an aortogram and the aortic annulus diameter measured by echocardiography is used to choose the balloon diameter. In more stable patients, aortography is performed using a pigtail or a side-hole catheter placed just above the aortic sinuses. The straight postero-anterior and lateral projections are usually adequate to profile the aortic valve annulus. The postero-anterior camera can be placed with a shallow left anterior oblique angulation to take the aortic valve off the spine and profile the aortic annulus. Poststenotic dilatation of the ascending aorta is frequently noted and its absence would suggest subaortic stenosis. The stenotic aortic valve domes during systole and a jet of unopacified blood can be seen passing through the narrowed valve orifice (Figure 22.2). It is helpful to remember the orientation of the jet in both projections when attempting to cross the valve with a guide wire. The hinge points of the aortic valve are usually easy to identify. The diameter of the aortic annulus is measured between the opposite hinge points on the projection where it is profiled the best (Figure 22.3). There is a fair correlation between the annulus angiographic diameter and the one measured by echocardiography on the long-axis parasternal view. A left ventricular angiogram can be performed when it is necessary to assess the size of the ventricle or identify associated anomalies such as discrete subaortic stenosis (Figure 22.4).

The pigtail catheter is then replaced with a 3 Fr or 4 Fr JR1 or JR2 catheter, although the pigtail can also be used as a directional catheter. A soft straight- or angle-tipped 0.018" or 0.021" guide wire (torque control or glide wire) is used to cross the valve. Reference images of the aortogram should be used to visualize the direction of the jet and the ostia of both the coronary arteries. The commissure between the left and the noncoronary cusps is the most common area of opening of the valve and the guide wire–catheter

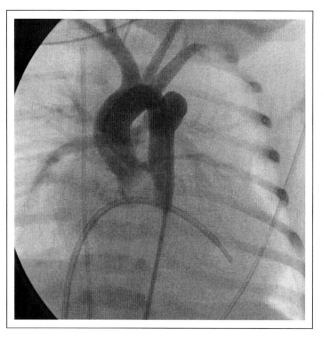

Figure 22.2 Ascending aorta angiogram in a patient with aortic stenosis showing an unopacified jet of blood through a doming aortic valve.

system should be pointed in that direction, which usually is toward the left and posterior aspect of the aortic root. The guide wire is gently advanced and pulled into the catheter to avoid perforation of the valve or damage to the coronary arteries. Before advancing the catheter, the position of the guide wire should be confirmed. A guide wire

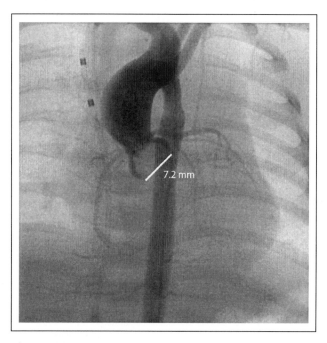

Figure 22.3 Measurement of aortic valve annulus diameter between opposite hinge points.

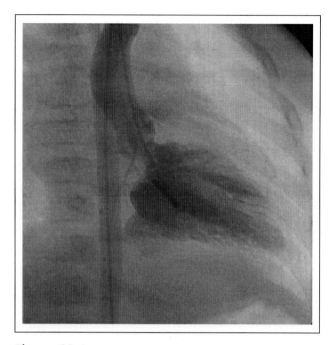

Figure 22.4 Left ventricular angiogram in a patient with aortic stenosis showing a doming aortic valve associated with discrete subaortic stenosis.

in the left coronary artery might occasionally be mistaken for being in the left ventricle, particularly on the postero-anterior projection. The guide wire position should then be compared with the two views of the left coronary artery in the aortogram before advancing the catheter. Following crossing of the valve, the balloon dilatation catheter can be advanced over the same guide wire used to cross the valve, if the internal diameter of the balloon catheter is the same size as the guide wire, and the guide wire is in a good position within the ventricle and has a stiff segment at the valve level. Otherwise, the guide catheter can be advanced into the ventricle and the guide wire exchanged for a J-tipped guide wire with a diameter appropriate for the balloon catheter. The intraventricular pressure can be measured at this time, if not done previously. A wide loop should be hand made on the J-tipped guide wire before advancing it into the ventricle to provide better guide wire position. The guide wire is positioned in the left ventricular apex anterior to the mitral valve. A posterior position of the guide wire should be avoided since it may result in mitral valve injury during balloon inflation if the guide wire is trapped in the mitral valve. Care should be taken not to accidentally pull the guide wire when the balloon is advanced in the aorta. If crossing of the valve has been unsuccessful within 20–30 min, antegrade approach is considered.

If sustained ventricular tachycardia or fibrillation develops when the valve is crossed with the guide wire, it should not be pulled out of the ventricle, since the chances of performing a successful resuscitation in a hemodynamically compromised patient are minimal. Instead, as resuscitation

is initiated, the balloon should be quickly advanced and the valve should be balloon dilated. This will immediately decrease the intraventricular pressure and improve myocardial ischemia.

A balloon with a diameter that is approximately 80–90% (0.8–0.9:1 ratio) of the annulus is chosen. We use the Tyshak Mini and the Tyshak II (NuMED, Hopkinton, NY) for the 3 Fr and 4 Fr systems, respectively. The use of balloons with diameters >100% (>1:1 ratio) of the valve annulus size has been associated with a higher incidence of significant aortic valve insufficiency.[9–12,23] Two-centimeter-long balloon catheters should be used to decrease the risk of mitral valve injury. If the guide wire is caught in the mitral valve apparatus, a longer balloon may be inadvertently inflated within the mitral valve chordae.

The balloon is first placed in the descending aorta, where it is carefully purged to remove all the air from it. We usually purge the balloon using a stopcock device with one port attached to the balloon and the other two attached to two syringes, one with 1/3 contrast and 2/3 normal saline solution, and the other one empty. Then, on the stopcock, we open the balloon toward the empty syringe and while aspirating we switch the stopcock to open the contrast syringe toward the balloon. The balloon is then inflated under fluoroscopy; if air is noticed, the procedure is repeated until no air remains in the system. This is usually achieved after 2–3 times. The balloon is advanced a little further into the ventricle than the desired position and then pulled back until it straddles the aortic valve. This is done to straighten the valve leaflets in case they are inadvertently folded when the balloon is advanced into the ventricle. Balloon inflation by hand or pressure indeflator is performed for a few seconds until the balloon is fully inflated or the waist disappears (Figure 22.5a and b). We usually repeat the inflation twice with each inflation–deflation cycle lasting no more than 5–7 s. Since small increases in balloon diameter can be achieved by increasing pressure, inflation should be gentle to avoid rupture or larger effective diameter, which may increase the risk of aortic regurgitation. Right ventricular pacing during balloon inflation is not usually necessary to facilitate balloon stabilization in neonates. Maintaining balloon position is easy in these patients due to high baseline heart rate and left ventricular dysfunction with low stroke volume.[24] The balloon is removed and hemodynamic measurements are repeated in similar fashion to predilatation. When the procedure is performed with a 4 Fr system, another approach is to use a multitrack catheter that uses the guide wire as a monorail to allow pressure monitoring and pullback gradient measurement without moving the guide wire. If the ductus arteriosus is not patent, a wide aortic differential pressure suggests significant residual aortic regurgitation. In order to avoid injury of the aortic or mitral valve, the guide wire is carefully pulled out with the catheter in the ventricle. In hemodynamically stable patients, an ascending aortogram is repeated to assess aortic valve

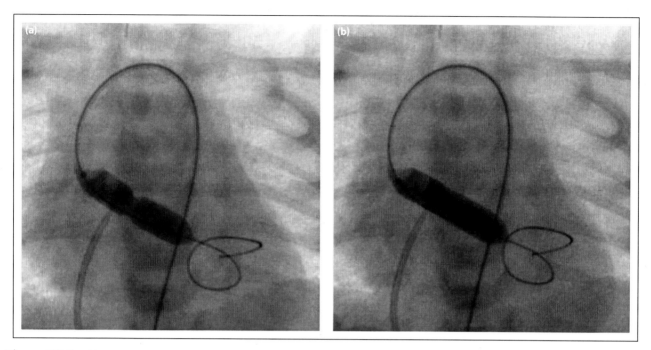

Figure 22.5   (a) Balloon waist during aortic valve balloon dilatation. Note the correct position of a looped J wire in the left ventricle. (b) Same patient as in (a); resolution of the balloon waist at full inflation.

competence, with the catheter positioned above the valve to avoid catheter-induced valve insufficiency. Otherwise, residual aortic regurgitation is assessed only by echocardiography. Provided that there is no or trivial aortic regurgitation, a successful result has been achieved if the residual peak gradient has been reduced more than 50% from the initial measurement. Other indirect signs of success are a fall in the left ventricular end-diastolic pressure and an increase in oxygen saturation in the lower extremities in patients with an open ductus arteriosus. When a significant residual gradient is present and there is no significant residual aortic regurgitation, valvuloplasty can be repeated with the next larger balloon size following the same sequence.

The right carotid artery approach to perform balloon aortic valvoplasty was first described in 1990 and its use has been advocated by different centers.[20,21,25] The procedure is performed in the catheterization laboratory with the aid of a surgeon who exposes the right carotid artery. Access into the vessel is achieved by an arteriotomy or with a 21 gauge needle. A 0.021" guide wire is introduced into the vessel and a 4 Fr or 5 Fr pediatric sheath is advanced over the guide wire into the ascending aort a. The use of a sheath with a smaller catheter allows simultaneous pressure measurement of the aorta and the left ventricle. Full heparinization (100 U/kg) is usually administered. Pressure recording and aortogram are performed through the sheath. A catheter (e.g., multipurpose) is then advanced into the ascending aorta and a floppy-tipped 0.018" guide wire is used to cross the valve. Alternatively, the balloon catheter can be used as a guide catheter.[26,27] An advantage of the carotid access is the direct angle of approach to the aortic valve, which makes crossing of the valve relatively easy. This procedure has been performed at the bedside using only transesophageal echocardiography for guidance.[19,28] The same floppy-tipped guide wire can be used to advance the balloon catheter or it can be exchanged for a stiffer Rosen guide wire with a handmade loop at the tip. The position of the guide wire with respect to the mitral valve should be assessed before balloon dilatation. The balloon is then positioned across the valve and inflated for a few seconds. Evaluation of residual aortic valve gradient or insufficiency is performed as described with the other approaches. At the conclusion of the procedure, the sheath is removed and the carotid artery is primarily repaired. The risk of neurologic events during the procedure is low. Right carotid artery patency is well preserved after neonatal surgical cutdown. Patients with mild residual stenosis at the site of the incision usually remain asymptomatic on midterm follow-up.[25]

Antegrade approach

The aortic valve is crossed from the left ventricle after entering the left atrium via a patent foramen ovale. The main advantage of this approach is that it reduces the risk of femoral arterial injury. Some authors have suggested that this approach also reduces the incidence of aortic regurgitation because the crossing of the aortic valve with a floppy-tipped guide wire from the left ventricle may decrease the risk of valve leaflet perforation. The disadvantages include the necessity of an atrial communication, the potential risk of mitral valve injury, and the risk of arrhythmias due to catheter manipulation within a compromised left ventricle.

A 5 Fr sheath is placed in a femoral vein or a 0.021" J guide wire is advanced through the umbilical venous catheter into the right atrium and then the umbilical catheter is exchanged with a 5 Fr pediatric sheath. A small 3 Fr catheter may be placed in the femoral artery for monitoring of the blood pressure. This is not necessary if an umbilical artery catheter is in place. If an ascending aortogram has not been performed, a 4 Fr or 5 Fr Berman angiographic catheter is advanced into the left atrium through the patent foramen ovale. In patients with an intact atrial septum, transseptal puncture is performed. The balloon is inflated carefully in the left atrium and advanced into the left ventricle. In order to point the tip of the catheter toward the mitral valve, we use the stiff end of a 0.021" J wire with a preshaped tight curve or a tip-deflecting guide wire. After measuring the left ventricular pressure, a low-volume, low-flow-rate angiogram is performed to measure the diameter of the aortic valve annulus. The Berman angiographic catheter is removed and a 4 Fr or 5 Fr end-hole catheter, preferably a balloon wedge catheter to avoid crossing the mitral valve through the chordae or the papillary muscle apparatus, is advanced in the left ventricular apex. Using the preformed curved stiff end of the 0.021" J wire or a tip-deflecting guide wire, the tip of the catheter is aimed toward the left ventricular outflow tract and advanced until it is positioned underneath the aortic valve. In patients in whom the catheter cannot be looped because of the small size of the left ventricle, a pigtail can be used to direct the guide wire. A soft-tipped guide wire (0.018" glide or torque guide wire) is used to cross the valve and is advanced into the descending aorta. The catheter is then advanced into the descending aorta and the 0.018" guide wire is exchanged for a Rosen guide wire, which exactly matches the inner diameter or the guide wire lumen of the balloon catheter. In this position, the guide wire pushes on the anterior leaflet of the mitral valve. In order to decrease the likelihood of mitral valve injury during balloon inflation,[29] a loop is formed with the guide wire within the left ventricle (Figure 22.6). The Rosen guide wire is hand shaped to allow for enough curve on it in the ventricular cavity. The appropriately sized balloon is advanced until it straddles the aortic valve and balloon inflation is performed. During inflation, the left ventricular contraction may push the balloon forward into the ascending aorta. Care should be taken not to pull on the guide wire in an attempt to maintain balloon position, since this may straighten the guide wire within the ventricle and damage the mitral valve.

Combined approach

In this approach, the aortic valve is crossed as in the antegrade approach and the guide wire snared in the aorta. The

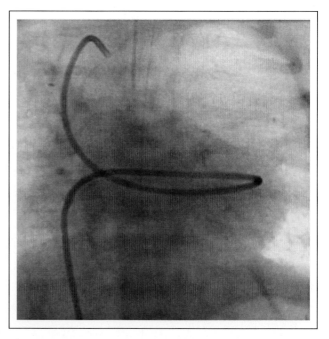

Figure 22.6 Antegrade approach technique with the tip of the catheter being advanced into ascending aorta. Note the wide catheter loop within the left ventricle.

guide wire is then gently pulled out through the femoral or umbilical artery. As it is pulled out, care should be taken to "feed" enough guide wire from the venous side to avoid putting tension on the mitral valve. Then a pigtail or right coronary artery catheter is advanced through the aorta into the left ventricle and the guide wire is pulled out. As in the retrograde approach, a J guide wire is advanced into the left ventricle and the catheter exchanged for a balloon catheter.

Complications

Morbidity and mortality in neonates undergoing balloon aortic valvuloplasty is higher than in older children but has decreased in recent years as proper selection of patients for single versus biventricular repair and neonatal surgical techniques have evolved. Procedure-related mortality occurs in 3.0–4.5% of the patients and, among early survivors, severe left ventricular dysfunction, a smaller left ventricle, and a smaller aortic annulus are associated with decreased long-term survival.[30–35]

Acute moderate or severe aortic regurgitation has been reported in 15–30% of neonates following balloon dilatation.[33,34,36–38] It remains the most feared complication as it may result in the need for emergency or early surgical reintervention.[33,38] Different studies have shown that the use of balloon/annulus ratios larger than 0.9:1.0 increase the risk of aortic regurgitation.[9,35,39,40] However, other studies have reported similar incidence of acute aortic regurgitation using balloons of up to 1.0:1.0 ratio.[41] Interestingly, the antegrade approach has been associated with a lower incidence of aortic regurgitation.[33,42] Aortic valve morphology has also been suggested as a contributor for procedural-related aortic regurgitation.[9,35] Unfortunately, no specific predictors have been identified and severe aortic regurgitation may occasionally occur following valvuloplasty with a low balloon/annulus ratio and a favorable valve anatomy (Figure 22.7).

Although the incidence of vascular injury is lower in the present era, it remains a concern in newborns undergoing transcatheter procedures. Femoral artery access in neonates is associated with arterial injury and pulse loss in 30–45% of procedures.[9,34,41–43] However, the risk of serious vascular injury resulting in vascular surgery or long-term sequelae such as growth retardation of the affected extremity is low.[10,35,41,44] In our practice, patients who have a cool, pale extremity and no palpable pulse 2–3 hours after the procedure are started on subcutaneous enoxaparin (1 mg/kg/dose) twice daily. If the extremity perfusion improves and pulses return within 12 hours, enoxaparin is discontinued. Otherwise, an arterial Doppler ultrasound of the affected extremity is performed and a 10-day course of enoxaparin is completed. Thrombolytic agents have proven beneficial but carry the risk of significant bleeding in small patients.[41,45] Although vascular injury with other forms of access is less common, it can potentially result in serious complications. Catheter manipulation in the umbilical artery has been associated with vessel disruption.[46] The transcarotid approach requires a cutdown and suture repair of the arteriotomy at the end of the procedure with the potential risk of thrombus formation on the catheter and embolization to the brain or residual stenosis of the right carotid artery.[21,25,28]

Aortic wall injury due to creation of an intimal flap has recently been described in 15% of neonates undergoing aortic balloon valvuloplasty via the retrograde approach as an often unrecognized and potentially lethal complication. The most common locations are the distal ascending aorta and transverse arch. Ventricular dysfunction, multiple balloon dilatations, and procedures performed by less experienced operators are associated with a higher risk.[38]

Most of the other reported complications, such as left ventricular wall or aortic valve cusp perforation, arrhythmias including complete atrioventricular block, or mitral valve injury, are considered preventable with the current catheterization technology.

Results and follow-up

Aortic valve stenosis is a lifelong disease and the parents of these patients should be informed about the palliative nature of the procedure. A gradient reduction of more than 50% is achieved in around 70% of the patients.[11–30] A low predilatation gradient and a small aortic annulus and aortic root have been identified as predictors of lower success rates. Most studies show survival rates of around 80–85% at 5 years and 70% at 10 years with most deaths occurring during the first year of life.[11,30,33,35,36]

Reinterventions on the aortic valve are common following neonatal aortic balloon valvuloplasty. Survival freedom from any aortic valve reintervention is 65% at 1 year and 50% at 5 years, with the highest risk during the first 6 months. Repeat balloon aortic valvuloplasty secondary to residual aortic stenosis is the most common reintervention during the first year after the initial procedure. Survival freedom from repeat balloon valvuloplasty is 95% at 1 month, 65% at 1 year, and 58% at 5 years. The risk factors include a higher predilatation aortic stenosis gradient and a higher residual gradient after balloon dilatation.[33] The early hazard for repeat balloon valvuloplasty is likely related to higher tolerance to residual gradients during the first procedure in order to avoid the risk of significant aortic regurgitation. Rapid patient growth and recovery from an initially depressed ventricular function may also be contributing factors.

Progression of aortic regurgitation is steady following balloon aortic valvuloplasty and is the most common indication for surgical intervention, followed by mixed lesions. Freedom from severe aortic regurgitation is 85% at 1 month, 77% at 1 year, and 65% at 5 years.[33,36,41,43] Coinciding with the progression of aortic regurgitation, the risk of surgical reintervention on the aortic valve becomes more prominent beyond the second year of life. Survival freedom from any surgical aortic valve reintervention is 90% at 1 year, 70% at 5 years, and 50–60% at 10 years.[33,36,38,41]

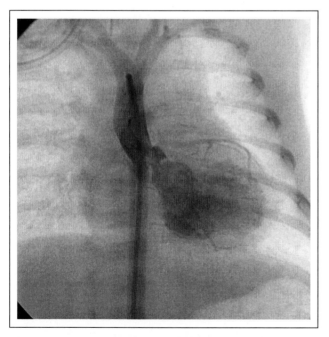

Figure 22.7 Ascending aortography demonstrating free aortic valve regurgitation following balloon aortic valvuloplasty with a 0.85:1 balloon:annulus ratio. The patient was referred for surgery.

The transvalvular gradient measured by Doppler is used to assess the residual severity and progression of both aortic stenosis and aortic regurgitation. In most centers, catheterization is recommended in asymptomatic patients with a peak gradient across the aortic valve of 70 mmHg or a mean gradient of 45 mmHg by Doppler echocardiography. Earlier reintervention should be considered in patients with symptoms or patients with moderate gradients by Doppler echocardiography and progressive left ventricular hypertrophy on the electrocardiogram.

References

1. Friedman WF. Aortic stenosis. In: Adams FH, Emmnouilides GC. Eds. *Heart Disease in Infants, Children and Adolescents Including the Fetus and Young Adult.* 5th ed. Baltimore: Williams & Wilkins; 1995.

2. Latson LA, Cheatham JP, Gutgesell HP. Relation of the echocardiographic estimate of left ventricular size to mortality in infants with severe left ventricular outflow obstruction. *Am J Cardiol* 1981; 48:887–91.

3. Hammon JW, Flavian LM, Maples MD, Merrill WH, Frist WH, Graham TP et al. Predictors of operative mortality in critical aortic stenosis presenting in infancy. *Ann Thorac Surg* 1988;45:537–40.

4. Parsons MK, Moreau GA, Graham TP, Johns JA, Boucek RJ. Echocardiographic estimation of critical left ventricular size in infants with isolated aortic valve stenosis. *J Am Coll Cardiol* 1991;18:1049–55.

5. Bu'Lock FA, Joffe HS, Jordan SC, Martin RP. Balloon dilatation (valvoplasty) as first line treatment for severe stenosis of the aortic valve in early infancy: Medium term results and determinants of survival. *Br Heart J* 1993;70:546–53.

6. Rhodes LA, Colan SD, Perry SB, Jonas RA, Sanders SP. Predictors of survival in neonates with critical aortic stenosis. *Circulation* 1991;84:2325–35.

7. Zeevi B, Keane JF, Castaneda AR, Perry SB, Lock JE. Neonatal critical valvar stenosis: A comparison of surgical and balloon dilation therapy. *Circulation* 1989;80:831–9.

8. Rupprath G, Neuhaus KL. Percutaneous balloon valvuloplasty for aortic valve stenosis in infancy. *Am J Cardiol* 1985;55:1655–6.

9. Sholler GF, Keane JF, Perry SB, Sanders SP, Lock JE. Balloon dilation of congenital aortic valve stenosis: Results and influence of technical and morphological features on outcome. *Circulation* 1988;78:351–60.

10. Egito EST, Moore P, O'Sullivan J, Colan S, Perry SB, Lock JE et al. Transvascular balloon dilation for neonatal critical aortic stenosis: Early and midterm results. *J Am Coll Cardiol* 1997;29:442–7.

11. Huhta JC, Carpenter RJ Jr, Moise KJ Jr, Deter RL, Ott DA, McNamara DG. Prenatal diagnosis and postnatal management of critical aortic stenosis. *Circulation* 1987;75(3):573–6.

12. Pass RH, Hellenbrand WE. Catheter intervention for critical aortic stenosis in the neonate. *Catheter Cardiovasc Interv* 2002;55(1):88–92.

13. Colan SD, McElhinney DB, Crawford EC, Keane JF, Lock JE. Validation and re-evaluation of a discriminant model predicting anatomic suitability for biventricular repair in neonates with aortic stenosis. *J Am Coll Cardiol* 2006;47(9):1858–65.

14. Lofland GK, McCrindle BW, Williams WG, Blackstone EH, Tchervenkov CI, Sittiwangkul R et al. Critical aortic stenosis in the neonate: A multi-institutional study of management, outcomes, and risk factors. Congenital Heart Surgeons Society. *J Thorac Cardiovasc Surg* 2001;121(1):10–27.

15. Hickey EJ, Caldarone CA, Blackstone EH, Lofland GK, Yeh T Jr, Pizarro C et al. Congenital Heart Surgeons' Society. Critical left ventricular outflow tract obstruction: The disproportionate impact of biventricular repair in borderline cases. *J Thorac Cardiovasc Surg* 2007;134(6):1429–36.

16. Eicken A, Georgiev S, Balling G, Schreiber C, Hager A, Hess J. Neonatal balloon aortic valvuloplasty-predictive value of current risk score algorithms for treatment strategies. *Catheter Cardiovasc Interv* 20101;76(3):404–10.

17. Feltes TF, Bacha E, Beekman RH 3rd, Cheatham JP, Feinstein JA, Gomes AS et al. American Heart Association Congenital Cardiac Defects Committee of the Council on Cardiovascular Disease in the Young; Council on Clinical Cardiology; Council on Cardiovascular Radiology and Intervention; American Heart Association. Indications for cardiac catheterization and intervention in pediatric cardiac disease: A scientific statement from the American Heart Association. *Circulation* 2011;123(22):2607–52.

18. Rao PS, Jureidini SB. Transumbilical venous, anterograde, snare-assisted balloon aortic valvuloplasty in a neonate with critical aortic stenosis. *Cathet Cardiovasc Diagn* 1998;45(2):144–8.

19. Weber HS, Mart CR, Kupferschmid J, Myers JL, Cyran SE. Transcarotid balloon valvuloplasty with continuous transesophageal echocardiographic guidance for neonatal critical aortic valve stenosis: An alternative to surgical palliation. *Pediatr Cardiol* 1998;19:212–7.

20. Maeno Y, Akagi T, Hashino K, Ishii M, Sugimura T, Takagi J et al. Carotid artery approach to balloon aortic valvuloplasty in infants with critical aortic valve stenosis. *Pediatr Cardiol* 1997;18:288–91.

21. Fischer DR, Ettedgui JA, Park SC, Siewers RD, del Nido PJ. Carotid artery approach for balloon dilation of aortic valve stenosis in the neonate: A preliminary report. *J Am Coll Cardiol* 1990;15:1633–6.

22. Alekyan BG, Petrosyan YS, Coulson JD, Danilov YY, Vinokurov AV. Right subscapular artery catheterization for balloon valvuloplasty of critical aortic stenosis in infants. *Am J Cardiol* 1995;76(14):1049–52.

23. Helgason H, Keane JF, Fellows KE, Kulik TJ, Lock JE. Balloon dilation of the aortic valve: Studies in normal lambs and in children with aortic stenosis. *J Am Coll Cardiol* 1987;9(4):816–22.

24. Mehta C, Desai T, Shebani S, Stickley J, DE Giovanni J. Rapid ventricular pacing for catheter interventions in congenital aortic stenosis and coarctation: Effectiveness, safety, and rate titration for optimal results. *J Interv Cardiol* 2010;23(1):7–13.

25. Borghi A, Agnoletti G, Poggiani C. Surgical cutdown of the right carotid artery for aortic balloon valvuloplasty in infancy: Midterm follow-up. *Pediatr Cardiol* 2001;22(3):194–7.

26. Fagan TE, Ing FF, Edens RE, Caldarone CA, Scholz TD. Balloon aortic valvuloplasty in a 1,600-gram infant. *Catheter Cardiovasc Interv* 2000;50(3):322–5.

27. Waight DJ, Hijazi ZM. Balloon aortic valvuloplasty: The single-wire technique. *J Interv Cardiol* 2004;17(1):21.

28. Weber HS, Mart CR, Myers JL. Transcarotid balloon valvuloplasty for critical aortic valve stenosis at the bedside via continuous transesophageal echocardiographic guidance. *Catheter Cardiovasc Interv* 2000;50(3):326–9.

29. Brierley JJ, Reddy TD, Rigby ML, Thanopoulous V, Redington AN. Traumatic damage to the mitral valve during percutaneous balloon valvotomy for critical aortic stenosis. *Heart* 1998;79(2):200–2.

30. Beekman RH, Rocchini AP, Andes A. Balloon valvuloplasty for critical aortic stenosis in the newborn: Influence of new catheter technology. *J Am Coll Cardiol* 1991;17(5):1172–6.

31. Kasten-Sportes CH, Piechaud JF, Sidi D, Kachaner J. Percutaneous balloon valvuloplasty in neonates with critical aortic stenosis. *J Am Coll Cardiol* 1989;13(5):1101–5.

32. Phillips RR, Gerlis LM, Wilson N, Walker DR. Aortic valve damage caused by operative balloon dilatation of critical aortic valve stenosis. *Br Heart J* 1987;57(2):168–70.

33. McElhinney DB, Lock JE, Keane JF, Moran AM, Colan SD. Left heart growth, function, and reintervention after balloon aortic valvuloplasty for neonatal aortic stenosis. *Circulation* 2005;111(4):451–8.

34. Rossi RI, Manica JL, Petraco R, Scott M, Piazza L, Machado PM. Balloon aortic valvuloplasty for congenital aortic stenosis using the femoral and the carotid artery approach: A 16-year experience from a single center. *Catheter Cardiovasc Interv* 2011;78(1):84–90.

35. Reich O, Tax P, Marek J, Rázek V, Gilík J, Tomek V et al. Long term results of percutaneous balloon valvoplasty of congenital aortic stenosis: Independent predictors of outcome. *Heart* 2004;90(1):70–6.

36. Fratz S, Gildein HP, Balling G, Sebening W, Genz T, Eicken A et al. Aortic valvuloplasty in pediatric patients substantially postpones the need for aortic valve surgery: A single-center experience of 188 patients after up to 17.5 years of follow-up. *Circulation* 2008;117(9):1201–6.

37. Han RK, Gurofsky RC, Lee KJ, Dipchand AI, Williams WG, Smallhorn JF et al. Outcome and growth potential of left heart structures after neonatal intervention for aortic valve stenosis. *J Am Coll Cardiol* 2007;50(25):2406–14.

38. Brown DW, Dipilato AE, Chong EC, Lock JE, McElhinney DB. Aortic valve reinterventions after balloon aortic valvuloplasty for congenital aortic stenosis intermediate and late follow-up. *J Am Coll Cardiol* 2010;56(21):1740–9.

39. McCrindle BW, Jones TK, Morrow WR, Hagler DJ, Lloyd TR, Nouri S et al. Acute results of balloon angioplasty of native coarctation versus recurrent aortic obstruction are equivalent. Valvuloplasty and Angioplasty of Congenital Anomalies (VACA) Registry Investigators. *J Am Coll Cardiol* 1996;28(7):1810–7.

40. Hawkins JA, Minich LL, Shaddy RE, Tani LY, Orsmond GS, Sturtevant JE et al. Aortic valve repair and replacement after balloon aortic valvuloplasty in children. *Ann Thorac Surg* 1996;61(5):1355–8.

41. Balmer C, Beghetti M, Fasnacht M, Friedli B, Arbenz U. Balloon aortic valvoplasty in paediatric patients: Progressive aortic regurgitation is common. *Heart* 2004;90(1):77–81.

42. Magee AG, Nykanen D, McCrindle BW, Wax D, Freedom RM, Benson LN. Balloon dilation of severe aortic stenosis in the neonate: Comparison of anterograde and retrograde catheter approaches. *J Am Coll Cardiol* 1997;30(4):10.

43. Ewert P, Bertram H, Breuer J, Dähnert I, Dittrich S, Eicken A et al. Balloon valvuloplasty in the treatment of congenital aortic valve stenosis—A retrospective multicenter survey of more than 1000 patients. *Int J Cardiol* 2011;149(2):182–5.

44. Peuster M, Freihorst J, Hausdorf G. Images in cardiology. Defective limb growth after retrograde balloon valvuloplasty. *Heart* 2000;84(1):63.

45. Bontadelli J, Moeller A, Schmugge M, Schraner T, Kretschmar O, Bauersfeld U et al. Enoxaparin therapy for arterial thrombosis in infants with congenital heart disease. *Intensive Care Med* 2007;33(11):1978–84.

46. Sasidharan P. Umbilical arterial rupture: A major complication of catheterization. *Indiana Med* 1985;78(1):34–5.

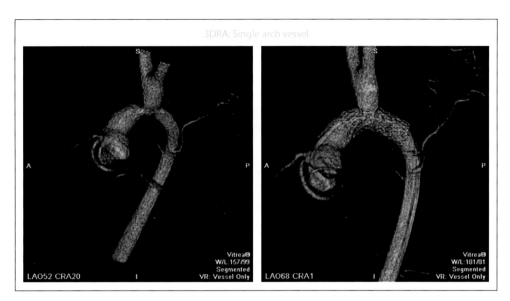

Figure 1.8 A 3-dimensional rotational angiogram (3DRA) nicely demonstrates a complex postoperative aortic arch obstruction before and after stent therapy.

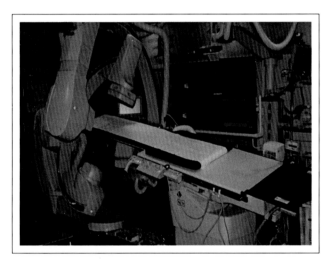

Figure 1.13 An integrated table in the cardiac catheterization suite with x-ray equipment is mandatory. The ability of the table to "cradle or roll" and be placed in the Trendelenburg and reverse Trendelenburg positions is very important to the cardiac surgeon … as demonstrated in this photograph.

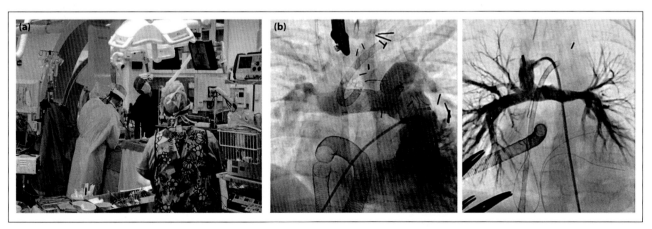

Figure 1.16 The Hybrid Cardiac Operating Suite was the next evolution in Hybrid therapies and is used in both CHD and SHD. This will accommodate all members of the Hybrid team (a). Exit angiography can now be easily performed to assess the operative procedure before the patient returns to the ICU, as seen in these two patients: after pulmonary valve replacement and intraoperative stents and after Comprehensive Stage II repair for HLHS (b).

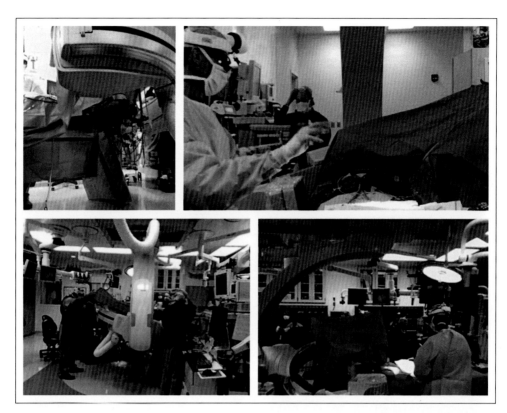

Figure 1.17   The newest technology that has been added to the Hybrid Cardiac Operating Suite is 3DRA, as shown here in the meticulous setup in our suite.

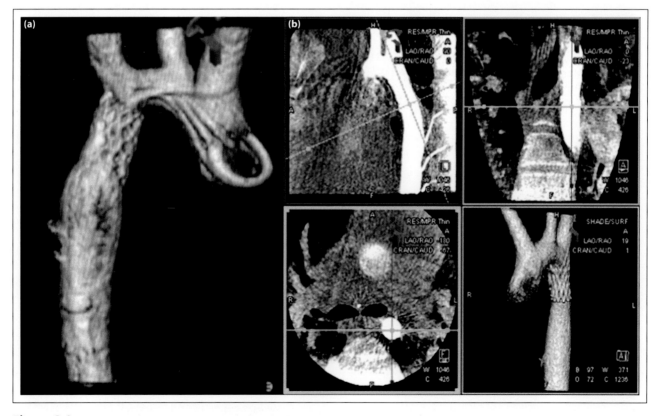

Figure 3.9   Left panel (a), a volume-rendered image of a stented arch coarctation obtained from a rotational angiogram. In panel (b), from the same acquisition, the CT soft tissue images in the axial, coronal, and sagittal planes.

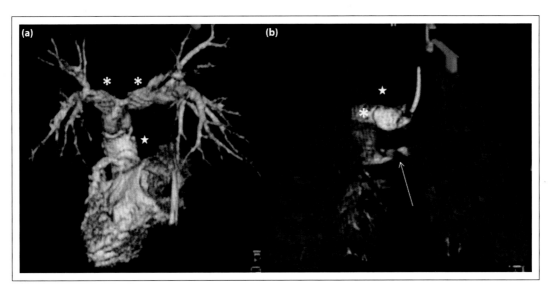

Figure 3.10 Panel (a) A three-dimensional rotational angiogram from an injection in the right ventricle, viewed from the back (a projection not available in standard two-dimensional angiography), showing two endovascular stents (*) and the right ventricle to pulmonary artery conduit (star). Panel (b) shows a volume-rendered image from a cavopulmonary vein injection (*), reconstructed to show the relationship of the trachea (star) and a stenosis in the left pulmonary artery (arrow).

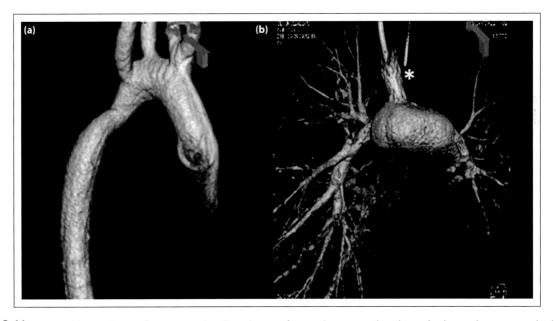

Figure 3.11 Panel (a) is an image from a rotational angiogram from prior to stenting the arch obstruction. It was obtained during rapid right ventricular pacing to allow the diluted contrast time to fill the vessel throughout the time of acquisition. In panel (b), a cavopulmonary injection (*) is made without pacing, as the blood flow is slow, allowing filling of the anastomosis, and the proximal and distal pulmonary arteries during acquisition.

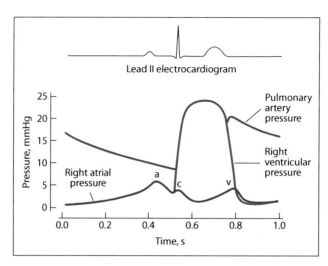

Figure 4.2 The right ventricular pressure tracing is similar to that generated by the left ventricle except that the pressures are lower. (Courtesy of McGraw Hill.)

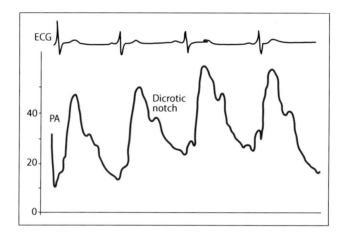

Figure 4.4 Example of a PA pressure tracing in a normal person. Note the variation in peak systolic and diastolic pressures with respiration. The dicrotic notch appears shortly after the end of ejection and the closure of the pulmonic valve.

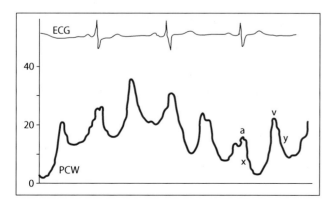

Figure 4.5 Example of PCWP tracing, reflecting the LA pressure, in a normal person.

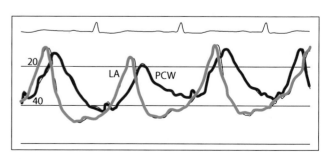

Figure 4.6 PCW tracing (red tracing) "approximates" actual LA tracing (blue tracing) but is slightly delayed since pressure wave is transmitted retrograde through pulmonary veins.

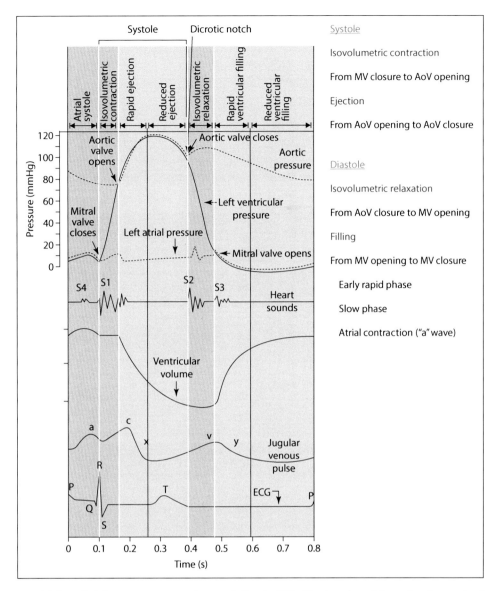

Figure 4.7 Normal left and right pressure waves in correlation to ECG. The isovolumetric contraction and relaxation times are shaded in pink.

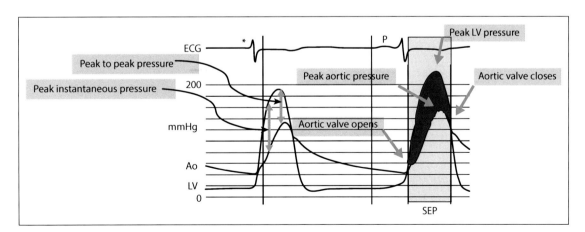

Figure 4.12 Simultaneously recorded pressures from the left ventricle (LV) and aorta (Ao) in a patient with aortic stenosis. There is a systolic pressure gradient (red shaded area) in which the LV systolic pressure is greater than that in the aorta. The pressure gradient and systolic ejection period (SEP, in s/beat) are used in the Gorlin formula to calculate the aortic valve area (aortic valve area = cardiac output ÷ [44.3 × SEP × HR × square root mean gradient]). The peak instantaneous gradient is the maximal pressure difference between Aorta and LV when the pressures are measured at the same moment. The peak-to-peak gradient is the difference between the maximal pressure in the aorta and the maximal pressure in LV. (Redrawn from Kern MJ (ed). *Cardiac Catheterization Handbook*, 2nd ed. St. Louis: Mosby-Year Book; 1995. With permission.)

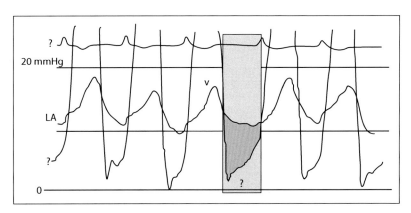

Figure 4.13 LA and LV pressure tracings in a patient with MS. Shaded area represents the mitral valve gradient. DFP = diastolic filling period. The planimetered area (green shaded) is used to calculate mean valve gradient (MVG).

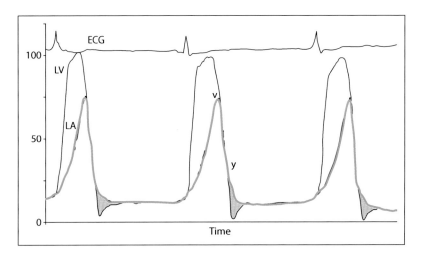

Figure 4.14 LV and LA pressure tracings in isolated, severe MR and atrial fibrillation. The "a" and "c" waves in the LA tracing (blue pressure tracing) are not evident and the "v" wave is accentuated.

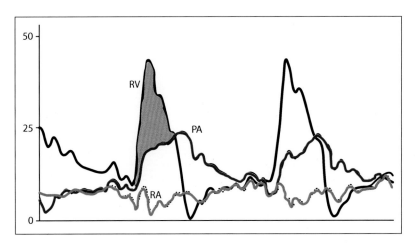

Figure 4.15 Simultaneous pressure recordings from RV, PA (red tracing), and RA (blue tracing) in a patient with pulmonic valve stenosis. The shaded area is the pulmonic valve stenosis gradient.

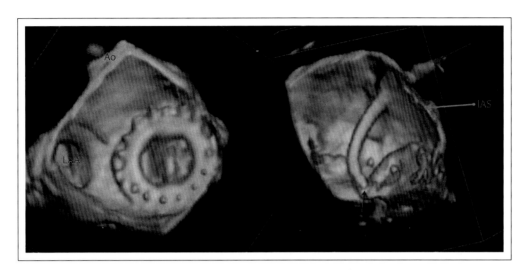

Figure 5.1   The standard clockface display of a paravalvar leak with aorta at 12 o'clock position and LAA at 9 o'clock position (on the right). Here, the intervention is performed through the transseptal approach. The sheath comes out through the transseptal puncture being guided to the regurgitant orifice (arrow on the left).

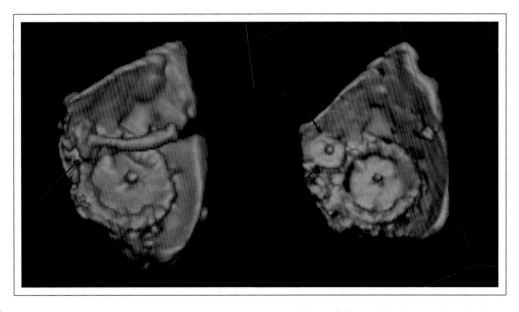

Figure 5.2   The LA disk of the PVL device being positioned under 3D guidance (left arrow) and postdevice deployment on the right (red arrows).

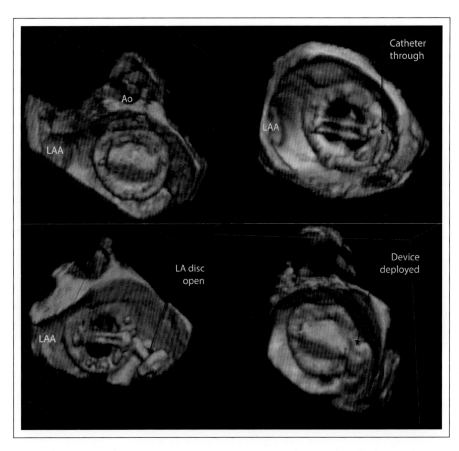

Figure 5.3 Mitral PVL medial lesion at 3 o'clock position shown in these 3DTEE images. The approach here was through the transapical route. Catheter positioning and device manipulation is shown through serial images from left to right. Left upper image shows the defect. Upper right image shows the catheter passing through the defect. The lower two images illustrate the device placement and release in final position.

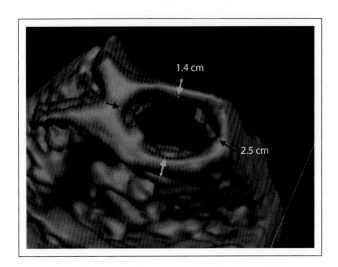

Figure 5.4 Asymmetry of the aortic valve "annulus" seen on 3DTEE imaging.

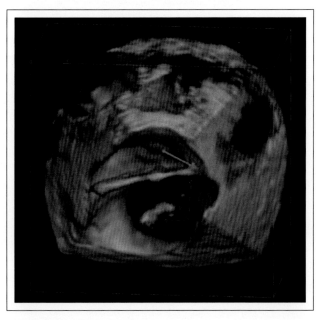

Figure 5.5 3D image of clot formation at the septal puncture site during LAA closure. Guide wire is through the transseptal puncture site (green arrow) and clot is attached to the interatrial septum (red arrow).

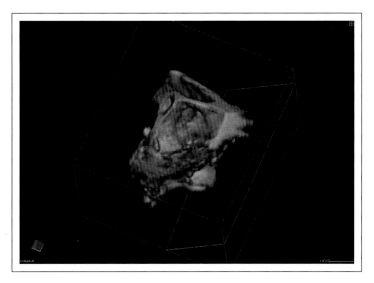

Figure 5.6 Small secundum ASD at the region of the oval fossa viewed from the LA.

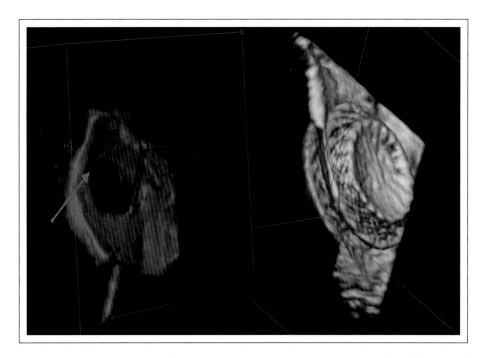

Figure 5.7 A large ASD with adequate margins (except deficient aortic rim) closed with an Occlutech™ device. The defect with catheter passing from the IVC to the LA on the left and the device in position on the right.

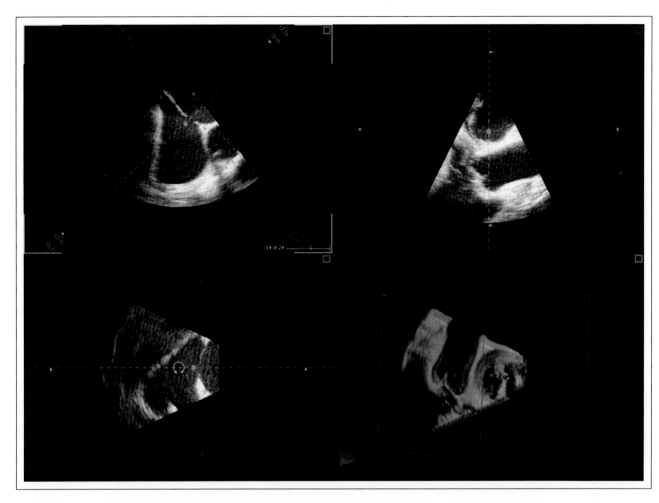

Figure 5.8 Two ASDs in parallel identified as single defect on 2DTEE but visualized as two separate defects in 3DTEE.

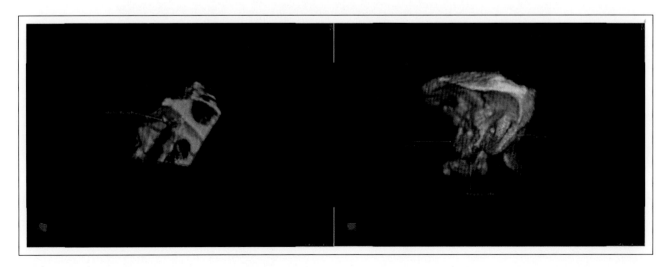

Figure 5.9 3DTEE showing two ASDs separated by a firm septum closed using two devices sitting comfortably, adjacent to each other with a small residual defect.

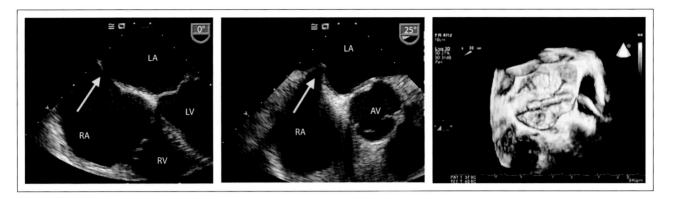

Figure 5.10 Transseptal puncture under 2DTEE and 3DTEE guidance.

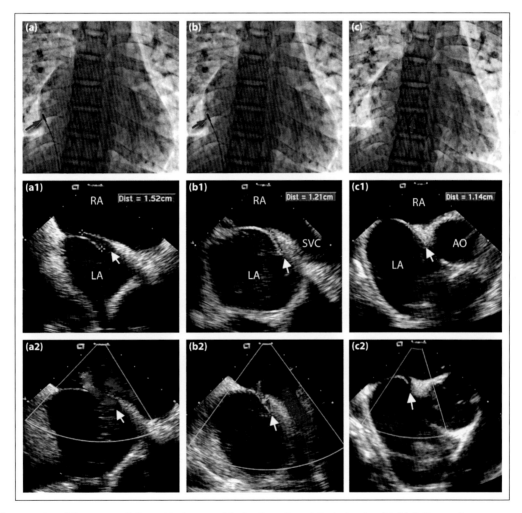

Figure 6.4 A series of images outlining PFO closure with the Gore Septal Occluder. (a–c) Initial diagnostic assessment of the PFO. (a–a2) The septal view of the atrial septum with and without color Doppler (demonstrating L–R shunt) with corresponding position of the ICE catheter on fluoroscopy outlined by the red arrow. (b–b2) The long-axis view (c–c2) demonstrating the short-axis view with the tunnel length measuring between 11 and 15 mm (a1, b1, c1). (d–f) Fluoroscopy images with ICE catheter position (red arrow) with the corresponding ICE image below. (d) R–L shunt of bubble contrast across the PFO with (e) clearly showing the wire crossing the defect and (f) balloon sizing of the defect, which is optional outside of most clinical trails. (g–i) Delivery of the HELEX device with corresponding fluoroscopy and ICE images in various views. (i) The left atrial component of the device deployed with (j, k) demonstrating the device pulled back to the septum and further deployment of the right atrial component of the device with it fully deployed in the long-axis (k) and short-axis views (l). (m, n) Release of the device on fluoroscopy with corresponding postdeployment ICE assessment with short-axis views and long-axis views with and without color (o1, o2, p1, p2).

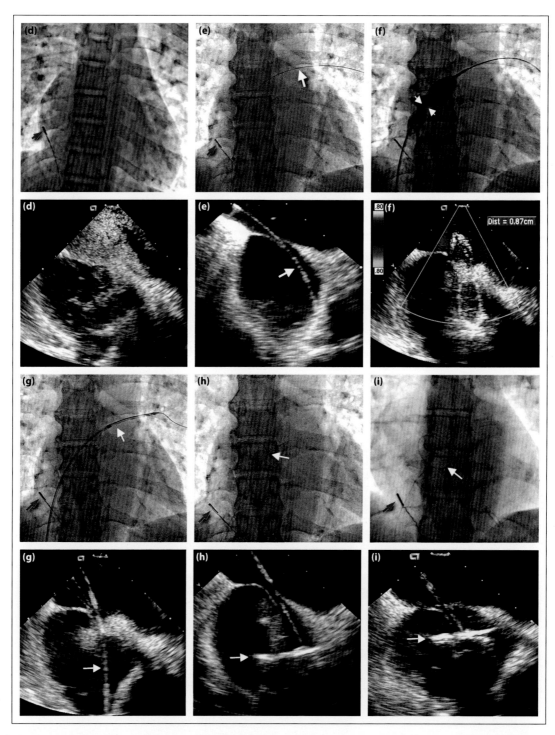

Figure 6.4 (continued) A series of images outlining PFO closure with the Gore Septal Occluder. (a–c) Initial diagnostic assessment of the PFO. (a–a2) The septal view of the atrial septum with and without color Doppler (demonstrating L–R shunt) with corresponding position of the ICE catheter on fluoroscopy outlined by the red arrow. (b–b2) The long-axis view (c–c2) demonstrating the short-axis view with the tunnel length measuring between 11 and 15 mm (a1, b1, c1). (d–f) Fluoroscopy images with ICE catheter position (red arrow) with the corresponding ICE image below. (d) R–L shunt of bubble contrast across the PFO with (e) clearly showing the wire crossing the defect and (f) balloon sizing of the defect, which is optional outside of most clinical trails. (g–i) Delivery of the HELEX device with corresponding fluoroscopy and ICE images in various views. (i) The left atrial component of the device deployed with (j, k) demonstrating the device pulled back to the septum and further deployment of the right atrial component of the device with it fully deployed in the long-axis (k) and short-axis views (l). (m, n) Release of the device on fluoroscopy with corresponding postdeployment ICE assessment with short-axis views and long-axis views with and without color (o1, o2, p1, p2).

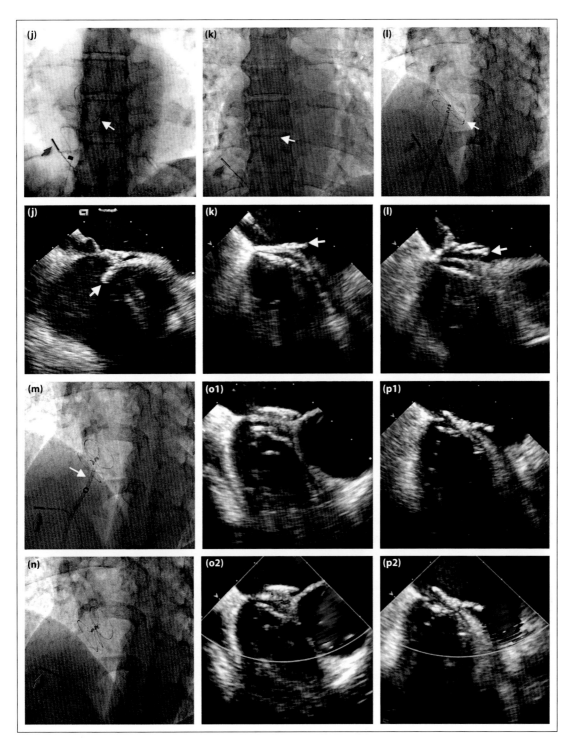

Figure 6.4 (continued) A series of images outlining PFO closure with the Gore Septal Occluder. (a–c) Initial diagnostic assessment of the PFO. (a–a2) The septal view of the atrial septum with and without color Doppler (demonstrating L–R shunt) with corresponding position of the ICE catheter on fluoroscopy outlined by the red arrow. (b–b2) The long-axis view (c–c2) demonstrating the short-axis view with the tunnel length measuring between 11 and 15 mm (a1, b1, c1). (d–f) Fluoroscopy images with ICE catheter position (red arrow) with the corresponding ICE image below. (d) R–L shunt of bubble contrast across the PFO with (e) clearly showing the wire crossing the defect and (f) balloon sizing of the defect, which is optional outside of most clinical trails. (g–i) Delivery of the HELEX device with corresponding fluoroscopy and ICE images in various views. (i) The left atrial component of the device deployed with (j, k) demonstrating the device pulled back to the septum and further deployment of the right atrial component of the device with it fully deployed in the long-axis (k) and short-axis views (l). (m, n) Release of the device on fluoroscopy with corresponding postdeployment ICE assessment with short-axis views and long-axis views with and without color (o1, o2, p1, p2).

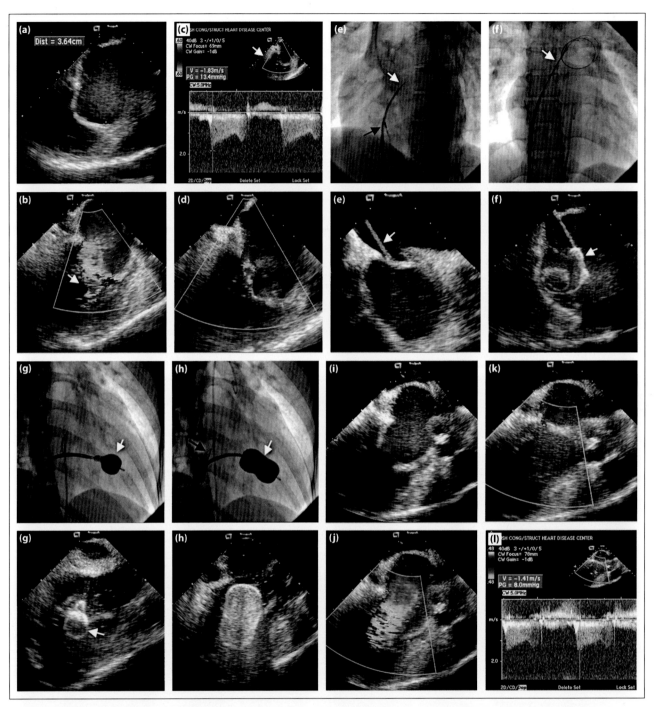

Figure 6.7 A series of images demonstrating ICE-guided balloon mitral valvuloplasty in a 36-year-old female with previous rheumatic heart disease. (a–d) Evaluation of the mitral annulus (a), stenosis (b), Doppler gradient (c), and degree of mitral regurgitation (d). (e) A fluoroscopy image outlining the transseptal needle position (white arrow) with the ICE catheter position outlined by the black arrow and corresponding ICE image below demonstrating tenting of the atrial septum in the long-axis view. (f) The wire across the atrial septum in the left atrium on fluoroscopy and ICE. (g, h) Fluoroscopy images of the various stages of inflation of the Inoue balloon (white arrows) with the ICE catheter position (black arrow (h)) and the corresponding ICE images. (i–l) Further ICE assessment of the mitral valve with significant improvement in valve opening both on 2-D (i) and color Doppler (j) imaging with trivial mitral regurgitation (k) and satisfactory reduction in mean transmitral Doppler gradient (l).

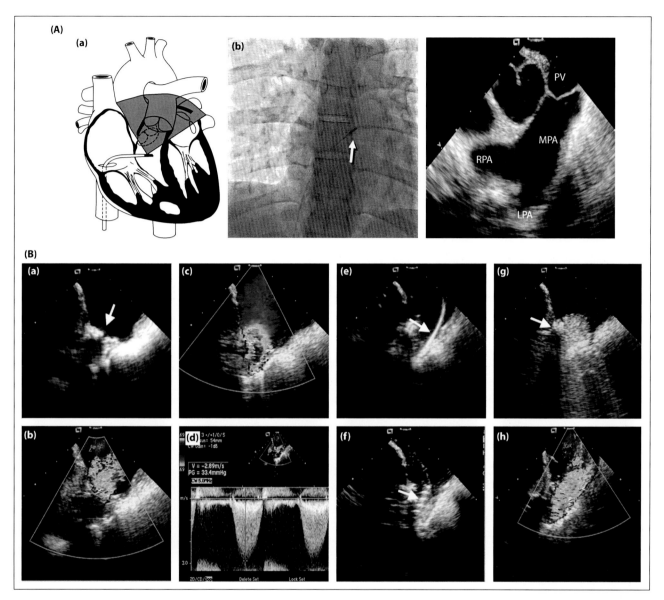

Figure 6.8 (A) (a, b) A diagrammatic representation with corresponding fluoroscopy image of the ICE catheter position within the RV with the transducer directed up toward the pulmonary valve. (c) The ICE image. (B) Series of images demonstrating transcatheter pulmonary valve replacement with the Edwards SAPIEN valve. (a) The thickened stenotic homograft valve (white arrow) with prominent pulmonary regurgitation (b). Color (c) and spectral Doppler (d) assessment confirm significant obstruction. (e) The wire across the valve (white arrow) with the predilated bare metal stent in position (white arrow (f)). Stent inflation (g) leads to free pulmonary regurgitation (h).

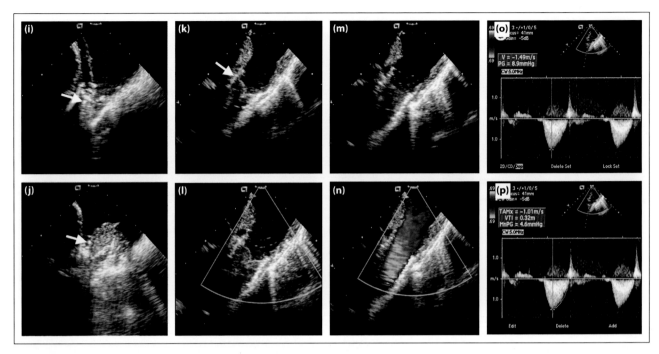

Figure 6.8 (continued) (i) Clear demonstration of the SAPIEN valve within the prestented RVOT, and following inflation (j), the functioning valve is clearly seen (k, m, n) with minimal pulmonary regurgitation (l). Repeat spectral Doppler confirms minimal estimated residual transvalvar Doppler gradient (o, p).

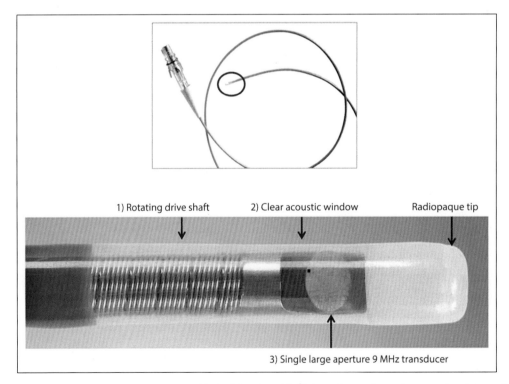

Figure 7.1 The distal end of the Ultra ICE catheter. (1) Flexible wire with high torsion and rotation capacity; (2) sonolucent window; (3) unique siliceous piezoelectric crystal with a frequency of 9 MHz.

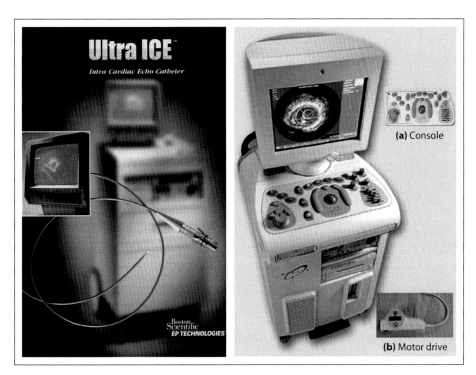

Figure 7.2 Dedicated review stations: ClearView Ultra System (left) and Galaxy System (right) with console (a) and motor drive unit (b). (From EP Technologies, Boston Scientific Corporation. With permission.)

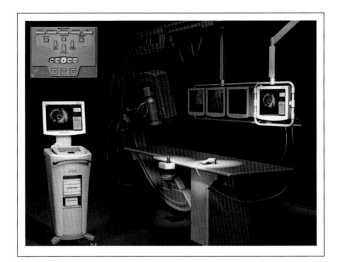

Figure 7.3 The Boston Scientific iLab System allows the option of fully integrating the hardware into the cardiac catheterization and electrophysiology laboratories, providing the integration of real-time fluoroscopic and echocardiographic images according to a modality immediately usable by operators; details of iLab System review station (top). (From EP Technologies, Boston Scientific Corporation. With permission.)

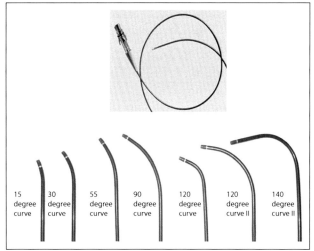

Figure 7.4 The Ultra ICE catheter is introduced through the femoral vein and advanced toward the right heart with an over-the-wire 8.5 Fr precurved introducer available in several lengths and curves.

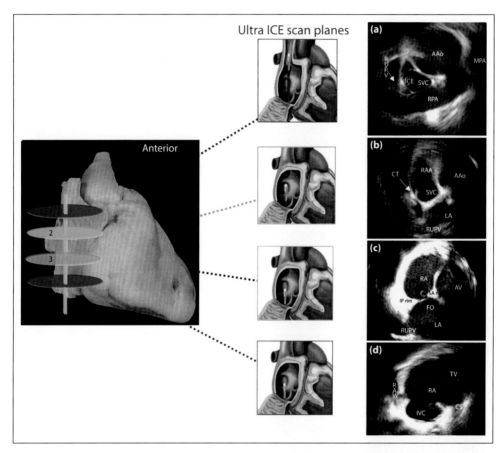

Figure 7.5 Intracardiac echocardiographic axial views: (a) *Great vessels axial plane*, SVC, superior vena cava; RUPV, right upper pulmonary vein; RPA, right pulmonary artery; AAo, ascending aorta; MPA, mean pulmonary artery; (b) *Superior vena cava–right atrium junction axial plane*, SVC, superior vena cava; RAA, right atrial auricle; CT, crista terminalis; RUPV, right upper pulmonary vein; Aao, ascending aorta; (c) *Aortic valve axial plane*: the aortic valve is viewed in its short axis astride the right and left atria, whereas the atrial septum is transversally scanned in its entirety and the fossa ovalis with its superior–anterior and inferior–posterior rims may be well appreciated, RA, right atrium; AV, aortic valve; LA, left atrium; RUPV, right upper pulmonary vein; FO, fossa ovalis; SA rim, superior–anterior rim; IP rim, inferior–posterior rim; (d) *Cavotricuspid isthmus axial plane*, RA, right atrium; TV, tricuspid valve; RAW, right atrial wall; CS, coronary sinus; IVC, inferior vena cava.

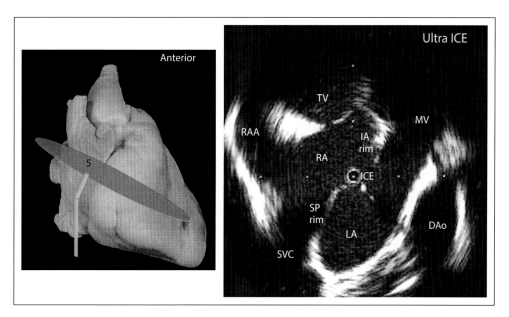

Figure 7.6 *Long-axis four-chamber plane*: The long-axis view is obtained with a 55° precurved introducer sheath advanced up to the end of the catheter and turned posterior and leftward, to longitudinally scan the atrial septum. On this plane, it is possible to visualize the right and left atria, right and left atrial auricles, tricuspid and mitral valves, and the descending aorta. Moreover, the atrial septum is longitudinally scanned and the fossa ovalis with its inferior–anterior and superior–posterior rims can be well appreciated. SVC, superior vena cava; RA, right atrium; RAA, right atrial auricle; FO, fossa ovalis; TV, tricuspid valve; MV, mitral valve; LA, left atrium; DAo, descending aorta; SP rim, superior–posterior rim; IA rim, inferior–anterior rim.

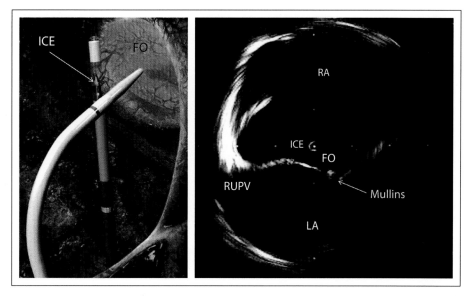

Figure 7.16 Ultra ICE permits continuous monitoring of the transseptal puncture showing the tip of Mullins transseptal sheath and the Brockenbrough needle seated against the middle of the fossa ovalis, causing a slight "tenting effect." RA, right atrium; LA, left atrium; ICE, intracardiac echocardiography probe; RUPV, right upper pulmonary vein; FO, fossa ovalis.

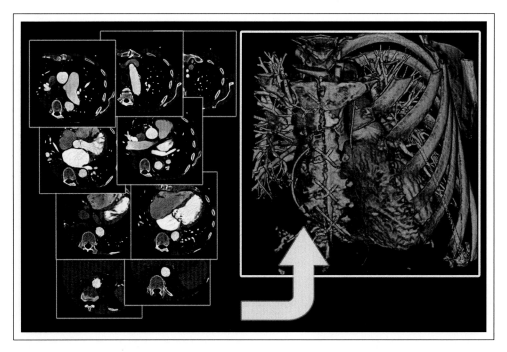

Figure 8.1 2-D data acquired from helical multidetector CT (MDCT) scanning can be reconstructed into 3-D volume-rendered images using postprocessing techniques.

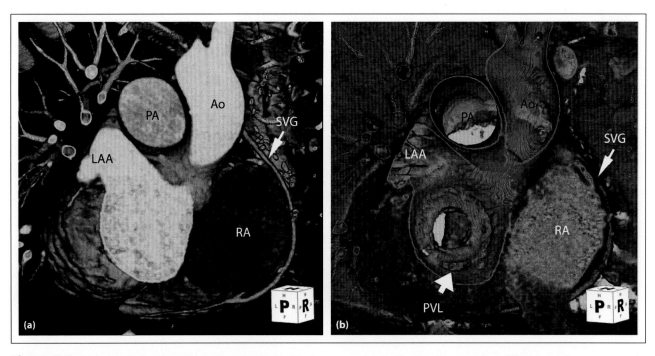

Figure 8.2 3-D reconstruction of a cardiac CTA study. The image can be manipulated to examine different cardiac structures by selectively changing the opacities of voxels with different densities. (a) The course of a patent saphenous vein graft (SVG, arrow) is clearly seen. (b) The same image in (a) after making high-density voxels more transparent. The SVG (thin arrow) is not seen as well as in (a), but a prosthetic mitral valve with a paravalvar leak (PVL, thick arrow) is now identified.

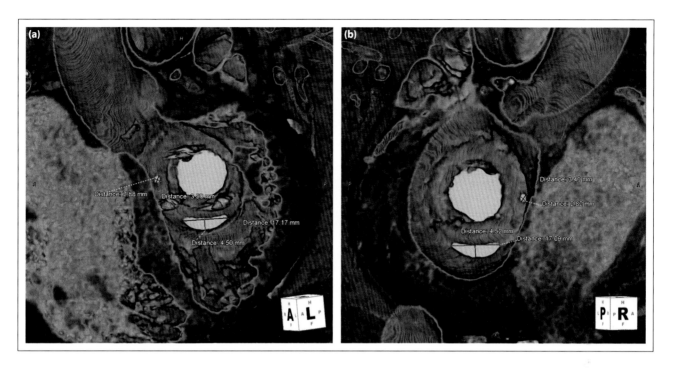

Figure 8.3 Volume-rendered CT images are useful for making accurate measurements of cardiac structures. In this case, the dimensions of two mitral paravalvar leaks are measured from the ventricular side (a) and the atrial side (b) prior to consideration of percutaneous PVL closure.

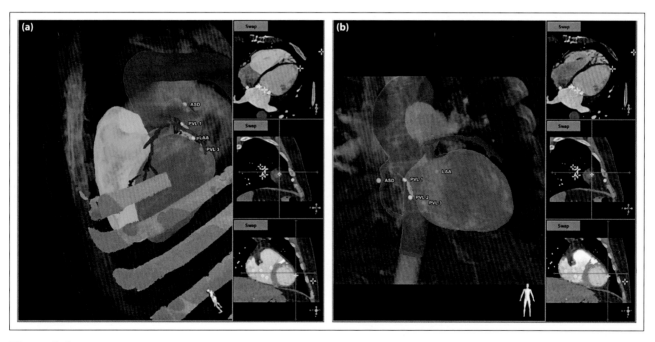

Figure 8.4 Segmentation of 3-D volume-rendered CT images for preprocedural planning. (a) The aorta and coronary arteries (red), right ventricle (green), left ventricle (purple), and ribs (tan) are segmented. The locations of an atrial septal defect (blue dot), three paravalvar leaks (PVL 1–3), and left atrial appendage (LAA) are marked (yellow dots). (b) The image in (a) is rotated to show the same structures in a different orientation. Segmented structures can be added or removed. In this case, the ribs were removed to better visualize the left ventricle.

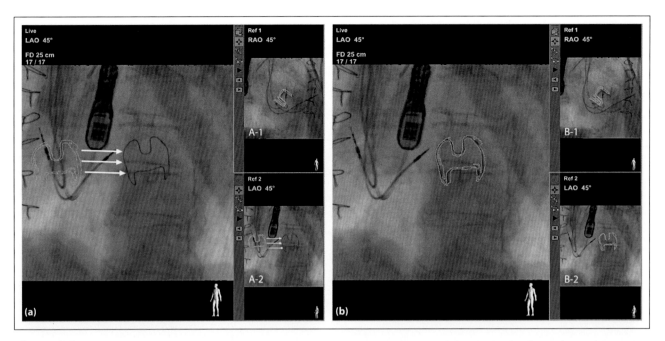

Figure 8.5 Registration of 3-D CTA data to live fluoroscopy. (a) The outline of a prosthetic mitral valve frame (orange) is overlaid onto the fluoroscopy screen. It is then adjusted to correspond to the same size, location, and orientation as the radiopaque frame seen on fluoroscopy using specialized software (Philips HeartNavigator, Best, Netherlands). (b) Once the CTA data are properly registered, the movement of the C-arm will be tracked, and the CT overlay images will automatically move and rotate accordingly (B-1 and B-2). Additional structures and landmarks from the CTA data can be added or removed as needed for procedural guidance.

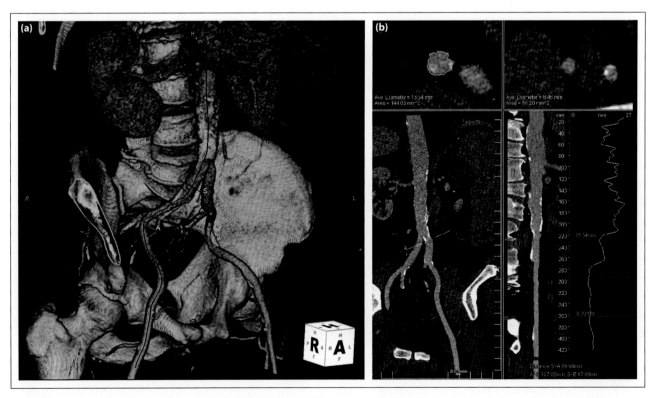

Figure 8.6 CTA images of the peripheral vasculature in a patient prior to transcatheter aortic valve replacement (TAVR). (a) 3-D volume-rendered CTA images can identify tortuosity and atherosclerotic disease that increase the risk of vascular complications. In this case, the iliofemoral vessels are mildly tortuous, and calcification of the descending aorta is present. (b) Curved multiplanar reconstruction (CMPR) in the same patient allows accurate measurements of the iliofemoral vessels. In this patient, TAVR was successfully performed using femoral artery access.

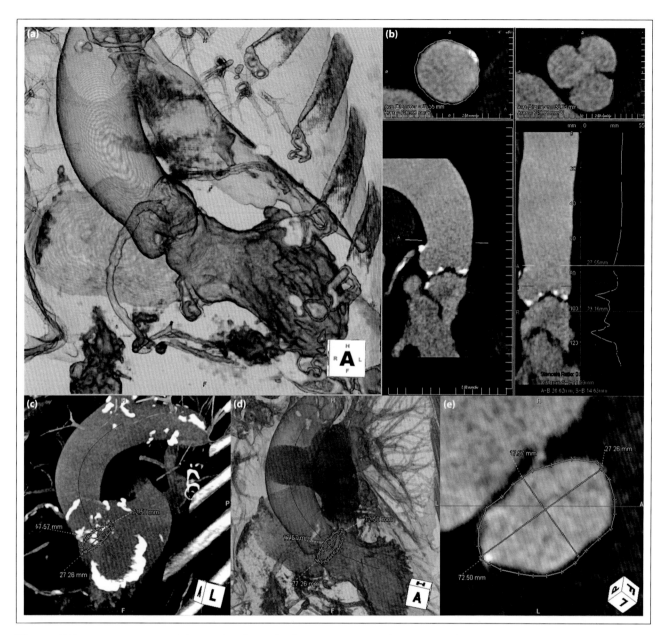

Figure 8.7 CTA assessment of the aortic valve and adjacent structures prior to transcatheter aortic valve replacement (TAVR). (a) 3-D volume-rendered CTA images provide an overview of the size and angulation of the ascending aorta during preprocedural planning for TAVR. (b) Curved multiplanar reconstruction (CMPR) of the ascending aorta is used to measure the aorta at the sinotubular junction (green outline, top left panel) and the sinus of Valsalva (red outline, top right panel). (c–e) Multiple images are used for the assessment of the aortic valve annulus. (c) Demonstrates surrounding calcium (white) in relationship to the aortic annular plane (green outline) using a maximum-intensity projection (MIP). (d) Demonstrates the spatial orientation of the aortic annular plane (green outline) in a volume-rendered image. (e) Shows a cross section of the annulus using CMPR to make accurate measurements of the aortic annulus perimeter and maximum and minimum diameters.

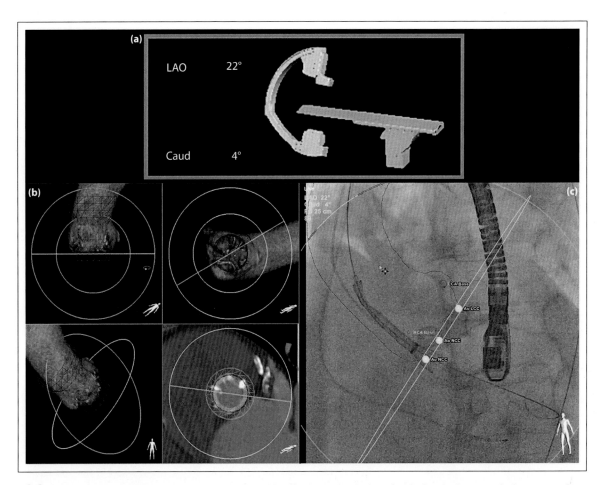

Figure 8.8 3-D volume-rendered CTA images are used to identify the optimal plane for device deployment during transcatheter aortic valve implantation (TAVR), in which all three aortic valve leaflets lie in a single plane. (a, b) The predicted C-arm angulation to achieve the desired orientation can be identified by CTA prior to the procedure. A volume-rendered CTA image of the aorta can be rotated to align the aortic valve leaflets, with the plane containing all three represented by the yellow circle (b). In this case, a model of a CoreValve is placed in the CTA image to identify the optimal device position. (c) A fluoroscopic view in the predetermined C-arm angulation during CoreValve deployment. The preacquired CTA images have been registered to the fluoroscopic images, and the outline of the aorta (red) and the base of each aortic valve leaflet (yellow dots) are overlaid onto the fluoroscopy screen. The plane of the leaflets is represented by the yellow circle.

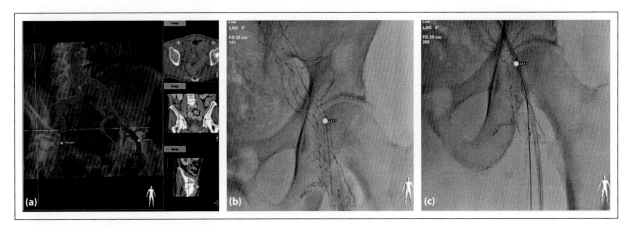

Figure 8.9 (a) The iliofemoral system is segmented after 3-D reconstruction of CTA data in a patient undergoing transcatheter aortic valve replacement (TAVR). The planned puncture sites of both femoral arteries are marked with yellow dots. (b) After the CTA data have been registered to the fluoroscopic images, CT overlay imaging is used to guide femoral artery access. The needle is guided toward the planned puncture site in the left femoral artery (yellow dot). (c) After accessing the femoral artery, the vessel is preclosed (Prostar XL, Abbott Vascular, Abbott Park, IL, USA) prior to insertion of the delivery sheath.

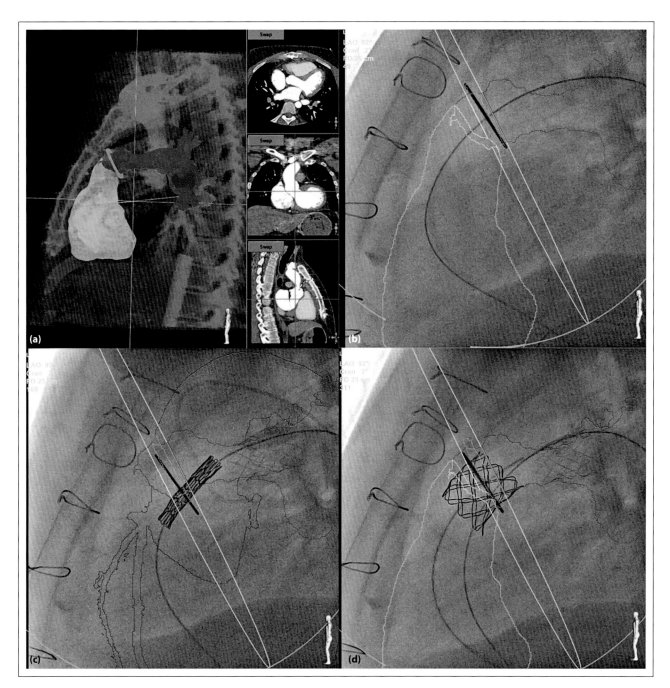

Figure 8.10 CT guidance during implantation of a transcatheter Melody valve (Medtronic, Minneapolis, MN, USA) in a patient with tetralogy of Fallot and severe pulmonary insufficiency of a right ventricular outflow tract conduit. The patient also had severe stenosis of the left main pulmonary artery. (a) 3-D volume-rendered CTA images identify the right ventricle (green) and proximal pulmonary vasculature (magenta). The pulmonary valve prosthesis in the RVOT conduit is also identified (orange). The CT data are then registered to fluoroscopy for CT overlay guidance. (b) A fluoroscopic image with CT–fluoroscopy fusion imaging used to mark the outline of the right ventricle (green) and pulmonary arteries (magenta). The plane of the pulmonary valve is identified with a yellow circle. (c) A fluoroscopic image with the Melody valve being positioned prior to deployment. CT–fluoroscopy fusion imaging is used to identify the left ventricle and left coronary artery (red outline) to assess for potential coronary compression during valve deployment. A stent is visible in the left pulmonary artery that was placed prior to deploying the Melody valve. (d) A fluoroscopic image showing the Melody valve in the final position.

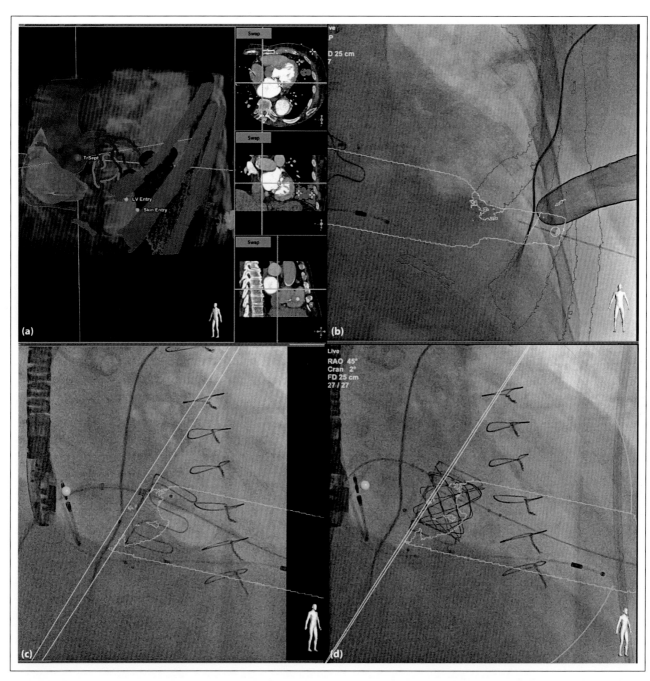

Figure 8.11 CT guidance for mitral valve-in-valve implantation in a patient with a degenerated bioprosthetic mitral valve using a Melody transcatheter valve. An antegrade transseptal approach was used to deliver the Melody valve, with transapical access used to snare and exteriorize the guide wire to create a "rail-wire" for secure device delivery. (a) 3-D volume-rendered CTA images are segmented to identify the aorta and coronary arteries (red), left atrium (orange), and ribs (magenta). The transapical skin and left ventricle entry points (green dots) and planned transseptal puncture site (gray dot) are marked. (b) A fluoroscopic image showing transapical access using CT overlay guidance. After the CTA data have been registered to fluoroscopy, the skin entry point (green dot) is placed on the fluoroscopic image for access guidance. A manually constructed cylinder coaxial to the mitral valve is overlaid onto the fluoroscopic image to guide the angle of needle entry. (c) The transseptal guide wire has been exteriorized through the transapical access site to create a rail-wire, and a catheter is advanced over the wire. The transseptal puncture site was marked for guidance (blue dot). (d) The Melody valve is deployed within the degenerated mitral bioprosthesis over the rail-wire.

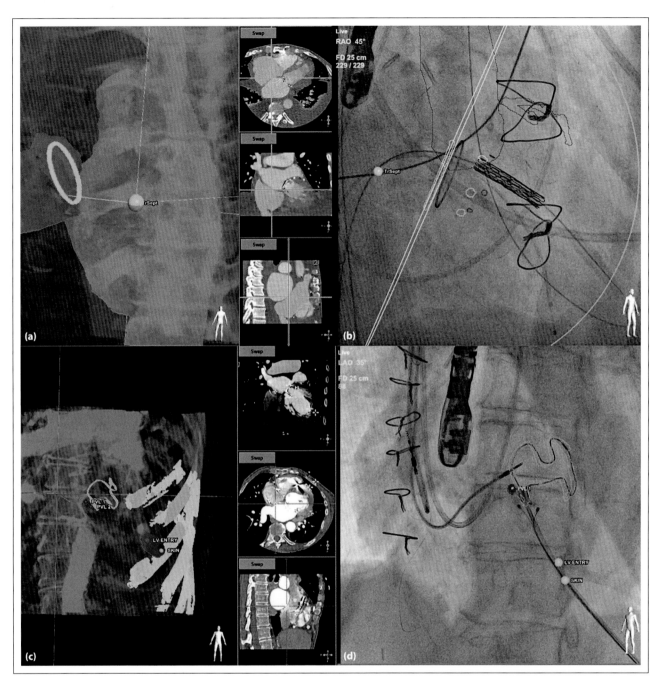

Figure 8.12 CT guidance for site-specific transseptal and transapical access. (a, b) CT guidance for transseptal access during a mitral valve-in-valve implantation procedure using a Melody transcatheter pulmonary valve (Medtronic, Minneapolis, MN, USA). The patient has a degenerated mitral bioprosthetic valve and was deemed to be inoperable. (a) Shows segmentation of the left atrium (orange) and the left ventricle (purple) from 3-D volume-rendered CTA images. The mitral valve prosthesis is marked (green circle). The ideal transseptal puncture site for delivery of the Melody valve is marked (blue dot). (b) Shows a fluoroscopic image during delivery of the Melody valve. Transseptal access was obtained and a rail-wire was snared in the aorta and exteriorized through the femoral artery to deliver the Melody valve. CT data were registered to fluoroscopic images, and CT overlay guidance was used for site-specific transseptal puncture (blue dot). (c, d) CT guidance for an aortic paravalvar leak (PVL) closure. (c) Shows segmentation of the prosthetic aortic valve (orange) and ribs (green). The PVL is marked (red dots) and the skin and left ventricular entry points are identified (green dots) at a safe distance from the lung, coronary arteries, and ribs. A manually constructed cylinder is placed between the skin and ventricular entry points to identify the angle of needle entry. (d) Shows a fluoroscopic image during the procedure, with a catheter extending through the left ventricular apex to the aortic valve, and two Amplatzer Vascular Plug II devices (St. Jude Medical, St. Paul, MN, USA) being deployed across the PVL (red dot).

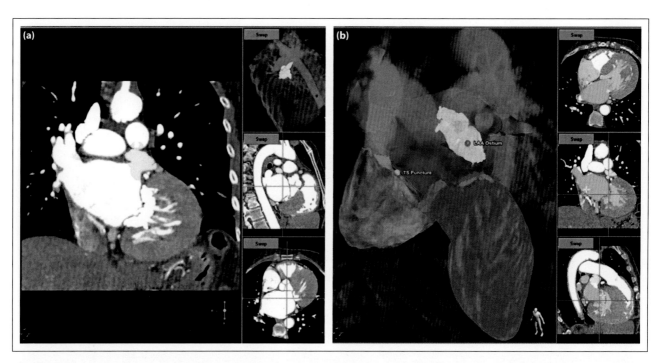

Figure 8.13 (a) The size, morphology, and orientation of the left atrial appendage (LAA, yellow shading) can be assessed by CTA prior to LAA exclusion. Improper sizing of an exclusion device may lead to perforation, incomplete exclusion, or device embolization. (b) For procedural guidance, the cardiac chambers and LAA are segmented on volume-rendered CT images. The planned transseptal (TS) puncture site is identified and marked with a blue dot. The images can then be registered to fluoroscopy and used for CT overlay guidance during the procedure.

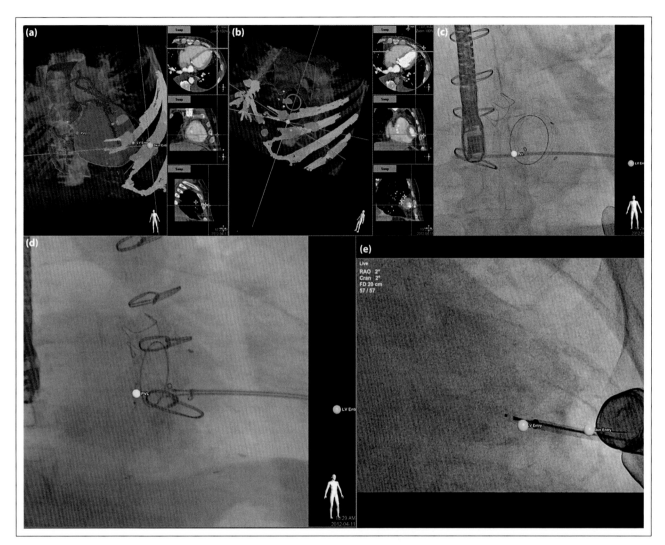

Figure 8.14 CT guidance for paravalvar leak (PVL) closure using transapical access. (a, b) Segmentation of volume-rendered CT images is used to identify the 3-D location of the PVL (yellow dot), as well as the skin and left ventricular puncture sites (blue dots), in relationship to surrounding structures. (c) After registering the CT data to fluoroscopic images, CT overlay guidance is used for crossing the PVL (yellow dot) with a guide wire and advancing a delivery sheath. The radiopaque portion of the mitral bioprosthesis used for registration is identified by the green circle. (d) Two Amplatzer Vascular Plug II devices (St. Jude Medical, St. Paul, MN, USA) are deployed across the PVL using CT overlay guidance. (e) An Amplatzer duct occluder device (St. Jude Medical, St. Paul, MN, USA) is used to close the left ventricular access site (blue dot).

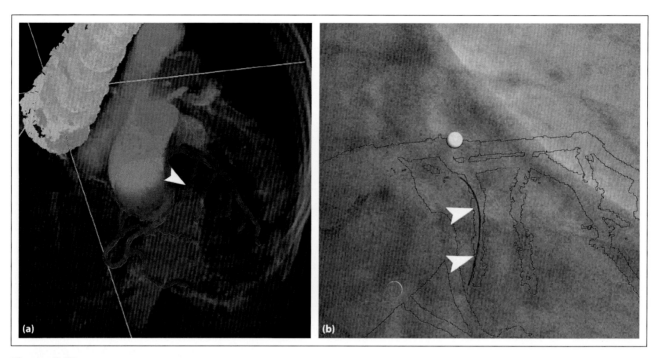

Figure 8.15 CT guidance for alcohol septal ablation in a patient with hypertrophic obstructive cardiomyopathy (HOCM). (a) Prior to performing an alcohol septal ablation procedure for HOCM, 3-D volume-rendered CTA images are used to segment the coronary arteries (red). The first septal perforator artery is identified (arrowhead). (b) CT overlay guidance for alcohol septal ablation. After registration of the CT data to fluoroscopic images, the coronary arteries are identified (red outline). The ostium of the first septal perforator is marked (yellow dot). A guide wire (white arrowheads) is advanced into the first septal perforator (arrowheads) using CT guidance and the position is confirmed by contrast angiography prior to injection of ethanol.

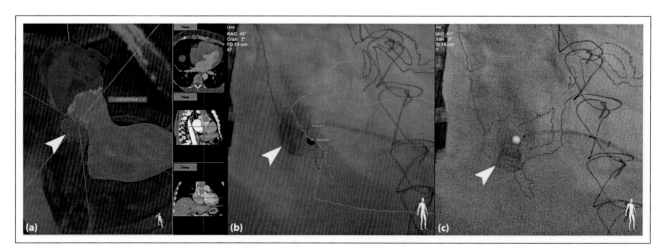

Figure 8.16 CT guidance for ventricular pseudoaneurysm closure. This patient developed a pseudoaneurysm in the left ventricular outflow tract (LVOT) after aortic valve replacement for endocarditis. (a) 3-D volume-rendered CTA images are segmented to identify the aorta and coronary arteries (red), left ventricle (purple), and a pseudoaneurysm in the LVOT (magenta). (b) A catheter is advanced into the pseudoaneurysm from a transapical approach, and contrast is injected into the pseudoaneurysm to confirm the catheter location. The pseudoaneurysm had two ostia communicating with the LVOT, identified as ostium 1 (purple circle) and ostium 2 (red dot). (c) Embolization coils (Cook Medical, Bloomington, IN, USA) are successfully deployed into the pseudoaneurysm using CT overlay guidance.

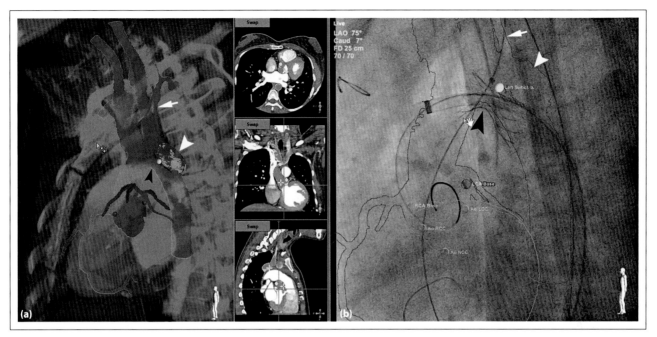

Figure 8.17 CT imaging guidance for aortic stent placement in a patient with coarctation of the aorta. This patient had coarctation repair in childhood and later had a left carotid artery to descending aorta graft placed. She developed symptomatic recurrent coarctation with a high gradient across the coarctation. CTA identified a severe ostial subclavian stenosis in addition. (a) Volume-rendered 3-D CTA images are segmented to show the aorta and location of the coarctation (black arrow), coronary arteries, left subclavian artery (white arrow) with ostial stenosis (yellow dot), and left carotid artery to descending aorta graft (white arrowhead). The length and diameter of the coarctation, distance from aortic arch branch vessels, and diameter of the proximal and distal aortic segments were measured on CTA images prior to the procedure. (b) A Palmaz XL 3110 stent (Johnson and Johnson, New Brunswick, NJ) was placed across the coarctation using fluoroscopy with CT overlay guidance. After registration of the CT data to fluoroscopic images, the outline of the aorta, coronary arteries, and left carotid artery to descending aorta graft are placed on the fluoroscopy screen for guidance (red outlines). The ostium of the stenotic left subclavian artery is identified (yellow dot). A subclavian artery stent was placed after implantation of the aortic stent.

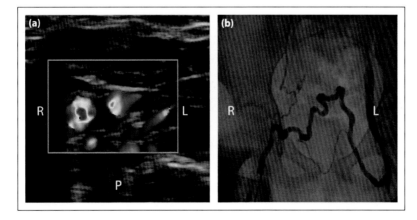

Figure 9.3 Right femoral vein cannulation. (a) Color Doppler is useful for confirming arterial and venous flow and can facilitate access. (b) Ultrasound-guided access often allows access to smaller vessels, although these may not be useful in securing a sheath for intervention as demonstrated here, where an angiogram through the access needle demonstrates right femoral vein occlusion. The left femoral vein appears patent.

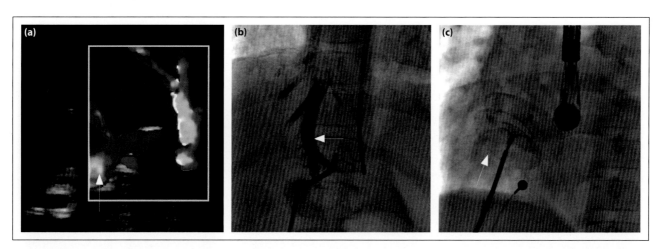

Figure 9.4 Transhepatic access for atrial septal defect closure in a patient with left atrial isomerism and interrupted inferior caval vein with azygous continuation. (a) Ultrasound is useful for identifying large hepatic venous vessels with a direct path toward the right atrium. (b) A hand angiogram through the needle is still performed to confirm flow toward the right atrium and that the vein is of sufficient caliber for the final sheath size intended (arrow). (c) Here, access has been secured and an 8 French sheath used to close a large atrial septal defect (arrow, Amplatz septal occluder). This procedure would have been difficult from either an internal jugular or subclavian vein approach.

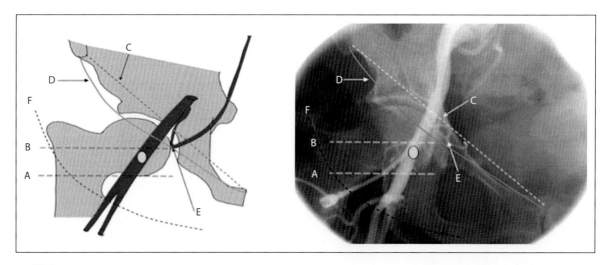

Figure 10.1 "Landing zone" for the placement of percutaneous femoral sheaths. (a) Lower margin of the femoral head. (b) Center point of the femoral head. (c) Line connecting the anterior superior iliac crest and symphysis pubis for approximation of inguinal ligament location. (d) Actual inguinal ligament location. (e) Point where the inferior epigastric artery descends below the inguinal ligament before turning cranial. (f) Inguinal crease. Yellow circle is the target for needle entry into common femoral artery. (Courtesy of Dr. Zultan Turi. With permission.)

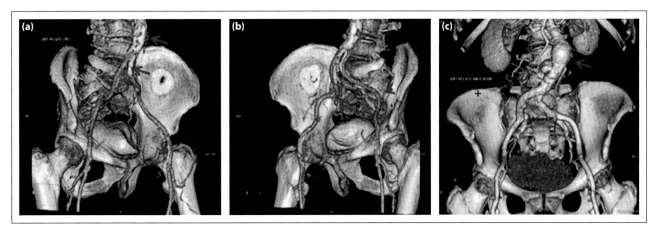

Figure 10.2 Three-dimensional reconstruction of CT angiogram for the evaluation of ileo-femoral arteries. (a) RAO projection demonstrating moderate calcification of the abdominal aorta and iliac bifurcation (large arrows) as well as mild calcification and narrowing of the left common femoral artery (small arrow). (b) LAO projection of the same patient demonstrating moderate tortuousity (arrowheads), which was not as well appreciated on the RAO view. (c) An AP projection of a patient with moderate abdominal aorta calcification and aneurysm (arrow).

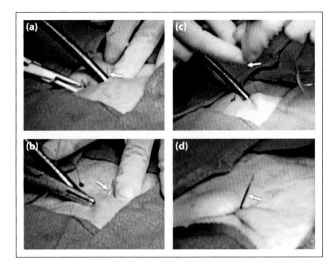

Figure 10.5 Figure-of-eight suture. (a) The first stitch is placed distal to the sheath deep in the subcutaneous tissue (arrow). (b) The second stitch is placed just above the sheath, more superficially than the first one (arrow), thereby creating a figure-of-eight. (c) The fisherman's knot is tied (arrow) and the suture is tightened as the sheath is removed. (d) The final appearance of the stitch, which compresses the femoral vein underneath to achieve hemostasis.

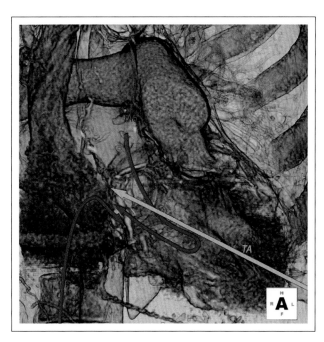

Figure 15.1 In this example, a 3-D volume-rendered CTA image depicts a target lesion near the mitral valve with unfavorable angles for wire crossing and device delivery through a retrograde aortic (TAo) or transseptal approach (TS) (red arrows). Alternatively, transapical access (TA) offers a more direct approach to the target lesion (green arrow).

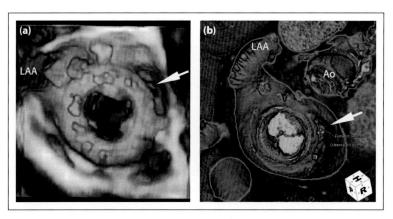

Figure 15.2 (a) 3-D TEE demonstrates the presence of a prosthetic mitral valve with a paravalvular leak (white arrow). Defect size, location in relation to the prosthetic valve, and relationship to surrounding structures are identified. The left atrial appendage (LAA) can be used as a reference point for identifying the location of the leak. (b) A 3-D volume-rendered CTA image in a similar projection as the TEE image in (a), showing the mitral paravalvular leak (white arrow) and surrounding structures. Measurements can be made for device selection and sizing. Based on the location of the defect, an access route can be chosen.

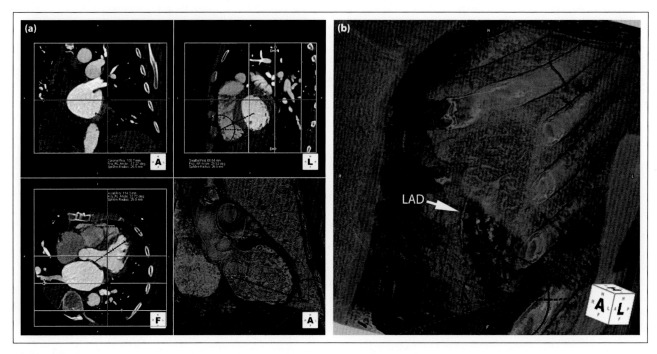

Figure 15.3 (a) Helical CTA images can be viewed in multiple planes and with 3-D reconstruction to identify an optimal puncture site and angle of entry that is coaxial to the target lesion. The distance from the skin surface to the left ventricle can be measured by CTA. The distance from the sternum to the planned puncture site can be measured as a reference for guiding access. (b) 3-D volume-rendered CTA images are used to assess the location of coronary arteries (left anterior descending artery, white arrow) and lung tissue to avoid inadvertent puncture during transapical access. The rib interspace through which the ventricle will be accessed can be identified.

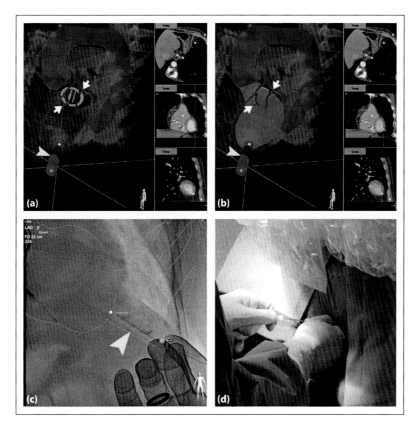

Figure 15.4 CT guidance for transapical access. (a) 3-D volume-rendered CT images are segmented to identify relevant structures: aorta and coronary arteries (red) and mitral valve prosthesis (orange). Two mitral paravalvular leaks (PVL) are marked (red dots). The skin and ventricular planned puncture sites are marked (skin—green dot, left ventricle—white dot). A cylinder is manually constructed to connect the skin and ventricular entry points (yellow arrow). (b) The left ventricle (purple) is added to the image to show the relationship of the ventricle to the skin and ventricular puncture sites. (c) After the CT data have been registered to the fluoroscopic images, an outline of the left ventricle and the cylinder containing the skin and ventricular puncture sites (skin—green dot, left ventricle—white dot) are overlaid onto the fluoroscopy screen and used for access guidance. (d) After a 0.018 inch guide wire has been advanced into the left ventricle, a sheath is advanced over the wire. In this case, a 4 Fr micropuncture sheath is being used to exchange the guide wire for a 0.035 inch guide wire, and a larger sheath will then be advanced over the 0.035 inch guide wire.

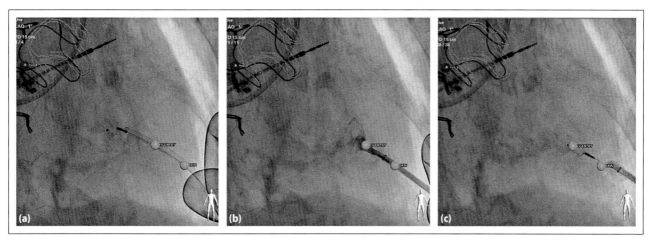

Figure 15.6 Transapical access closure using a 6-4 Amplazter ductal occluder device (ADO). (a) The ADO device is advanced through the sheath into the left ventricle. The skin and left ventricular entry points (green dots) are identified using CT overlay imaging, as are the mitral prosthetic valve frame (orange) and the mitral paravalvular leak with closure devices in place (red dot). (b) The sheath and ADO are withdrawn until the sheath is in the pericardial space and the disk of the ADO device is secure against the inner wall of the myocardium. The position of the sheath is confirmed by contrast injection. (c) After the device is properly positioned, the sheath is withdrawn and the ADO is released.

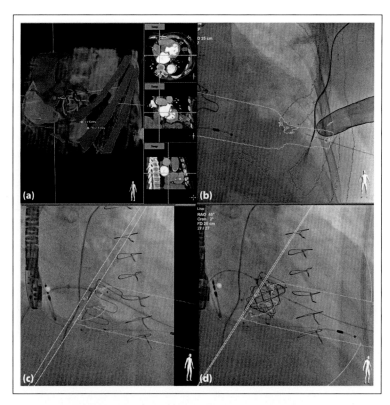

Figure 15.7　Transapical access for a mitral valve-in-valve implantation in a patient with a degenerated mitral valve prosthesis. (a) 3-D volume-rendered CTA images are segmented to identify the aorta and coronary arteries (red), left atrium (orange), ribs (magenta), and partial left lung (blue). The planned transseptal puncture location (gray dot) and LV and skin entry points (green dots) are marked. The frame of the mitral valve prosthesis is identified (green outline). (b) After the CTA images are registered to fluoroscopy, transapical access is obtained with a micropuncture needle at the previously identified skin entry site (green dot), at an angle coaxial to the mitral valve. A manually constructed cylinder from the CTA data (green outline) connecting the skin entry to the mitral valve is overlaid onto the fluoroscopy screen and used to guide LV puncture. (c) After obtaining transseptal and transapical access (blue dot—transseptal puncture site), a guide wire is snared and exteriorized. A catheter is advanced over the rail-wire across the mitral valve. (d) A Melody transcatheter valve (Medtronic, Minneapolis, MN, USA) is successfully deployed within the frame of the degenerated mitral valve prosthesis over the rail-wire.

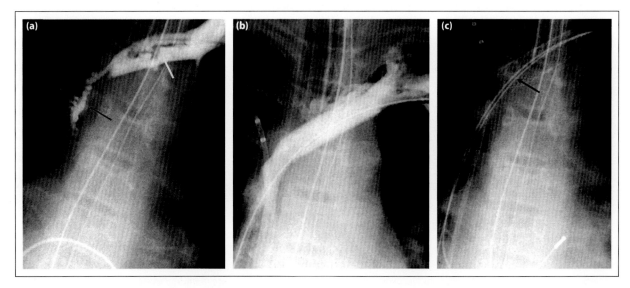

Figure 16.14　(a) Following removal of a transvenous pacing wire, an innominate vein angiogram shows complete occlusion of the vessel as it enters into the SVC (red arrow). Proximally, thrombus is noted along the vessel (yellow arrow). (b) Angiogram taken following stent implantation showing wide patency of the innominate vein into the SVC. (c) New pacing wires (black arrow) are passed across the stented innominate vein.

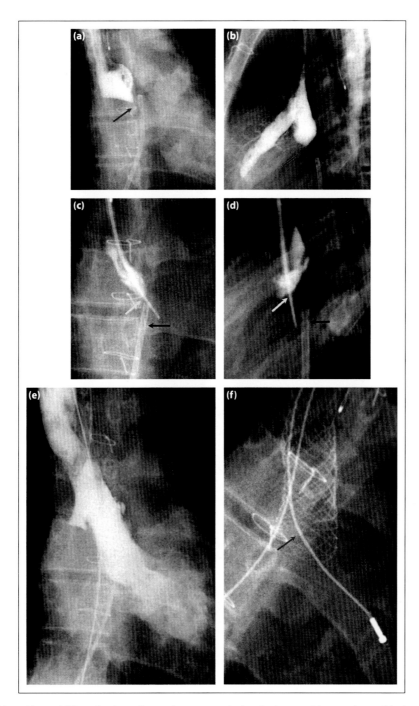

Figure 16.15 AP (a) and lateral (b) projection of complete SVC occlusion (red arrows) in a patient with d-transposition of the great arteries s/p Mustard repair. AP (c) and lateral (d) projection of successful transseptal needle puncture across the occluded segment (yellow arrows). A catheter was inserted from the femoral vein and positioned below the occluded site in the right atrium to act as a target (black arrows) for the transseptal needle. (e) Angiogram post-SVC baffle stent showing wide patency of flow into the "neo-right atrium." (f) New transvenous pacing wires placed through the stented SVC baffle.

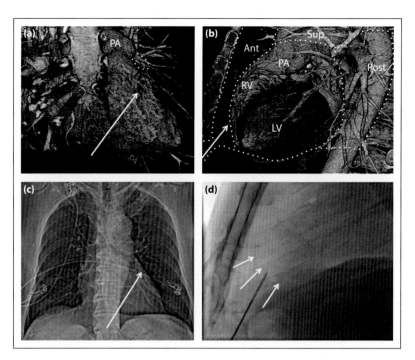

Figure 17.1 The orientation of the pericardial access for LAA ligation utilizing the LARIAT™ suture delivery device. Pericardial access for LAA ligation utilizing the LARIAT suture delivery device requires an anterior access approach into the pericardial space. As seen in the anteroposterior view (AP) of the 3D reconstruction of the CT angiogram (a), the LAA (delineated by the dashed line) is lateral to the pulmonary artery (PA) and appears to be in front of the hilum. The needle is directed (direction of the arrow) just lateral to the LAA, which is generally toward the left shoulder. In the fluoroscopic image, the needle (arrow) would be directed just lateral to the hilum (c). The lateral view of the 3D reconstruction of the CT angiogram (b) demonstrates the virtual space of the anterior mediastinal space (Ant). The needle (arrow) is directed through the sternocostal triangle that allows for the needle to pass under the xiphoid process and above the diaphragm into the anterior mediastinal space, thus avoiding damage to the diaphragm and avoiding abdominal organs. The 90° left lateral fluoroscopic view allows for the needle to be advanced to the myocardial border (d). Ant: anterior mediastinal space, Sup: superior mediastinal space, Post: posterior mediastinal space. RV: right ventricle, PA: pulmonary artery, LV: left ventricle.

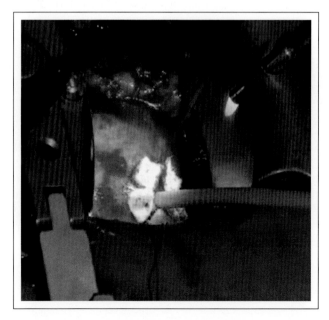

Figure 18.1 Surgical access to the ascending aorta as used in the transaortic approach. An incision in the right 2nd intercostal space is made, the aorta exposed, and a pledgeted purse-string suture placed. The sheath for valve deployment is introduced from the cranial aspect of the patient and directed toward the aortic valve.

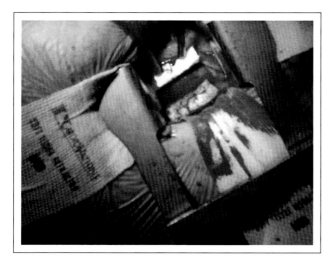

Figure 18.2 Surgical access to the apex of the left ventricle as used in the transapical approach. An incision in the left 5th intercostal space is made, the apex and left anterior descending artery exposed, and a purse-string suture placed. A soft tissue retractor facilitates access and exposure to the apex. In this figure, a parallel U-stitch technique is used as a purse-string, secured with two pledgets and tourniquets.

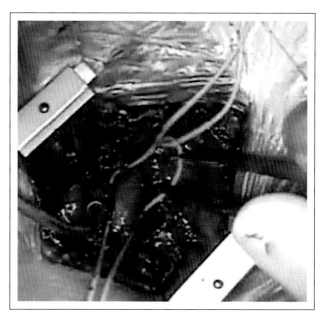

Figure 18.4 Surgical access to the axillary artery as used in the subclavian approach. The incision is made in the lateral portion of the clavicle. The pectoral muscle above the artery is split and the vessel and its side branches are snared with vessel loops.

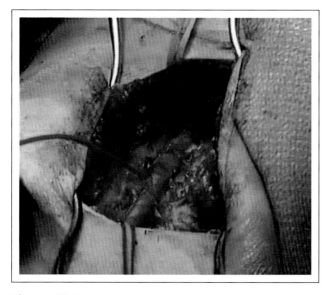

Figure 18.3 Surgical access to the common femoral artery as used in the transfemoral approach. The vessel and its side branches are snared with vessel loops.

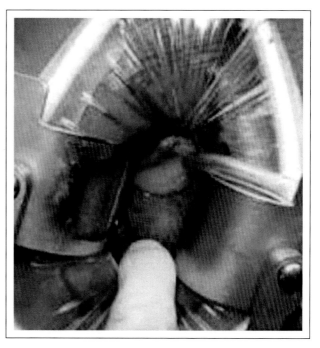

Figure 18.5 Surgical access to the right atrium as used in the transatrial approach. An incision in the right 4th intercostal space is made, the aorta exposed, and a purse-string suture placed. The sheath for valve deployment is introduced from the cranial aspect of the patient and directed toward the aortic valve.

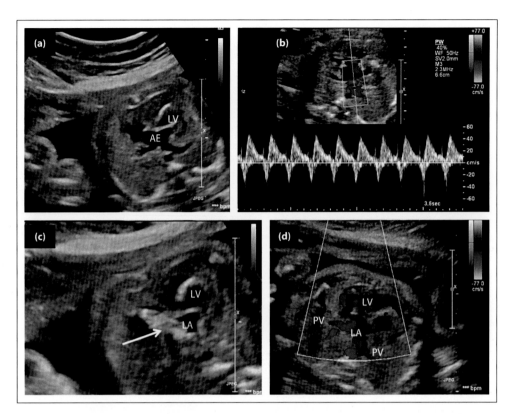

Figure 19.4 Fetal atrial septostomy in a patient with hypoplastic left heart syndrome and restrictive atrial septal defect. Echocardiographic views. (a) The left atrium and the pulmonary veins are dilated. (b) Doppler pattern in the pulmonary vein showing bidirectional flow due to a prominent "a" wave. (c) Balloon (arrow) inflated across the interatrial septum after transseptal puncture. (d) Immediate result after fetal atrial septostomy showing reduction in left atrial size and an unobstructed flow across the interatrial septum on color flow mapping (red color). LA: left atrium; LV: left ventricle; PV: pulmonary vein.

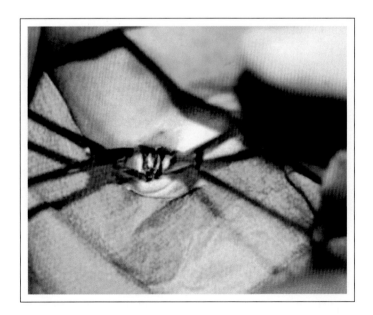

Figure 20.2 Recommendations for axillary artery cutdown.

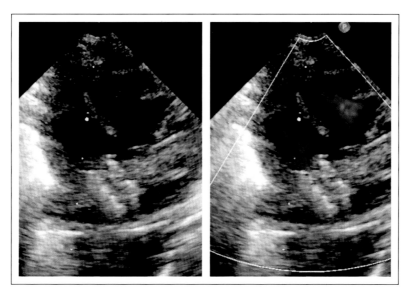

Figure 20.31 TTE 2D (left) and color Doppler (right) images of the stent position after implantation.

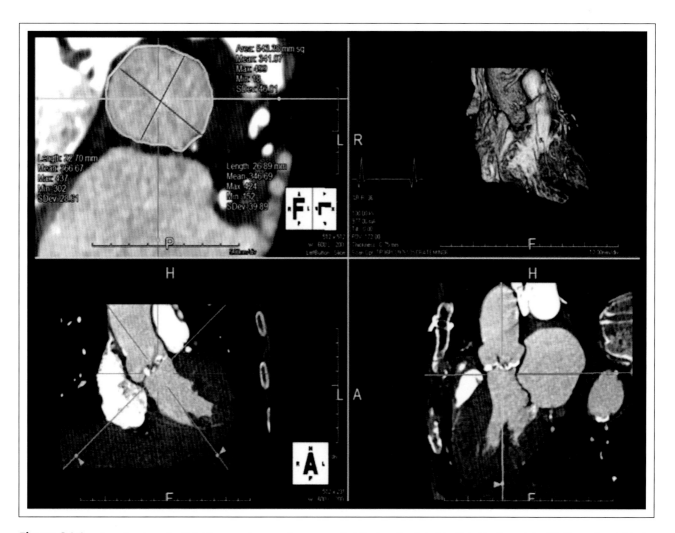

Figure 24.1 Annular sizing by CTA. The annulus area is measured at the basal point of leaflet attachment. In this figure (top left), the annulus area is 563 mm² and measures 26.9 mm × 22.7 mm.

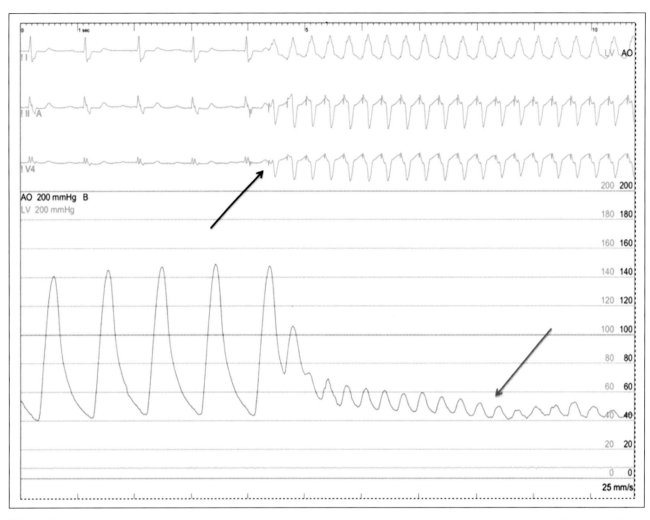

Figure 24.3 Rapid pacing. The patient is in sinus rhythm at the beginning of the tracing. Rapid pacing is begun (black arrow) and over the ensuing 10 beats, the pulse pressure narrows to about 10 mmHg and the mean pressure decreases to about 50 mmHg.

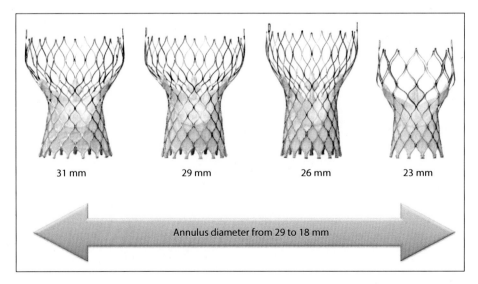

Figure 26.1 Medtronic CoreValve Revalving System in four different sizes covering an aortic annulus diameter from 18 to 29 mm. (Courtesy of Medtronic, MN, USA. With permission.)

Valve size (mm)	Mean diameter (mm)	Perimeter (mm)	Cover index (%)
31	28	88	10
31	27	85	13
31	26	82	16
31	25	79	19
29	26	82	10
29	25	79	14
29	24	75	17
29	23	72	21
26	23	72	11
26	22	69	15
26	21	66	19
23	20	63	13
23	19	60	17
23	18	57	22

Figure 26.3 CoreValve sizing according to computed tomography measurements.

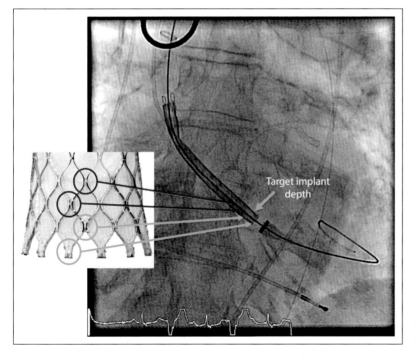

Figure 26.4 CoreValve implantation starting at a target implantation depth of 4–6 mm.

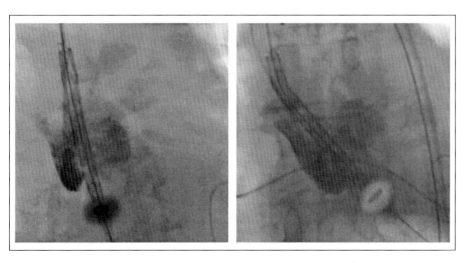

Figure 26.5 Perfect implantation position is achieved when the radiopaque catheter marker ring near the nose cone appears as a straight line.

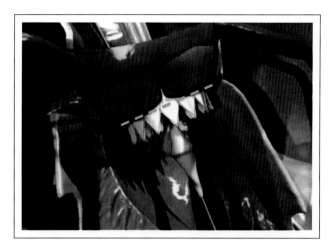

Figure 26.8 Target implantation depth of 4–6 mm. (Courtesy of Medtronic, MN, USA. With permission.)

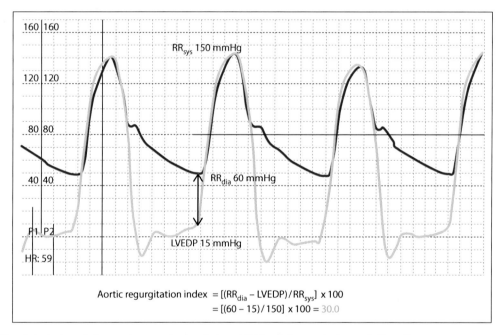

Aortic regurgitation index $= [(RR_{dia} - LVEDP)/RR_{sys}] \times 100$
$= [(60 - 15)/150] \times 100 = 30.0$

Figure 26.12 Calculation of the aortic regurgitation index. LVEDP = left ventricular end-diastolic pressure; RR_{dia} = diastolic blood pressure in the aorta; RR_{sys} = systolic blood pressure in the aorta.

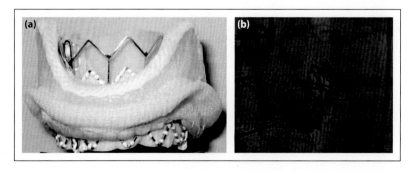

Figure 27.3 Demonstration of *in vitro* (a) and *in vivo* implantation (b) of an Edwards THV within a Carpentier–Edwards bioprosthesis.

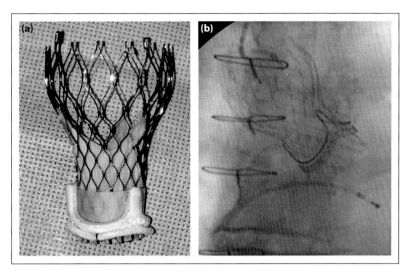

Figure 27.4 Demonstration of *in vitro* (a) and *in vivo* implantation (b) of a CoreValve THV within a Carpentier–Edwards bioprosthesis.

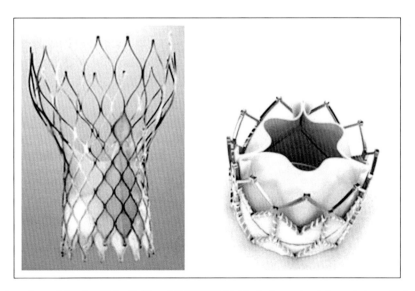

Figure 28.1 Current iterations of the CoreValve (left) and SAPIEN XT (right). Both can be delivered via an 18 Fr system.

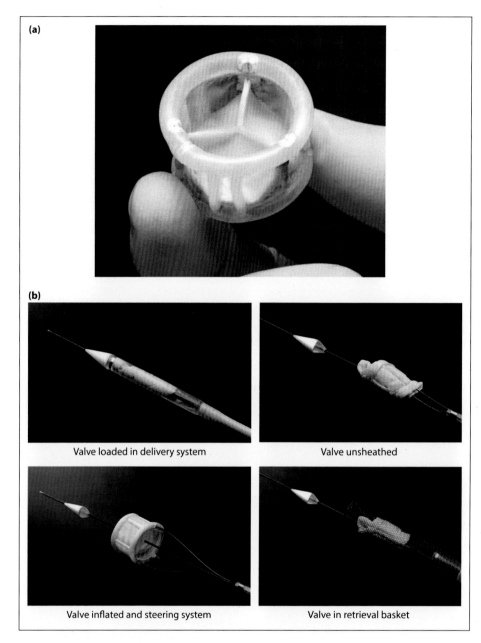

Figure 28.2 (a) DirectFlow valve. (b) Deployment sequence of the DirectFlow valve.

Valve loaded in delivery system

Valve unsheathed

Valve inflated and steering system

Valve in retrieval basket

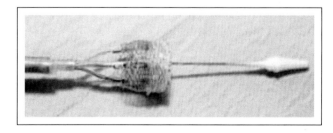

Figure 28.3 The Boston Scientific Lotus valve.

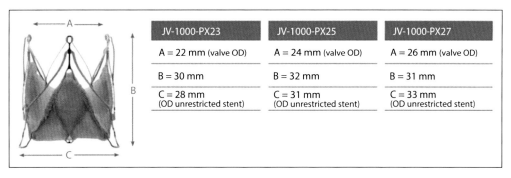

JV-1000-PX23	JV-1000-PX25	JV-1000-PX27
A = 22 mm (valve OD)	A = 24 mm (valve OD)	A = 26 mm (valve OD)
B = 30 mm	B = 32 mm	B = 31 mm
C = 28 mm (OD unrestricted stent)	C = 31 mm (OD unrestricted stent)	C = 33 mm (OD unrestricted stent)

Figure 28.4 The JenaValve.

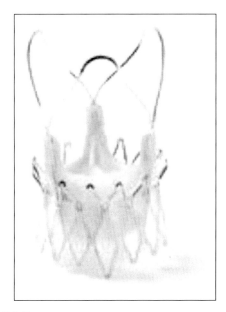

Figure 28.5 The Symetis valve.

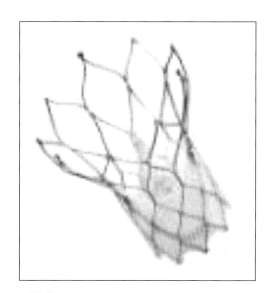

Figure 28.6 The Portico valve.

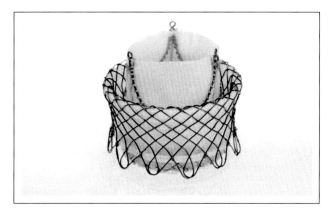

Figure 28.7 The Heart Leaflet Technology valve. (Courtesy of HLT Inc., 2012.)

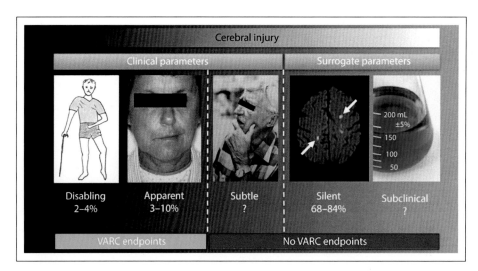

Figure 29.2 Cerebral injury presents in different *shades of gray*. Clinical, imaging, and serological parameters can objectify cerebral injury related to transcatheter aortic valve implantation (TAVI). Obvious and apparent deficits have an incidence of up to 10%. They are detected clinically and account as cerebrovascular events (CVE). Yet little is known on the mechanism and the incidence of cognitive deterioration after TAVI, which is reflected as subtle clinical changes, for example, impairment of memory function or constructional skills. Nonclinical measures of cerebral injury encompass imaging and serology. Silent cerebral injury is detected by diffusion-weighted magnetic resonance imaging (DW-MRI), transcranial Doppler sonography or serology but does not count as a clinical endpoint of the Valve Academic Research Consortium (VARC). The effects of embolic protection devices on clinical and surrogate endpoints are currently being investigated in randomized, controlled studies.

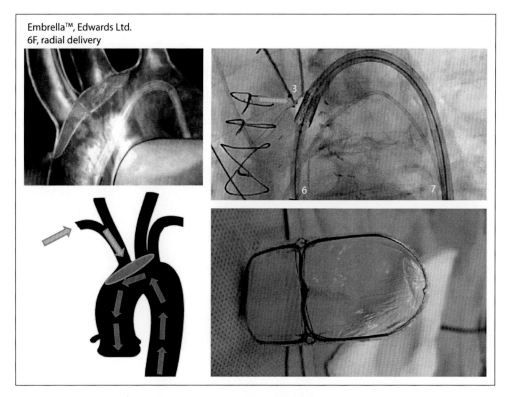

Figure 29.4 Embrella—Distal embolic protection device. The Embrella embolic protection device is delivered over a 0.014″ guide wire from a left-radial sheath (6 F). The deflection shield is deployed in the aortic arch covering the ostia of the brachiocephalic, the right common carotid artery, and, in most cases, also the ostium of left subclavian artery (from where the left-posterior brain perfusion originates) is shielded. The shield is retracted to the origins of the supra-aortic arteries to achieve maximal coverage (blue arrows indicate the delivery route of the protection device [blue circles], the pathway of a transfemoral valve delivery is indicated with gray arrows). 3—Common brachiocephalic trunk, 6—ascending aorta, 7—descending aorta. (Reproduced from Edwards Medical, Inc. With permission.)

23

Aortic stenosis in the elderly: Background, indication for transcatheter treatment, and clinical trial results

Sameer Gafoor, Jennifer Franke, Stefan Bertog, and Horst Sievert

Background

Etiology and prevalence

Valvular aortic stenosis (AS) is most likely due to calcific disease, rheumatic valvular disease, or congenitally abnormal valve (unicuspid or bicuspid) with additional calcification. In Europe and North America, the most common causes are calcific heart disease and congenitally abnormal aortic valve (AV), followed by rheumatic heart disease (which is most common worldwide). Other causes include metabolic diseases such as Fabry's disease, systematic lupus erythematosus, Paget's disease, and alkaptonuria.

The prevalence of calcific AS increases with age. In a study of over 5000 elderly individuals, the prevalence of AS was 2% overall for those over the age of 65 and 2.6% for those over the age of 75.[1] The increase in age may also be associated with an increase in severity, as seen in a group of over 500 elderly individuals where the prevalence of critical AS increased from 1% to 2% in those who were 75–76 years of age to almost 6% in those who were over 86 years of age.[2]

A bicuspid AV is present in almost 2% of the general population.[3] When AS is the only valvular disease, bicuspid AS is more likely to be the underlying etiology.[4,5] Nearly all bicuspid valves progress to AS,[6] with an increased likelihood of progression to aortic regurgitation (often correlated with an ascending aortic aneurysm) or a combined state.[7–9]

Pathogenesis

On gross pathology, calcific stenotic AVs show thickening and calcification (Figure 23.1). This is due to lipid accumulation, inflammation, and calcification. Multiple pathologic mechanisms are involved,[10] including the accumulation of low-density lipoprotein (LDL) and L(a), inflammatory cell infiltrate with T-lymphocytes and macrophages,[11,12] local calcification-promoting proteins,[13–17] the production of angiotensin-converting enzyme,[18,19] the presence of interleukin-1-beta and transforming growth factor beta-1,[20,21] adhesion molecule upregulation,[22] and matrix metalloproteinase activity alteration.[23] In later stages, AVs can show heterotopic ossification, leading to active cartilage and bone formation.[14] AS is also associated with atherosclerosis[24] and genetic factors (such as mutations or polymorphisms in NOTCH1, interleukin-10, vitamin D receptor, and angiotensin-converting enzyme).[25–30] Patients with

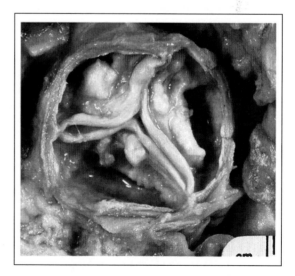

Figure 23.1 Pathological specimen of aortic stenosis. This heavily calcified aortic valve in aortic stenosis shows the gross pathology of endothelial and fibrous damage. Thickening moves from the raphe laterally into the cusps and reduces aortic valve annulus. (Image courtesy of Dr. Renu Virmani, CVPath Inc., Maryland, USA.)

combined hypercholesterolemia, Paget's disease, or end-stage renal disease may have an earlier progression to AS.

Rheumatic heart disease is caused by interleaflet commissural fusion. The changes in histology are similar to rheumatic disease, and many patients have coincident mitral stenosis and/or mitral regurgitation. Antibodies against Group A streptococcus cross-react with host antigens due to a molecular mimicry. Streptococcal M protein and N-acetyl-beta-D-glucosamine (NABG) share epitopes with myosin,[31-35] and rodent studies have shown that this may lead to myositis and valvulitis.

Risk factors

Multiple risk factors for calcific AS have been identified. These include age (each 10-year increase in age doubles risk), male gender (twice as common as female), current cigarette smoking (35% increase in risk), and a history of hypertension (20% increase in risk).[1]

AV thickening, or sclerosis, can also progress to AS. Like AS, this increases with age (26% of those over the age of 65 and 37% of those over the age of 75).[1] The overall incidence of AV calcium has been reported as 1.7% per year, with risk factors of older age, male gender, higher body mass, current smoking, and antihypertensive medications,[36] which are similar to AS. Aortic sclerosis can progress to significant stenosis in one of eight patients and to severe stenosis in one of 64 patients.[37]

As mentioned earlier, bicuspid valves can also progress to stenosis.[6] Risk factors for progression include anatomic and genetic criteria. Anatomic criteria include a greater likelihood in those with anterior/posterior valves[38] and asymmetric cusps (due to increased hemodynamic stress that stretches valve leaflets).[39] There may be a genetic component to bicuspid AVs, as seen in studies of first-degree relatives of nonrelated patients with bicuspid AVs. The prevalence in first-degree relatives is roughly 9%, spread over one-third of the families.[40,41] This has led to screening recommendations for family members of individuals with bicuspid AVs.[42]

Pathophysiology

As the opening of the AV decreases, there is an obstruction to the left ventricular (LV) ejection. When gradual in nature, the LV adapts by increasing systolic pressure. This happens through concentric hypertrophy to maintain normal wall stress. This allows the preservation of cardiac output and left ventricular end-diastolic volume (LVEDV).

Over time, the LV is unable to adapt to the decreased AV orifice. LV end-diastolic pressure increases and there is abnormal diastolic function. Abnormalities in systolic function may exist due to regional wall motion abnormalities, fibrosis, or subendocardial ischemia.[43] Eventually, the LV cannot develop enough pressure to overcome the valvular obstruction, causing a decrease in stroke volume, a decrease in cardiac output, and the onset of heart failure.

Clinical symptoms

Early symptoms of AS include dyspnea on exertion or decreased exercise tolerance. This occurs because of diastolic dysfunction and an inability to increase cardiac output during exercise. End-stage symptoms include exertional dizziness and syncope. The causes for this include exercise-induced vasodilation due to the fixed obstruction, transient bradyarrhythmia after exertion, baroreceptor response abnormalities, or arrhythmia. Angina can happen due to coronary artery disease (CAD), increased LV oxygen demand, coronary artery compression due to compression, reduced diastolic coronary perfusion time during tachycardia, and reduced coronary flow reserve.[44]

Generally, the onset of the symptom correlates with the presence of severe AS, as defined by the valve area <1 cm², jet velocity over 4.0 m/s, and/or mean transvalvular gradient exceeding 40 mm Hg. However, patients can have symptoms earlier or later than this mark. Of note, the progression to symptoms is often before the LV systolic dysfunction.

Diagnosis

On physical examination, AS leads to a turbulent crescendo–decrescendo ejection murmur (starting after the first-heart sound S1 and ending before the second-heart sound S2), originating from the base of the heart and transmitting to the carotid arteries. A louder or late-peaking murmur correlates with stenosis severity. After S1, an ejection click may be associated with a congenital bicuspid valve. S2 is softer because A2 due to AV closure is delayed and is simultaneous with P2. The presence of S4 before S1 can be due to vigorous left atrial contraction. Carotid pulse can be weak and rise slowly, also known as "parvus et tardus." The impulse at the cardiac apex can be displaced laterally late in aortic regurgitation. A simultaneous louder murmur that radiates to the apex may be mitral regurgitation, also known as the Gallavardin phenomenon. A review of clinical studies showed that three findings were best for ruling in AS: a slow rate of rise in the carotid pulse, mid-to-late peak in murmur intensity, and reduced intensity of the second-heart sound.[45,46] AS may also be associated with cardiac arrhythmias (atrial or ventricular fibrillation), endocarditis (especially with congenitally bicuspid AVs),[47] and tendency to bleeding (especially chronic gastric bleeding due to angiodysplasia and bleeding at skin and mucosal sites).[48,49]

The electrocardiogram (ECG) and chest x-ray provide an additional input to help diagnose AS, but findings are nonspecific. On the ECG, the findings are often due to LV hypertrophy (LVH), and include increased QRS voltage, ST-T wave abnormalities, and left atrial hypertrophy. Interventricular or atrioventricular conduction abnormalities may be due to extension of calcium from the valve ring into the interventricular septum. Ventricular arrhythmias can go along with LV dysfunction, and atrial fibrillation may be seen in heart failure. The chest x-ray may show a rounding of the ventricular apex (LVH), and dilatation of the ascending aorta due to root dilatation.

On cardiac catheterization, a transvalvular gradient is essential to diagnose AS. This requires simultaneous measurement of aortic pressure (often with a pigtail catheter above the valve) and LV pressure (with dual-arterial catheters, an additional venous transseptal catheter, or a high-fidelity transducer catheter). With this information, Gorlin's formula can be used to calculate valve area

$$AVA = (SV \div SEP) \div (44.3 \times [\sqrt{\Delta P}])$$

where SV = stroke volume (mL per beat), SEP = systolic ejection period (s per beat), and the change in pressure is the transvalvular gradient.[50] Coronary angiography can also identify the coincident CAD.

Echocardiography has largely replaced cardiac catheterization in diagnosing AS. A complete examination includes direct valve imaging (to evaluate thickening, calcification, reduced excursion, and number of leaflets), evaluation of LV chamber size and thickness (to diagnose LVH), LV diastolic and systolic function (with emphasis on wall motion abnormalities that may predict coronary ischemia), Doppler echocardiography (calculate jet velocity, LV–aortic gradient, and therefore valve area), pulmonary artery pressures (to evaluate for pulmonary hypertension), concurrent valvular disease (especially aortic and mitral regurgitation), and aortic root dilatation. Both flow-dependent indices and flow-independent indices should be used.[51] Figure 23.2 shows two basic views of the AVs.

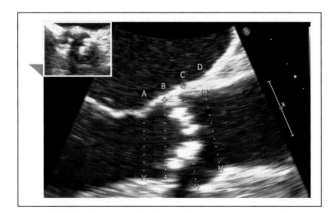

Figure 23.2 Echocardiographic evaluation of aortic stenosis. Transesophageal echocardiogram shows 30° short-axis (inset) and 125° long-axis (main picture) views of the aortic valve. Four measurements can be made. These include hinge-point of mitral valve to subannular aortic thickening (A), aortic valve annulus (B), sinus of Valsalva (C), and sinotubular junction (D). (Images courtesy of Dr. Ilona Hofmann, CVC Frankfurt.)

The European (ESC/EACTS 2012 guidelines[52]) as well as American (ACC/AHA 2006 guidelines in collaboration with SCA, SCAI, and STS[53]) societies have published guidelines for echocardiographic determination of AS severity. The ESC describes severe valve stenosis as aortic area <1.0 cm^2, indexed valve area <0.6 cm^2/m^2, mean gradient >40 mm Hg, maximum jet velocity >4.0 m/s, and velocity ratio of <0.25.[52] The ACC/AHA guidelines also describe the values for mild (area >1.5 cm^2, gradient <25 mm Hg, and jet velocity <3.0 m/s), moderate (area $1.0–1.5$ cm^2, gradient $25–40$ mm Hg, and velocity $3.0–4.0$ m/s), and critical AS (area <0.6 cm^2).[53]

Exercise testing is contraindicated in symptomatic patients with AS, but can be recommended in physically active patients who are subclinically symptomatic or at for risk stratification.[54,55] Special attention should be paid to abnormal blood pressure response, increase in mean pressure gradient, and changes in LV function with exercise.[54,56]

The European and American societies differ in guidelines for serial echocardiographic testing. According to the European 2012 guidelines, serial clinical testing for asymptomatic severe AS should be every 6 months and yearly for mild and moderate AS with calcification. For younger patients with mild AS and no calcification, intervals can be every 2–3 years.[52] The American 2006 guidelines recommend reevaluation every year for severe AS, every 1–2 years for moderate AS, and every 3–5 years for mild AS.[57]

Cardiovascular magnetic resonance (CMR) and computed tomography (CT) can also be useful for the evaluation of AS. In CMR, the anatomic valve area can be measured by flow planimetry in short-axis views[58,59] and the velocity can be measured in an angle-independent manner by velocity-encoded imaging.[60] Midwall fibrosis may help to risk stratify patients with AS.[61] For CT, both electron-beam and rapid multislice chest tomography can quantify valve calcification, which can correlate with stenosis severity and clinical outcomes.[62,63] An example of AV evaluation by CT can be seen in Figure 23.3.

To add to diagnostic complexity, the classic findings of a high transvalvular gradient may not be present, such as in patients with low-gradient AS where the low gradient is secondary to low transvalvular flow. This is due to the combined development of LV systolic dysfunction and heart failure, but can also be seen in some patients with normal ejection fraction.[64,65] Clinically defined as severe AS (valve area <1.0 cm) with a transvalvular pressure gradient of <30 mm Hg, it can be divided into patients with low-gradient low-flow AS (where the low gradient is due to severe AS and secondary LV dysfunction), and pseudostenosis (where the low gradient is due to moderate AS and low cardiac output). Unfortunately, the Gorlin equation, which is flow dependent, suggests that at low transvalvular flows (<175 mL/s), the mean gradient will be <20 mm Hg independent of AV area suggesting only mild AS.[50,66,67] This can be differentiated by calculation of aortic resistance,[68]

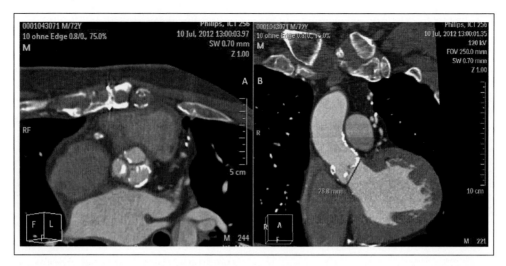

Figure 23.3   Computerized tomography (CT) evaluation of aortic stenosis. Part A shows the extensive calcification of the aortic valve at the level of the sinotubular junction. Part B shows the long-axis view with measurement at the level of the aortic annulus. (Images courtesy of Dr. Nina Hofmann and Dr. Grigorius Korosoglou, Department of Cardiology, University Hospital, Heidelberg.)

dobutamine echocardiography, and/or cardiac catheterization with dobutamine infusion.[57] In truly severe AS, low-dose dobutamine echocardiography would show only small changes in valve area (increase <0.2 cm² and remaining <1 cm²) with increasing flow rate, but a significant increase in gradients (mean gradient >40 mm Hg). In pseudosevere AS, there would be a marked increase in valve area but only a minor change in the gradient.[69] This can also detect the flow reserve (also termed contractile reserve), defined by an increase >20% of the stroke volume, which can lead to changes in prognosis.[69,70]

A low gradient can occur in patients with normal LV ejection fraction, called "paradoxical low-flow, low-gradient AS," and can have worse outcomes compared to those patients with AS and higher gradients.[71] Flows present with a stroke volume index <35 mL/m² with a mean gradient of <40 mm Hg with preserved left ventricular ejection fraction (LVEF).[72] The typical patient is usually elderly and has a small ventricular size, marked LVH, and a history of hypertension. The reasons for this include Doppler misunderestimation of flows, small body size, and inconsistent gradient cutoffs. More detailed measurements and the use of other diagnostic modalities may be helpful for further elucidation in this population.[52]

Natural history and prognosis

Patients can remain asymptomatic for long periods of time, which can vary between individuals. Sudden cardiac death can happen but is rare during the asymptomatic period.[73–76] Asymptomatic patients with severe AS have a reported 2-year event-free survival of 20–50%, but these figures also include asymptomatic patients who went on to surgery.[73–76] This involves an average increase in jet velocity of 0.3 m/s per year, increase in mean pressure gradient

of 7 mm Hg per year, and a decrease in AVA of 0.1 cm² per year.[77–80] As mentioned earlier, patients with aortic sclerosis can progress to AS. After a long latent period, symptoms develop (especially late symptoms such as angina, syncope, and heart failure). After this point, the average survival is 2–3 years with a high risk of sudden death.[81–83] At 5 years, the survival rate is between 15% and 50%.

Medical management

No known medical treatments prevent or delay AV stenosis. Small retrospective studies suggest that lipid-lowering therapy may be of some benefit,[84–87] but this has not been shown in large prospective, randomized trials.[88,89] Statin therapy should not be used in patients with AS unless it is for secondary prevention of atherosclerosis. Coincident hypertension should be treated and the maintenance of sinus rhythm is important.[52] Stenosis severity can also dictate serial testing and restrictions on participation in competitive sports.[52,53]

Surgical management

Surgical aortic valve replacement (SAVR) is the gold standard therapy for AS. Operative mortality for AS is reported as 1–3% in patients younger than 70 years and 4–8% in older adults.[90,91] Risk factors for operative mortality include older age, comorbidities, female gender, higher functional class, emergency operation, LV dysfunction, pulmonary hypertension, coexisting CAD, and previous bypass or valve surgery.[52] In-hospital mortality is higher for elderly patients (14% for those ≥80 years of age and 4% for those 65–70 years of age), which some have argued was due to the higher frequency of New York Heart Association (NYHA) functional class III or IV in the older group (86% vs. 36%).[92] The risk of SAVR increases if other procedures are combined, such as other valve replacements or aneurysm repair (30-day mortality of 5.2% for SAVR alone and 27.7% for the combined procedure).[93]

Long-term survival, symptoms, and quality of life (QOL) are improved in elderly patients after SAVR.[92–96] For older patients, long-term survival is similar to age-matched controls; for younger patients, it can be slightly less. Risk of late death is increased with age, comorbidities, severe symptoms, LV dysfunction, ventricular arrhythmias, and untreated CAD.[52] Even patients over 80 years of age can have a longer and improved QOL.[97–100] One study of outcome after SAVR in 1100 patients ≥80 years of age showed a 30-day cardiac mortality of 4%, 30-day all-cause mortality of 6.6%, and actuarial survival at 1, 5, and 8 years of 89%, 69%, and 46%, respectively. The deaths at the 30-days postoperative mark were mostly due to noncardiac causes (70% of all deaths due to mostly malignancy, stroke, or pneumonia).[95]

Elderly patients also have unique issues concerning the type of valve prosthesis (bioprosthesis versus mechanical valves). Bioprostheses and mechanical valves are prone to valve degeneration and thromboembolism/bleeding from anticoagulation, respectively.[101] Although early mortality and actuarial survival are similar, there is a difference in valve failure. At 15-year follow-up, bioprostheses can have structural deterioration of up to 63% (for age 40–49 years) and 10% (for age >70 years). This difference is partly due to decreased activity in older patients.[102] The Veterans Affairs health study showed 26% valve failure at 15 years in those <65 years of age down to 9% in those over 65 years of age.[103] Therefore, an octogenarian has a life expectancy that is shorter than the functional life of a bioprosthetic valve, making it the best choice in this population.[93,95,102,104,105]

Some elderly patients with a small aortic annulus (especially elderly women) who undergo SAVR have received a small aortic prosthesis that resulted in a residual transprosthetic gradient, also known as a patient–prosthesis mismatch.[106–108] This can lead to less functional improvement, higher in-hospital mortality, increased late mortality, and a rise in the risk of sudden cardiac death.[106,109–113] The risk of negative outcomes is higher in patients aged <70 years and in patients with decreased ejection fraction but not in obese patients.[114] Options include accepting the mismatch, implanting a mechanical valve instead (smaller transvalvular gradients and better hemodynamics),[93] enlarging the aortic annulus (which can raise operative mortality from 3.5% to 7.1%),[115] and using a stentless bioprosthetic valve (long-term data still unknown).[116,117]

Transcatheter treatment

Balloon valvuloplasty

Percutaneous balloon aortic valvuloplasty (BAV) involves balloon expansion of the aortic leaflets by fracturing calcific deposits within the valve leaflets and separating the calcified commissures. After emerging in the 1990s as a less-invasive technique to help those who are too old and sick to have AVR,[118] it has emerged as a possible bridge to transcatheter aortic valve replacement (TAVR) or SAVR. The basic technique includes a common retrograde or the less-used antegrade approach, crossing the AV, switching for a stiff wire, and advancing a balloon over the wire to the AV for deployment. In 2000, rapid ventricular pacing was introduced to stabilize cardiac movement, which allowed a more effective valvuloplasty.

Results of the procedure are not permanent (rarely exceeding 1.0 cm²) and serious complications can occur in 10–20% of patients historically.[119–123] Restenosis often happens within 6–12 months, without a change in long-term mortality.[121,124] At that time, repeat balloon valvuloplasty can be performed, but these patients also usually have a return to symptoms and a decrease in valve area after 6 months.[125]

Indications for balloon valvuloplasty are similar in the European and American guidelines. The ESC/EACTS 2012 guidelines recommend BAV as a bridge to surgery or TAVR in hemodynamically unstable patients or those who require noncardiac surgery. Nonoperative patients can benefit from palliative BAV.[52] The 2006 ACC/AHA valve disease guidelines recommend BAV as a bridge to surgery in hemodynamically unstable patients or those who are nonoperative candidates.[53]

Transcatheter AV implantation/ transcatheter AV replacement: The history of the procedure

The history of transcatheter aortic valve implantation (TAVI) or TAVR started with an *in vivo* canine procedure done by Davies in 1965.[126] This involved femoral arterial access and a parachute-like valve. In 1971, Moulopoulos et al.[127] showed three different transcatheter valve systems in dogs for traumatic aortic regurgitation, followed by a similar system by Phillips et al.[128] in 1976, who used a single-cusp valve mounted on a catheter. These animal studies were mostly designed to treat aortic regurgitation. In 1992, Andersen et al.[129] reported permanent subcoronary implantation of a transaortic valve in pigs, which not only led to a decrease in the peak-to-peak gradient but also a decrease in coronary flow. At this time, there were still significant issues with securing the valve to the aortic annulus and permitting blood flow into the coronaries.[130] After Bonhoeffer et al.[131,132] implanted a percutaneous pulmonary valve in man in 2000, the door was open for TAVI. In 2002, Cribier et al. performed the first-in-human TAVI using an antegrade approach through the femoral vein. The first study showed procedural success in five out of six patients, with an increase in the AV area from 0.5 ± 0.1 cm² to 1.70 ± 0.03 cm². Two out of five developed severe paravalvular aortic regurgitation and three patients died in the first 5 months due to noncardiac causes. Two patients were alive at 8 weeks without heart failure.[133]

The next step forward came from Webb et al.[133] in Vancouver, who developed a feasible retrograde transarterial version of the procedure in 2006. Originally requiring surgical cut down, the use of arterial-closure devices allowed this to be a fully percutaneous procedure. The first self-expandable valve implanted in the aortic position was reported by Grube et al.[134] in Germany in 2005. Other means of vascular access with the year of publication include transapical access (median sternotomy on-bypass in Leipzig and intercostal approach off-bypass in Vancouver in 2006 and 2007),[135,136] transaortic implantation through a mini-sternotomy in 2009,[137] subclavian access in 2010,[138] transaxillary access (in Munich in 2007),[139] and left carotid artery access in 2010.[140]

Transcatheter AV implantation/transcatheter AV replacement: The procedure

The TAVI procedure requires careful patient selection that in turn requires an assessment of surgical risk, comorbidities, and anatomic criteria. Before the case, anatomic criteria are judged by a combination of echocardiography, aortic root angiography, and computerized tomography (CT). Echocardiography provides information about morphology, vegetations, calcifications, gradient, presence of regurgitation, annulus size, and valve area. Angiography of the aortic root defines a radiologic angle perpendicular to the plane of the AV, aortic root measurement, and measurement of distance from coronary ostium to annulus; low abdominal aorta angiography defines the diameter and calcification of the iliac vessels for possible transfemoral access. CT provides additional information about valve and aortic calcification, tortuosity, AV area, and examination of the iliac vessels for calcification, size, and tortuosity. On the basis of these measurements, the access site and valve size are determined.

The procedure itself involves multiple steps. After choosing an access route (transfemoral, transaortic, transapical, subclavian, and axillary), the valve is crossed and a gradient is measured across the valve with attention to the diastolic pressures (for later evaluation of possible regurgitation). If not already present, a pacemaker is placed for rapid ventricular pacing. Balloon valvuloplasty is performed. Hemodynamic angiographic and echocardiographic criteria are used to evaluate the response to BAV and pacing as a way to predict the response to TAVR. The valve is advanced to the appropriate position and deployed with rapid pacing. After retrograde arterial access has been obtained, it is secured with preclosure devices if necessary. Repeat angiography and continued echocardiography assesses the position of the valve, patency of the coronary ostia, and presence of regurgitation.

The development of percutaneous heart valve technology has refocused attention on the "heart team" approach. The 2012 ACCF/AATS/SCAI/STS Expert Consensus Document describes the importance of the heart team and specific roles. Patient selection requires the health-care team approach, where the patient's individual risks are assessed and discussed to better inform and share expectations about the QOL. Candidacy for TAVR should be determined by both the surgeon and cardiologist, with preference for a structural heart disease clinic. During the procedure, the various procedural tasks should be discussed and shared between the two individuals. Each case should have a specific team leader, usually the cardiovascular surgeon, for surgical aspects of transapical and transaortic procedures and the interventional cardiologist for transfemoral procedures. Communication is vital, as well as planning for potential complications. After the procedure, postprocedure care can benefit from a multispecialty team service.[141]

This document also specifies recommendations for physical infrastructure and equipment. Suggested equipment includes a fixed overhead or floor-mounted system with possible biplane imaging and capacity for transesophageal echocardiogram (TEE) image integration. It should have full catheterization hemodynamic capability. Other equipment includes cardiopulmonary bypass machines, perfusionists, and related ancillary supplies for complication management. These include BAV, coronary equipment for coronary occlusion, peripheral balloons for iliac rupture, and a variety of vascular closure devices. Anesthesia equipment should also be available, including equipment for advanced airway management, general anesthesia, full hemodynamic monitoring, and administration of vasoactive agents. This requires coordination between team members, especially lab and Office of Research (OR) staff and personnel.[141]

Indications for treatment with TAVR

In 2012, the European guidelines for treatment of valvular heart disease addressed the topic of TAVI. Only hospitals with cardiac surgery on-site should perform surgery, with a multidisciplinary heart team to assess the patient. TAVI is recommended in patients with severe symptomatic AS who are unsuitable for surgery because of severe comorbidities. For high-risk operative candidates, the decision with individualized, EuroSCORE >20%, or STS score >10% may be used. Frailty, prior bypass, and prior radiation are other criteria that can make a patient less suitable for SAVR.[52]

Significant absolute contraindications to TAVR in the European guidelines include clinical (estimated life expectancy <1 year, comorbidities that would not allow improvement in the QOL, and severe primary disease of other valves that can be treated only by surgery) and anatomical contraindications (inadequate annulus size (<18 mm, >29 mm), LV thrombus, active endocarditis, elevated risk of coronary obstruction (asymmetric valve calcification, short distance between annulus and coronary ostium, and small aortic sinus), plaque with mobile thrombi in the ascending aorta or arch, and inadequate vessel access for transfemoral approach). Relative contraindications include bicuspid or noncalcified valves, untreated CAD requiring revascularization, hemodynamic instability, LVEF <20%, or in the case of transapical approach, severe pulmonary disease or an inaccessible LV apex.[52]

The 2012 American Expert Consensus Document allows inclusion of patients with echocardiographically derived severe AS (mean gradient >40 mm Hg or jet velocity >4.0 m/s and initial AVA of 0.8 cm^2 or indexed BOA <0.5 cm^2/m^2 within 45 days of the procedure). The cardiac team consists of a cardiac interventionalist and two experienced cardiothoracic surgeons who would have to say that the patient is inoperative on high surgical risk based on risk scores. The medical and anatomic factors would be included, as well as the STS score. The patient must be symptomatic from AS, and this should be differentiated from other chronic conditions.[142]

Exclusion criteria include evidence of a nontricuspid valve, or a mixed aortic disease with aortic regurgitation >3+. The patient should not have acute myocardial infarction <1 m before treatment, hemodynamic instability (requiring inotropic support, mechanical ventilation, or mechanical heart assistance within 30 days of screening), and need for emergency surgery. Other exclusion criteria include severe mitral regurgitation, hypertrophic cardiomyopathy, LVEF <20%, severe pulmonary hypertension, or echocardiographic evidence of intracardiac mass, thrombus, or vegetation. Significant comorbidities include stroke or transient ischemic attack (TIA) within 6 months (confirmed by magnetic resonance imaging [MRI]), severe incapacitating dementia, estimated life expectancy <1 year, renal insufficiency (Cr > 3.0 mg/dL), and/or end-stage renal dialysis at the time of screening. Those with thoracic or abdominal aortic aneurysm >5 cm, marked tortuosity, aortic arch atheroma, or narrowing were also excluded, as well as those who could not tolerate anticoagulation.[142]

Echocardiographic evaluation recommendations were published in 2011 by the European (EAE) and American (ASE) societies. Transthoracic echocardiogram (TTE) evaluation requires measurement of valve area, velocity, and mean gradient. Other important criteria include annular dimension (method detailed in the document) and detailed anatomic characteristics of the AV, including number, mobility, thickness of cusps, and extent and distribution of calcium. LV and right ventricular dimensions and function, aortic regurgitation, and other valves should also be assessed. Postprocedure patient-prosthetic mismatch should be evaluated. For transapical access, TTE is useful in guiding the thoracotomy.[143]

TEE may be performed preprocedure or as part of intra-procedural monitoring. This involves the long- and short-axis views to better describe the AV as well as the distance from the aortic annulus to the ostium of the coronary arteries. In addition, the ascending aorta, aortic arch, and descending thoracic aorta should be evaluated for atheroma. Periprocedural TEE can be helpful in balloon or prosthesis positioning and detecting postballoon or post-prosthesis aortic regurgitation.[143]

There are many postprocedural complications that can be detected by echocardiography. These include aortic prosthesis misplacement (embolization, too high, or too low), aortic regurgitation (central or paravalvular), mitral regurgitation (aortic prosthesis impinging on the anterior mitral leaflet, or damage to the subvalvular mitral apparatus caused by the wire), new wall motion abnormalities (possible coronary occlusion), and cardiac tamponade (possible ventricular rupture or aortic dissection). Three-dimensional (3D) TEE has unique applications including capturing the whole aortic root. Echocardiography can also be used for postimplantation follow-up.[143]

CT is recommended during the initial evaluation for TAVI/TAVR. Optimal data-acquisition protocol involves an ECG-synchronized, low-slice-thickness (<1.0 mm) scan for cardiac structures, and a nongated scan for the aorta and peripheral vessels. Contrast and radiation-sparing techniques should be used whenever possible. Access site measurement should involve manual multiplanar reformation or semiautomated centerline reconstruction to achieve the cross-sectional visualization measurement of vessel dimension. Sheath–femoral-artery ratio (SFAR), vascular tortuosity, and calcification can be used to predict vascular access-related complications and 30-day mortality.[144] The aorta should be imaged and evaluated to look for elongation, kinking, dissection, and obstruction.[145]

The aortic annulus can be measured with CT, and often provides larger aortic annulus dimensions than echocardiography. The oval nature of the AV can be overcome with planimetry and measurement of both small and large diameters on a plane exactly aligned with aortic cusp hinge points. This also can lead to lower "worse-than-mild" paravalvular leak.[146] Other important measurements include the distance of coronary ostia to the valve plane, aortic cusp length, width of the aortic sinus, width of the sinotubular junction, and width of the ascending aorta. Deployment can be assisted by CT prediction of the annular plane and location of AV calcification.[147]

The United States Center for Medicaid Services (CMS) has published a list of criteria for TAVR reimbursement (CAG-00430-N). These include a Food and Drug Administration (FDA) indication, two cardiac surgeons being involved with direct patient evaluation, and care under a heart team. There are requirements for the hospital (on-site heart valve surgery program, catheterization lab or hybrid lab with fixed radiographic imaging system, noninvasive imaging, sufficient space, intensive-care unit, and appropriate volume requirements). For those without TAVR experience, the hospital, cardiac surgeon, and interventional cardiologist procedural requirements are more stringent compared to those with TAVI experience. In addition, the heart team and hospital must participate in a prospective, national, and audited registry that specifies outcomes including mortality, stroke, TIA, major vascular events, acute kidney injury, repeat AV procedures, and QOL.[148]

The Valve Academic Research Consortium (VARC) 2011 document defines uniform outcomes for studies regarding heart valve therapy to help pool data.[149] However, the document required refinement, especially in areas of defining postprocedural valve area indexed to body surface area, reporting of procedure-related and nonprocedure-related blood loss, and standardizing echocardiographic definitions of paravalvular leak.[150] This was addressed in the VARC definition update, also known as VARC-2. This provided more concrete individual and composite definitions, comprehensive echocardiography recommendations for prosthetic valve dysfunction, and definitions for QOL assessments.[151]

Clinical trial results

Registry data

The main registries for the Edwards-SAPIEN valve and CoreValve are the SOURCE (SAPIEN Aortic Bioprosthesis European Outcome)[152] and the CoreValve registries, respectively. These patients are usually not eligible for randomized controlled trials because of strict selection criteria. However, standardized endpoint definitions are often not used and endpoints are not prospectively adjudicated.

Registry data for transfemoral SAPIEN include the SOURCE,[152] REVIVE/REVIVAL/PARTNER EU,[153] French,[154] Belgian,[155] and Canadian[156] registries. The age of patients was roughly 83, with EuroSCORE above 20 and mostly NYHA III/IV. 30-day mortality ranged from 7.5% to 10.4%, with 1-year mortality of 19–24%. Stroke occurred in roughly 3.0–5.0% of patients, with major vascular complications in between 11.4% and 27.9% of patients. A permanent pacemaker was used in 1.8–8.5% of patients.[142]

Multiple CoreValve registries[157–162] exist, with most patients from Tamburino et al.[160] The baseline information as far as age and gender was similar, with some patients having a lower EuroSCORE and lower prevalence of NYHA class III/IV. The procedural success was over 90% in almost all studies, with a 30-day mortality of 2.2–15.2%. One-year mortality ranged from 15% to 38.1%, with a stroke rate of 2.2–4.5% and a major vascular complication rate of 2.0–21.3%. Pacemaker placement was higher in this group, ranging from 2.0% to 21.3%.[142]

Randomized controlled trials

The PARTNER trial[100,163] was a prospective unblended randomized controlled multicenter trial to evaluate the Edwards-SAPIEN valve. The cohorts were Cohort A (high-risk-operable patients) or Cohort B (inoperable patients). The patients in each cohort were randomized to TAVR or SAVR (Cohort A) or medical therapy (Cohort B).

High risk for Cohort A[100] was defined as predicted operative mortality of ≥15% and/or an STS risk score of >10%. In Cohort A, the patients who did not qualify for transfemoral TAVR were evaluated for transapical TAVR and this was appropriately randomized to transapical TAVR or SAVR.[100] Inoperability in Cohort B[163] was defined as patients with " >50% predicted probability of mortality or serious irreversible complication by 30 days by 1 cardiologist and 2 cardiothoracic surgeons." In Cohort B, those who did not qualify for transfemoral TAVR were removed from the study because transapical TAVR was too risky for surgery.[163]

The demographics of the study showed a mean age of roughly 83, with slightly more female patients in Cohort B and slightly more male patients in Cohort A. Over 90% were NYHA III/IV, and 60% had prior coronary artery bypass surgery/percutaneous coronary intervention (CABG/PCI). Systolic function was mostly normal. Cohort B had other conditions that led to nonoperability, including porcelain aorta (15.1%), chest-wall deformity or prior chest-wall irradiation (13.1%), oxygen-dependent respiratory insufficiency (23.5%), or frailty (23.1%).[163]

There was an improvement in mortality for Cohort B and Cohort A patients. For inoperable patients, the results of the trial showed a reduction in all-cause mortality by 50% (30-day 5% vs. 9% ($p = 0.41$),[163] 1-year 30.7% vs. 50.7% ($p < 0.001$),[163] and 2-year 43.3% vs. 68.7% ($p < 0.001$)).[164] For operative patients, mortality was equivalent at 30 days (TAVI 3.4% vs. SAVR 6.5%, $p = 0.07$),[100] 1 year (TAVI 24.2% vs. SAVR 26.8%, $p = 0.44$),[100] and 2 years (TAVI 33.9% vs. SAVR 35.0%, $p = 0.78$).[165] The results of QOL and complications will be discussed separately.

In relation to mortality, there were a few unexpected findings from the PARTNER trial. AVR mortality at 30 days (6.5%) was lower than expected (11.8%). This could be due to the expertise of the surgeons in the trial, general increase in the overall surgical outcomes over time, or specific issues dealing with AS patients in terms of the risk scores used. The SOURCE registry mortality of 8.4% was higher than the 30-day mortality of 3.4% in PARTNER high-risk-operative patients and 5.0% in PARTNER nonoperative patients.

Early results from the PARTNER II valve with SAPIEN XT in nonoperable patients were reported at ACC 2013. All-cause mortality at 30 days for the SAPIEN XT was equivalent to the SAPIEN valve (22.5% vs. 23.7%, respectively).[166] Of note, this is a decrease from the nonoperative cohort in PARTNER I, where the 30-day mortality was 30.7%.

Quality of life

QOL has been measured with multiple metrics, including the Short Form-36 Health Questionnaire (SF-36), Short Form-12 Health Questionnaire (SF-12), EuroQOL (EQ-5D), Kansas City Cardiomyopathy Questionnaire (KCCQ), Minnesota Living with Heart Failure Questionnaire (MLHF), and with symptoms such as NYHA class and 6-min walk. However, the NYHA class is limited by the discrete nature of the scale; so it often cannot detect clinically relevant changes, making it more an assessment of functional status than QOL. MLHF and KCCQ have the advantage of having a continuous scale, which improves responsiveness and sensitivity. The VARC-2 recommendations are that patients have both a comprehensive measure (e.g., KCCQ or MLHF) and one or more generic measures (SF-12, SF-36, or EQ-5D). These should be performed at 2 weeks, 1, and 3 months to assess early recovery. Later time points such as 1–5 years would benefit from heart-failure-specific measurements as well as assessments of cognitive function.[151] One must be aware that attrition of the oldest subjects can lead to a positive bias in later reporting, which can be countered by reporting combination endpoints (e.g., survival and improvement of QOL endpoints) or endpoints that integrate survival and QOL (e.g., quality-adjusted life expectancy) for the entire study cohort as well as the surviving patients.[151]

Short- and mid-term outcomes of functional status show positive results. Randomized controlled trial data include the PARTNER B and PARTNER A trials. Compared to medical therapy, patients receiving TAVI in the PARTNER B trial showed increased NYHA class I and II with TAVR at 1 year (74.8% vs. 42.0%),[163] improved 6-min walk at 1 year, and fewer hospitalizations at 1 year. The PARTNER A trial showed incremental differences with NYHA class at 30 days that were not present at 1 year; this was paralleled by a similar trend in 6-min walk time. There was a shorter length of hospital stay with TAVR.[100]

QOL has also improved in these patients. Studies with short-term data report an enhancement in MLHF[167] and an increase in physical functioning, bodily pain, general health, and vitality.[168] At 5 and 6 months, an increase was seen in all eight health components of the SF-12v2[169] and SF-36,[170] respectively. Mid-term (roughly 11–12-month) data showed significant improvement in all domains and summary scores,[171] MLHFQ score,[172] postprocedural summary scores at the level of the general population,[173] and also KCCQ and SF-12.[174]

Stroke

Standard definitions for stroke and TIA have been well defined in the VARC criteria, including appropriate studies, evaluation by a specialist, and Rankin score criteria.[151] Stroke occurs between 2.9% and 3.2% at 30 days,[150] with a minor stroke of 1.0%, TIA 1.2%, and all strokes of 5.7%. At 1 year, the stroke rate was 5.2 ± 3.4%, which was significantly lower in those with transapical TAVI (2.7 ± 1.4%).[175] Stroke may be caused by thromboembolism from the valve site, ulcerative aortic plaque dislodged by the catheter, hypotension during the procedure, or due to acceleration of stroke caused by other risk factors such as age, hypertension, diabetes, or atrial fibrillation.[176] However, most strokes happen during the first 30 days, making them, most likely, procedure related.[177] Smaller delivery systems, anticoagulation, and embolic protection devices may help push this number downward.[142]

Conduction defects

Although conduction defects after TAVR are thought due to local trauma or suture placement in proximity of the AV node or bundle, TAVR can contribute to conduction effects by mechanical pressure from the valve.[142] This has led to recommendations for 72 hours of continuous rhythm monitoring after the procedure.[151] Permanent pacemaker implantation ranges from 19% to 22%. Risk factors include those with preexisting right bundle-branch block,[178] the CoreValve device (rate of 19.2–42.5% compared with SAPIEN rate of 1.8–8.5% or SAVR rate of 1–10%),[142,175,179] and transarterial compared to transapical (15.6% vs. 5.8%).[179] However, this is not associated with a decrease in survival at 30 days or 1 year.[142,180]

Vascular complications

Vascular access site complications are the highest prevalence of complications after TAVR, and have been well defined as major complications, minor complications, and percutaneous device failure.[151] Risk factors for major vascular complications include center/operator experience, degree and location of vascular calcification, vascular tortuosity, and SFAR, with an SFAR >1.05 predicting complications and 30-day mortality.[181,182] The rate of major vascular complications is 2–26% for transfemoral access and 5–7% for transapical access.[153,159,160,183,184] VARC definition studies showed major and minor complications to be present in 11.9% and 9.7% of patients, for a total of 18.8% of all patients as reported in 14 of 16 studies.[150] For transfemoral TAVI, these were more likely with the SAPIEN valve as opposed to CoreValve (22.3% vs. 10.8%); however, this may be due to the larger sheath requirements for the early SAPIEN valve.[179] The SAPIEN XT valve was found to have less vascular events in nonoperative patients compared to the SAPIEN valve (9.6% vs. 15.5% at 30 days, $p = 0.04$), with less perforations and dissections.[166] Smaller sheath sizes, better recognition of difficult vascular anatomy, and periprocedural vascular protection techniques may lead to improvements in the future.[142]

Paravalvular leak

Paravalvular leak, which can affect long-term valve durability and dysfunction, has been defined by the VARC-2 definitions with central regurgitation as part of a combined volume load on the LV. Multiple quantitative and semiquantitative measurements in multiple echocardiographic windows are used to quantify the leak. The PARTNER trial and other Edwards registries found moderate/severe periventricular leukomalacia (PVL) in 12% of patients,[100,163] which was higher than that reported by CoreValve registries (9–21%).[158,160–162,185,186] PVL progression is controversial: progression was noted in the PARTNER trial in 22% of patients,[184] stability was shown at 30 days and 1 year by follow-up,[187] and Ussia et al.[188] showed a decrease in mild and moderate PVL at 3 years (53–47% and 15–10%, respectively). Differences in measurement can account for some of these changes.

Various risk factors and treatment strategies have been suggested for PVL.

PVL can predict a 10-year mortality in SAVR patients (184), which leads credence to the increased in-hospital mortality (15.1% vs. 6.7%) (185), 1-year mortality (175, 186, and 187), and 2-year mortality with moderate–severe PVL (188). Risk factors for PVL include (1) incomplete prosthesis apposition due to calcification[178,189–191] or an eccentric annulus,[192] (2) device undersizing,[193–195] (3) device malposition,[196] and specifically for CoreValve, the depth of implantation as well as the angle between the aorta and LV outflow tract,[197,198] as described by Genereux et al.[199] in a recent review. Treatment strategies have included balloon dilatation[200] and snare repositioning of the valve,[201,202] which carry risks of cerebrovascular events[200] and damage to the ascending aorta, respectively.[201,202] Valve in valve has shown good safety and efficacy at 1-year follow-up[203,204] and has been performed even with a different valve.[205] Upcoming strategies to reduce PVL may benefit from increased CT attention to the oval shape of the AV[145,206–210] as well as future valve technologies that include a sealing cuff or mechanisms to control better valve deployment, repositioning, or removal.[199]

References

1. Stewart BF, Siscovick D, Lind BK et al. Clinical factors associated with calcific aortic valve disease. Cardiovascular Health Study. *J Am Coll Cardiol* 1997;29:630–4.
2. Lindroos M, Kupari M, Heikkila J, Tilvis R. Prevalence of aortic valve abnormalities in the elderly: An echocardiographic study of a random population sample. *J Am Coll Cardiol* 1993;21:1220–5.
3. Roberts WC. The congenitally bicuspid aortic valve. A study of 85 autopsy cases. *Am J Cardiol* 1970;26:72–83.
4. Roberts WC, Ko JM. Frequency by decades of unicuspid, bicuspid, and tricuspid aortic valves in adults having isolated aortic valve replacement for aortic stenosis, with or without associated aortic regurgitation. *Circulation* 2005;111:920–5.
5. Subramanian R, Olson LJ, Edwards WD. Surgical pathology of pure aortic stenosis: A study of 374 cases. *Mayo Clin Proc* 1984;59:683–90.
6. Lewin MB, Otto CM. The bicuspid aortic valve: Adverse outcomes from infancy to old age. *Circulation* 2005;111:832–4.
7. Keane MG, Wiegers SE, Plappert T, Pochettino A, Bavaria JE, Sutton MG. Bicuspid aortic valves are associated with aortic dilatation out of proportion to coexistent valvular lesions. *Circulation* 2000;102:III35–9.
8. Sadee AS, Becker AE, Verheul HA, Bouma B, Hoedemaker G. Aortic valve regurgitation and the congenitally bicuspid aortic valve: A clinico-pathological correlation. *Brit Heart J* 1992;67:439–41.
9. Roberts WC, Morrow AG, McIntosh CL, Jones M, Epstein SE. Congenitally bicuspid aortic valve causing severe, pure aortic regurgitation without superimposed infective endocarditis. Analysis of 13 patients requiring aortic valve replacement. *Am J Cardiol* 1981;47:206–9.
10. Freeman RV, Otto CM. Spectrum of calcific aortic valve disease: Pathogenesis, disease progression, and treatment strategies. *Circulation* 2005;111:3316–26.
11. Otto CM, Kuusisto J, Reichenbach DD, Gown AM, O'Brien KD. Characterization of the early lesion of "degenerative" valvular aortic stenosis. Histological and immunohistochemical studies. *Circulation* 1994;90:844–53.
12. Olsson M, Dalsgaard CJ, Haegerstrand A, Rosenqvist M, Ryden L, Nilsson J. Accumulation of T lymphocytes and expression of interleukin-2 receptors in nonrheumatic stenotic aortic valves. *J Am Coll Cardiol* 1994;23:1162–70.
13. Kaden JJ, Bickelhaupt S, Grobholz R et al. Expression of bone sialoprotein and bone morphogenetic protein-2 in calcific aortic stenosis. *J Heart Valve Dis* 2004;13:560–6.
14. Mohler ER, III, Gannon F, Reynolds C, Zimmerman R, Keane MG, Kaplan FS. Bone formation and inflammation in cardiac valves. *Circulation* 2001;103:1522–8.
15. Mohler ER, III, Adam LP, McClelland P, Graham L, Hathaway DR. Detection of osteopontin in calcified human aortic valves. *Arterioscler Thromb Vasc Biol* 1997;17:547–52.
16. Zhao FY, Saito K, Yoshioka K et al. Subtypes of tachykinin receptors on tonic and phasic neurones in coeliac ganglion of the guinea-pig. *Br J Pharmacol* 1995;115:25–30.
17. Nakayama K, Morimoto K, Nozawa Y, Tanaka Y. Calcium antagonistic and binding properties of semotiadil (SD-3211), a benzothiazine derivative assessed in cerebral and coronary arteries. *J Cardiovasc Pharmacol* 1992;20:380–91.
18. Helske S, Lindstedt KA, Laine M et al. Induction of local angiotensin II-producing systems in stenotic aortic valves. *J Am Coll Cardiol* 2004;44:1859–66.
19. O'Brien KD, Shavelle DM, Caulfield MT et al. Association of angiotensin-converting enzyme with low-density lipoprotein in aortic valvular lesions and in human plasma. *Circulation* 2002;106:2224–30.
20. Kaden JJ, Dempfle CE, Grobholz R et al. Interleukin-1 beta promotes matrix metalloproteinase expression and cell proliferation in calcific aortic valve stenosis. *Atherosclerosis* 2003;170:205–11.
21. Jian B, Narula N, Li QY, Mohler ER, III, Levy RJ. Progression of aortic valve stenosis: TGF-beta1 is present in calcified aortic valve cusps and promotes aortic valve interstitial cell calcification via apoptosis. *Ann Thorac Surg* 2003;75:457–65; discussion 65–6.
22. Jian B, Jones PL, Li Q, Mohler ER, III, Schoen FJ, Levy RJ. Matrix metalloproteinase-2 is associated with tenascin-C in calcific aortic stenosis. *Am J Pathol* 2001;159:321–7.
23. Ghaisas NK, Foley JB, O'Briain DS, Crean P, Kelleher D, Walsh M. Adhesion molecules in nonrheumatic aortic valve disease: Endothelial expression, serum levels and effects of valve replacement. *J Am Coll Cardiol* 2000;36:2257–62.
24. Agmon Y, Khandheria BK, Meissner I et al. Aortic valve sclerosis and aortic atherosclerosis: Different manifestations of the same disease? Insights from a population-based study. *J Am Coll Cardiol* 2001;38:827–34.

25. McKellar SH, Tester DJ, Yagubyan M, Majumdar R, Ackerman MJ, Sundt TM, III. Novel NOTCH1 mutations in patients with bicuspid aortic valve disease and thoracic aortic aneurysms. *J Thorac Cardiovasc Surg* 2007;134:290–6.

26. Garg V, Muth AN, Ransom JF et al. Mutations in NOTCH1 cause aortic valve disease. *Nature* 2005;437:270–4.

27. Ertas FS, Hasan T, Ozdol C et al. Relationship between angiotensin-converting enzyme gene polymorphism and severity of aortic valve calcification. *Mayo Clin Proc* 2007;82:944–50.

28. Ortlepp JR, Schmitz F, Mevissen V et al. The amount of calcium-deficient hexagonal hydroxyapatite in aortic valves is influenced by gender and associated with genetic polymorphisms in patients with severe calcific aortic stenosis. *Eur Heart J* 2004;25:514–22.

29. Novaro GM, Sachar R, Pearce GL, Sprecher DL, Griffin BP. Association between apolipoprotein E alleles and calcific valvular heart disease. *Circulation* 2003;108:1804–8.

30. Ortlepp JR, Hoffmann R, Ohme F, Lauscher J, Bleckmann F, Hanrath P. The vitamin D receptor genotype predisposes to the development of calcific aortic valve stenosis. *Heart* 2001;85:635–8.

31. Galvin JE, Hemric ME, Ward K, Cunningham MW. Cytotoxic mAb from rheumatic carditis recognizes heart valves and laminin. *J Clin Invest* 2000;106:217–24.

32. Cunningham MW, McCormack JM, Fenderson PG, Ho MK, Beachey EH, Dale JB. Human and murine antibodies cross-reactive with streptococcal M protein and myosin recognize the sequence Gln–Lys–Ser–Lys–Gln in M protein. *J Immunol* 1989;143:2677–83.

33. Cunningham MW, McCormack JM, Talaber LR et al. Human monoclonal antibodies reactive with antigens of the group A streptococcus and human heart. *J Immunol* 1988;141:2760–6.

34. Dale JB, Beachey EH. Epitopes of streptococcal M proteins shared with cardiac myosin. *J Exp Med* 1985;162:583–91.

35. van de Rijn I, Zabriskie JB, McCarty M. Group A streptococcal antigens cross-reactive with myocardium. Purification of heart-reactive antibody and isolation and characterization of the streptococcal antigen. *J Exp Med* 1977;146:579–99.

36. Owens DS, Katz R, Takasu J, Kronmal R, Budoff MJ, O'Brien KD. Incidence and progression of aortic valve calcium in the Multi-Ethnic Study of Atherosclerosis (MESA). *Am J Cardiol* 2010;105:701–8.

37. Cosmi JE, Kort S, Tunick PA et al. The risk of the development of aortic stenosis in patients with "benign" aortic valve thickening. *Arch Intern Med* 2002;162:2345–7.

38. Beppu S, Suzuki S, Matsuda H, Ohmori F, Nagata S, Miyatake K. Rapidity of progression of aortic stenosis in patients with congenital bicuspid aortic valves. *Am J Cardiol* 1993;71:322–7.

39. Edwards JE. The congenital bicuspid aortic valve. *Circulation* 1961; 23:485–8.

40. Huntington K, Hunter AG, Chan KL. A prospective study to assess the frequency of familial clustering of congenital bicuspid aortic valve. *J Am Coll Cardiol* 1997;30:1809–12.

41. Cripe L, Andelfinger G, Martin LJ, Shooner K, Benson DW. Bicuspid aortic valve is heritable. *J Am Coll Cardiol* 2004;44:138–43.

42. Warnes CA, Williams RG, Bashore TM et al. ACC/AHA 2008 guidelines for the management of adults with congenital heart disease: A report of the American College of Cardiology/American Heart Association Task Force on Practice Guidelines (writing committee to develop guidelines on the management of adults with congenital heart disease). *Circulation* 2008;118:e714–833.

43. Jin XY, Pepper JR, Gibson DG. Effects of incoordination on left ventricular force-velocity relation in aortic stenosis. *Heart* 1996;76:495–501.

44. Julius BK, Spillmann M, Vassalli G, Villari B, Eberli FR, Hess OM. Angina pectoris in patients with aortic stenosis and normal coronary arteries. Mechanisms and pathophysiological concepts. *Circulation* 1997;95:892–8.

45. Etchells E, Glenns V, Shadowitz S, Bell C, Siu S. A bedside clinical prediction rule for detecting moderate or severe aortic stenosis. *J Gen Intern Med* 1998;13:699–704.

46. Etchells E, Bell C, Robb K. Does this patient have an abnormal systolic murmur? *J Am Med Assoc* 1997;277:564–71.

47. Gersony WM, Hayes CJ, Driscoll DJ et al. Bacterial endocarditis in patients with aortic stenosis, pulmonary stenosis, or ventricular septal defect. *Circulation* 1993;87:I121–6.

48. Vincentelli A, Susen S, Le Tourneau T et al. Acquired von Willebrand syndrome in aortic stenosis. *N Engl J Med* 2003;349:343–9.

49. Pareti FI, Lattuada A, Bressi C et al. Proteolysis of von Willebrand factor and shear stress-induced platelet aggregation in patients with aortic valve stenosis. *Circulation* 2000;102:1290–5.

50. Gorlin R, Gorlin SG. Hydraulic formula for calculation of the area of the stenotic mitral valve, other cardiac valves, and central circulatory shunts. I. *Am Heart J* 1951;41:1–29.

51. Baumgartner H, Hung J, Bermejo J et al. Echocardiographic assessment of valve stenosis: EAE/ASE recommendations for clinical practice. *J Am Soc Echocardiogr* 2009;22:1–23; quiz 101–2.

52. Vahanian A, Alfieri O, Andreotti F et al. Guidelines on the management of valvular heart disease (version 2012). *Eur Heart J* 2012;33:2451–96.

53. Bonow RO, Carabello BA, Chatterjee K et al. ACC/AHA 2006 guidelines for the management of patients with valvular heart disease: A report of the American College of Cardiology/American Heart Association Task Force on Practice Guidelines (writing committee to revise the 1998 guidelines for the management of patients with valvular heart disease) developed in collaboration with the Society of Cardiovascular Anesthesiologists endorsed by the Society for Cardiovascular Angiography and Interventions and the Society of Thoracic Surgeons. *J Am Coll Cardiol* 2006; 48:e1–148.

54. Picano E, Pibarot P, Lancellotti P, Monin JL, Bonow RO. The emerging role of exercise testing and stress echocardiography in valvular heart disease. *J Am Coll Cardiol* 2009;54:2251–60.

55. Rafique AM, Biner S, Ray I, Forrester JS, Tolstrup K, Siegel RJ. Meta-analysis of prognostic value of stress testing in patients with asymptomatic severe aortic stenosis. *Am J Cardiol* 2009;104:972–7.

56. Lancellotti P, Lebois F, Simon M, Tombeux C, Chauvel C, Pierard LA. Prognostic importance of quantitative exercise Doppler echocardiography in asymptomatic valvular aortic stenosis. *Circulation* 2005;112:I377–82.

57. Bonow RO, Carabello BA, Chatterjee K et al. Focused update incorporated into the ACC/AHA 2006 guidelines for the management of patients with valvular heart disease: A report of the American College of Cardiology/American Heart Association Task Force on Practice Guidelines (writing committee to revise the 1998 guidelines for the management of patients with valvular heart disease): Endorsed by the Society of Cardiovascular Anesthesiologists, Society for Cardiovascular Angiography and Interventions, and Society of Thoracic Surgeons. *Circulation* 2008;118:e523–661.

58. John AS, Dill T, Brandt RR et al. Magnetic resonance to assess the aortic valve area in aortic stenosis: How does it compare to current diagnostic standards? *J Am Coll Cardiol* 2003;42:519–26.

59. Friedrich MG, Schulz-Menger J, Poetsch T, Pilz B, Uhlich F, Dietz R. Quantification of valvular aortic stenosis by magnetic resonance imaging. *Am Heart J* 2002;144:329–34.

60. Kilner PJ, Manzara CC, Mohiaddin RH et al. Magnetic resonance jet velocity mapping in mitral and aortic valve stenosis. *Circulation* 1993;87:1239–48.

61. Dweck MR, Joshi S, Murigu T et al. Midwall fibrosis is an independent predictor of mortality in patients with aortic stenosis. *J Am Coll Cardiol* 2011;58:1271–9.

62. Messika-Zeitoun D, Aubry MC, Detaint D et al. Evaluation and clinical implications of aortic valve calcification measured by electron-beam computed tomography. *Circulation* 2004;110:356–62.

63. Shavelle DM, Budoff MJ, Buljubasic N et al. Usefulness of aortic valve calcium scores by electron beam computed tomography as a marker for aortic stenosis. *Am J Cardiol* 2003;92:349–53.

64. Carabello BA, Green LH, Grossman W, Cohn LH, Koster JK, Collins JJ, Jr. Hemodynamic determinants of prognosis of aortic valve replacement in critical aortic stenosis and advanced congestive heart failure. *Circulation* 1980;62:42–8.

65. Smith N, McAnulty JH, Rahimtoola SH. Severe aortic stenosis with impaired left ventricular function and clinical heart failure: Results of valve replacement. *Circulation* 1978;58:255–64.

66. Burwash IG, Thomas DD, Sadahiro M et al. Dependence of Gorlin formula and continuity equation valve areas on transvalvular volume flow rate in valvular aortic stenosis. *Circulation* 1994;89:827–35.

67. Cannon SR, Richards KL, Crawford M. Hydraulic estimation of stenotic orifice area: A correction of the Gorlin formula. *Circulation* 1985;71:1170–8.

68. Ford LE, Feldman T, Chiu YC, Carroll JD. Hemodynamic resistance as a measure of functional impairment in aortic valvular stenosis. *Circ Res* 1990;66:1–7.

69. Monin JL, Quere JP, Monchi M et al. Low-gradient aortic stenosis: Operative risk stratification and predictors for long-term outcome: A multicenter study using dobutamine stress hemodynamics. *Circulation* 2003;108:319–24.

70. Levy F, Laurent M, Monin JL et al. Aortic valve replacement for low-flow/low-gradient aortic stenosis operative risk stratification and long-term outcome: A European multicenter study. *J Am Coll Cardiol* 2008;51:1466–72.

71. Hachicha Z, Dumesnil JG, Bogaty P, Pibarot P. Paradoxical low-flow, low-gradient severe aortic stenosis despite preserved ejection fraction is associated with higher afterload and reduced survival. *Circulation* 2007;115:2856–64.

72. Minners J, Allgeier M, Gohlke-Baerwolf C, Kienzle RP, Neumann FJ, Jander N. Inconsistencies of echocardiographic criteria for the grading of aortic valve stenosis. *Eur Heart J* 2008;29:1043–8.

73. Otto CM, Burwash IG, Legget ME et al. Prospective study of asymptomatic valvular aortic stenosis. Clinical, echocardiographic, and exercise predictors of outcome. *Circulation* 1997;95:2262–70.

74. Rosenhek R, Binder T, Porenta G et al. Predictors of outcome in severe, asymptomatic aortic stenosis. *N Engl J Med* 2000;343:611–7.

75. Pellikka PA, Sarano ME, Nishimura RA et al. Outcome of 622 adults with asymptomatic, hemodynamically significant aortic stenosis during prolonged follow-up. *Circulation* 2005;111:3290–5.

76. Rosenhek R, Zilberszac R, Schemper M et al. Natural history of very severe aortic stenosis. *Circulation* 2010;121:151–6.

77. Otto CM, Pearlman AS, Gardner CL. Hemodynamic progression of aortic stenosis in adults assessed by Doppler echocardiography. *J Am Coll Cardiol* 1989;13:545–50.

78. Roger VL, Tajik AJ, Bailey KR, Oh JK, Taylor CL, Seward JB. Progression of aortic stenosis in adults: New appraisal using Doppler echocardiography. *Am Heart J* 1990;119:331–8.

79. Faggiano P, Ghizzoni G, Sorgato A et al. Rate of progression of valvular aortic stenosis in adults. *Am J Cardiol* 1992;70:229–33.

80. Brener SJ, Duffy CI, Thomas JD, Stewart WJ. Progression of aortic stenosis in 394 patients: Relation to changes in myocardial and mitral valve dysfunction. *J Am Coll Cardiol* 1995;25:305–10.

81. Ross J, Jr., Braunwald E. Aortic stenosis. *Circulation* 1968;38:61–7.

82. Kelly TA, Rothbart RM, Cooper CM, Kaiser DL, Smucker ML, Gibson RS. Comparison of outcome of asymptomatic to symptomatic patients older than 20 years of age with valvular aortic stenosis. *Am J Cardiol* 1988;61:123–30.

83. Iivanainen AM, Lindroos M, Tilvis R, Heikkila J, Kupari M. Natural history of aortic valve stenosis of varying severity in the elderly. *Am J Cardiol* 1996;78:97–101.

84. Aronow WS, Ahn C, Kronzon I, Goldman ME. Association of coronary risk factors and use of statins with progression of mild valvular aortic stenosis in older persons. *Am J Cardiol* 2001;88:693–5.

85. Novaro GM, Tiong IY, Pearce GL, Lauer MS, Sprecher DL, Griffin BP. Effect of hydroxymethylglutaryl coenzyme a reductase inhibitors on the progression of calcific aortic stenosis. *Circulation* 2001;104:2205–9.

86. Shavelle DM, Takasu J, Budoff MJ, Mao S, Zhao XQ, O'Brien KD. HMG CoA reductase inhibitor (statin) and aortic valve calcium. *Lancet* 2002;359:1125–6.

87. Pohle K, Maffert R, Ropers D et al. Progression of aortic valve calcification: Association with coronary atherosclerosis and cardiovascular risk factors. *Circulation* 2001;104:1927–32.

88. Palta S, Pai AM, Gill KS, Pai RG. New insights into the progression of aortic stenosis: Implications for secondary prevention. *Circulation* 2000;101:2497–502.

89. Rajamannan NM, Otto CM. Targeted therapy to prevent progression of calcific aortic stenosis. *Circulation* 2004;110:1180–2.

90. Vahanian A, Otto CM. Risk stratification of patients with aortic stenosis. *Eur Heart J* 2010;31:416–23.

91. Gummert JF, Funkat A, Beckmann A et al. Cardiac surgery in Germany during 2009. A report on behalf of the German Society for Thoracic and Cardiovascular Surgery. *Thorac Cardiovasc Surg* 2010;58:379–86.

92. Olsson M, Granstrom L, Lindblom D, Rosenqvist M, Ryden L. Aortic valve replacement in octogenarians with aortic stenosis: A case-control study. *J Am Coll Cardiol* 1992;20:1512–6.

93. Elayda MA, Hall RJ, Reul RM et al. Aortic valve replacement in patients 80 years and older. Operative risks and long-term results. *Circulation* 1993;88:II11–6.

94. Kvidal P, Bergstrom R, Horte LG, Stahle E. Observed and relative survival after aortic valve replacement. *J Am Coll Cardiol* 2000;35:747–56.

95. Asimakopoulos G, Edwards MB, Taylor KM. Aortic valve replacement in patients 80 years of age and older: Survival and cause of death based on 1100 cases: Collective results from the UK Heart Valve Registry. *Circulation* 1997;96:3403–8.

96. Akins CW, Daggett WM, Vlahakes GJ et al. Cardiac operations in patients 80 years old and older. *Ann Thorac Surg* 1997;64:606–14; discussion 14-5.

97. Brown JM, O'Brien SM, Wu C, Sikora JA, Griffith BP, Gammie JS. Isolated aortic valve replacement in North America comprising 108,687 patients in 10 years: Changes in risks, valve types, and outcomes in the Society of Thoracic Surgeons National Database. *J Thorac Cardiovasc Surg* 2009;137:82–90.

98. ElBardissi AW, Shekar P, Couper GS, Cohn LH. Minimally invasive aortic valve replacement in octogenarian, high-risk, transcatheter aortic valve implantation candidates. *J Thorac Cardiovasc Surg* 2011;141:328–35.

99. Chukwuemeka A, Borger MA, Ivanov J, Armstrong S, Feindel CM, David TE. Valve surgery in octogenarians: A safe option with good medium-term results. *J Heart Valve Dis* 2006;15:191–6; discussion 6.

100. Smith CR, Leon MB, Mack MJ et al. Transcatheter versus surgical aortic-valve replacement in high-risk patients. *N Engl J Med* 2011;364:2187–98.

101. Kvidal P, Bergstrom R, Malm T, Stahle E. Long-term follow-up of morbidity and mortality after aortic valve replacement with a mechanical valve prosthesis. *Eur Heart J* 2000;21:1099–111.

102. Yun KL, Miller DC, Moore KA et al. Durability of the Hancock MO bioprosthesis compared with standard aortic valve bioprostheses. *Ann Thorac Surg* 1995;60:S221–8.

103. Hammermeister K, Sethi GK, Henderson WG, Grover FL, Oprian C, Rahimtoola SH. Outcomes 15 years after valve replacement with a mechanical versus a bioprosthetic valve: Final report of the Veterans Affairs randomized trial. *J Am Coll Cardiol* 2000;36:1152–8.

104. Rahimtoola SH. Choice of prosthetic heart valve for adult patients. *J Am Coll Cardiol* 2003;41:893–904.

105. Cohn LH. Use of heart valves in older patients. *Circulation* 2005;111:2152–3.

106. Pibarot P, Dumesnil JG, Lemieux M, Cartier P, Metras J, Durand LG. Impact of prosthesis–patient mismatch on hemodynamic and symptomatic status, morbidity and mortality after aortic valve replacement with a bioprosthetic heart valve. *J Heart Valve Dis* 1998; 7:211–8.

107. Franzen SF, Huljebrant IE, Konstantinov IE, Nylander E, Olin CL. Aortic valve replacement for aortic stenosis in patients with small aortic root. *J Heart Valve Dis* 1996;5(Suppl 3): S284–8.

108. Arom KV, Goldenberg IF, Emery RW. Long-term clinical outcome with small size standard St Jude Medical valves implanted in the aortic position. *J Heart Valve Dis* 1994;3:531–6.

109. Adams DH, Chen RH, Kadner A, Aranki SF, Allred EN, Cohn LH. Impact of small prosthetic valve size on operative mortality in elderly patients after aortic valve replacement for aortic stenosis: Does gender matter? *J Thorac Cardiovasc Surg* 1999;118:815–22.

110. Medalion B, Lytle BW, McCarthy PM et al. Aortic valve replacement for octogenarians: Are small valves bad? *Ann Thorac Surg* 1998;66:699–705; discussion-6.

111. Sawant D, Singh AK, Feng WC, Bert AA, Rotenberg F. Nineteen-millimeter aortic St. Jude Medical heart valve prosthesis: Up to sixteen years' follow-up. *Ann Thorac Surg* 1997;63:964–70.

112. Kratz JM, Sade RM, Crawford FA, Jr., Crumbley AJ, III, Stroud MR. The risk of small St. Jude aortic valve prostheses. *Ann Thorac Surg* 1994;57:1114–8; discussion 8–9.

113. Barner HB, Labovitz AJ, Fiore AC. Prosthetic valves for the small aortic root. *J Card Surg* 1994;9:154–7.

114. Mohty D, Dumesnil JG, Echahidi N et al. Impact of prosthesis-patient mismatch on long-term survival after aortic valve replacement: Influence of age, obesity, and left ventricular dysfunction. *J Am Coll Cardiol* 2009;53:39–47.

115. Sommers KE, David TE. Aortic valve replacement with patch enlargement of the aortic annulus. *Ann Thorac Surg* 1997;63:1608–12.

116. David TE. Aortic valve replacement with stentless porcine bioprostheses. *J Card Surg* 1998;13:344–51.

117. David TE, Puschmann R, Ivanov J et al. Aortic valve replacement with stentless and stented porcine valves: A case-match study. *J Thorac Cardiovasc Surg* 1998;116:236–41.

118. Cribier A, Savin T, Saoudi N, Rocha P, Berland J, Letac B. Percutaneous transluminal valvuloplasty of acquired aortic stenosis in elderly patients: An alternative to valve replacement? *Lancet* 1986;1:63–7.

119. Nietlispach F, Wijesinghe N, Wood D, Carere RG, Webb JG. Current balloon-expandable transcatheter heart valve and delivery systems. *Catheter Cardiovasc Interv* 2010;75:295–300.

120. Klein A, Lee K, Gera A, Ports TA, Michaels AD. Long-term mortality, cause of death, and temporal trends in complications after percutaneous aortic balloon valvuloplasty for calcific aortic stenosis. *J Interv Cardiol* 2006;19:269–75.

121. Lieberman EB, Bashore TM, Hermiller JB et al. Balloon aortic valvuloplasty in adults: Failure of procedure to improve long-term survival. *J Am Coll Cardiol* 1995;26:1522–8.

122. Percutaneous balloon aortic valvuloplasty. Acute and 30-day follow-up results in 674 patients from the NHLBI Balloon Valvuloplasty Registry. *Circulation* 1991;84:2383–97.

123. Nishimura RA, Holmes DR, Jr., Reeder GS. Percutaneous balloon valvuloplasty. *Mayo Clin Proc* 1990;65:198–220.

124. Litvack F, Jakubowski AT, Buchbinder NA, Eigler N. Lack of sustained clinical improvement in an elderly population after percutaneous aortic valvuloplasty. *Am J Cardiol* 1988;62:270–5.

125. Ferguson JJ, Garza RA. Efficacy of multiple balloon valvuloplasty procedures. The Mansfield Scientific Aortic Valvuloplasty Registry Investigators. *J Am Coll Cardiol* 1991;17:1430–5.

126. Davies H, Lessof MH, Roberts CI, Ross DN. Homograft replacement of the aortic valve: Follow-up studies in twelve patients. *Lancet* 1965;1:926–9.

127. Moulopoulos SD, Anthopoulos L, Stamatelopoulos S, Stefadouros M. Catheter-mounted aortic valves. *Ann Thorac Surg* 1971;11: 423–30.

128. Phillips SJ, Ciborski M, Freed PS, Cascade PN, Jaron D. A temporary catheter-tip aortic valve: Hemodynamic effects on experimental acute aortic insufficiency. *Ann Thorac Surg* 1976;21:134–7.

129. Andersen HR, Knudsen LL, Hasenkam JM. Transluminal implantation of artificial heart valves. Description of a new expandable aortic valve and initial results with implantation by catheter technique in closed chest pigs. *Eur Heart J* 1992;13:704–8.

130. Boudjemline Y, Bonhoeffer P. Steps toward percutaneous aortic valve replacement. *Circulation* 2002;105:775–8.

131. Bonhoeffer P, Boudjemline Y, Saliba Z et al. Percutaneous replacement of pulmonary valve in a right-ventricle to pulmonary-artery prosthetic conduit with valve dysfunction. *Lancet* 2000;356: 1403–5.

132. Cribier A, Eltchaninoff H, Bash A et al. Percutaneous transcatheter implantation of an aortic valve prosthesis for calcific aortic stenosis: First human case description. *Circulation* 2002;106:3006–8.

133. Webb JG, Chandavimol M, Thompson CR et al. Percutaneous aortic valve implantation retrograde from the femoral artery. *Circulation* 2006;113:842–50.

134. Grube E, Laborde JC, Zickmann B et al. First report on a human percutaneous transluminal implantation of a self-expanding valve prosthesis for interventional treatment of aortic valve stenosis. *Catheter Cardiovasc Interv* 2005;66:465–9.

135. Lichtenstein SV, Cheung A, Ye J et al. Transapical transcatheter aortic valve implantation in humans: Initial clinical experience. *Circulation* 2006;114:591–6.

136. Walther T, Falk V, Borger MA et al. Minimally invasive transapical beating heart aortic valve implantation—Proof of concept. *Eur J Cardiothorac Surg* 2007;31:9–15.

137. Bauernschmitt R, Schreiber C, Bleiziffer S et al. Transcatheter aortic valve implantation through the ascending aorta: An alternative option for no-access patients. *Heart Surg Forum* 2009;12:E63–4.

138. Petronio AS, De Carlo M, Bedogni F et al. Safety and efficacy of the subclavian approach for transcatheter aortic valve implantation with the CoreValve Revalving System. *Circ Cardiovasc Interv* 2010;3:359–66.

139. Asgar AW, Mullen MJ, Delahunty N et al. Transcatheter aortic valve intervention through the axillary artery for the treatment of severe aortic stenosis. *J Thorac Cardiovasc Surg* 2009;137:773–5.

140. Modine T, Lemesle G, Azzaoui R, Sudre A. Aortic valve implantation with the CoreValve ReValving System via left carotid artery access: First case report. *J Thorac Cardiovasc Surg* 2010;140:928–9.

141. Holmes DR, Jr., Mack MJ, Kaul S et al. ACCF/AATS/SCAI/STS Expert Consensus Document on transcatheter aortic valve replacement: Developed in collabration with the American Heart Association, American Society of Echocardiography, European Association for Cardio-Thoracic Surgery, Heart Failure Society of America, Mended Hearts, Society of Cardiovascular Anesthesiologists, Society of Cardiovascular Computed Tomography, and Society for Cardiovascular Magnetic Resonance. *J Thorac Cardiovasc Surg* 2012;144:e29–84.

142. Holmes DR, Jr., Mack MJ, Kaul S et al. ACCF/AATS/SCAI/STS Expert Consensus Document on transcatheter aortic valve replacement. *J Am Coll Cardiol* 2012;59:1200–54.

143. Zamorano JL, Badano LP, Bruce C et al. EAE/ASE recommendations for the use of echocardiography in new transcatheter interventions for valvular heart disease. *J Am Soc Echocardiogr* 2011;24:937–65.

144. Toggweiler S, Gurvitch R, Leipsic J et al. Percutaneous aortic valve replacement: Vascular outcomes with a fully percutaneous procedure. *J Am Coll Cardiol* 2012;59:113–8.

145. Jabbour A, Ismail TF, Moat N et al. Multimodality imaging in transcatheter aortic valve implantation and post-procedural aortic regurgitation: Comparison among cardiovascular magnetic resonance, cardiac computed tomography, and echocardiography. *J Am Coll Cardiol* 2011;58:2165–73.

146. Jilaihawi H, Kashif M, Fontana G et al. Cross-sectional computed tomographic assessment improves accuracy of aortic annular sizing for transcatheter aortic valve replacement and reduces the incidence of paravalvular aortic regurgitation. *J Am Coll Cardiol* 2012;59: 1275–86.

147. Achenbach S, Delgado V, Hausleiter J, Schoenhagen P, Min JK, Leipsic JA. SCCT Expert Consensus Document on computed tomography imaging before transcatheter aortic valve implantation (TAVI)/transcatheter aortic valve replacement (TAVR). *J Cardiovasc Comput Tomogr* 2012;6:366–80.

148. Services CfMaM. Decision memo for transcatheter aortic valve replacement (TAVR) (CAG-00430N). 2012.

149. Leon MB, Piazza N, Nikolsky E et al. Standardized endpoint definitions for transcatheter aortic valve implantation clinical trials: A consensus report from the Valve Academic Research Consortium. *J Am Coll Cardiol* 2011;57:253–69.

150. Genereux P, Head SJ, Van Mieghem NM et al. Clinical outcomes after transcatheter aortic valve replacement using Valve Academic Research Consortium definitions: A weighted meta-analysis of 3,519 patients from 16 studies. *J Am Coll Cardiol* 2012;59:2317–26.

151. Kappetein AP, Head SJ, Genereux P et al. Updated standardized endpoint definitions for transcatheter aortic valve implantation: The Valve Academic Research Consortium-2 consensus document. *J Am Coll Cardiol* 2012;60:1438–54.

152. Thomas M, Schymik G, Walther T et al. One-year outcomes of cohort 1 in the Edwards SAPIEN Aortic Bioprosthesis European Outcome (SOURCE) Registry: The European registry of transcatheter aortic valve implantation using the Edwards SAPIEN valve. *Circulation* 2011;124:425–33.

153. Lefevre T, Kappetein AP, Wolner E et al. One year follow-up of the multi-centre European PARTNER transcatheter heart valve study. *Eur Heart J* 2011;32:148–57.

154. Gilard M, Eltchaninoff H, Iung B et al. Registry of transcatheter aortic-valve implantation in high-risk patients. *N Engl J Med* 2012;366:1705–15.

155. Bosmans JM, Kefer J, De Bruyne B et al. Procedural, 30-day and one year outcome following CoreValve or Edwards transcatheter aortic valve implantation: Results of the Belgian national registry. *Interact Cardiovasc Thorac Surg* 2011;12:762–7.

156. Rodes-Cabau J, Webb JG, Cheung A et al. Transcatheter aortic valve implantation for the treatment of severe symptomatic aortic stenosis in patients at very high or prohibitive surgical risk: Acute and late outcomes of the multicenter Canadian experience. *J Am Coll Cardiol* 2010;55:1080–90.

157. Avanzas P, Munoz-Garcia AJ, Segura J et al. Percutaneous implantation of the CoreValve self-expanding aortic valve prosthesis in patients with severe aortic stenosis: Early experience in Spain. *Rev Esp Cardiol* 2010;63:141–8.

158. Buellesfeld L, Gerckens U, Schuler G et al. 2-year follow-up of patients undergoing transcatheter aortic valve implantation using a self-expanding valve prosthesis. *J Am Coll Cardiol* 2011;57:1650–7.

159. Godino C, Maisano F, Montorfano M et al. Outcomes after transcatheter aortic valve implantation with both Edwards-SAPIEN and CoreValve devices in a single center: The Milan experience. *JACC Cardiovasc Interv* 2010;3:1110–21.

160. Tamburino C, Capodanno D, Ramondo A et al. Incidence and predictors of early and late mortality after transcatheter aortic valve implantation in 663 patients with severe aortic stenosis. *Circulation* 2011;123:299–308.

161. Zahn R, Gerckens U, Grube E et al. Transcatheter aortic valve implantation: First results from a multi-centre real-world registry. *Eur Heart J* 2011;32:198–204.

162. Moat NE, Ludman P, de Belder MA et al. Long-term outcomes after transcatheter aortic valve implantation in high-risk patients with severe aortic stenosis: The U.K. TAVI (United Kingdom Transcatheter Aortic Valve Implantation) Registry. *J Am Coll Cardiol* 2011;58:2130–8.

163. Leon MB, Smith CR, Mack M et al. Transcatheter aortic-valve implantation for aortic stenosis in patients who cannot undergo surgery. *N Engl J Med* 2010;363:1597–607.

164. Makkar RR, Fontana GP, Jilaihawi H et al. Transcatheter aortic-valve replacement for inoperable severe aortic stenosis. *N Engl J Med* 2012;366:1696–704.

165. Kodali SK, Williams MR, Smith CR et al. Two-year outcomes after transcatheter or surgical aortic-valve replacement. *N Engl J Med* 2012;366:1686–95.

166. Wood S. PARTNER 2: New SAPIEN XT matches first TAVR device, with lower complications. *theheartorg:* (2013, accessed March 17, 2013).

167. Gotzmann M, Hehen T, Germing A et al. Short-term effects of transcatheter aortic valve implantation on neurohormonal activation, quality of life and 6-minute walk test in severe and symptomatic aortic stenosis. *Heart* 2010;96:1102–6.

168. Krane M, Deutsch MA, Bleiziffer S et al. Quality of life among patients undergoing transcatheter aortic valve implantation. *Am Heart J* 2010;160:451–7.

169. Ussia GP, Mule M, Barbanti M et al. Quality of life assessment after percutaneous aortic valve implantation. *Eur Heart J* 2009;30:1790–6.

170. Bekeredjian R, Krumsdorf U, Chorianopoulos E et al. Usefulness of percutaneous aortic valve implantation to improve quality of life in patients >80 years of age. *Am J Cardiol* 2010;106:1777–81.

171. Georgiadou P, Kontodima P, Sbarouni E et al. Long-term quality of life improvement after transcatheter aortic valve implantation. *Am Heart J* 2011;162:232–7.

172. Gotzmann M, Bojara W, Lindstaedt M et al. One-year results of transcatheter aortic valve implantation in severe symptomatic aortic valve stenosis. *Am J Cardiol* 2011;107:1687–92.

173. Ussia GP, Barbanti M, Cammalleri V et al. Quality-of-life in elderly patients one year after transcatheter aortic valve implantation for severe aortic stenosis. *EuroIntervention* 2011;7:573–9.

174. Reynolds MR, Magnuson EA, Lei Y et al. Health-related quality of life after transcatheter aortic valve replacement in inoperable patients with severe aortic stenosis. *Circulation* 2011;124:1964–72.

175. Erkapic D, De Rosa S, Kelava A, Lehmann R, Fichtlscherer S, Hohnloser SH. Risk for permanent pacemaker after transcatheter aortic valve implantation: A comprehensive analysis of the literature. *J Cardiovasc Electrophysiol* 2012;23:391–7.

176. Goldstein LB, Bushnell CD, Adams RJ et al. Guidelines for the primary prevention of stroke: A guideline for healthcare professionals from the American Heart Association/American Stroke Association. *Stroke* 2011;42:517–84.

177. Ghanem A, Muller A, Nahle CP et al. Risk and fate of cerebral embolism after transfemoral aortic valve implantation: A prospective pilot study with diffusion-weighted magnetic resonance imaging. *J Am Coll Cardiol* 2010;55:1427–32.

178. Koos R, Mahnken AH, Aktug O et al. Electrocardiographic and imaging predictors for permanent pacemaker requirement after transcatheter aortic valve implantation. *J Heart Valve Dis* 2011;20:83–90.

179. Khatri PJ, Webb JG, Rodes-Cabau J et al. Adverse effects associated with transcatheter aortic valve implantation: A meta-analysis of contemporary studies. *Ann Intern Med* 2013;158:35–46.

180. D'Ancona G, Pasic M, Unbehaun A, Hetzer R. Permanent pacemaker implantation after transapical transcatheter aortic valve implantation. *Interact Cardiovasc Thorac Surg* 2011;13:373–6.

181. Kahlert P, Al-Rashid F, Weber M et al. Vascular access site complications after percutaneous transfemoral aortic valve implantation. *Herz* 2009;34:398–408.

182. Hayashida K, Lefevre T, Chevalier B et al. Transfemoral aortic valve implantation new criteria to predict vascular complications. *JACC Cardiovasc Interv* 2011;4:851–8.

183. Thomas M, Schymik G, Walther T et al. Thirty-day results of the SAPIEN Aortic Bioprosthesis European Outcome (SOURCE) Registry: A European registry of transcatheter aortic valve implantation using the Edwards SAPIEN valve. *Circulation* 2010;122:62–9.

184. Kodali SK, O'Neill WW, Moses JW et al. Early and late (one year) outcomes following transcatheter aortic valve implantation in patients with severe aortic stenosis (from the United States REVIVAL trial). *Am J Cardiol* 2011;107:1058–64.

185. Gotzmann M, Pljakic A, Bojara W et al. Transcatheter aortic valve implantation in patients with severe symptomatic aortic valve stenosis–predictors of mortality and poor treatment response. *Am Heart J* 2011;162:238–45 e1.

186. Eltchaninoff H, Prat A, Gilard M et al. Transcatheter aortic valve implantation: Early results of the FRANCE (FRench Aortic National CoreValve and Edwards) registry. *Eur Heart J* 2011;32:191–7.

187. Webb JG, Altwegg L, Boone RH et al. Transcatheter aortic valve implantation: Impact on clinical and valve-related outcomes. *Circulation* 2009;119:3009–16.

188. Ussia GP, Barbanti M, Petronio AS et al. Transcatheter aortic valve implantation: 3-Year outcomes of self-expanding CoreValve prosthesis. *Eur Heart J* 2012;33:969–76.

189. Haensig M, Lehmkuhl L, Rastan AJ et al. Aortic valve calcium scoring is a predictor of significant paravalvular aortic insufficiency in transapical–aortic valve implantation. *Eur J Cardiothorac Surg* 2012;41:1234–40; discussion 40-1.

190. Colli A, D'Amico R, Kempfert J, Borger MA, Mohr FW, Walther T. Transesophageal echocardiographic scoring for transcatheter aortic valve implantation: Impact of aortic cusp calcification on postoperative aortic regurgitation. *J Thorac Cardiovasc Surg* 2011;142:1229–35.

191. Yared K, Garcia-Camarero T, Fernandez-Friera L et al. Impact of aortic regurgitation after transcatheter aortic valve implantation: Results from the REVIVAL trial. *JACC Cardiovasc Imaging* 2012;5:469–77.

192. Unbehaun A, Pasic M, Dreysse S et al. Transapical aortic valve implantation: Incidence and predictors of paravalvular leakage and transvalvular regurgitation in a series of 358 patients. *J Am Coll Cardiol* 2012;59:211–21.

193. Buzzatti N, Maisano F, Latib A et al. Computed tomography-based evaluation of aortic annulus, prosthesis size and impact on early residual aortic regurgitation after transcatheter aortic valve implantation. *Eur J Cardiothorac Surg* 2013;43:43–50; discussion-1.

194. Schultz CJ, Tzikas A, Moelker A et al. Correlates on MSCT of paravalvular aortic regurgitation after transcatheter aortic valve implantation using the Medtronic CoreValve prosthesis. *Catheter Cardiovasc Interv* 2011;78:446–55.

195. Detaint D, Lepage L, Himbert D et al. Determinants of significant paravalvular regurgitation after transcatheter aortic valve: Implantation impact of device and annulus discongruence. *JACC Cardiovasc Interv* 2009;2:821–7.

196. Block PC. Leaks and the "great ship" TAVI. *Catheter Cardiovasc Interv* 2010;75:873–4.

197. Takagi K, Latib A, Al-Lamee R et al. Predictors of moderate-to-severe paravalvular aortic regurgitation immediately after CoreValve implantation and the impact of postdilatation. *Catheter Cardiovasc Interv* 2011;78:432–43.

198. Sherif MA, Abdel-Wahab M, Stocker B et al. Anatomic and procedural predictors of paravalvular aortic regurgitation after implantation of the Medtronic CoreValve bioprosthesis. *J Am Coll Cardiol* 2010;56:1623–9.

199. Genereux P, Head SJ, Hahn R et al. Paravalvular leak after transcatheter aortic valve replacement: The new Achilles' heel? A comprehensive review of the literature. *J Am Coll Cardiol* 2013;61(11):1125–36.

200. Nombela-Franco L, Rodes-Cabau J, DeLarochelliere R et al. Predictive factors, efficacy, and safety of balloon post-dilation after transcatheter aortic valve implantation with a balloon-expandable valve. *JACC Cardiovasc Interv* 2012;5:499–512.

201. Majunke N, Doss M, Steinberg DH et al. How should I treat a misplaced self-expanding aortic bioprosthetic valve? *EuroIntervention* 2010;6:537–42.

202. Vavuranakis M, Vrachatis D, Stefanadis C. CoreValve aortic bioprosthesis: Repositioning techniques. *JACC Cardiovasc Interv* 2010;3:565; author reply-6.

203. Gerckens U, Latsios G, Mueller R et al. Procedural and mid-term results in patients with aortic stenosis treated with implantation of 2 (in-series) CoreValve prostheses in 1 procedure. *JACC Cardiovasc Interv* 2010;3:244–50.

204. Ussia GP, Barbanti M, Ramondo A et al. The valve-in-valve technique for treatment of aortic bioprosthesis malposition an analysis of incidence and 1-year clinical outcomes from the Italian CoreValve registry. *J Am Coll Cardiol* 2011;57:1062–8.

205. Schleger S, Kasel M, Vogel J et al. Successful transapical implantation of an Edwards SAPIEN valve within an insufficient aortic CoreValve prosthesis: An initial experience. *Ann Thorac Surg* 2013;95:1070–2.

206. Hamdan A, Guetta V, Konen E et al. Deformation dynamics and mechanical properties of the aortic annulus by 4-dimensional computed tomography: Insights into the functional anatomy of the aortic valve complex and implications for transcatheter aortic valve therapy. *J Am Coll Cardiol* 2012;59:119–27.

207. Schultz CJ, Moelker AD, Tzikas A et al. Cardiac CT: Necessary for precise sizing for transcatheter aortic implantation. *EuroIntervention* 2010;6(Suppl G):G6–13.

208. Ng AC, Delgado V, van der Kley F et al. Comparison of aortic root dimensions and geometries before and after transcatheter aortic valve implantation by 2- and 3-dimensional transesophageal echocardiography and multislice computed tomography. *Circ Cardiovasc Imaging* 2010;3:94–102.

209. Schultz CJ, Weustink A, Piazza N et al. Geometry and degree of apposition of the CoreValve ReValving System with multislice computed tomography after implantation in patients with aortic stenosis. *J Am Coll Cardiol* 2009;54:911–8.

210. Tops LF, Wood DA, Delgado V et al. Noninvasive evaluation of the aortic root with multislice computed tomography implications for transcatheter aortic valve replacement. *JACC Cardiovasc Imaging* 2008;1:321–30.

24

Aortic valve stenosis in the elderly: Balloon aortic valvuloplasty

John L. Parks and Daniel H. Steinberg

Introduction and background

The natural history of aortic stenosis is well established. Once moderate disease is present (defined as a jet velocity greater than 3.0 m/s, Table 24.1), the expectation is gradual progression of approximately 0.3 m/s or 1 cm²/year.[1,2] For patients with severe aortic stenosis (valve area <1 cm², jet velocity >4 m/s, or mean gradient >40 mmHg), the cardinal symptoms of cardiac syncope, angina, or exertional dyspnea portend a very poor prognosis if untreated.[3] Surgical aortic valve replacement (AVR) has long been recognized as the standard treatment modality, with favorable long-term outcomes extending beyond 30 years. The American College of Cardiology/American Heart Association and European Society of Cardiology guidelines both recommend surgical AVR for patients with severe, symptomatic aortic stenosis and for those with asymptomatic disease with coexisting left ventricular dysfunction or undergoing cardiac surgery for another reason.[4,5]

While most patients with symptomatic, severe aortic stenosis are appropriate candidates for surgical valve replacement, many patients, particularly those of advanced age, have issues placing them at elevated surgical risk. Comorbid conditions such as chronic lung disease, peripheral vascular or cerebrovascular disease, diabetes, renal insufficiency, and left ventricular dysfunction all figure into a patient's individual risk for surgery. These and other factors have become part of objective risk stratification tools, such as the Society of Thoracic Surgery (STS) or EuroSCORE, that aim to quantify risk and identify those who would likely not have an overall benefit from surgery. Other conditions, such as liver disease and frailty, are not necessarily included in traditional risk stratification, but they are often a part of the subjective evaluation of surgical risk stratification.

For patients at prohibitive surgical risk, options have traditionally been quite limited. With the introduction of percutaneous transluminal aortic valvuloplasty (PTAV) by Cribier in 1985,[6] an option arose for patients with aortic stenosis and prohibitive risk of surgical AVR. By fracturing leaflet calcification and, to a lesser extent, stretching valve tissue and splitting of commissures, PTAV is associated with a 30–50% acute reduction in the transvalvular gradient, improvements in aortic valve area of 0.3–0.4 cm², and symptomatic improvement.[7–9]

Unfortunately, PTAV has important limitations that have tempered initial enthusiasm. First, procedural complications are not uncommon, ranging from 16% to 30%.[7,8,10] Second, the acute improvements in mean gradient and valve area are not long-lasting. Indeed, restenosis rates (defined as >50% loss of acute gain) of up to 80% were reported at 15 month follow-up.[10] Additionally, and most importantly, long-term survival is no better than the natural history of untreated disease with survival rates of 50–60% at one year and only 20–25% at 3 years.[11–13] As a result, PTAV had largely become a palliative or bridging procedure beneficial in only a few clinical situations, and was recognized as a class IIb or even a class III recommendation in prior guidelines.[4]

The advent of transcatheter aortic valve replacement (TAVR) has rekindled interest in PTAV, particularly in its role as a bridging procedure. As TAVR provides the potential for curative AVR in patients at prohibitive risk for surgical AVR,[14] PTAV has gained an important place in patient selection and management in the pre-TAVR evaluation. This chapter focuses on PTAV in its current role. The details of TAVR are discussed in additional chapters.

Table 24.1 Severity of AS		
Indicator	Moderate	Severe
Jet velocity	3.0–4.0 m/s	Greater than 4.0 m/s
Mean gradient	25–40 mmHg	Greater than 40 mmHg
Valve area	1.0–1.5 cm²	Less than 1.0 cm²

Indications for PTAV

Isolated PTAV

Current guidelines suggest valvuloplasty is reasonable in patients with severe, symptomatic aortic stenosis combined with hemodynamic instability, using PTAV as a bridge to surgical AVR.[4] This is most appropriate in those patients with high risk of complications with surgical replacement, as PTAV may help lower some perioperative risks. Those patients with lower surgical risk should proceed directly to AVR once optimized as much as able, even if complicated by hemodynamic instability or refractory pulmonary edema. PTAV is also reasonable in patients with severe AS for palliation of symptoms if not candidates for surgical AVR. Valvuloplasty may also help optimize patients planned for noncardiac surgery if symptomatic AS exists (Table 24.2). It should be clear that PTAV is not to be considered an alternative to surgical AVR in the adult patient unless contraindications exist.

As a bridge to AVR or TAVR

As noted earlier, contemporary use of PTAV has significantly increased with the introduction of TAVR into clinical practice as this procedure has revolutionized the treatment of elderly patients with severe AS and significant comorbidities or contraindications to surgery.[14,15] PTAV may be used as a technique to help "triage" this cohort of patients. The patient with significant lung disease and aortic stenosis can be evaluated for symptomatic improvement after PTAV, potentially providing evidence for efficacy of additional interventions. The critically ill patient with aortic stenosis and cardiogenic shock may require temporizing PTAV, allowing more time for evaluation by a referral center. These contemporary applications can be crucial in this complex, critically ill population.

Palliation

Despite providing significant symptomatic relief, PTAV does not lead to lasting results when compared with AVR or TAVR. However, PTAV can still play a role in palliation for critically ill patients who are not (and will not) be candidates for surgical or transcatheter AVR. In certain circumstances, PTAV may be repeated for further palliation. It remains clear that patients undergoing palliative PTAV often have poor outcomes. This is likely related to the realization that if there was a definitive surgical or transcatheter option, PTAV would be performed with bridging intent.

Procedural considerations

Access

Depending on the type and diameter of the valvuloplasty balloon, arterial access ranges from 8 F to 14 F. Based on the patient's peripheral anatomy, the operator may choose to "preclose" the vessel with a suture-based closure device. Options include the braided suture 10F ProSTAR device or 2 prolene suture 6F PerClose devices (both by Abbott Vascular, Abbott Park, IL, USA). Venous access is usually obtained for both the transvenous pacemaker wire (discussed later) and/or a PA catheter. In our practice, we place two sheaths (6F and 7F) in the same femoral vein ipsilateral to the femoral arterial sheath.

Balloon sizing

Classically, a balloon diameter/LVOT ratio of 1–1.1 to 1 was considered standard practice with the option of employing a larger balloon if gradient reductions were suboptimal. Over the last few years, coincident with the advent of TAVR, there is increased focus on sizing the aortic annulus to help optimize balloon sizing. Although this has primary

Table 24.2 Indication for PTAV		
Indication	**Recommendation**	**Guideline**
Hemodynamically unstable, high risk for AVR	IIa Evidence level C	STS 2013
Symptom palliation not candidate for AVR	IIb Evidence level C	STS 2013
Severe AS without calcific disease in the young adult	IIa Evidence level C	ACC/AHA 2008
Severe symptomatic AS before urgent noncardiac surgery	IIb Evidence level C	STS 2013
Bridge until evaluation for AVR or TAVR if likely candidate	IIa Evidence level C	STS 2013
Evaluation for symptomatic improvement if questionable benefit from repair	IIa Evidence level C	STS 2013

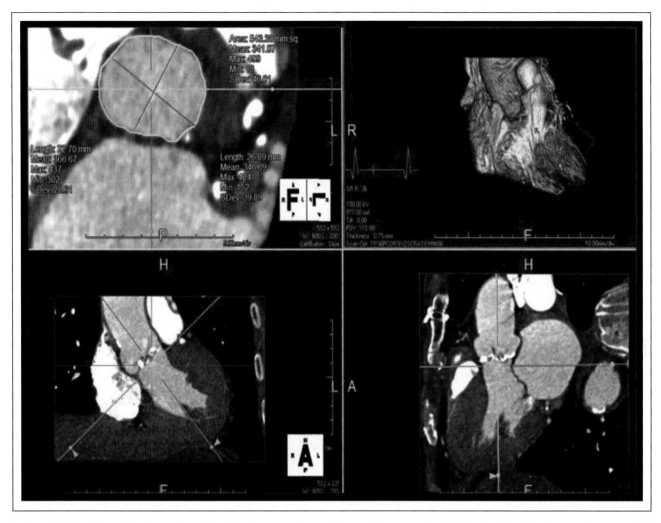

Figure 24.1 **(See color insert.)** Annular sizing by CTA. The annulus area is measured at the basal point of leaflet attachment. In this figure (top left), the annulus area is 563 mm² and measures 26.9 mm × 22.7 mm.

relevance to valve sizing in TAVR, it may also be useful in PTAV. Sizing can be done prior to the procedure by computed tomography (Figure 24.1) or it can be done during PTAV by aortography at the time of balloon inflation. In the latter case, assessment of periballoon aortic insufficiency occurs during inflation (Figure 24.2) with larger balloons selected for subsequent dilation as indicated.

Rapid pacing

Rapid right ventricular pacing (RP) as an aid for precise balloon positioning during valvuloplasty was originally described by Ing et al. in 2002 in pediatric patients with congenital aortic stenosis. It was adopted for use in calcific aortic stenosis after proving to be a safe technique, and was widely adopted by operators as a more stable method for balloon positioning.[16,17] RP has been typically described as right ventricular pacing using a temporary venous pacing wire, usually at rates of 160–200 beats per minute. Our practice has been to use a trial pacing run before the actual

balloon inflation, adjusting pacing rates for a goal mean arterial pressure of 40–50 mmHg and a pulse pressure under 10 mmHg (Figure 24.3). It should be recognized that while this method is widely accepted as common practice, RP has not been shown to provide mortality benefit or significantly change postvalvuloplasty valve area.

Valvuloplasty techniques

PTAV should be carried out under conscious (moderate) sedation, although anesthesia support is occasionally required. Procedural staff should be primed to deal with a rapidly decompensating patient, with preparations made to be ready for immediate resuscitation. We recommend intraprocedural pulmonary artery catheter monitoring and defibrillator pads readily available.

PTAV has traditionally been described using femoral arterial access and intervening using a retrograde approach.[6] Occasionally, peripheral vascular disease will prevent femoral arterial access and either upper extremity

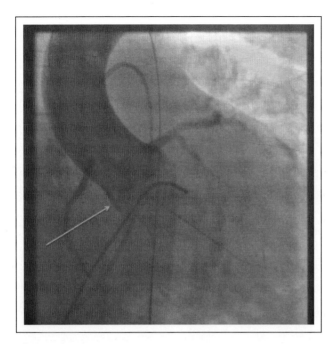

Figure 24.2   Under conditions of rapid pacing, a 25 mm × 4 cm balloon is inflated. Aortography demonstrates incomplete seal as evidenced by aortic insufficiency (arrow).

retrograde or an antegrade approach (via femoral venous access and transseptal puncture) may be required.[18] Upper extremity access has been described utilizing the axillary artery (via a cutdown) or the brachial artery. More recently, even radial artery access has been described as a possible access site, depending on the valvuloplasty balloon used.

Retrograde approach

Once access is obtained and appropriate diagnostics such as a hemodynamic valve study or coronary angiography are performed, arterial access is upgraded to support the desired balloon catheter. The valve is crossed by standard techniques, and many operators have their own preferences. In our practice, we typically employ a Judkins right or an Amplatz left 1 with a 0.038 inch straight-tipped Glidewire (Terumo, Somerset, NJ). Upon successfully crossing the valve, heparin is administered, and the coronary catheter is exchanged over the wire for dual lumen pigtail catheter. The Glidewire is then exchanged for a stiff 0.035 inch J-tipped wire (usually an Amplatz Extra Stiff Guidewire, Boston Scientific, Miami, FL). The balloon catheter is advanced into position, and under conditions of rapid pacing the balloon is inflated. The focus should be on precise positioning in order to ensure adequate valve expansion, with inflation times of approximately 5 s. Minimal pacing runs provide less risk of hemodynamic compromise. Following withdrawal of the balloon catheter, hemodynamics are assessed and ideally the procedure is concluded. Access closure is at the discretion of the operator, with the option of closure-assist devices as previously described.

Antegrade approach

For patients with anatomy unsuitable for the retrograde approach, the PTAV may be performed antegrade from venous access and a transseptal puncture. Potential advantages of this approach include relative ease of crossing the valve from the ventricular side and balloon stability during inflation (with less need for pacing). However, this approach is not usually favored because of the inherent added complexity of a transseptal puncture. Nevertheless, it remains a viable alternative in certain situations.

Complications and postprocedure care

The incidence of adverse events with PTAV has been described as approximately 16% in the modern era.[11] Vascular injury is the most commonly described event (requiring intervention or transfusion, 6.9%), followed by acute stroke with identifiable deficit (1.9%), and intraprocedural death (1.6%). Less common complications include acute, severe aortic insufficiency, requirement for permanent pacing, dissection or occlusion of a coronary artery, renal failure, need for acute hemodynamic resuscitation, and rarely tamponade. A decrease in the rate of complications (from approximately 30% in the early, larger groups) is likely attributed to PTAV being commonly performed by more experienced operators in referral centers (Table 24.3). It may also be that PTAV is not being offered to those patients with such advanced comorbidities that their overall prognosis is grim, even with an improvement in aortic stenosis.

In the immediate postprocedure state, the left ventricle is undergoing significant changes in hemodynamics. With the rapid unloading of a ventricle accustomed to a fixed obstruction and high filling pressures, supporting preload with fluid resuscitation may be needed. Our experience has led to the practice of matching postprocedure urine output with volume resuscitation for the first 24 hours, expecting a degree of autodiuresis. Early mobilization is an important lesson taken from postoperative experiences, with practical consideration given to ensure access site hemostasis. Emphasis on pulmonary toilet is commonly needed given the high incidence of concomitant lung disease.

Current perspective and future directions

With the introduction of TAVR into clinical practice, PTAV has seen renewed interest. Surgical AVR has still been recognized as the standard therapy for severe AS, but TAVR may begin to play a more prominent treatment role in the future. While TAVR is currently reserved for those deemed "high-risk" for surgical AVR, there is significant

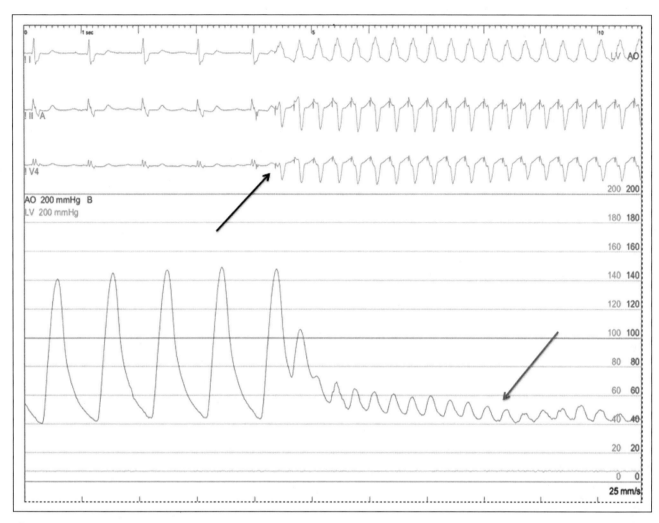

Figure 24.3 **(See color insert.)** Rapid pacing. The patient is in sinus rhythm at the beginning of the tracing. Rapid pacing is begun (black arrow) and over the ensuing 10 beats, the pulse pressure narrows to about 10 mmHg and the mean pressure decreases to about 50 mmHg.

belief that this paradigm will shift. TAVR has promising initial data, and PTAV may be used as a bridge until evaluation for TAVR or to see if symptoms at least temporarily improve. Those patients that have significant symptomatic benefit with PTAV should be referred for potential TAVR unless clear contraindications exist.

In 2013, the Society of Thoracic Surgeons introduced an Executive Summary update regarding aortic valve disease and its treatment. While continuing to recognize that PTAV is not an ideal therapy, it remains an important option for the elderly patient with prohibitive surgical risk. Specifically, these newest guidelines emphasize PTAV's

Table 24.3 PTAV outcomes

Reference	Number of patients	Major periprocedural complications (%)	Vascular injury (%)	Stroke or TIA (%)	In-hospital mortality (%)
NHLBI Registry, 1991[7]	674	31	7	3	10
Mansfield Registry, 1991[8]	492	20.5	11	2.2	7.6
Letac et al., 1988[20]	218	32	13	1.8	4.6
Agarwal et al., 2005[21]	212	30	13.5	1.1	8
Klein et al., 2006[22]	78	22	20	1	1.2
Berland et al., 1989[23]	55	20	12.7	1.8	5

role in delineating reversible symptoms related to AS (vs. advanced lung disease, etc.) or its use as a bridge to surgical or transcatheter AVR. These guidelines update PTAV as a IIa recommendation for these two indications, while the other previously mentioned applications remain a IIb recommendation.[19]

In summary, PTAV is an established, relatively safe procedure best utilized as a bridge to surgical or transcatheter AVR. The procedure also has a role in helping establish anticipated benefit of AVR in certain high-risk patients with competing comorbid conditions. As the long-term results are not favorable and the procedure does not extend life, PTAV used purely as a palliative treatment should be carefully considered, with realistic expectations discussed with patients and families. PTAV remains an important treatment option for the modern interventional cardiologist, and continues to have a fundamental role in the treatment of severe aortic stenosis.

References

1. Otto CM, Pearlman AS, Gardner CL. Hemodynamic progression of aortic stenosis in adults assessed by Doppler echocardiography. *J Am Coll Cardiol* 1989;13(3):545–50.

2. Rosenhek R et al. Predictors of outcome in severe, asymptomatic aortic stenosis. *N Engl J Med* 2000;343(9):611–7.

3. Ross J Jr., Braunwald E. Aortic stenosis. *Circulation* 1968; 38(1 Suppl):61–7.

4. Bonow RO et al. Focused update incorporated into the ACC/AHA 2006 guidelines for the management of patients with valvular heart disease: A report of the American College of Cardiology/American Heart Association Task Force on Practice Guidelines (Writing Committee to revise the 1998 guidelines for the management of patients with valvular heart disease). Endorsed by the Society of Cardiovascular Anesthesiologists, Society for Cardiovascular Angiography and Interventions, and Society of Thoracic Surgeons. *J Am Coll Cardiol* 2008;52(13):e1–142.

5. Vahanian A et al. Guidelines on the management of valvular heart disease: The Task Force on the Management of Valvular Heart Disease of the European Society of Cardiology. *Eur Heart J* 2007; 28(2):230–68.

6. Cribier A et al. Percutaneous transluminal valvuloplasty of acquired aortic stenosis in elderly patients: An alternative to valve replacement? *Lancet* 1986;1(8472):63–7.

7. Percutaneous balloon aortic valvuloplasty. Acute and 30-day follow-up results in 674 patients from the NHLBI Balloon Valvuloplasty Registry. *Circulation* 1991;84(6):2383–97.

8. McKay RG. The Mansfield Scientific Aortic Valvuloplasty Registry: Overview of acute hemodynamic results and procedural complications. *J Am Coll Cardiol* 1991;17(2):485–91.

9. Letac B, Gerber LI, Koning R. Insights on the mechanism of balloon valvuloplasty in aortic stenosis. *Am J Cardiol* 1988;62(17):1241–7.

10. Letac B et al. Evaluation of restenosis after balloon dilatation in adult aortic stenosis by repeat catheterization. *Am Heart J* 1991;122(1 Pt 1): 55–60.

11. Ben-Dor I et al. Complications and outcome of balloon aortic valvuloplasty in high-risk or inoperable patients. *JACC Cardiovasc Interv* 2010;3(11):1150–6.

12. O'Keefe JH Jr et al. Natural history of candidates for balloon aortic valvuloplasty. *Mayo Clin Proc* 1987;62(11):986–91.

13. Otto CM et al. Three-year outcome after balloon aortic valvuloplasty. Insights into prognosis of valvular aortic stenosis. *Circulation* 1994;89(2):642–50.

14. Leon MB et al. Transcatheter aortic-valve implantation for aortic stenosis in patients who cannot undergo surgery. *N Engl J Med* 2010; 363(17):1597–607.

15. Smith CR et al. Transcatheter versus surgical aortic-valve replacement in high-risk patients. *N Engl J Med* 2011;364(23):2187–98.

16. Sack S et al. Revival of an old method with new techniques: Balloon aortic valvuloplasty of the calcified aortic stenosis in the elderly. *Clin Res Cardiol* 2008;97(5):288–97.

17. Witzke C et al. Impact of rapid ventricular pacing during percutaneous balloon aortic valvuloplasty in patients with critical aortic stenosis: Should we be using it? *Catheter Cardiovasc Interv* 2010; 75(3):444–52.

18. Block PC, Palacios IF. Comparison of hemodynamic results of anterograde versus retrograde percutaneous balloon aortic valvuloplasty. *Am J Cardiol* 1987;60(8):659–62.

19. Svensson LG et al. Aortic valve and ascending aorta guidelines for management and quality measures. *Ann Thorac Surg* 2013;95(6 Suppl):S1–66.

20. Letac B et al. Results of percutaneous transluminal valvuloplasty in 218 adults with valvular aortic stenosis. *Am J Cardiol* 1988;62(9):598–605.

21. Agarwal A et al. Results of repeat balloon valvuloplasty for treatment of aortic stenosis in patients aged 59 to 104 years. *Am J Cardiol* 2005; 95(1):43–7.

22. Klein A et al. Long-term mortality, cause of death, and temporal trends in complications after percutaneous aortic balloon valvuloplasty for calcific aortic stenosis. *J Interv Cardiol* 2006;19(3): 269–75.

23. Berland J et al. Percutaneous balloon valvuloplasty in patients with severe aortic stenosis and low ejection fraction. Immediate results and 1-year follow-up. *Circulation* 1989;79(6):1189–96.

25

Aortic valve stenosis in the elderly: Transcatheter aortic valve implantation—Edwards SAPIEN valve

Sa'ar Minha, Ron Waksman, and Augusto D. Pichard

Introduction

Aortic stenosis in the elderly is one of the most common valvular diseases and is associated with increased risk for morbidity and mortality. For decades, surgery was the standard therapeutic option for symptomatic patients with severe aortic stenosis. Transcatheter aortic valve replacement (TAVR) has evolved to be an acceptable therapeutic alternative for specific patient populations with severe symptomatic aortic stenosis. After successful animal experiences, the first TAVR in man was performed by Cribier et al. in 2002,[1] which initiated the research and development of various TAVR systems.

Edwards SAPIEN transcatheter heart valve

The SAPIEN transcatheter heart valve (THV) is composed of a stainless-steel stent, valve tissue (trileaflet bovine pericardium), and a polyethylene terephthalate fabric cuff, and is available in two sizes—23 and 26 mm. Prior to a procedure, the valve is manually mounted over a designated delivery system (RetroFlex 3 for transfemoral/Ascendra for transapical). This delivery system includes a catheter ("pusher") with a steerable distal portion that enables delivery though the aortic arch and a balloon catheter within it. The valve is mounted and crimped over this balloon at the tip of the catheter. The system also includes a designated hydrophilically coated sheath with two sheath sizes 22 F (for the 23 mm valve) and 24 F (for the 26 mm valve). Currently, the SAPIEN valve is the only valve approved for clinical use in the United States for inoperable or high-risk patients. SAPIEN XT is the successor of the SAPIEN valve. It also includes trileaflet bovine pericardium with improved durability and hemodynamic profile mounted on a cobalt–chromium frame. This device utilized the NovaFlex delivery system. In this system, the valve is crimped off the balloon, which allows a smaller profile, and the actual mounting over the balloon is performed prior to delivery *in vivo*. The SAPIEN XT system has 23, 26, and 29 mm valve sizes (and on a limited basis, a 20-mm valve), and is delivered through e-sheaths 16/18/20 F respectively. The SAPIEN 3 (balloon-expandable) and Centera (self-expanding) valves are the most recent versions of the Edwards THV system. These can be delivered through a 14F expandable sheath (e-sheath), and have a special skirt around the valve designated to minimize or eliminate perivalvular leak (PVL).[2]

Patient selection

Ample scientific data exist to support the use of these valve systems to treat specific patient subsets (see Chapter 23). Patient selection is an essential part of any TAVR program. Meticulous screening may assist in determining eligibility, access route, and complication avoidance. The initial screening process should focus on assessing the patient's overall risk and the likelihood of the patient returning to active life once aortic stenosis is no longer present. Although equivocal in their ability to predict outcome in TAVR, the Society of Thoracic Surgeons (STS) score and LogisticEuro score are both validated means of assessing the risk of a specific patient and should be calculated for every patient to create a common baseline for defining the patient as low, intermediate, or high risk. This is usually followed by a thorough evaluation by a heart team. Cardiac surgeons, interventional cardiologists, clinical cardiologists, and members from other disciplines are involved in the risk definition process. The "eyeball" test (the ability to predict the outcome by looking at the patient's nutritional and functional status) is an important test for correctly defining the risk, and is not reflected in the STS/LogisticEuro scores. Other frailty indices (e.g., 15 foot walk test, average grip strength) are also routinely used in the overall assessment. The trials have shown that there is a group of patients with multiple comorbidities that do not benefit from TAVR, and remain disabled by their other comorbidities. Those should be excluded from this therapy.

The next step of assessing for eligibility includes multiple imaging modalities. Echocardiography has been used as the gold standard for defining the severity of aortic stenosis and is confirmed by hemodynamic evaluation. Coronary angiography, left ventriculography, and aortography are also performed. A 4F pigtail is left in the abdominal aorta and the patient is then sent to the CT suite for a CT of the abdominal aorta/iliac vessels: this is performed with 10 cc of diluted contrast injected through the pigtail; excellent images are obtained with minimal contrast use.[3] Transfemoral eligibility assessment routinely begins by observing the noncontrast images. This allows appreciation of the degree, extent, and distribution of calcification. External and internal iliac bifurcation should be carefully evaluated since this is usually a nonmobile segment prone for dissection and perforation. Artery diameter is then evaluated in small cross sections from the aorta down to the femoral arteries. Even if the diameters seem adequate, tortuosity and calcification affect the final decision for safe femoral access. If noncalcified severe tortuosity is straightened by a wire, it usually signifies the possibility to use such a vessel for transfemoral access. We have learned to be very conservative on the assessment of iliac dimensions for percutaneous access. If sheath advancement meets significant resistance, we abort that site for access to prevent possible vascular complication. Puncture site should also be planned with 2D and 3D CT analysis: we choose a relatively long segment of the common femoral arteries, free of anterior calcification and branches.

For years, intraprocedural transesophageal echocardiography (TEE) was used to make the final decision regarding the valve size. The determination of valve size was based on the diameter of the annulus that was best visualized on TEE. Data accumulated over the years had demonstrated that the aortic valve annulus is an oval structure in at least 40% of patients, which makes a single annulus diameter measurement unreliable. This explains why some patients would end up with significant paravalvular leak or rarely with annular rupture. Nowadays, the gold standard is to measure the annulus dimensions, including area, diameters, and perimeter by CT, MRI, or 3D TEE, and the data have confirmed improved outcomes by selecting the valve size based on these measurements. All these initial screening assessment steps are performed in a day and a consensus decision of the heart team is completed that day or the following morning.

"Tips and tricks" in delivering the SAPIEN system

Catheterization lab setup

The "cath" lab should be set up with a designated space for an anesthesiologist, transesophageal echo, and a cardiopulmonary bypass machine. Hybrid rooms are ideal for this purpose, but not always available and so are large-sized detectors. Multiple display monitors allow for simultaneous displays of fluoroscopy alongside hemodynamic tracings, electrocardiography, echo, road maps, anesthesia parameters, and so on. The cath lab should be equipped with "emergency tool kits"—this includes a backup pacemaker, kit for emergent thoracotomy, vascular balloons and covered stents, pericardiocentesis kit, and coronary stent for emergent revascularization. TAVR can be safely performed under conscious sedation without the need for general anesthesia, leading to a shorter stay in the intensive care unit and shorter hospitalization.[4] Most times, a cardiac anesthesiologist manages the conscious sedation, and is prepared for intubation in the rare occasion of a complication; this avoids the complications of general anesthesia while maintaining the ability to get some feedback from the patient; for instance, severe abdominal pain felt by the patients while advancing the dilators or sheath usually signifies an impending vascular complication and one should not advance the catheter further.

Gaining access: Transfemoral approach

Vascular access-related issues are one of the most common complications of TAVR. Prevention of vascular complication dictates meticulous screening, procedure planning, and constant intraprocedural awareness. Access is first obtained from the contralateral side by utilizing the micropuncture technique under angiographic guidance and a 7 F sheath is introduced into the common femoral artery. After crossover to the ipsilateral side, a steelcore (Abbott Vascular, Abbott Park, IL, USA) or V-18 control wire (Boston Scientific, Natick, MA, USA) (0.018) is placed distal to the designated potential puncture site. These wires may be used for occluding balloons, stent grafts, or other techniques to handle vascular complications.

After crossover, an injection into the contralateral femoral is performed with digital subtraction. This "road map" is used to puncture the vessel at the ideal site. After initial access to the artery with a micropuncture, a J-tipped Terumo wire is advanced in the aorta and closure devices are applied. We mostly use two ProGlides but ProStar can also be utilized successfully. Prior to the introduction of the first dilator, the skin and subcutaneous tissues should be dilated with scalpel and hemostat; some vascular experts recommend that one should be able to insert the pinkie finger into the incision site. A set of dilators is then used to create a suitable track for sheath. After the first dilator, the Terumo wire is replaced by a superstiff wire—Amplatzer wire (Boston Scientific, Natick, MA, USA). Special care must be taken in patients with severely calcified and torturous arteries. If there is resistance advancing a dilator, fluoroscopy should be used to ensure that it is not displacing the entire iliac/aorta as it encounters calcification: if this is noted, a different access route needs to be chosen. Temporary pacing wire is placed through the femoral vein or the internal jugular vein. Either a balloon-tipped or a screw-in pacemaker may be used. In either case, the catheter is advanced in the right anterior oblique (RAO) projection toward the right ventricle; then left anterior oblique (LAO) projection is used to ensure that the pacer tip is pointing toward the interventricular septum and not the right ventricle (RV) free wall;[5] this simple maneuver prevents potential tamponade from RV perforation by the pacemaker.

Sinus alignment, valve crossing, and valvuloplasty

We perform a rotational aortogram to define the optimal projection for sinus alignment. The goal is to find the angulation that aligns all three valve leaflets (Figure 25.1). Diluted contrast (25 cc) is injected during RV pacing, and

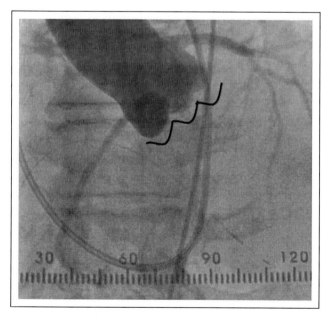

Figure 25.1 Leaflet alignment on an angiography. The three coronary leaflets are aligned by using rotational aortography. This is usually achieved on caudal RAO projection.

the detector is rotated from about 20° RAO to 20° LAO in 12° of caudal projection (Video 25.1). Several other options are available (prior CT, Paieon, Navigator, etc.) to determine optimal sinus alignment. Magnified straight RAO projection is used to direct a catheter to be 1 inch above the valve. FR catheter is the initial catheter followed by AL1 and AR1. A straight Terumo wire is directed toward the valve opening prior to crossing attempts. By watching for wire vibration during systole, the valve opening is identified, and the wire is advanced during systole, ideally without having touched the valve (Video 25.2). This minimized the risk of damage to the calcified aortic valve and the risk of mobilizing particles. In the case of bradycardic patients, pacing the patient to 80 beats/min can also assist in crossing the valve by shortening diastole. After successful crossing, the catheter is advanced down to the left ventricle (LV) and the stiff Amplatzer wire is placed in the LV. This often requires a pigtail for optimal location in the LV cavity. Both valvuloplasty and valve deployment are performed over this stiff wire looped in the LV; Amplatzer extrastiff or Superstiff (Boston Scientific) are commonly used. A large loop in the LV or a smaller loop at the apex can be used (Figure 25.2). Valvuloplasty has been performed in most cases before implantation of the stent valve, but recent data suggest that it may not always be necessary. The benefit is usually seen in extremely critical stenosis, in which the valvuloplasty balloon assists crossing with the prosthesis, and further allows adequate blood flow around the device during positioning. We use 20 mm balloons and avoid larger sizes. Contrast injection during valvuloplasty is occasionally utilized to assess the potential sealing with a specific balloon size. It is also used to evaluate for possible coronary obstruction in cases with long leaflets and bulky calcification.

Valve deployment

Prior to deployment, the valve is crimped over the balloon (SAPIEN) or proximal to the balloon (XT and S3) *ex vivo* and advanced over the stiff wire. Slow retroflection of the delivery catheter is used to facilitate atraumatic advancement through the arch and crossing the valve. We usually compress the common carotids while the valve assembly crosses the arch and the valve to minimize particle embolization to the brain (Video 25.3). New deflectors and filters are now being evaluated to protect the cerebral circulation. Thanks to the newer valve system nose cones, crossing the valve became easier. Extreme force should not be applied during native valve crossing since this may lead to annulus rupture. When the prosthesis is engaged in between leaflets and cannot be further advanced into the LV, we inflate the distal end of the balloon with 1 cc, to "disengage" and assist in crossing. The recommendation

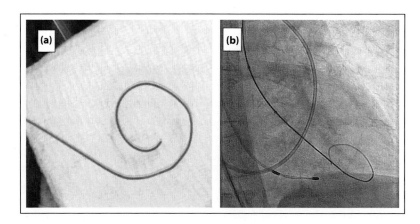

Figure 25.2 Stiff-wire shaping. (a) Small loop is shaped at the tip of the stiff wire. (b) Wire position at the apex.

for deployment of the Edwards valve is (in percentage) 50/50 above and below the annulus and we did this for the first few years. More recently, we chose to place the valve 70/30 or 80/20 above and below the annulus. This way the valve is well anchored in the calcified annulus, and does not stent the LV outflow tract. Low valve deployment is more hazardous than high as each diastole continues to push the valve toward the LV and could lead to embolization. Inflation of the balloon and valve deployment is performed using a "two-step deployment";[6] first, the patient is paced at 180/min to achieve blood pressure <40–50 mm Hg. The valve is inflated partially, the aorta is filled with contrast, and final adjustment of the valve position is obtained while inflation is slowly completed (Video 25.4). Full balloon inflation is maintained for 5 s to obtain maximal expansion. Pacing is not stopped until the balloon is fully deflated so as to prevent the balloon ejecting the valve. While the wire is still positioned at the apex and the system is retracted to the ascending aorta, TEE images are obtained for confirming the position of the valve and, more importantly, evaluating the degree of PVL. If no significant PVL exists, the wire is pulled to allow better echocardiographic assessment of the valve function. The wire is pulled out of the LV earlier if there is persistent hypotension. We have found that the stiff wire can push on the MV apparatus, induce severe MR, and facilitate severe hypotension. Even a mild degree of PVL leak may be associated with an increased risk for mortality; thus, efforts are made to minimize those leaks. Consensus exists regarding the need to treat significant PVL.[7] This can be accomplished by reballooning (utilizing the readily available SAPIEN balloon). If PVL is severe, and attributed to malposition of the valve, a second valve within the first implanted valve (valve-in-valve procedure) becomes necessary. Aortic insufficiency index ((aortic end diastolic pressure – left ventricular end diastolic pressure)/aortic end systolic pressure) >25 signifies

adequate function, while an index <25 suggests significant AR beyond valve function. Echocardiography at this point (ideally, TEE) is utilized to exclude new wall motion abnormalities and pericardial effusion. Postprocedural gradients are then recorded by cautiously crossing the prosthetic valve.

Vascular access closure

Vascular access closure is initiated by pulling the sheath and tying both perclose knots, with a Terumo wire still in the vessel. There is also a crossover wire placed at the beginning of the procedure from the other femoral. Manual pressure is applied if bleeding persists. If this still persists, we often add a single Angio-seal (St. Jude Medical, St. Paul, MN, USA). This approach usually leads to hemostasis. A final femoral angiography is then performed to exclude perforation or stenosis. If perforation is noted, a peripheral angioplasty balloon is brought over the crossover wire and left inflated for 3–5 min, with excellent results most of the time. If bleeding persists, a covered stent may be deployed to treat this complication.[8] We no longer use protamine due to the risk for thrombosis. In the case of a significant, flow-limiting stenosis, an attempt to improve flow should be pursued with the peripheral balloon and, if needed, a stent should be further deployed.

References

1. Cribier A, Eltchaninoff H, Bash A et al. Percutaneous transcatheter implantation of an aortic valve prosthesis for calcific aortic stenosis: First human case description. *Circulation* 2002;106(24):3006–8.
2. Binder RK, Rodes-Cabau J, Wood DA, et al. Transcatheter aortic valve replacement with the SAPIEN 3: A new balloon-expandable transcatheter heart valve. *JACC Cardiovasc Interv* 2013;6(3):293–300.
3. Joshi SB, Mendoza DD, Steinberg DH, et al. Ultra-low-dose intra-arterial contrast injection for iliofemoral computed tomographic angiography. *JACC Cardiovasc Imaging* 2009;2(12):1404–11.

4. Ben-Dor I, Looser PM, Maluenda G et al. Transcatheter aortic valve replacement under monitored anesthesia care versus general anesthesia with intubation. *Cardiovasc Revasc Med: Including Mol Interv* 2012;13(4):207–10.

5. Barbash IM, Waksman R, Pichard AD. Prevention of right ventricular perforation due to temporary pacemaker lead during transcatheter aortic valve replacement. *JACC Cardiovasc Interv* 2013;6(4):427.

6. Nijhoff F, Agostoni P, Samim M et al. Optimisation of transcatheter aortic balloon-expandable valve deployment: The two-step inflation technique. *EuroIntervention: J EuroPCR Collab Working Group Interv Cardiol Eur Soc Cardiol* 2013;9(5):555–63.

7. Hayashida K, Lefevre T, Chevalier B et al. Impact of post-procedural aortic regurgitation on mortality after transcatheter aortic valve implantation. *JACC Cardiovasc Interv* 2012;5(12):1247–56.

8. Toggweiler S, Leipsic J, Binder RK et al. Management of vascular access in transcatheter aortic valve replacement: Part 2: Vascular complications. *JACC Cardiovasc Interv* 2013;6(8):767–76.

26

Aortic valve stenosis in the elderly: Transcatheter aortic valve implantation—CoreValve

Eberhard Grube, Georg Nickenig, Nikos Werner, and Jan-Malte Sinning

Introduction

The Medtronic CoreValve ReValving System (Medtronic, Minneapolis, MN, USA) consists of a self-expanding niti-nol frame, which is implanted in a sutureless fashion using oversizing to anchor the prosthesis at the level of the aortic annulus. The nitinol stent frame holds a trileaflet porcine pericardial tissue valve. The current third generation of the CoreValve is available in four sizes (23, 26, 29, and 31 mm) for annulus diameters from 18 to 29 mm (Figure 26.1) and is delivered using an 18 French implantation catheter.

The noncylindrical frame design of the CoreValve incorporates three different parts (Figure 26.2): the lower part (inflow portion) exerts a high radial force to anchor the prosthesis in the annulus of the native aortic valve and to mitigate paravalvular aortic regurgitation (PAR) by adaption to the native annulus. The middle part of the CoreValve holds the valve leaflets in a supra-annular position to

ensure proper valve functioning even if the inflow part of the valve is noncircular. The concave, hourglass-like shape of the frame avoids the coronary artery ostia and allows unimpeded coronary blood flow. The upper part (outflow portion) sits with low radial force in the ascending aorta and ensures an optimal alignment of the prosthesis during deployment.

The first human transcatheter aortic valve implantation (TAVI) using the self-expanding CoreValve was success-fully performed by Eberhard Grube in 2005 in a 73-year-old female patient who was declined surgical aortic valve replacement because of comorbidities.[1] While the first-generation CoreValve consisted of bovine pericardial tis-sue and had to be delivered via a 24 French transfemoral sheath with surgical cutdown, nowadays, the third-gen-eration porcine pericardial tissue CoreValve is implanted via an 18 French sheath in a completely percutaneous fash-ion—predominantly via transfemoral access. However, in

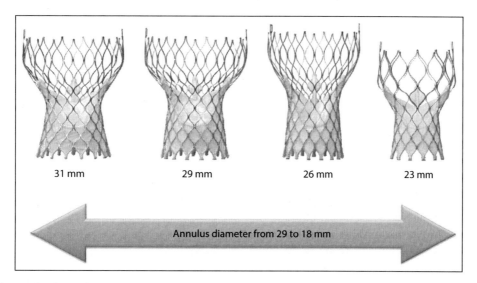

Figure 26.1 (**See color insert.**) Medtronic CoreValve Revalving System in four different sizes covering an aortic annulus diameter from 18 to 29 mm. (Courtesy of Medtronic, MN, USA. With permission.)

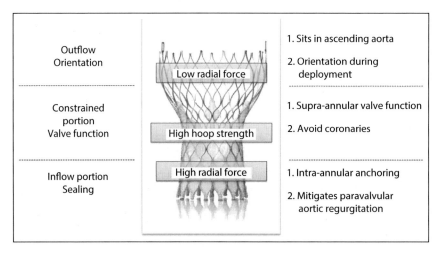

Figure 26.2   Different parts of the CoreValve system. (Courtesy of Medtronic, Minneapolis, MN, USA. With permission.)

patients with unsuitable transfemoral access, a CoreValve implantation can also be performed via transsubclavian or direct aortic access.

ADVANCE study

The results of the postmarket ADVANCE registry, in which 1015 extreme or high-risk patients with aortic stenosis undergoing TAVI with use of the Medtronic CoreValve prosthesis were enrolled from 44 centers in 12 countries between March 2010 and July 2011, were presented at the EuroPCR 2013 in Paris. All participating centers conducted at least 40 procedures prior to the study and had a heart team in place. This prospective registry showed a high procedural success rate of 97.5%.[2] At 30 days and 1 year, mortality rates were 4.5% and 17.9%, respectively. After TAVI, only 1.3% of the patients had to undergo emergent cardiac surgery or percutaneous reintervention during the first 30 days. A stroke after 30 days and 1 year occurred in 3.0% and 4.5% of the patients, respectively. At discharge, 16% of the patients suffered from more than mild PAR. In these patients, a trend toward higher 1-year mortality (21.2%; $p = 0.07$) was found.

Annulus sizing and valve selection

The dilemma before each TAVI procedure is the appropriate sizing of the dimensions of the aortic annulus and the choice not only of the correct size but also the transcatheter heart valve type (self-expanding vs. balloon expandable) that fits the given anatomy best. As oversizing plays a pivotal role for the fixation of the CoreValve in the annulus of the native valve, implantation depth and prosthesis size are

essential to reduce the rate and the severity of PAR. Thus, preprocedural three-dimensional imaging techniques are needed for detailed and accurate assessment of the aortic annulus and proper prosthesis sizing. Multislice computed tomography (MSCT) is the current gold standard for three-dimensional imaging of the aortic root and the annulus of the native aortic valve, as it in addition allows an assessment of the access vessels. A larger prosthesis size might improve postprocedural results in patients with a borderline annulus with lower risk for annular rupture than in balloon-expandable transcatheter heart valves (THVs). With respect to the mean diameter (preferably CT perimeter-based), an oversizing by more than 10% for the CoreValve seems to be associated with a lesser extent of PAR (Figure 26.3). If the stent frame of the valve is not fully expanded due to heavily calcified cusps of the native aortic valve, postdilation with a balloon aortic valvuloplasty catheter helps to reduce the severity of PAR in most cases.[3]

Valve size (mm)	Mean diameter (mm)	Perimeter (mm)	Cover index (%)
31	29	91	6
31	28	88	10
31	27	85	13
31	26	82	16
31	25	79	19
29	27	85	8
29	26	82	10
29	25	79	14
29	24	75	17
29	23	72	21
26	24	75	8
26	23	72	11
26	22	69	15
26	21	66	19
23	21	66	9
23	20	63	13
23	19	60	17
23	18	57	22

Figure 26.3   **(See color insert.)** CoreValve sizing according to computed tomography measurements.

CoreValve TAVI procedure

Before starting the procedure, a temporary pacing lead is advanced, preferably over the jugular vein of the patient, into the right ventricle to induce rapid ventricular pacing for balloon aortic valvuloplasty (BAV) during the procedure and to treat conduction disturbances after TAVR. For transfemoral access, both common femoral arteries have to be punctured: one for the introduction of the delivery catheter and the contralateral one for hemodynamic monitoring, aortic root angiography, and the placement of a pigtail catheter as landmark for the aortic annulus plane in the noncoronary sinus. After placement of a ProStar XL closure device (Abbott Vascular Laboratories, Abbott Park, IL, USA) or two ProGlide 10 French suture-mediated closure devices (Abbott Vascular Laboratories) for vessel closure after the procedure, an 18 French (inner diameter) sheath is inserted over an Amplatz Super Stiff wire. The Amplatz Super Stiff wire should be preshaped to the contours of the patient's left ventricle (LV) and should be placed over a pigtail catheter into the ventricle under fluoroscopic surveillance to prevent ventricular perforation. Then, the CoreValve bioprosthesis, which is crimped on an 18 French delivery catheter, can be advanced retrogradely across the native aortic valve.

For correct positioning and proper placement of the CoreValve, perpendicular alignment of the native aortic annulus with visualization of all three sinuses on a single plane is essential. A pigtail catheter, which is placed in the nadir of the noncoronary cusp, is used as reference target for the positioning and deployment of the valve and allows correct valve implantation even in the absence of calcium. Since the inflow part of the prosthesis, which is going to be placed into the aortic annulus and partly into the left ventricular outflow tract, is covered by a pericardial skirt with a height of 12 mm, the target implantation depth of the prosthesis should be between 4 and 6 mm (Figure 26.4). An implantation depth beyond 12 mm would lead to significant PAR.[3] In case of a too low implant ("too ventricular") of the CoreValve, the prosthesis is deployed at a depth that exceeds the height of its tissue skirt; the PAR jet passes above the skirt ("supra-skirt" PAR), from within the aortic portion of the stent frame into the paravalvular space and the left ventricular outflow tract (LVOT). In case of a too high implant ("too aortic"), the prosthesis is deployed partially above the native annulus; the PAR jet passes from the paravalvular space across the irregular inflow edge of the prosthesis into the LVOT ("infra-skirt" PAR). In addition, an implantation depth between 4 and 6 mm of the CoreValve prosthesis is associated with less occurrence of conduction disturbances and a significantly lower pacemaker rate after the procedure.

The current manufacturer recommend instructions for use of the BAV before crossing the native aortic valve with the delivery catheter and implanting the CoreValve device. However, clear evidence supporting BAV as mandatory part of the TAVI procedure is missing. A pilot trial has shown that TAVI without balloon predilation is feasible and safe and might be a promising approach not only to simplify the procedure but also to help prevent distal embolizations with subsequent stroke as well as atrioventricular conduction disturbances.[4]

The delivery catheter with the crimped CoreValve is advanced a few millimeters across the plane of the native aortic annulus as indicated by the pigtail catheter placed in the noncoronary sinus. Then, the C-arm angulation should

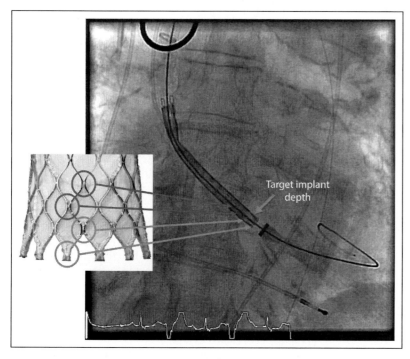

Figure 26.4 (See color insert.) CoreValve implantation starting at a target implantation depth of 4–6 mm.

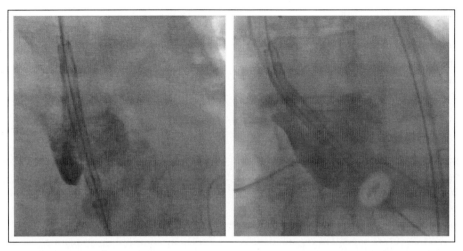

Figure 26.5 **(See color insert.)** Perfect implantation position is achieved when the radiopaque catheter marker ring near the nose cone appears as a straight line.

be adjusted to ensure that the valve is aligned coaxially within the annulus and is perpendicular to the basal plane. The perfect position is achieved when the radiopaque catheter marker ring near the nose cone appears as a straight line (Figure 26.5). However, another option is to stay in the plane, in which the three cusps of the native aortic valve are fully aligned. The implantation of the CoreValve should be started at a depth between the first and second marker band of the crimped CoreValve, which as the radiopaque lines indicate, are the joints of the diamond cell design of the nitinol frame and, thus, represent the first 4 mm of the prosthesis (Figure 26.4).

The implanter has to anticipate slight movement of the CoreValve toward the ventricle during the first third of the deployment—especially when the inflow portion of the prosthesis starts to flare (Figure 26.6). Therefore, one should release the valve very slowly during this first third in order to be able to precisely adjust the starting depth and to reposition the delivery catheter before full annular engagement of the CoreValve (Figure 26.7). In the initial phase of the flaring, there is no drop in blood pressure, since the blood flow across the native aortic valve is not completely obstructed at first. For the CoreValve 31 mm prosthesis, a very slow release is recommended during this step with frequent pauses to release radial force, which otherwise might pull the prosthesis down into the LVOT. Inspection of the relation of the lower-most "diamonds" of the nitinol frame and the pigtail in the nadir of the noncoronary cusp allows the operator to correct the position of the frame. The blood pressure will go down when the frame reaches the opposite side of the aortic root and gets full annular contact. Then, the deployment has to be continued more quickly to allow pressure recovery, while avoiding the CoreValve embolizing into the ascending aorta ("parachuting effect") during this step, which predominantly occurs with use of the CoreValve 31 mm prosthesis and in patients with a very hypertrophied LV. The

achievement of the optimal implantation depth of 4–6 mm especially depends on this part of the procedure (Figure 26.8). When the blood pressure has stabilized again, the position of the valve can be rechecked by aortic root angiography (Figure 26.9). If the CoreValve is too low, the first operator may exert gentle traction on the delivery catheter.

In larger anatomies, greater movement of the CoreValve during deployment has to be appreciated and pacing at a heart rate of 90–130 bpm can be considered. Controlled pacing might be helpful to increase valve stability during CoreValve deployment by controlling heart rhythm and especially preventing extrasystolic beats.

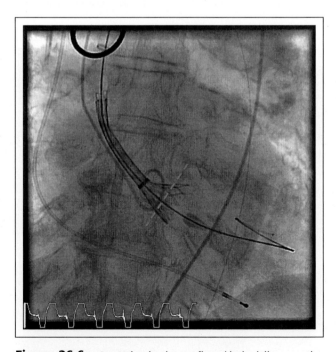

Figure 26.6 CoreValve begins to flare (dashed line = native aortic annulus plane).

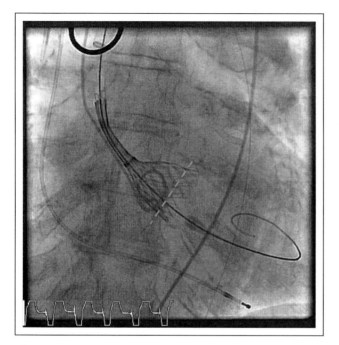

Figure 26.7 Full annular engagement of the CoreValve with consecutive low blood pressure.

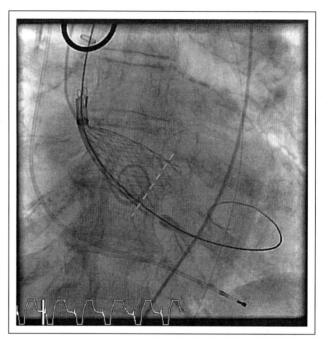

Figure 26.9   Pressure recovery after deployment of two-thirds of the CoreValve.

During deployment of the CoreValve, it is also important to understand foreshortening of the released nitinol frame as a potential contributor to minor movements, as it may cause the inflow portion of the frame to move up (2–3 mm) and it may pull the delivery catheter down (4–5 mm), creating tension in the system during the remainder of the deployment (Figure 26.10), when the frame is detached from the catheter. The position of the delivery catheter along the inner curvature of the aortic arch indicates the presence of tension in the system (Figure 26.10). If tension is present, it should be released just prior to the final valve release from the catheter by

releasing tension on the guide wire and slightly pushing on the catheter. After final release of the CoreValve with deattachment of both hooks from the delivery catheter, the catheter should be carefully removed without any force by gently pulling on the guide wire in order not to risk valve embolization by catheter retrieval.

Assessing paravalvular aortic regurgitation after corevalve implantation

The final position of the CoreValve and the degree of PAR can be assessed by aortography (Figure 26.11) (25–30 mL at a flow rate of 14–20 mL/s) and/or transesophageal echocardiography. In addition, aortography is important to verify the appearance of the coronary arteries to rule out unexpected coronary occlusion.

PAR can be classified according to the visually estimated density of opacification of the LV into three degrees adapted to the VARC-2 criteria: mild (reflow of contrast in the outflow tract and middle portion of the LV but clearing with each beat), moderate (reflow of contrast in the whole left ventricular cavity with incomplete washout in a single beat and faint opacification of the entire LV over several cardiac cycles), and severe (opacification of the entire LV with the same intensity as in the aorta and persistence of the contrast after a single beat). Using transesophageal echocardiography (TEE), it is desirable to measure the

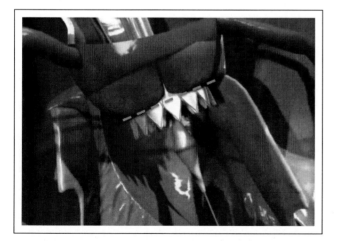

Figure 26.8 **(See color insert.)** Target implantation depth of 4–6 mm. (Courtesy of Medtronic, MN, USA. With permission.)

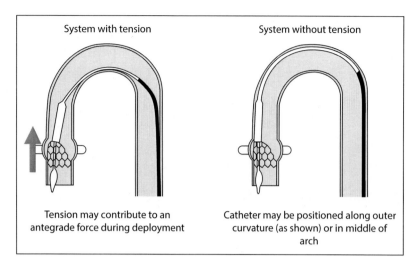

System with tension   System without tension

Tension may contribute to an   Catheter may be positioned along outer
antegrade force during deployment   curvature (as shown) or in middle of
                                       arch

Figure 26.10 Release of tension before full deployment of the CoreValve. (Courtesy of Medtronic, Minneapolis, MN, USA. With permission.)

circumferential extent of the jet in the short-axis view to identify patients with clinically significant PAR (<10%: mild, 10–29%: moderate, and ≥30%: severe PAR).[3]

In addition, the determination of hemodynamics after the procedure in the form of the aortic regurgitation (AR) index can be helpful to further evaluate the severity of PAR, especially in borderline cases.[5] The so-called AR index is the ratio of the transvalvular gradient between diastolic blood pressure (RR_{dia}) in the aorta and left ventricular end-diastolic pressure (LVEDP) to systolic blood pressure (RR_{sys}) in the aorta: $[(RR_{dia}–LVEDP)/RR_{sys}] \times 100$ (Figure 26.12). The AR index shows an inverse proportion to the severity of PAR and differentiates between patients suffering from mild, moderate, or severe PAR immediately after the procedure. A cutoff value of 25 independently predicts the associated 1-year mortality risk.[5]

The AR index cutoff value can be used as part of standardized algorithm to assess and treat PAR after TAVR: If no PAR is present, no other measures have to be taken. In all other cases with mild to severe PAR, the determination of the AR index is helpful to more precisely quantify the extent of PAR and to have a point of reference before corrective measures are taken. In patients with more-than-mild PAR and/or an AR index <25, the evaluation of PAR by echocardiography, preferably TEE, is recommended to elucidate the etiology of PAR and its mechanism. When corrective measures have been taken in patients with clinically significant PAR, the severity of PAR can be reevaluated by imaging modalities and the AR index.[3]

Corrective measures to reduce PAR after corevalve implantation

Several corrective measures have been proposed to overcome significant residual PAR following TAVR. However, data on these measures predominantly originate from small series or case reports and the impact of corrective measures for the reduction of PAR on long-term outcome and especially valve durability still has to be clarified in future studies.

Balloon postdilation is an option to reduce the degree of PAR by obtaining a better expansion of the prosthesis stent frame and a better sealing of the paravalvular space if the CoreValve has been deployed at correct implantation depth. The size of the balloon for postdilation should conform to the aortic annulus dimension and not exceed the maximum diameter of the native aortic valve. For the CoreValve prosthesis, a straight valvuloplasty balloon with a maximum

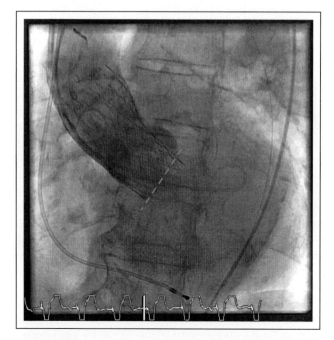

Figure 26.11 Aortography after full release of the CoreValve to assess the degree of paravalvular aortic regurgitation after TAVI and to check whether the coronary artery ostia are obstructed.

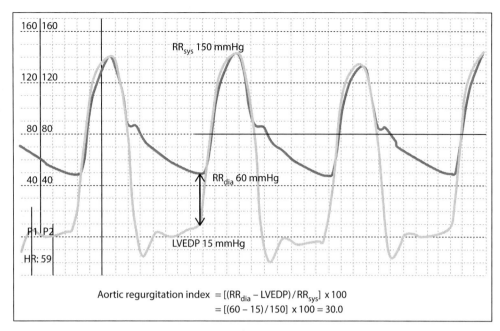

Figure 26.12 (**See color insert.**) Calculation of the aortic regurgitation index. LVEDP = left ventricular end-diastolic pressure; RR_{dia} = diastolic blood pressure in the aorta; RR_{sys} = systolic blood pressure in the aorta.

diameter of 22, 25, 28, and 29 mm is recommended for the 23, 26, 29, and 31 mm CoreValve, respectively.[3]

The Snare technique represents an option worth considering for a too deeply implanted CoreValve (too "ventricular" placement of the prosthesis). In this case, correction of the device position may be achieved by engaging one of the anchoring hooks and pulling with a snare catheter. To increase the leverage effect, the snaring maneuver can be performed via transbrachial access. However, this corrective maneuver is not without hazards (e.g., aortic dissection) and bears the potential risk of CoreValve embolization into the ascending aorta.[3]

For a malpositioned CoreValve with too shallow ("too aortic") or too deep ("too ventricular") implantation of the prosthesis, valve-in-valve implantation is a viable treatment strategy to reduce significant PAR and to prevent bailout cardiac surgery. The second valve can be deployed in a way that the sealing pericardial skirts of both valves overlap and the second CoreValve ensures sealing with the native valve annulus. Thus, initial procedural failure can be converted into procedural success in up to 90% of the attempts, and valve-in-valve implantation results in comparable hemodynamic results with satisfactory short- and midterm outcomes. In addition, the valve-in-valve technique is a viable treatment option for significant transvalvular AR due to severe prosthetic leaflet dysfunction and has important implications for patients who develop late failure of THVs, also in case of restenosis, as a "re-do" procedure. However, one major drawback of THV-in-THV implantation with the CoreValve is the restricted access

to the coronary ostia. In the near future, repositionability and retrievability will be addressed by the next generation CoreValve Evolut R and help to reduce the occurrence of malpositioning.[3]

Future TAVI improvements will be driven by improved procedural technique and postprocedure patient management, product innovations such as the repositionable CoreValve Evolut R, and expansion to new patient populations such as valve-in-valve implantation for degenerated surgical aortic valves and TAVI in patients with pure AR without stenosis and calcified degeneration of the native aortic valve. The ADVANCE registry showed that the CoreValve can be used for TAVI in real world (high-risk) patients with a high procedural success rate. The results of the randomized CoreValve US Pivotal Trial are eagerly awaited and might help to further expand the indications for treatment with the CoreValve.

Conclusions

- Annulus sizing is one of the most important steps for CoreValve implantation.
- Direct TAVI (no BAV) may be associated with fewer complications (stroke, pacemaker implantation rate, cardiac failure).
- Always aim at a high implantation in order to decrease the risk for pacemaker implantation and PAR.
- Careful assessment and treatment of PAR is mandatory to improve outcome of patients.

References

1. Grube E, Laborde JC, Zickmann B, Gerckens U, Felderhoff T, Sauren B et al. First report on a human percutaneous transluminal implantation of a self-expanding valve prosthesis for interventional treatment of aortic valve stenosis. *Catheter Cardiovasc Interv.* 2005;66:465–9.

2. Linke A, Bleiziffer S, Bosmans J, Gerckens U, Wenaweser P, Brecker S et al. on behalf of the ADVANCE Investigators. One Year Outcomes in Real World Patients Treated with Transcatheter Aortic Valve Implantation. The ADVANCE Study. EuroPCR 2013, Paris, France.

3. Sinning JM, Vasa-Nicotera M, Chin DT, Hammersting C, Ghanem A, Bence J et al. Evaluation and management of paravalvular aortic regurgitation after transcatheter aortic valve replacement. *J Am Coll Cardiol.* 2013;62:11–20.

4. Grube E, Naber C, Abizaid A, Sousa E, Mendiz O, Lemos P et al. Feasibility of transcatheter aortic valve implantation without balloon pre-dilation. *JACC Cardiovasc Interv.* 2011;4:751–7.

5. Sinning JM, Hammerstingl C, Vasa-Nicotera M, Adenauer V, Lema Cachiguango SJ, Scheer AC et al. Aortic regurgitation index defines severity of peri-prosthetic regurgitation and predicts outcome in patients after transcatheter aortic valve implantation. *J Am Coll Cardiol.* 2012;59:1134–41.

27

Aortic valve stenosis in the elderly: Valve-in-valve implantations

Azeem Latib and Antonio Colombo

Bioprosthetic heart valves are increasingly being used in preference to a mechanical valve in younger adult patients, and have been associated with comparable long-term survival.[1-6] The major advantage of tissue valves is that there is no need for long-term anticoagulation with its inherent risks of bleeding and thromboembolism.[2,3,5,6] However, the trade-off is an increased risk of late reoperation due to structural degeneration, which progressively increases with time.[1,3,6,7] Reoperation is the current standard of care for bioprosthetic failure but can be associated with significant risk, which is escalated further by older age and the concomitant comorbidity often associated with these patients, such as left ventricular dysfunction, renal insufficiency, pulmonary hypertension, and the need for a concurrent cardiac procedure. The operative mortality for an elective redo aortic valve surgery is reported to range from 2% to 7%, but this percentage can increase to more than 30% in high-risk patients.[8,9] Furthermore, redo surgery can be associated with significant morbidity such as blood transfusions, renal failure, wound infection, postoperative pain, and delayed recovery.[1,10] As more younger patients are successfully treated with tissue valves and their life expectancy continues to increase, we will be faced with a growing number of degenerated bioprostheses requiring reoperation.[11]

Transcatheter heart valve (THV) implantation with the valve-in-valve (VIV) technique is emerging as a feasible, reproducible, and low-risk treatment option in high-risk or inoperable patients with degenerated tissue valves.[1-4,11] The VIV technique consists of implanting an Edwards SAPIEN THV (Edwards Lifesciences, Irvine, California) or Medtronic CoreValve Revalving System (Medtronic, Minneapolis, Minnesota) inside the degenerated surgical bioprosthesis. Although not primarily designed for this application, percutaneous VIV implantation offers a minimally invasive alternative to conventional redo surgery, by avoiding redo sternotomy, cardiotomy, valve excision, and cardiopulmonary bypass.[1,3] It also results in considerable hemodynamic improvement, including an immediate decrease in valve gradients and aortic regurgitation grade. As will be explained in detail in this chapter, the VIV procedure is potentially a technically simpler TAVI procedure because the existing bioprosthesis provides a well-defined circular landing zone of known diameter, is often radiopaque and thus the procedure can be performed without contrast media, and there is a limited risk of conduction disorder or paravalvular leak. However, the successful outcome of this procedure is highly dependent on patient selection, a thorough understanding of the design and structure of the degenerated bioprosthesis, anticipation of complications, procedural planning, and a multidisciplinary team approach. It is presumed that the team performing a VIV procedure is experienced in TAVI and thus the general aspects of THV implantation will not be discussed in this chapter.

Primer on surgical bioprostheses and their mechanisms of failure

Identifying the type and size of bioprosthesis is mandatory for planning and ensuring an optimal outcome of a VIV procedure. Knowledge of the type and dimensions of the bioprosthesis will determine the landing zone, implantation technique, risk of complications, and the size of the implanted THV. As a general rule, surgical bioprosthetic valves may be either stented or stentless. Valve leaflets can be of xenograft (specifically, porcine aortic valve or bovine pericardium) or homograft origin.

Stented valves: Stented valves are typically constructed using a base ring that is covered by a fabric sewing cuff and from which a stent or frame (with three struts or stent posts) arises at a right angle to support the valve leaflets.[1,12] The support structures are composed of various alloys or plastics (which may or may not be radiopaque) that are designed to absorb the forces on the leaflets and maintain structural integrity. The base (sewing) ring may be circular or scalloped-shaped and is sutured to the native aortic annulus at an intra- or supra-annular position during surgical implantation. This circular ring provides the most reliable anchor to the THV device and determines how much a THV can expand.[1,8,12]

Manufacturer sizing and labeling of surgical bioprostheses are not standardized and vary by manufacturer. Indeed, even internal diameters vary for a given labeled size. As a result, in Table 27.1, we have attempted to summarize the dimensions of all the commonly available stented valves. For stented valves, there are three important dimensions to consider as regards VIV procedures: (1) the manufacturer's label size corresponds to the outer stent diameter; (2) the inner stent diameter is the most relevant for VIV as it determines the size of the THV chosen; and

(3) prosthesis height in order to predict the risk of coronary occlusion and location of a nonradiopaque sewing ring. However, it should be remembered that the internal diameter provided by the manufacturer is the diameter before the valve leaflets are sewn in. Thus, the "actual internal diameter" of a given bioprosthesis will be always lower than the internal diameter provided. As pointed out by Bapat et al., the actual internal diameter measured by a Hegar dilator is 1–3 mm smaller than the internal diameter on the chart depending on the make and model.[8,12] Calcification of the leaflets and pannus ingrowth may further reduce the internal diameter. These factors need to be taken into consideration when choosing a THV device for a VIV procedure.

Stentless valves: Stentless valves, as the name implies, do not have a stent/frame or base ring and are sutured to the root in the position of a native valve. Although stentless valves have more laminar flow and lower postoperative

Table 27.1 Manufacturer, model, label size, and corresponding internal diameter and height of surgical stent bioprostheses

Stented bioprostheses		Internal diameter across labeled sizes/valve height (mm)						
Manufacturer	Model/labeled size	19	21	23	25	27	29	31
Medtronic	Mosaic®	17.5/13.5	18.5/15.0	20.5/16.0	22.5/17.5	24/18.5	26/20.0	
Medtronic	Hancock® II		18.5/15.0	20.5/16.0	22.5/17.5	24/18.5	26/20.0	
Medtronic	Hancock® Modified Orifice (M.O.) 250	16/17	18/18.5	20/19.5	21.8/21.25			
Medtronic	Hancock® Porcine Bioprosthesis "Standard"			20/17.25	21.8/18.75	22.3/20	24.1/21.25	26/22.75
Edwards	Perimount 2700	18/13	20/14	22/15	24/16	26/17	28/18	
Edwards	Perimount 2800/2900	18/14	20/15	22/16	24/17	26/18	28/19	
Edwards	Perimount Magna 3000	18/14	20/15	22/16	24/17	26/18	28/19	
Edwards	Perimount Magna Ease 3300	18/13	20/14	22/15	24/16	26/17	28/18	
Edwards	Carpentier–Edwards Porcine Bioprosthesis 2625	17/15	19/16	21/16	23/18	25/18	27/19	29/19
Edwards	Carpentier–Edwards S.A.V.[a]	17[a]/14	19/15	21/16	23/17	25/17	27[a]/18	
Sorin	Mitroflow LX	15.4/11	17.3/13	19/14	21/15	22.9/16		
Sorin	Mitroflow Model 12	15.4/11	17.3/13	19/14	21/15	22.9/16	24.7[a]/16.4	
SJM	Biocor		19/14	21/15	23/16	25/17	27/19	
SJM	Biocor Supra[b]	19/14	21/15	23/16				
	Epic		19/14	21/15	23/16	25/17	27/19	
	Epic Supra[b]	19/14	19/14	21/15	23/16	25/17	27/19	
SJM	Trifecta	17/15	19/16	21/17	23/18	25/19		
		20	21	23	25	27		
Vascutek	Aspire[a]	18.2/16	19.2/16	21/17	23/118	25/18		
		18	20	22	24	26	28	
Sorin	Soprano[a,b]	17.8/12	19.8/14	21.7/15	23.7/16	25.6/18	27.6/19	

[a] Not available in the United States.
[b] Labeled size taken from internal diameter.

gradients, they have not been associated with better clinical outcomes as compared with stented valves.[5] Also, some stentless valves can be associated with excessive calcification of the aortic root, thus increasing the complexity of reoperation. Generally, the labeled size of a stentless valve corresponds to its outer diameter. In the absence of a rigid base ring or stent, the only relevant dimensions are its inner and outer diameters. Furthermore, the lack of a frame for anchoring the THV and the absence of radiopaque markers makes VIV procedures for stentless valves more challenging.

Correct positioning and deployment of a THV inside a surgical bioprosthesis requires correct radiographic recognition. Stented valves are identified by recognizing the radiopaque components of the base ring and/or stent on fluoroscopy.[1,12] The fluoroscopic appearance of all the commercially available surgical bioprostheses has been extensively described by Piazza et al. and Bapat et al. and can now be downloaded as smartphone apps.[1,12] Stentless valves, on the other hand, do not have any radiopaque components. With either valve type, calcifications may help with identifying the margins and location of the prosthesis. However, attention needs to be given to the exact location of the calcifications as they may not always identify the annulus or valve ring.

Bioprosthetic valve failure can be the result of calcification, wear and tear, pannus formation, thrombosis, and/or endocarditis.[1,10] Leaflet tissue deterioration, whether calcific or noncalcific, is the major cause of bioprosthetic valve failure. In general, failure due to calcification, pannus formation, or thrombus results in valvular stenosis, and failure due to leaflet destruction (endocarditis) or paravalvular leak results in regurgitation. In failure due to wear and tear, which is frequently associated with calcification and abnormal leaflet coaptation, mixed stenosis/regurgitation is common.[5] The mechanism of degeneration may have an impact on THV sizing. A regurgitant valve with torn leaflets may have a larger internal diameter as compared with a stenotic valve with prominent pannus or calcification. Finally, the mechanism of degeneration will determine the implantation technique (if regurgitant, then rapid pacing is mandatory even for CoreValve) and possibly even long-term outcome (stenosis worse than regurgitation).

Preprocedural screening and planning

We recommend multimodality imaging, including echocardiography and particularly multislice computed tomography (MSCT), in all patients to evaluate (1) the severity and mode of bioprosthetic failure; (2) the peripheral vasculature in order to determine the implantation approach; (3) the aortic root anatomy and bioprosthesis dimensions to facilitate sizing, positioning, and strategic planning of the THV implantation; and (4) anatomic location of coronary vessels or bypass grafts and the relation of the coronary and graft ostia to the bioprosthesis.

THV sizing and the prediction of complications such as malposition or coronary occlusion are particularly relevant for VIV implantation. In particular, the operator needs to take into account the reported internal diameter, bulkiness of the degenerated valve, nature of the valve failure, and finally the location of calcification, pannus, leaflets, and stent posts in relation to the coronary ostia. MSCT is essential to evaluate these factors as demonstrated in the example in Figure 27.1. In cases such as the example with a low coronary height shown in Figure 27.1, it is essential to evaluate the dimensions of the aortic sinuses. A low coronary height may not be an exclusion for VIV if the sinuses are large, as they will not occlude despite displacement of the bioprosthetic leaflets. We also always measure the internal diameter of the bioprosthesis on MSCT in order to (1) quantify discrepancies between the *in vitro* and *in vivo* internal diameter particularly in cases with excessive calcification, leaflet thickening, and/or pannus in growth, (2) exclude major discrepancies in valve size to that reported in the patient's medical file or when the specific model or size is unknown, and (3) determine the annular dimensions in cases of stentless valves.

In general, the THV size is chosen with a nominal external diameter matching or exceeding the reported internal diameter of the failed prosthesis to allow for secure fixation and sealing as well as prevent embolization. It is important to consider that excess VIV oversizing may be associated with significant underexpansion of the newly implanted valve, resulting in high residual gradients and possibly limited durability. Furthermore, excessive oversizing may result in forward valve advancement during implantation and malposition, especially with self-expanding THVs. In general, the THV size is chosen using the same sizing ranges as those used to size in native anatomy, with a maximum range of 5–10% oversizing.

Procedure and implantation technique

The choice of general anesthesia versus conscious sedation is based on the team's preference or the access site. The initial aortic VIV procedures were performed via the transapical route because of the possible advantages of direct access to the valve, better control of device deployment, and coaxial positioning. However, VIV procedures have now been performed via multiple access sites (transfemoral, subclavian, direct aortic) with such excellent results that there is no preferable route for aortic VIV procedures. The access site should be chosen based on patient anatomy and the skill of the TAVI team. As compared with a TAVI procedure of a native valve, there are certain technical aspects of VIV procedures that should be highlighted: (1) predilatation is

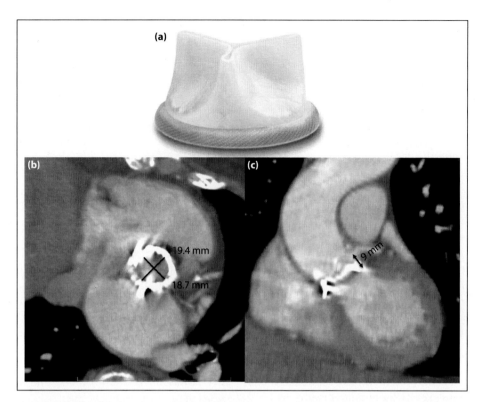

Figure 27.1 A Sorin Mitroflow valve demonstrating that the leaflets are mounted externally over the stent rather than internally (a). MSCT evaluation of a patient with a degenerated 23 mm Mitroflow with an internal diameter of 19 mm and a height of 14 mm. Axial view (b) confirms that actual internal diameter (19.4 × 18.7 mm) is similar to the manufacturer's reported diameter. On the oblique view (c), the left coronary height is only 9 mm and the valve completely fills the narrow aortic sinuses, thus suggesting that this patient would be at risk for coronary occlusion during VIV implantation.

usually unnecessary; (2) the angiographic projection should be perpendicular to the sewing ring; (3) coaxial positioning of THV within the bioprosthesis; (4) implantation depth is less than native valves; and (5) rapid pacing during deployment for self-expanding valves.

Balloon valvuloplasty is not routinely performed before VIV implantation, even in stenotic bioprostheses. In comparison to native leaflets, surgical valves may tear or disintegrate with balloon dilatation, thus resulting in torrential regurgitation, debris embolization, and stroke. However, it is essential to make an attempt to cross the valve with a valvuloplasty balloon that is uninflated or inflated at low pressure (2–3 atm) prior to insertion of the Edwards delivery system. Depending on the version of Edwards delivery system, the system may not be retrieved without implanting the valve (Edwards SAPIEN and Retroflex) or has to be discarded after retrieving the nonimplanted valve (SAPIEN XT and Novaflex). Preimplantation valvuloplasty may however be useful in evaluating the risk of coronary occlusion by injecting contrast above the inflated balloon and observing coronary flow and the movement of the bioprosthetic leaflets. In cases where there are concerns about coronary occlusion, a "protection" coronary guide wire or even a coronary angioplasty balloon can be positioned in the coronary artery during valve implantation (Figure 27.2).

Accurate positioning requires coaxial positioning of the THV and thus it is essential to find the angiographic view perpendicular to the bioprosthesis in order to minimize foreshortening. If the radiographic marker for implantation is the basal sewing ring, then this should appear as a straight line on the correct implantation view. The typical aortic valve is directed slightly to the right and posterior, such that left anterior oblique-cranial views are often helpful.[5] For radiolucent stented or stentless valves, aortography with a pigtail catheter in the noncoronary cusp or transesophageal echocardiography is essential. Lack of coaxial alignment has been thought to be one of the most important reasons for THV embolization during these procedures. It is also why many centers prefer the transapical approach for VIV. In our VIV experience, which is predominantly via the transfemoral approach,[3] we always attempt to coaxially align the THV within the failed bioprosthesis, but this is not always possible. We have found that ensuring complete coaxiality may not always be necessary because this step occurs almost spontaneously at the time of slow balloon inflation during rapid pacing.

As mentioned above, the success of a VIV procedure is highly dependent on a good understanding of the failing bioprostheses, as the THV should ideally be positioned to overlap the surgical valve's sewing ring. This crucial step

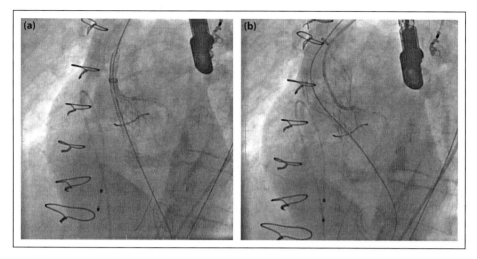

Figure 27.2   Fluoroscopic images of a patient with a 21 mm Mitroflow that was at risk for left coronary occlusion. During implantation of a 23 mm CoreValve, the left coronary artery was protected by a guide wire in the coronary artery and an angioplasty balloon in the left main (a, b).

secures deployment without embolization. This not only includes knowledge of the device design but also its fluoroscopic appearance and how it correlates with the implanted valve. Some valves may have radiopaque markers or rings at the basal portion close to the anatomic sewing ring, whereas in others, the markers may be close to the tip of the stent posts or there may be no radiopaque markers at all.

The ideal position will be one that achieves good anchorage and at the same time covers the leaflets. Insufficient overlap of the sewing ring may result in the stent posts of the bioprosthesis being splayed during deployment with distal embolization of the THV. For balloon-expandable valves, the aim is to place at least 20% of the valve below the sewing ring, whereas for self-expanding valves, the target depth is 4–6 mm. In particular for the CoreValve, implantation depth should be as high as possible in order to take advantage of the supra-annular position of the THV leaflets, with improved hemodynamics because the THV is not constrained by the unexpandable sewing ring. Examples of a CoreValve and Edwards THV implanted in a Carpentier–Edwards surgical bioprosthesis are shown in Figures 27.3 and 27.4.

Finally, severe prosthetic aortic valve regurgitation can be associated with large stroke volumes, thus making

accurate VIV positioning difficult unless rapid pacing is performed during deployment.[1] This is important to consider during the implantation of self-expanding THVs that are not routinely implanted with rapid pacing.

Complications specific to VIV

All the complications that can occur during a TAVI procedure may also occur during a VIV procedure. However, there are certain complications that are more or less frequent or that are specific to these procedures.

Although paravalvular leaks are common after TAVI for native aortic valve stenosis, regurgitation post-VIV appears to be absent or mild in most published reports probably explained by the fact that the circular and symmetrical sewing ring of the bioprosthesis facilitates intervalvular sealing.[1,3,5,10] In the context of VIV procedures, residual aortic regurgitation should be reported as paravalvular (between failed bioprosthesis and native annulus), intervalvular (between failed bioprosthesis and THV), or transvalvular (through the newly implanted THV). Similarly, permanent pacemaker implantation has been less frequent with VIV procedures, probably because the rigid ring of

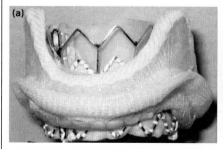
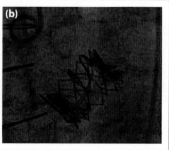

Figure 27.3   (**See color insert.**) Demonstration of *in vitro* (a) and *in vivo* implantation (b) of an Edwards THV within a Carpentier–Edwards bioprosthesis.

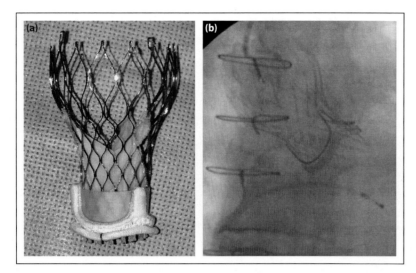

Figure 27.4 (**See color insert.**) Demonstration of *in vitro* (a) and *in vivo* implantation (b) of a CoreValve THV within a Carpentier–Edwards bioprosthesis.

the surgical valve protects the conduction system from compression by the THV.[1,2,5]

As opposed to paravalvular leaks, coronary obstruction appears to be more frequent with VIV as compared with native valve procedures.[3,4] This may be particularly related to design of certain stented bioprostheses such as the Sorin Mitroflow (Sorin Group, Milan, Italy) and St. Jude Trifecta (St. Jude, St. Paul, MN) that have leaflets mounted outside the stent to maximize orifice area. As these leaflets are not constrained by stent posts, they may be pushed toward the aortic wall and obstruct the coronary arteries during VIV implantation. Coronary obstruction has also been observed with certain stentless prostheses that may bring the coronary ostia closer to the annulus either due to design or the technique of implantation. As mentioned above, it is essential to carefully evaluate the relationship of the coronary ostia to the failed valve (Figure 27.1) and in high-risk cases it may be useful to consider placing a safety wire in the coronary artery (Figure 27.2). Probably the most relevant issue related to VIV procedures is underexpansion of a THV in a nondistensible rigid sewing ring, especially when treating bioprostheses with an internal diameter <20 mm (Figure 27.5). Underexpanded THVs may function suboptimally, resulting in increased transvalvular pressure gradients and impaired coaptation of leaflets with central aortic regurgitation in some cases.[4] This leaflet distortion may increase stress on the leaflets and limit the durability of the THV.[2] Furthermore, until recently, there have been limited THV sizes with an absence of smaller sizes, and implantation of an oversized THV in a small bioprosthesis has also resulted in higher transvalvular gradients. Indeed patient–prosthesis mismatch may inevitably occur after VIV in patients with small bioprostheses along with the negative effects seen after as regards left ventricular mass regression, cardiac failure, and perioperative and long-term mortality. Potential solutions to reduce patient–prosthesis

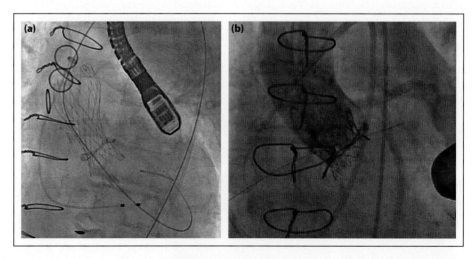

Figure 27.5 Demonstration of the underexpansion of a CoreValve (a) and Edwards (b) THV as a result of implanting an oversized THV within a small bioprosthesis.

mismatch include the availability of smaller-sized THVs and increased usage of supra-annular THVs, in which the leaflets are situated above the bioprosthesis to maximize available orifice area.

Clinical data: The Global Valve-in-Valve Registry

The published literature as regards VIV implantation has been limited to case reports or small case series, usually involving only one type of THV. The best clinical information that we currently have comes from the Global Valve-in-Valve Registry.[4] The registry currently includes over 400 patients and the data on the first 202 patients enrolled have recently been published. The mechanism of bioprosthetic failure was stenosis in 42.1%, regurgitation in 33.7%, and combined stenosis/regurgitation in 24.3%. A majority of the surgical valves were stented (76.7%). The VIV procedure was performed with a CoreValve in 61% and an Edwards in 39%. Adverse procedural outcomes included initial device malposition in 15.3% of cases and ostial coronary obstruction in 3.5%, which appeared to be more frequent in the Mitroflow and Freedom stentless valve (Sorin). Although procedural success was high (93.1%), Valve Academic Research Consortium (VARC)-defined device success was relatively low (58.9%), primarily due to high postprocedural gradients. Indeed, high post-VIV gradients (mean ≥20 mmHg) were observed in 28.4% of patients and were higher after Edwards SAPIEN than after CoreValve implantation (40% vs. 21.3%: $p < 0.0001$). High postprocedural gradients were particularly noticeable for VIV procedures with an Edwards THV implanted inside a small bioprosthesis with an internal diameter <20 mm (58.8% vs. 20% in CoreValve). This difference is probably due to the intra-annular location of the leaflets with Edwards as compared with the supra-annular location with CoreValve. The 1-year survival of 85.5% is comparable to that found with TAVI in native aortic valve stenosis.

Conclusions

The VIV procedure is a clinically effective therapeutic alternative to redo surgery for a failed bioprosthesis in high-risk patients or possibly even in younger patients in whom delaying replacement with a mechanical valve may be desirable. In experienced centers, the procedure may be technically easier than TAVI in a native valve provided that certain procedural challenges specific to VIV implantation are taken into account. Ensuring excellent procedural and follow-up outcomes requires a true heart team approach and a thorough understanding of the failing surgical bioprosthesis and its relationship to the patient's anatomy. Important unanswered questions that remain are the impact of higher postprocedural gradients on long-term outcomes, THV durability, and the feasibility and number of repeat procedures that can be performed.

Acknowledgments

The authors would like to thank John C. Hay for his invaluable contribution to this chapter by collecting and providing all the data in Table 27.1. The authors would also like to thank Dr. Jean-Claude Laborde, MD, for providing many of the images in this chapter.

References

1. Piazza N, Bleiziffer S, Brockmann G et al. Transcatheter aortic valve implantation for failing surgical aortic bioprosthetic valve: From concept to clinical application and evaluation (Part 1). *J Am Coll Cardiol Interv* 2011;4:721–32.
2. Azadani AN, Tseng EE. Transcatheter heart valves for failing bioprostheses. *Circ Cardiovasc Interv* 2011;4:621–8.
3. Latib A, Ielasi A, Montorfano M et al. Transcatheter valve-in-valve implantation with the Edwards SAPIEN in patients with bioprosthetic heart valve failure: The Milan experience. *EuroIntervention* 2012;7:1275–84.
4. Dvir D, Webb J, Brecker S et al. Transcatheter aortic valve replacement for degenerative bioprosthetic surgical valves: Results from the global valve-in-valve registry. *Circulation* 2012;126:2335–44.
5. Gurvitch R, Cheung A, Ye J et al. Transcatheter valve-in-valve implantation for failed surgical bioprosthetic valves. *J Am Coll Cardiol* 2011;58:2196–209.
6. Hammermeister K, Sethi GK, Henderson WG et al. Outcomes 15 years after valve replacement with a mechanical versus a bioprosthetic valve: Final report of the Veterans Affairs randomized trial. *J Am Coll Cardiol* 2000;36:1152–8.
7. Hammermeister KE, Sethi GK, Henderson WG et al. A comparison of outcomes in men 11 years after heart-valve replacement with a mechanical valve or bioprosthesis. Veterans Affairs cooperative study on valvular heart disease. *N Engl J Med* 1993;328:1289–96.
8. Bapat V, Attia R, Redwood S et al. Use of transcatheter heart valves for a valve-in-valve implantation in patients with degenerated aortic bioprosthesis: Technical considerations and results. *J Thorac Cardiovasc Surg* 2012;144:1372–80.
9. Chan V, Malas T, Lapierre H et al. Reoperation of left heart valve bioprostheses according to age at implantation. *Circulation* 2011;124:S75–80.
10. Piazza N, Bleiziffer S, Brockmann G et al. Transcatheter aortic valve implantation for failing surgical aortic bioprosthetic valve: From concept to clinical application and evaluation (Part 2). *J Am Coll Cardiol Interv* 2011;4:733–42.
11. Webb JG, Wood DA, Ye J et al. Transcatheter valve-in-valve implantation for failed bioprosthetic heart valves. *Circulation* 2010;121:1848–57.
12. Bapat V, Mydin I, Chadalavada S et al. A guide to fluoroscopic identification and design of bioprosthetic valves: A reference for valve-in-valve procedure. *Catheter Cardiovasc Interv* 2013;81:853–61.

28

Aortic valve stenosis in the elderly: New percutaneous aortic valves

Peter C. Block

Introduction

Any review of "new" transcatheter valves must begin with the latest iteration of the "old" valves. To date, two transcatheter aortic valves have been widely used in Europe, Canada, and the United States: the balloon-expandable Edwards valve (including the initial Cribier–Edwards valve,[1,2] the second-generation Edwards SAPIEN, and the third-generation Edwards SAPIEN XT [Edwards Lifesciences Corporation, Irvine, CA, USA] versions—and the self-expandable CoreValve [Medtronic, St. Paul, MN]) system. The Edwards SAPIEN valve, used in the PARTNER I Trials,[3,4] is now commercially available in the United States. However, its design has evolved into the lower-profile SAPIEN XT (Figure 28.1) and its 18 Fr NovaFlex transfemoral delivery system, which is in clinical trials (PARTNER 2) in the United States. The transcatheter SAPIEN XT valve received the CE mark in March 2010, and is commercially available outside the United States.

The CoreValve, commercially available in Europe and Canada, is also in clinical trials both in the United States and Europe. It has had minor design changes and maintains its lowest-profile 18 Fr introducer system (Figure 28.1).[5,6] Both valves have extensive track records with numerous publications of benefit, risk, complications, and so on, and will be the benchmark against which all other "new" valves will be gauged.

Other, new percutaneous transcatheter aortic valves have now advanced beyond safety and efficacy trials. Some have achieved, or await, CE mark approval in Europe, and early trials in the United States are anticipated. The new valves share a number of common features: reduced profile, ability to reposition, and ability to recapture and replace if needed before final deployment. Their usefulness will also depend on whether they address the major deficiencies of first-generation valves, which include perivalvar leak and pacemaker need for heart block.

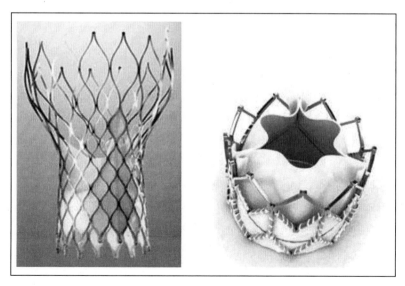

Figure 28.1 **(See color insert.)** Current iterations of the CoreValve (left) and SAPIEN XT (right). Both can be delivered via an 18 Fr system.

DirectFlow Medical valve

The DirectFlow Medical (Santa Rosa, CA) transcatheter aortic valve utilizes a unique nonmetallic valve design on a flexible 18 Fr delivery system (Figure 28.2). The valve is stentless, and has a fabric cuff, which is inflatable. The purpose of the design is to provide adjustable placement of the valve within the annulus and minimize postplacement aortic regurgitation (AR). After transfemoral insertion and crossing the stenotic native valve, the distal ring is deployed with saline inflation and positioned just below the aortic annulus by gentle withdrawal of the delivery system. Once the distal ring is inflated, the valve begins to function so that cardiac output is maintained during positioning. Burst ventricular pacing is not needed for deployment. Three tethers attached to the valve, which can be individually advanced or retracted, allow adjustment of coaxial position of the distal valve ring. The proximal ring is then inflated and the hemodynamics of the valve evaluated (including the amount of AR). If the position is not adequate or there is AR, the valve can be "deflated," repositioned, or retrieved.[7]

The DISCOVER CE mark study ($n = 33$ patients) presented at TCT 2012 was a multicenter study with a primary endpoint of freedom from all-cause mortality from procedure to 30 days. All patients had severe, symptomatic aortic stenosis with a mean aortic valve gradient >40 mmHg *or* peak jet velocity >4.0 m/s and aortic valve area (AVA)

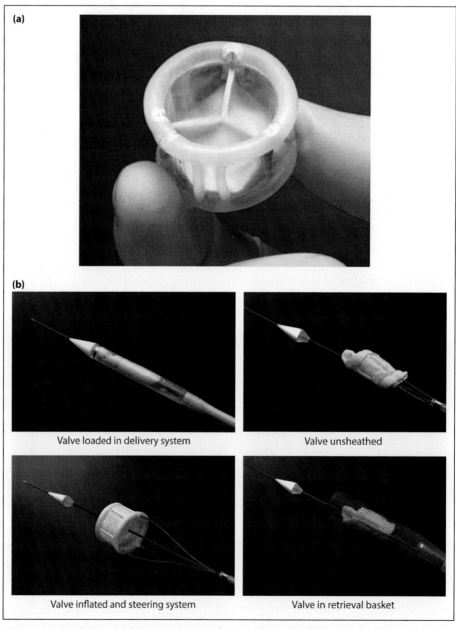

(a)

(b)

Valve loaded in delivery system

Valve unsheathed

Valve inflated and steering system

Valve in retrieval basket

Figure 28.2 **(See color insert.)** (a) DirectFlow valve. (b) Deployment sequence of the DirectFlow valve.

≤0.8 cm^2 *or* AVA index ≤0.5 cm^2/m^2. The native valve annulus diameter was >19 mm or <26 mm (by CT) and only 25 mm and 27 mm valves were deployed. Patients had a logistic EuroScore >20 or comorbidities such as severe chronic obstructive pulmonary disease, porcelain aorta, or previous thoracic irradiation. In the study, one patient died at 12 days after the procedure resulting in a freedom from all-cause mortality within 30 days of 97%. All patients had successful device secondary endpoints, which included successful vascular access, positioning of the device in the proper location, and delivery, deployment, and retrieval of the delivery system. During the study, three patients had valves successfully retrieved and replaced with larger-sized valves. The valve was ultimately implanted in the proper location in 100% of the patients. Intended performance of the valve (mean gradient <20 mmHg or peak velocity <3 m/s, without moderate or severe AR) was achieved in all but one patient. Mean gradient assessment by a Core laboratory showed a reduction of the aortic valve gradient from 46 mmHg preprocedure to 13.6 mmHg at discharge and 12.9 mmHg at 30 days. Ninety-eight percent of the valves demonstrated no/trace or only mild AR postprocedure. The conclusion of the study was that the valve achieved 97% freedom from all-cause mortality and 100% freedom from cardiovascular mortality at 30 days; could safely and effectively be used to treat high- and extreme surgical risk patients with aortic stenosis; provided hemodynamic stability during implantation; allowed controlled positioning, repositioning, and safe retrieval; and virtually eliminated aortic regurgitation. Safety and efficacy studies are anticipated in the United States in 2013.

Lotus™ valve

The Lotus valve (Boston Scientific, Los Gatos, CA) prosthesis is self-expanding and is composed of a nitinol continuous-braid frame with bovine pericardial leaflets. It is repositionable and covered by a flexible membrane to seal perivalvar gaps due to aortic annular irregularity (Figure 28.3). The 19 Fr catheter is placed across the stenotic native aortic valve and the prosthesis is then unsheathed. The self-expanding prosthesis shortens as it expands with low radial force, allowing the prosthetic valve to begin functioning during deployment. When the position is optimal

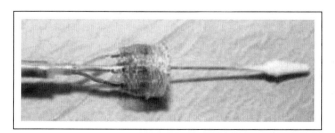

Figure 28.3 **(See color insert.)** The Boston Scientific Lotus valve.

within the native aortic annulus, the nitinol frame is further actively shortened and secured in position. The valve is attached to the deployment catheter by three "arms," allowing the device to be collapsed and retrieved if positioning is not ideal. If the prosthetic valve is in good position, it is then released from the delivery catheter. A report of the first-in-man use[8] described a retrograde approach for insertion of the 21 Fr Lotus catheter loaded with the valve prosthesis via surgical cutdown to the external iliac artery. The prosthesis was successfully inserted and deployed within the calcified native valve. Echocardiography immediately after device deployment showed a significant reduction of the transaortic mean pressure gradient from 32 to 9 mmHg, and a final valve area of 1.7 cm^2 without evidence of residual aortic regurgitation. The postprocedural clinical status improved from New York Heart Association (NYHA)-IV to NYHA-II and these results remained unchanged at 3 month follow-up. The Lotus valve has achieved CE mark status in Europe and initial clinical trials are anticipated in the United States in 2013.

JenaValve

The JenaValve is made from a porcine aortic root including the porcine aortic valve mounted within a self-expanding nitinol frame. The self-expanding stent has three "feelers," which allow placement within the native aortic sinuses (Figure 28.4). The valve is delivered antegrade from a transapical approach and the "feelers" positioned so that they lie in the native aortic valve sinuses. The prosthetic valve is first freed from the delivery catheter, which superimposes the prosthetic valve commissures on the native commissures. The valve begins to function during this early stage of deployment so that cardiac output is maintained during deployment. Rapid pacing is not required. The valve is anchored by freeing the lower portion of the JenaValve nitinol stent, which becomes a "clip" with the already deployed "feelers" within the native sinuses. This "clipping" mechanism anchors the valve within the native aortic valve, which does not allow migration of the prosthesis and produces a tight anchor with the native aortic annulus. During positioning and before final deployment, the JenaValve can be repositioned and can be retrieved if needed.[9] The JenaValve comes in three sizes: 23, 25, and 27 mm, allowing treatment of patients with aortic annuli from 21 to 27 mm in diameter. The JenaValve received CE mark approval in Europe in 2011. Data were collected from 73 patients with severe symptomatic aortic valve stenosis at seven German study sites between October 2010 and July 2011. The primary endpoint of the trial was the 30-day mortality rate. A secondary endpoint was the rate of successful implantation. The results of the study's primary endpoint were presented at the TCT scientific meeting in October 2012. Data were included on 67 patients implanted with this valve, from July 2010 to July 2011. The

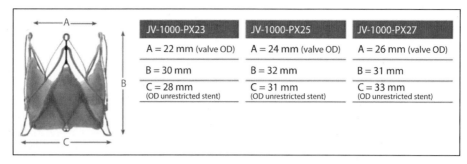

Figure 28.4 **(See color insert.)** The JenaValve.

mean age of the patients was 83 years. In conforming with earlier transcatheter aortic valve trials, all patients had severe aortic stenosis. Ninety-two percent of patients were in NYHA class 3 or higher heart failure and were considered to be inoperable or at high risk for conventional aortic valve surgery. Procedural success occurred in 90% of patients. Thirty-day mortality, the primary endpoint of the study, was 7.6%. Two patients had complications of stroke, two deaths were cardiac-related, and four patients were converted to open-heart surgery. No myocardial infarctions were reported. Pacemaker implantation was necessary in six patients (9%).[10] Clinical benefit in this initial study was evidenced by most patients improving by 1 or more NYHA classes. At 1 year follow-up, freedom from cardiac death was 85% and all-cause death 68%.

Symetis Acurate valve

The Symetis Acurate valve is a self-expandable nitinol porcine valve, delivered transapically to a subcoronary position. It is designed for rotation during implantation to align with the native commissures (Figure 28.5). It is available in three sizes and can be used in patients with native annular sizes of 21–27 mm. The valve has two unique features: a stabilization arch, meant to prevent tilting of the valve during deployment, and a so-called "upper crown," the most distal part of the stent body, which is unsheathed during step one of the deployment and then provides tactile feedback to aid positioning. Partial release first exposes the stabilization arches and then the upper crown. The upper crown engages the cusps of the native leaflets. By gently pulling the valve down toward the left ventricle, the operator can feel proper placement at the annulus. With gentle downward pressure, the Acurate is released, leaving the lower crown fully expanded. The stabilization arches act as a pivot providing axial alignment and a polyethylene terephthalate (PET) skirt provides an annular seal, reducing perivalvar leak.[11,12] First-in-man data were reported at the European Association for Cardiothoracic Surgery (EACTS) meeting in 2011 on 40 patients. Their average age was 83 years and all were NYHA class 3 or 4. Six-month survival was 82.5%. Functional status of

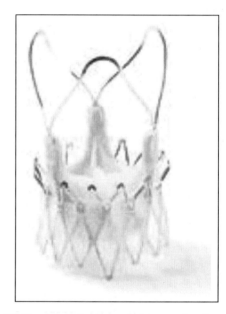

Figure 28.5 **(See color insert.)** The Symetis valve.

90% of the patients was improved to NYHA class 1 or 2 at 6 months. Importantly, 97% of patients had no or only trace perivalvar leak after the Acurate implantation. Three patients required pacemaker implantation; two patients had stroke. The Acurate valve has received CE mark approval in Europe on the basis of the above study and an earlier pilot study of 50 additional patients. A postmarket surveillance study is under way (the Symetis Aortic Valve Implantation Registry [SAVI]). A 15-center pivotal trial comprising 150 patients is planned in the United States.

Portico valve

The Portico valve is made of bovine pericardial tissue. It can be placed via a transapical or transfemoral route (Figure 28.6). Importantly, it can be completely resheathed and repositioned at the implant site before being released from the delivery system. The resheathing feature also allows retrieval of the valve, if needed. Recently, St. Jude Medical announced the CE mark approval of the Portico valve and transfemoral delivery system. Early data from 10 patients

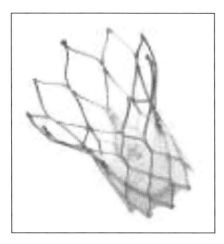

Figure 28.6 (**See color insert.**) The Portico valve.

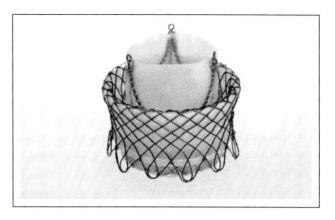

Figure 28.7 (**See color insert.**) The Heart Leaflet Technology valve. (Courtesy of HLT Inc., 2012.)

(all women) presented at the Congenital and Structural Interventions Symposium in Frankfurt, Germany in 2012 showed that patients had a mean age of 86 years, with high frailty indices and relatively moderate Society of Thoracic Surgery (STS) risk of 6.5 and Logistic Euroscore of 18.9. All cases were performed percutaneously with local anesthesia using an 18 Fr introducer system. Two valves required resheathing. At 30 days after implantation, there were no deaths or strokes. Four patients had new left bundle branch block but none required pacemaker insertion. Mean gradients were reduced from 40.7 mmHg to 7.8 mmHg at 30 days and 9.1 mmHg at 6 months. Seven patients had no or trivial AR and the remaining patients had only mild AR at 30 days and 6 months postprocedure. All 10 patients moved from NYHA class 2 or 3 to NYHA class 1 at 30 days and 6 months. The Portico transcatheter aortic heart valve, the transapical delivery system, and the transfemoral delivery system are not yet approved for use in the United States. Plans are underway for a safety and efficacy trial in the United States.

Heart Leaflet Technologies valve

The Heart Leaflet Technologies (HLT) valve uses porcine, pericardial tissue that is mounted on a flexible, nitinol wire form. The wire form, which is designed to reduce tissue stress throughout the cardiac cycle, is attached to an outer support structure and is intended to allow the leaflets to maintain a circular geometry and preserve flow area even in an eccentric, diseased annulus (Figure 28.7). The HLT valve utilizes an 18 Fr delivery system that allows it to be fully repositioned or retrieved. Once delivered to the native annulus, the performance of the fully functioning valve can be assessed. If needed, the valve can be fully retrieved until final release from the delivery system. An early feasibility study to evaluate the HLT transcatheter valve included six patients with critical aortic stenosis enrolled at the University Herzzentrum in Leipzig,

Germany. All patients were female with a mean age 84 ± 3 years, an NYHA functional class of 3.0 ± 0.0, an STS score of 11.6 ± 4.2, a Logistic EuroScore of 27.5 ± 13.6, and an left ventricular ejection fraction (LVEF) of 54 ± 9%. In five of six patients, valve placement was successfully accomplished and mean gradients (as evaluated by a Core Lab) were reduced from a baseline value of 29.6 ± 9.6 to 5.5 ± 1.9 mmHg at 1 month with an associated improvement in NYHA class to 1.3 ± 0.5. Residual aortic insufficiency was grade 0.4 (range 0–0.5) at 1 month. This early study revealed that the delivery system had the potential to cause ventricular injury. As a result, changes to the delivery system were initiated to prevent this possibility. The modified delivery system is being finalized prior to continuation of the clinical study.

Other transcatheter valves, both transfemoral and transapical (Innovare, Engager, etc.) are under development, in early clinical trials, or are in process of design modifications. All of the new valves will have to be used in extensive clinical trials (probably randomized in the future against the SAPIEN valve or CoreValve) so that a larger number of patients treated with them can be evaluated. It is likely that acceptance and use of the new valves will depend on the clinical data generated by such trials. However, if there are early signs that perivalvar leak and/or pacemaker need are significantly decreased with their use, acceptance will likely be more rapid.

References

1. Cribier A et al. Percutaneous transcatheter implantation of an aortic valve prosthesis for calcific aortic stenosis. First human case description. *Circulation* 2002;106:3006–8.
2. Cribier A et al. Early experience with percutaneous transcatheter implantation of heart valve prosthesis for the treatment of end-stage inoperable patients with calcific aortic stenosis. *J Am Coll Cardiol* 2004;43:698–703.
3. Leon MB et al. Transcatheter aortic-valve implantation for aortic stenosis in patients who cannot undergo surgery. *N Engl J Med* 2010;363:1597–607.

4. Smith CR et al. Transcatheter versus surgical aortic-valve replacement in high-risk patients. *N Engl J Med* 2011;364:2187–98.

5. Grube E et al. Percutaneous aortic valve replacement for severe aortic stenosis in high-risk patients using the second- and current third-generation self-expanding CoreValve prosthesis. *J Am Coll Cardiol* 2007;50:69–76.

6. Piazza N et al. Procedural and 30-day outcomes following transcatheter aortic valve implant using the third generation (18F) CoreValve revalving system: Results from the multicentre, expanded evaluation registry 1-year following CE mark approval. *EuroIntervention* 2008;4:242–9.

7. Schofer J et al. Aortic stenosis: A first-in-man retrograde transarterial implantation of a non-metallic aortic valve prosthesis. *Circ Cardiovasc Interv* 2008;1:126–33.

8. Buellesfeld L, Gerckens U, Grube E. Percutaneous implantation of the first repositionable aortic valve prosthesis in a patient with severe aortic stenosis. *Cathet Cardiovasc Interv* 2008;71:579–84.

9. Kempfert J, Rastan AJ, Mohr FW, Walther T. A new self-expanding transcatheter aortic valve for transapical implantation—First in man implantation of the JenaValve. *Eur J Cardiothorac Surg* 2011;40:761–3.

10. Kempfert J, Treede H, Rastan AJ, Schönburg M, Thielmann M, Sorg S, Mohr FW, Walther T. Transapical aortic valve implantation using a new self-expandable bioprosthesis (ACURATE TA™): 6-month outcomes. *Eur J Cardiothorac Surg.* 2013;43(1):52–6; Epub 2012 Apr 4.

11. Falk V et al. New anatomically oriented transapical aortic valve implantation. *Ann Thorac Surg* 2009;87:925–6.

12. Falk V et al. Transapical aortic valve implantation with a self-expanding anatomically oriented valve. *Eur Heart J* 2011;32:878–87.

29

Aortic valve stenosis in the elderly: Embolic protection during transcatheter aortic valve implantation

Alexander Ghanem and Eberhard Grube

Introduction

Transcatheter aortic valve implantation (TAVI) has emerged as a therapeutic option in elderly patients with aortic stenosis. However, numerous challenges need to be addressed in order to further improve the outcome of this distinct cohort, one of which is the risk of cerebrovascular events (CVE) related to TAVI. Individual stroke risk cumulates in aged patients with severe aortic stenosis resulting in an annual event rate of up to 4.5%.[1,2] The prevalence of CVEs is mainly related to patient age and comorbidities, reaching up to 15% in healthy octogenarians, and exceeding this number in aged patients with aortic stenosis.[3] These numbers characterize the high baseline stroke risk of patients eligible for TAVI.

The results of the Partner trials offered prospective, randomized controlled data on stroke risk in patients with aortic stenosis undergoing conservative, interventional, or surgical treatment. In the cohort of patients without surgical option (Partner IB), TAVI resulted in a significant decrease of mortality.[1] However, these encouraging results were at the cost of an increased stroke rate early after TAVI (30 days: 6.7% vs. 1.7%, $p = 0.02$), persisting for up to 2 years in patients with excessive surgical risk (1 year: 11.2% vs. 5.5%, $p = 0.06$; 2 years: 13.8% vs. 5.5%, $p = 0.01$).[4] Also the patient cohort with a surgical option (Partner IA) demonstrated significantly higher stroke rates in the TAVI group after the first (8.7% vs. 4.3%, $p = 0.03$) and second year (11.2% vs. 6.5%, $p = 0.05$).[5] Interestingly, the latest data presented at this year's annual meeting of the American College of Cardiology (ACC) demonstrated that stroke rates, which diverged early, were not different in prevalence at 3 years after TAVI (8.2% in the TAVI group vs. 9.3% in the surgical group). Since approximately half of the CVEs occur subacute and late, and therefore are not directly related to the procedure itself, neuroprotective approaches need to be tailored according to the underlying mechanisms (see Figure 29.1).

In a multicenter registry encompassing 1061 patients, Nombela-Franco et al. demonstrated that the history of cerebrovascular (carotid stenosis, prior endarterectomy, prior CVE) and peripheral vascular disease each independently doubled the risk of TAVI-related, early CVEs. Further, chronic atrial fibrillation was found to independently increase the risk of late CVEs (>30 days after TAVI) almost by a factor of three.[6] Likewise, the extent of aortic arch atheroma was predictive for cerebral embolism.[7] Hence, with respect to comorbidities, atherosclerotic disease burden and chronic atrial fibrillation seem to be the key independent predictors of acute CVEs related to TAVI.

Since aortic valve stenosis is of degenerative origin, it is conceivable that each and every manipulation within the aortic arch and the stenosed, calcified valve needed for this complex intervention (valvuloplasty, passage of a large bore catheter, valve positioning and deployment, postdilatation) could potentially lead to embolic dislodgement of thrombotic and/or atheromatous and/or calcific debris. The impact of the access route and the valve type on the occurrence of CVEs has not yet been elucidated. We and others were not surprised that passing the semirigid, large-bore delivery catheter containing the folded bioprothesis through the aortic arch and into the stenosed valve led to silent and apparent cerebral embolism in 73–84% and 3–10%, respectively.[8–10] Studies utilizing transcranial Doppler sonography (TCD) demonstrated that the positioning and the deployment of the prosthesis within the calcified valve are the most critical steps of the TAVI procedure.[11] In a multicenter registry, postdilatation of the valve prothesis and valve dislodgment/embolization were identified as independent predictors of CVEs, increasing the event rate 2.5- and 4.4-fold, respectively.[6] Thus, the manipulative burden on the prosthesis is directly associated with the risk of CVEs.

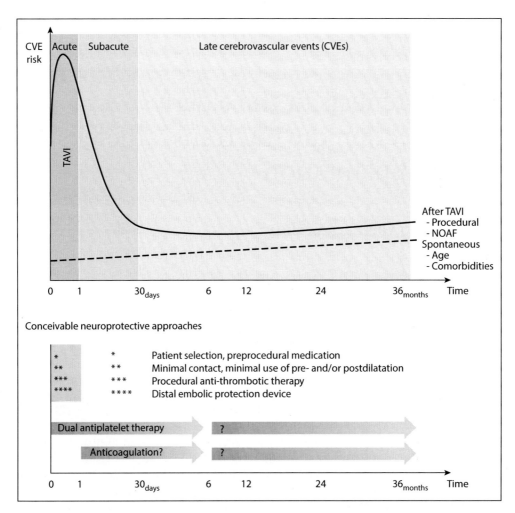

Figure 29.1 Risk of cerebrovascular events according to time after TAVI risk of cerebrovascular events (CVEs) related to the time after transcatheter aortic valve implantation (TAVI, solid line). The dotted line indicates the baseline risk of an age-, sex-, and risk factor-matched population with aortic stenosis. Embolic protection during TAVI could reduce cerebral embolic burden during the procedure. Neuroprotective approaches targeting subacute and late events encompass patient allocation to therapeutic strategy, anticoagulation in case of new onset of atrial fibrillation (NOAF), as well as management of antithrombotic therapy. (Modified from Stortecky S and Windecker S. *Circulation* 2012;126:2921–4.)

Cerebral injury, in analogy to myocardial injury, is not always clinically apparent and is reflected in different shades of gray (see Figure 29.2). CVEs are known to cause focal neurological deficits and disability and are dreaded for their excessive morbidity and mortality. For repetitive, standardized assessment of CVEs, the National Institutes of Health Stroke Scale (NIHSS) is often recommended. Besides focal neurological deficits, which can be obtained straightforwardly by a physician without dedicated neurological training, cerebral injury can be present as "minor change," such as neurocognitive decline or dependency in activities of daily living. Several investigators examined cognitive function after TAVI utilizing the mini-mental state examination (MMSE), which is a crude cognitive test, and found stable cognitive performance for up to 3 months after TAVI.[8,10] In our experience, no subclinical parameter of brain injury was related to lifestyle or to activities of daily living 1 year after TAVI.[12]

Cerebral embolic events have been prospectively investigated with several imaging modalities, such as CT, TCD, and diffusion-weighted magnetic resonance imaging (DW-MRI). In contrast to the tomographic modalities, TCD identified valve positioning and deployment as critical intraprocedural steps with respect to cerebral embolism[11] (see Figure 29.3). Besides classification, quantification, and localization of CVEs, DW-MRI allows the detection of noncortical, cortical microembolic, and cortical territorial events. Fortunately, TAVI-related embolic lesions in DW-MRI were associated neither with focal neurological deficits nor with decay of crude neurocognitive function after 3 months. Moreover, clinically silent microembolism has no effect on self-sufficiency in lifestyle,[12] HRQoL,[7] and mortality.[12] However, the contribution of

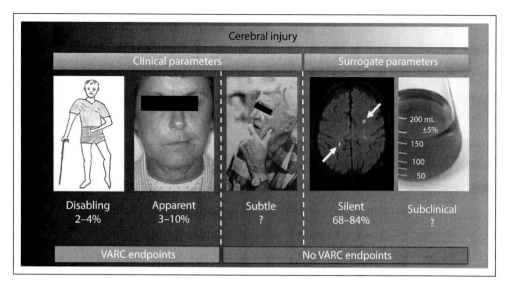

Figure 29.2   **(See color insert.)** Cerebral injury presents in different *shades of gray*. Clinical, imaging, and serological parameters can objectify cerebral injury related to transcatheter aortic valve implantation (TAVI). Obvious and apparent deficits have an incidence of up to 10%. They are detected clinically and account as cerebrovascular events (CVE). Yet little is known on the mechanism and the incidence of cognitive deterioration after TAVI, which is reflected as subtle clinical changes, for example, impairment of memory function or constructional skills. Nonclinical measures of cerebral injury encompass imaging and serology. Silent cerebral injury is detected by diffusion-weighted magnetic resonance imaging (DW-MRI), transcranial Doppler sonography or serology but does not count as a clinical endpoint of the Valve Academic Research Consortium (VARC). The effects of embolic protection devices on clinical and surrogate endpoints are currently being investigated in randomized, controlled studies.

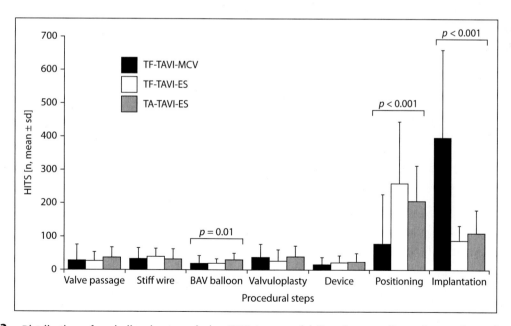

Figure 29.3   Distribution of emboligenic steps during TAVI transcranial Doppler recordings allow periprocedural monitoring of cerebral embolism by detection of high-intensity transient signals (HITS). As reported by Philipp Kahlert and colleagues,[13] most HITS occurred on manipulation of the calcified aortic valve during positioning and implantation of the stent valves. Although the balloon-expandable Edwards SAPIEN (ES) prosthesis caused significantly more HITS during positioning, the self-expandable Medtronic CoreValve (MCV) prosthesis caused more HITS during implantation. TF—transfemoral, TA—transapical approach, BAV—balloon aortic valvuloplasty. (Courtesy of Kahlert P et al. *Circulation* 2012;126:1245–55.)

cerebral embolism to neurocognitive decline, mild cognitive impairment, and vascular dementia remains to be elucidated in long-term follow-up studies.[13]

Patients suffering from early CVEs after TAVI demonstrated a significantly higher mortality rate as compared with patients without. In-hospital mortality was reported to be as high as 21%, irrespective of the embolic mechanism.[14] Major, disabling stroke was associated with higher 30-day (7.4-fold) and late (1.75-fold) mortality.[6] Also large-scale meta-analyses reported on a 3.5-fold increase of mortality after CVE.[15] Several measures of subclinical cerebral injury have been reported to be associated with TAVI, but only apparent CVEs seem to have an adverse impact on prognosis.[12]

Prevention of cerebrovascular events with dedicated embolic protection devices

Recent data indicate that additional preprocedural administration of antithrombotic and lipid-lowering drugs have proved beneficial with respect to periprocedural CVEs in patients undergoing carotid artery stenting (CAS).[16] Therefore, optimized medical therapy should always be considered as a potential neuroprotective approach. Although, prevention of acute CVEs can be tackled in the preprocedural setting, several preventive measures can be considered during the intervention (Table 29.1). On the one hand, improvements in the design of delivery catheters, such as smaller size and steerability, can reduce contact with vulnerable lesions. On the other hand, recent

TCD studies have demonstrated that cerebral embolism occurs throughout the multistep TAVI procedure, but cumulate predominantly during valve positioning and deployment within the calcified native valve.[11] Hence, the "no contact," "minimal contact," or "direct" TAVI approaches, without preparatory balloon valvuloplasty to minimize the dislodgment of calcified atherosclerotic emboli, have been proposed to reduce the risk of periprocedural stroke.[17] Precise sizing of the annulus and the correct valve selection is of pivotal importance to avoid valve dislodgement and malposition, as well as consecutive aortic regurgitation and the need of manipulation, postdilatation, or deployment of a second valve, each of which might increase the risk of CVEs. Hence, a meticulous planning and swift performance of the procedure is crucial.

Systematic reviews indicated that the use of cerebral protection devices decreases the risk of perioperative stroke with CAS.[18] By analogy to CAS, distal cerebral embolic protection devices have been developed, all of which consist of a filter membrane placed either in the aortic arch to deflect debris toward the descending aorta (TriGuard™ Cerebral Protection Device, Keystone Heart Ltd.; Embrella™, Edwards) or in the innominate and common carotid arteries (Montage™, Claret Medical) to either deflect (TriGuard, Embrella) or capture (Montage) embolic debris during the procedure (see Figures 29.4 through 29.6).

The TriGuard system is delivered via femoral access requiring a 9 F sheath. This device is placed within the aortic arch and covers the trifurcation, including the left subclavian artery supplying the left posterior cerebral perfusion. The TriGuard, also known as an SMT device, demonstrated a reduction of embolic burden within a case series of 15 patients.[19] The Edwards Embrella is delivered

Table 29.1 Pre- and periprocedural variables with potential neuroprotective effects

	Embolic cerebral injury
Preprocedural	Mechanisms:
	Incomplete valve endothelialization and high thrombocytic residual platelet activity early after TAVI
	Cholesterol embolization
	Conceivable interventions:
	Standardized antiplatelet protocol, for example, 600 mg clopidogrel "loading dose" 12 h prior to TAVI
	Lipid-lowering drug protocol, for example, statin "reloading"
Intraprocedural	Mechanisms:
	Thromboembolism
	Embolism of valvular debris by predilatation, valve positioning, repositioning, postdilatation, and valve-in-valve implantation
	Conceivable interventions:
	Standardized anticoagulation protocol
	Minimal touch implantation or direct TAVI
	Meticulous imaging work-up and valve sizing
	Utilization of a distal embolic protection device

TAVI—transcatheter aortic valve implantation.

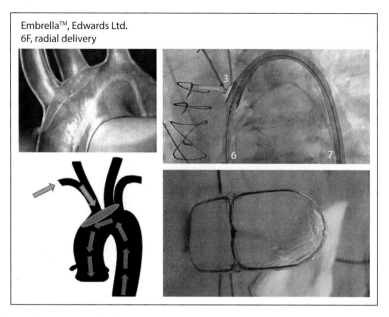

Figure 29.4 **(See color insert.)** Embrella—Distal embolic protection device. The Embrella embolic protection device is delivered over a 0.014″ guide wire from a left-radial sheath (6 F). The deflection shield is deployed in the aortic arch covering the ostia of the brachiocephalic, the right common carotid artery, and, in most cases, also the ostium of left subclavian artery (from where the left-posterior brain perfusion originates) is shielded. The shield is retracted to the origins of the supra-aortic arteries to achieve maximal coverage (blue arrows indicate the delivery route of the protection device [blue circles], the pathway of a transfemoral valve delivery is indicated with gray arrows). 3—Common brachiocephalic trunk, 6—ascending aorta, 7—descending aorta. (Reproduced from Edwards Medical, Inc. With permission.)

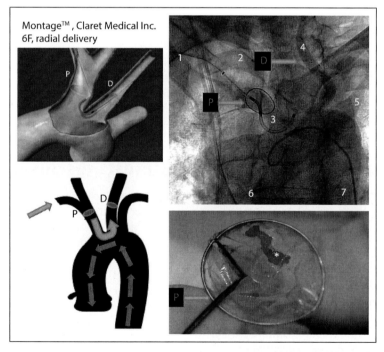

Figure 29.5 **(See color insert.)** Montage—Distal embolic protection device. Embolic protection devices are developed to prevent transcatheter aortic valve implantation (TAVI)-related embolism into the brain supplying vessels. The Montage dual-filter embolic protection device is delivered over a 0.014″ guide wire from a left-radial approach (6 F). The proximal filter (P) is placed within the innominate artery; the distal filter (D) is to be delivered into the left common carotid artery (blue arrows indicate the delivery route of the protection device [blue circles], the pathway of a transfemoral valve delivery is indicated with gray arrows). This system allows retrieval of embolic debris (asterisk, "*"). 1—Right subclavian artery, 2—right common carotid artery, 3—common brachiocephalic trunk/anonymous artery, 4—left common carotid artery, 5—left subclavian artery, 6—ascending aorta, 7—descending aorta. (Reproduced from Claret Medical, Inc. With permission.)

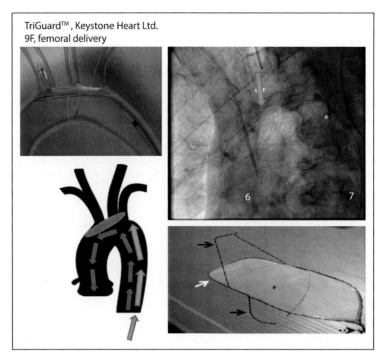

Figure 29.6   **(See color insert.)** TriGuard—Distal embolic protection device. The Keystone TriGuard embolic protection device is delivered from a femoral approach (9 F) and deployed in the aortic arch. The deflection shield allows coverage of the ostia of the arch vessels (blue arrows indicate the delivery route of the protection device [blue circle], the pathway of a transfemoral valve delivery is indicated with gray arrows). The nitinol frame (white arrow) holds a nitinol mesh (white asterisk) which is kept in place by upper and lower stabilizers (black arrows), to achieve maximal coverage of the aortic trifurcation throughout the intervention. 6—Ascending aorta, 7—descending aorta. (Reproduced from Europa Digital & Publishing. With permission.)

through an brachial 6 F shuttle sheath without a guide wire.[20] The device demonstrated its safety and feasibility in an initial study; efficacy is currently being investigated in the PROTAVI trial.

The only currently commercially available system to allow retrieval of debris without deflection into the descending aorta is the Claret embolic protection device (Montage Dual Filter Device, Claret Medical). First-in-man data showed safety and feasibility; efficacy has been proven by capture of embolic debris in 75% of the used filters.[21] Overall, thrombotic material and tissue fragments compatible with aortic valve leaflet or aortic wall origin were obtained in 52% of patients.[22]

Therefore, the use of dedicated embolic protection devices during TAVI could emerge as preventive method to reduce cerebral embolic burden. However, efficacy data of the PROTAVI trial demonstrated embolic events in every patient undergoing TAVI with an employed Embrella.[10] Peri-interventional TCD confirmed embolic potential of device placement and manipulation within the aortic arch. Thus, TCD seems to be an appropriate safety measure to weight the embolic risk of protection devices against the risk of TAVI itself. On the other hand, DW-MRI is the most sensitive and specific method to objectify the cerebral embolic burden of TAVI. This readout is a key prerequisite for the investigation of neuroprotective approaches in randomized,

controlled trials with a reasonable sample size and adequate statistical power. Hence, randomized data on the preventive efficacy of all three devices are of paramount interest.

Financial and competing interests disclosure

Dr. Eberhard Grube is a proctor for CoreValve/Medtronic. All other authors have no relevant affiliations or financial involvement with any organization or entity with a financial interest in or financial conflict with the subject matter or materials discussed in the manuscript. This includes employment, consultancies, honoraria, stock ownership or options, expert testimony, grants or patents received or pending, or royalties. No writing assistance was utilized in the production of this manuscript.

References

1. Leon MB, Smith CR, Mack M et al. Transcatheter aortic-valve implantation for aortic stenosis in patients who cannot undergo surgery. *N Engl J Med* 2010;363:1597–607.
2. Smith CR, Leon MB, Mack MJ et al. Transcatheter versus surgical aortic-valve replacement in high-risk patients. *N Engl J Med* 2011;364:2187–98.

3. Roger VL, Go AS, Lloyd-Jones DM et al. Heart disease and stroke statistics—2012 update: A report from the American Heart Association. *Circulation* 2012;125:e2–e220.

4. Makkar RR, Fontana GP, Jilaihawi H et al. Transcatheter aortic-valve replacement for inoperable severe aortic stenosis. *N Engl J Med* 2012;366:1696–704.

5. Kodali SK, Williams MR, Smith CR et al. Two-year outcomes after transcatheter or surgical aortic-valve replacement. *N Engl J Med* 2012;366:1686–95.

6. Nombela-Franco L, Webb JG, de Jaegere PP et al. Timing, predictive factors, and prognostic value of cerebrovascular events in a large cohort of patients undergoing transcatheter aortic valve implantation. *Circulation* 2012;126:3041–53.

7. Fairbairn TA, Mather AN, Bijsterveld P et al. Diffusion-weighted MRI determined cerebral embolic infarction following transcatheter aortic valve implantation: Assessment of predictive risk factors and the relationship to subsequent health status. *Heart* 2012;98:18–23.

8. Kahlert P, Knipp SC, Schlamann M et al. Silent and apparent cerebral ischemia after percutaneous transfemoral aortic valve implantation: A diffusion-weighted magnetic resonance imaging study. *Circulation* 2010;121:870–8.

9. Ghanem A, Müller A, Nähle CP et al. Risk and fate of cerebral embolism after transfemoral aortic valve implantation: A prospective pilot study with diffusion-weighted magnetic resonance imaging. *J Am Coll Cardiol* 2010;55:1427–32.

10. Rodes-Cabau J, Dumont E, Boone RH et al. Cerebral embolism following transcatheter aortic valve implantation: Comparison of transfemoral and transapical approaches. *J Am Coll Cardiol* 2011;57:18–28.

11. Kahlert P, Al-Rashid F, Dottger P et al. Cerebral embolization during transcatheter aortic valve implantation: A transcranial Doppler study. *Circulation* 2012;126:1245–55.

12. Ghanem A, Muller A, Sinning JM et al. Prognostic value of cerebral injury following transfemoral aortic valve implantation. *EuroIntervention* 2013;8:1296–306.

13. Vermeer SE, Prins ND, den HT et al. Silent brain infarcts and the risk of dementia and cognitive decline. *N Engl J Med* 2003;348:1215–22.

14. Amat-Santos IJ, Rodes-Cabau J, Urena M et al. Incidence, predictive factors, and prognostic value of new-onset atrial fibrillation following transcatheter aortic valve implantation. *J Am Coll Cardiol* 2012;59:178–88.

15. Eggebrecht H, Schmermund A, Voigtlander T et al. Risk of stroke after transcatheter aortic valve implantation (TAVI): A meta-analysis of 10,037 published patients. *EuroIntervention* 2012;8:129–38.

16. Patti G, Tomai F, Melfi R et al. Strategies of clopidogrel load and atorvastatin reload to prevent ischemic cerebral events in patients undergoing protected carotid stenting. Results of the randomized ARMYDA-9 CAROTID (Clopidogrel and Atorvastatin Treatment during Carotid Artery Stenting) study. *J Am Coll Cardiol* 2013;61:1379–87.

17. Grube E, Naber C, Abizaid A et al. Feasibility of transcatheter aortic valve implantation without balloon pre-dilation: A pilot study. *J Am Coll Cardiol Cardiovasc Interv* 2011;4:751–7.

18. Garg N, Karagiorgos N, Pisimisis GT et al. Cerebral protection devices reduce periprocedural strokes during carotid angioplasty and stenting: A systematic review of the current literature. *J Endovasc Ther* 2009;16:412–27.

19. Onsea K, Agostoni P, Samim M et al. First-in-man experience with a new embolic deflection device in transcatheter aortic valve interventions. *EuroIntervention* 2012;8:51–6.

20. Nietlispach F, Wijesinghe N, Gurvitch R et al. An embolic deflection device for aortic valve interventions. *J Am Coll Cardiol Cardiovasc Interv* 2010;3:1133–8.

21. Naber CK, Ghanem A, Abizaid AA et al. First-in-man use of a novel embolic protection device for patients undergoing transcatheter aortic valve implantation. *EuroIntervention* 2012;8:43–50.

22. Van Mieghem NM, Schipper ME, Ladich E et al. Histopathology of embolic debris captured during transcatheter aortic valve replacement. *Circulation* 2013;127:2194–201.

23. Stortecky S and Windecker S. Stroke: An infrequent but devastating complication in cardiovascular interventions. *Circulation* 2012;126:2921–4.

30

Pulmonary valve disease: Pulmonary regurgitation—Background, indications for treatment, and clinical trial results

Hitesh Agrawal, Damien Kenny, and Ziyad M. Hijazi

Background

Pulmonary regurgitation (PR) has evolved into the "silent assassin" of congenital heart disease. Rare as an isolated congenital lesion outside of absent pulmonary valve syndrome, it is usually iatrogenic, occurring as a consequence of infantile balloon pulmonary valvuloplasty (BPV) or corrective surgery for tretralogy of Fallot (TOF). Chronic PR usually results in right ventricular volume overload and potential for subsequent right and left ventricular dysfunction (in up to 21% of patients) and the devastating consequences of ventricular arrhythmia and sudden cardiac death (SCD).[1] Its management represents one of the great challenges of treating patients with congenital heart disease in ensuring that the consequences of our interventions in early life do not lead to significant pathology in adolescence or adulthood. This chapter will review in detail the causes, consequences, and the evolving treatment guidelines and clinical options for PR.

Precipitants

Tetralogy of Fallot

The association between TOF repair and PR is based upon the perceived need for patching across the hypoplastic pulmonary annulus. This leads to an unobstructed right ventricular outflow at the expense of pulmonary valvar function. Appreciation of the longer-term detrimental consequences of chronic PR has led to a move toward "valve-sparing" repairs; however, this is more challenging to achieve in smaller infants. A contemporary review of trends in surgical management from the Society for Thoracic Surgeons (STS) database evaluating 3059 operations between 2002 and 2007 demonstrated approximately 10% of patients requiring palliative surgery prior to full repair.[2] The majority of primary repair surgeries (63%) were performed between 3 months and 1 year with only a small fraction occurring in neonatal life (6%). Over 50% of the total primary repairs underwent a transannular patch, with 82% of those undergoing repair during the neonatal period reported to have a transannular repair, suggesting that neonatal repair is possible but is associated with higher risk of neutralizing valvar function. Interestingly, primary neonatal repair was also associated with a mortality of 7.8%. This needs to be balanced against a significant reported risk for mortality for surgical palliation in this population (6.2–7.9% in the first 3 months).[2]

In another series of 56 cyanotic tetralogy infants operated at less than 6 months of age, those that underwent initial palliation ($n = 15$) had a transannular patching rate of 13% when they ultimately underwent complete repair. In contrast, a transannular patch was required in 56% of patients that underwent primary repair at a median of 2.9 months. Initial palliation lead to an increase in the pulmonary annulus size at the time of definitive repair (mean difference z value = 2.2 ± 1.6 standard deviation; $p = 0.006$).[3] More recent surgical approaches with a pulmonary annulus preservation strategy including pulmonary valve leaflet plasty with autologous pericardium at a median age of 6.5 months had transannular patch rates as low as 5% and improved midterm outcomes.[4] Other strategies including intraoperative balloons[5] have been reported in an attempt to optimize valve-sparing surgery; however, success to date has been limited.

Balloon pulmonary valvuloplasty

BPV has been widely used to relieve pulmonary stenosis in patients with isolated pulmonary valve abnormalities and is one of the most effective interventional procedures performed consistently over the past 30 years in patients with congenital heart disease. Classical perception is that both rates of reintervention and development of progressive PR are low. However, there are contemporary studies suggesting that balloon valvuloplasty may predispose a reasonable percentage of patients to the fate of significant chronic PR over time. Harrild et al.[6] studied 41 patients with cardiac magnetic resonance (CMR) and cardiopulmonary exercise testing (CPET) at a median of 13.1 years from balloon dilation. Fourteen patients (34%) had PR fraction >15%; 7 (17%) had PR fraction >30%. Higher PR fraction was associated with younger age at dilation and larger balloon:annulus ratio (BAR); BAR > 1.4 was associated with a significantly higher risk of PR fraction >15%. Right ventricle (RV) dilation (z score ≥2) was present in 40% (14 of 35 patients). A PR fraction >15% was associated with lower peak VO$_2$, suggesting that isolated PR and consequent RV dilation may lead to impaired cardiopulmonary function.

Pathophysiology

In the setting of pulmonary valve dysfunction, the degree of PR is influenced by the diastolic pressure difference between the pulmonary artery and the RV.[7] These variables in turn are influenced by a number of different factors both acutely and chronically, namely, pulmonary vascular resistance, branch pulmonary artery (BPA) size, and ventricular compliance. In the immediate postoperative period, intermittent positive pressure ventilation can increase the right ventricular afterload and thereby worsen PR,[8] while negative pressure ventilation reduces the PR by reducing the mean airway pressure.[9]

In the long run, the dynamic interplay between BPA diastolic compliance and right ventricular stiffness determines the degree of PR. In patients with BPA stenosis, there is a relatively higher regurgitant fraction coming from the larger contralateral artery as it has relatively increased pulmonary vascular resistance. In the absence of disparity in BPA size, there appears to be a preferential contribution from the left pulmonary artery (LPA), which may be due to a higher LPA vascular impedance possibly related to a smaller left lung with further compromise by an enlarged heart impinging upon the left lung.[10] Either way, relief of BPA stenosis has been shown to cause a dramatic reduction in PR and RV dilation (Figure 30.1) with an improvement in right ventricular function also seen,[11] and aggressive management is advised. Other sources of right-sided volume loading, including residual atrial septal defects, should also be sought out and treated, as these are likely to exacerbate the degree of PR. Once LV dysfunction becomes established, higher left atrial pressures may also impact upon pulmonary artery pressures and further exacerbate PR.

Right ventricular stiffness is also a key player in determining RV end-diastolic pressure and the consequent diastolic pressure differential with the pulmonary arteries. In the setting of TOF, this is caused by myocardial hypertrophy

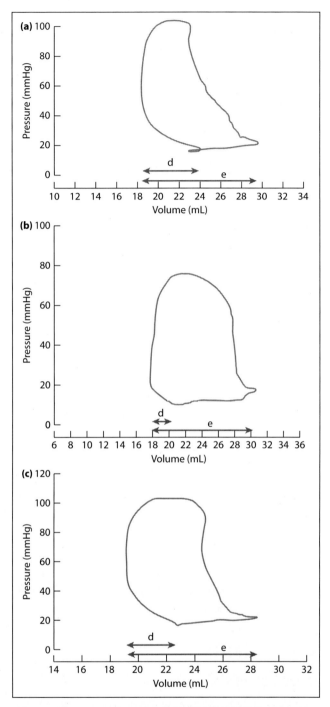

Figure 30.1 Stent insertion decreases pulmonary regurgitation in a patient with repaired tetralogy of Fallot with left pulmonary artery stenosis. In the baseline condition (a), pulmonary regurgitant fraction is 38%, and after stent deployment (b), pulmonary regurgitant fraction has decreased to 24%. Inflation of a balloon within the left pulmonary artery stent (c) results in an increase in pulmonary regurgitant fraction to 42%. The indentation in the bottom left-hand corner of the right ventricular pressure–volume loops is caused by pulmonary regurgitation, increasing right ventricular volume during "isovolumic" relaxation. Pulmonary regurgitant fraction is taken as the ratio d/e. (Reprinted from Chaturvedi RR, Redington AN. *Heart* 2007;93:880–9.)

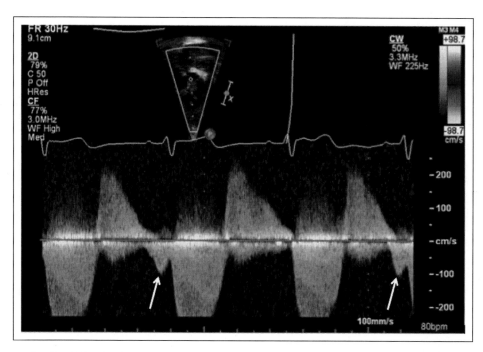

Figure 30.2   Doppler signal showing intermittent diastolic "a" wave in the main pulmonary artery marked by vertical arrows. The stiff right ventricle acts as a passive conduit and allows the conduction of atrial "a" wave into the main pulmonary artery.

or fibrosis as a consequence of the developmental outflow tract obstruction; however, it is unclear why this "restrictive physiology" is more pronounced in some patients than in others. Whether the upregulation of some genes related to the degree of accompanying cyanosis impact upon calcium hemostasis within the myocardium and consequent ventricular compliance has yet to be elucidated.[12] This restrictive RV physiology is detectable by Doppler as antegrade diastolic flow in the pulmonary artery during atrial systole (Figure 30.2)[13] and is thought to be a protective factor against RV dilation in the setting of chronic PR.

Consequences of PR

LV dysfunction

Right ventricular dilation and dysfunction appear to have consequences for left ventricular (LV) function. LV dysfunction has been reported in 21% of repaired tetralogy patients with significant PR, particularly in those with significant RV dysfunction and arrhythmia.[1] The exact mechanisms underlying the LV dysfunction are not clear, but ventricular diastolic interaction, along with prolonged abnormal electrical remodeling may be involved.[14] In the context of severe PR, surgical pulmonary valve replacement (PVR) resulted in significant overall improvement in left ventricular ejection fraction (LVEF) (n = 39) but this effect was dependent on the preoperative status of the left ventricle with those with the most pronounced LV dysfunction (LVEF ≤ 45%), demonstrating the most significant improvements.[14] Similarly, transcatheter PVR (tPVR) in the setting of severe PR has

demonstrated small but significant increases in LVEF.[15,16] It is unclear if this represents a beneficial effect of earlier intervention, which may otherwise lead to lack of complete RV remodeling and continue to influence left ventricular filling properties. The other possibility is the impact of tPVR on concomitant stenosis. Relief of stenosis in this setting with tPVR has been shown to increase left ventricular end-diastolic volumes.[17] Further work by the same group demonstrated that improved left ventricular filling dynamics were secondary to reduction in interventricular mechanical delay (caused by leftward bowing of the interventricular septum), which may impede left ventricular filling.[18] Either way, the impact on the LV is unlikely to be related solely to RV dilation as similar deterioration in LV function has not been seen in patients with chronic volume overload as a consequence of atrial septal defects.[19]

Arrhythmia

RV dilation and stretch slows interventricular conduction and creates a mechanoelectrical substrate for reentry circuits, predisposing to sustained ventricular tachycardia. QRS duration >180 ms has been associated with a 42-fold increased risk of developing sustained ventricular tachycardia and a 2.2-fold increased risk of SCD in a 10-year follow-up.[20] While QRS lengthening, seen immediately after repair, reflects surgical injury to the myocardium and on the right bundle, late QRS prolongation almost universally reflects RV dilatation. Interval change in QRS duration, thus, may have a greater prognostic value for sustained ventricular tachycardia and SCD than absolute QRS measurements at any point in time.[20]

Assessment

Echocardiography

With the evolution of CMR imaging, there has been a debate as to the place of transthoracic echocardiography for assessment of PR. However, given the widespread availability and the simplicity of the procedure, it has been used in the long-term follow-up of these patients. The assessment of PR by echocardiography has been largely qualitative, although multiple attempts to better quantify PR have been made[21] (Table 30.1).

Recent data from the US Melody® valve clinical trial comparing echocardiographic right heart assessment with that of CMR suggested that assessment of PR using a 3-point severity scale showed good correlation with CMR-derived pulmonary regurgitant fraction. Moreover, RV apical diastolic area was highly reproducible and had an excellent correlation with CMR-derived RV end-diastolic volume and all patients with RV apical diastolic areas $\geq$30 cm^2/m^2 had CMR RV end-diastolic volumes $\geq$160 mL/m^2. However, standard TTE was less effective at determining a quantitative assessment of RV function.[22]

Table 30.1 Echocardiographic assessment parameters for assessment of PR

- The vena contracta: The diameter of the narrowest portion of the PR jet as it crosses the pulmonary valve varies with severity proportionally.
- Volume of RVOT occupied with regurgitation and the degree of retrograde jet penetration.
- Pulmonary regurgitant index: The ratio between the duration of PR and total diastole (severe PR will have a dense jet that rapidly decelerates so that regurgitant flow ends around middiastole while mild to moderate PR flow persists throughout diastole).
- Velocity of flow is not proportional to or indicative of severity (higher velocities suggested by aliasing of color Doppler signal or by continuous wave peak velocity reflect higher pressure gradients between RVOT and pulmonary circulation)
- Tricuspid regurgitant velocity facilitates measurement of the RV pressure
- Indexed RV end-diastolic diameter and right atrial size
- Diastolic to systolic time velocity integral ratio (DSTVI): The ratio between the regurgitant (diastolic) time-velocity integral to the antegrade (systolic) time-velocity integral correlates linearly with regurgitant fraction on CMR.
- Pulsatility index of the branch pulmonary arteries: Ratio of systolic to diastolic diameter of the branch pulmonary arteries. Higher values suggest worse PR.

Source: Mercer-Rosa L et al. *Circ Cardiovasc Imaging* 2012;5:637–43; Schiller NB, Ristow B, Kulkarni A. *Echocardiographic Evaluation of the Pulmonic Valve and Pulmonary Artery.* In: Manning WJ, Gaasch WH. Ed. UpToDate 2011.

Cardiac magnetic resonance

CMR has become the gold standard for the quantification of PR and the assessment of RV size and systolic function. The accurate measurement of pulmonary regurgitant fraction/volume, RV ejection fraction, and the RV end-diastolic volume by CMR has paved the way to better understanding of this entity and is beginning to form the basis of recommendations for the treatment of PR (Figure 30.3). However, PR fraction should be interpreted with caution, as the expression of a percentage does not allow one to appreciate the magnitude of the numerator or the denominator. Clinicians should be comfortable interpreting both PR_{volume} and $PR_{fraction}$, although indexed PR_{volume} may be the more sensitive and accurate expression of significant pulmonary incompetence when compared with expression of PR burden as a $PR_{fraction}$.[23] Further addition to the technology is phase-contrast angiography that provides a noninvasive three-dimensional measure of blood flow and is very useful for accurate measurement of PR_{volume} and $PR_{fraction}$.

CT angiography

Computed Tomography angiography (CTA) provides an alternative to CMR assessment of the right heart. Although significantly less time-consuming for the patient, accurate quantification of RV size, function, and pulmonary regurgitant fraction has not yet been established, although evolving reports suggest this may be achievable.[24] Furthermore, the anatomic and dynamic variability that exists within the RVOT makes this technique useful particularly in determining the relationship of the RVOT to the origin of the left main and left anterior descending coronary arteries. The technique may also be preferable to MRI to assess stent geometry following valve replacement or in the setting of previous pacemaker or implantable defibrillator placement where CMR may not be feasible.

Diagnostic cardiac catheterization

With the advent of CMR in the setting of PR, diagnostic cardiac catheterization is often reserved for preoperative assessment of coronary arteries in older patients due for cardiopulmonary bypass or assessment of pulmonary vascular resistance. More often, cardiac catheterization is reserved for intervention on BPA stenosis, which may significantly impact upon the degree of PR as discussed above. Occasionally, assessment of the RVOT diameter with a compliant balloon may be carried out to determine if the patient is suitable for transcatheter valve implantation (Figure 30.4). This test is of paramount importance in determining the proximity of the RVOT to the coronary artery (Figure 30.5). From a hemodynamic point of view, pressure tracing in the PAs may confirm the severity of the PR.

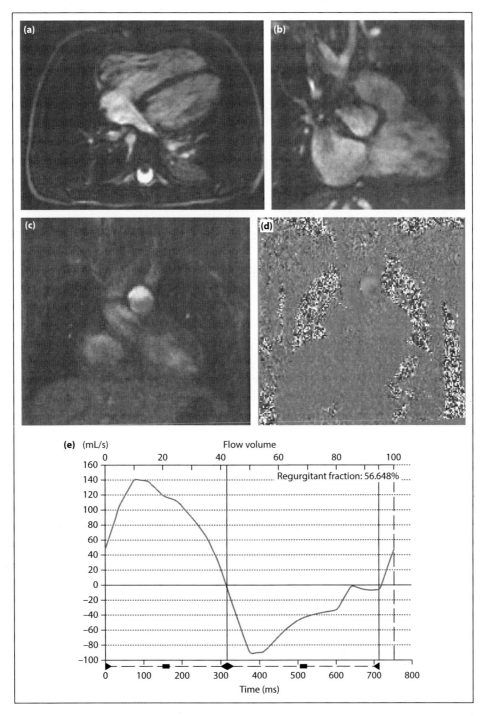

Figure 30.3   Series of CMR images outlining assessment of a child with significant pulmonary regurgitation following previous TOF repair. (a) Axial view of the RV demonstrating RV dilation with marked trabeculations. (b) Coronal view of the RV confirming the dilation. (c, d) Phase-contrast images used to evaluate pulmonary regurgitation with (e) the flow volume loops confirming severe pulmonary regurgitation with an RF of 57%.

Cardiopulmonary exercise testing

Exercise capacity can be affected by the degree of right ventricular dysfunction and by the amount of PR. Hence, CPET can identify those patients with severe PR and right ventricular dysfunction and stratify them according to risk of both hospitalization and death.[25] Patients with peak oxygen uptake ≤36% of predicted value and those with ventilation per unit of carbon dioxide production (VE/VCO_2) slopes greater than 39 have been shown to be at greater

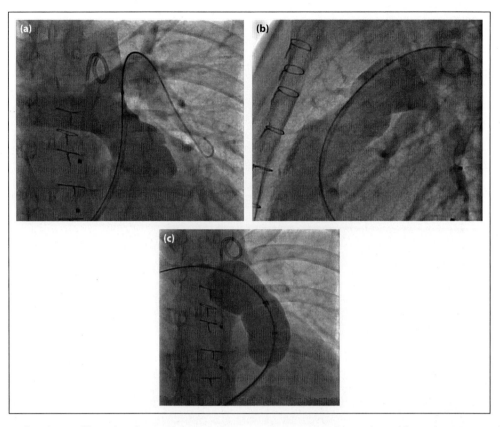

Figure 30.4   Series of AP and lateral angiographic images demonstrating severe PR in a patient with previous TOF repair (a,b). Balloon inflation in the RVOT with a compliant sizing balloon to determine the size and compliance of the RVOT and suitability for transcatheter valve implantation (c).

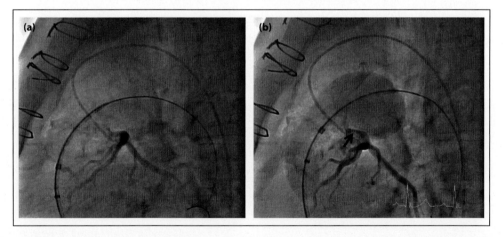

Figure 30.5   Angulated view demonstrating selective coronary artery injection in a patient with a previous Ross operation. (a) Demonstration of the left coronary artery and (b) demonstration of the distinct compression of the left mainstem coronary (arrow) with balloon inflation in the RVOT. Further IVUS imaging confirmed coronary artery compression when the RVOT was stretched with a balloon and stenting of the RVOT was abandoned.

risk for cardiac-related death.[26] CPET may be useful in patients with PR being evaluated for tPVR when there is a question regarding symptoms, thus providing an objective assessment of exercise capacity. However, it is unclear whether CPET should be routinely used after tPVR to demonstrate improvement.

Indications for treatment

In the context of chronic PR, there is reasonable consensus that PVR should be offered to symptomatic individuals.[27] However, the optimal timing for intervention in asymptomatic patients remains under debate (Table 30.2). With

Table 30.2 Indications for treatment of pulmonary regurgitation in asymptomatic individuals

MRI indices

Right ventricular end-diastolic volume index >150 mL/m^2

Right ventricular regurgitant fraction >40%

Right ventricular ejection fraction <40%

QRS duration >180 ms

LV dysfunction

advancement in CMR availability, attempts have been made to define right ventricular volumes above which normalization of RV volumes cannot be established following the insertion of a competent pulmonary valve.[28–30] Reported right ventricular end-diastolic volume indexes (RVEDVI) for optimal outcome have fallen from an initial report by Therrien et al.[28] of ≤170 mL/m^2 to ≤160 mL/m^2 by Oosterhov et al.,[29] to ≤150 mL/m^2 by Frigiola et al.[30] The American Heart Association (AHA)/American College of Cardiology (ACC) guidelines for repeat surgery in this setting are not so explicit.[27] With lack of guideline consensus on the optimal cutoff, early intervention with RVEDVI >150 mL/m^2 seems reasonable, as it leads to the normalization of RV volumes, improvement in biventricular function, and submaximal exercise capacity.[30] Whether the introduction of tPVR will influence earlier timing of intervention with the potential for further valve-in-valve procedures has yet to be seen. AHA/ACC guidelines for tPVR are even less clear-cut, advocating tPVR in a patient with an RV-to-pulmonary artery conduit with associated moderate-to-severe PR or stenosis provided the patient meets inclusion/exclusion criteria for the available valve.[31] Indeed, it is possible that these mixed lesions with moderate degrees of both stenosis and regurgitation may have an additive detrimental effect on the RV and intervention should be considered at lower regurgitant volumes or Doppler gradients than when exclusive regurgitation or stenosis is present. As the procedure becomes more acceptable, it is likely that indications will be more prescriptive.

Two important indications for intervention should not be overlooked, namely, QRS duration ≥180 ms with risk for longer-term arrhythmia/SCD and progressive left ventricular dysfunction as discussed above. Importantly, both surgical and transcatheter PVR significantly reduces QRS duration[32,33] and also improves LV dynamics by increasing LVEF.[15]

Clinical trials and outcomes

Pulmonary valve replacement: Surgical and transcatheter

The relevant clinical outcomes relate to procedural success, that is, placing a well-functioning valve in the desired location, number, and extent of procedural complications, and longer-term freedom from valvar dysfunction and reintervention. There are no direct comparative trials evaluating outcomes in patients undergoing surgical versus tPVR. Often, the cohorts are not comparable and whether this will be achievable in the future with newer transcatheter valve systems (see Chapter 36) designed specifically for native outflow tracts remains to be seen. Data from the largest most recently published studies evaluating attempted tPVR (Melody and SAPIEN™) in 500 patients are outlined in Table 30.3. Procedural success is generally high, with mean valve deployment of 95%. Procedural complications vary according to definition, but in those studies reporting exclusively major complications, the mean procedural complication rate was just greater than 4%. Coronary artery compression in this setting has been associated with mortality and may present after the procedure;[15] therefore, if there is any doubt, valve deployment should not be attempted. Conduit rupture has also been reported[34] and risk factors associated with this complication need to be elucidated. Overall mean freedom from reintervention was 86% over a mean follow-up of 26 months. Stent fracture remains an important event with the Melody valve despite prestenting (5–16%) and is the most common reason for reintervention; however, the extent of stent fracture is also relevant to clinical outcomes. Type I stent fractures are likely to occur initially, and only 56% of patients are free from type II fractures at 2 years from initial diagnosis of stent fracture and therefore require careful monitoring.[35] Stent fracture has not been reported to date with the SAPIEN valve. The other notable outcome variable is the risk of infective endocarditis, which has been reported consistently at between 1% and 4% with the Melody valve. Reported data are not available for the SAPIEN valve in the pulmonary position.

A recent single institutional study retrospectively compared the outcomes of SAPIEN (N = 20) and Melody (n = 13) valves in the pulmonary position. Both valves demonstrated similar midterm valve function except that follow-up mean pulmonary Doppler gradients were higher with the SAPIEN cohort (18.43 ± 9.06 mmHg [S] and 11.17 ± 5.24 mmHg [M], p = 0.016). Greater residual gradients with the SAPIEN valve may represent a more conservative early presenting approach with this valve.[36] Larger and blinded trials with longer follow-up periods are required to demonstrate the true efficacy of one transcatheter valve over the other.

The most contemporary large data set evaluating valve dysfunction and reintervention in adolescent patients undergoing surgical PVR (n = 254) revealed mean freedom from valvar dysfunction of 72% and mean freedom from reintervention of 90% at 5 years with no difference between homograft and bioprosthetic valve cohorts.[37] In contrast, Fiore et al.[38] reviewed the performance of the mosaic porcine, bovine pericardial, and homograft valves for PR and found that late valve dysfunction was highest with homografts (54%), followed by porcine (19%) and pericardial

Table 30.3	Procedural outcomes from clinical studies				
Author	**N**	**Success**	**Complics**	**Fracture**	**FFR (follow-up)**
Lurz[41]	163 pts	155 pts (95%)	7 pts (4.5%)	21%	70% (70 months)
McElhinney[42]	136 pts	124 pts (91%)	8 pts (6%)	22%	93.5% (12 months)
Eicken[15]	102 pts	100%	2 pts (2%)	5%	89% (12 months)
Kenny[43]	36 pts	33 pts (92%)	7 pts[a] (20.5%)	0	97% (6 months)
Butera[44]	63 pts	61 pts (97%)	9 pts[a] (14%)	16%	81.4% (30 months)

[a] Includes major and minor complications.
Complics: procedural complications; FFR: freedom from reintervention.

valves (5.5%). In this report, the pulmonary homograft demonstrated a comparatively higher degree of dysfunction secondary to early valve insufficiency, and freedom from reoperation at 6 years was as low as 35%. Furthermore, Geva et al.[39] investigated whether the addition of surgical RV remodeling with removal of scar tissue along with PVR would result in better RV function as compared with PVR alone and they found no significant difference.

Conclusions

Chronic PR has significant longer-term consequences and requires serial accurate evaluation to determine appropriate timing of intervention. Aggressive management of precipitating factors is indicated. The current challenge lies in finding unanimous indices to guide the therapeutic approach for optimal outcome given the finite life span of any available valve. Transcatheter PVR is a significant advancement in itself, but is still evolving and its long-term fate needs to be elucidated. Development of living autologous valves and especially those with potential to grow *in vivo* still remain areas of uncharted territory.

References

1. Broberg CS, Aboulhosn J, Mongeon FP et al. Alliance for Adult Research in Congenital Cardiology (AARCC). Prevalence of left ventricular systolic dysfunction in adults with repaired tetralogy of fallot. *Am J Cardiol* 2011;107:1215–20.
2. AlHabib HF, Jacobs JP, Mavroudis C et al. Contemporary patterns of management of tetralogy of Fallot: Data from the Society of Thoracic Surgeons Database. *Ann Thorac Surg* 2010;90:813–9.
3. Sousa Uva M, Lacour-Gayet F, Komiya T et al. Surgery for tetralogy of Fallot at less than six months of age. *J Thorac Cardiovasc Surg* 1994;107:1291–300.
4. Hua Z, Li S, Wang L, Hu S, Wang D. A new pulmonary valve cusp plasty technique markedly decreases transannular patch rate and improves midterm outcomes of tetralogy of Fallot repair. *Eur J Cardiothorac Surg* 2011;40:1221–6.
5. Robinson JD, Rathod RH, Brown DW et al. The evolving role of intraoperative balloon pulmonary valvuloplasty in valve-sparing repair of tetralogy of Fallot. *J Thorac Cardiovasc Surg* 2011;142:1367–73.
6. Harrild DM, Powell AJ, Tran TX et al. Long-term pulmonary regurgitation following balloon valvuloplasty for pulmonary stenosis risk factors and relationship to exercise capacity and ventricular volume and function. *J Am Coll Cardiol* 2010;55:1041–7.
7. Chaturvedi RR, Redington AN. Pulmonary regurgitation in congenital heart disease. *Heart* 2007;93:880–9.
8. Chaturvedi RR, Kilner PJ, White PA et al. Increased airway pressure and simulated branch pulmonary artery stenosis increase pulmonary regurgitation after tetralogy of Fallot. Real-time analysis with a conductance-catheter technique. *Circulation* 1997;95:643–9.
9. Shekerdemian LS, Shore DF, Lincoln C, Bush A, Redington AN. Negative pressure ventilation improves cardiac output after right heart surgery. *Circulation* 1996;94:49–55.
10. Harris MA, Whitehead KK, Gillespie MJ et al. Differential branch pulmonary artery regurgitant fraction is a function of differential pulmonary arterial anatomy and pulmonary vascular resistance. *J Am Coll Cardiol Cardiovasc Imaging* 2011;4:506–13.
11. Petit CJ, Gillespie MJ, Harris MA et al. Relief of branch pulmonary artery stenosis reduces pulmonary valve insufficiency in a swine model. *J Thorac Cardiovasc Surg* 2009;138:382–9.
12. Ghorbel MT, Cherif M, Jenkins E et al. Transcriptomic analysis of patients with tetralogy of Fallot reveals the effect of chronic hypoxia on myocardial gene expression. *J Thorac Cardiovasc Surg* 2010;140:337–345.e26.
13. Cullen S, Shore D, Redington A. Characterization of right ventricular diastolic performance after complete repair of tetralogy of Fallot. Restrictive physiology predicts slow postoperative recovery. *Circulation* 1995;91:1782–9.
14. Tobler D, Crean AM, Redington AN et al. The left heart after pulmonary valve replacement in adults late after tetralogy of Fallot repair. *Int J Cardiol* 2012;160:165–70.
15. Eicken A, Ewert P, Hager A et al. Percutaneous pulmonary valve implantation: Two-centre experience with more than 100 patients. *Eur Heart J* 2011;32:1260–5.
16. Vezmar M, Chaturvedi R, Lee KJ et al. Percutaneous pulmonary valve implantation in the young 2-year follow-up. JACC. *Cardiovasc Interv* 2010;3:439–48.
17. Coats L, Khambadkone S, Derrick G et al. Physiological and clinical consequences of relief of right ventricular outflow tract obstruction late after repair of congenital heart defects. *Circulation.* 2006;113:2037–44.
18. Lurz P, Puranik R, Nordmeyer J et al. Improvement in left ventricular filling properties after relief of right ventricle to pulmonary artery conduit obstruction: Contribution of septal motion and interventricular mechanical delay. *Eur Heart J* 2009;30:2266–74.
19. Dragulescu A, Grosse-Wortmann L, Redington A et al. Differential effect of right ventricular dilatation on myocardial deformation in patients with atrial septal defects and patients after tetralogy of Fallot repair. *Int J Cardiol* 2013;168:803–10.

20. Gatzoulis MA, Balaji S, Webber SA et al. Risk factors for arrhythmia and sudden cardiac death late after repair of tetralogy of Fallot: A multicentre study. *Lancet* 2000;356:975–81.

21. Mercer-Rosa L, Yang W, Kutty S et al. Quantifying pulmonary regurgitation and right ventricular function in surgically repaired tetralogy of Fallot: A comparative analysis of echocardiography and magnetic resonance imaging. *Circ Cardiovasc Imaging* 2012;5:637–43.

22. Brown DW, McElhinney DB, Araoz PA et al. Reliability and accuracy of echocardiographic right heart evaluation in the U.S. Melody valve investigational trial. *J Am Soc Echocardiogr* 2012;25:383–92.

23. Wald RM, Redington AN, Pereira A et al. Refining the assessment of pulmonary regurgitation in adults after tetralogy of Fallot repair: Should we be measuring regurgitant fraction or regurgitant volume? *Eur Heart J* 2009;30:356–61.

24. Raman SV, Cook SC, McCarthy B, Ferketich AK. Usefulness of multidetector row computed tomography to quantify right ventricular size and function in adults with either tetralogy of Fallot or transposition of the great arteries. *Am J Cardiol* 2005;95:683–6.

25. Giardini A, Specchia S, Coutsoumbas G et al. Impact of pulmonary regurgitation and right ventricular dysfunction on oxygen uptake recovery kinetics in repaired tetralogy of Fallot. *Eur J Heart Fail* 2006;8:736–743.

26. Giardini A, Specchia S, Tacy TA et al. Usefulness of cardiopulmonary exercise to predict long-term prognosis in adults with repaired tetralogy of Fallot. *Am J Cardiol* 2007;99:1462–7.

27. Warnes CA, Williams RG, Bashore TM et al. ACC/AHA 2008 Guidelines for the Management of Adults with Congenital Heart Disease: A report of the American College of Cardiology/American Heart Association Task Force on Practice Guidelines (writing committee to develop guidelines on the management of adults with congenital heart disease). *Circulation* 2008;118:e714–e833.

28. Therrien J, Provost Y, Merchant N, Williams W, Colman J, Webb G. Optimal timing for pulmonary valve replacement in adults after tetralogy of Fallot repair. *Am J Cardiol* 2005;95:779–82.

29. Oosterhof T, van Straten A, Vliegen HW et al. Preoperative thresholds for pulmonary valve replacement in patients with corrected tetralogy of Fallot using cardiovascular magnetic resonance. *Circulation* 2007;116:545–51.

30. Frigiola A, Tsang V, Bull C et al. Biventricular response after pulmonary valve replacement for right ventricular outflow tract dysfunction: Is age a predictor of outcome? *Circulation* 2008;118:182–90.

31. Feltes TF, Bacha E, Beekman RH 3rd et al. Indications for cardiac catheterization and intervention in pediatric cardiac disease: A scientific statement from the American Heart Association. *Circulation* 2011;123:2607–52.

32. Plymen CM, Bolger AP, Lurz P et al. Electrical remodeling following percutaneous pulmonary valve implantation. *Am J Cardiol* 2011;107:309–14.

33. van Huysduynen BH, van Straten A, Swenne CA et al. Reduction of QRS duration after pulmonary valve replacement in adult Fallot patients is related to reduction of right ventricular volume. *Eur Heart J* 2005;26:928–32.

34. Sosnowski C, Kenny D, Hijazi ZM. Bailout use of the Gore excluder following pulmonary conduit rupture during transcatheter valve replacement. *Catheter Cardiovasc Interv* 2013;81:331–4.

35. McElhinney DB, Cheatham JP, Jones TK et al. Stent fracture, valve dysfunction, and right ventricular outflow tract reintervention after transcatheter pulmonary valve implantation: Patient-related and procedural risk factors in the US Melody Valve Trial. *Circ Cardiovasc Interv* 2011;4:602–14.

36. Faza N, Kenny D, Kavinsky C et al. Single center comparative outcomes of the Edwards Sapien and medtronic melody transcatheter heart valves in the pulmonary position. *Catheter Cardiovasc Interv* 2013;82:E535–41.

37. Batlivala SP, Emani S, Mayer JE et al. Pulmonary valve replacement function in adolescents: A comparison of bioprosthetic valves and homograft conduits. *Ann Thorac Surg* 2012;93:2007–16.

38. Fiore AC, Rodefeld M, Turrentine M et al. Pulmonary valve replacement: A comparison of three biological valves. *Ann Thorac Surg* 2008;85:1712–8.

39. Geva T, Gauvreau K, Powell AJ et al. Randomized trial of pulmonary valve replacement with and without right ventricular remodeling surgery. *Circulation.* 2010;122:201–8.

40. Schiller NB, Ristow B, Kulkarni A. *Echocardiographic Evaluation of the Pulmonic Valve and Pulmonary Artery.* In: Manning WJ, Gaasch WH. Ed. Up To Date 2011.

41. Lurz P, Coats L, Khambadkone S et al. Percutaneous pulmonary valve implantation: Impact of evolving technology and learning curve on clinical outcome. *Circulation* 2008;117:1964–72.

42. McElhinney DB, Hellenbrand WE, Zahn EM et al. Short- and medium-term outcomes after transcatheter pulmonary valve placement in the expanded multicenter US melody valve trial. *Circulation* 2010;122:507–16.

43. Kenny D, Hijazi ZM, Kar S et al. Percutaneous implantation of the Edwards SAPIEN transcatheter heart valve for conduit failure in the pulmonary position: Early phase 1 results from an international multicenter clinical trial. *J Am Coll Cardiol* 2011;58:2248–56.

44. Butera G, Milanesi O, Spadoni I et al. Melody transcatheter pulmonary valve implantation. Results from the registry of the Italian Society of Pediatric Cardiology (SICP). *Catheter Cardiovasc Interv* 2013;81:310–6.

31

Pulmonary valve disease: Pulmonary valve stenosis

P. Syamasundar Rao

Introduction

Transcatheter therapy of valvar pulmonary stenosis is one of the first, if not the first, catheter intervention that has facilitated the application of this technology for children so that many of them can benefit by less invasive treatment for structural congenital heart defects. In this chapter, transcatheter management of pulmonary stenosis (PS) will be discussed.

Anatomy and pathophysiology

The pathologic features of the stenotic pulmonary valve vary.[1] The most commonly observed pathology is what is described as a "dome-shaped" pulmonary valve. The fused pulmonary valve leaflets protrude from their attachment into the pulmonary artery as a conical, windsock-like structure. The size of the pulmonary valve orifice varies from a pinhole to several millimeters, usually central in location, but can be eccentric. Raphae, presumably fused valve commissures, extend from the stenotic orifice to a variable distance down into the base of the dome-shaped valve. The number of the raphae may vary from zero to seven. Less common variants are unicuspid (unicommissural), bicuspid, and tricuspid valves. Thickening of the valve leaflets is seen, which may be due to an increase in valve spongeosa or due to excessive fibrous, collagenous, myxomatous, and elastic tissue. The valve annulus is abnormal in most cases with partial or complete lack of fibrous backbone, thus, a "true" annulus may not be present.

Pulmonary valve ring hypoplasia and dysplastic pulmonary valves may be present in a small percentage of patients. Pulmonary valve dysplasia is characterized by thickened, nodular, and redundant valve leaflets with minimal or no commissural fusion, valve ring hypoplasia, and lack of poststenotic dilatation of the pulmonary artery.[2] The obstruction is mainly related to thickened, myxomatous immobile pulmonary valve cusps and valve-ring hypoplasia.

Changes secondary to pulmonary valve obstruction do occur and include right ventricular muscle hypertrophy, proportional to the degree and duration of obstruction[3]

and dilatation of the main pulmonary artery, independent of the severity of obstruction, presumably related to a high-velocity jet across the stenotic valve.[4]

Clinical features

The majority of children with valvar PS are asymptomatic and are detected because of a cardiac murmur heard on routine examination, although they can present with signs of systemic venous congestion (usually interpreted as congestive heart failure) due to severe right ventricular dysfunction or cyanosis because of right-to-left shunt across the atrial septum.

The right ventricular and the right ventricular outflow tract impulses are increased and a heave may be felt at the left lower and left upper sternal borders. A thrill may be felt at the left upper sternal border and/or in the suprasternal notch. The second heart sound is variable, depending upon the degree of obstruction. An ejection systolic click is heard in most cases of valvar stenosis. The click is heard best at the left lower-, mid-, and upper sternal borders and varies with respiration (decreases or disappears with inspiration). An ejection systolic murmur is heard best at the left upper sternal border and it radiates into infraclavicular regions, axillae, and back. The intensity of the murmur may vary between grades II and V/VI; the intensity of the murmur is not necessarily related to the severity of the stenosis but rather its duration and time of peaking; the longer the murmur and the later it peaks, the more severe is the PS.

Indications for balloon pulmonary valvuloplasty

It is generally believed that indications for balloon pulmonary valvuloplasty are similar to those used for surgical pulmonary valvotomy, that is, a moderate degree of pulmonary valve stenosis with a peak-to-peak gradient ≥50 mmHg with normal cardiac index.[5] Some workers, including the American Heart Association Committee[6] on guidelines, use lesser gradients (gradient of 40 mmHg or right ventricular pressure of 50 mmHg) for intervention. Careful examination of all the available studies[5] suggested that (1) there is only marginal reduction of right ventricular pressure if mild stenoses are dilated, (2) natural history studies revealed trivial and mild stenoses (<50 mmHg gradient) are likely to remain mild at follow-up,[7] and (3) an increase in gradient can easily be quantified by echo-Doppler studies at follow-up examination. If an increase in gradient is documented, the patient could then undergo balloon dilatation. Based on these observations, the author continue to advocate[8,9] that balloon dilatation should be performed only in patients with a peak-to-peak gradient >50 mmHg.

More recently, the interventional procedures are increasingly performed under general anesthesia and the gradients are usually lower with general anesthesia than with conscious sedation. Consequently, the same criteria should not be applied. Therefore, the Doppler gradients (discussed in the echocardiography section) should be used in making the decision regarding balloon pulmonary valvuloplasty.

Some workers have suggested that balloon dilatation should not be undertaken for very severe stenosis with right ventricular systolic pressure twice that in the left ventricle. In our own series,[10] 16 (23%) of 71 patients had right ventricular pressure twice that in the left ventricle and these children underwent successful balloon valvuloplasty. Therefore, it is believed that extreme stenosis is not a contraindication for balloon dilatation.

Pulmonary valve dysplasia has been considered by some workers as a relative contraindication for balloon dilatation. Based on our own experience[11] and that of others,[12] balloon valvuloplasty is the initial treatment of choice. Balloons that are 1.4–1.5 times the pulmonary valve annulus should probably be used in patients with dysplastic valves to achieve a good result.[11] But, more importantly, the determinant of a favorable result is the presence of commissural fusion.

In adult subjects with moderate to severe stenosis without symptoms, some authors were hesitant to recommend intervention.[13] But, based on a poor response to exercise[14] and the potential for development of myocardial fibrosis, I believe it is prudent to provide catheter-directed relief of the obstruction in all patients, including adults, with moderate to severe stenosis, irrespective of the symptoms.[15]

Surgical therapy

Until the early 1980s, surgical pulmonary valvotomy under cardiopulmonary bypass was the only treatment available. At the present time, relief of pulmonary valve obstruction can be accomplished by balloon pulmonary valvuloplasty. Indeed, presently, balloon pulmonary valvuloplasty is the treatment of choice. Occasionally, surgical intervention

may become necessary when there is severe supravalvar stenosis, significant valve annulus hypoplasia, severely dysplastic pulmonary valves, or persistent and severe infundibular narrowing (most of this resolves spontaneously or with beta-blocker therapy[3,16]) despite successful balloon pulmonary valvuloplasty.

Historical aspects of balloon pulmonary valvuloplasty

The first attempt to relieve pulmonary valve obstruction by transcatheter methodology, to my knowledge, was in the early 1950s by Rubio-Alverez et al.[17,18] In 1979, Semb and his associates[19] employed a balloon-tipped angiographic (Berman) catheter to produce rupture of pulmonary valve commissures by rapidly withdrawing the inflated balloon across the pulmonary valve. More recently, Kan and her associates[20] applied the technique of Gruntzig et al.[21] to relieve pulmonary valve obstruction by the radial forces of balloon inflation of a balloon catheter positioned across the pulmonary valve.

Technique

The diagnosis and assessment of pulmonary valve stenosis are made by the usual clinical, radiographic, electrocardiographic, and echo-Doppler data. Once a moderate to severe obstruction is diagnosed, cardiac catheterization and cineangiography are performed percutaneously to confirm the clinical impression and to consider balloon dilatation of the pulmonary valve. It is important that a full explanation of the balloon dilatation procedure is given to the patients/parents, along with the potential complications. Such informed consent is essential, especially in view of the fact that acute complications can occur and long-term results are limited. The technique of balloon pulmonary valvuloplasty involves positioning of a balloon angioplasty catheter across the stenotic valve, usually over an extra-stiff exchange-length guide wire and inflating the balloon, thus producing valvotomy. Details of the technique will be discussed in the ensuing sections.

Preintervention noninvasive studies
Echo-Doppler studies

Two-dimensional echocardiographic precordial short-axis and subcostal views are most useful in the evaluation of the pulmonary valve leaflets. Thickening and doming of the pulmonary valve leaflets can often be visualized.[22] Markedly thickened, nodular, and immobile pulmonary valve leaflets, suggestive of dysplastic pulmonary valves, may also be recognized. The pulmonary valve annulus can also be visualized and measured; the latter can be compared with normal values (z score) to determine if the annulus is hypoplastic (z score ≤2). Such measurements are also useful in the selection of balloon diameter for balloon valvuloplasty. Poststenotic dilatation of the pulmonary artery can be imaged and the right ventricular size, wall thickness, and function can be evaluated by the two-dimensional technique.

Pulsed, continuous-wave, and color Doppler evaluation in conjunction with two-dimensional echocardiography is most useful in confirming the clinical diagnosis and in quantifying the degree of obstruction. Pulsed Doppler interrogation of the right ventricular outflow tract with the sample volume moved across the pulmonary valve demonstrates an abrupt increase in peak Doppler flow velocity, suggesting pulmonary valve obstruction. In addition, the flow pattern in the main pulmonary artery is turbulent instead of being laminar. Color Doppler imaging will also show smooth, laminar subpulmonary flow (blue) with some flow acceleration (red) immediately beneath the pulmonary valve and turbulent (mosaic) flow beginning immediately distal to the pulmonary valve leaflets. Furthermore, a narrow jet of color-flow disturbance can be visualized, which should be used to align the continuous-wave ultrasound beam to record maximum velocity. The angle of incidence between ultrasound beam and color jet should be kept to a minimum. Two-dimensional and color flow-directed continuous-wave Doppler recordings from multiple transducer positions, including the precordial short axis, high parasternal and subcostal, should be performed for documenting the maximum velocity. Several studies have demonstrated the usefulness of peak Doppler velocities in predicting the catheter-measured peak-to-peak gradients across the pulmonary valve. The peak instantaneous Doppler gradient may be calculated using a modified Bernoulli equation:

$$\Delta P = 4\ V^2$$

where ΔP is the pressure gradient and V is the peak Doppler flow velocity in the main pulmonary artery.

Continuous-wave and color Doppler interrogation for the tricuspid regurgitant jet is important to further confirm high right ventricular pressure. The right ventricular peak systolic pressure (RVP) may be estimated by using a modified Bernoulli equation

$$RVP = 4\ V^2 + ERAP$$

where V is the peak tricuspid regurgitant jet velocity and ERAP is the estimated right atrial pressure (5–10 mmHg).

It is important that the Doppler study is performed when the patient is quiet and in a resting state; young children and patients who are extremely anxious may have to be mildly sedated. It should be remembered that Doppler measurements represent peak instantaneous gradients, whereas

catheterization gradients are peak-to-peak gradients. It was initially thought that the peak instantaneous gradient is reflective of the peak-to-peak systolic gradient measured during cardiac catheterization; however, the peak instantaneous gradient overestimates the peak-to-peak gradient, presumably related to pressure recovery phenomenon.[23] In our experience, the catheter peak-to-peak gradient is somewhere in between Doppler peak instantaneous and mean gradients.

Color Doppler and pulsed Doppler interrogation of the atrial septum is useful and may reveal left-to-right or right-to-left shunt. Because of high sensitivity of color Doppler, contrast echocardiography to document right-to-left shunt is not routinely utilized.

Other noninvasive studies

Computed tomographic (CT) scans and magnetic resonance imaging (MRI) may demonstrate pulmonary valve stenosis, but the current state-of-the-art echo-Doppler studies are more useful in diagnosing and quantifying pulmonary valve obstruction. Myocardial energy demands and perfusion may be evaluated by magnetic resonance spectroscopy and positron emission tomography but, at this time, clinical utility of these techniques in the management of pulmonary stenosis has not been established.

Sedation and anesthesia

Balloon pulmonary valvuloplasty may be performed with the patient sedated with a mixture of meperidine, promethazine, and chlorpromazine, given intramuscularly. If necessary, this is supplemented with intermittent doses of midazolam (versed) (0.05–0.1 mg/kg IV) and/or Fentanyl (0.5–1.0 µg/kg IV). General anesthesia with endotracheal ventilation is used in infants below the age of 3 months. Others use katamine or general anesthesia for all interventional cases. However, institutional practices should be respected with regard to the type of sedation used and whether general anesthesia is employed.

Vascular access

The percutaneous femoral venous route is the most preferred entry site for balloon pulmonary valvuloplasty and should be used routinely. However, other sites such as axillary[24] or jugular[25] venous or transhepatic[26] routes have been successfully used in the absence of femoral venous access. A #5 to #7 French sheath is inserted into the vein depending upon the age and size of the patient as well as the anticipated size of the balloon dilatation catheter.

An arterial line (#3 French in infants, #4 French in children, and #5 French in adolescents and adults) is inserted percutaneously into the femoral artery to continuously monitor the arterial blood pressure and to intermittently monitor oxygen saturation.

Hemodynamic assessment

The measurement of right ventricular (RV) and pulmonary artery pressures along with the peak-to-peak gradient across the pulmonary valve is performed. This peak-to-peak gradient is used to assess the severity of pulmonary valve obstruction. Calculation of the pulmonary valve area by the Gorlin formula[27] has been advocated by some workers, but because of multiple assumptions that must be made during calculation and because of limitations in applying this formula to calculate pulmonary valve area, we do not routinely calculate the pulmonary valve area. Instead, we utilize peak-to-peak pulmonary valve gradients to assess the severity of obstruction after ensuring that the cardiac index is within normal range.

If it is not possible to advance the Berman angiographic catheter into the pulmonary artery across the pulmonary valve, the catheter is exchanged with either a multipurpose catheter or right coronary artery catheter to obtain the pulmonary valvar gradients. Some cardiologists use a cobra catheter for this purpose. Whereas recording pressure pullbacks is considered important, sometimes, when it is extremely difficult to cross the pulmonary valve, it may not be prudent to perform such a pullback tracing. In such instances, the separately recorded RV and pulmonary arterial pressures are used to calculate the gradient.

A simultaneous recording of the right ventricular and femoral artery pressures is also undertaken. This also helps assess the severity of pulmonary valve obstruction; right ventricular peak systolic pressure ≥75% of peak systolic systemic pressure is considered significant.

Recordings are made of heart rate, systemic pressure, and cardiac index to ensure that a change in transpulmonary gradient after valvuloplasty is not related to a change in cardiac output, but is indeed related to balloon pulmonary valvuloplasty. During the initial phases of the development of this procedure, we were diligent to record cardiac index either by the thermodilution technique or by the Fick technique with measured oxygen consumption. We no longer undertake these, but rely on the Fick technique without measuring oxygen consumption.

Angiography

Biplane RV cineangiogram in a sitting-up (anterio-posterior camera tilted to 15° LAO and 35° cranial) and lateral view (Figures 31.1a and 31.2a) are performed to confirm the site of obstruction, to evaluate the size and function of the right ventricle, and to measure pulmonary valve annulus, preparatory to balloon pulmonary valvuloplasty. We use a Berman angiographic catheter for the right ventriculogram, with the inflated balloon positioned in the right ventricular apex.

Additional cineangiograms from other locations are not necessary unless the echocardiographic and hemodynamic

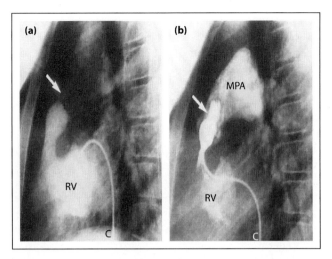

Figure 31.1 Selected frames from lateral views of right ventricular (RV) cineangiograms before (a) and after (b) balloon pulmonary valvuloplasty. Note the extremely thin jet (arrow) prior to balloon dilatation (a), which increased to a much wider jet (arrow) after valvuloplasty (b) opacifying the main pulmonary artery (MPA). (c) Catheter. (Reproduced from Rao PS. *Current Problems in Cardiology*. Chicago: Year Book Medical Publishers, Inc; 1989. Vol. 14(8), pp. 417–500, with permission from the publisher.)

data require exclusion of other abnormalities. Selective left ventricular angiography and coronary arteriography may be performed in patients older than 50 years, depending on the institutional policy or in patients with suspected coronary artery disease.

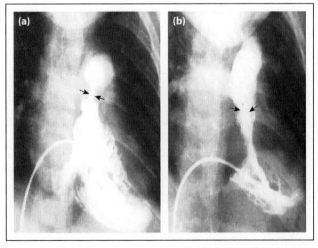

Figure 31.2 Selected cineangiographic frames from a "sitting-up" view (15° left anterior oblique and 35° cranial) of a right ventricular angiogram prior to (a) and 15 min following (b) balloon pulmonary valvuloplasty. Note the thin jet of contrast material passing through the narrowed pulmonary valve (arrows in (a)), which has marked increased after valvuloplasty (arrows in (b)). (Reproduced from Rao PS. *Current Problems in Cardiology*. Chicago: Year Book Medical Publishers, Inc; 1989. Vol. 14(8), pp. 417–500, with permission from the publisher.)

Catheters/wires preparatory to balloon dilatation

Positioning a guide in the distal right or left pulmonary artery or in the descending aorta in neonates is a necessary prerequisite for undertaking balloon valvuloplasty. If the balloon angiographic (Berman) catheter easily crosses the pulmonary valve, we replace this catheter with the same French size balloon wedge catheter and advance it across the pulmonary valve. If the balloon angiographic (Berman) catheter was not easily advanced across the pulmonary valve, a #4 or #5 French multipurpose (multi A2—Cordis) catheter is positioned in the right ventricular outflow tract and a soft-tipped guide wire is used to cross the pulmonary valve. My personal preference is a 0.035-inch Benston straight guide wire (Cook). In neonates and young infants, a 0.014-inch coronary guide wire with a floppy end is used to cross the pulmonary valve. Instead of the multipurpose catheter, a #4 or #5 French right coronary artery catheter, #4 French angled Glidecath catheter or a cobra catheter may be used to cross the pulmonary valve. Once the guide wire is across the pulmonary valve, the catheter is advanced into the distal right or left pulmonary artery or into the descending aorta via the patent ductus arteriosus. A reference image of the RV cineangiogram is helpful in this regard. The catheter is then advanced over the guide wire, again into the distal right or left pulmonary artery or into the descending aorta. The catheter is left in place and the guide wire is removed slowly and replaced with a guide wire (extra-stiff, exchange length Amplatz, Platinum Plus, or others) that is suited to position the balloon dilatation catheter.

Balloon dilatation catheters

A variety of balloon angioplasty catheters have been used in the past. Initially, balloon angioplasty catheters manufactured by Medi-Tech (Watertown, MA, USA), Mansfield Scientific (Boston, MA, USA), Surgimed (Oakland, NJ, USA), Cook Inc. (Bloomington, IN, USA), and Schneider-Medintag (Zurich, Switzerland) were utilized for balloon dilatation, depending on the availability at a given institution. Subsequently, specifically designed catheters such as XXL, Ultrathin, and Diamond (Boston Scientific, Natick, MA); Marshal (Meditech, Watertown, MA); Maxi LD, Opta LP, Opta Pro, PowerFlex (Cordis Endovascular, Warren, NJ); Tyshak I and II, Tyshak-mini, Z-Med, Z-Med II and Mullins catheters (NuMed, Hopkinton, NY), and others have been used. Currently, most cardiologists, including our group, use Tyshak II balloon angioplasty catheters for balloon pulmonary valvuloplasty because of their low profile, allowing their passage through small-sized sheaths and the ease with which they track over the guide wire. A number of other balloon dilatation catheters, including Tyshak X, Z-Med X, Z-Med II X, and Mullins X (NuMed) have since been designed and are available commercially. The cited theoretical advantages of these catheters, however, have not been validated. The Inoue balloon has been used in adults with success.[28] The major advantage of the Inoue balloon over conventional balloons is its adjustable diameter, which makes stepwise dilation possible. The diameter and length of the balloon and number of balloons used for valvuloplasty are important and are discussed below.

Balloon diameter

The initial recommendations were to use a balloon that is 1.2–1.4 times the pulmonary valve annulus. These recommendations are formulated on the basis of immediate,[29] and immediate as well as follow-up[30–32] results. Balloons larger than 1.5 times the pulmonary valve annulus should not be used because of the damage to right ventricular outflow tract such large balloons may produce.[33] Furthermore, such large balloons do not have any advantage beyond that produced by balloons that are 1.2–1.4 times the annular size.[31,32]

While the recommendation to use balloons 1.2–1.4 times the annulus are generally followed, recent reports of pulmonary insufficiency at late follow-up[34–38] raised concerns regarding the balloon size.[39–41] Based on detailed analysis of all the available data,[39–41] I recommended that we strive for a balloon/annulus ratio of 1.2–1.25 instead of the previously recommended 1.2–1.4. Such smaller balloons are likely to result in good relief of pulmonary valve obstruction while at the same time may help to prevent significant pulmonary insufficiency at late follow-up.

The results of balloon pulmonary valvuloplasty for patients with dysplastic pulmonary valves are generally poor with the use of conventional balloon pulmonary valvuloplasty techniques. The use of large balloons, up to 150% of pulmonary valve annulus,[10] or high-pressure balloons[42] may increase the effectiveness of balloon therapy and avoid the need for surgery.

Balloon length

We generally use 20-mm-long balloons in neonates and infants, 30-mm-long balloons in children and 40- or 50-mm-long balloons in adolescents and adults. There are no data either from our own series or from the literature to assess whether a given length of balloon is better than other lengths in producing a more successful relief of obstruction. With shorter balloons, it is difficult to maintain the balloon center across the pulmonary valve annulus during balloon inflation. Longer balloons may impinge upon the tricuspid valve, causing tricuspid insufficiency,[43] or on the conduction system, causing heart block.[44] Consequently, the use of 20-, 30-, and 40/50-mm-long balloons for neonates and infants, children, and adolescents and adults, respectively, appears reasonable.

Number of balloons

When the pulmonary valve annulus is too large to dilate with a single balloon, valvuloplasty with simultaneous inflation of two balloons across the pulmonary valve (Figure 31.3) may be performed. When two balloons are utilized, the following formula may be used to calculate the effective balloon size:[30]

$$\frac{D_1 + D_2 + \Pi\,(D_1/2 +\ D_2/2)}{\Pi}$$

where D_1 and D_2 are diameters of the balloons used. This formula has been further simplified:[45] Effective balloon diameter = 0.82 $(D_1 + D_2)$.

Some cardiologists advocate the use of double-balloon valvuloplasty instead of single balloon valvuloplasty,[46] especially for adult patients. We have compared the results of single-balloon with double-balloon valvuloplasty.[47] When equivalent balloon/valve annulus ratios are used, the results of double-balloon valvuloplasty, though excellent, are comparable to, but not superior to those observed with single-balloon valvuloplasty.[47,48] Furthermore, the double-balloon technique does indeed prolong the procedure and involves an additional femoral venous site and the attendant potential complications. In addition, the availability of large-diameter balloons carried on catheters with relatively small shaft sizes facilitates the use of a single balloon instead of two balloons. However, the double-balloon technique in some cases may be more effective in maintaining a stable balloon position across the pulmonary valve, particularly adolescents and adults.

Bifoil and trefoil balloons

Because of the complete obstruction of the right ventricle with a single balloon during balloon inflation, there is necessarily systemic hypotension (Figure 31.4). But, during a double-balloon procedure, the right ventricular output may continue in between the balloons; this is one of the postulated reasons for recommending double-balloon technique, in that it produces less hypotension.[46] Bifoil and trefoil balloon catheters[49–51] may serve this purpose in that they may allow (at least theoretically) RV output during balloon inflation. But because of the fact that we use balloons larger than the pulmonary valve annulus, the theoretical advantage cited by these authors[46,49–51] does not exist in that there is no space between the balloons and the pulmonary valve annulus. Furthermore, the bifoil and trefoil balloon catheter shafts are bulky, making it difficult to position the catheters across the pulmonary valve. In addition, our limited experience (Figure 31.5) suggests that the advantage of less hypotension during valvuloplasty is minimal.[48,52,53] Instead, we suggest a short period (5 s) of balloon inflation so that the hypotension is less severe and recovers faster (Figure 31.6).[52,53]

Pressure, number, and duration of balloon inflation

The recommendations for balloon inflation pressure (2.0–8.5 atm), number of inflations (1–4), and duration inflation (5–60 s) varied from one investigator to the other, but

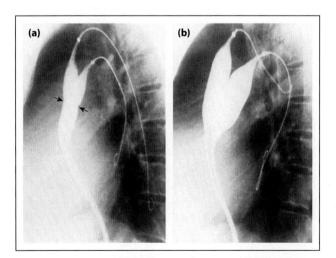

Figure 31.3 Selected cine frames of two balloon catheters placed across the pulmonary valve showing "waisting" of the balloons (arrows in (a) during the initial phases of balloon inflation, which was completely abolished after complete inflation of the balloons (b). (Reproduced from Rao PS. *Current Problems in Cardiology*. Chicago: Year Book Medical Publishers, Inc; 1989. Vol. 14(8), pp. 417–500, with permission from the publisher.)

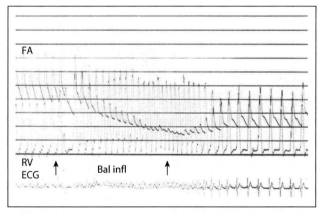

Figure 31.4 Simultaneous recording of the right ventricular (RV) and femoral artery (FA) pressures during balloon dilatation of the stenotic pulmonary valve. Note marked increase in RV pressure, presumably related to complete obstruction of the RV. There is a simultaneous fall in FA pressure, again related to complete obstruction of the RV during balloon valvuloplasty. Following deflation of the balloon, the FA pressure returns toward normal. The 10 s period of balloon inflation (Bal Infl) is marked with arrows. (Reproduced from Rao PS. *Current Problems in Cardiology*. Chicago: Year Book Medical Publishers, Inc; 1989. Vol. 14(8), pp. 417–500, with permission from the publisher.)

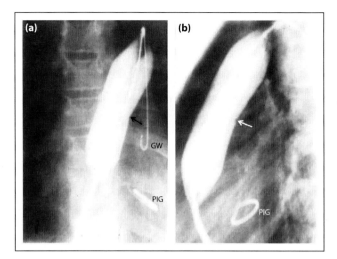

Figure 31.5 Trefoil balloon across the pulmonary valve in posterio-anterior (a) and lateral views is shown. Note the indentation of the balloon (arrows) produced by the pulmonary valve annulus. Guide wire (GW) in the left pulmonary artery and pigtail (PIG) catheter in the left ventricle are seen. (Reproduced from Rao PS. *Current Problems in Cardiology*. Chicago: Year Book Medical Publishers, Inc; 1989. Vol. 14(8), pp. 417–500, with permission from the publisher.)

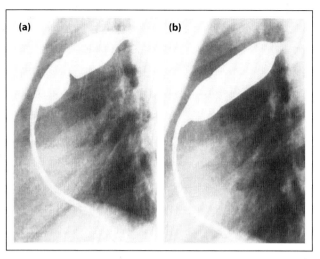

Figure 31.7 Selected cineradiographic frames of a balloon dilatation catheter placed across a stenotic pulmonary valve. Note "waisting" of the balloon during the initial phases of the balloon inflation (a), which was almost completely abolished during the later phases of balloon inflation (b). (Reproduced from Rao PS. *Current Problems in Cardiology*. Chicago: Year Book Medical Publishers, Inc; 1989. Vol. 14(8), pp. 417–500, with permission from the publisher.)

without much data to support such contentions. We have examined these parameters from our study subjects.[48,52] The balloon inflation characteristics in the group with good results were compared with those with poor results. No significant differences were found, suggesting that the outcome of valvuloplasty is not related to the balloon inflation characteristics. We have also scrutinized the data[48,52] with arbitrary division of maximum pressure, number of

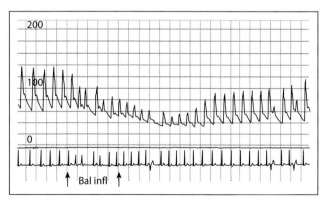

Figure 31.6 Femoral artery pressure during balloon inflation for pulmonary valvuloplasty in which a 5 s balloon inflation is used. Note the fall in femoral artery pressure, but the decrease in systemic pressure is not as severe as with 10 s inflation (Figure 31.4). Also, the return of pressure toward normal is not as slow as with 10 s inflation (Figure 31.4). The 5 s balloon inflation (Bal Infl) is marked with arrows. (Reproduced from Rao PS. *Current Problems in Cardiology*. Chicago: Year Book Medical Publishers, Inc; 1989. Vol. 14(8), pp. 417–500, with permission from the publisher.)

balloon inflations, and duration of balloon inflation, and determined that higher pressure, larger number of inflations, and longer duration of balloon inflation did not favorably influence residual gradients at follow-up, especially when the effect of balloon/annulus ratio is removed.

Based on these and other considerations, we would recommend balloon inflation at or below the level of balloon burst pressure stated by the manufacturer, and will continue balloon inflation until the waisting of the balloon disappears (Figure 31.7). The duration of inflation is kept as short as possible, usually just until after the waisting disappears. Shorter balloon inflation cycles produce less hypotension and more rapid return of pressures toward normal (Figures 31.4 and 31.6). We usually perform one more balloon inflation after the disappearance of waisting is demonstrated, to ensure adequate valvuloplasty.

Balloon valvuloplasty procedure (step-by-step)

1. Clinical and echocardiographic diagnosis of moderate to severe valvar pulmonary stenosis.
2. Informed consent.
3. Confirmation of the severity of the stenosis by hemodynamic measurements: gradients across the pulmonary valve and/or comparison of the RV systolic pressure with systemic pressure.
4. RV angiography in sitting-up (15° LAO and 35° cranial) and straight lateral views.

5. Measurement of pulmonary valve annulus is undertaken in both views and an average of these is calculated. If the valve annulus could not clearly be identified, the echocardiographic measurement of the valve annulus may be used.

6. Selection of the balloon catheter to be used is made. An inflated diameter is selected such that it is 1.2–1.25 times the pulmonary valve annulus, as detailed in the preceding section. The length of the balloon should be 20–40/50 mm depending upon the patient's age and size, also as discussed in the preceding section.

7. If a femoral arterial line is not in place, an arterial line is placed into the femoral artery (#3 French in neonates and infants; #4 French in children and #5 French in adolescents and adults) for monitoring of arterial pressure continuously. Heart rate, blood pressure, respirations, and pulse oximetry are also continuously monitored throughout the procedure.

8. We do not routinely administer additional heparin for pulmonary valve dilatations, but, if there is an intracardiac communication (patent foramen ovale or an atrial septal defect), we administer heparin (100 units/kg intravenously) and monitor activated clotting times (ACTs) and maintain between 200 and 250 s.

9. A #4 to #6 French multipurpose (multi A-2 [Cordis]) catheter is introduced into the femoral venous sheath and advanced across the pulmonary valve and the tip of the catheter is positioned in the distal left (preferable) or right pulmonary artery. In neonates and young infants, the catheter may be positioned in the descending aorta via the ductus; this will increase the stability of the wire and may make it easier to pass the balloon catheter across the pulmonary valve. The type of catheter used for crossing the pulmonary valve varies— balloon wedge, right coronary artery catheter, cobra catheter, or other—depending upon the operator's choice and the patient's anatomy. If the stenosis is only moderate, it is easy to pass a catheter across the pulmonary valve. In very severe or critical obstructions, reference images from RV cineangiogram may help guide the passage of catheters/guide wires across the stenotic valve. The use of soft-tipped guide wires to assist crossing the pulmonary valve was alluded to in the preceding section.

10. A 0.014–0.035 inch J-tipped, exchange-length, extra-stiff guide wire is passed through the catheter already in place and the catheter is removed. The selection of the wire diameter is dependent upon the selected balloon dilatation catheter. In difficult cases, a super-stiff, short, soft-tipped Amplatzer guide wire (Meditech) may be used.

11. If the size of the sheath in the femoral vein does not accommodate the selected balloon angioplasty catheter, the sheath may be upsized to the appropriate size at this point. Alternatively, this may be undertaken

prior to positioning the catheter across the pulmonary valve.

12. The selected balloon angioplasty catheter is advanced over the guide wire, but within the sheath and positioned across the pulmonary valve. The bony landmarks, namely, ribs, sternum, or other fixed landmarks, are used for this purpose. A frozen video frame of the RV cineangiogram displayed on the screen is helpful in this regard.

13. At times, it may be difficult to cross and position an appropriate-sized balloon angioplasty catheter across the severely stenotic pulmonary valve, especially in neonates. In such instances, we use smaller 3–6 mm diameter balloon catheters initially to predilate and then use larger, more appropriate-sized balloon catheters (Figure 31.8).

14. The balloon is inflated with diluted contrast material (1 in 4) using any of the commercially available inflators, while monitoring the pressure of inflation. The inflation pressure is gradually increased up to the manufacturer-recommended pressure or until disappearance of the

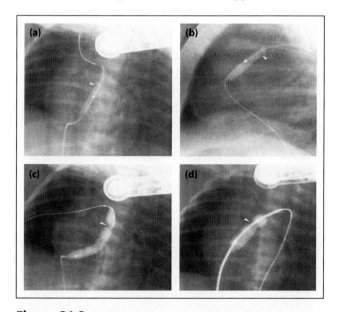

Figure 31.8 Selected cineradiographic frames demonstrating use of progressively larger balloons in a 1-day-old infant with critical pulmonary stenosis. Initially, a 0.014" coronary guide wire was advanced into the pulmonary artery via a #5 French multi-A2 catheter (Cordis) positioned in the right ventricular outflow tract. A #3.5 French catheter carrying a 4-mm-diameter balloon was positioned across the pulmonary valve. Posterio-anterior (a) and lateral (b) view cine frames showing waisting (arrows) of the balloon during initial phases of balloon inflation. After two balloon inflations, this balloon catheter was replaced with a #5 French catheter carrying a 6-mm-diameter balloon (c) and finally a #5 French catheter (d) carrying an 8-mm-diameter balloon. (Reproduced from Rao PS. Balloon angioplasty and valvuloplasty in infants, children and adolescents. *Current Problems in Cardiology*. Chicago: Year Book Medical Publishers, Inc; 1989. Vol. 14(8), pp. 417–500, with permission from the publisher.)

balloon waist. If the balloon is not appropriately centered across the pulmonary valve, the position of the catheter is readjusted and balloon inflation repeated. Once satisfactory balloon inflation is achieved, one more balloon inflation may be performed as per the operator's preference.

15. Sometimes, it may be difficult to maintain the position of the balloon across the pulmonary valve during balloon inflation; the use of an appropriate-length balloon, depending upon the age of the patient, and holding the balloon catheter tight to prevent its movement is likely to resolve this issue. The use of the double-balloon technique, particularly in adolescents and adults, has been useful. Others use adenosine-induced transient cardiac standstill[54] or rapid right ventricular pacing[55] to achieve a stable position of the balloon during valvuloplasty. A nucleus balloon (NuMed) with a "barbell" configuration may keep the balloon across the valve. However, there are no known reports of its use and these catheters are bulky, requiring large sheaths.

16. The balloon catheter is removed, leaving the guide wire in place.

Postballoon protocol

Following balloon valvuloplasty, the measurement of pressure gradient across the pulmonary valve, pulmonary and femoral arterial oxygen saturations, and simultaneous femoral artery and right ventricular pressures are undertaken to assess the result of valvuloplasty. Either a multi-Track catheter[56] or a Tuohy-Borst is used to record the pressure gradients across the pulmonary valve, so that the guide wire is left in place across the pulmonary valve while evaluating the results of valvuloplasty. If the result is not satisfactory (peak-to-peak valvar gradient in excess of 30 mmHg), a repeat dilatation with a larger balloon (2 mm larger than the first) is undertaken. Finally, the catheter and guide wire are removed and Berman angiography catheter is repositioned in the right ventricular apex and an angiogram is performed to evaluate the mobility of the pulmonary valve leaflets, to visualize the jet of contrast across the dilated pulmonary valve (Figures 31.1 and 31.2), to detect infundibular stenosis, and to discern any complications such as tricuspid insufficiency. We do not routinely perform echocardiography in the catheterization laboratory.

Pitfalls, problems, and complications

Problems

The balloon may not be truly across the pulmonary valve during balloon inflation. It is important to ensure that the balloon is indeed across the valve. The waisting of the balloon may be produced by supravalvar stenosis or infundibular constriction. When in doubt, centering the balloon

at various locations across the right ventricular outflow region may become necessary.

Acute complications

Complications during and immediately after balloon valvuloplasty have been remarkably minimal; the VACA registry reported a 0.24% death rate and 0.35% major complication rate[57] from the 822 balloon pulmonary valvuloplasty procedures from 26 institutions, attesting to the relative safety of the procedure. The study group involved initial experiences of many centers participating in the data collection; with increased experience, the complication rate should even be lower at the present time.

Transient bradycardia, premature beats, and a fall in systemic pressure during balloon inflation have been uniformly noted by all workers. These abnormalities rapidly return to normal following balloon deflation (Figures 31.4 and 31.6). Systemic hypotension may be minimal in the presence of a patent foramen ovale[58] because a right-to-left shunt across it fills the left ventricle. The use a the double-balloon technique or the use of bifoil or trefoil balloons has been suggested to circumvent this problem, but as discussed in the preceding section, the use of a short period of balloon inflation may help to reduce the degree and duration of hypotension.

Blood loss requiring transfusion has been reported, but with better catheter/sheath systems that are currently available, the blood loss is minimal. Complete right bundle branch block, transient or permanent heart block, cerebrovascular accident, loss of consciousness, cardiac arrest, convulsions, balloon rupture at high balloon-inflation pressures, rupture of tricuspid valve papillary muscle, and pulmonary artery tears, though rare, have been reported. Some of these complications may be unavoidable. However, meticulous attention to the technique, use of appropriate diameter and length of the balloon, avoiding high balloon-inflation pressures, and short inflation/deflation cycles may prevent or reduce the complications.

The development of severe infundibular obstruction has been reported. Infundibular gradients occur in nearly 30% of patients; the higher the age and higher the severity of obstruction, the greater is the prevalence of infundibular reaction.[3] When the residual infundibular gradient is ≥50 mmHg, beta-blockade therapy is generally recommended.[3,16] Infundibular obstruction regresses to a great degree at follow-up (Figures 31.9 and 31.10), just as demonstrated for infundibular reaction following surgical valvotomy, with a rare patient requiring surgical intervention. Issues related to the significance of infundibular obstruction and its management are discussed in greater detail elsewhere.[3,16,59]

Transient prolongation of the QTc and development of premature ventricular contractions following balloon pulmonary valvuloplasty have been reported, causing concern that R-on-T phenomenon may develop and produce ventricular arrhythmia. Rare cases of ventricular arrhythmia have been reported; however, none of the patients from our large series and many other studies were known to develop significant ventricular arrhythmia. Nonetheless, patient monitoring following balloon valvuloplasty is warranted.

Complications at follow-up

Femoral venous occlusion and development of restenosis and pulmonary insufficiency have been noted. Seven to nineteen percent of the patients may develop femoral venous obstruction;[60] the femoral venous obstruction is more likely in small infants. Recurrent pulmonary valve obstruction may occur in about 8% of patients and repeat balloon valvuloplasty may help relieve the residual or recurrent obstruction.[61] The causes of restenosis have been identified.[62] If the issues related to the technique are the reason for recurrence, repeat balloon valvuloplasty is useful. If the substrate (dysplastic valves without commissural fusion, supravalvar pulmonary artery stenosis, or severe fixed infundibular obstruction) is the problem, surgical intervention may become necessary. Long-term follow-up data of balloon pulmonary valvuloplasty (reviewed in detail elsewhere[3,39,41]) indicate the development of pulmonary insufficiency (PI); the frequency and severity of PI increases with time. From our study group, 70 of 80 (88%) had PI at long-term follow-up, while only 10% had PI prior to balloon valvuloplasty.[34] Similar experiences documenting high incidence of PI have been reported by other workers in the field.[35,41] Although none of our patients[34] or other patients reported by several other cardiologists[35,40] required pulmonary valve replacement for PI, 6% of patients followed by Berman et al.[36] developed severe PI, requiring (or requiring consideration for) pulmonary valve replacement. The development of substantial PI at late follow-up

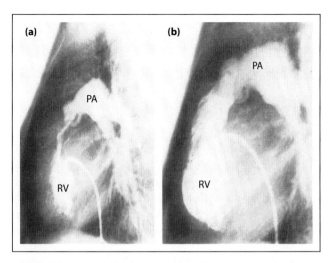

Figure 31.10 Selected frames from lateral view of the right ventricular (RV) cineangiogram showing severe infundibular stenosis (a) immediately following balloon valvuloplasty (corresponding Figure 31.9, center). At 10 months after balloon valvuloplasty, the right ventricular outflow tract (b) is wide open and corresponds to Figure 31.9, right. Peak-to-peak pulmonary valve gradient was 20 mmHg and there was no infundibular gradient. PA, pulmonary artery. (Reproduced from Thapar MK, Rao PS. *Am Heart J* 1989;118:99–103, with permission from the publisher.)

is an important observation and attempts to discern causes of late PI, devise methods to prevent such problems, and careful long-term follow-up studies to confirm these observations are warranted.

Postcatheter management

We usually perform an electrocardiogram and an echocardiogram on the morning following the procedure. Clinical, electrocardiographic, and echo-Doppler evaluation at 1, 6, 12, 24, and 60 months after the procedure, and every 5 years thereafter is generally recommended. Regression of RV hypertrophy on the electrocardiogram following balloon dilatation has been well documented[63] and the electrocardiogram is a useful adjunct in the evaluation of follow-up results. However, electrocardiographic evidence for hemodynamic improvement does not become apparent until 6 months after valvuloplasty. Doppler gradient is generally reflective of the residual obstruction and is a useful and reliable noninvasive monitoring tool.[15,34,52,53]

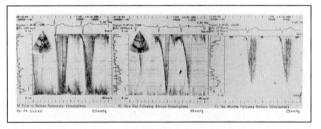

Figure 31.9 Doppler flow velocity recordings from the main pulmonary artery prior to (left) and 1 day (center) and 10 months (right) after successful balloon pulmonary valvuloplasty. Note that there is no significant fall in the peak flow velocity on the day after balloon procedure, but there is a characteristic triangular pattern, indicative of infundibular obstruction. At 10 month follow-up, the flow velocity decreased, suggesting resolution of infundibular obstruction. (Reproduced with permission from Thapar MK, Rao PS. *Am Heart J* 1989;118:99–103, with permission from the publisher.)

References

1. Gikonyo BM, Lucus RV, Edwards JE. Anatomic features of congenital pulmonary valvar stenosis. *Pediat Cardiol* 1987;8:109–15.
2. Koretzky ED, Moller JH, Korns ME et al. Congenital pulmonary stenosis resulting from dysplasia of the valve. *Circulation* 1969;60:43–53.
3. Thapar MK, Rao PS. Significance of infundibular obstruction following balloon valvuloplasty for valvar pulmonic stenosis. *Am Heart J* 1989;118:99–103.

4. Rodbard S, Ikeda K, Montes M. Mechanisms of post-stenotic dilatation. *Circulation* 1963;28:791–8.
5. Rao PS. Indications for balloon pulmonary valvuloplasty. *Am Heart J* 1988;116:1661–2.
6. Feltes TF, Bacha E, Beekman RH 3rd et al. for American Heart Association Congenital Cardiac Defects Committee of the Council on Cardiovascular Disease in the Young; Council on Clinical Cardiology; Council on Cardiovascular Radiology and Intervention; American Heart Association. Indications for cardiac catheterization and intervention in pediatric cardiac disease: A scientific statement from the American Heart Association. *Circulation* 2011;123:2607–52.
7. Nugent EW, Freedom RM, Nora JJ et al. Clinical course of pulmonic stenosis. *Circulation* 1977;56 (Suppl I):I-18–47.
8. Rao PS. Balloon pulmonary valvuloplasty (Letter). *Catheter Cardiovasc Diagn* 1997;40:427–8.
9. Rao PS. Percutaneous balloon pulmonary valvuloplasty: State of the art. *Catheter Cardiovasc Interv* 2007;69:747–63.
10. Rao PS. Percutaneous balloon pulmonary valvuloplasty. In: Cheng T. Ed. *Percutaneous Balloon Valvuloplasty*. New York: Igaku-Shion Med Publishers, 1992. pp. 365–420.
11. Rao PS. Balloon dilatation in infants and children with dysplastic pulmonary valves: Short-term and intermediate-term results. *Am Heart J* 1988;116:1168–73.
12. Marantz PM, Huhta JC, Mullins CE et al. Results of balloon valvuloplasty in typical and dysplastic pulmonary valve stenosis: Doppler echocardiographic follow-up. *J Am Coll Cardiol* 1988;12:476–9.
13. Johnson LW, Grossman W, Dalen JE, Dexter L. Pulmonary stenosis in the adult: Long-term follow-up results. *New Engl J Med* 1972;287:1159–63.
14. Krabill KA, Wang Y, Einzid S, Moller JH. Rest and exercise hemodynamics in pulmonary stenosis: Comparison of children and adults. *Am J Cardiol* 1985;36:360–5.
15. Rao PS. Pulmonary valve disease. In: Alpert JS, Dalen JE, Rahimtoola S. Eds. *Valvular Heart Disease*. 3rd ed. Philadelphia, PA: Lippincott Raven, 2000. pp. 339–76.
16. Fontes VF, Esteves CA, Eduardo J, et al., Regression of infundibular hypertrophy after pulmonary valvotomy for pulmonic stenosis. *Am J Cardiol* 1988;62:977–9.
17. Rubio-Alvarez V, Limon-Lason R, Soni J. Valvulotomias intracardiacas por medio de un cateter. *Arch Inst Cordiol Mexico* 1952;23:183–92.
18. Rubio V, Limon-Lason R. Treatment of pulmonary valvular stenosis and tricuspid stenosis using a modified catheter (abst), Second World Congress of Cardiology, Washington, DC, Program Abstract, 1954;II:205.
19. Semb BKH, Tijonneland S, Stake G et al. Balloon valvotomy of congenital pulmonary valve stenosis with tricuspid valve insufficiency. *Cardiovasc Radiol* 1979;2:239–41.
20. Kan JS, White RJ, Jr, Mitchell SE, Gardner TJ. Percutaneous balloon valvuloplasty: A new method for treating congenital pulmonary valve stenosis. *New Engl J Med* 1982;307:540–2.
21. Gruntzig AR, Senning A, Siegothaler WE. Non-operative dilatation of coronary artery stenosis: Percutaneous transluminal coronary angioplasty. *New Engl J Med* 1979;301:61–8.
22. Weyman AE, Hurwitz RA, Girod DA. Cross-sectional echocardiographic visualization of the stenotic pulmonary valve. *Circulation* 1977;56:769–74.
23. Singh GK, Balfour IC, Chen S, Ferdman B, Jureidini SB, Fiore AC, Rao PS. Lesion specific pressure recovery phenomenon in pediatric patients: A simultaneous Doppler and catheter correlative study (abst). *J Am Coll Cardiol* 2003;41:493A.
24. Sideris EB, Baay JE, Bradshaw RL et al. Axillary vein approach for pulmonary valvuloplasty in infants with iliac vein obstruction. *Cathet Cardiovasc Diagn* 1988;15:61–3.
25. Chaara A, Zniber L, Haitem NE et al. Percutaneous balloon valvuloplasty via the right internal jugular vein for valvar pulmonic stenosis with severe right ventricular failure. *Am Heart J* 1989;117:684–5.
26. Shim D, Lloyd TR, Cho KJ et al. Transhepatic cardiac catheterization in children: Evaluation of efficacy and safety. *Circulation* 1995;92:1526–30.
27. Gorlin R, Gorlin SG. Hydraulic formula for calculation of the area of the stenotic mitral valve, other valves and central circulatory shunts. *Am Heart J* 1951;41:1–29.
28. Bahl VK, Chandra S, Goel A et al. Versatility of Inoue balloon catheter. *Int J Cardiol* 1997;59:75–83.
29. Radhke W, Keane JF, Fellows KE et al. Percutaneous balloon valvotomy of congenital pulmonary stenosis using oversized balloons. *J Am Coll Cardiol* 1986;8:909–15.
30. Rao PS. Influence of balloon size on short-term and long-term results of balloon pulmonary valvuloplasty. *Texas Heart Institute J* 1987;14:57–61.
31. Rao PS. How big a balloon and how many balloons for pulmonary valvuloplasty? *Am Heart J* 1988;116:577–80.
32. Rao PS. Further observations on the effect of balloon size on the short-term and intermediate-term results of balloon dilatation of the pulmonary valve. *Br Heart J* 1988;60:507–11.
33. Ring JC, Kulik TT, Burke BA et al. Morphologic changes induced by dilatation of pulmonary valve annulus with over-large balloons in normal newborn lamb. *Am J Cardiol* 1986;52:210–4.
34. Rao PS, Galal O, Patnana M, Buck SH, Wilson AD. Results of three-to-ten-year follow-up of balloon dilatation of the pulmonary valve. *Heart* 1998;80:591–5.
35. Rao PS. Long-term follow-up results after balloon dilatation of pulmonic stenosis, aortic stenosis and coarctation of the aorta: a review. *Progr Cardiovasc Dis* 1999;42:59–74.
36. Berman W, Jr, Fripp RR, Raiser BD, Yabek SM. Significant pulmonary valve incompetence following oversize balloon pulmonary valvuloplasty in small infants: A long-term follow-up study, *Catheter Cardiovasc Interv* 1999;48:61–5.
37. Abu Haweleh A, Hakim F. Balloon pulmonary valvuloplasty in children: Jordanian experience. *J Saudi Heart J* 2003;15:31–4.
38. Garty Y, Veldtman G, Lee K, Benson L. Late outcomes after pulmonary valve dilatation in neonates, infants and children. *J Invasive Cardiol* 2005;17:318–22.
39. Rao PS. Late pulmonary insufficiency after balloon dilatation of the pulmonary valve (Letter). *Catheter Cardiovasc Interv* 2000;49:118–9.
40. Rao PS. Balloon pulmonary valvuloplasty. *J Saudi Heart Assoc* 2003;15:1–4.
41. Rao PS. Balloon pulmonary valvuloplasty in children. *J Invasive Cardiol* 2005;17:323–5.
42. Moguillansky D, Schneider HE, Rome JJ, Kreutzer J. Role of high-pressure balloon valvotomy for resistant pulmonary valve stenosis. *Congenit Heart Dis* 2010;5:134–40.
43. Attia I, Weinhaus L, Walls JT, Lababidi Z. Rupture of tricuspid papillary muscle during balloon pulmonary valvuloplasty, *Am Heart J* 1987;114:1233–4.
44. Lo RNS, Lau KC, Leung MP. Complete heart block after balloon dilatation of congenital pulmonary stenosis. *Br Heart J* 1988;59:384–6.
45. Narang R, Das G, Dev V et al. Effect of the balloon-annulus ration on the intermediate and follow-up results of pulmonary balloon valvuloplasty. *Cardiology* 1997;88:271–6.
46. Al Kasab S, Riberiro PA, Al Zaibag M et al. Percutaneous double-balloon pulmonary valvotomy in adults: One-to-two year follow-up. *Am J Cardiol* 1988;62:822–5.
47. Rao PS and Fawzy ME. Double-balloon technique for percutaneous balloon pulmonary valvuloplasty: Comparison with single balloon technique. *J Interv Cardiol* 1988;1:257–62.
48. Rao PS. Balloon pulmonary valvuloplasty: A review. *Clin Cardiol* 1989;12:55–72.
49. Meier B, Friedli B, Oberhaensli I et al. Trefoil balloon for percutaneous valvuloplasty. *Cathet Cardiovasc Diag* 1986;12:277–81.

50. van den Berg EJM, Niemyeyer MG, Plokker TWM et al. New triple-lumen balloon catheter for percutaneous (pulmonary) valvuloplasty. *Cathet Cardiovasc Diag* 1986;12:352–6.

51. Meier B, Friedli L, von Segesser L. Valvuloplasty with trefoil and bifoil balloons and the long sheath technique. *Herz* 1988;13:1–13.

52. Rao PS. Balloon angioplasty and valvuloplasty in infants, children and adolescents. *Current Problems in Cardiology*. Chicago: Year Book Medical, 1989. Vol. 14(8), pp. 417–500.

53. Rao PS. Balloon pulmonary valvuloplasty for isolated pulmonic stenosis. In: Rao PS. Ed. *Transcatheter Therapy in Pediatric Cardiology*. New York: Wiley-Liss, 1993. pp. 59–104.

54. De Giovanni JV, Edgar RA, Cranston A. Adenosine induced transient cardiac standstill in catheter interventional procedures for congenital heart disease. *Heart* 1998; 80:330–3.

55. Daehnert I, Rotzsch C, Wiener M, Schneider P. Rapid right ventricular pacing is an alternative to adenosine in catheter interventional procedures for congenital heart disease. *Heart* 2004;90:1047–50.

56. Bonnhoeffer P, Piechaud J, Stumper O et al. The multi-track angiography catheter: A new tool for complex catheterization in congenital heart disease. *Heart* 1996;76:173–7.

57. Stranger P, Cassidy SC. Girod DA et al. Balloon pulmonary valvuloplasty: Results of the valvuloplasty and angioplasty of congenital anomalies registry. *Am J Cardiol* 1990;65:775–83.

58. Shuck JW, McCormick DJ, Cohen IS et al. Percutaneous balloon valvuloplasty for pulmonary valve: Role of right to left shunt through patent foramen ovale. *J Am Coll Cardiol* 1984;4:132–5.

59. Rao PS, Thapar MK. Balloon pulmonary valvuloplasty (Letter). *Am Heart J* 1991;121:1839.

60. Rao PS, Pulmonary valve in children. In: Sigwart U, Bertrand M, Serruys PW. Eds. *Handbook of Cardiovascular Interventions*. New York, NY: Churchill Livingstone, 1996. pp. 273–310.

61. Rao PS, Galal O, Wilson AD. Feasibility and effectiveness of repeat balloon dilatation of restenosed obstructions following previous balloon valvuloplasty/angioplasty. *Am Heart J* 1996;132:403–7.

62. Rao PS, Thapar MK, Kutayli F. Causes of restenosis following balloon valvuloplasty for valvar pulmonic stenosis, *Am J Cardiol* 1988;62:979–82.

63. Rao PS, Solymar L. Electrocardiographic changes following balloon dilatation of valvar pulmonic stenosis. *J Interv Cardiol* 1988;1:189–97.

32

Pulmonary valve disease: Pulmonary atresia

Zaheer Ahmad, Marhisham Che Mood, and Mazeni Alwi

Introduction

Pulmonary atresia more commonly occurs as part of a complex cyanotic congenital cardiac malformation such as tetralogy of Fallot with pulmonary atresia (TOF-PA), and hearts with single ventricle physiology. The focus of this chapter is transcatheter management of pulmonary atresia with intact ventricular septum (PAIVS), a less common cyanotic heart disease.

Although the designation of PAIVS suggests a simple lesion characterized by complete obstruction of the right ventricular (RV) outflow, the disease encompasses a wide range of morphologic abnormalities of the RV, from the tricuspid valve (TV) to the RV body and the outflow tract (RVOT).[1,2] In a small proportion of cases, the disease is associated with abnormal connections between the RV and coronary arteries, whereas in the most severe form, the coronary bed is dependent on the high RV pressure for perfusion (RV-dependent coronary circulation, RVDCC) because of interruptions or severe stenoses in the proximal coronary arteries. The pulmonary blood flow is ductus dependent; hence, intervention in the neonatal period is required. The anatomy of the RV dictates the management of PAIVS, with a goal toward a two-ventricle circulation in those with favorable anatomic substrate whereas in those with diminutive RV the single ventricle track is a more realistic goal.[3,4] Surgery used to be the principal means of treatment.

In the current era, percutaneous interventional techniques have gained wide acceptance as the method of choice in the initial management.[5-7] Some discussion of the anatomy of the RV and RVOT is necessary for formulating management strategies, patient selection, and planning of the procedure and techniques.

Anatomy, initial evaluation, and patient selection

An important characteristic of PAIVS is the morphologic heterogeneity of the RV, which represents a continuum.

At one end of this morphologic spectrum is the RV that is near normal, having mild hypoplasia of the cavity with all three parts—inlet, apex, and infundibulum—present and well developed, with membranous atresia of the pulmonary valve (PV) as the principal abnormality. At the other end is the RV cavity that is diminutive, with much of it obliterated by muscles, including the RVOT (muscular atresia), except for a very small inlet guarded by an equally small TV (Figure 32.1). The TV, apart from being smaller than the mitral valve, may also be abnormal and dysplastic, causing varying degrees of tricuspid regurgitation (TR). Outside this continuum is a small proportion of patients with severe Ebstein's malformation of the TV, with a dilated, thin-walled RV and RVOT, but small pulmonary valve annulus and main pulmonary artery (MPA). Communications between the cavity of the right ventricle and the coronary arteries is a peculiar association with pulmonary atresia with an intact ventricular septum, which is seen most often in those with a diminutive RV cavity.

Given the spectrum of morphologic abnormality that also dictates the initial procedure as part of overall management strategy, a detailed evaluation of the anatomy at presentation is essential. 2D and Doppler echocardiography provide a general idea of the RV cavity size, the RVOT, nature of the atresia as well as an excellent assessment of the TV anatomy and severity of TR and RV systolic pressure. Measurement of the TV annulus, other parameters of RV dimensional Z scores, and the ratio of tricuspid to mitral annulus, provides some degree of objective evaluation of the RV size and guide management.[8-11] However, details of the RV, RVOT, and pulmonary arteries may be best obtained by angiography, which also allows direct measurement of the hemodynamics. As patent ductus arteriosus (PDA) stenting has become an important part in the initial management, angiographic evaluation of the PDA morphology is also essential.[12] In cases with RV–coronary fistulous connections, it is important to look for the presence of stenoses or interruptions of these connections, as their presence strongly suggests RVDCC.

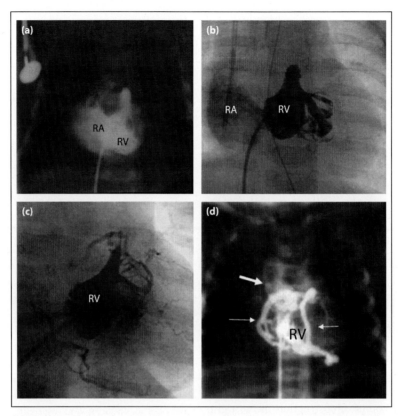

Figure 32.1 The RV in PAIVS—RV angiogram in AP projection. (a) Tripartite RV with inlet, infundibulum, and apical parts of the RV cavity present. The infundibulum is well developed. No RV–coronary connections. Moderate TR and dilated RA. (b) Bipartite RV with well-developed infundibulum and inlet. The apical part is obliterated by muscles except for intertrabecular spaces. No RV–coronary connections. Mild TR. (c) Bipartite RV but the infundibulum near the atretic valve is small with numerous minor RV–coronary connections. The apical part is completely obliterated. No TR. (d) Diminutive RV with only a small inlet part. Two major RV–coronary connections opacifying the aortic root. Valve perforate and balloon dilation may be performed in (a) with additional PDA stenting in (b), (c) not appropriate for (d). RV: right ventricle; PAIVS: pulmonary atresia with intact ventricular septum; AP: antero-posterior; RA: right atrium; TR: tricuspid regurgitation; PDA: patent ductus arteriosus.

If this is found to be the case, the RV decompression that follows successful perforation and dilation of the atretic pulmonary valve may be injudicious because of the risk of inducing myocardial ischemia.

Patients who are suitable for transcatheter valvotomy and balloon dilation

1. Membranous atresia, tripartite RV, mild RV hypoplasia   This is the most favorable morphologic subgroup of PAIVS and is seen in about 50–60% cases. The inlet, trabecular, and infundibular components are well developed, and the pathologic abnormality is a membranous imperforate valve. This may be considered as the extreme end of the critically stenotic pulmonary valve. Nevertheless, the RV size is seldom "normal," as hypertrophy of the RV myocardium causes some degree of hypoplasia of the RV cavity (Figure 32.1a).
   The TV is often normal although dysplasia with regurgitation is not uncommon. The TV annulus Z

score is generally >−2.0 based on the normogram by Rowlatt.[8] RV; coronary connections are uncommon.

The RVOT is generally well developed with a smooth outline, but occasionally fixed, subvalvar muscular obstruction by an abnormal muscle bundle occurs below the atretic valve. The atretic pulmonary valve membrane is very thin (<0.3 mm), with a good annulus size. The well-developed MPA and sinuses "cup" over the blind-ending RVOT (Figure 32.2a). Low complication rates and an excellent outcome with immediate RV decompression can be expected with valve perforation and balloon dilation, with subsequent normal RV growth. In adult life, pulmonary regurgitation resulting from the procedure and TR from a dysplastic valve may require attention.[13] Uncommonly, poor RV compliance consequent on severe right ventricular hypertrophy (RVH) and a rather contracted right ventricular cavity may cause persistence of severe hypoxia and PGE1 dependence from right-to-left shunt despite there being efficient relief of obstruction.[14] A surgically modified Blalock–Taussig (mBT) shunt or PDA stenting would be subsequently required

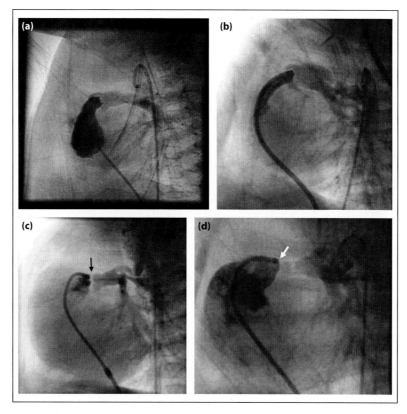

Figure 32.2 The RVOT in PAIVS. Simultaneous injections in the RVOT and the aorta opposite the PDA are performed in the lateral projection to view the infundibulum, pulmonary valve annulus and valve plate, and the MPA. (a) Smooth, good-sized infundibulum and pulmonary annulus with thin valve plate in a patient with bipartite RV. Well-developed MPA and sinuses "cupping" over a blind-ending RVOT. (b) PAIVS with smaller infundibulum but also with thin valve plate and well-developed MPA and sinuses. (c) The valve plate is thick, measuring 1 mm (arrow) and the MPA sinuses are not well developed. Absence of "cupping" over the RVOT. (d) PAIVS with severe Ebstein's anomaly and severe TR. Markedly dilated RVOT, small MPA with no sinuses, and thick valve plate (arrow). Perforation presents the highest success rate and lowest risk in (a) and (b), as the valve plate is thin and the MPA sinuses cup over the RVOT. Perforation in (c) was feasible, but required higher energy due to the thick valve plate. A risk of perforation due to the poorly developed sinuses. In (d), risk of perforation is high and retrograde perforation from the MPA is preferable. This patient received an mBT shunt and subsequent repair of the TV and RVOT reconstruction. RVOT: right ventricular outflow tract; PAIVS: pulmonary atresia with intact ventricular septum; PDA: patent ductus arteriosus; MPA: main pulmonary artery; RV: right ventricle; TR: tricuspid regurgitation; mBT: modified Blalock Taussig; TV: tricuspid valve.

in this case. This makes elective PDA stenting at the time of valvotomy and balloon dilation an attractive strategy in patients with borderline RV size.

2. **Membranous atresia with moderate RV hypoplasia or bipartite RV (intermediate)** In some patients, the three components of the RV are moderately hypoplastic due to muscular overgrowth that significantly reduces the overall RV cavity size (Figure 32.1c). However, quite commonly, the major reduction in the RV cavity is mainly limited to obliteration of the apical part (except for slits or intertrabecular spaces), that is, a bipartite RV (Figure 32.1b). The infundibulum and pulmonary annulus remain well developed though the inlet and TV may be moderately small (TV Z score between −2.5 and −5.0). Unlike group (i), the morphology of the infundibulum, pulmonary valve, and MPA is more variable. In some patients, the infundibulum is well developed with thin

membranous atresia, good-sized annulus, and well-developed MPA and sinuses "cupping" over the blind-ending RVOT as in group (i) (Figure 32.2a and b). In others, the infundibulum, the valve annulus, and MPA are more hypoplastic with the absence of "cupping" over the RVOT. The atretic valve plate may also be thicker (>1.0 mm) (Figure 32.2c). Minor RV–coronary connections are not uncommon but major connections may also be seen (Figure 32.3a).

In this subgroup of patients, we recommend perforation and balloon dilation, and additionally "prophylactic" PDA stenting at the same time, as the smaller RV cavity and poor RV compliance from the marked RVH is unlikely to be able to take the entire preload, hence the likelihood of persistence of hypoxia and the need for PGE1 even after complete relief of RV outflow obstruction. Patients in this subgroup are also likely to

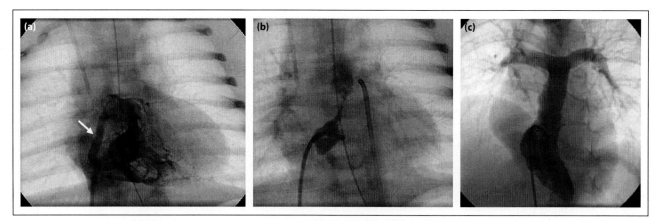

Figure 32.3 The fate of an RV–coronary connection and the RV. (a) RV angiogram in AP projection showing a bipartite RV with well-developed infundibulum. The apical part is almost obliterated except for intertrabecular spaces. A large RV–RCA connection is present with no stenosis or interruption (arrow). (b) Immediate post-balloon dilation. The RV–coronary connection disappears. The RV went into spasm and the patient became severely hypoxic. The PDA was stented. (c) RV angiogram in LAO cranial projection 4 years post-procedure. RVH has regressed and RV cavity is near normal with well-formed apical part. Normal RV pressure and SaO$_2$ 94%. The PDA stent has occluded spontaneously. RV: right ventricle; AP: antero-posterior; RCA: right coronary artery; LAO: left anterior oblique; RVH: right ventricular hypertrophy; PDA: patent ductus arteriosus.

require additional surgical procedures such as RVOT reconstruction and the bidirectional Glenn shunt as the RV may remain small.[4,15]

Patients in whom transcatheter valvotomy and balloon dilation is inappropriate or contraindicated

Patients with muscular atresia where the RVOT is obliterated by muscles are obviously unsuitable for perforation and valvuloplasty of the pulmonary valve (Figure 32.1d). Usually, these are patients with unipartite RV, who have only a diminutive inlet cavity and are commonly associated with major RV–coronary connections. These patients are destined for the Fontan pathway, and the initial management, if surgical, would be the creation of a systemic pulmonary shunt. Our institutional practice, based on the fact that the PDA in PAIVS tends to be amenable to stent implantation, is to stent the arterial duct as initial palliation in this subgroup. Associated branch pulmonary artery stenosis is rare in this context, but its presence would direct us to the surgical shunt palliation as an alternative.

In the rare patient with membranous atresia and definite RVDCC, RV decompression may cause myocardial ischemia and is therefore contraindicated. Major RV–coronary connections without "dependency" is not a contraindication. These will usually regress following balloon dilation and RV decompression (Figure 32.3).

In patients with severe Ebstein's anomaly where the thin-walled RVOT is dilated and the pulmonary annulus is small, accurate catheter placement for valve perforation is extremely difficult. Retrograde perforation via the PDA

and MPA may be considered (Figure 32.2d). Our preference is initial palliation with PDA stenting or systemic–pulmonary shunt, followed by extensive surgical repair of the TV and RVOT at 3–4 months of age.

Procedure and techniques

Except for patients with unipartite RV in whom PDA stenting is contraindicated, most patients undergo cardiac catheterization under one of three groups: for perforation and balloon dilation only for patients with good RV size (group i), valvotomy + balloon dilation and PDA stenting for group (ii) (intermediate), or PDA stenting only as first stage palliation for group (iii) patients in whom balloon dilation is inappropriate.

The procedure should be performed under general anesthesia and the patient returned to the ICU postprocedure. Cardiac catheterization should be performed with biplane fluoroscopy. An ultrasound machine is placed on standby in the catheter lab. Unless not tolerated, PGE1 infusion should be stopped 6 h before the procedure especially if PDA stenting is planned electively. Hemodynamics and angiography are initially performed to obtain further morphologic details of the RV, RVOT, pulmonary artery, and PDA.

Preintervention baseline study

1. The femoral vein is cannulated with a 5 F sheath and femoral artery with 4 F sheath. Baseline aortic pressure is recorded. Arterial blood gas is checked and any metabolic acidosis is corrected. Heparin 50 units/kg is given.
2. Right heart catheterization is performed using an NIH or multipurpose-shaped catheter to obtain RA and RV pressure, and to perform an RV angiogram.

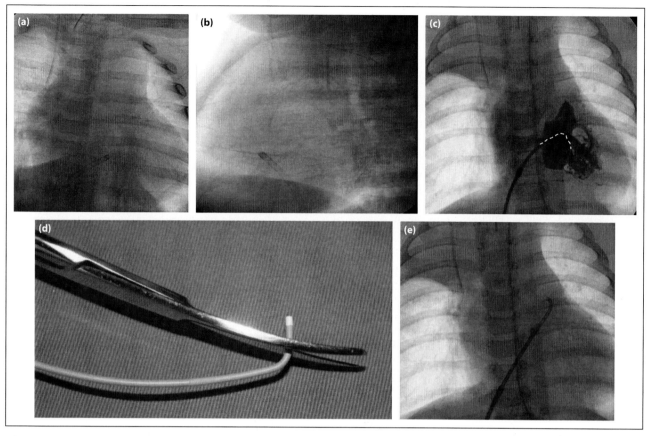

Figure 32.4   Details of the technique (i). (a), (b), and (c) A 5 F Mullins sheath with its tip facing the TV facilitates entering the RV or RVOT with the JR catheter. Dotted lines show the tip of the catheter in the RV obscured by contrast. Because of the shallow RV and heavy trabeculations, manipulating the JR tip into the RVOT may be difficult. (d) and (e) Cutting back the tip toward the distal curve may facilitate this maneuver. RV: right ventricle; RVOT: right ventricular outflow tract; JR: Judkins' right.

Sometimes, it may be difficult to enter the RV, particularly with a Judkins' right (JR) catheter in cases where there is severe TR and the RA is markedly dilated. This may be facilitated by replacing the short venous sheath with a 5 F Mullins sheath (Cook, Bloomingdale, IN, USA) with its tip in the RA facing the TV (Figure 32.4a and b). A hand-shot angiogram would be sufficient to assess the RV size, and the inlet, apical, and infundibular parts of the RV, the degree of TR, and the presence or otherwise of RV–coronary connections. If stenoses or interruptions are suspected in the proximal coronary arteries, aortic root angiography should be performed to confirm this. Hypotension and ST-T changes may occur in this clinical setting.

3.   For the assessment of the RVOT, pulmonary valve plate, and MPA, the 5 F NIH catheter is replaced with a 5 F JR catheter. The terminal tip of the catheter may need to be cut just beyond the terminal curve (Figure 32.4c and d) to facilitate manipulation of the catheter in a shallow and heavily trabeculated RV into the infundibulum and positioning below the valve plate. A cobra catheter may also suit this purpose. Simultaneous hand-shot injections with the JR catheter and the pigtail catheter facing the PDA ampulla will opacify the infundibulum and the MPA. The size of the infundibulum and the MPA, the pulmonary annulus, and thickness of the valve plate can be assessed (Figure 32.2). With a well-formed infundibulum, annulus, and thin valve plate, the MPA and sinuses are usually well developed and are seen "cupping" over the blind-ending infundibulum (Figure 32.2a and b). On the other hand, in less favorable anatomy, all three structures may be small with no pulmonary sinuses and the valve plate is thick (Figure 32.2c). In such cases, higher energy is required for perforation, which carries with it a risk of myocardial perforation outside the heart. The aortogram via the pigtail enables assessment of the PDA morphology.

Valvotomy and balloon dilation

1.   *Mechanical perforation.*   Mechanical perforation using the sharp, stiff end of the 0.014 inch coronary guide wire was used before radio-frequency (RF)

wires and generators became available. There is a tendency for this stiff wire to straighten the JR catheter and displace its tip from the valve plate.[16] This can lead to perforation of the RV free wall and may cause tamponade. This is not a recommended technique, and like the laser wire, has become largely obsolete. However, in the more straightforward cases with a thin valve plate and pulmonary sinuses cupping over the RVOT, the use of stiffer coronary wires (9–12 g tip load)—generally used for recanalization of chronic total occlusion in coronary interventions—is feasible and helps simplify the procedure (Figure 32.5d).[17]

2. *RF perforation.* RF perforation and balloon dilation has gained wide acceptance in the management of PAIVS with membranous atresia, as the generator is small, portable, easy to use, and inexpensive. Its efficacy and safety has been well demonstrated.

The Baylis radio-frequency coaxial system (Baylis Medical Company [BMC], Montreal, Canada) with its generator and wires has been specifically designed for perforation of the atrial septum, but it is also the most widely used system for perforation of the membranous atretic pulmonary valve. It consists of the BMC radio-frequency perforation generator and the Nykanen radio-frequency perforation catheter (wire). The active tip diameter of the wire is 0.012 inch and body diameter is 0.024 inch.

The Baylis system has largely superseded the older Osypka system (Dr. Osypka GmBH, Rheinfelden, Germany) with its Cereblate PA 120 wire (diameter 0.018") and the HAT 300 generator. In the more challenging cases, our preference is to use the Cereblate wire, but with the Baylis BMC generator as we find the smaller-diameter Osypka wire more flexible and perhaps has less tendency to cause tamponade in case of misperforation.

The Baylis system has the advantage that it comes with a fine coaxial catheter, which can be advanced over the wire once valve perforation is achieved. The RF wire is then removed and replaced with a 0.014 inch coronary guide wire for graded balloon dilation. However, with the Osypka system, one can pass a medium-stiffness coronary guide wire, for example, Choice PT extra support, tip load 3 g (Boston Scientific, Miami, FL, USA) alongside the RF perforating wire into the pulmonary artery (Figure 32.5c). The RF wire is then removed and graded dilation is similarly performed.

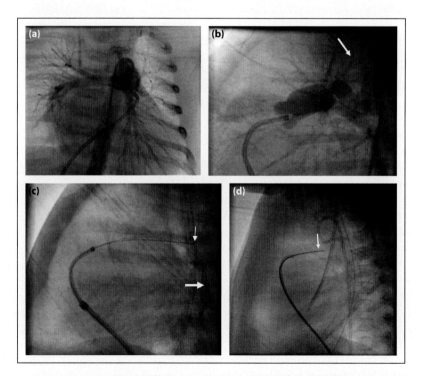

Figure 32.5 Details of the technique (ii). (a) and (b) Once perforation with RF wire is achieved, the energy is switched off and the wire pushed distally. An aortogram is performed opposite the PDA. The RF wire position in the upper-lobe RPA is verified (arrow). (c) A moderately stiff coronary guide wire (Choice PT extra support, large arrow) is passed along the perforating Nykanen wire (small arrow) and anchored in a distal PA branch. The RF wire is then removed and graded balloon dilation performed. (d) In this patient, perforation was performed using a stiffer coronary guide wire generally used for total chronic coronary occlusion (arrow). Graded balloon dilation may be performed over the same wire. RF: radio-frequency; PDA: patent ductus arteriosus; RPA: right pulmonary artery; PA: pulmonary artery.

Perforation

Once all the diagnostic angiograms have been achieved, the RF wire is inserted via a y-connector into the JR catheter with its tip beneath the atretic valve.

Before RF energy is applied, repeat hand-shots through the side port of the y-connector should be done in anteroposterior (AP) and lateral projections to ensure that the catheter tip is still in the desired position. For cases with a thin valve plate, an energy of 3–5 W and set for 2 s is usually sufficient. As the generator is activated, the RF wire is pushed forward under lateral fluoroscopy. The RF administration should be stopped once the valve is crossed or when inappropriate perforation is suspected. For a thick valve plate, an energy of 10–15 W may be administered. It is crucial that the RF wire is verified in the pulmonary artery before proceeding with balloon dilation. This is best done by contrast injection with the pigtail opposite the PDA to opacify pulmonary arteries (Figure 32.5a and b). Perforation into the pericardial space will show the wire following the outline of the cardiac silhouette.

Graded balloon dilation

The Nykanen or Osypka wire is replaced with a medium-stiffness coronary guide wire and the JR catheter is removed.

A 3-mm-diameter 2.0-cm-long coronary balloon may be used for the initial dilation. Difficulty in tracking the balloon over the wire in the right ventricle and right ventricular outflow tract may cause the balloon catheter and wire to loop in the right atrium and risk loss of wire position. Our practice is to replace the initial JR catheter (lumen 0.038″) with a 5 F JR guiding catheter for a

smooth balloon delivery to the right ventricular outflow tract and across the valve (Figure 32.6). Alternatively, the coronary guide wire may be parked in the descending aorta, but this is not always possible without snaring it out of the MPA.

The final balloon size should be 150–200% of the annulus size, and for a 3kg neonate; this is usually an 8-mm-diameter 2.0-cm-long Tyshak balloon (Numed Canada, Cornwall, Ontario, Canada) that can be tracked over the same coronary guide wire.

Following this, the hemodynamic measurement is repeated and a right ventricle angiogram may be repeated if the hemodynamic data are unsatisfactory. This may be due to insufficient dilation, spasm of the infundibulum, or presence of a muscle bundle causing fixed obstruction (Figure 32.7). In patients with RV–coronary connections, the right ventricle angiogram will show the immediate disappearance of these vessels (Figure 32.3).

One may then proceed to PDA stenting if this is already planned or deemed necessary at the end of the procedure.

During the procedure, close monitoring of the blood pressure, heart rate, blood gases, and ST-T segment of the ECG is essential, and any related abnormalities accordingly. Quite often, the procedure is performed with intravenous dopamine support using intermittent small, diluted boluses of epinephrine to maintain satisfactory hemodynamics.

Complications

The major complication related to the procedure is tamponade following perforation into the pericardial space. Perforation is more commonly seen in less straightforward

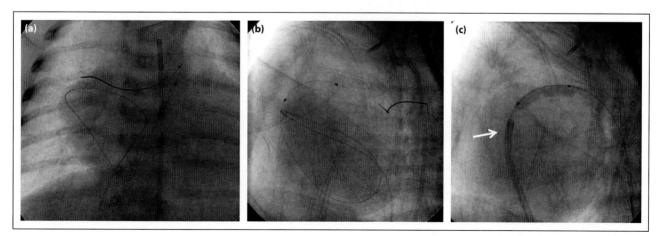

Figure 32.6 Details of the technique (iii). (a) and (b) AP and lateral projection. The coronary catheter and guide wire may loop in the RA while advancing the coronary balloon especially when the RA is dilated due to severe TR. (c) A 5 F JR guiding catheter placed in the RVOT facilitated tracking of coronary balloon across the perforated valve. AP: antero-posterior; RA: right atrium; TR: tricuspid regurgitation; JR: Judkins' Right; RVOT: right ventricular outflow tract.

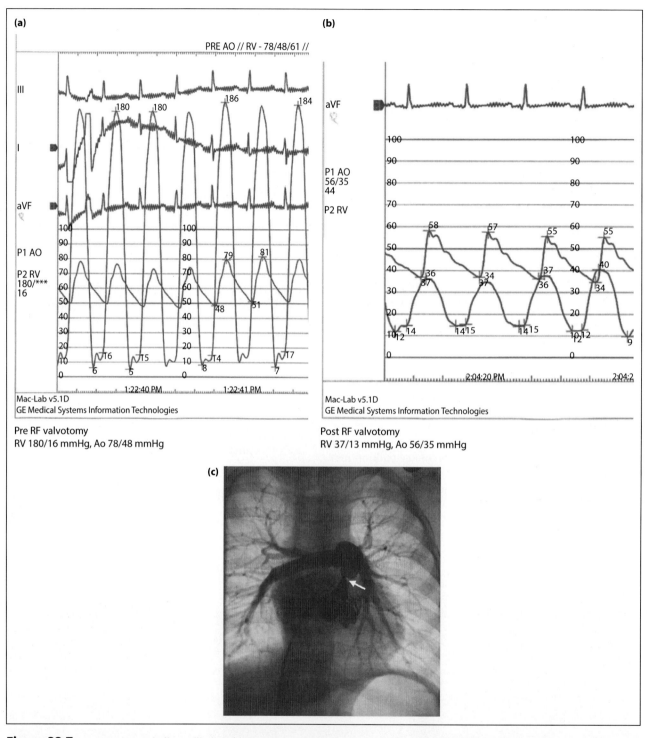

Figure 32.7 A response to balloon dilation. (a) RV pressure 180/16, Ao pressure 78/48 mmHg before balloon dilation. (b) RV systolic pressure came down to 36 mmHg systolic though there was mild hypotension immediate post-dilation. (c) A patient with fixed subvalvar obstruction (arrow). The RV pressure did not drop with balloon dilation. The RV is also small (bipartite). Oxygen saturation remained low and the PDA was stented. RV: right ventricle; PDA: patent ductus arteriosus.

cases where the pulmonary valve annulus is small, pulmonary sinuses are poorly developed, and the valve plate is thick. However, tamponade is relatively uncommon, though echocardiography should be performed immediately if this is suspected. Tamponade may be relieved by draining with a 22 G cannula and needle; most operators replace the aspirated blood by autotransfusion. Protamine may be given to reverse any heparinization. If bleeding into the pericardium cannot be controlled, surgical intervention is recommended.

In patients with RV–coronary connections, ischemic changes may occur with catheter manipulation in the RV. Hypotension and bradycardia are not uncommon, as these are often sick neonates and inotropic support may be required. As end-hole catheters like the JR are frequently used in a small-cavity RV, care should be taken to prevent air embolism. If blood does not bleed back spontaneously, avoid aspiration; repositioning may be prudent. Atrial tachycardia is another well-known complication.

Postprocedure care

The patient is returned to the ICU for continued ventilation and care, often with intropic support. Arterial blood pressure, heart rate, oxygen saturation, acid–base balance, and urine output are monitored and any abnormalities corrected.

In patients who did not undergo PDA stenting, PGE1 may need to be restarted if the oxygen saturation drops below 80%. PDA stenting or a surgical shunt should be considered if the patient remains PGE1 dependent and a protracted stay is expected.

Follow-up

Clinical progress and echocardiographic examination are important aspects of follow-up, looking at RV growth, progression of TR and its effects, valvar restenosis, and so on. Patients with the most favorable anatomy often have excellent medium- to long-term outcome but reinterventions for tricuspid or pulmonary regurgitation in early adult life may be required. Surgery is the mainstay of reintervention, but transcatheter therapies are likely to have an important role in the future.

A significant proportion of patients require reinterventions in the short and medium term for a number of problems such as repeat balloon dilation for valvar restenosis, RVOT reconstruction for fixed subvalve obstruction, repair of the TV for severe TR, and bidirectional Glenn shunt as part of the so-called one and a half ventricle repair. In patients in whom RV growth and biventricular circulation has been achieved, shunt through the ASD may be closed with a device. The stented PDA tends to occlude spontaneously in the months following the procedure.

Summary

In PAIVS with membranous atresia, RF perforation and balloon dilation has become the initial procedure of choice. Stiffer coronary guide wires may also be used for perforation in the more straightforward cases. A detailed assessment by echocardiography and angiography is advised for case selection and planning of the procedure.

Elective PDA stenting at the time of balloon dilation avoids the need for unplanned early reintervention in those with a smaller-cavity RV. The medium- to long-term survival has improved significantly in many PAIVS patients but reinterventions—surgical or transcatheter—are commonly required in a significant proportion of patients. It is likely that interventional techniques for valve replacement and repair will play a bigger role in reinterventions in the future.

References

1. Freedom RM, Nykanen DG. Pulmonary atresia and intact ventricular septum. In: Allen HD, Clark EB, Gutgesell HP, Driscoll DJ. Eds. *Moss and Adams Heart Disease in Infant, Children and Adolescents: Including the Fetus and Young Adult.* New York: Lippincott Williams and Wilkins, 2000. p. 845.
2. Daubeney PEF, Delany DJ, Anderson RH et al. Pulmonary atresia with intact ventricular septum. Range of morphology in a population-based study. *J Am Coll Cardiol* 2002;39:1670–9.
3. Alwi M. Management algorithm in pulmonary atresia with intact ventricular septum. *Catheter Cardiovasc Interv* 2006;67:679–86.
4. Ashburn DA, Blackstone EH, Wells WJ et al. Determinants of mortality and type of repair in neonates with pulmonary atresia and intact ventricular septum. *J Thorac Cardiovasc Surg* 2004;127:1000–8.
5. Alwi M, Geetha K, Bilkis AA et al. Pulmonary atresia with intact ventricular septum percutaneous radiofrequency-assisted valvotomy and balloon dilation versus surgical valvotomy and Blalock Taussig shunt. *J Am Coll Cardiol* 2000;35:468–76.
6. Agnoletti G, Piechaud JF, Bonhoeffer P et al. Perforation of the atretic pulmonary valve. *J Am Coll Cardiol* 2003;41:1399–403.
7. Humpl T, Söderberg B, McCrindle BW et al. Percutaneous balloon valvotomy in pulmonary atresia with intact ventricular septum—Impact on patient care. *Circulation* 2003;108:826–32.
8. Rowlatt JF, Rimoldi MJA, Lev M. The quantitative anatomy of the normal child's heart. *Pediatr Clin North Am* 1963;10:499–588.
9. Hanseus K, Bjorkhem G, Lundstrom NR. Dimensions of cardiac chambers and great vessels by cross-sectional echocardiography in infants and children. *Pediatr Cardiol* 1988;9:7–15.
10. Daubeney PEF, Blackstone EH, Weintraub RG et al. Relationship of the dimension of cardiac structures to body size: An echocardiographic study in normal infants and children. *Cardiol Young* 1999;9:402–10.
11. Minich LL, Tani LY, Ritter S et al. Usefulness of the preoperative tricuspid/mitral valve ratio for predicting outcome in pulmonary atresia with intact ventricular septum. *Am J Cardiol* 2000;85:1325–8.
12. Chubb H, Pesonen E, Sivasubramanian S et al. Long-term outcome following catheter valvotomy for pulmonary atresia with intact ventricular septum. *J Am Coll Cardiol* 2012;59:1468–76.
13. John AS, Warnes CA. Clinical outcomes of adult survivors of pulmonary atresia with intact ventricular septum. Article in press—published online, *Int J Cardiol* 2011.

14. Gibbs JL, Blackburn ME, Uzun D et al. Laser valvotomy with balloon valvuloplasty for pulmonary atresia with intact ventricular septum: Five years experience. *Heart* 1997;77:225–8.

15. Alwi M, Choo KK, Radzi NAM et al. Concomitant stenting of the patent ductus arteriosus and radiofrequency valvotomy in pulmonary atresia with intact ventricular septum and intermediate right ventricle: Early in-hospital and medium-term outcomes. *J Thorac Cardiovasc Surg* 2011;141:1355–61.

16. Justo RN, Nykanen DG, Williams WG et al. Transcatheter perforation of the right ventricular outflow tract as initial therapy for pulmonary valve atresia and intact ventricular septum in the newborn. *Catheter Cardiovasc Diagn* 1997;40:408–13.

17. Alwi M, Budi RR, Che Mood M et al. Pulmonary atresia with intact septum: The use of Conquest Pro coronary guidewire for perforation of atretic valve and subsequent interventions. *Cardiol Young* 2012, published online: 29 May 2012.

33

Pulmonary valve disease: Pulmonary valve in cyanotic heart defects with pulmonary oligemia

P. Syamasundar Rao

Introduction

Cyanotic congenital heart defects, as a group, constitute up to 20–25% of all congenital heart defects. In cyanotic heart defects, the arterial oxygen desaturation is secondary to right-to-left shunting at the atrial, ventricular, or great artery level or transposition of the great arteries in which the deoxygenated blood recirculates through the body. In the latter group, balloon and/or blade atrial septostomy may be useful in augmenting mixing of blood at the atrial level. These procedures have been described elsewhere in this book and will not be dealt with in this chapter. In the former group, obstruction to pulmonary blood flow by a stenotic or atretic pulmonary valve is an integral part of the cardiac malformation causing right-to-left shunting. The most common type of defect in this group is tetralogy of Fallot. Other defects include transposition of the great arteries, double outlet right (or left) ventricle, single ventricle, tricuspid atresia, ventricular inversion (corrected transposition of the great arteries), and other types of univentricular hearts, all with nonrestrictive interventricular communication and severe pulmonary valve stenosis. These patients usually present with symptoms in the neonatal period or early in infancy. The degree of cyanosis and the level of hypoxemia determine the symptomatology. Physical findings and laboratory data (chest x-ray, electrocardiogram, and echocardiogram) depend on the defect complex and are reasonably characteristic for each defect. The majority of cyanotic heart defects with pulmonary oligemia can be surgically treated. Total surgical correction may not be possible in some patients because of anatomic complexity. Yet, they may require palliation to augment pulmonary blood flow and to improve systemic arterial oxygen saturation. Surgical aortopulmonary shunts have conventionally been utilized in these situations. Since the introduction of transluminal balloon dilatation techniques in children by Kan et al.,[1] we and others[2–5] have utilized balloon pulmonary valvuloplasty

to augment pulmonary blood flow instead of a systemic-to-pulmonary artery shunt and have successfully relieved pulmonary oligemia and systemic arterial hypoxemia.

The management of cyanotic defects with pulmonary atresia is discussed elsewhere in the book and will not be reviewed in this chapter.

Indications for balloon pulmonary valvuloplasty

The indications for balloon valvuloplasty that we have used[4,6] were cardiac defects not amenable to surgical correction at the age and size at the time of presentation, but required palliation for pulmonary oligemia. Symptoms related to hypoxemia and erythrocytosis (polycythemia) are indications for intervention. Hypoplasia of the pulmonary valve ring—main and/or branch pulmonary arteries—is another indication, even if symptoms are not present. The presence of two or more sites of obstruction (Figure 33.1) is considered a prerequisite when using balloon valvuloplasty,[4] because if valvar stenosis is the sole obstruction, relief of such an obstruction may result in a marked increase in pulmonary blood flow and elevation of pulmonary artery pressure and resistance.

Technique

The technique of balloon pulmonary valvuloplasty is similar to that used for isolated valvar pulmonary stenosis, described in Chapter 32. Following the decision to proceed with balloon valvuloplasty, a 4 or 5 French multipurpose A-2 catheter (Cordis) is advanced across the pulmonary valve and is positioned in the left or right pulmonary artery. An appropriately sized (0.014–0.035") flexible tip J guide wire is positioned in the distal left or right pulmonary artery via the catheter already in place and

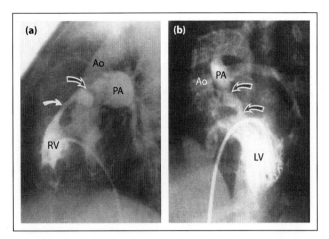

Figure 33.1 Selected cineangiographic frames from patients with tetralogy of Fallot (a) and d-transposition of the great arteries (b), demonstrating two sites of pulmonary outflow obstruction (two arrows). When the pulmonary valve obstruction is relieved by balloon valvuloplasty, the subvalvar obstruction remains and prevents flooding of the lungs. Ao, aorta; LV, left ventricle; PA, pulmonary artery; RV, right ventricle. (Reproduced with permission from the authors and publisher. Rao PS et al. *Catheter Cardiovasc Diagn* 1992;25:16–24.)

the catheter is removed. A balloon angioplasty catheter is then positioned across the pulmonary valve and the balloon is inflated (Figure 33.2). The diameter of the balloon is selected to be 1.2–1.25 times the pulmonary valve annulus, as discussed in Chapter 32 on pulmonary valve stenosis. One or more balloon inflations are usually performed. Ten to fifteen minutes following valvuloplasty, systemic arterial saturation, oxygen saturation data to calculate systemic and pulmonary flows, pulmonary artery and/or right ventricular angiography and pressure

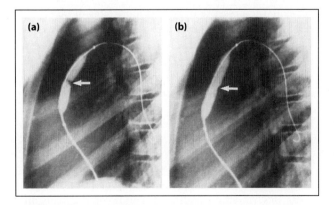

Figure 33.2 Selected cineradiographic frames of a balloon dilatation catheter placed across the pulmonic valve in an infant with tetralogy of Fallot. Note waisting of the balloon during the initial phases of balloon inflation (a), which is almost completely abolished during the later phases of balloon inflation. (Reproduced with permission from the authors and publisher. Rao PS et al. *Catheter Cardiovasc Diagn* 1992;25:16–24.)

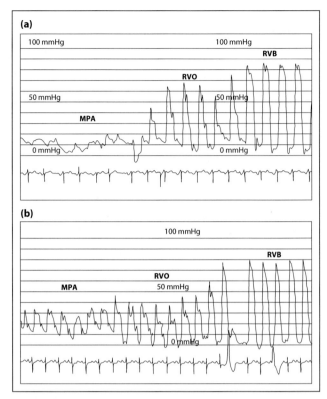

Figure 33.3 Pressure pullback tracings across the pulmonary valve and right ventricular outflow tract before (a) and 15 min after (b) balloon pulmonary valvuloplasty in a patient with tetralogy of Fallot. Note that the pulmonary valve gradient disappeared, whereas the infundibular gradient persisted after balloon pulmonary valvuloplasty. (Reproduced with permission from the authors and publisher. Rao PS, Brais M. *Am Heart J* 1988;115:1105–10.)

pullback across the pulmonary valve and infundibulum (Figure 33.3) are all recorded.

Improvements in systemic arterial oxygen saturation, increases in pulmonary blood flow and Qp:Qs and decreases in pulmonary valve gradients (Figure 33.3) have been observed[4,6–8] following balloon valvuloplasty. However, infundibular and total right ventricular outflow gradients remain unchanged (Figure 33.3).

Complications

Complications during and immediately after the procedure have been relatively low. A transient fall in systemic arterial saturation while the balloon is inflated is seen, but improves rapidly following balloon deflation. Hypotension during balloon inflation so commonly seen in isolated pulmonary valve dilatations is not seen in these patients, presumably due to the flow through the ventricular septal defect. Surprisingly, cyanotic spells following balloon valvuloplasty have not been a problem, presumably due to the improvement of pulmonary blood flow following the procedure. However, increase in cyanosis has been reported by some workers.[5]

Discussion

An increase in the size of the pulmonary arteries (Figure 33.4) and of the left atrium/ventricle at follow-up occurred such that some patients who were thought to have uncorrectable defects became good candidates for surgical correction.[4–10] More recently, this technique has been extended[11] successfully to a group of children with truly diminutive pulmonary arteries. While most workers have favorable results, some investigators were unable to document the benefit. Battistessa and associates[12] examined the results of prior balloon valvuloplasty at the time of surgical correction of tetralogy of Fallot; they did not see evidence of significant growth of the pulmonary valve annulus in the 27 patients that they evaluated. They also determined that the need for transannular patch was not abolished at the time of intracardiac repair. Therefore, they were not supportive of balloon pulmonary valvuloplasty as a palliative procedure. However, it should be noted that 15 of the 27 patients were previously reported by Qureshi et al.[5] and were included in Battistessa's study as well. Also, Battistessa's patients form a subgroup of a larger experience reported by Sreeram et al.[10] These latter authors[5,10] documented favorable results. The increase in the pulmonary valve annulus size is shown in the larger group of patients[10] that included Battistessa's patients. Furthermore, the increased size ($p < 0.001$) of the pulmonary valve annulus was demonstrated in 24 patients who

also had improved their systemic arterial oxygen saturation following balloon pulmonary valvuloplasty; this increase in the size of the pulmonary valve annulus was greater ($p < 0.005$) than expected from normal growth.[10] The improvement in pulmonary artery size documented by several authors[3–10] is similar to that observed following the Brock procedure[13,14] and systemic-to-pulmonary artery shunts.[15–18] In view of these varied observations as well as the current state-of-art with feasibility of surgical repair at a younger age, it would seem prudent that the balloon pulmonary valvuloplasty procedure be performed in selected patients with tetralogy of Fallot or other cyanotic defects. Not all cyanotic heart defect patients with pulmonary stenosis are candidates for balloon pulmonary valvuloplasty. Based on our experience and that reported by others, we[6,8,19] recommended this procedure be performed in selected patients. The selection criteria recommended are (1) the infant/child requires palliation of pulmonary oligemia, but is not a candidate for total surgical correction because of the size of the patient, the type of the defect, or other anatomic variants; (2) valvar obstruction is a significant component of the right ventricular outflow tract obstruction; and (3) multiple obstructions in a series are present so that there is residual subvalvar obstruction after relief of pulmonary valvar obstruction such that flooding of the lungs is prevented. Other indications are any type of contraindication for open-heart surgery or refusal by parents/guardians for open-heart surgical correction.

References

1. Kan JS, White RJ, Jr, Mitchell SE, Gardner TJ. Percutaneous balloon valvuloplasty: A new method for treating congenital pulmonary valve stenosis. *New Engl J Med* 1982;307:540–42.
2. Rao PS. Balloon pulmonary valvuloplasty for complex cyanotic heart defects. Presented at the Pediatric Cardiology International Congress, Vienna, Austria, February 21–25, 1987.
3. Boucek MM, Webster HE, Orsmond GS, Ruttenberg HD. Balloon pulmonary valvotomy: Palliation for cyanotic heart disease. *Am Heart J* 1988;115:318–22.
4. Rao PS, Brais M. Balloon pulmonary valvuloplasty for congenital cyanotic heart defects. *Am Heart J* 1988;115:1105–10.
5. Qureshi SA, Kirk CR, Lamb RK, Arnold R, Wilkinson JL. Balloon dilatation of the pulmonary valve in the first year of life in patients with tetralogy of Fallot: A preliminary study. *Br Heart J* 1988;60:232–35.
6. Rao PS, Wilson AD, Thapar MK, Brais M. Balloon pulmonary valvuloplasty in the management of cyanotic congenital heart defects. *Catheter Cardiovasc Diagn* 1992;25:16–24.
7. Rao PS. Transcatheter management of cyanotic congenital heart defects: A review. *Clin Cardiol* 1992;15:483–96.
8. Rao PS. Role of balloon dilatation and other transcatheter methods in the treatment of cyanotic congenital heart defects. In: Rao PS. Ed. *Transcatheter Therapy in Pediatric Cardiology*. New York: Wiley-Liss; 1993. pp. 229–53.
9. Parsons JM, Laudusans EJ, Qureshi SA, Growth of pulmonary artery after neonatal balloon dilatation of the right ventricular outflow tract in an infant with tetralogy of Fallot and atrioventricular septal defect. *Br Heart J* 1989;62:65–8.

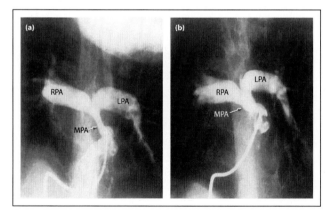

Figure 33.4 Selected frames from a pulmonary artery cineangiogram in a sitting-up view in a patient with tetralogy of Fallot patient prior to (a) and 12 months following (b) balloon pulmonary valvuloplasty. Note significant improvement in the size of the valve annulus and main and branch pulmonary arteries at follow-up. LPA, left pulmonary artery; MPA, main pulmonary artery; RPA, right pulmonary artery. (Reproduced with permission from the authors and publisher. Rao PS et al. *Catheter Cardiovasc Diagn* 1992;25:16–24.)

10. Sreeram N, Saleem M, Jackson M, Pearl I, McKay R, Arnold R et al. Results of balloon pulmonary valvuloplasty as a palliative procedure in tetralogy of Fallot. *J Am Coll Cardiol* 1991;8:159–65.

11. Kreutzer J, Perry SB, Jonas RA, Mayer JE, Castaneda AR, Lock JE. Tetralogy of Fallot with diminutive pulmonary arteries: Preoperative pulmonary valve dilatation and transcatheter rehabilitation of pulmonary arteries, *J Am Coll Cardiol* 1996;27:1741–7.

12. Battistessa SA, Robles A, Jackson M et al. Operative findings after percutaneous pulmonary balloon dilatation of right ventricular outflow tract in tetralogy of Fallot. *Br Heart J* 1990;64:321–4.

13. Brock RC. Late results of palliative operations for Fallot's tetralogy. *J Thorac Cardiovasc Surg* 1974;67:511–8.

14. Mathews HR, Belsey RHR. Indications for Brock's operation in the current treatment of tetralogy of Fallot. *Thorax* 1973;28:1–9.

15. Kirklin JW, Bargeron LM, Pacifico AD. The enlargement of small pulmonary arteries by preliminary palliative operations. *Circulation* 1977;56:612–7.

16. Gale AW, Arciniegas E, Green EW et al. Growth of pulmonary valve annulus and pulmonary arteries after the Blalock-Taussig shunt. *J Thorac Cardiovasc Surg* 1979;77:459–65.

17. Alfieri O, Blackstone EH, Parenzan L. Growth of pulmonary annulus and pulmonary arteries after the Waterston anastomosis. *J Thorac Cardiovasc Surg* 1979;78:440–4.

18. Guyton RA, Owens JE, Waumett JD et al. The Blalock–Taussig shunt: Low risk effective palliation, and pulmonary artery growth. *J Thorac Cardiovasc Surg* 1983;85:917–22.

19. Rao PS. Interventional pediatric cardiology: State of the art and future directions. *Pediat Cardiol* 1998;19:107–24.

34

Pulmonary valve disease: Transcatheter pulmonary valve implantation with the Melody valve

Sachin Khambadkone and Philipp Bonhoeffer

Anatomy/pathophysiology

The most common indication for pulmonary valve replacement (PVR) is a residual lesion after repair of congenital heart disease. Residual right ventricular outflow tract (RVOT) lesions can be stenotic, regurgitant, or mixed. Usually they are seen after surgical repair of

- Pulmonary atresia, ventricular septal defect (VSD)
- Tetralogy of Fallot
- Absent pulmonary valve syndrome
- Common arterial trunk (truncus arteriosus)
- Rastelli-type repair of transposition, VSD with pulmonary stenosis, or pulmonary atresia
- Homograft in the pulmonary outflow, for example, after Ross operation

Stenosis results from

- Insertion of a conduit in a young patient, which fails to grow
- Residual narrowing due to angulation, kinking, or twist of the conduit
- Intimal proliferation
- Degenerative calcification

Regurgitation may be due to

- Resection of the valve leaflets during surgery in the native RVOT
- Degeneration of valvular mechanism (e.g., homograft degeneration)
- Calcified outflow tracts may lead to severe stenosis.

Regurgitation may be caused by a transannular patch and usually leads to aneurysmal dilatation of the RVOT (most common with autologous pericardial patch).

Indications of pulmonary valve replacement

These are not clearly defined. Consensus indications include[1]

1. Symptomatic patients with severe pulmonary regurgitation (PR) with right ventricular (RV) dysfunction and/or dilatation
2. Patients with symptomatic arrhythmias and severe PR with RV dysfunction/dilatation
3. Severe PR and evidence of RV dysfunction (on echo/magnetic resonance imaging (MRI)/radionuclide angiography) and objective evidence of decreased exercise tolerance in asymptomatic patients
4. Patients with moderate or severe PR and additional lesions (residual VSD, branch pulmonary artery (PA) stenosis, tricuspid regurgitation (TR)), needing intervention, with or without symptoms

The indications have been expanded to include patients with right ventricular outflow tract patch repairs and residual lesions after percutaneous interventions on the native pulmonary valve with dimensions that are suitable for anchoring the Melody valve

Class IIa

It is reasonable to consider percutaneous PVR in a patient with an RV-to-PA conduit with associated moderate-to-severe pulmonary regurgitation or stenosis, provided the patient meets inclusion/exclusion criteria for the available valve (level of evidence: B).[2]

History

Transcatheter replacement of the pulmonary valve was first described by Bonhoeffer et al. in 2000.[3] The first eight cases in Paris were reported to have no regurgitation and relief of stenosis.[4] Over 3500 patients worldwide have now received the Melody implant with a low procedural mortality.[5–9]

Precatheter assessment

This includes history, including New York Heart Association (NYHA) functional class assessment, electrocardiogram (ECG) to assess right ventricular hypertrophy (RVH), QRS duration, and Holter monitoring for asymptomatic ventricular or supraventricular arrhythmias. Echocardiography is needed to assess RV and right atrial (RA) dilatation, to look for associated lesions, for example, severe TR or residual VSD, TR jet interrogation by CW Doppler to assess RV pressure on four-chamber and RV inflow view on parasternal long-axis planes, and RVOT Doppler velocity. Continuous-wave Doppler may indicate the level of right ventricular outflow tract obstruction (RVOTO). MRI assessment is mandatory to help in decision making.

Tips for case selection

1. Low-velocity TR jet (V_{max} <3 m/s on CW Doppler) indicates absence of significant stenosis despite a RVOT Doppler velocity suggesting stenosis
2. Assessment of calcification of the RVOT
3. Assessment of the dynamic nature of the RVOT in patients with aneurysmal RVOT
4. Chest x-ray/computed tomography to assess calcification of RVOT

Case selection

RV-to-PA conduit of any type (circumferential conduit) of a minimum diameter ≥16 mm and maximum diameter of ≤22 mm at the time of surgery or at the time of consideration of the catheter intervention is an important selection criterion. There have been successful implantations in patients with nonconduit outflow tracts, where a good landing zone is created by presenting of the outflow tract to appropriate dimensions to implant a Melody valve.

It is important to have an appropriate length to the conduit well away from the PA bifurcation. The Melody valve is mounted on a 34 mm 8-zig Cheatham-platinum (CP) stent that shortens by 13.5% to 28.8 mm at 18 mm balloon inflation, and by 26% to 24.6 mm at 22 mm balloon inflation.

The risk of coronary artery compression by stent implantation must be ruled out. The procedure is performed under general anesthesia and femoral venous and arterial access are obtained. However, the procedure has been performed through the internal jugular vein. Furthermore, hybrid implantation of the Melody valve through per-ventricular access through the right ventricle has been performed, especially in those patients who may have a tricuspid valve prosthesis.

It is best to start with a large venous sheath, such as 10 Fr sheath and a 5–7 Fr arterial sheath, the latter for monitoring of the systemic pressure and to assess hemodynamics as well as for aortography, coronary angiography, or other concomitant arterial interventions.

The steps for the procedure are

1. Right heart catheterization is performed for hemodynamic assessment with JR 3.5 or any other catheter with a curved tip. The tricuspid valve is crossed with a balloon-tipped catheter or with a convex curve of a catheter with a right atrial loop to prevent getting this caught in the chordae tendinae. A hydrophilic-coated guide wire (Terumo 0.035") is used to obtain a good distal position in the right or left PA followed by a good distal position of the catheter. The catheter is exchanged with a stiff exchange wire (Amplatz 0.035" Ultra Stiff 260 cm, or Lunderqvist or Back-up Meier wire). A curve is made on the wire to match the curve of the RVOT and branch PAs. A multitrack angiographic catheter is passed over the stiff guide wire to obtain hemodynamics and assess gradients on pull-back.
2. Angiography is performed in the RVOT and branch PA anatomy is assessed to rule out any distal obstruction, if MRI or CT has not been performed beforehand to assess PA bifurcation and anatomy.

    The angiographic projections for the RVOT are AP/lateral, lateral with caudal tilt (10–20), and right anterior oblique (RAO) to open up length of stenosis.

    For PA bifurcation, a four-chamber projection (left anterior oblique (LAO)/cranial 60/40) is used.

    Rotational angiography with three-dimensional reconstruction can provide good spatial orientation in complex cases to evaluate the bifurcation and the relationship of the coronary artery to the RVOT.
3. It is mandatory to perform aortography or selective coronary arteriography with simultaneous angiography of the RVOT and balloon inflation in the RVOT to rule out the risk of coronary artery occlusion, if the coronary artery anatomy has not been delineated in relationship to the Melody implantation site.

    The choice of the balloon should be at least the same diameter, if not 1–2 mm larger, than the implant diameter of the Melody valve (outer balloon diameter of the Ensemble delivery system).
4. Presenting of the RVOT is now accepted as standard before a Melody valve implantation. This relieves stenosis of the tight RVOT to facilitate delivery of the Melody valve, reduces risk of stent fractures,[10] and by using covered stents that cover both the proximal and distal anastomosis of a very calcified conduit, reduces the risk of catastrophic bleeding from conduit rupture. In patients with a nonconduit outflow tract, presenting provides a good landing zone for the Melody valve. In patients with noncompliant dilated outflow tracts, presenting can be performed a few months prior to valve implantation with either bare-metal stents or covered stents that could be left to endothelialize for a few months.

Prestenting is performed with established techniques of using large stents, balloon-in-balloon (BIB) catheters through large long sheaths (Mullins) over stiff guide wires (Amplatz Ultra Stiff, Back-up Meier, Lunderqvist). The stents are dilated to no more than the implanting diameter of the Melody valve.

Prestenting may cause conduit rupture in patients with severely stenosed and calcified conduits, although this event is not predictable. Signs of this include hypotension that persists after deflation of the balloon and may require intravenous fluids, opacification of the hemithorax on fluoroscopy, hemodynamic compromise, or angiographic demonstration of rupture on an RVOT angiogram after predilatation.

If there are concerns about conduit rupture or dissection, both the proximal and distal anastomosis of the conduit should be protected with a covered stent during prestenting.

5. If the patient is suitable for percutaneous pulmonary valve implantation (PPVI), the Melody valve is opened to rinse off the glutaraldehyde preservative. The valve is then washed in two normal saline washes for 1 min each. It is important to avoid handling or manipulating the valve leaflets and that the label on the valved stent is not removed too early (Figure 34.1).

6. During the washing of the valve, the Multitrack catheter and the introducer sheath are removed, and the femoral vein is dilated with 14 Fr and 22 Fr dilators to provide easy entry of the delivery system through the skin.

7. The valve-delivery Ensemble system is prepared by flushing the guide wire lumen, and the side arm of the outer shaft of the delivery system (Figure 34.2).

8. The **i**nner (color **i**ndigo) and **o**uter (color **o**range) balloons are prepared after deairing with one-fifth strength contrast diluted with saline. A 10 mL (Luer Lock syringe) is used to inflate the inner balloon and a 20 mL for the outer balloon.

9. After removal from the second saline wash, the valve is crimped down on a 2 mL syringe by a symmetrical squeezing and elongating (milking) action, until it loosely fits in the body of the syringe.

10. Ensure the correct orientation of the valve while crimping and subsequent loading onto the BIB balloon by checking the label, which indicates the "distal" end of the valve and by matching the sutures in the valve stent with the delivery system.

Tips: The blue suture matches the blue "carrot"-shaped dilator of the delivery system, which is the distal end of the BIB balloon, and the white suture matches the white of the proximal end of the BIB balloon catheter. This should be checked and signed off by lab personnel not scrubbed for the procedure (nurse, radiographer, anesthetist) and recorded (Figure 34.3).

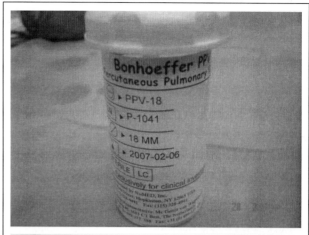
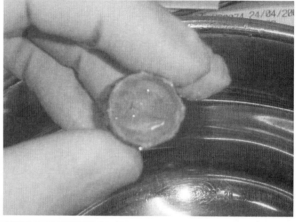

Figure 34.1 (**See color insert.**) Bonhoeffer PPV.

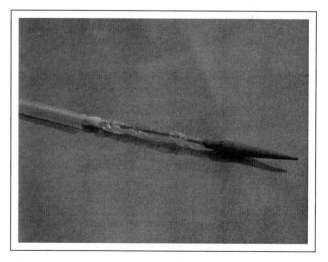

Figure 34.2 (**See color insert.**) Delivery system with BIB balloon and outer sheath.

11. The valve is loaded onto the BIB balloon of the delivery system, which should be uncovered by withdrawing the outer sheath. The valve is crimped over the BIB balloon with the same symmetrical squeezing and elongating

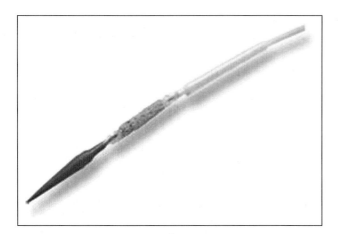

Figure 34.3 **(See color insert.)** Appropriate loading of the PPV on the BIB balloon of the delivery system.

action with thumb and fingers of both hands, pulling away from the center to proximal and distal ends of the valve stent.

12. The position of the stent should be on the center of the BIB.
13. The stent–valve assembly is covered by the outer sheath such that all the proximal struts of the stent are covered by the outer sheath. which covers the stent from its proximal end and does not move it from the center of the balloon as it reaches to cover the distal end.
14. The side arm of the outer shaft is flushed as it covers the BIB/valve/stent assembly and engages the proximal end of the dilator tip (the carrot).
15. The delivery system is now loaded with the assembly.
16. The 22 Fr dilator is removed, a small incision is made on the skin with a blade, and the delivery system is advanced over the stiff guide wire and tracked to reach the RVOT in projections that are deemed most suitable for implantation.

17. Manipulation of the delivery system over the stiff wire may require manipulation of both to advance the system into tortuous and stenosed RVOTs. Standard rules of guide wire/balloon catheter/sheath manipulation apply. For example, to facilitate advancement of the delivery system, pull on the guide wire without losing position of the distal end, or pull the guide wire away from the wall of the RVOT and try to keep the guide wire in the center of the lumen with optimum tension.
18. Predilatation may be required for severely stenosed and calcified conduits to facilitate advancement of the delivery system for prestenting. Beware of dissection and rupture of the conduit during predilatation (Figure 34.4a and b).
    Signs to look out for are
    a. Hypotension remains sustained after deflation of the balloon and may require intravenous fluids
    b. Opacification of hemithorax on fluoroscopy
    c. Hemodynamic compromise
    d. Angiographic diagnosis—on RVOT angiogram after predilatation
19. The following rules should be used for the site of valve implantation:
    a. Away from the bifurcation
    b. Stent does not lie in the muscular RVOT.
    c. The length of the stenosis in the conduit is covered by the stent without a and b.
    Tip: Sternal wires, clips on shunts, an ET tube, and a pigtail catheter in the aortic root could be used to mark the implantation site.
20. Once the site of implantation is reached, the valve is uncovered. The previously implanted bare metal stent provides a good marker for the implantation site. The valve is uncovered by withdrawing the outer shaft of the delivery system over the shaft of the balloon

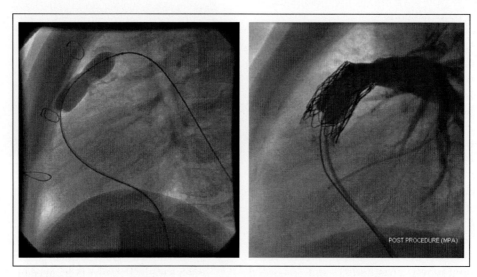

Figure 34.4 (a) Predilatation of a calcified conduit. (b) Prestenting for severely stenosed RVOT.

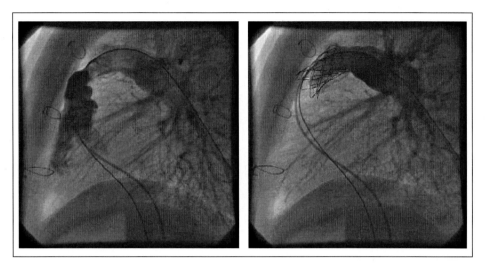

Figure 34.5   Before and after percutaneous pulmonary valve implantation.

catheter to the black double-ring marker on the shaft. The distal end of the outer sheath is not radiopaque and uncovering would be seen only as a change in the alignment of the valve–stent assembly. It is important to pull back on the shaft of the outer sheath and not on the side-arm.

21. Angiography can be performed from the sidearm of the outer sheath to reassess the position of the valve.
22. Once a good position is achieved, the balloons are inflated in sequence. The inner balloon is inflated and its position confirmed; checking angiography can be repeated, if required.
23. With the inner balloon inflated, the second operator inflates the outer balloon to its full dimension to implant the valve/stent assembly.
24. Both balloons are deflated simultaneously.
25. The delivery system is removed while holding the guide wire in the center of the valve with appropriate tension.
26. Careful manipulation of the delivery system is needed during its withdrawal through the implanted valve to prevent dislodgement.
27. The multitrack catheter is advanced over the guide wire for hemodynamics (RA, RV, PA pressure, RVOT gradient).
28. If acceptable, angiography is performed above the valve to assess valvar and paravalvar regurgitation.
29. If a residual gradient of more than 25 mmHg is present, a high-pressure balloon (e.g., Mullins balloon) of the same size as the outer diameter of the BIB is advanced over the guide wire and inflated with an indeflator to 10 atmosphere pressure.
30. Hemodynamics and angiography are repeated (Figure 34.5).
31. If all are acceptable, any catheter or guide wire across the valve is removed under screening.
32. Hemostasis and local anesthesia are applied to the groin.

Choice of delivery system

Although the currently available delivery systems are 18, 20, and 22 mm (these indicate the size of the outer balloon of the BIB), the choice of the delivery system is based on the implantation diameter of the Melody valve being nearly equal to the outer diameter of the Ensemble system.

Unusual anatomy

1. Coronary anatomy should be delineated before the procedure from the previous catheterization procedure, MRI, or operative notes. The relationship to the RVOT and the impact of stent implantation on the coronary arteries should be considered (Figure 34.6).
2. If the coronary anatomy is unusual or unknown, selective coronary arteries with balloon inflation in the RVOT is performed. ST segment changes and hemodynamic compromise during balloon inflation should be noted.
3. Extra-anatomic conduits (Rastelli procedure for TGA, VSD, PS, or pulmonary atresia with conduits) usually require difficult manipulation to achieve a good position (Figure 34.7).
4. Retrosternal conduits with calcifications may not allow expansion of the stent to its full diameter and so may leave residual stenosis (Figure 34.8).
5. In RVOTs that are appropriately sized but have a very elastic/dynamic nature, a sizing balloon may be helpful to assess the dimensions of the RVOT.

Postprocedure

After other interventional catheterization procedures, other routine observations are indicated.

Echocardiography should be performed to evaluate the presence of any pericardial effusion and worsening of TR in

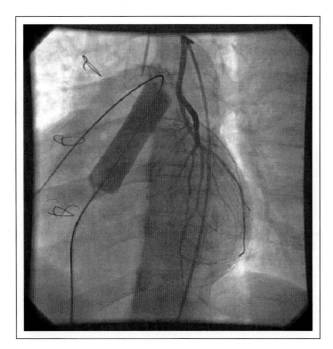

Figure 34.6 Simultaneous balloon inflation in the RVOT with coronary angiography in an unusual coronary anatomy—a case of ALCAPA repair.

order to assess hemodynamics, TR velocity, RVOT velocity, severity of PR, and the position of the valve.

A chest x-ray in PA and lateral projections are performed the following day. Aspirin, if not contraindicated, is prescribed life-long. The patient may need pain control overnight and, very occasionally, opiates are needed.

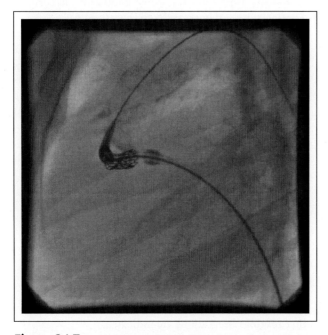

Figure 34.7 A difficult course of the delivery system in extra-anatomic conduit in the right ventricle.

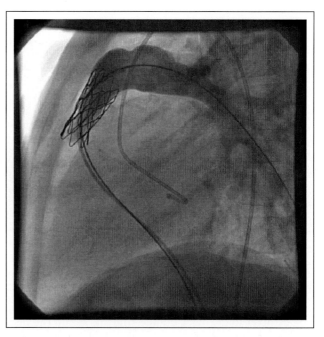

Figure 34.8 Residual stenosis in a retrosternal conduit.

Febrile episodes may occur similar to those seen after surgical homograft placements, with elevated inflammatory markers but negative blood cultures, and so may need anti-inflammatory medications.

Follow-up

The patients require clinical follow-up and echocardiography to assess hemodynamics, RVOT gradient, and grade of PR.

Chest x-rays are routinely needed to rule out any stent fractures or if there are other clinical concerns, particularly in patients with important residual stenosis and compression of the stents with cardiac cycle. Antibiotic prophylaxis against infective endocarditis should be given.

References

1. Davlouros PA, Karatza AA, Gatzoulis MA, Shore DF. Timing and type of surgery for severe pulmonary regurgitation after repair of tetralogy of Fallot. *Int J Cardiol* 2004;97(Suppl 1):91–101.
2. Feltes TF, Bacha E, Beekman RH, 3rd, Cheatham JP, Feinstein JA, Gomes AS et al. Indications for cardiac catheterization and intervention in pediatric cardiac disease: A scientific statement from the American Heart Association. *Circulation.* 2011;123:2607–52.
3. Bonhoeffer P, Boudjemline Y, Saliba Z, Merckx J, Aggoun Y, Bonnet D et al. Percutaneous replacement of pulmonary valve in a right-ventricle to pulmonary-artery prosthetic conduit with valve dysfunction. *Lancet* 2000;356(9239):1403–5.
4. Bonhoeffer P, Boudjemline Y, Qureshi SA, Le Bidois J, Iserin L, Acar P et al. Percutaneous insertion of the pulmonary valve. *J Am Coll Cardiol* 2002;39(10):1664–9.

5. Khambadkone S, Coats L, Taylor A, Boudjemline Y, Derrick G, Tsang V et al. Percutaneous pulmonary valve implantation in humans: Results in 59 consecutive patients. *Circulation* 2005;112(8):1189–7.

6. Lurz P, Coats L, Khambadkone S, Nordmeyer J, Boudjemline Y, Scheivano S et al. Percutaneous pulmonary valve implantation: Impact of evolving technology and learning curve on clinical outcome. *Circulation* 2008;117:1964.

7. McElhinney et al. Short and medium term outcomes after transcatheter pulmonary valve placement in the expanded multicenter US Melody valve trial. *Circulation* 2010;122:507.

8. Butera G, Milanese O, Spadoni I, Piazza L, Donti A, Ricci C et al. Melody transcatheter pulmonary valve implantation. Results from the Registry of Italian Society of pediatric cardiology. *Catheter Cardiovasc Interv* 2013;81(2):310–6.

9. Eicken A, Ewert P, Hager A, Peters B, Fratz S, Kuehne T et al. Percutaneous pulmonary valve implantation—Two center experience in more than 100 patients *Eur Heart J* 2011;32(10):1260–5.

10. Nordmeyer J, Khambadkone S, Coats L, Schievano S, Lurz P, Parenzan G et al. Risk stratification, systematic classification and anticipatory management strategies for stent fractures after percutaneous pulmonary valve implantation Circulation *Circulation* 2007;115(11):1392–7.

35

Pulmonary valve disease: Transcatheter pulmonary valve implantation with the Edwards SAPIEN valve

Noa Holoshitz and Ziyad M. Hijazi

Introduction

Transcatheter pulmonic valve implantation (tPVR) was first described by Philipp Bonhoeffer et al. in 2000. In this initial report, a fresh bovine jugular vein containing a native biological valve was attached to a platinum iridium stent and implanted in a sheep model.[1] Only 2 months after this animal trial, the first report of implantation of the valve in a human was published by the same group.[2] These initial reports marked the beginning of a new era in congenital and structural interventional cardiology. Bonhoeffer's valve design showed very successful clinical outcomes[3–6] and was later acquired by Medtronic and renamed the Melody valve (Medtronic, Minneapolis, MN, USA).

Edwards SAPIEN THV

Two years following Bonhoeffer's report, Cribier et al. described the first percutaneous transcatheter implantation of an aortic valve prosthesis in a 57-year-old patient with calcific aortic stenosis.[7] This valve was the predecessor to the Edwards SAPIEN transcatheter heart valve (THV) (Edwards Lifesciences, Irvine, CA, USA). Although it was initially developed as a percutaneous substitute to surgical valve replacement for aortic stenosis,[8,9] it has emerged as an alternative to the Melody valve in the pulmonic position as well. It has been used successfully in right ventricular (RV) to pulmonary artery (PA) conduits since 2005.[10]

Valve design

The SAPIEN THV is made up of three equal-sized bovine pericardial leaflets, which are hand-sewn to a stainless-steel, balloon-expandable stent (Figure 35.1). There is a fabric cuff covering the lower end of the stent to enable a seal with the calcified conduit and prevent paravalvular leak. The valve has been designed to reduce leaflet stress and maximize coaptation. The pericardial tissue is processed with the Thermafix anticalcification treatment that is utilized in the Carpentier–Edwards PERIMOUNT Magna surgical valve. It is available in 23 and 26 mm diameters with heights of 14.5 and 16 mm, respectively.[11] It can therefore be used in conduits up to 24 mm at the time of transcatheter valve replacement. The delivery system is the Retroflex III, with a tapered nose cone-shaped balloon catheter and a deflectable guiding catheter that requires either a 22 or 24 Fr hydrophilic sheath for the 23 and 26 mm valves, respectively. The hub of the guiding catheter has a control knob, which can deflect the catheter through passage into the right ventricular outflow tract (RVOT) (Figure 35.2).

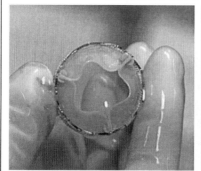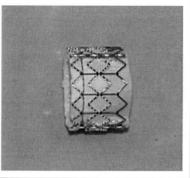

Figure 35.1 (See color insert.) The Edwards SAPIEN transcatheter heart valve. The valve (shown *en face* on the left and from the side on the right) is available in 23 mm or 26 mm diameter. It consists of three bovine pericardial cusps mounted into a stainless-steel, balloon-expandable stent.

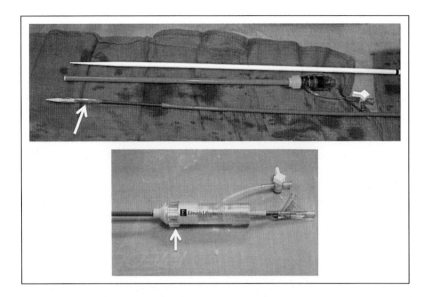

Figure 35.2 **(See color insert.)** The delivery system that includes the 35-cm-long delivery sheath and dilator and the RetroFlex delivery catheter that has a tapered steerable tip (shown in the top panel), which facilitates valve crossing; white arrow indicates the location of the valve on the catheter. The handle of the Retroflex catheter (shown in the bottom panel) has a nob (arrow) to steer the tip of the catheter.

Currently, the next generation of the SAPIEN THV, the SAPIEN XT, is being evaluated for use in the aortic position in the PARTNER II trial.[12] In the updated valve, the stent material has changed from stainless steel to a cobalt chromium alloy, which allows for a smaller delivery profile and sheath. In addition, the valve is now available in a 29 mm diameter (outside the United States). There is no available data for the SAPIEN XT valve in the pulmonic position.

There are multiple differences between the Edwards SAPIEN valve and the Melody valve, which are listed in Table 35.1. The SAPIEN THV is available in larger sizes than the current Melody valve, and therefore may be appropriate for placement in larger conduits, which are usually found in older patients. The SAPIEN THV also has a shorter height, which is beneficial in certain anatomy. The Melody delivery system, however, is less bulky and the retractable sheath protects the valve until it is deployed in the desired location. The bulkier delivery system of the SAPIEN THV makes it potentially more difficult to implant, especially in patients with a tortuous RVOT. Careful consideration must be given to the likelihood of procedural success before attempting valve implantation because the SAPIEN THV system does not use a covering sheath; therefore, once it exits its delivery sheath (35 cm long) it may be difficult to retract into the sheath.

Indications

Since it was first described over a decade ago, the field of tPVR has made great strides and the procedure has become much more widely used. The 2010 American Heart Association statement on the Indications for Cardiac Catheterization and Intervention in Pediatric Cardiac Disease was expanded to include a class IIa indication for tPVR.[13] It recommends: "It is reasonable to consider percutaneous pulmonary valve replacement in a patient with an RV-to-PA conduit with associated moderate to severe pulmonary regurgitation or stenosis provided the patient meets inclusion/exclusion criteria for the available valve. (Level of Evidence: B)."

The inclusion and exclusion criteria for the SAPIEN valve trial are summarized in Table 35.2. These criteria were based on surgical indications for RVOT revision. However, it is important to note that there is some controversy regarding the optimal timing of surgery to prevent irreversible RV damage. A study published in 2008[14] suggests that an indexed RV end-diastolic volume <150 mL/m^2 at the time of surgery leads to improved RV function as well as normalization of RV volumes. Yet, the current ACC/AHA guidelines for repeat surgery in RV-to-PA conduits are fairly vague and are based primarily on symptoms and subjective assessments.[15]

Procedural details

tPVR is performed under general endotracheal anesthesia. The femoral vein is the preferred route of delivery; however, it is also possible to perform the procedure through

Table 35.1 Comparison of the Melody and SAPIEN valves		
Characteristic	**Melody valve**	**SAPIEN valve**
Stent material	Iridium 10%, platinum 90%	Stainless steel
Valve material	Bovine jugular vein	Bovine pericardium treated with Thermafix
Available size (diameter)	18–22 mm	23 mm, 26 mm (SAPIEN XT available in 29 mm outside the United States)
Stent height	34 mm	14.5 mm, 16 mm
Delivery sheath size	22 French	22 French, 24 French

Table 35.2 Inclusion and exclusion criteria for the edwards SAPIEN valve trial

Inclusion criteria

Weight >35 kg

In situ conduit ≥16 mm and ≤24 mm

Dysfunctional RVOT conduit:
- ≥ 3+ PR by transthoracic echocardiography
- Pulmonary regurgitant fraction ≥40%
- With or without pulmonic stenosis

Exclusion criteria[a]

Active infection requiring antibiotics

History of, or active endocarditis

Intravenous drug abuse

Preexisting prosthetic heart valve in any position

Pregnancy

Severe chest wall deformity

Echocardiographic evidence of intracardiac mass, thrombus, or vegetation

Known intolerance for aspirin or heparin

[a] Multiple exclusion criteria; see http://clinicaltrials.gov for full list.

the internal jugular vein. A 7 French sheath is used initially and is later upsized to a larger sheath, based on the size of the valve chosen. In addition, arterial access is obtained (5 or 6 French) for aortic root or selective coronary angiography. Once access is obtained, the patient is given intravenous heparin for a goal activated clotting time (ACT) of >200 s. The research protocols also include starting the patients on 81 mg of aspirin (for adult patients) the night prior to the procedure. All patients should be given antibiotic prophylaxis per protocol.

1. Standard right heart catheterization is performed to assess the preprocedural hemodynamics and the pressure gradient across the dysfunctional conduit.
2. Angiographic assessment of the RV–PA conduit is performed through a side-hole catheter with biplane angiography to assess the degree of pulmonary regurgitation (Figure 35.3a).
3. The minimum diameter of the conduit is evaluated by inflating a sizing balloon across the pulmonic valve (Figure 35.3b).
4. Aortic root angiography or selective coronary angiography is performed with simultaneous balloon inflation in the RVOT to assess for possible coronary artery compression (Figure 35.3c). This step is extremely important due to the presence of coronary artery origin anomalies in some patients with congenital heart disease. The operator has to make sure that a final conduit diameter will not impinge on the coronary flow. Therefore, some operators even suggest inflating a balloon that is used for the final diameter to insure safe distance from the conduit to the origin of the coronary arteries. Others are satisfied with inflation of sizing

balloons and assuring presence of at least 10 mm from the edge of the inflated balloon to the origin of the coronary arteries.
5. Owing to the short height of the Edwards SAPIEN THV, stent implantation (prestenting) as a landing zone is routinely performed. The bare-metal stent is deployed on a BiB (balloon-in-balloon) catheter (NuMED, Hopkinton, NY, USA) over a stiff guide wire placed in either pulmonary artery, preferably in the left pulmonary artery (Figure 35.3d–g). General recommendations are to inflate the balloon to a diameter of up to 2 mm less than the original conduit size in stenotic conduits or slightly larger in conduits with no stenosis.[16]
6. The final valve size is guided by the size of the bare-metal stent used for presenting. It is important to measure the fully expanded stent diameter in two dimensions (utilizing biplane fluoroscopy) to ensure symmetrical stent expansion. In general, we implant the 23 mm valve to be no less than 21 mm in diameter and the 26 mm valve to be no less than 23 mm in diameter. The valve has been tested for durability and functionality for these diameters.
7. The valve stent is crimped symmetrically using a specialized crimping tool onto a 30-mm-long presized balloon catheter (Figure 35.4).
8. The valve is delivered across the prestented outflow tract over a very stiff guide wire (Meier wire or Lunderquist). Multiple angiograms are performed prior to balloon inflation to ensure proper position of the valve/stent (Figure 35.3h–j).
9. Valve performance is evaluated by angiography (Figure 35.3K) and/or intracardiac echocardiography. Continuous-wave Doppler as well as color Doppler across the valve is used to evaluate the gradient and assess for any paravalvular or valvular regurgitation (Figure 35.5).
10. It is recommended that venous hemostasis be achieved by utilization of a vascular closure device such as two Perclose sutures (Abbott Vascular, Abbott Park, IL, USA) placed at the beginning of the procedure.[16] However, we also have utilized the "figure-of-8" suture effectively.[17]

Patients are usually kept for observation overnight and discharged home the following day on 81 mg aspirin for 1 year. Follow-up examination and echocardiography is performed at 1, 6, and 12 months and yearly thereafter. A chest radiograph is obtained before discharge and at 6 months to look for valve/stent position and any potential stent fracture.

Complications

Serious complications that are associated with tPVR are rare, but can be devastating when they do occur. In the US multicenter SAPIEN study (COMPASSION), the rate of

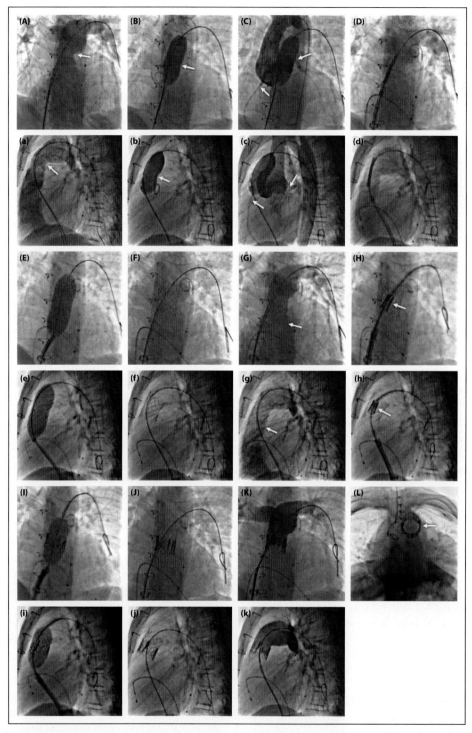

Figure 35.3 Angiographic stepwise approach to TPVR. *Uppercase letters indicate AP projection and lowercase letters indicate lateral projection.* (A,a) Angiography of degenerated conduit showing pulmonic regurgitation and narrowing (arrow). (B,b) Balloon inflation in the conduit for sizing, arrow indicating residual waist. (C,c) Simultaneous balloon inflation and aortic root injection to assess distance from the conduit to the coronary arteries (arrows). (D,d) Positioning of the bare-metal stent in the conduit. (E,e) Deployment of the bare-metal stent in the conduit. (F,f) Bare-metal stent following deployment demonstrating no residual waist and long landing zone. (G,g) Angiography in the RVOT demonstrating free pulmonic regurgitation (arrow) following prestenting. (H,h) Positioning of the Edwards SAPIEN valve (arrow) in the RVOT. (I,i) Deployment of the Edwards SAPIEN valve. (J,j) Final positioning of the valve in the RVOT following deployment. (K,k) Angiography in the RVOT following valve deployment demonstrating no narrowing and no pulmonic insufficiency. (L) *En face* view of the stent and valve showing uniform expansion.

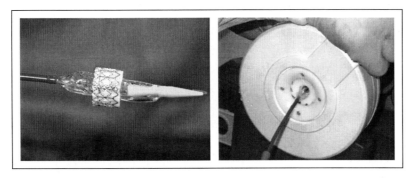

Figure 35.4 (**See color insert.**) Left: The valve is positioned on the delivery balloon, green suture line lined up away from the yellow tip. Right: Valve being crimped using the crimping tool.

serious complications was as high as 19.4% in the initial 36 procedures attempted.[16] These included three cases of stent mitration, two cases of pulmonary hemorrhage, one stent migration to the right ventricle, and one patient with ventricular fibrillation. The European multicenter registry reported a major complication rate of 13.6% in the first 22 procedures performed.[18] These complications included one patient in whom the valve could not be delivered from the femoral vein and had to be deployed in the inferior vena

cava, one valve migration, and one cerebral plexus palsy secondary to patient positioning. We expect this complication rate to become much lower as operators become more experienced with the use of the SAPIEN valve in the pulmonic position. In 2008, Bonhoeffer's group published a study evaluating the learning curve for tPVR using the Melody valve since it was first performed in 2001. They reported that after their initial 50 patients, the incidence of procedural complications fell to 2.9%.[4]

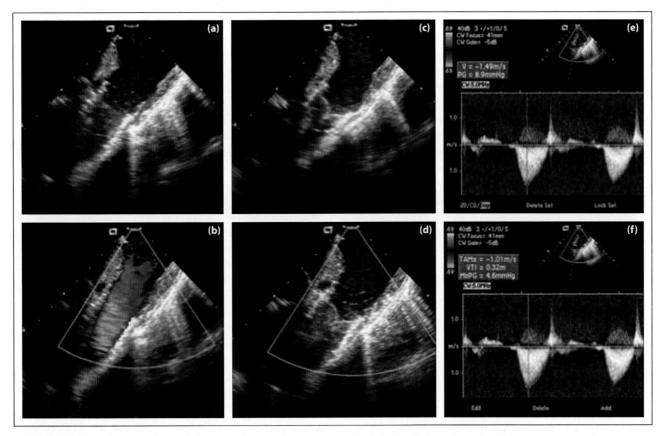

Figure 35.5 (**See color insert.**) Intracardiac echocardiography. (a) After prestenting the RVOT, (b) color Doppler demonstrates free pulmonic insufficiency. (c) After deployment of Edwards SAPIEN valve, (d) color Doppler demonstrates trivial pulmonic insufficiency. (e) Continuous-wave Doppler across the RVOT at baseline showing significant gradient. (f) Continuous-wave Doppler across the RVOT following valve implantation showing reduction in gradient.

1. *Vascular complications:* Given the large caliber of the delivery sheath of the SAPIEN valve, there is potential for serious vascular complications, including femoral vein thrombosis or hematoma. Using a vascular closure device such as the Perclose (two sutures placed at the beginning of the case) has been advocated as a way to reduce access site complications. Some groups also propose using a venous cutdown and repair of the vessel at the end of the procedure. What was the rate of vascular complications in the COMPASSION trial? There were no reported vascular complications in the COMPASSION trail or the European cohort.[16,18]

2. *Coronary artery compression:* This is not an uncommon problem, with a recent study showing that as many as 4.4% of the US Melody valve cohort had unsuitable anatomy and therefore did not undergo valve implantation.[6] This complication can be avoided by CT/MRA prior to the procedure to assess the distance between the conduit and the coronary artery. In addition, simultaneous nonselective aortic root angiography or selective coronary angiography with the balloon inflated in the RVOT has become a routine part of the tPVR procedure and should prevent this catastrophic complication. Three-dimensional rotational angiography can also be used during the procedure to more accurately assess the distance from the RVOT to the coronary ostia.

3. *Conduit rupture:* This is a serious life-threatening complication, which may necessitate converting to an open surgery. However, utilization of covered stents as a bailout is an effective way to avoid surgery in this situation.[19] We believe that laboratories performing tPVR should have the appropriate-sized covered stents available.

4. *Valve embolization:* Given the shorter height of the SAPIEN valve compared to the Melody valve, embolization is a possibility. Stent migration and embolization are typically successfully treated with percutaneous device retrieval and redeployment or surgery. Bailout perventricular pulmonary valve implantation following failed percutaneous attempt with stent migration has also been reported.[20] The rate of valve migration in the COMPASSION trial was 8.8% and 4.5% in the European cohort.[16,18]

5. *Pulmonary artery obstruction:* It is possible to obstruct either pulmonary artery by stent placement or by the SAPIEN valve. It is very important to evaluate the landing zone angiographically prior to stent placement and assess the position of the valve fully before deployment. Deploying the stent or valve across either pulmonary artery can lead to decreased flow and difficulty in accessing the branch pulmonary arteries for future interventions if needed.

6. *Pulmonary artery hemorrhage due to perforation:* Very careful attention must be paid to the tip of the guide wire during the procedure. Perforation of the pulmonary artery with either a hydrophilic wire or a stiff guide wire can easily occur, especially when the arteries have been subjected to high pressure and have become more friable. Most bleeding is self-limited and manifests as blood in the endotracheal tube. However, major pulmonary artery bleeding can lead to hemodynamic compromise necessitating an open thoracotomy and is associated with a high mortality rate. A cardiothoracic surgeon with experience in congenital heart disease should always be available on site in case of such complications.

7. *Stent fracture:* This has been a major limitation of the Melody valve, with rates of stent fracture reported to be between 12% and 28%.[3–6] Prestenting of the RVOT with a bare-metal stent is thought to reduce the rate of stent fracture.[21,22] There have not been any stent fractures reported with the Edwards SAPIEN valve, most likely because of the shorter stent height.

8. *Endocarditis:* In one study, five patients (3.2%) were diagnosed with endocarditis over a mean follow-up of 5 months.[4] The updated AHA guidelines recommend continuing life-long endocarditis prophylaxis for patients who have a conduit.[23]

Literature review

As tPVR with the SAPEIN valve is a relatively new procedure, there have not been as many studies published on it as compared to the Melody valve. In 2011, the Congenital Multicenter Trial of Pulmonic Valve Regurgitation Studying the SAPIEN Interventional THV (COMPASSION) trial demonstrated an effective reduction of RVOT gradient with reduction in clinical symptoms and maintenance of pulmonary valve competence at 6 months follow-up.[16] The study included 36 patients recruited from four centers (three from the United States, one from Europe). In two patients, valve deployment was not attempted because of unfavorable anatomy in one and stent embolization (used for prestenting) in the other. In the remaining 34 patients, implantation was successful in 33 (97.1%). Valve migration occurred in three patients with two requiring surgical retrieval. Perventricular valve implantation and retrieval was performed in one of those patients after surgical retrieval without the use of cardiopulmonary bypass. In the third patient, the valve was successfully deployed in the inferior vena cava. Additional complications included pulmonary hemorrhage ($n = 2$), ventricular fibrillation, and stent migration. Right ventricular/aortic pressure ratio decreased from 0.6 ± 0.2 to 0.4 ± 0.1 ($p < 0.001$). At 6 month follow-up, there were no deaths and pulmonary regurgitation was <2+ in 97% of the patients. One patient required elective placement of a second valve due to conduit-induced distortion of the initial implant.

The most recent data on the SAPIEN valve in the pulmonic position are the initial results in 22 European patients.[18] They reported a 95.5% procedural success rate (21 or 22 patients). There were three reported complications, including the inability to pass the valve past the inferior vena cava due to severe occlusion, one stent embolization, and one cerebral plexus injury due to positioning. RV systolic pressure decreased from 61.2 mmHg ± 23.1 to 41.2 mmHg ± 8.6. There was substantial reduction of the pulmonary regurgitation with only one patient having mild pulmonic regurgitation following valve implantation.

Future directions

Over a decade has passed since the first report of tPVR, and in that time period, huge strides have been made in this emerging field in interventional cardiology. Patients who in the past have required multiple open-heart surgeries with cardiopulmonary bypass can now prolong the life spans of their conduits with a minimally invasive procedure and go home the following day! The Edwards SAPIEN valve has recently emerged as an alternative to the Melody valve and short-term follow-up is promising.[16,18] We expect to continue seeing clinical benefits when longer follow-up is available.

Current indications for the SAPIEN valve include only dysfunctional RV-to-PA conduits. However, case reports of the valve used off-label in an expanded patient population are starting to surface. These include implantation of the valve into a pulmonary bioprosthesis (valve-in-valve)[24,25] and the use in a patient with tetralogy of Fallot without an RV-to-PA conduit (RVOT patch repair) and pulmonic regurgitation.[26] In addition, there is a report of use of the 26 mm Edwards SAPIEN valve in a native pulmonary artery with an annulus of 26 mm in a woman with a history of membranous pulmonary atresia who had undergone valvotomy of her pulmonic valve and presented with severe pulmonic valve regurgitation and right ventricular dysfunction.[27] With the availability of the 29 mm SAPIEN XT valve, we expect that the patient population we can treat will expand even further. Additionally, as previously placed transcatheter pulmonic valves start to fail, it may be possible to insert a new transcatheter valve (valve-in-valve) and therefore delay additional surgery even further.

Acknowledgment

The authors wish to thank Dr. Qi-Ling Cao for providing the figures and the entire catheterization laboratory staff at the Rush Center for Congenital & Structural Heart Disease for their hard work.

References

1. Bonhoeffer P, Boudjemline Y, Zakhia S et al. Transcatheter implantation of a bovine valve in pulmonary position: A lamb study. *Circulation* 2000;102:813–6.
2. Bonhoeffer P, Boudjemline Y, Saliba Z et al. Percutaneous replacement of pulmonary valve in a right-ventricle to pulmonary-artery prosthetic conduit with valve dysfunction. *Lancet* 2000;356:1403–5.
3. Khambadkone S, Coats L, Tahlor A et al. Percutaneous pulmonary valve implantation in humans results in 59 consecutive patients. *Circulation* 2005;112:1189–97.
4. Lurz P, Coats L, Khambadkone S et al. Percutaneous pulmonary valve implantation impact of evolving technology and learning curve on clinical outcomes. *Circulation* 2008;117(15):1964–72.
5. Zahn EM, Hellenbrand WE, Lock JE et al. Implantation of the Melody transcatheter pulmonary valve in patients with a dysfunctional right ventricular outflow tract conduit. *J Am Coll Cardiol* 2009;54:1722–9.
6. McElhinney DB, Hellenbrand WE, Zahn EM et al. Short- and medium-term outcomes after transcatheter pulmonary valve placement in the expanded multicenter US Melody valve trial. *Circulation* 2010;122:507–16.
7. Cribier A, Eltchaninoff H, BashA, Borenstein N. Percutaneous transcatheter implantation of an aortic valve prosthesis for calcific aortic stenosis. *Circulation* 2002;106:3006–8.
8. Webb JB, Chandavimol M, Thompson CR et al. Percutaneous aortic valve implantation retrograde from the femoral artery. *Circulation* 2006;113:842–50.
9. Leon MD, Smith CR, Mack M et al. PARTNER trial investigators. Transcatheter aortic-valve implantation for aortic stenosis in patients who cannot undergo surgery. *N Engl J Med* 2010;363:1597–607.
10. Garay F, Webb J, Hijazi ZM. Percutaneous replacement of pulmonary valve using the Edwards-Cribier percutaneous heart valve: First report in a human patient. *Catheter Cardiovasc Interv* 2006;67:659–62.
11. Boone RH, Webb JG, Horlick E et al. Transcatheter pulmonary valve implantation using the Edwards SAPIEN™ transcatheter heart valve. *Catheter Cardiovasc Interv* 2010;75:286–94.
12. Webb JG, Altwegg L, Masson J et al. A new transcatheter aortic valve and percutaneous valve delivery system. *J Am Coll Cardiol* 2009;53:1855–8.
13. Feltes TF, Bacha E, Beekman RH 3rd et al. Indications for cardiac catheterization and intervention in pediatric cardiac disease: A scientific statement from the American Heart Association. *Circulation* 2011;123:2607–52.
14. Frigiola A, Tsang V, Bull C et al. Biventricular response after pulmonary valve replacement for right ventricular outflow tract dysfunction: Is age a predictor of outcome? *Circulation* 2008;118 (suppl):S182–90.
15. Warnes CA, Williams RB, Bashore TM et al. ACC/AHA 2008 Guidelines for the management of adults with congenital heart disease: A report of the American College of Cardiology/American Heart Association task force on practice guidelines. *Circulation* 2008;118:714–833.
16. Kenny D, Hijazi ZM, Kar S et al. Percutaneous implantation of the Edwards SAPIEN transcatheter heart valve for conduit failure in the pulmonary position: Early phase 1 results from an international multicenter clinical trial. *J Am Coll Cardiol* 2011;58:2248–56.
17. Cilingiroglu M, Salinger M, Zhao D et al. Technique of temporary "Figure-of-eight" sutures to achieve hemostasis after removal of large-caliber femoral venous sheaths. *Catheter Cardiovasc Interv* 2011;78:155–60.
18. Haas NA, Moysich A, Neudorf U et al. Percutaneous implantation of the Edwards SAPIEN pulmonic valve: Initial results in the first 22 patients. *Clin Res Cardiol* 2012;102(2):119–28.

19. Sosnowski CR, Kenny D, Hijazi ZM. Bail out use of the gore excluder following pulmonary conduit rupture during transcatheter pulmonary valve replacement. *Catheter Cardiovasc Interv* 2013;81(2):331–4.
20. Cubeddu R, Hijazi ZM. Bailout perventricular pulmonary valve implantation following failed percutaneous attempt using the Edwards Sapien transcatheter heart valve. *Catheter Cardiovasc Interv* 2011;77:276–80.
21. Demkow M, Biernacka EK, Spiewak M et al. Percutaneous pulmonary valve implantation preceded by routine presenting with a bare-metal stent. *Catheter Cardiovasc Interv* 2011;77:381–89.
22. Nordmeyer J, Lurz P, Khambadkone S et al. Pre-stenting with a bare-metal stent before percutaneous pulmonary valve implantation: Acute and 1-year outcomes. *Heart* 2011;97:118–23.
23. Wilson W, Taubert KA, Gewitz M et al. Prevention of infective endocarditis: Guidelines from the American Heart Association. *Circulation* 2007;116:1736–54
24. MacDonald ST, Carminati M, Butera G. Percutaneous implantation of an Edwards SAPIEN valve in a failing pulmonary bioprosthesis in palliated tetralogy of Fallot. *Eur Heart J* 2011;32:1534.
25. Lombardi M, Violini R, Fiorella A et al. Percutaneous implantation of Edwards-SAPIEN valve into pulmonary bioprosthesis (valve-in-valve). *J Cardiovasc Med* 2012;13:74–5.
26. Lauten A, Hoyme M, Figulla HR. Severe pulmonary regurgitation after tetralogy of Fallot repair: Transcatheter treatment with the Edwards SAPIEN XT heart valve. *Heart* 2012;98:623–24
27. Bertels RA, Blom NA, Schalij MJ. Edwards SAPIEN transcatheter heart valve in native pulmonary valve position. *Heart* 2010;96:661.

36

Pulmonary valve disease: New percutaneous pulmonary valves

Damien Kenny, Massimo Caputo, and Ziyad M. Hijazi

Introduction

Great strides in a short time period have been made with transcatheter pulmonary valve replacement (tPVR). The original report of percutaneous delivery of a valved stent into a 12-year-old boy with stenosis and insufficiency of a prosthetic conduit from the right ventricle to the pulmonary artery was published in 2000,[1] and in the space of 12 years, over 4000 transcatheter pulmonary valve implants have been carried out worldwide. The procedure has evolved from selective placement within a dysfunctional conduit to placement within failing bioprosthetic valves and the native right ventricular outflow tract.[2–6] The impact of the hostile environment of the right ventricular outflow tract (RVOT) on valve stent integrity and durability has been studied in detail.[7,8] As a consequence, RVOT prestenting evolved and has significantly reduced stent fracture rates,[9,10] which is the leading cause for valve dysfunction and reintervention.[8,11] Smaller patients with evolving delivery approaches have also been described (Figure 36.1). The next significant hurdle is clinical testing of a valved stent appropriate for the large variety of native outflow tracts seen in patients with predominant pulmonary regurgitation.[12] However, further challenges exist to overcome the degenerative processes that occur and lead to slow destruction of nonautologous tissue and consequent valve dysfunction. This chapter will outline some of these challenges and discuss novel approaches to overcoming them with evolving valve technologies.

Anatomical Variability

Although transcatheter valve replacement has now been described for all four cardiac valves, the varied etiologies and subsequent anatomical consequences of surgically induced pulmonary valve dysfunction continue to provide a challenge for the ideal transcatheter pulmonary valve system. To some extent, the success of transcatheter aortic valve replacement

has been based on the remarkable consistency of the pathological substrate. We are not so fortunate with the RVOT. Scar tissue, conduit calcification, outflow tract aneurysm, compressive forces from the sternum anteriorly, as well as the potential for significant posterior angulation from the native or replaced pulmonary valve toward bifurcating branch pulmonary arteries, the distance between which is extremely variable, are just part of the challenge. The impact of some of these variants in relation to pulmonary valve dysfunction and replacement has been studied. Nordmeyer et al.[12] evaluated the impact of surgical homograft geometry on pulmonary valve function at 1 year and found that alterations in *in situ* homograft geometry were associated with the likelihood of developing significant valve incompetence, which was present in one-sixth of patients. Three factors were associated with more pronounced pulmonary regurgitation (PR), namely, an eccentric pulmonary forward flow pattern, a more acute homograft distortion angle (Figure 36.2), and a larger prehomograft RVOT diameter. Although balloon-expandable stent–valve systems provide a more rigid support system, avoiding mechanical kinking or distortion, anterior compression from the sternum has been shown to impact upon stent geometry with consequent valve dysfunction.[8] The challenges are even greater with the native outflow. Schievano et al.[13] evaluated the variations in postoperative RVOT morphology in 83 patients using cardiac mitral regurgitation (MR), assessing the implications for percutaneous pulmonary valve implantation. Five different morphological subtypes were identified and although type I morphology (Figure 36.3) was most commonly seen with those undergoing transannular patch, type II–V morphologies were also seen within this subgroup. The pyramidal shape of type I morphologies may provide challenges for a self-expanding system (currently under development for the native RVOT) as the diameters of the proximal and distal portions of the stent may be very variable and the implications of this asymmetry for valve function/distortion (similar to geometrical kinking of surgical homografts)

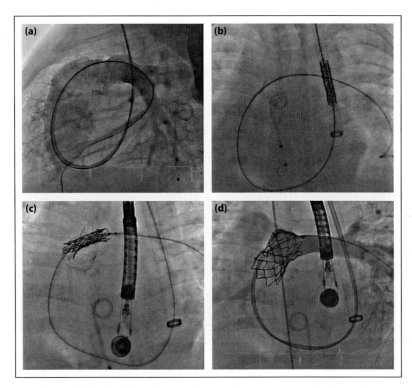

Figure 36.1 Series of fluoroscopic images in a 14-kg infant with mirror-image dextrocardia and previous repair of tetralogy of Fallot and complete atrioventricular septal defect undergoing Melody valve implantation from the left internal jugular vein (LIJV). The patient had developed significant RVOT narrowing following a valve-sparing repair and had undergone a previous RVOT stent. (a) MPA angiogram in the lateral view demonstrates the previously placed stent and free PR. (b) A 20 Fr sheath is paced in the LIJV and the Melody valve is seen as it is advanced through the sheath. (c) Angulated frontal projection demonstrating the Melody valve advanced out of the sheath and across the previously paced stent. (d) Final main pulmonary artery angiogram demonstrates the expanded functioning Melody valve in position with no pulmonary incompetence seen.

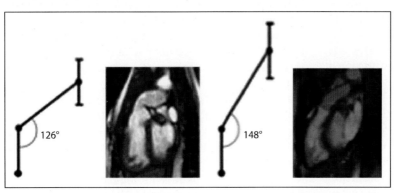

Figure 36.2 Parasagittal cardiac MR angiogram of the RVOT demonstrating the variation in homograft angle that may be seen. This has been shown to impact on homograft function on 1-year follow-up. (From Nordmeyer J. *Eur Heart J* 2009;30:2147–54.)

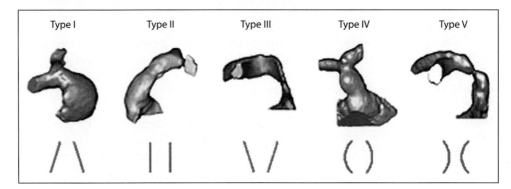

Figure 36.3 Classification of RVOT morphologies that may be encountered in patients with previous surgical intervention on the RVOT.

are unclear. It is also worth noting that any transcatheter system will not be able to overcome the potentially negative impact of the aneurysmal/akinetic RVOT on both right and left ventricular function and potential for ventricular arrhythmia;[14,15] however, more recent randomized results suggest that RVOT remodeling is less important at least for short-term outcomes following PVR.[16] Other anatomical challenges provided by short-segment main pulmonary artery (MPA) or distal MPA/proximal branch PA narrowing have also been overcome with stenting across the relevant branch PA with an open-cell stent. Further dilation of the area of the stent covering the ostium of the contralateral branch PA with a high-pressure balloon may then be carried out to ensure that access to this vessel is maintained.[17] This approach has also been used to apply a balloon-expandable valve system to a dilated outflow tract.[6,17]

New and developing transcatheter pulmonary valve systems

Clinical experience to date has been with two balloon-expandable systems, namely, the Melody valve (Medtronic, Minneapolis, MN) with the Ensemble delivery system and the SAPIEN valve (Edwards Lifesciences, Irvine, CA) using the Retroflex delivery system. Both systems have undergone clinical trials[11,18] and the specifics of these valves, the delivery systems, and the outcome data are extensively covered in other chapters.

Prior to discussing new valve systems, it is important to cover newer applications of preexisting valves. Both the Melody and the SAPIEN valves have been used in native outflow tracts with good success.[4,19] Limitations to extended application of these valves have generally centered on the size of the patient and of the RVOT. The 22 Fr delivery system used most commonly with both the Melody and SAPIEN valves has limited transfemoral delivery to children over 20 kg; however, other options

are available. The internal jugular vein may be used in these smaller patients and experience with this approach is evolving (Figure 36.1). An alternative approach is valve delivery directly through the heart (perventricular) via a sheath placed in the right ventricular free wall. Extended applications of the valve relate not only as an alternative to elective surgical valve replacement but also in establishing valvar competence in those patients who may not otherwise be surgical candidates. Lurz et al.[20] described successful tPVR in seven patients with significant pulmonary hypertension and severe pulmonary regurgitation. Following valve implantation, there was improvement in patient symptoms with an increase in right ventricular stroke volumes, and oxygen saturations and a decrease in right ventricular volumes. The valve has functioned well at median follow-up of 20 months despite near systemic pulmonary artery pressures in some. Attempts to extend the application of preexisting valves to dilated outflow tracts have also included preplacement of an intravascular reducer (Figure 36.4).[21] This is a novel self-expanding nitinol stent with a central constriction. The device shortens as both extremities curve backward during deployment, which provides more stability within the dilated RVOT. The device has a PTFE covering to assure sealing of the device and prevent paravalvar leaks. Once deployed, a balloon-expandable system may be placed within. Further approaches with telescoping stents from the branch pulmonary arteries to provide a landing zone in the dilated native RVOT may also provide greater stability with marginal RVOTs (24–26 mm); however, one might question

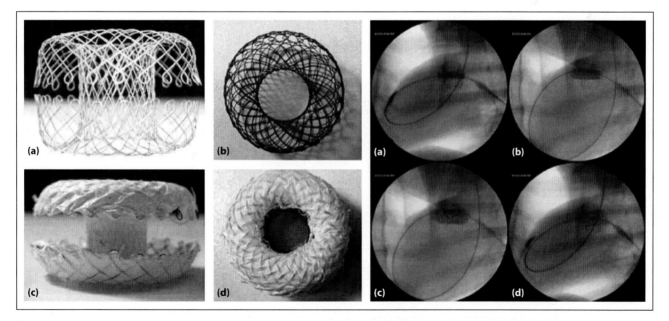

Figure 36.4 Panel 1—Series of images outlining the novel self-expanding nitinol stent with a central constriction. The device is shortened as both extremities curve backward, which also provides more stability. (a, b) Demonstration of the device in two different views. (c, d) Demonstration of the device with PTFE covering to assure sealing of the device and prevent paravalvar leak. Panel 2—Series of fluoroscopic images outlining deployment of the Melody valve within a native RVOT with the novel self-expanding stent at place. (From Mollet A et al. *Pediatr Res* 2007;62:428–33.)

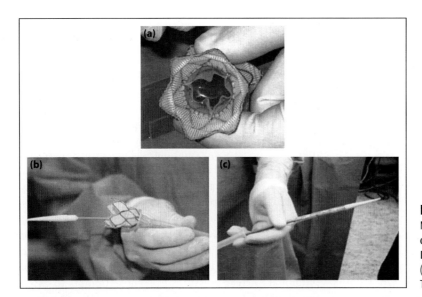

Figure 36.5 (**See color insert.**) A new Medtronic self-expanding valve, currently in development, is being designed for native RVOTs. (a) Demonstration of the short-axis view of the valve. (b) Loading the valve into the delivery system. (c) The valve fully loaded and ready for delivery.

the widespread application of this approach and a definitive system for the dilated RVOT is required. Although the Melody has been dilated up to 24 mm with an outer diameter of 26 mm, and a 29 mm SAPIEN valve may be available in the near future for the pulmonic position, it is unlikely that the solution to the dilated RVOT will be provided by a balloon-expandable system.

Evolving systems: Self-expanding transcatheter systems

Clinical reports of a new valve sewn into a self-expanding nitinol frame have been described (Figure 36.5).[23] The valve design consists of a cylindrical hourglass shape with the valve in the central portion. The stent is composed of six nitinol rings interwoven with polyester fabric. The two outer rings are nested inside the adjacent rings while the other rings are connected to each other with point-to-point sutures. Clinical experience to date has been limited to a case report[23] with a follow-up computational evaluation of the valve *in vivo*.[24] Medtronic is planning to perform a small feasibility study in 20 patients with significant pulmonary regurgitation and right heart dilation ($\geq$150 mL/m^2) with or without symptoms to determine the performance of the valve in the native outflow. The valve will require a 25 Fr delivery system; however, further data on the system are limited.

Other self-expanding valve systems are in development (Figure 36.6). The Lifetech Scientific valve (Shenzhen, China) is a porcine pericardial trileaflet valve mounted on a self-expanding nitinol frame, intended for use in patients with a regurgitant or stenotic outflow tract $\geq$16 mm in diameter. It is delivered with a 16–18 Fr retrievable catheter

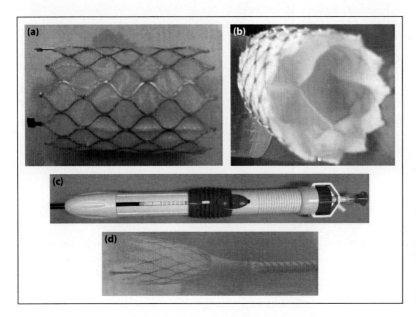

Figure 36.6 (**See color insert.**) Series of images outlining the Lifetech self-expanding pulmonary valve system. (a) Demonstration of the long-axis view of the expanded valve. (b) Demonstration of the short-axis view of the outflow end of the valve with the three tissue leaflets seen clearly. (c) The delivery system allows for rapid or slow deployment with (d) a superelastic reinforced end to allow flaring and recovery after over two-thirds of the device is deployed.

delivery system. The stent has a diamond cell configuration and is completely covered with porcine pericardium. It is available in three sizes (20, 24, and 28 mm) with expanded lengths of 39, 36, and 32 mm, respectively.

The Venus P Valve

The Venus Pulmonary Valve (Venus Medtech, Shanghai, China) is a self-expandable Nitinol multi-level support frame with a tri-leaflet porcine pericardial tissue valve (Figure 36.7a) with a 14–22 Fr delivery catheter (Figure 36.7b). The entire stent is covered (except the distal cells) by porcine pericardial tissue. The valve tissue is fabricated from three equal sections of porcine pericardium that have been preserved in low concentration solutions of buffered glutaraldehyde to fully crosslink the tissue, while preserving its flexibility and strength. A flared uncovered outflow end secures anchoring at the distal (pulmonary artery bifurcation) end with radiopaque markers indicating the distal anchoring position and the valve location. The proximal end is also flared but covered allowing conformability with the dilated RVOT. Stent valve diameters range from 20 to 32 mm (in 2 mm increments) with each diameter available in 20 and 30 mm straight section lengths. The crimper is a nonpatient contacting, compression device that symmetrically reduces the overall diameter/profile of the bioprosthesis when loaded inside the catheter (Figure 36.7c). Once crimped in ice-water the valve maintains its shape (Figure 36.7d) and is loaded onto the delivery system (Figure 36.7e) which varies from 14 to 22 Fr depending on valve size, and deployed with a controlled release handle. Early clinical experience is promising with excellent early valve function and RV remodeling reported.[25]

Evolving systems: Injectable valves

Initial clinical experience with an injectable self-expanding pulmonary valve system (Shelhigh, Union, NJ) was reported in 2006.[26] Further clinical studies followed and the valve has undergone modifications and is now CE marked under the management of BioIntegral Surgical. The tissue valve is mounted on a self-expanding stent, the No-React Injectable BioPulmonic (BioIntegral Surgical, Toronto, Canada) (Figure 36.8), and allows the valve to be implanted through the right ventricle without using cardiopulmonary bypass, thereby avoiding its adverse side effects. The Injectable BioPulmonic prosthesis is currently available in sizes up to a diameter of 31 mm. MPA reduction/plication is advised in outflow tracts greater than 29 mm and the valve may also be fixed to the RVOT with sutures following deployment to augment stability. Data from a small nonrandomized comparative trial are outlined in Table 36.1 and demonstrate significant

advantages in morbidity over open surgical valve replacement; however, longer-term follow-up data are required to assess valve durability.

Evolving systems: Smaller delivery systems

While work on these newer valve systems is ongoing, attempts to miniaturize delivery systems so that smaller children with dysfunctional conduits/bioprosthetic valves may be treated percutaneously require further work. The newer generation of the SAPIEN valve (the SAPIEN XT) requires a smaller delivery system of 18–19 Fr (NovaFlex). However, this system has not been evaluated in clinical trials yet for deployment in the pulmonary position. Also, newer lower-profile pulmonary valves are being evaluated in animal models. One such new valve is the Colibri Heart Valve (Colibri Heart Valve, Broomfield, CO) (Figure 36.9). This valve has been tested in a swine model and it requires 12–16 Fr delivery system for valves ranging in size from 20 to 30 mm. The stent is made of stainless steel and a special porcine pericardium tissue processing has permitted a dry membrane valve configuration that reduces the overall delivery profile. The system is fully integrated in a prepackaged delivery system and ready to use directly without any predelivery washing.

Tissue engineering

The last endeavor should be to merge these approaches with tissue-engineering technologies to provide living autologous valve replacements with regenerative and growth potential. This approach involves seeding cells in three-dimensional matrices to form living tissue products having structural and functional properties that can be used to restore, maintain, or improve tissue function. The repopulation of a decellularized matrix with a patient's own stem cells before surgery can potentially create a living structure with subsequent long-term preservation of mechanical and biological properties (Figure 36.10). This approach has already been used to transplant a tissue-engineered airway in a human subject.[27] Tissue-engineered pulmonary valves have been implanted in an ovine model[28] and multiple laboratories are evaluating the optimal scaffold and cell line to create a viable living tissue alternative.

Conclusions

Considering the evolutionary pace of transcatheter valve replacement, it is likely that a complete transcatheter solution to native pulmonary outflow tract disease will be available in the near future. Challenges exist with optimizing this technology. Further endeavors to implant pulmonary valves and conduits that will "grow" with infants and children though seeding of native cell lines may be some way off as yet.

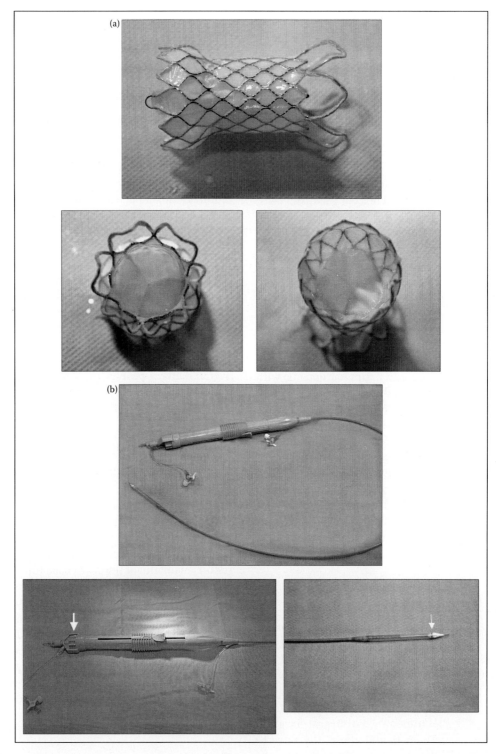

Figure 36.7 (a) Long (above) and short axis (below—from both ends) views of the Venus P valve with the covered configuration internal to the stent (apart from the distal end) and the trileaflet nature of the porcine pericardial valve. (b) The proximal and distal ends of the valve delivery system demonstrating the tapered distal end (below right—white arrow) and the proximal controlled release handle (below left) facilitating both slow (white arrow) and fast valve deployment. (c) The triangular crimping device facilitates a symmetrical and controlled valve crimping which when performed in ice-cold water ensures the valve maintains its crimped state for loading. (d) The crimped valve is then loaded through a short plastic funnel to facilitate loading onto the delivery catheter. (e) Demonstrates loading of the valve onto the delivery catheter with the finally prepared valve (large white arrow) seen covered by the transparent distal end of the delivery system with the tapered carrot (smaller white arrow).

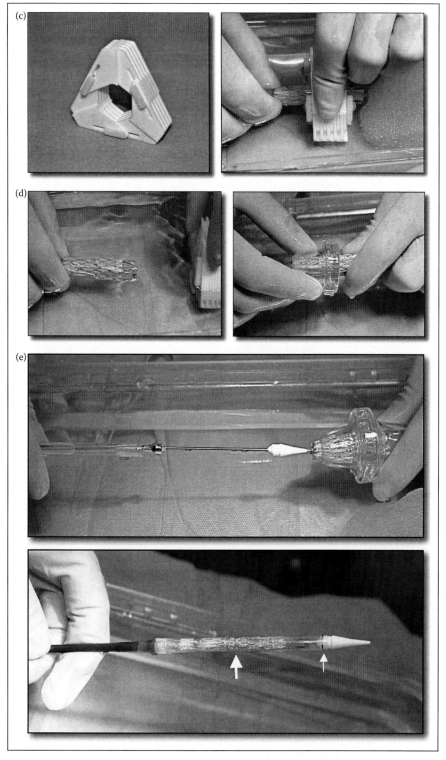

Figure 36.7 (continued) (a) Long (above) and short axis (below—from both ends) views of the Venus P valve with the covered configuration internal to the stent (apart from the distal end) and the trileaflet nature of the porcine pericardial valve. (b) The proximal and distal ends of the valve delivery system demonstrating the tapered distal end (below right—white arrow) and the proximal controlled release handle (below left) facilitating both slow (white arrow) and fast valve deployment. (c) The triangular crimping device facilitates a symmetrical and controlled valve crimping which when performed in ice-cold water ensures the valve maintains its crimped state for loading. (d) The crimped valve is then loaded through a short plastic funnel to facilitate loading onto the delivery catheter. (e) Demonstrates loading of the valve onto the delivery catheter with the finally prepared valve (large white arrow) seen covered by the transparent distal end of the delivery system with the tapered carrot (smaller white arrow).

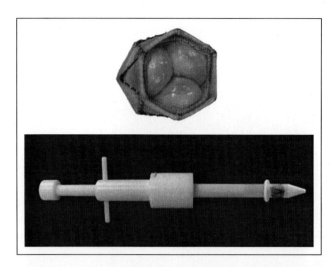

Figure 36.8 **(See color insert.)** The No-React Injectable BioPulmonic valve with the perventricular delivery catheter seen in the bottom panel.

Table 36.1 Comparative data on the injectable pulmonary valve versus conventional surgery in patients with dominant PR undergoing pulmonary valve replacement

Variables	Injectable valve ($n = 8$)	Conventional ($n = 8$)	p value
Age (years)	28.2 ± 21 (12–62)	23.4 ± 13 (10–46)	0.6
Body surface area (m²)	1.86 ± 0.37 (1.38–2.39)	1.02 ± 0.22 (1.31–1.89)	0.2
Diagnosis at initial operation			0.1
Tetralogy of Fallot	6	7	
Isolated pulmonary stenosis	1	1	
Pulmonary atresia/intact septum	1	0	
RVEDVI (mL/m²)	131.6 ± 26.7 (95–270)	136.7 ± 28.7 (92–281)	0.2
RVESVI (mL/m²)	67.4 ± 8.7 (56–75.9)	69.4 ± 8.9 (51–79.9)	0.1
RVEF (%)	46.5 ± 11.4 (30–56)	48.5 ± 14.4 (32–58)	0.5
Size of valve (mm)	26.6 ± 1.9 (25–29)	23.3 ± 1.3 (21–25)	<0.05
Operating time (mins)	165.7 ± 43.3 (110–240)	298.6 ± 57.4 (221–375)	<0.001
CPU time (mins)	0	108.5 ± 47.4	<0.001
Pre-op Hb (g/dL)	14.5 ± 0.7 (13.9–15.7)	13.4 ± 2.0 (10.2–15.5)	0.2
Post-op Hb (g/dL)	13.4 ± 1.7 (11.4–15.6)	9.8 ± 1.7 (6.6–11.7)	<0.001
Chest drainage (mls)	83.3 ± 28.6 (50–120)	527.1 ± 485.3 (210–1150)	<0.05
Blood products used (units)	0	3.6 ± 3.9 (2–11)	<0.05
Intubation time (h)	7.5 ± 6.2 (1.5–16)	21.2 ± 26.3 (5–79)	0.2
ICU stay (days)	1.8 ± 1.1 (1–4)	2.3 ± 1.2 (1–4)	0.5
Hospital stay (days)	6.0 ± 3.0 (3–11)	6.9 ± 1.3 (6–9)	0.5
Mortality	0	0	

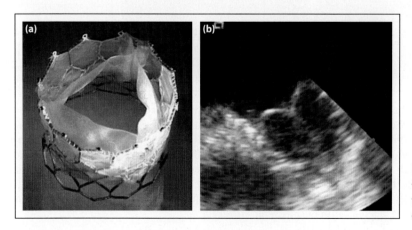

Figure 36.9 **(See color insert.)** (a) The Colibri valve. (b) Intracardiac echocardiographic image of the valve following deployment in the RVOT in a canine model.

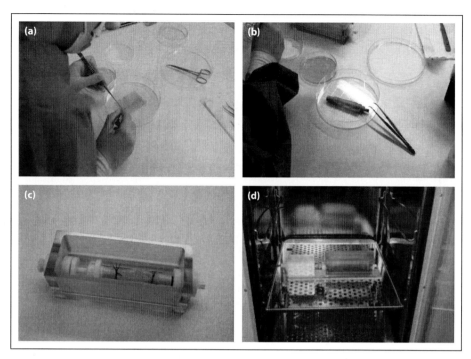

Figure 36.10   (**See color insert.**) Series of images outlining the development of a core-matric scaffold for seeding of stem cells and the ultimate development of a tissue-engineered scaffold. Human cord blood stem cell-derived smooth muscle cells were seeded onto a core scaffold and incubated for 2 days before the assembly of the conduit. (a) Sewing the two pieces of scaffold together as a cylinder. (b) The core column is sheathed in tissue-engineered conduit, before being installed on the bioreactor. (c) Tissue-engineered conduit, installed and fixed in the bioreactor. (d) Tissue-engineered conduit incubating in the bioreactor at 37°C incubator.

References

1. Bonhoeffer P, Boudjemline Y, Saliba Z et al. Percutaneous replacement of pulmonary valve in a right-ventricle to pulmonary-artery prosthetic conduit with valve dysfunction. *Lancet* 2000;356:1403–5.
2. Khambadkone S, Coats L, Taylor A et al. Percutaneous pulmonary valve implantation in humans: Results in 59 consecutive patients. *Circulation* 2005;112:1189–97.
3. Nordmeyer J, Coats L, Lurz P et al. Percutaneous pulmonary valve-in-valve implantation: A successful treatment concept for early device failure. *Eur Heart J* 2008;29:810–5.
4. Momenah TS, El Oakley R, Al Najashi K et al. Extended application of percutaneous pulmonary valve implantation. *J Am Coll Cardiol* 2009;53:1859–63.
5. Asoh K, Walsh M, Hickey E et al. Percutaneous pulmonary valve implantation within bioprosthetic valves. *Eur Heart J* 2010;31:1404–9.
6. Boudjemline Y, Brugada G, Van-Aerschot I et al. Outcomes and safety of transcatheter pulmonary valve replacement in patients with large patched right ventricular outflow tracts. *Arch Cardiovasc Dis* 2012;105:404–13.
7. Nordmeyer J, Khambadkone S, Coats L et al. Risk stratification, systematic classification, and anticipatory management strategies for stent fracture after percutaneous pulmonary valve implantation. *Circulation* 2007;115:1392
8. McElhinney DB, Cheatham JP, Jones TK et al. Stent fracture, valve dysfunction, and right ventricular outflow tract reintervention after transcatheter pulmonary valve implantation: Patient-related and procedural risk factors in the US Melody Valve Trial. *Circ Cardiovasc Interv* 2011;4:602–14.
9. Eicken A, Ewert P, Hager A et al. Percutaneous pulmonary valve implantation: Two-centre experience with more than 100 patients. *Eur Heart J* 2011;32:1260–5.
10. Nordmeyer J, Lurz P, Khambadkone et al. Pre-stenting with a bare metal stent before percutaneous pulmonary valve implantation: Acute and 1-year outcomes. *Heart* 2011;97:118–23.
11. McElhinney DB, Hellenbrand WE et al. Short- and medium-term outcomes after transcatheter pulmonary valve placement in the expanded multicenter US melody valve trial. *Circulation* 2010;122:507–16.
12. Nordmeyer J, Tsang V, Gaudin R et al. Quantitative assessment of homograft function 1 year after insertion into the pulmonary position: Impact of *in situ* homograft geometry on valve competence. *Eur Heart J* 2009;30:2147–54.
13. Schievano S, Coats L, Migliavacca F et al. Variations in right ventricular outflow tract morphology following repair of congenital heart disease: Implications for percutaneous pulmonary valve implantation. *J Cardiovasc Magn Reson* 2007;9:687–95.
14. Davlouros PA, Kilner PJ, Hornung TS et al. Right ventricular function in adults with repaired tetralogy of Fallot assessed with cardiovascular magnetic resonance imaging: Detrimental role of right ventricular outflow aneurysms or akinesia and adverse right-to-left ventricular interaction. *J Am Coll Cardiol* 2002;40:2044–52.
15. Uebing A, Gibson DG, Babu-Narayan SV et al. Right ventricular mechanics and QRS duration in patients with repaired tetralogy of Fallot: Implications of infundibular disease. *Circulation* 2007;116:1532–9.
16. Geva T, Gauvreau K, Powell AJ et al. Randomized trial of pulmonary valve replacement with and without right ventricular remodeling surgery. *Circulation* 2010;122(11 Suppl):S201–8.

17. Boudjemline Y, Legendre A, Ladouceur M et al. Branch pulmonary artery jailing with a bare metal stent to anchor a transcatheter pulmonary valve in patients with patched large right ventricular outflow tract. *Circ Cardiovasc Interv* 2012;5:e22–5.

18. Kenny D, Hijazi ZM, Kar S et al. Percutaneous implantation of the Edwards SAPIEN transcatheter heart valve for conduit failure in the pulmonary position: Early phase 1 results from an international multicenter clinical trial. *J Am Coll Cardiol* 2011;58:594–8.

19. Guccione P, Milanesi O, Hijazi ZM, Pongiglione G. Transcatheter pulmonary valve implantation in native pulmonary outflow tract using the Edwards SAPIEN™ transcatheter heart valve. *Eur J Cardiothorac Surg* 2012;41:1192–4.

20. Lurz P, Nordmeyer J, Coats L, Taylor AM, Bonhoeffer P, Schulze-Neick I. Immediate clinical and haemodynamic benefits of restoration of pulmonary valvar competence in patients with pulmonary hypertension. *Heart* 2009;95:646–50.

21. Law KB, Phillips KR, Butany J. Pulmonary valve-in-valve implants: How long do they prolong reintervention and what causes them to fail? *Cardiovasc Pathol* 2012;21:519–21.

22. Mollet A, Basquin A, Stos B, Boudjemline Y. Off-pump replacement of the pulmonary valve in large right ventricular: A transcatheter approach using an intravascular infundibulum reducer. *Pediatr Res* 2007;62:428–33.

23. Schievano S, Taylor AM, Capelli C et al. First-in-man implantation of a novel percutaneous valve: A new approach to medical device development. *EuroIntervention* 2010;5:745–50.

24. Biglino G, Capelli C, Binazzi A et al. Virtual and real bench testing of a new percutaneous valve device: A case study. *EuroIntervention* 2012;8:120–8.

25. Cao QL, Kenny D, Zhou D, Pan W, Guan L, Ge J, Hijazi ZM. Early clinical experience with a novel self-expanding percutaneous stent-valve in the native right ventricular outflow tract. *Catheter Cardiovasc Interv.* 2014.

26. Schreiber C, Bauernschmitt R, Augustin N et al. Implantation of a prosthesis mounted inside a self-expandable stent in the pulmonary valvar area without use of cardiopulmonary bypass. *Ann Thorac Surg* 2006;81:1–3.

27. Macchiarini P, Jungebluth P, Asnaghi MA et al. Clinical transplantation of a tissue-engineered airway. *Lancet* 2008;372:2023–30.

28. Schmidt D, Dijkman PE, Driessen-Mol A et al. Minimally-invasive implantation of living tissue engineered heart valves: A comprehensive approach from autologous vascular cells to stem cells. *J Am Coll Cardiol* 2010;56:510–20.

37

Mitral and tricuspid valve stenosis: Percutaneous mitral valvuloplasty

Igor F. Palacios and Guilherme V. Silva

Since its introduction in 1984 by Inoue et al.,[1] percutaneous mitral balloon commissurotomy (PMV) has been used successfully as an alternative to open or closed surgical mitral commissurotomy in the treatment of patients with symptomatic rheumatic mitral stenosis.[2-18] PMV produces good immediate hemodynamic outcome, low complication rate, and clinical improvement in the majority of patients with mitral stenosis.[2-18] PMV is safe and effective, and provides sustained clinical and hemodynamic improvement in patients with rheumatic mitral stenosis. The immediate and long-term results appear to be similar to those of surgical mitral commisssurotomy.[2-18] Today, PMV is the preferred form of therapy for relief of mitral stenosis for a selected group of patients with symptomatic mitral stenosis.

Technique of PMV

PMV should be performed in the fasting state under mild sedation. Antibiotics (dicloxacillin 500 mg p.o. q/6 h for 4 doses) are started before the procedure or cefalotin 1 gram *iv* at the time of the procedure is given. Patients allergic to penicillin should receive vancomycin 1 gram *iv* at the time of the procedure.

All patients carefully chosen as candidates for mitral balloon valvuloplasty should undergo diagnostic right and left and transseptal left heart catheterization. Following transseptal left heart catheterization, systemic anticoagulation is achieved by the intravenous administration of 100 units/kg of heparin. In patients older than 40 years, coronary arteriography should also be performed.

Hemodynamic measurements, cardiac output, and cine left ventriculography are performed before and after PMV. Cardiac output is measured by thermodilution and Fick method techniques. Mitral valve calcification and angiographic severity of mitral regurgitation (Seller's classification) are graded qualitatively from 0 grade to 4 grades as previously described.[3] An oxygen diagnostic run is performed before and after PMV to determine the presence of left-to-right shunt after PMV.

There is not a unique technique of percutaneous mitral balloon valvuloplasty. Most of the techniques of PMV require transseptal left heart catheterization and use of the antegrade approach. Antegrade PMV can be accomplished using single-[2,3,6] or double-balloon techniques.[3-5,7] In the latter approach, the two balloons could be placed through a single femoral vein and single transseptal punctures[3,5,7] (using the Multi-Track balloon system) or through two femoral veins and two separate atrial septal punctures.[4] In the retrograde technique of PMV, the balloons dilating the catheters are advanced percutaneously through the right and left femoral arteries over guide wires that have been snared from the descending aorta.[19] These guide wires have been advanced transseptally from the right femoral vein into the left atrium, the left ventricle, and the ascending aorta. A retrograde nontransseptal technique of PMV has also been described.[20,21]

Antegrade double-balloon technique

In performing PMV using the antegrade double-balloon technique (Figure 37.1), a 7 F flow-directed balloon catheter is advanced through the transseptal sheath across the mitral valve into the left ventricle.[22-32] The catheter is then advanced through the aortic valve into the ascending aorta and then the descending aorta. A 0.035- or 0.038-inch, 260-cm-long Teflon-coated exchange wire is then passed through the catheter. The sheath and the catheter are removed, leaving the wire behind. A 5-mm balloon-dilating catheter is used to dilate the atrial septum.[34,36] A second exchange guide wire is passed parallel to the first guide wire through the same femoral vein and atrial septum punctures using a double-lumen catheter. The double-lumen catheter is then removed, leaving the two guide wires across the mitral valve in the ascending and descending aorta. During these maneuvers, care should be taken to maintain large and smooth loops of the guide wires in the left ventricular cavity to allow appropriate placement

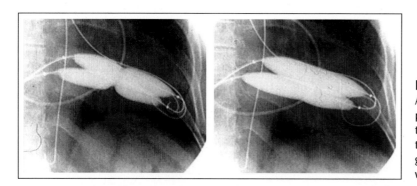

Figure 37.1 Double-balloon technique of PMV. An indentation on the balloons is seen in the right panel. Full inflation of the balloons is achieved in the left panel. One of the guide wires is placed in the ascending and descending aorta and a second guide wire is placed in the left ventricular cavity with its curlew tip at the apex.

of the dilating balloons. If a second guide wire cannot be placed into the ascending and descending aorta, a 0.038-inch Amplatz-type transfer guide wire with a preformed curlicue at its tip can be placed at the left ventricular apex. In patients with aortic valve prosthesis, both guide wires with preformed curlew tips should be placed at the left ventricular apex. When one or both guide wires are placed in the left ventricular apex, the balloons should be inflated sequentially. Care should be taken to avoid forward movement of the balloons and guide wires to prevent left ventricular perforation. Two balloon-dilating catheters, chosen according to the patient's body surface area, are then advanced over each one of the guide wires and positioned across the mitral valve parallel to the longitudinal axis of the left ventricle. The balloon valvotomy catheters are then inflated by hand until the indentation produced by the stenotic mitral valve is no longer seen. Generally one, but occasionally two or three inflations are performed. After complete deflation, the balloons are removed sequentially. The double-balloon technique of PMV is effective but demanding, and carries the risk of left ventricular perforation

by the guide wires or the tip of the balloons. The Multi-Track system introduced by Bonhoeffer shares the advantages of the traditional double-balloon technique. It is safer, reducing the risk of accidental balloon displacement. The procedure is easier to perform as it only requires the presence of a single guide wire and therefore procedure time is reduced. The system is versatile and can be used in other indications. With this technique two separate balloons are introduced over a single guide wire. The first catheter, with only a distal guide wire lumen, is introduced into the vein and then advanced into the mitral orifice. Subsequently, a rapid exchange balloon catheter running on the same guide wire is inserted and lined up with the first catheter so the two are positioned side by side. Both balloons are then inflated simultaneously.

Inoue Technique of PMV

PMV is more frequently performed using the Inoue technique (Figure 37.2).[1,15–17] The Inoue balloon is a 12 F shaft, coaxial, double-lumen catheter. The balloon is made of

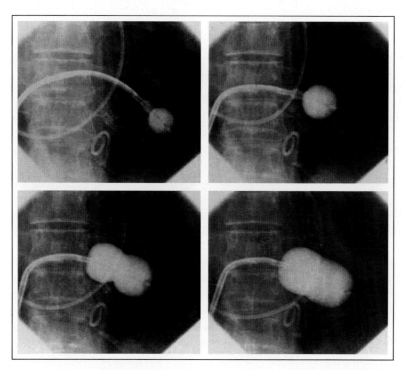

Figure 37.2 Mitral balloon valvuloplasty with the Inoue balloon. Sequential balloon inflation from the left ventricle and across the mitral valve.

a double layer of rubber tubing with a layer of synthetic micromesh in between.

Following transseptal catheterization, a stainless-steel guide wire is advanced through the transseptal catheter and placed with its tip coiled into the left atrium and the transseptal catheter removed. A 14 F dilator is advanced over the guide wire and is used to dilate the femoral vein and the atrial septum. A balloon catheter chosen according to the patient's height is advanced over the guide wire into the left atrium. The distal part of the balloon is inflated and advanced into the left ventricle with the help of the spring wire stylet, which has been inserted through the inner lumen of the catheter. Once the catheter is in the left ventricle, the partially inflated balloon is moved back and forth inside the left ventricle to assure that it is free of the chordae tendinae. The catheter is then gently pulled against the mitral plane until resistance is felt. The balloon is then rapidly inflated to its full capacity and then deflated quickly. During inflation of the balloon, an indentation should be seen in its midportion. The catheter is withdrawn into the left atrium and the mitral gradient and cardiac output measured. If further dilations are required, the stylet is introduced again and the sequence of steps described above repeated at a larger balloon volume. After each dilation, its effect should be assessed by pressure measurement, auscultation, and 2D echocardiography. If mitral regurgitation occurs, further dilation of the valve should not be performed.

Equally important during the Inoue PMV is the careful evaluation of the shape of the Inoue balloon in each of the balloon inflations. We should keep in mind that the Inoue balloon is associated with only 25% of bicommissural splitting. Therefore, if one of the balloon borders becomes flat during a given inflation, it is likely that the balloon has successfully split one of the commissures and serious consideration should be given to stop the procedure then, as further increases in balloon volume more likely would result in damage of the mitral leaflets and the appearance of severe postballoon mitral regurgitation (Figure 37.3). Our criteria for stopping the procedure are complete opening of at least one of the commissures with a valve area >1 cm^2/m^2 body surface area or >1.5 cm^2, or the appearance of regurgitation or its increase by 25%.

Percutaneous mitral valvotomy with a metal dilator

Alan Cribier described an alternative technique of PMV using a newly designed metallic valvulotome (Figure 37.4). The device consists of a detachable metallic cylinder with two articulated bars screwed onto the distal end of a disposable catheter whose proximal end is connected to activating pliers. Squeezing the pliers opens the bars up to a maximum of 40 mm. The results with this device are at least comparable to those of the other balloon techniques of PMV. However, multiple uses after sterilization should markedly decrease procedural costs.

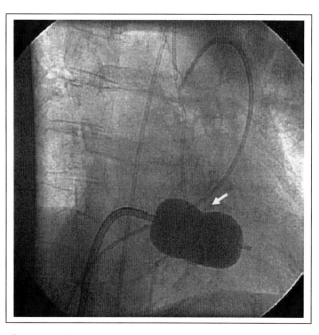

Figure 37.3   The Inoue balloon technique of PMV. Once the catheter is in the left ventricle, the partially inflated balloon is moved back and forth inside the left ventricle to assure that it is free of the chordae tendinae. The catheter is then gently pulled against the mitral plane until resistance is felt. The balloon is then rapidly inflated to its full capacity and then deflated quickly.

Double-balloon versus Inoue balloon techniques of PMV

Today, the Inoue approach of PMV is the technique more widely used. There was controversy as to whether the double-balloon or the Inoue technique provided superior immediate and long-term results. We compared the immediate procedural and the long-term clinical outcomes after PMV using the double-balloon technique ($n = 659$) and the Inoue technique ($n = 233$).[66] There were no statistically significant differences in baseline clinical and morphological characteristics between the double-balloon and Inoue patients. Although the post-PMV mitral valve area was larger with the double-balloon technique (1.94 ± 0.72 vs. 1.81 ± 0.58; $p = 0.01$), success rate (71.3% vs 69.1%; $p = NS$), incidence of $\geq 3+$ mitral regurgitation (9% vs 9%), in-hospital complications, and long-term and event-free survival were similar with both techniques. In conclusion, both the Inoue and the double-balloon techniques are equally effective techniques for PMV, and the procedure of choice should be performed based on the interventionist experience in the technique.

Patient selection

Selection of patients for PMV should be based on symptoms, physical examination, and two-dimensional and Doppler echocardiographic findings.[57] PMV is usually performed electively. However, emergency PMV can be

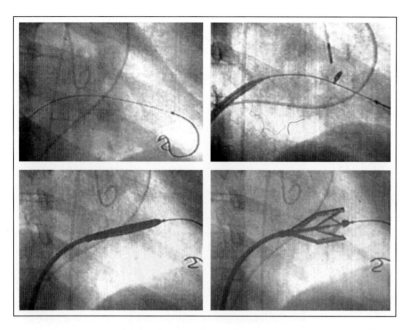

Figure 37.4 The Cribier metallic dilator technique. The device is advanced over a guide wire with its tip curlew in the ventricular apex. Squeezing the pliers opens the bars up to a maximum of 40 mm.

performed as a life-saving procedure in patients with mitral stenosis and severe pulmonary edema refractory to medical therapy and/or cardiogenic shock. Patients considered for PMV should be symptomatic (NYHA ≥ II) and should have no recent thromboembolic events, less than 2 grades of mitral regurgitation by contrast ventriculography using the Seller's classification,[35] and no evidence of left atrial thrombus on 2D and transesophageal echocardiography (Table 37.1). Transthoracic and transesophageal echocardiography should be performed routinely before PMV.

Patients in atrial fibrillation and patients with previous embolic episodes should be anticoagulated with warfarin with a therapeutic International Normalized Ratio (INR) for at least 3 months before PMV. Patients with left atrium thrombus on 2D echocardiography should be excluded. However, PMV could be performed in these patients if left atrium thrombus has resolved after warfarin therapy.

The echocardiographic examination of the mitral valve can accurately characterize the severity and extent of the pathological process in patients with rheumatic mitral

Table 37.1 Recommendations for percutaneous mitral valvuloplasty[a]

Current indication	Class	Level of evidence
Symptomatic patients (NYHA functional class II, III, or IV), moderate or severe mitral stenosis (area <1.5 cm²), and valve morphology favorable for percutaneous balloon valvuloplasty in the absence of left atrial thrombus or moderate to severe mitral regurgitation.	I	Grade A
Asymptomatic patients with moderate or severe mitral stenosis (area <1.5 cm²) and valve morphology favorable for percutaneous balloon valvuloplasty who have pulmonary hypertension (pulmonary artery systolic pressure >50 mmHg at rest or 60 mmHg with exercise) in the absence of left atrial thrombus or moderate to severe mitral regurgitation.	IIa	Grade C
Patients with NYHA functional class III–IV, moderate or severe mitral stenosis (area <1.5 cm²), and a nonpliable calcified valve who are at a high risk for surgery in the absence of left atrial thrombus or moderate to severe mitral regurgitation.	IIa	Grade B
Asymptomatic patients, moderate or severe mitral stenosis (area <1.5 cm²), and valve morphology favorable for percutaneous balloon valvuloplasty who have new onset of atrial fibrillation in the absence of left atrial thrombus or moderate to severe mitral regurgitation.	IIb	Grade B
Patients in NYHA functional class III–IV, moderate or severe mitral stenosis (area <1.5 cm²), and a nonpliable calcified valve who are low-risk candidates for surgery.	IIb	Grade C
Patients with mild mitral stenosis.	III	Grade C

[a] Adapted from current American College of Cardiology/American Heart Association and European guidelines for the management of patients with valvular heart disease.

Table 37.2 Echocardiographic score

Grade	Leaflet mobility	Valvular thickening	Valvular calcification	Subvalvular thickening
0	Normal	Normal	Normal	Normal
1	Highly mobile valve with restriction of only the leaflet tips	Leaflet near normal (4–5 mm)	A single area of increased echo brightness	Minimal thickening of chordal structures just below the valve
2	Middle portion and base of leaflets have reduced mobility	Midleaflet thickening, marked thickening of the margins	Scattered areas of brightness confined to leaflet margins	Thickening of chordae extending up to one-third of chordal length
3	Valve leaflets move forward in diastole mainly at the base	Thickening extending through the entire leaflets (5–8 mm)	Brightness extending into the midportion of leaflets	Thickening extending to the distal third of the chordae
4	No or minimal forward movement of the leaflets in diastole	Marked thickening of all leaflet tissue (>8–10 mm)	Extensive brightness throughout most of the leaflet tissue	Extensive thickening and shortening of all chordae extending down to the papillary muscles

Note: Echocardiographic grading of the severity and extent of the anatomic abnormalities in patients with mitral stenosis. The total score is the sum of each of these echocardiographic features (maximum 16).

stenosis. The most utilized score to identify the anatomic abnormalities of the stenotic mitral valve is that described by Wilkins et al. (Table 37.2, Figure 37.5).[49] This echocardiographic score is an important predictor of the immediate and long-term outcome of PMV. In this morphologic score, each of the following—leaflet rigidity, leaflet thickening, valvular calcification, and subvalvular disease—are scored from 0 to 4. A higher score would represent a heavily calcified, thickened, and immobile valve with extensive thickening and calcification of the subvalvular apparatus. The increase in mitral valve area with PMV is inversely related to the echocardiographic score. The best outcomes with PMV occur in those patients with echocardiographic scores ≤8. The increase in mitral valve area is significantly greater in patients with echocardiographic scores ≤8 than in those with echocardiographic score >8. Among the four components of the echocardiographic score, valve leaflet

thickening and subvalvular disease correlate the best with the increase in mitral valve area produced by PMV.[33] Therefore, suboptimal results with PMV are more likely to occur in patients with valves that are more rigid and more thickened, and with more subvalvular fibrosis and calcification (Figures 37.6 and 37.7). The Wilkins score not only predicts success but also predicts long-term prognosis in patients undergoing percutaneous mitral valvuloplasty. The Wilkins score, however, cannot accurately predict the development of severe mitral regurgitation as a complication of PMV.

Padial and colleagues, in a seminal study, developed an echocardiographic score that anatomically predicts the development of severe mitral regurgitation post-PMV.[67] Studies of surgically excised mitral valves of patients who developed severe mitral regurgitation after percutaneous mitral valvulotomy had consistently shown three anatomic

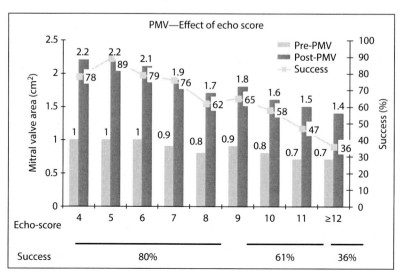

Figure 37.5 (See color insert.) Relationship between the echo score, the pre- and post-PMV MVA, and immediate success after PMV.

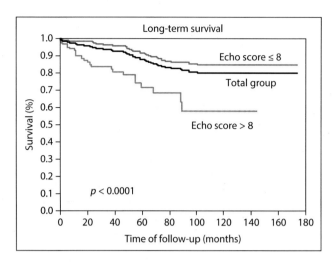

Figure 37.6   Fifteen-year survival for all patients, and for patients with echocardiographic score ≤8 and >8, undergoing percutaneous mitral balloon valvuloplasty at the Massachusetts General Hospital.

characteristics: (1) heterogeneously thickened mitral valves with thick areas coexisting with thin or almost normal zones; (2) severe and extensive fusion, thickening, and foreshortening of the mitral subvalvular apparatus; and (3) calcium in one or both commissures.[68] Based on those surgical studies, Padial and colleagues then developed a score that took into account the valvular thickening of the anterior and posterior leaflets separately, commissural calcification, and subvalvular disease. The Padial score was studied in 566 consecutive patients with rheumatic mitral stenosis who underwent PMV at Massachusetts General Hospital. Interestingly, no differences were noted between the Wilkins scores of patients with and without severe mitral regurgitation following percutaneous mitral valvulotomy.

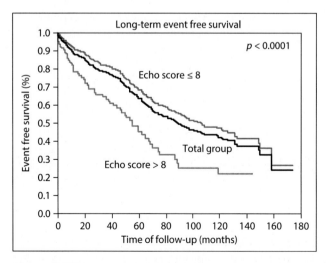

Figure 37.7   Fifteen-year event-free survival for all patients, and for patients with echocardiographic score ≤8 and >8, undergoing percutaneous mitral balloon valvuloplasty at the Massachusetts General Hospital.

When using a cutoff of a Padial score of greater or equal to 10, the sensitivity of the echocardiographic score for detecting patients with severe mitral regurgitation was $90\% \pm 5\%$, its specificity was $97\% \pm 3\%$, and its accuracy was $94\% \pm 3\%$. The positive predictive value was $97\% \pm 3\%$, and the negative predictive value was $91\% \pm 5\%$.

When considering patients for PMV, the clinician clearly needs to take into account the Wilkins and the Padial echocardiographic scores. Those scores, nonetheless, do not include patient characteristics that could influence the success and long-term prognosis of the procedure. A multifactorial score derived from clinical, anatomic/echocardiographic, and hemodynamic variables would predict procedural success and clinical outcome.[56] Demographic data, echocardiographic parameters (including echocardiographic score, Figure 37.8), and procedure-related variables recorded from 1085 consecutive patients who underwent PMV at the Massachusetts General Hospital (MGH) and their long-term clinical follow-up (death, mitral valve replacement, redo PMV) were used to derive this clinical score. Multivariate regression analysis of the first 800 procedures was performed to identify independent predictors of procedural success. Significant variables were formulated into a risk score and validated prospectively. Six independent predictors of PMV success were identified: age less than 55 years, New York Heart Association classes I and II, pre-PMV mitral area of 1 cm² or greater, pre-PMV mitral regurgitation grade less than 2, echocardiographic score of 8 or less, and male sex.[56] A score was constructed from the arithmetic sum of variables present per patient. Procedural success rates increased incrementally with increasing score (0% for 0/6, 39.7% for 1/6, 54.4% for 2/6, 77.3% for 3/6, 85.7% for 4/6, 95% for 5/6, and 100% for 6/6; $p < 0.001$). In a validation cohort ($n = 285$ consecutive procedures), the multifactorial score remained a significant predictor of PMV success ($p < 0.001$). Comparison between the new

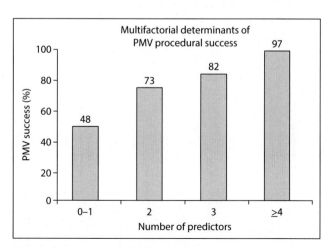

Figure 37.8   A multifactorial score derived from clinical, anatomic/echocardiographic, and hemodynamic variables would predict procedural success and clinical outcome.

score and the echocardiographic score confirmed that the new index was more sensitive and specific ($p < 0.001$). This new score also predicts long-term outcomes ($p < 0.001$). Clinical, anatomic, and hemodynamic variables predict PMV success and clinical outcome and may be formulated in a scoring system that would help to identify the best candidates for PMV.

Mechanism of PMV

The mechanism of successful PMV is splitting of the fused commissures toward the mitral annulus, resulting in commissural widening. This mechanism has been demonstrated by pathological, surgical, and echocardiographic studies.[58–62] In addition, in patients with calcific mitral stenosis, the balloons could increase mitral valve flexibility by the fracture of the calcified deposits in the mitral valve leaflets.[62] Although rare, undesirable complications such as leaflet tears, left ventricular perforation, tear of the atrial septum, and rupture of chordae, mitral annulus, and papillary muscle could also occur.

Complications

Table 37.3 shows the complications reported by several investigators after PMV.[63,64] Mortality and morbidity with PMV are low and similar to surgical commissurotomy. Overall, there is a less than 1% procedural mortality. Severe mitral regurgitation (4 grades by angiography) has been reported in 1–5.2% of the patients, with some of these patients required in hospital mitral valve replacement. Thromboembolic episodes and stroke have been reported in 0–3.1% and pericardial tamponade in 0.2–4.6% of cases in these series. Pericardial tamponade can occur from transseptal catheterization and more rarely from ventricular

perforation. PMV is associated with a 3–16% incidence of left-to-right shunt documented by oxymetry immediately after the procedure. However, the pulmonary to systemic flow ratio is ≥2:1 in only a minimum number of patients.

We have demonstrated that severe mitral regurgitation (4 grades by angiography) occurs in about 3% of patients undergoing PMV. An undesirable increase in mitral regurgitation (≥2 grades by angiography) occurred in 10.1% of patients. This undesirable increase in mitral regurgitation is well tolerated in most patients. Furthermore, more than half of them have less mitral regurgitation at follow-up cardiac catheterization. We have demonstrated that the ratio of the effective balloon-dilating area to body surface area (EBDA/BSA) is a predictor of increased mitral regurgitation after PMV.[65,66–69] The EBDA is calculated using standard geometric formulas. The incidence of mitral regurgitation is lower if balloon sizes are chosen so that EBDA/BSA is ≤4.0 cm²/m². The single-balloon technique results in a lower incidence of mitral regurgitation but provides less relief of mitral stenosis than the double-balloon technique. Thus, there is an optimal EBDA between 3.1 and 4.0 cm²/m², which achieves a maximal mitral valve area with a minimal increase in mitral regurgitation. An echocardiographic score for the mitral valve that can predict the development of severe mitral regurgitation following PMV has also been described.[8]

This score takes into account the distribution (even or uneven) of leaflet thickening and calcification, the degree and symmetry of commissural disease, and the severity of subvalvular disease (Table 37.4).

Left-to-right shunt through the created atrial communication determined by oxymetry occurred in 3–16% of the patients undergoing PMV. The size of the defect is small as reflected in the pulmonary to systemic flow ratio of <2:1 in the majority of patients. Older age, fluoroscopic evidence of mitral valve calcification, higher echocardiographic

Table 37.3   Complications following percutaneous mitral valvuloplasty

Author	Number of patients	Mortality (%)	Tamponade (%)	Severe MR (%)	Embolism (%)
Palacios et al.	879	0.6	1.0	3.4	1.8
Vahanian et al.	1514	0.4	0.3	3.4	0.3
Hernández et al.	561	0.4	0.6	4.5	
Stefanadis et al.	438	0.2	0.0	3.4	0.0
Chen et al.	4832	0.1	0.8	1.4	0.5
NHLBI	738	3.0	4.0	3.0	3.0
Inoue et al.	527	0.0	1.6	1.9	0.6
Inoue Registry	1251	0.6	1.4	3.8	0.9
Ben Farhat et al.	463	0.4	0.7	4.6	2.0
Arora et al.	600	1.0	1.3	1.0	0.5
Cribier et al.	153	0.0	0.7	1.4	0.7

MR, mitral regurgitation.

Table 37.4 Echocardiographic score for severe mitral regurgitation after percutaneous mitral valvulotomy

Grade	Valvular thickening of the anterior leaflet	Valvular thickening of the posterior leaflet	Commissural calcification	Subvalvular disease
0	Normal	Normal	Normal	Normal
1	Leaflet near normal (4–5 ram) or with only a thick segment	Leaflet near normal (4–5 ram) or with only a thick segment	Fibrosis and/or calcium in only one commissure	Minimal thickening of chordal structures just below the valve
2	Leaflet fibrotic and/or calcified evenly; no thin areas	Leaflet fibrotic and/or calcified evenly; no thin areas	Both commissures mildly affected	Thickening of chordae extending up to one-third of chordal length
3	Leaflet fibrotic and/or calcified with uneven distribution; thinner segments are mildly thickened (5–8 mm)	Leaflet fibrotic and/or calcified with uneven distribution; thinner segments are mildly thickened (5–8 mm)	Calcium in both commissures, one markedly affected	Thickening to the distal third of the chordae
4	Leaflet fibrotic and/or calcified with uneven distribution; thinner segments are near normal (4–5 mm)	Leaflet fibrotic and/or calcified with uneven distribution; thinner segments are near normal (4–5 mm)	Calcium in both commissures, both markedly affected	Extensive thickening and shortening of all chordae extending down to the papillary muscle

Source: Modified from Luis RP, *JACC* 1996;27(5):1225–31.

Note: The total score is the sum of each of these echocardiographic features (maximum 16).

score, pre-PMV lower cardiac output, and higher pre-PMV NYHA functional class are the factors that predispose patients to develop left-to-right shunt post-PMV.[67] Clinical, echocardiographic, surgical, and hemodynamic follow-up of patients with post-PMV left-to-right shunt demonstrated that the defect closed in approximately 60%. Persistent left-to-right shunt at follow-up is small (QP/QS < 2:1) and clinically well tolerated. In the series from the Massachusetts General Hospital, there is one patient in whom the atrial shunt remained hemodynamically significant at follow-up. This patient underwent percutaneous transcatheter closure of her iatrogenic residual atrial defect with a clamshell device. Desideri et al. reported atrial shunting determined by color flow transthoracic echocardiography in 61% of 57 patients immediately after PMV. The shunt persisted in 30% of patients at 19 ± 6 (range 9–33) months follow-up.[70] They identified the magnitude of the post-PMV atrial shunt (QP/QS > 1.5:1), use of Bifoil balloon (2 balloons on 1 shaft), and smaller post-PMV mitral valve area as independent predictors of the persistence of atrial shunt at long-term follow-up.

Clinical follow-up

Long-term follow-up studies after PMV are encouraging. Following PMV, the majority of patients have marked clinical improvement and become NYHA class I or II. The symptomatic, echocardiographic, and hemodynamic improvement produced by PMV persists in intermediate and long-term follow-up. The best long-term results are seen in patients with echocardiographic scores ≤8. When PMV produces a good immediate outcome in this group of patients, restenosis is unlikely to occur at follow-up. Although PMV can result in a good outcome in patients with echocardiographic scores >8, hemodynamic and echocardiographic restenosis is frequently demonstrated at follow-up despite ongoing clinical improvement. Table 37.5 shows long-term follow-up results of patients undergoing PMV at different institutes. We reported an estimated 12-year survival rate of 74% in a cohort of 879 patients undergoing PMV at the Massachusetts General Hospital (Figure 37.5). Death at follow-up was directly

Table 37.5 Clinical long-term follow-up after percutaneous mitral valvuloplasty

Author	Number of patients	Age	Follow-up (years)	Survival (%)	Event-free survival (%)
Palacios et al.	879	55	12	74	33
Iung et al.	1024	49	10	85	56
Hernández et al.	561	53	7	95	69
Orrange et al.	132	44	7	83	65
Ben Farhat et al.	30	29	7	100	90
Stefanadis et al.	441	44	9	98	75

related to age, post-PMV pulmonary artery pressure, and pre-PMV NYHA functional class IV. In the same group of patients, the 12-year event-free survival (alive and free of mitral valve replacement or repair and redo PMV) was 33% (Figure 37.6). Cox regression analysis identified age (risk ratio (R.R.) 1.02; C.I. 1.01–1.03; $p < 0.0001$), pre-PMV NYHA functional class IV (R.R. 1.35; C.I. 1.00–1.81; $p = 0.05$), prior commissurotomy (R.R. 150; C.I. 1.16–1.92; $p = 0.002$), the echocardiographic score (R.R. 1.31; C.I. 1.02–1.67; $p = 0.003$), pre-PMV mitral regurgitation ≥2+ (R.R. 1.56; C.I. 1.09–2.22; $p = 0.02$), post-PMV mitral regurgitation ≥3+ (R.R. 3.54; C.I. 2.61–4.72; $p < 0.0001$), and post-PMV mean pulmonary artery pressure (R.R. 1.02; C.I. 1.01–1.03; $p < 0.0001$) as independent predictors of combined events at long-term follow-up.

Actuarial survival and event-free survival rates throughout the follow-up period were significantly better in patients with echocardiographic scores ≤8. Survival rates were 82% for patients with echocardiographic score ≤8 and 57% for patients with score >8 at a follow-up time of 12 years ($p < 0.0001$). Event-free survival (38% vs. 22%; $p < 0.0001$) at 12-year follow-up were also significantly higher for patients with echocardiographic score ≤8. Similar follow-up studies have been reported in other series with the double-balloon technique and with the Inoue technique of PMV.[69] Over 90% of young patients with pliable valves, in sinus rhythm, and with no evidence of calcium under fluoroscopy remain free of cardiovascular events at an approximate follow-up of 5 years.[71,72]

Functional deterioration at follow-up is late and related primarily to mitral restenosis.[14] The incidence of restenosis, as assessed by sequential echocardiography, is approximately 40% after 7 years.[14] Repeat PMV can be proposed if recurrent stenosis leads to symptoms. At the moment, we have only a small number of series available on redo PMV. They show encouraging results in selected patients with favorable characteristics when restenosis occurs several years after an initially successful procedure and if the predominant mechanism of restenosis is commissural refusion.[10]

Percutaneous tricuspid balloon valvuloplasty

Percutaneous balloon valvuloplasty has revolutionized the treatment of mitral stenosis as described above. In rheumatic heart disease, mitral stenosis sometimes coexists with tricuspid stenosis. As such, tricuspid stenosis is most commonly of rheumatic etiology; though other rare causes of flow obstruction at the level of the tricuspid valve include congenital atresia or stenosis of the valve, right atrial, or metastatic tumors. Carcinoid syndrome can also cause tricuspid stenosis but tricuspid regurgitation is more common. Bacterial endocarditis, particularly in association with a permanent pacemaker lead or a prosthetic valve, can also present as tricuspid stenosis.

In cases of rheumatic heart disease with tricuspid valve stenosis, the majority of cases present with tricuspid regurgitation or a combination of regurgitation and stenosis and associated mitral and/or aortic valve disease. Echocardiographic features of tricuspid stenosis include limited mobility of the leaflets, reduced separation of the leaflet tips, a reduction in the diameter of the tricuspid annulus, and diastolic doming of the valve. Although leaflet thickening is seen, the degree of thickening and calcification is generally less pronounced than in rheumatic mitral stenosis. Doppler echocardiography reveals high-velocity turbulent diastolic flow across the stenotic orifice and prolonged pressure half-time. A tricuspid valve area less than 1.0 cm² indicates severe tricuspid stenosis. It is important to assess the presence and severity of tricuspid regurgitation, since this can influence the decision to proceed with balloon valvuloplasty.

For tricuspid stenosis with signs and symptoms of systemic venous hypertension and congestion, one should consider an invasive treatment such as surgical commissurotomy or percutaneous valvuloplasty. Percutaneous tricuspid valvuloplasty is performed with a technique similar to that utilized in mitral valvuloplasty. Both the double-balloon technique and the Inoue technique have been used with good results (Figure 37.9). There is far less experience with tricuspid valvuloplasty than with mitral valvuloplasty.

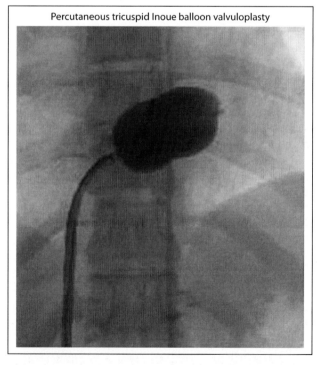
Percutaneous tricuspid Inoue balloon valvuloplasty

Figure 37.9 Successful tricuspid balloon valvuloplasty using the Inoue balloon catheter. With valvuloplasty, the tricuspid gradient decreased from 8 to 2 mmHg and the mean right atrium pressure decreased from 11 to 4 mmHg. (From Sharief S et al. *J Invas Cardiol* 2005;17.)

Transvalvular pressure gradients as low as 3 mmHg and valve areas less than 1.5 cm² can indicate serious, but treatable, stenosis. Valve areas generally increase from less than 1 to almost 2 cm². While some stenosis persists, this change in area is sufficient to produce a significant reduction in the transvalvular pressure gradient and a decrease in right atrial pressure.

Tricuspid regurgitation that is greater than mild is generally thought to be a contraindication to valvuloplasty, but a few patients with moderate regurgitation have been successfully treated with this technique. Tumor masses, vegetations, and thrombi are contraindications to valvuloplasty.

In summary, percutaneous balloon tricuspid valvuloplasty for tricuspid stenosis seems to be effective and associated with a low morbidity. Thus, if symptoms of systemic venous hypertension and congestion are not adequately controlled with diuretics and angiotensin-converting enzymes (ACE) inhibitors or angiotensin receptor antagonists, balloon valvuloplasty of the stenotic tricuspid valve should be considered. Otherwise, surgical correction of the stenotic lesion should be limited to those patients whose valve is not treatable with balloon techniques.

Conclusions

PMV should be the procedure of choice for the treatment of patients with rheumatic mitral stenosis who are, from the clinical and morphological points of view, optimal candidates for PMV. Patients with echocardiographic scores ≤8 have the best results, particularly if they are young, are in sinus rhythm, and have no pulmonary hypertension, and there is no evidence of calcification of the mitral valve under fluoroscopy. The immediate and long-term results of PMV in this group of patients are similar to those reported after surgical mitral commissurotomy. Patients with echocardiographic scores >8 have only a 50% chance to obtain a successful hemodynamic result with PMV, and long-term follow-up results are less good than those from patients with echocardiographic scores ≤8. In patients with echocardiographic scores ≥12, it is unlikely that PMV could produce good immediate or long-term results. They preferably should undergo open-heart surgery. PMV could be performed in these patients if they are non/high-risk surgical candidates. Finally, much remains to be done in refining indications for patients with few or no symptoms and those with unfavorable anatomy. However, surgical therapy for mitral stenosis should actually be reserved for patients who have ≥2 grades of Seller's mitral regurgitation by angiography, which can be better treated by mitral valve repair and for those patients with severe mitral valve thickening and calcification or with significant subvalvular scarring to warrant valve replacement.

References

1. Inoue K, Owaki T, Nakamura T, Kitamura F, Miyamoto N. Clinical application of transvenous mitral commissurotomy by a new balloon catheter. *J Thorac Cardiovasc Surg* 1984;87:394–402.
2. Lock JE, Kalilullah M, Shrivastava S, Bahl V, Keane JF. Percutaneous catheter commissurotomy in rheumatic mitral stenosis. *N Engl J Med* 1985;313:1515–8.
3. Palacios I, Block PC, Brandi S et al. Percutaneous balloon valvotomy for patients with severe mitral stenosis. *Circulation* 1987;75:778–84.
4. Al Zaibag M, Ribeiro PA, Al Kassab SA, Al Fagig MR. Percutaneous double balloon mitral valvotomy for rheumatic mitral stenosis. *Lancet* 1986;1:757–61.
5. Vahanian A, Michel PL, Cormier B et al. Ascar J: Results of percutaneous mitral commissurotomy in 200 patients. *Am J Cardiol* 1989;63:847–52.
6. Mc Kay RG, Lock JE, Safian RD et al. Grossman W. Balloon dilatation of mitral stenosis in adults patients: Postmortem and percutaneous mitral valvuloplasty studies. *J Am Coll Cardiol* 1987;9:723–31.
7. Mc Kay CR, Kawanishi DT, Rahimtoola SH. Catheter balloon valvuloplasty of the mitral valve in adults using a double balloon technique. Early hemodynamic results. *JAMA* 1987;257:1753–61.
8. Abascal VM, O'Shea JP, Wilkins GT et al. Prediction of successful outcome in 130 patients undergoing percutaneous balloon mitral valvotomy. *Circulation* 1990;82:448–56.
9. Herrman HC, Wilkins GT, Abascal VM, Weyman AE, Block PC, Palacios IF. Percutaneous balloon mitral valvotomy for patients with mitral stenosis: Analysis of factors influencing early results. *J Thorac Cardiovasc Surg* 1988;96:33–8.
10. Rediker DE, Block PC, Abascal VM, Palacios IF. Mitral balloon valvuloplasty for mitral restenosis after surgical commissurotomy. *J Am Coll Cardiol* 1988;2:252–56.
11. Palacios IF, Block PC, Wilkins GT, Weyman AE. Follow-up of patients undergoing percutaneous mitral balloon valvotomy: Analysis of factors determining restenosis. *Circulation* 1989;79:573–79.
12. Abascal VM, Wilkins GT, Choong CY, Palacios IF, Block PC, Weyman AE. Echocardiographic evaluation of mitral valve structure and function in patients followed for at least 6 months after percutaneous balloon mitral valvuloplasty. *J Am Coll Cardiol* 1988;12:606–15.
13. Block PC, Palacios IF, Block EH, Tuzcu EM, Griffin B. Late (two year) follow-up after percutaneous mitral balloon valvotomy. *Am J Cardiol* 1992;69:537–41.
14. Tuzcu EM, Block PC, Griffin BP, Newell JB, Palacios IF. Immediate and long term outcome of percutaneous mitral valvotomy in patients 65 years and older. *Circulation* 1992;85:963–71.
15. Nobuyoshi M, Hamasaki N, Kimura T et al. Indications, complications, and short term clinical outcome of percutaneous transvenous mitral commissurotomy. *Circulation* 1989;80:782–92.
16. Chen CR, Cheng TO, Chen JY, Zhou YL, Mei J, Ma TZ. Percutaneous mitral valvuloplasty with the Inoue balloon catheter. *Am J Cardiol* 1992;70:1455–58.
17. Hung JS, Chern MS, Wu JJ et al. Short and long term results of catheter balloon percutaneous transvenous mitral commissurotomy. *Am J Cardiol* 1991;67:854–62.
18. Cribier A, Eltchaninoff H, Koning R et al. Percutaneous mechanical mitral commissurotomy with a newly designed metalic valvulotome. *Circulation* 1999;99:793–99.
19. Ross J Jr, Braunwald E, Morrow AG. Transseptal left atrial puncture: New technique for the measurement of left atrial pressure in man. *Am J Cardiol* 1959;3:653–5.
20. Cope C. Technique for transseptal catheterization of the left atrium: Preliminary report. *J Thorac Surg* 1959;37:482–6.

21. Brockenbrough EC, Braunwald E, Ross J Jr. Transseptal left heart catheterization: A review of 450 studies and description of an improved technic. *Circulation* 1962;25:15–21.
22. Mullins CE. Transseptal left heart catheterization: Expeience with a new technique in 520 pediatric and adult patients. *Pediatr Cardiol* 1983;4:239–246.
23. Dunn M. Is Transseptal Catheterization Necessary? *J Am Coll Cardiol* 1985;5:1393–4.
24. Swan HJC, Ganz W, Forrester J, Marcus H, Diamond G, Chonette D. Catheterization of the heart in man with use of a flow directed balloon-tipped catheter. *N Engl J Med* 1970;283:447–51.
25. Schoonmaker FW, Vijay NK, Jantz RD. Left atrial and ventricular transseptal catheterization review: Losing skills? *Catheter Cardiovas Diag* 1987;13:233–38.
26. Lundqvist CB, Olsson SB, Varnauskas E. Transseptal left heart catheterization: A review of 278 studies. *Clin Cardiol* 1986;9:21–6.
27. Baim DS, Grossman W. Percutaneous approach, including transseptal catheterization and apical left ventricular puncture in cardiac catheterization. *Angiogr Interv* 1991.
28. Clugston R, Lau FYK, Ruiz C. Transseptal catheterization update 1992. *Catheter Cardiovasc Diag* 1992;26:266–74.
29. Roelke M, Smith AJC, Palacios IF. The technique and safety of transseptal left heart catheterization. The massachusetts general hospital experience with 1,279 procedures. *Catheter Cardiovasc Diag* 1994;32:332–9.
30. Schoenfield MH, Palacios IF, Jutter AM, Jacoby SS, Block PC. Underestimation of prosthetic mitral valve areas: Role of transseptal catheterization in avoiding unnecessary repeat mitral valve surgery. *J Am Coll Cardiol* 1985;5:1387–92.
31. O'Keefe JH, Vlietstra MB, Hanley PC, Seward JB. Revival of the transseptal aproach for catheterization of the left atrium and ventricle. *Mayo Clin Proc* 1985;60:790–5.
32. Carabello BA, Barry WH, Grossman W. Changes in arterial pressure during left heart pullback in patients with aortic stenosis: A sign of severe aortic stenosis. *Am J Cardiol* 1979;44:424–7.
33. Palacios IF. Techniques of balloon valvotomy for mitral stenosis. In: Robicsek F. Ed. *Cardiac Surgery: State of the Art Reviews.* Philadelphia, PA: Hanley R Belfus; 1991. pp. 229–38.
34. Block PC, Palacios I. Comparison of hemodynamic results of antegrade versus retrograde percutaneous balloon aortic valvuloplasty. *Am J Cardiol* 1987;60:659–62.
35. Rashkind WJ. Transcatheter treatment of congenital heart disease. *Circulation* 1983;67:711–6.
36. Saul JP, Hulse JE, Hulse E et al. Catheter ablation of accessory atrioventricular pathways in young patients: Use of long vascular sheaths, the transseptal approach, and a retrograde left posterior parallel approach. *J Am Coll Cardiol* 1993;21:571–83.
37. Lindeneg O, Hansen AT. Complication in transseptal left heart catheterization. *Acta Med Scand* 1966;180:395–9.
38. Adrouny AZ, Sutherland DW, Griswold HE, Ritzman LW. Complications with transseptal left heart catheterization. *Am Heart J* 1963;65:327–33.
39. Braunwald E. Transseptal left heart catheterization. *Circulation* 1968;37(Suppl III):74–9.
40. Nixon PGF, Ikram H. Left heart catheterization with special reference of the transeptal method. *Br Heart J* 1965;28:835–41.
41. Croft CH, Lipscomb K. Modified technique of transseptal left heart catheterization. *J Am Coll Cardiol* 1985;5:904–10.
42. Doorey AJ, Goldenberg EM. Transseptal catheterization in adults: Enhanced efficiency and safety by low-volume operators using a 'non-standard' technique. *Catheter Cardiovasc Diag* 1991;8:535–42.
43. Ali Khan MA, Mulins CE, Bash SE, Al Yousef S, Nihill MR, Sawyer W. Transseptal left heart catheterisation in infants, children, and young adults. *Catheter Cardiovasc Diag* 1989;17:198–201.
44. Singleton RT, Scherlis L. Transseptal catheterization of the left heart: Observations in 56 patients. *Am Heart J* 1960;60(6):879–85.
45. Folland ED, Oprian C, Giancomini J et al. Complications of cardiac catheterization and angiography in patients with valvular heart disease. *Catheter Cardiovasc Diag* 1989;17:15–21.
46. Kronzon I, Glassman E, Cohen M, Winer H. Use of Two-dimensional echocardiography during transseptal cardiac catheterization. *J Am Coll Cardiol* 1984;4(2):425–8.
47. Libanoff AJ, Silver AW. Complications of transseptal left heart catheterization. *Am J Cardiol* 1965;16:390–93.
48. Peckham GB, Chrysohou A, Aldridge H, Wigle ED. Combined percutaneous retrograde aortic and transseptal left heart catheterization. *Br Heart J* 1964;26:460–468.
49. Wilkins GT, Weyman AE, Abascal VM, Block PC, Palacios IF. Percutaneous mitral valvotomy: An analysis of echocardiographic variables related to outcome and the mechanism of dilatation. *Br Heart J* 1988;60;299–308.
50. Henderson MA. Transseptal left atrial catheterization(letter). *Catheter Cardiovasc Diag* 1990;21:63.
51. Laskey WK, Kusiak V, Unkreter WJ, Hirshfield JW Jr. Transseptal left heart catheterization: Utility of a sheath technique. *Catheter Cardiovasc Diag* 1982;8:535542.
52. Weiner RI, Maranhao V. Development and application of transseptal left heart catheterization. *Catheter Cardiovasc Diag* 1988;15:112–20.
53. Wyman RM, Safian RD, Portway V, Skillman JJ, Mckay RG, Baim DS. Current complications of diagnostic and therapeutic cardiac catheterization. *J Am Coll Cardiol* 1988;12:1400–6.
54. Leon MN, Harrell LC, Simosa HF et al. Comparison of immediate and long-term results of mitral balloon valvotomy with the double-balloon versus Inoue techniques. *Am J Cardiol* 1999;83(9):1356–63.
55. Palacios IF, Sanchez PL, Harrell LC, Weyman AE, Block PC. Which patients benefit from percutaneous mitral balloon valvuloplasty? Prevalvuloplasty and postvalvuloplasty variables that predict long-term outcome. *Circulation* 2002;105:1465–71.
56. Desideri A, Vanderperren O, Serra A et al. Long term (9 to 33 months) echocardiographic follow-up after successful percutaneous mitral commissurotomy. *Am J Cardiol* 1992;69:1602–6.
57. Sanchez PL, Rodríguez-Alemparte M, Inglessis I, Palacios IF. The impact of age in the immediate and long-term outcomes of percutaneous mitral balloon valvuloplasty. *J Invasive Cardiol* 2005;18(4):217–25.
58. Sutaria N, Elder AT, Shaw TR. Long term outcome of percutaneous mitral balloon valvotomy in patients aged 70 and over. *Heart* 2000;83:433–8.
59. Tuzcu EM, Block PC, Griffin B, Dinsmore R, Newell JB, Palacios IF. Percutaneous Mitral Balloon Valvotomy in Patients With Calcific Mitral Stenosis: Immediate and Long Term Outcome. *J Am Coll Cardiol* 1994;23:1604–9.
60. Williams JA, Littmann D, Warren R. Experience with the surgical treatment of mitral stenosis. *N Engl J Med* 1958;258:623–30.
61. Scannell JG, Burke JF, Saidi F, Turner JD. Five-year follow-up study of closed mitral valvotomy. *J Thorac Cardiovasc Surg* 1960;40:723–30.
62. Tuzcu EM, Block PC, Griffin BP, Newell JB, Palacios IF. Immediate and long term outcome of percutaneous mitral valvotomy in patients 65 years and older. *Circulation* 1992;85:963–71.
63. Vahanian A, Palacios IF. Percutaneous approaches to valvular disease. *Circulation* 2004;109:1572–79.
64. Davidson CJ, Bashore TM, Mickel M, Davis K. Balloon mitral commissurotomy after previous surgical commissurotomy. The National Heart, Lung, and Blood Institute Balloon Valvuloplasty Registry participants. *Circulation* 1992;86:91–9.
65. Jang IK, Block PC, Newell JB, Tuzcu EM, Palacios IF. Percutaneous mitral balloon valvotomy for recurrent mitral stenosis after surgical commissurotomy. *Am J Cardiol* 1995;75:601–5.
66. Luis RP, Nelmacy F, Alex S et al. Echocardiography can predict which patients will develop severe mitral regurgitation after percutaneous mitral valvulotomy. *J Am Coll Cardiol* 1996;27(5):1225–31.

67. Kaplan JD, Isner JM, Karas RH et al. *In vitro* analysis of mechanisms of balloon valvuloplasty of stenotic mitral valves. *Am J Cardiol* 1987;59:318–23.

68. Lau KW, Ding ZP, Gao W, Koh TH, Johan A. Percutaneous balloon mitral valvuloplasty in patients with mitral restenosis after previous surgical commissurotomy. A matched comparative study. *Eur Heart J* 1996;17:1367–72.

69. Eltchaninoff H, Tron C, Cribier A. Effectiveness of percutaneous mechanical mitral commissurotomy using the metallic commissurotome in patients with restenosis after balloon or previous surgical commissurotomy. *Am J Cardiol* 2003;91:425–8.

70. Turi ZG, Reyes VP, Raju BS et al. Percutaneous balloon versus surgical closed commissurotomy for mitral stenosis: A prospective, randomized trial. *Circulation* 1991;83:1179–85.

71. Ben Farhat M, Ayari M, Maatouk F et al. Percutaneous balloon versus surgical closed and open mitral commissurotomy: Seven-year follow-up results of a randomized trial. *Circulation* 1998;97:245–50.

38

Mitral and tricuspid valve stenosis: Percutaneous tricuspid valvuloplasty

R. Arora

Tricuspid valve anatomy

Tricuspid valve

The tricuspid valve is located between the right atrium and right ventricle and has a valve area of 4–6 cm^2.[1]

The tricuspid valvular apparatus consists of (Figure 38.1)[2]

1. *Tricuspid valve annulus.*
   a. Tricuspid valve annulus is a fibrous ring that constitutes the anatomical junction between the ventricle and the right atrium, and serves as an insertion site for the leaflet tissue.
   b. Tricuspid valve leaflets.
2. *Three cusps.* The tricuspid valve consists of three triangular cusps:
   a. The anterior or *infundibular* cusp is the largest cusp.
   b. The *posterior* or *marginal* cusp is in relation to the right margin of the ventricle.
   c. The *medial* or *septal* cusp is in relation to the ventricular septum.
3. *Chordae tendineae.*
4. *Papillary muscles.* There are three papillary muscles: anterior, posterior, and septal.
   a. The *anterior* is the larger, and its chordae tendineae are connected with the anterior and posterior cusps of the valve.
   b. The *posterior* papillary muscle sometimes consists of two or three parts; its chordae tendineae are connected with the posterior and medial cusps.
   c. The *septal* papillary muscles are small papillary muscles arising from the septal wall. The chordae tendineae are attached to the septal and anterior cusps.[2]

Tricuspid stenosis

Causes and pathophysiology

Tricuspid stenosis results from alterations in the structure of the tricuspid valve that precipitate inadequate excursion of the valve leaflets.[4] The most common etiology is rheumatic fever. Other causes of obstruction to right atrial emptying are unusual and include congenital tricuspid atresia, right atrial tumors that may produce a clinical picture suggesting rapidly progressive tricuspid stenosis (TS), and the carcinoid syndrome, which more frequently produces tricuspid regurgitation (TR). Rarely, obstruction to the right ventricle (RV) inflow can be caused by endomyocardial fibrosis, tricuspid valve vegetations, a pacemaker lead, or extracardiac tumors.[5]

Most patients with rheumatic tricuspid valve disease present with TR or a combination of TS and TR. Isolated rheumatic TS is uncommon and almost never occurs as an isolated lesion, but generally accompanies mitral valve disease. A mean pressure gradient as low as 2 mmHg is sufficient to establish the diagnosis of tricuspid stenosis. Since the pressures in the right-sided cardiac chambers are usually low, even a gradient as small as 5 mmHg can be sufficient to elevate the mean right atrial pressure. As a result, most patients with significant tricuspid stenosis have systemic venous congestion with jugular venous distension, ascites, and peripheral edema.[6]

Epidemiology

Tricuspid stenosis is found in approximately 3% of the international population. It is more prevalent in areas with a high incidence of rheumatic fever. The general mortality rate is approximately 5%. It is observed more commonly in women than in men, similar to mitral stenosis of rheumatic origin. The congenital form of the disease has a slightly higher male predominance.[7]

Clinical presentation

Symptoms

Obstruction to tricuspid flow limits cardiac output, causes fatigue, and produces signs of systemic venous

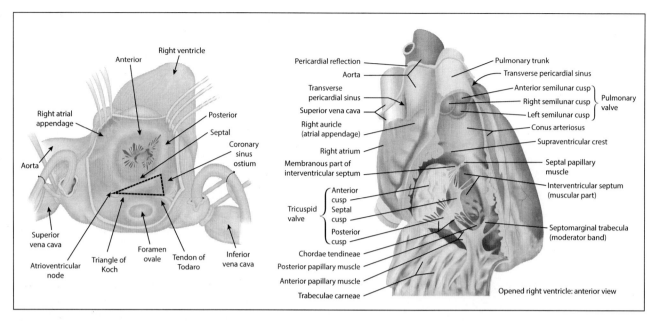

Figure 38.1   (**See color insert.**) Anatomy of TV and subvalvular apparatus. (From Gray H, Standring S. Eds. *Gray's Anatomy: The Anatomical Basis of Clinical Practice*. 39th ed. Edinburgh, UK: Churchill Livingstone Elsevier, 2005. pp. 1003–4.)

hypertension. Such patients often complain of abdominal discomfort, which is due to hepatomegaly and hepatic congestion. Some patients may sense a fluttering discomfort in the neck, caused by tall "a" waves in the jugular venous pulse.[8]

Physical examination

The findings seen on physical examination in patients with tricuspid stenosis are similar to those of mitral stenosis. Since these two lesions often coexist, the diagnosis of tricuspid stenosis may be missed.

An obstruction to the flow across the tricuspid valve produces an increase in right atrial and jugular venous pressure. Jugular venous pulsations often exhibit a prominent presystolic "a" wave, which may be confused with an arterial pulsation. The "y" descent is slow and barely appreciated.

The lungs are usually clear, despite the presence of jugular venous distension, hepatomegaly and hepatic pulsations, ascites, peripheral edema and, occasionally, anasarca. A right ventricular parasternal lift is usually not obvious.[8]

Auscultation

An opening snap of the tricuspid valve may be heard but, when mitral stenosis is also present, it may be difficult to distinguish from the opening snap of mitral stenosis. The tricuspid opening snap usually follows the opening snap of the mitral valve and is localized to the lower left sternal border. A low-frequency diastolic murmur is heard at the lower left sternal border in the fourth intercostal space; it

is usually softer, higher pitched, and shorter in duration than the murmur of mitral stenosis. The intensity of the murmur and opening snap in tricuspid stenosis increases with maneuvers that increase blood flow across the tricuspid valve, especially with inspiration (Carvallo sign) and also with leg raising, inhalation of amyl nitrate, squatting, or isotonic exercise.[8]

Diagnostic evaluation modalities

Electrocardiography

There are no tall right atrial P waves and no right ventricular hypertrophy in the absence of atrial flutter (AF). The P wave amplitude in leads II and V_1 exceeds 0.25 mV. Because most patients with TS have mitral valvular disease, the electrocardiographic signs of biatrial enlargement are commonly found.[9]

Radiography

A dilated right atrium without enlarged pulmonary artery segment (i.e., prominence of the right heart border), which extends into a dilated superior vena cava and azygos vein.[9]

Echocardiography

Echocardiographic features of tricuspid stenosis (Figure 38.2) include limited mobility of the leaflets, reduced separation of the leaflet tips, a reduction in the diameter of the tricuspid annulus, and diastolic doming of the valve. Although leaflet thickening is seen, the degree of

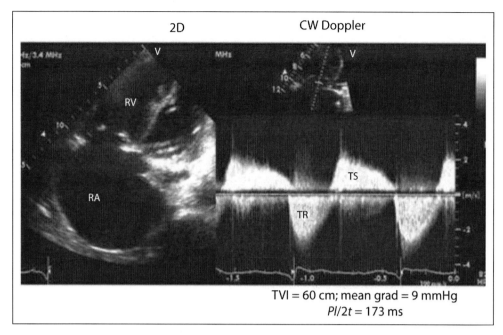

Figure 38.2   The left panel illustrates a 2D echocardiographic image of a stenotic tricuspid valve obtained in a modified apical four-chamber view during diastole. The right panel shows a CW Doppler recording through the tricuspid valve. (From Helmut B, Judy H, Javier B et al. *Eur J Echocardiogr* 2009;10:1–25.)

thickening and calcification is generally less pronounced than in rheumatic mitral stenosis.[10]

Doppler echocardiography reveals high-velocity turbulent diastolic flow across the stenotic orifice and prolonged pressure half-time. A tricuspid valve area less than 1.0 cm^2 indicates severe tricuspid stenosis.[11,12]

Cardiac catheterization

This may be required prior to surgery in older patients to assess for concomitant coronary artery disease. Right heart catheterization can be used to determine the gradient across the valve and valve area (i.e., severity of stenosis) and assess the presence of associated congenital defects (e.g., septal defects, intracardiac shunts, anomalous veins) if present. Assessment of aortic and mitral valves via left heart catheterization is useful in patients with rheumatic disease.[13]

Management

Intervention on the tricuspid valve is usually carried out at the time of intervention on the other valves in patients who are symptomatic despite medical therapy. According to anatomy and surgical expertise in valve repair, conservative surgery or valve replacement is preferred to balloon commissurotomy; however, there is a lack of data on the evaluation of long-term results.[14]

A large bioprosthesis is preferred to a mechanical prosthesis in the tricuspid position because of the high risk of

thrombosis of the latter and the longer durability of bioprostheses in the tricuspid than in the mitral or aortic positions.[15]

Patient selection for valvotomy

Patients with signs and symptoms of systemic venous hypertension and congestion should be considered for balloon valvotomy. Transvalvular pressure gradients as low as 3 mmHg and valve areas less than 1.5 cm^2 can indicate serious, but treatable, stenosis. Tricuspid regurgitation that is greater than mild is generally thought to be a contraindication to valvotomy, but a few patients with moderate regurgitation have been successfully treated with this technique. Tumor masses, vegetations, and thrombi are contraindications to valvotomy.[13]

Pregnancy

It is not infrequent that signs and symptoms of rheumatic heart disease first occur during pregnancy, when the cardiac output increases because of a dramatic rise in blood volume and heart rate. There is little experience with balloon valvotomy during pregnancy, but it appears to be effective in patients with refractory systemic venous congestion. Isolated balloon tricuspid valvotomy and concurrent balloon valvotomy of mitral and tricuspid valves have been successfully performed during pregnancy.[16,17] Great care must be taken to limit radiation exposure.

Techniques of tricuspid balloon valvotomy

Tricuspid double balloon valvotomy (Figure 38.3)

Ribeiro et al.[18] studied percutaneous balloon valvotomy in tricuspid stenosis. An 18-gauge cannula was inserted into the right femoral artery for pressure monitoring. A 7 French catheter was passed from each femoral vein to measure the pressure gradient across the tricuspid valve and to perform a right ventricular angiogram before and after balloon inflation. After calibration and the recording of identical simultaneous right atrial pressure tracings from both catheters, one catheter was advanced to the right ventricular cavity. Ten consecutive cardiac cycles were recorded at a paper speed of 100 mm/s to measure the gradient across the tricuspid valve. The mean tricuspid gradient was only accepted after two identical simultaneous right atrial pressure traces had been recorded after the withdrawal of the right ventricular catheter back into the right atrium. The 0.038 inch Teflon-coated exchange guide wires (250 cm long) with curved tips were advanced through two 7 French pigtail catheters, which previously had been inserted percutaneously in each femoral vein. The curved end of each wire was positioned at the apex of the right ventricle (Figure 38.3). A 9 French balloon catheter (Meditech; 15-mm diameter, 3-cm length) was advanced percutaneously over each guide wire and positioned across the tricuspid valve under fluoroscopic control in the 10 degrees right anterior oblique projection. The balloons were correctly positioned across the tricuspid valve with the aid of contrast media injections into the right atrium, and the positioning was confirmed by fluoroscopic detection of balloon indentation during inflation. The balloons were inflated simultaneously on three occasions to a maximum pressure of 5 atmospheres. There

was no reduction in the tricuspid gradient and no balloon indentation occurred during these inflations. Therefore, we replaced one of the 15-mm-diameter balloon catheters with a 20-mm-diameter balloon that was slid over the exchange guide wire, which was left in position. The balloons were inflated three more times. During the third inflation, proper balloon alignment was achieved, with indentation of one balloon (Figure 38.3). Disappearance of this indentation, together with the subsequent considerable reduction in the gradient, was taken to indicate a successful result.

The Inoue balloon for dilatation of the tricuspid valve (Figure 38.4)

Shaw[19] studied the Inoue balloon for dilatation of the tricuspid valve: a modified over-the-wire approach. The design of the Inoue balloon is unique. Its walls contain a network of synthetic nylon fibers, which give different compliance characteristics to its distal, proximal, and middle segments, so that at inflation the distal portion of the balloon enlarges first, allowing this portion to be drawn back against the stenosed orifice. On further inflation, the proximal segment enlarges, holding the balloon at the valve orifice, which is then dilated as the middle segment expands at full inflation. The short length of the Inoue balloon and its blunt distal point reduce the risk of perforating the myocardial wall. The deflated Inoue balloon does not have a low profile, and to allow passage through the skin (and though the atrial septum for dilatation of the mitral valve), a metal stretching tube is included in the balloon equipment set. This is inserted into the balloon catheter lumen and causes the deflated balloon to be stretched into a lower, more rigid shape. The Inoue balloon catheter has no intrinsic curve and when it is used to dilate the mitral valve, a curved stylet wire is inserted to arc the

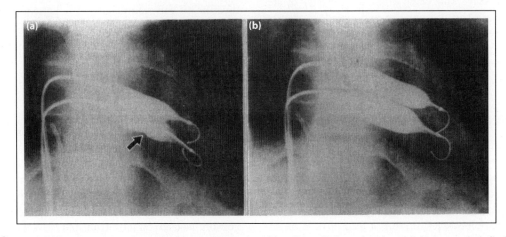

Figure 38.3 Two balloons positioned across the tricuspid valve. (a) Balloon indentation (arrow) during early inflation. (b) Loss of balloon indentation after successful double balloon tricuspid valvotomy. (From Ribeiro PA, Al Zaibag M, Al Kasab S et al. *Am J Cardiol* 1988;61:660.)

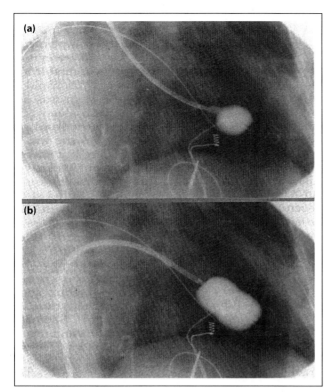

Figure 38.4 Inoue balloon dilatation at the tricuspid valve. (a) The distal portion of the balloon has been dilated. (b) The balloon catheter has been pulled back to engage the distal portion of the orifice and the balloon has beautifully dilated. A 0.035 inch guide wire also lies across the tricuspid valve. An epicardial pacemaker system is *in situ* and an F6 pigtail catheter lies in the descending aorta to monitor systemic pressure. (From Shaw TR. The Inoue balloon for dilatation of the tricuspid valve: A modified over-the-wire approach. *Br Heart J* 1992;67(3):263–5.)

balloon toward the mitral valve. The Inoue balloon, with its metal stretching tube inserted could be advanced over a 0.025 inch guide wire; the stretching tube was essential for passing the balloon percutaneously to reach the right atrial cavity. Once the stretching tube was removed, the Inoue balloon followed by an over-the-wire approach to the tricuspid orifice. The Inoue stylet was unable to direct the balloon to the orifice with such a giant right atrium. This over-the-wire approach might also be applicable in occasional cases of mitral stenosis where there is difficulty in crossing the mitral orifice.

Results of balloon valvotomy

The feasibility of tricuspid balloon valvuloplasty has been demonstrated and this procedure may be combined with mitral balloon valvuloplasty, but there is far less experience with tricuspid valvotomy than with mitral valvotomy.[14] Valve areas generally increase from less than 1 to almost 2 cm². While some stenosis persists, this change in area is sufficient to produce a significant reduction in the transvalvular pressure gradient and a decrease in right atrial pressure.

- In a report of four patients, tricuspid valvotomy performed with two balloons produced a rise in the valve area from a mean of 0.8 to 1.8 cm².[18] There was no increase in the severity of tricuspid regurgitation. A follow-up at 8–20 weeks showed persistence of the early beneficial effects; the valve area was 1.9 cm² and cardiac output was significantly higher at rest and during exercise. Symptomatic improvement was reported in all four patients.
- Another study evaluated the use of one, two, and three balloons to perform valvotomy.[20] The single patient treated with one balloon did not show improvement, but the three treated with two balloons and the one treated with three balloons all exhibited significant improvement in valve area and symptoms without increase in tricuspid regurgitation. The authors concluded that the combined use of two balloons (23–25 mm) is adequate for most patients. Later experience with the Inoue balloon indicated that single-balloon techniques may be as effective as the previous double-balloon techniques.[21]

Similar beneficial results have been described when balloon valvotomy is used to treat combined mitral and tricuspid stenosis, as well as in cases of combined aortic, mitral, and tricuspid stenosis.[22,23]

Risks

Balloon valvuloplasty can have serious complications. For example, the valve can become misshapen so that it does not close completely, which makes the condition worse. Embolism, where either clots or pieces of valve tissue break off and travel to the brain (in the presence of patent foramen ovale [PFO]) or the lungs causing blockage, is another possible risk. If the procedure causes severe damage to the valve leaflets, immediate valve replacement is required. Less frequent complications are bleeding and hematoma (a local collection of clotted blood) at the puncture site, abnormal heart rhythms, reduced blood flow, cardiac arrest, heart puncture, infection, and circulatory problems.[24]

Recommendations

Recognizing that there are no published studies that compare percutaneous balloon valvotomy with surgical valvuloplasty, and that only limited long-term results have been published,[22] limited conclusions are appropriate. The available data indicate that balloon valvotomy for tricuspid stenosis is effective and is associated with a low morbidity. Thus, if symptoms of systemic venous hypertension and congestion are not adequately controlled with diuretics and angiotensin converting enzyme (ACE) inhibitors or angiotensin receptor antagonists, balloon valvotomy of the stenotic tricuspid valve should be performed. Surgical correction of the stenotic lesion is indicated in patients whose valve is not treatable with balloon techniques.[13]

References

1. Rogers JH, Bolling SF. The tricuspid valve: Current perspective and evolving management of tricuspid regurgitation. *Circulation* 2009;119(20):2718–25.
2. Joudinaud TM, Flecher EM, Duran CM. Functional terminology for the tricuspid valve. *J Heart Valve Dis* 2006;15:382–8.
3. Gray H, Standring S. Eds. *Gray's Anatomy: The Anatomical Basis of Clinical Practice.* 39th ed. Edinburgh, UK: Churchill Livingstone Elsevier, 2005. pp. 1003–4.
4. Wafae N, Hayashi H, Gerola LR, Vieira MC. Anatomical study of the human tricuspid valve. *Surg Radiol Anat* 1990;12(1):37–41.
5. Daniels SJ, Mintz GS, Kotler MN. Rheumatic tricuspid valve disease: Two-dimensional echocardiographic, hemodynamic, and angiographic correlations. *Am J Cardiol* 1983;51:492.
6. Waller BF. Morphological aspects of valvular heart disease: Part I. *Curr Probl Cardiol* 1984;9(7):1–66.
7. Waller BF. Morphological aspects of valvular heart disease: Part II. *Curr Probl Cardiol* 1984;9(8):1–74.
8. Shah PM et al. Tricuspid and pulmonary valve disease evaluation and management. *Rev Esp Cardiol* 2010;63(11):1349–65.
9. Robert O. Bonow, Douglas L. Mann, Douglas P. Zipes et al. *Braunwald's Heart Disease. A Textbook of Cardiovascular Medicine.* 9th ed. 2011. 66, p. 1515.
10. Zaroff JG, Picard MH. Transesophageal echocardiographic (TEE) evaluation of the mitral and tricuspid valves. *Cardiol Clin* 2000;18:731.
11. Bonow RO, Carabello BA, Chatterjee K et al. Focused update incorporated into the ACC/AHA 2006 guidelines for the management of patients with valvular heart disease: A report of the American College of Cardiology/American Heart Association Task Force on Practice Guidelines (Writing Committee to Revise the 1998 Guidelines for the Management of Patients with Valvular Heart Disease): Endorsed by the Society of Cardiovascular Anesthesiologists, Society for Cardiovascular Angiography and Interventions, and Society of Thoracic Surgeons. *Circulation* 2008;118:e523.
12. Helmut B, Judy H, Javier B et al. Echocardiographic assessment of valve stenosis: EAE/ASE recommendations for clinical practice. *Eur J Echocardiogr* 2009;10:1–25.
13. http://www.uptodate.com/contents/tricuspid-stenosis-clinical-features-diagnosis-and-percutaneous-tricuspid-balloon-valvotomy.
14. Yeter E, Ozlem K, Kilic H et al. Tricuspid balloon valvuloplasty to treat tricuspid stenosis. *J Heart Valve Dis* 2010;19:159–60.
15. Unger P, Rosenhek R, Dedobbeleer C, Berrebi A, Lancellotti P. Management of multiple valve disease. *Heart* 2011;97:272–7.
16. Gamra H, Betbout F, Ayari M et al. Recurrent miscarriages as an indication for percutaneous tricuspid valvuloplasty during pregnancy. *Cathet Cardiovasc Diagn* 1997;40:283.
17. Bahl VK, Chandra S, Mishra S. Concurrent balloon dilatation of mitral and tricuspid stenosis during pregnancy using an Inoue balloon. *Int J Cardiol* 1997;59:199.
18. Ribeiro PA, Al Zaibag M, Al Kasab S et al. Percutaneous double balloon valvotomy for rheumatic tricuspid stenosis. *Am J Cardiol* 1988;61:660.
19. Shaw TR. The Inoue balloon for dilatation of the tricuspid valve: A modified over-the-wire approach. *Br Heart J* 1992;67(3):263–5.
20. Orbe LC, Sobrino N, Arcas R et al. Initial outcome of percutaneous balloon valvuloplasty in rheumatic tricuspid valve stenosis. *Am J Cardiol* 1993;71:353.
21. Patel TM, Dani SI, Shah SC et al. Tricuspid balloon valvuloplasty: A more simplified approach using Inoue balloon. *Cathet Cardiovasc Diagn* 1996;37:86.
22. Sancaktar O, Kumbasar SD, Semiz E et al. Late results of combined percutaneous balloon valvuloplasty of mitral and tricuspid valves. *Cathet Cardiovasc Diagn* 1998;45:246.
23. Sobrino N, Calvo Orbe L, Merino JL et al. Percutaneous balloon valvuloplasty for concurrent mitral, aortic and tricuspid rheumatic stenosis. *Eur Heart J* 1995;16:711.
24. Emilio R. Giuliani et al. *Mayo Clinic Practice of Cardiology: Balloon Valvuloplasty.* 3rd ed. Mosby, 1996.

39

Mitral valve insufficiency: Background and indications for treatment

Sameer Gafoor, Jennifer Franke, Stefan Bertog, and Horst Sievert

Etiology and pathology

There are two broad categories of mitral regurgitation, which are organic and functional mitral regurgitation. The first classification, by Carpentier et al., classified mitral regurgitation into four types based on leaflet and chordal motion. Normal leaflet motion is type I. This occurs often with annular dilatation with dilated cardiomyopathy, endocarditis leading to leaflet perforation, degenerative due to annular calcification, or congenital cleft leaflet. Leaflet prolapse or excessive motion is type II. This can be seen in degenerative valve disease, such as mitral valve prolapse or flail leaflet, as well as endocarditis with ruptured chords or ischemic cardiomyopathy with papillary muscle rupture. Type III is based on leaflet restriction. This can occur in diastole (IIIa) or systole (IIIb). Examples of type IIIa include rheumatic valve disease, iatrogenic disease (radiation or drugs), and inflammatory diseases such as lupus. Type IIIb can occur with dilated cardiomyopathy, myocarditis, or functional ischemic cardiomyopathy.[1]

Another classification based on etiology includes organic and functional regurgitation. Organic mitral regurgitation is broadly defined as a structural abnormality of the mitral valve apparatus that prevents competent valve closure. Causes include degenerative valve disease, rheumatic valve disease, endocarditis, and congenital mitral valve disease. Functional mitral regurgitation occurs where the mitral valve complex is normal, but there is an underlying myocardial process that leads to mitral regurgitation. This includes both dilated cardiomyopathy and ischemic heart disease. An overview of both classifications can be seen in Table 39.1.

Table 39.1 Etiology of mitral regurgitation

		Mechanism			
		Organic			Functional
		Type I	Type II	Type IIIa	Type I/IIIb
Cause	Ischemic		Ruptured papillary muscle		Functional ischemic (three vessel or left main disease)
	Nonischemic	1. Endocarditis (perforation) 2. Degenerative (mitral annular calcification 3. Congenital (cleft leaflet)	1. Degenerative (flail leaflet), mitral valve prolapse) 2. Endocarditis (ruptured chords)	1. Rheumatic 2. Iatrogenic (radiation/ drug) 3. Inflammatory (lupus)	1. Cardiomyopathy 2. Myocarditis 3. Left ventricular dysfunction

Source: Adapted from Pedrazzini GB. *Swiss Med Weekly* 2010;140(3–4):36–43.
Note: The cause of mitral regurgitation may be ischemic or nonischemic (*y*-axis) with the mechanism being either organic or functional (*y*-axis). The Carpentier classifications are also included.

Degenerative mitral disease

Degenerative mitral disease is often due to myxomatous degeneration. Genetically, this is associated with abnormalities in collagen I, collagen III, and fibrillin. Mitral valve prolapse is an abnormal systolic motion of one or both leaflets toward the left atrium (≥2 mm beyond annulus) and occurs in 5–6% of adult subjects with a female predominance.[2] This may occur due to chordal rupture and prolapse of one segment or prolapse of multiple segments.

Diffuse myxomatous degeneration, also known as Barlow's disease, has diffuse excess tissue. This is associated with a large valve size, diffuse chordal elongation, chordal rupture, severe annular dilatation, annular calcification, subvalvular fibrosis, calcified papillary muscles, and multiple jets of regurgitation.[3]

Rheumatic mitral disease

Rheumatic mitral disease is the most common cause of mitral regurgitation worldwide. The leaflets often fuse at the commissures, leading to restricted leaflet motion in diastole (leading to stenosis) and systole (leading to regurgitation). There is often subvalvular disease with fibrosis, papillary muscle scarring, and thickening/foreshortening of the chordae tendinae.[4]

Endocarditis

Endocarditis in native valves often occurs with *Staphylococcus aureus*, and is often in valves with prior bacteremia, for example, indwelling lines or intravenous drugs. Valves with myxomatous degeneration are prone to less virulent organisms such as *Streptococcus viridans*. As the valve destructs, it can lead to severe regurgitation.

Functional mitral regurgitation

This is a state when the valve apparatus in not affected primarily; this is secondary to an underlying myocardial process. In global dysfunction or dilated cardiomyopathy, the annulus is dilated and the papillary muscles are spread apart. In ischemic dysfunction, the leaflet ipsilateral to the wall motion abnormality is tethered. After inferior–posterior myocardial infarction, the posterior leaflet is tethered and the mitral regurgitation is anteriorly directed. In hypertrophic obstructive cardiomyopathy, flow acceleration through the left ventricular outflow tract leads to anterior leaflet drag, which then leads to malcoaptation and a posteriorly directed mitral regurgitation jet.[5]

Pathophysiology

Acute mitral regurgitation occurs from a variety of reasons (papillary muscle rupture, chordal rupture, or leaflet destruction from endocarditis) and results in an acute increase in preload and decrease in afterload. This increase in end-diastolic volume (EDV) and end-systolic volume (ESV) results in an increase in total stroke volume (TSV). However, the forward stroke volume (FSV) is decreased as most of the flow goes retrograde to the low-pressure left atrium, resulting in an increase in left atrial pressure (LAP). In the acute setting, the atrium is noncompliant and, therefore, this increase in LAP may result in pulmonary edema, heart failure, and cardiogenic shock.

Chronic compensated mitral regurgitation occurs as the left atrium and left ventricle dilate to accommodate the increased volume. Therefore, LAP is normal or only minimally elevated. Left ventricular dilatation occurs via eccentric hypertrophy, and through this TSV and FSV are maintained. The wall stress increases according to Laplace's law as the radius of the left ventricular cavity increases, but left ventricular end diastolic pressure (LVEDP) remains normal. During this time period, the ejection fraction is actually increased, as more volume enters and leaves the left ventricle. As the left ventricle enlarges, the mitral annulus also stretches, worsening mitral regurgitation and left ventricular dilatation. Mitral regurgitation, therefore, begets mitral regurgitation. Pulmonary vascular resistance also increases as a consequence of the chronic increase in LAP.

Chronic decompensated mitral regurgitation occurs as the left ventricle starts to fail. There are increases in EDV and ESV, with a concomitant fall in ejection fraction. The FSV falls and the regurgitant fraction (RF) increases. Atrial fibrillation may also occur, causing a loss of atrial kick to preload. With this also comes an elevation of LAP and LVEDP, resulting in pulmonary edema, heart failure, and cardiogenic shock. The risk of sudden cardiac death also increases.

Mitral regurgitation worsens with time. The severity increases with the regurgitant volume (RV) at a rate of 7.4 mL/year, associated with an increase in the regurgitant fraction (RF) of 2.9% per year. The regurgitant orifice area (ROA) grows at a rate of 5.9 mm^2/year.[6]

Clinical evaluation

Symptoms and physical examination

Patients with chronic mitral regurgitation often remain asymptomatic with ventricular adaptation. Symptoms can occur with increased physical activity. These consist of pulmonary congestion, weakness, and dyspnea on exertion. Over time, right-sided heart failure can also occur with hepatomegaly and peripheral edema. Palpitations can indicate the onset of atrial fibrillation, which is more likely with advanced mitral regurgitation and stretch of the left atrium. Acute mitral regurgitation may result in sudden onset of dyspnea and pulmonary edema, that can result in heart failure, cardiogenic shock, and/or death.

On physical examination, the cardiac impulse is displaced to the left. S1 is usually diminished with a prominent S2. This may be widely split from the shortening of LV systole and early closure of the aortic valve. The murmur of mitral regurgitation is holosystolic, blowing a moderately harsh murmur that radiates to the axilla. When chordae of the posterior leaflet are ruptured, the mitral regurgitation jet is directed anteriorly, which can disrupt the atrial septum near the base of the aorta and radiate the murmur to the neck. When chordae of the anterior leaflet are affected, the jet is angulated toward the posterior left atrial wall and the murmur is best heard posteriorly. Patients with mitral valve prolapse have a midsystolic click that occurs as the valve chordae tighten to their maximum. This is followed by a late systolic murmur.[7]

Echocardiography

Echocardiography provides the ability to find multiple key pieces of data to characterize mitral regurgitation. These include the etiology, location, and severity of mitral regurgitation as well as degree of calcification. Examples of mitral regurgitation evaluation by echocardiography can be seen in Figures 39.1 through 39.3. This can be performed through qualitative and quantitative measures.

Qualitative measures include a color-flow jet area, density of the continuous-wave Doppler signal, and pulmonary vein flow pattern. Quantitative measures include an effective regurgitant orifice area (EROA), RV, and a regurgitant fraction (RF). Various articles have been published to quantify mitral regurgitation based on these parameters.[5,8] RV and RF can be quantified using various volumetric methods. These are all dependent on the ability to completely visualize the regurgitant jet, the lack of rhythm irregularities, and a clear visualization of aortic jets to calculate FSV. Other limitations include apex foreshortening, failure to align with true LV center, and the inability to trace the true endocardial border.

3D and transesophageal echocardiograms add extra information. A transesophageal echocardiogram provides better imaging quality and adds information when a transthoracic echocardiogram is suboptimal or when complex calcified or endocarditic lesions are suspected. 3D echocardiography provides superior assessment of regurgitant mitral valve morphology and pathology, as well as identifying individual segment/prolapse of the mitral valve. It is also useful for volumetric measurement. However, this is also now prone to image artifacts over three dimensions.

The 2003 ASE guidelines[9] provide important information to characterize severe mitral regurgitation:

1. A vena contracta width ≥7 mm
2. A regurgitant orifice area ≥0.40 cm^2
3. A regurgitant volume ≥60 mL

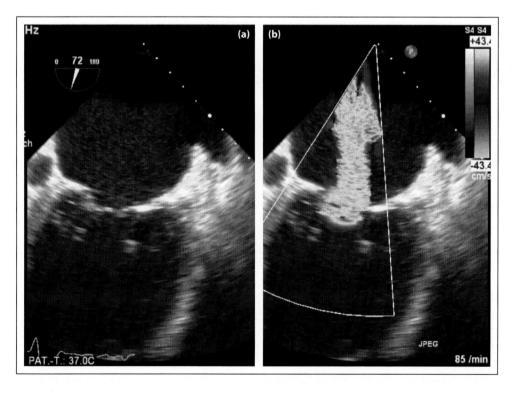

Figure 39.1 (**See color insert.**) Mitral regurgitation, type I: annulus dilatation. As seen in (a), the annulus is dilated, leading to the central wide color flow pattern seen in (b).

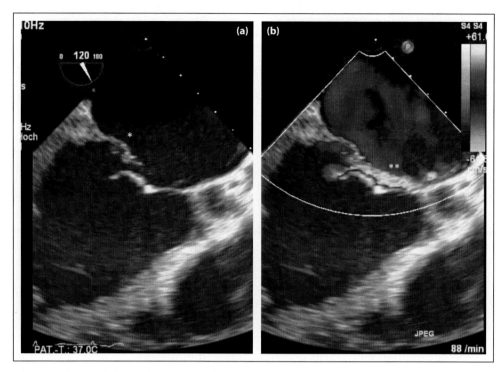

Figure 39.2 Mitral regurgitation, type II: mitral valve prolapse. As seen in (a), there is a significant prolapse of the posterior leaflet (marked by single asterisk). This allows regurgitant flow in an anterior direction (marked by double asterisk) (b).

4. A regurgitant fraction ≥50%
5. A jet area >40% of left atrial area, but this is not so reproducible and less often used

Exercise testing

The "asymptomatic" patient may be sedentary or masking symptoms that may be unmasked with exercise. Exercise testing determines functional testing and defines changes in LV systolic function, ROA, and pulmonary artery pressure. Negative outcomes are associated with the failure of left ventricular ejection fraction (LVEF) to increase, the increase in EROA, and increased pulmonary artery pressure with exercise.[10]

Cardiac catheterization

Coronary angiography provides management for patients over 35 years of age. Right heart catheterization with wedge pressure assessment or transseptal evaluation of the LAP may reveal a characteristic "v" wave of mitral regurgitation. Severity of mitral regurgitation can be estimated by LA opacification during angiography.[8]

Magnetic resonance imaging

Cardiac magnetic resonance (CMR) has additional strengths for evaluation of mitral regurgitation. This includes determination of left and right ventricular volumes, left and right ventricular function, aortic flow volume, and in ischemic mitral regurgitation, assessment of myocardial function and viability. Steady-state free procession sequences provide information on mitral valve anatomy, while gradient echo cine pulse sequences are better for localization and sizing of regurgitant jets. The regurgitant volume helps quantify mitral regurgitant severity, under the assumption that there is no other valvular disease or intracardiac shunt that would make RV and LV stroke volumes unequal.[11]

Treatment rationale, options, and timing of therapy

Natural history of mitral regurgitation

There is a risk of increased mortality with mitral regurgitation. Ling et al.[12] showed a 10-year mortality of 6.3% with a risk of 63% and atrial fibrillation of 30%. Enriquez-Sarano et al.[13] evaluated asymptomatic patients with an ERO >40 mm². At 5 years, cardiac mortality was 36% with an event rate of 62%.

Serial monitoring

Patients with mild MR and no evidence of LV enlargement, LV dysfunction, or pulmonary hypertension should be seen yearly. Yearly echocardiography is not necessary unless there is clinical evidence of worsening MR. Those

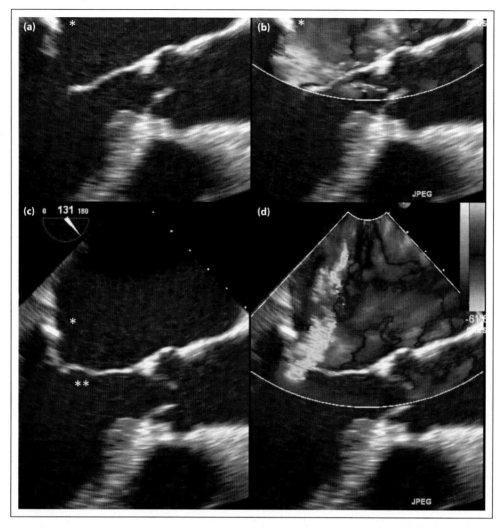

Figure 39.3   (See color insert.) Mitral regurgitation, type III: restrictive leaflets. The posterior leaflet in diastole is seen without color in (a) and with color in (b), marked by the single asterisk. (c) The patient in systole, where the posterior leaflet has not moved due to restriction (single asterisk). Of note, the anterior leaflet has risen to meet the posterior leaflet (double asterisk), but there is still significant regurgitation (d).

with moderate MR should have a clinical visit and echocardiography every year (ACC/AHA guidelines) or every 2 years (ESC guidelines 2012). Those with severe MR should be seen 6–12 months or sooner if symptoms with repeat TTE to evaluate for conformity to echo cutoffs.

Physical activity and exercise

Patients with mild–moderate MR in sinus rhythm, normal LV size and function, and normal PA pressure can participate in all competitive sports. Those with mild–moderate MR who also have mild LV enlargement can participate in low and moderate static, and all dynamic competitive sports. Those with severe MR and definite LV enlargement, pulmonary hypertension, or LV systolic dysfunction at rest should not participate in any competitive sports. There are no restrictions on asymptomatic patients

in sinus rhythm, with normal LV and LA dimensions, and normal PA pressure.[14]

Atrial fibrillation

Patients that undergo surgery after atrial fibrillation has persisted for 1 year show continued persistence of atrial fibrillation after surgery.[15] Normal LA size is associated with a higher rate of return to normal sinus rhythm.

Medical therapy

For degenerative acute mitral regurgitation, nitrates and diuretics reduce filling pressure. In the case of hypotension, inotropes and intra-aortic balloon pump may be used. For chronic degenerative mitral regurgitation without heart failure, there is no evidence for vasodilators. In the case of heart failure, ACE inhibitors can be used in advanced mitral regurgitation and severe symptoms, with beta-blockers and spironolactone when appropriate. For those patients with primary mitral regurgitation and symptoms, preload reduction will not change the ROA, so systolic pressure reduction is the goal.[16]

For secondary mitral regurgitation, heart failure management is paramount. This includes ACE inhibitors, beta-blockers, and possibly aldosterone antagonists. If there is fluid overload, diuretics may be required. Symptomatic patients who are not candidates for surgery may benefit from chronic vasodilator therapy.[16]

Cardiac resynchronization therapy

Cardiac resynchronization therapy (CRT) may be useful in patients with moderate–severe functional mitral regurgitation. This points to atrial-synchronized biventricular or left ventricular stimulation. For responders, CRT may reduce mitral regurgitation (MR) severity by (1) increasing closing force and papillary muscle resynchronization[15] and (2) reduction in tethering force due to LV reverse modeling.[16] There was a significant improvement in mitral regurgitation in 49% of patients who survived to 8-month follow-up; this was more likely in nonischemic-cause patients and the benefits disappear in patients when CRT is discontinued.[17]

Surgical approaches

There are a variety of surgical approaches to mitral regurgitation, beyond the scope of this chapter. Anatomic approaches are mostly through the left atrium, but there is also the transapical approach for the percutaneous valve in failed bioprosthesis, mitral chordae replacement, and also in patients having concomitant left ventriculotomy for aneurysm. Surgical incisions vary from median sternotomy, lateral thoracotomy, or percutaneous access. There are also endoscopic approaches and robotic assistance. Surgical mitral repair techniques include therapy for annulus, leaflets, chords, and ventricle.[18]

Mitral annuloplasty can be complete or partial, suture or ring, and even within-ring annuloplasty, rigid or flexible. A partial or suture annuloplasty is important for children as the annulus grows over time. For prolapse and myxomatous mitral valves, flexible rings allow the base to contract and rigid rings help with central regurgitation. For functional mitral regurgitation, a complete rigid ring is better than a flexible one.[18]

Leaflets can be resected in case of myxomatous disease, patched in case of perforation, or closed in case of cleft leaflet. Chords are also a target for surgery, especially if ruptured, elongated, or shortened. Chords can be transferred or new chords can be made, for example, polytetrafluoroethylene suture chords.[19]

The edge-to-edge repair describes when the anterior leaflet is sutured to the posterior leaflet to prevent systolic anterior motion of the anterior leaflet. This is often done with annuloplasty, except in cases of hypertrophic cardiomyopathy, where it can worsen outflow tract obstruction. Relative contraindications include patients with rheumatic leaflets, stiffened leaflets, or small annulus where stenosis can result.[20]

Repair of the ventricle includes posterior wall plication and papillary muscle approximation. In addition, surgical mitral valve replacement has also been used for mitral regurgitation.[18]

Percutaneous approaches

Various percutaneous approaches exist for repair of mitral regurgitation that affect multiple areas of the mitral valve complex. Leaflet therapies include edge-to-edge repair (E-Valve or MitraClip), space occupier (PercuPro, Cardiosolutions), and leaflet ablation (ThermoCool, Biosense Webster). Annuloplasty can be indirect, such as the coronary sinus approach (Monarc from Edwards LifeSciences, Carillon from Cardiac Dimensions, Viacor) or an asymmetrical approach (St. Jude device, NIH Cerclage). Annuloplasty can also be direct, such as mechanical cinching (Mitralign, Accucinch, Millipede), energy-mediated cinching (QuantumCor and Recor), or a hybrid approach (MitralSolutions from MitraSolutions and MiCardia from MiCardia/ValCare). Chordal implants can also be placed percutaneously via a transapical (Neochord, Mitraflex) and transseptal (Babic) approach. LV remodeling approaches also exist through the Coapsys and iCoapsys systems. Percutaneous mitral valve replacement has also been developed, with the Endovalve-Herrmann (Endovalve) and CardiAQ (CardiAQ) being two notable examples.

Data behind mitral valve repair and replacement

Multiple outcome measures for surgery after mitral regurgitation exist, including early and late survival, recurrence of mitral regurgitation, and the need for reoperation. These depend on preoperative factors such as age, symptoms, LV function, atrial fibrillation, MR etiology, and the presence of CAD. The ability to repair or replace the valve also plays an important role. Adverse surgical outcomes are associated with older age, NYHA III/IV symptoms, LVEF <60%, preexisting atrial fibrillation, and associated coronary artery disease. Mitral valve repair is found to be "more physiologic" than mitral valve replacement, leading to certain indications for repair and different ones for replacement.

Durability of repair at 20–25 years is in roughly 90% of patients.[21,22] Patients more likely to have reoperation include those who were more likely to have replacement in the first place, including anterior or bileaflet pathology, rheumatic/infectious/ischemic etiology, in addition to lack of ring annuloplasty. In addition, low surgeon/center volume were predictors of replacement over repair.[23] After 10 years, myxomatous valve repair usually ends with moderate mitral regurgitation in 15–30% of patients and severe in 5–10% of patients.[24,25] For functional/ischemic mitral valve repair the rate was 20–30% at 1–5 years,[26] which sparked changes in technique. A recent meta-analysis showed that repair was often better than replacement with short-term odds ratio of 2.67 and a 6-month hazard ratio of 1.4.[27]

Mitral valve repair allows the ability to avoid anticoagulation, and has long-term durability over a bioprosthesis, less ventricular function impairment, less posterior wall rupture, and less early and late mortality. However, mitral valve replacement can eliminate mitral regurgitation better and has better durability for elderly patients and better results in patients with hypertrophic cardiomyopathy. The overall durability of bioprosthetic heart valves, especially in patients <60 years of age, is limited to 50% freedom from structural valve deterioration or reoperation after 17 years.[28] The overall mortality for isolated mitral valve replacement is 6%.[23]

Adams et al.[29] raised important points about issues with trials that study mitral regurgitation. First, various definitions for mitral regurgitation exist, including ones that are based on etiology, dysfunction, and lesion severity. Second, there is often variation in surgical techniques, which can lead to different "acceptable" early results for mitral valve repair. Third, echocardiographic data is often not available pre- and postoperation. Fourth, studies often have significant methodologic limitations, such as low case volume, long study periods, bias by era, and the reliance on retrospective studies. Fifth, there are often evolving technology and protocols within institutions. Sixth, there are statistical limitations, such as competing outcomes (death vs. reoperation vs. transplant), qualitative grading (mild, moderate, and severe), and irregular echocardiographic follow-up.

Controversies: Surgical coronary artery disease and moderate–severe ischemic mitral regurgitation

What is the role of surgery in ischemic mitral regurgitation? Options include coronary artery bypass graft (CABG) alone, CABG with mitral valve repair, and CABG with mitral valve replacement.

CABG alone may lead to higher perioperative mortality and reduced survival, especially in those with impaired LV function,[30] but this is controversial.[31] However, 47% of patients with moderate-to-severe mitral valve regurgitation that had CABG alone went on to being hospitalized for congestive heart failure.[32]

CABG with mitral repair is another option. Large series have shown 50% residual or recurrent moderate-to-severe mitral regurgitation at 6 months,[33] but the use of outdated techniques have sparked new studies that contradict this finding. The Randomized Ischemic Mitral Evaluation (RIME) study showed that adding mitral annuloplasty to CABG in patients with moderate ischemic MR with LVEF >30% may improve functional capacity, left ventricular reverse modeling, and MR severity at 1 year.[34] The STICH trial enrolled patients with LVEF ≤35% and coronary artery disease. A comparison of mitral valve surgery and CABG to CABG alone in 120 patients with moderate-to-severe mitral regurgitation resulted in early morbidity but late survival.[35] The one randomized trial to compare mitral valve restrictive annuloplasty plus coronary bypass grafting versus coronary bypass grafting alone for moderate ischemic mitral regurgitation was not powered to predict survival and only showed the benefits of functional class, ejection function, and left ventricular diameter in the short term.[36]

CABG with mitral valve replacement has been studied, but no randomized controlled trials exist. In addition, patients referred to replacement were higher risk, including salvage redo operations as well as acute ischemic mitral regurgitation due to papillary muscle rupture.[37] Poor outcome may also have to do with lack of sparing of the subvalvar apparatus, which is a known risk factor for low cardiac output, poor perioperative mortality, and long-term survival. Older bioprostheses have more issues with hemorrhage and thrombosis. In addition, redo salvage replacement after mitral valve repair has the added issue of having to place a valve inside an annulus with prior annuloplasty, increasing the rate of mitral valve stenosis.

Controversies: Moderate-to-severe mitral valve regurgitation and congestive heart failure

Patients with heart failure have mitral regurgitation often due to left ventricular dilatation and incomplete coaptation. There is significant controversy as to whether mitral valve surgery will help these patients. A small sample size study by Wu et al. showed no mortality benefit for patients with significant MR and severe left ventricular dysfunction.[38] A few retrospective studies showed benefit, for example, DeBonis et al. showed a hospital mortality of 2.3% for repair and 12.5% for replacement with a 2.5-year survival of 92% for repair and 73% for replacement.[39] The STICH trial showed a hazard ratio of 0.41 comparing mitral repair and CABG to CABG alone in patients with ischemic mitral regurgitation and decreased left ventricular systolic function.[35] Overall, if the patient has no capacity for revascularization, one can consider repair if comorbidity is low. Other options include medical therapy with cardiac synchronization therapy, ventricular assist devices, cardiac restraint devices, or heart transplantation. The use of percutaneous mitral clip procedure in nonoperative patients with severe LV dysfunction is another option.

Indications for therapy in patients with primary mitral regurgitation

Primary mitral regurgitation is when there are intrinsic lesions of the mitral valve apparatus. Predictive outcomes for primary mitral regurgitation include age, atrial fibrillation, pulmonary hypertension, and repair of the valve. A cutoff of 45 mm exists for the flail leaflet and LVESD ≥ 40 mm (≥22 mm/m² BSA) is associated with increased mortality with medical treatment.[40]

An overview of the 2012 ESC guidelines flowsheet is seen in Figure 39.4. According to the 2012 ESC guidelines, the indications for mitral valve surgery in chronic primary mitral regurgitation include

1. For acute severe mitral regurgitation, urgent surgery is indicated. Papillary muscle rupture requires stabilization (intra-aortic balloon pump [IABP], inotropic agents, vasodilators when possible) and urgent surgical treatment, most likely with valve replacement.[41]
2. Mitral valve repair is preferred when it is expected to be durable (class I, LOE C).
3. Symptomatic patients with LVEF >30% and LVESD <55 mm should go to surgery (class I, LOE B).
4. Asymptomatic patients with preserved LVEF

a. New onset of atrial fibrillation or pulmonary hypertension (PASP at rest >50 mmHg) should go to surgery (class IIa, LOE C)[42]
b. High likelihood of durable repair, low surgical risk, and flail leaflet and LVESD ≥ 40 mm (class IIa, LOE C)
c. High likelihood of durable repair, low surgical risk and
   i. LA dilatation and sinus rhythm—(Class IIb, LOE C)[43]
   ii. Pulmonary hypertension on exercise (SPAP ≥ 60 mmHg at exercise)—(class IIb, LOE C)[44]
5. Severe LV dysfunction (LVEF <30% and/or LVESD >55 mm) refractory to medical therapy with high likelihood of durable repair and low comorbidity (class IIa, LOE C)
6. If inoperable or considered high risk by the "heart team," have life expectancy >1 year, symptomatic and fulfill echo criteria of eligibility, can get percutaneous edge-to-edge repair (class IIb, LOE C)

Indications for therapy in patients with secondary mitral regurgitation

Operative mortality and long-term prognosis is worse in secondary mitral regurgitation than primary mitral regurgitation. Surgery for coronary artery disease is often performed, but does not necessarily provide survival benefit. Repair is often better than replacement according to a meta-analysis, but no randomized data exist. Percutaneous

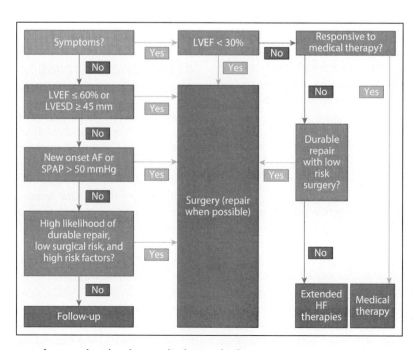

Figure 39.4 Management of severe chronic primary mitral regurgitation.

therapy with the EVEREST trial and from observational study show feasibility if there is no severe tethering and may provide beneficial in functional condition and left ventricular function.[45]

Therefore, the indications for mitral valve surgery in chronic secondary mitral regurgitation include

1. Severe MR considered in patients going to bypass surgery (class I, LOE C)
2. Surgery should be considered if patients with moderate MR are having CABG.
   a. If patients are capable of exercising, exercise echocardiography should be considered and exercise-induced dyspnea and large increase in MR severity and systolic pulmonary artery pressure favor combined surgery
3. Surgery should be considered in symptomatic patients with severe MR, LVEF <30%, option for revascularization, and evidence of viability (class IIa, LOE C).
4. Surgery may be considered if patients with severe MR, LVEF >30% who are symptomatic despite optimal medical management (including CRT if indicated) and have low comorbidity, when revascularization is not indicated (level IIb, LOE C).
5. Percutaneous mitral clip can be considered in patients with symptomatic severe secondary MR despite optimal medical therapy (including CRT if indicated), who fulfill the echocardiographic criteria of eligibility, are inoperable or high surgical risk, and have life expectancy greater than 1 year (level IIb, LOE C).

References

1. Carpentier A. Cardiac valve surgery—The "French correction". *J Thorac Cardiovasc Surg* 1983;86:323–37.
2. Barlow JB, Pocock WA. Mitral valve prolapse, the specific billowing mitral leaflet syndrome, or an insignificant non-ejection systolic click. *Am Heart J* 1979;97:277–85.
3. Anyanwu AC, Adams DH. Etiologic classification of degenerative mitral valve disease: Barlow's disease and fibroelastic deficiency. *Semin Thorac Cardiovasc Surg* 2007;19:90–6.
4. Atalay S, Ucar T, Ozcelik N, Ekici F, Tutar E. Echocardiographic evaluation of mitral valve in patients with pure rheumatic mitral regurgitation. *Turk J Pediatr* 2007;49:148–53.
5. Foster E. Evaluation of mitral valve regurgitation: Implications for percutaneous mitral valve repair. 2005;2013:7.
6. Enriquez-Sarano M, Basmadjian AJ, Rossi A, Bailey KR, Seward JB, Tajik AJ. Progression of mitral regurgitation: A prospective Doppler echocardiographic study. *J Am Coll Cardiol* 1999;34:1137–44.
7. Perloff JK, Harvey WP. Auscultatory and phonocardiographic manifestations of pure mitral regurgitation. *Prog Cardiovasc Dis* 1962;5:172–94.
8. Grayburn PA, Weissman NJ, Zamorano JL. Quantitation of mitral regurgitation. *Circulation* 2012;126:2005–17.
9. Zoghbi WA, Enriquez-Sarano M, Foster E et al. Recommendations for evaluation of the severity of native valvular regurgitation with two-dimensional and Doppler echocardiography. *J Am Soc Echocardiogr* 2003;16:777–802.
10. Bonow RO, Carabello BA, Chatterjee K et al. ACC/AHA 2006 guidelines for the management of patients with valvular heart disease: A report of the American College of Cardiology/American Heart Association Task Force on Practice Guidelines (writing Committee to Revise the 1998 guidelines for the management of patients with valvular heart disease) developed in collaboration with the Society of Cardiovascular Anesthesiologists endorsed by the Society for Cardiovascular Angiography and Interventions and the Society of Thoracic Surgeons. *J Am Coll Cardiol* 2006;48:e1–148.
11. Chan KM, Wage R, Symmonds K et al. Towards comprehensive assessment of mitral regurgitation using cardiovascular magnetic resonance. *J Cardiovasc Magn Reson* 2008;10:61.
12. Ling LH, Enriquez-Sarano M, Seward JB et al. Clinical outcome of mitral regurgitation due to flail leaflet. *N Engl J Med.* 1996;335(19):1417–23.
13. Enriquez-Sarano M, Tajik AJ. Natural history of mitral regurgitation due to flail leaflets. *Eur Heart J.* 1997;18(5):705–7.
14. Bonow RO, Cheitlin MD, Crawford MH, Douglas PS. Task Force 3: Valvular heart disease. *J Am Coll Cardiol* 2005;45:1334–40.
15. Reed D, Abbott RD, Smucker ML, Kaul S. Prediction of outcome after mitral valve replacement in patients with symptomatic chronic mitral regurgitation. The importance of left atrial size. *Circulation* 1991;84:23–34.
16. Vahanian A, Alfieri O, Andreotti F et al. Guidelines on the management of valvular heart disease (version 2012). *Eur Heart J* 2012;33:2451–96.
17. van Bommel RJ, Marsan NA, Delgado V et al. Cardiac resynchronization therapy as a therapeutic option in patients with moderate-severe functional mitral regurgitation and high operative risk. *Circulation* 2011;124:912–9.
18. Glower DD. Surgical approaches to mitral regurgitation. *J Am Coll Cardiol* 2012;60:1315–22.
19. Frater RW, Vetter HO, Zussa C, Dahm M. Chordal replacement in mitral valve repair. *Circulation* 1990;82:IV125–30.
20. Alfieri O, De Bonis M. The role of the edge-to-edge repair in the surgical treatment of mitral regurgitation. *J Card Surg* 2010;25:536–41.
21. Mohty D, Orszulak TA, Schaff HV, Avierinos JF, Tajik JA, Enriquez-Sarano M. Very long-term survival and durability of mitral valve repair for mitral valve prolapse. *Circulation* 2001;104: I1–I7.
22. Braunberger E, Deloche A, Berrebi A et al. Very long-term results (more than 20 years) of valve repair with Carpentier's techniques in nonrheumatic mitral valve insufficiency. *Circulation* 2001;104:I8–11.
23. Bolling SF, Li S, O'Brien SM, Brennan JM, Prager RL, Gammie JS. Predictors of mitral valve repair: Clinical and surgeon factors. *Ann Thorac Surg* 2010;90:1904–11; discussion 12.
24. Salvador L, Mirone S, Bianchini R et al. A 20-year experience with mitral valve repair with artificial chordae in 608 patients. *J Thorac Cardiovasc Surg* 2008;135:1280–7.
25. Lawrie GM, Earle EA, Earle N. Intermediate-term results of a non-resectional dynamic repair technique in 662 patients with mitral valve prolapse and mitral regurgitation. *J Thorac Cardiovasc Surg* 2011;141:368–76.
26. McGee EC, Gillinov AM, Blackstone EH et al. Recurrent mitral regurgitation after annuloplasty for functional ischemic mitral regurgitation. *J Thorac Cardiovasc Surg* 2004;128:916–24.
27. Vassileva CM, Boley T, Markwell S, Hazelrigg S. Meta-analysis of short-term and long-term survival following repair versus replacement for ischemic mitral regurgitation. *Eur J Cardiothorac Surg* 2011;39:295–303.
28. Rizzoli G, Mirone S, Ius P et al. Fifteen-year results with the Hancock II valve: A multicenter experience. *J Thorac Cardiovasc Surg* 2006;132:602–9, 9 e1–4.
29. Adams DH, Anyanwu A. Pitfalls and limitations in measuring and interpreting the outcomes of mitral valve repair. *J Thorac Cardiovasc Surg* 2006;131:523–9.

30. Grossi EA, Crooke GA, DiGiorgi PL et al. Impact of moderate functional mitral insufficiency in patients undergoing surgical revascularization. *Circulation* 2006;114:I573–6.

31. Diodato MD, Moon MR, Pasque MK et al. Repair of ischemic mitral regurgitation does not increase mortality or improve long-term survival in patients undergoing coronary artery revascularization: A propensity analysis. *Ann Thorac Surg* 2004;78:794–9; discussion -9.

32. Mallidi HR, Pelletier MP, Lamb J et al. Late outcomes in patients with uncorrected mild to moderate mitral regurgitation at the time of isolated coronary artery bypass grafting. *J Thorac Cardiovasc Surg* 2004;127:636–44.

33. Calafiore AM, Di Mauro M, Gallina S et al. Mitral valve surgery for chronic ischemic mitral regurgitation. *Ann Thorac Surg* 2004;77:1989–97.

34. Chan KM, Punjabi PP, Flather M et al. Coronary artery bypass surgery with or without mitral valve annuloplasty in moderate functional ischemic mitral regurgitation: Final results of the Randomized Ischemic Mitral Evaluation (RIME) trial. *Circulation* 2012;126:2502–10.

35. Deja MA, Grayburn PA, Sun B et al. Influence of mitral regurgitation repair on survival in the surgical treatment for ischemic heart failure trial. *Circulation* 2012;125:2639–48.

36. Fattouch K, Guccione F, Sampognaro R et al. POINT: Efficacy of adding mitral valve restrictive annuloplasty to coronary artery bypass grafting in patients with moderate ischemic mitral valve regurgitation: A randomized trial. *J Thorac Cardiovasc Surg* 2009;138:278–85.

37. Grossi EA, Goldberg JD, LaPietra A et al. Ischemic mitral valve reconstruction and replacement: Comparison of long-term survival and complications. *J Thorac Cardiovasc Surg* 2001;122:1107–24.

38. Wu AH, Aaronson KD, Bolling SF, Pagani FD, Welch K, Koelling TM. Impact of mitral valve annuloplasty on mortality risk in patients with mitral regurgitation and left ventricular systolic dysfunction. *J Am Coll Cardiol* 2005;45:381–7.

39. De Bonis M, Ferrara D, Taramasso M et al. Mitral replacement or repair for functional mitral regurgitation in dilated and ischemic cardiomyopathy: Is it really the same? *Ann Thorac Surg* 2012;94:44–51.

40. Tribouilloy C, Grigioni F, Avierinos JF et al. Survival implication of left ventricular end-systolic diameter in mitral regurgitation due to flail leaflets a long-term follow-up multicenter study. *J Am Coll Cardiol* 2009;54:1961–8.

41. Russo A, Suri RM, Grigioni F et al. Clinical outcome after surgical correction of mitral regurgitation due to papillary muscle rupture. *Circulation* 2008;118:1528–34.

42. Camm AJ, Lip GY, De Caterina R et al. 2012 focused update of the ESC Guidelines for the management of atrial fibrillation: An update of the 2010 ESC Guidelines for the management of atrial fibrillation. Developed with the special contribution of the European Heart Rhythm Association. *Eur Heart J* 2012;33:2719–47.

43. Le Tourneau T, Messika-Zeitoun D, Russo A et al. Impact of left atrial volume on clinical outcome in organic mitral regurgitation. *J Am Coll Cardiol* 2010;56:570–8.

44. Magne J, Lancellotti P, Pierard LA. Exercise-induced changes in degenerative mitral regurgitation. *J Am Coll Cardiol*. 2010;56:300–9.

45. Feldman T, Foster E, Glower DD et al. Percutaneous repair or surgery for mitral regurgitation. *N Engl J Med* 2011;364:1395–406.

40

Mitral valve insufficiency: Mitral valve repair with the MitraClip

Mamoo Nakamura and Saibal Kar

Introduction

Mitral valve (MV) insufficiency (or regurgitation) is one of the most common valvular heart diseases, particularly in the aging population.[1] As the aging population increases, the clinical impact of this pathology becomes more significant. In patients with severe symptomatic mitral regurgitation (MR), surgical repair of MV is considered a mainstream therapy to improve quality of life and/or prognosis. However, owing to higher risk, the surgical MV repair tends to be underutilized in the elderly population and those with abnormal cardiac function who potentially benefit from this invasive modality.[2] The MitraClip (Abbott Vascular, Menlo Park, CA, USA) is a catheter-based device that enables the repair of severe MR by clipping anterior and posterior leaflets with minimum invasiveness. This novel device simulates the surgical edge-to-edge repair of MV that was originally described by Alferi,[3] and has been demonstrated to effectively reduce MR severity, thereby improving hemodynamics and quality of life of treated patient. The MitraClip was available for use in the United States as of October 24, 2013, for patients with degenerative MR who are at a prohibitive surgical risk for MV surgery. This is determined by a heart valve team that includes a cardiac surgeon experienced in MV surgery and a cardiologist experienced in MV disease and patients in whom existing comorbidities would not preclude the expected benefit of the MV regurgitation reduction; in Europe, this is for both functional and degenerative MR. It is the most widely used catheter-based device for MV repair with nearly 11,000 patients (2000 of them have been enrolled in prospective clinical trials) treated as of October 2013. In this chapter, clinical indication, procedural steps, and a recent perspective from a published study regarding the MitraClip are reviewed.

Indication of mitral valve repair with MitraClip

Although there is no consensus-specific guideline for MV repair with MitraClip, clinical indication for surgical repair is well documented in the guidelines published by academic organizations such as the American Heart Association, American College of Cardiology, and European Society of Cardiology.[4,5] Generally, patients with symptomatic severe MR are well accepted for MV repair for symptom relief and potential survival benefit. Additionally, anatomic suitability of MV has to be assessed on consideration of the MitraClip. These include (1) a coaptation length of at least 2 mm and depth of no more than 11 mm for a functional MR, and (2) a flail gap and width less than 10 and 15 mm, respectively, for MR due to flail leaflet. A regurgitant jet originated at the A2 to P2 segment is also considered a favorable anatomic feature for the MitraClip.[6,7] Patients who have untreated and active endocarditis, rheumatic valvular heart disease, and mitral stenosis are generally considered for contraindication of the MitraClip. Given its less invasive and well-tolerated nature, together with surgical MV repair being considered a gold standard approach for operative patients, currently, the MitraClip procedure is more qualified for patients with a high surgical risk who develop symptomatic MR with suitable anatomy for this procedure.

MitraClip device system

The MitraClip system is a triaxial catheter system, consisting of two main components: the steerable guide catheter and the clip delivery system (CDS) (Figure 40.1a) The steerable guide catheter is a 24-French in the proximal portion with a 22-French tip that is placed in the left atrium through the interatrial septum. There is a knob on its proximal shaft that is used to deflect its tip. The CDS is a delivery catheter with the steerable sleeve that is equipped with two knobs to adjust its tip to medial–lateral and anterior–posterior direction. The mitral clip is attached on the tip of the delivery catheter and is a cobalt–chromium implant that has two arms and two grippers (Figure 40.1b). Each arm is 5-mm wide and 9-mm long and is covered in a polyester fabric that facilitates tissue ingrowth.[8] The CDS catheter is

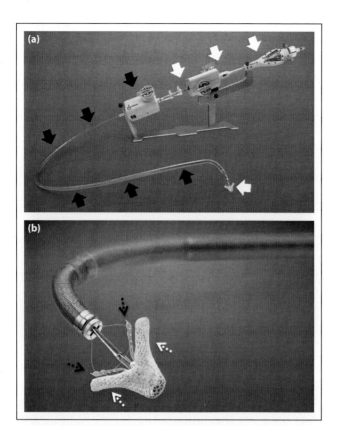

Figure 40.1   (**See color insert.**) The MitraClip device system. (a) Two main components of the MitraClip system. Black arrows indicate the steerable guide catheter and white arrows the clip delivery system that is advanced through the steerable guide catheter. (b) The MitraClip attached on the tip of the clip delivery catheter has two arms (white broken arrows) and two grippers (black broken arrows).

introduced into the left atrium through the steerable guide catheter in order to properly position an implantable clip by manipulation and advancement of the steerable sleeve and the delivery catheter.

Procedural steps; keys and tips for a successful MitraClip procedure

The MitraClip procedure is performed by using both transesophageal echocardiogram (TEE) and fluoroscopic guidance. General anesthesia is usually conducted for patient comfort and breath control to achieve precise deployment of the clip on the target portion of the leaflets. Owing to procedural complexity, a multidisciplinary team consisting of one to two interventional cardiologists, an anesthesiologist, and an echocardiographer are generally involved. The right femoral vein is used for the device access site. Since the MitraClip procedure requires placement of a large-caliber sheath, preclosure of the venous access using

a vascular closure device may facilitate hemostasis with a reduction of excessive bleeding on conclusion of the procedure. The other central venous access and an arterial access should also be obtained to monitor hemodynamics during the MitraClip procedure.

There are several crucial steps for a successful MitraClip procedure. These include (1) MR evaluation, (2) site-specific transseptal puncture, and (3) optimal positioning/deployment of the MitraClip. Immediately prior to the MitraClip procedure, TEE should be performed to assess baseline MR severity using color Doppler and pulmonary vein flow pattern, a mean pressure gradient across the MV, and a location and direction of the MR jet in relation to MV anatomy. These measurements should be repeated on each MV clip deployment.

On obtaining vascular accesses and baseline MR and hemodynamic assessment, the transseptal puncture is performed (Figure 40.2). In order to optimize positioning of the clip, site selection of septal puncture is crucial. Generally, transseptal puncture should be performed aiming at the posterior/superior aspect of the atrial septum; entering through this site is likely to facilitate directionality and positioning of the MitraClip to the target MV leaflets. Bicaval (superior/inferior location) and a short-axis (anterior/posterior) image of TEE is vigorously used to optimize the position of the septal puncture system (Figure 40.2a and b). Prior to the septal puncture, using a four-chamber view of TEE, a distance from the projected puncture site and the coaptation site of MV should be measured and adjusted by approximately 3.5–4.5 cm (Figure 40.2c).

On successful septal puncture and following administration of anticoagulation, the steerable guide catheter is advanced via femoral venous access over the 0.035 inch stiff wire and its 22-French tip is placed across the interatrial septum into the left atrium. Careful attention should be paid to minimize excessive trauma to the atrial septum on advancement of the tip of the steerable guide catheter. On advancement of the catheter, real-time short-axis view of TEE is used to confirm appropriate positioning of the guide catheter tip (Figure 40.3a). Then the CDS system is inserted through the steerable guide catheter and introduced into the left atrium (Figure 40.3b). The direction of the clip is adjusted by manipulation of the guide catheter either clockwise or counterclockwise and rotating the knobs of the CDS sleeve in the medial–lateral or anterior-posterior direction as appropriate. A short-axis, intercommissural two-chamber and left ventricle out track (LVOT) view of TEE is used to determine the direction of the clip toward the LV apex (Figure 40.4). The direction of the clip shaft is optimized to where the projected clip deployment splits the regurgitation jet in two equal amounts while maintaining trajectory of the clip shaft on the perpendicular angle to mitral annulus (and/or coaptation of MV) in the intercommissural two-chamber and LVOT view of

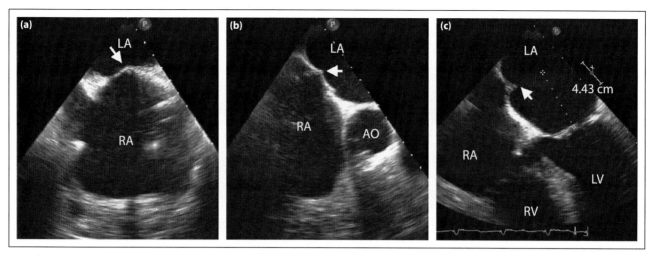

Figure 40.2   Transesophageal echocardiogram (TEE)-guided septal puncture. (a) Bicaval view showed tenting by the sheath (indicated by the white arrow) in midlevel of atrial septum. (b) Under short-axis view, the septal puncture system is directed to the posterior aspect of the atrial septum. (c) Once the septal puncture site is determined, the distance between the projected puncture site and the mitral valve coaptation is measured to confirm appropriateness of this length for optimal clip delivery system manipulation.

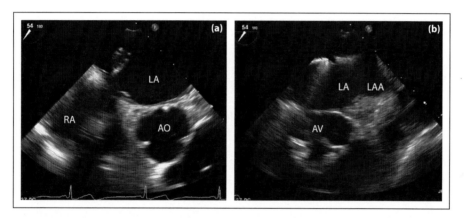

Figure 40.3   Following the placement of the steerable guide catheter in the left atrium (a), the clip delivery system (CDS) is introduced into the left atrium using TEE short-axis view (b).

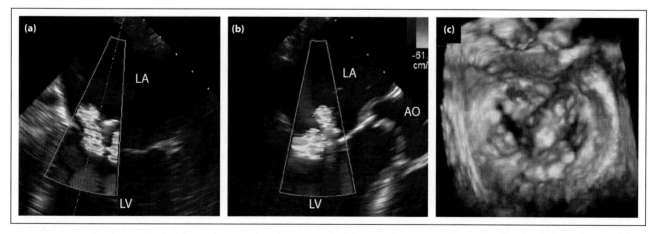

Figure 40.4   (**See color insert.**) The direction of the clip shaft is optimized by the manipulation of the steerable guide catheter and clip delivery system. Following the opening of the MitraClip in the left atrium, under a intercommissural two-chamber view, the clip shaft is directed to divide the regurgitation jet (a). The direction of the clip shaft is adjusted so that the shaft is perpendicular to the mitral annulus both in intercommissural two-chamber (a) and LVOT view (b). On determination of clip shaft trajectory, it is rotated to position the clip arm perpendicular to the commissure. Three-dimensional reconstruction of TEE image facilitates this maneuver (c).

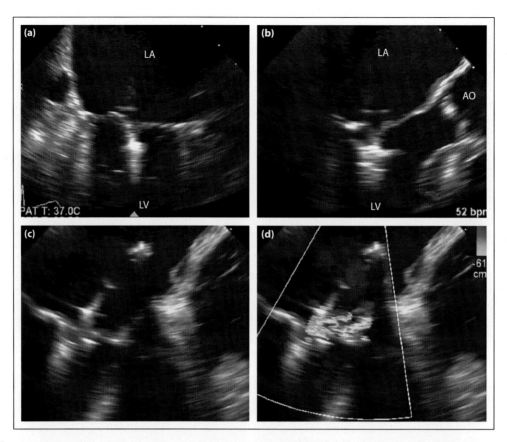

Figure 40.5 **(See color insert.)** The clip delivery system is slowly advanced into the left ventricle with real-time TEE guidance using an intercommissural two-chamber (a) and LVOT view (b). On final confirmation of the clip arm position, the clip delivery system is slowly pulled back immediately under the mitral valve leaflet to grasp. The LVOT view is the standard view, as this allows slight adjustment of clip arm in anterior–posterior direction (c). Using color Doppler, the clip arm is completely closed to confirm the reduction of regurgitation jet (d).

the TEE (Figure 40.4a and b). A fluoroscopic right anterior oblique (RAO) caudal view is also used to assist a process to determine the appropriate trajectory of the clip shaft. Following this, the clip and gripper are opened and rotated to position the arm perpendicular to the line of coaptation (Figure 40.4c). The clip is then advanced into the LV while maintaining an open angle and deployed to the target portion of the MV if an adequate position to the coaptation line is maintained (Figure 40.5a and b). The LVOT view of TEE is generally used in order to confirm appropriate gripping and closure of the clip at the target anterior and posterior leaflet (Figure 40.5c and d). If a location of the clip is suboptimal, it can be retrieved and repositioned unless it is completely released from the CDS. Furthermore, if further MR reduction is required, more than one clip can be used. In this case, advancement of the clip into the LV has to be performed with the clip remaining closed.

Prior to the complete release of the clip, it is crucial to assess a successful reduction of MR without an increase of the transmitral gradient (no more than a mean gradient of 4 mmHg). A comprehensive TEE assessment of mitral function should be performed. Then, the clip is released

from the clip delivery shaft and a final TEE assessment is carried out (Figure 40.6).

Potential complications and postprocedure care

Potential serious complications include access site bleeding; procedural associated cardiac trauma, including cardiac tamponade and significant residual interatrial shunt at septal puncture site; and device embolization. Generally, the latter three events are exceptionally rare, but if one occurs, prompt treatment is required. Access site bleeding that is likely associated with the placement of a large-caliber guide catheter (24-French) can cause serious clinical sequelae and is potentially life-threatening. However, this may be reduced by application of a preclosure approach using vascular closure devices. Alternatively, some operators apply the "figure 8" stitch with good results.

In an uneventful case of the MitraClip procedure, a recovery process after procedure is generally fast even

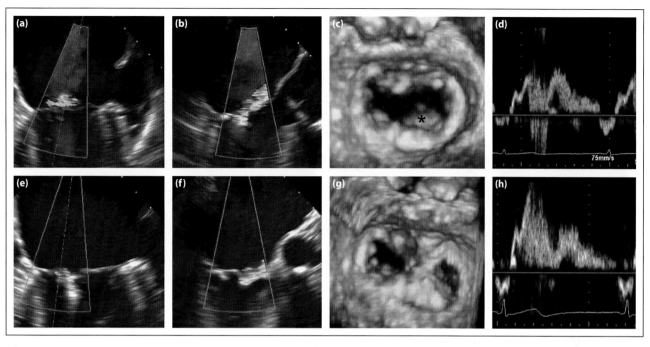

Figure 40.6   (**See color insert.**) A case of successful repair with the MitraClip in a patient with mitral regurgitation due to flail posterior leaflet. Baseline TEE showed significant eccentric mitral regurgitation (a and b) due to frail P2 posterior leaflet (asterisk in c). A Doppler of a pulmonary vein showed systolic flow reversal (d). Following deployment of the mitral clip, successful improvement of MR was observed (e and f). Three-dimensional reconstruction of the TEE image showed successful deployment of the MitraClip at the target portion of mitral valve (g) and systolic flow reversal of pulmonary vein also improved (h).

in high-risk cases. Following a successful procedure, the patient can be observed in the telemetry floor for monitoring and then can be discharged the next day if the hospital course is uneventful. Prior to discharge from the hospital, a follow-up transthoracic echocardiogram may be performed to evaluate the stability of the deployed clip and to confirm consistent reduction of MR by the MitraClip.

Safety, feasibility, and clinical outcomes

Tables 40.1 and 40.2 provide a summary of clinical outcomes in major published trials of the MitraClip. The MitraClip procedure is a generally safe and well-tolerated procedure in a wide spectrum of patients with respect to surgical risk and comorbidities. In the EVEREST and EVEREST II trials, early mortality rate after the MitraClip procedure was extremely low in the surgical cohort (~1%) and even in the high-risk cohort, the 30-day mortality was 7.7%.[6,7,9] A low, early mortality rate was consistently observed in subsequent European registries that enrolled larger numbers of patients with a higher risk for surgery.[10,11] The most frequent adverse event related to the MitraClip is blood transfusion, with an incidence ranging from 5% to 17% of the studied patients. Yet, an occurrence of a blood transfusion was significantly less in the patient with

MitraClip than in those with surgical MV repair. Cardiac tamponade and significant septal defect at the septal puncture site is a rare complication associated with the MitraClip procedure with occurrence in 1–2% of the studied population. A successful clip deployment rate at the MV is generally very high and ≥90% throughout the published studies. Device embolization is extremely rare.

Based on the EVEREST II trial, the surgical MV repair is generally more effective in the reduction of MR severity compared to the MitraClip. In prespecified subgroup analysis, younger age (less than 70 years old), degenerative MR, and normal left ventricular ejection fraction (>60%) are associated with a less favorable outcome with a MitraClip procedure.[7] Nonetheless, the MitraClip constantly demonstrated that it can improve overall MR severity, albeit to a lesser degree in this diverse patient subset with respect to surgical risk and medical comorbidities. Furthermore, a successful MitraClip procedure results in immediate hemodynamic improvement as well as a sustained and improved quality of life, left ventricular function and dimension during the clinical follow-up up to 2 years.[7,9–12] These favorable functional and anatomical effects are potentially associated with the reduction of admission to the hospital due to heart failure exacerbation.[9] It appears that the successful and effective immediate MR reduction following a MitraClip procedure is the likely key to successful and favorable clinical outcomes

Table 40.1 Summary table of clinical outcomes in patient treated with MitraClip from clinical trials

Trial	Trial design	Number of patients	[a]Patient characteristics	Study results
EVEREST/ EVEREST II pivotal	Prospective, multicenter, single-arm study	107	Mean age—71 Baseline NYHA III/IV—46% Functional MR—21%	Acute procedure success with reduction in MR ≤ grade 2 in 74% of patients (n = 79) No procedure-related death Surgery free in 70% of patient (75 of 107) after a median follow-up of 680 days [b]The primary composite endpoint for efficacy—66%
EVEREST II (surgical cohort)	International multicenter, randomized comparison (2:1 to MitraClip: Surgery)	184 in MitraClip arm (a total of 279 patients)	Mean age—67 Baseline NYHA III/IV—52% Functional MR—27%	Acute procedure success of MitraClip with reduction in MR ≤ grade 2 in 77% of patients (137 of 178 patients) [c]Superior primary endpoint for safety in MitraClip arm (15% vs. 48% in surgical arm, p < 0.001), driven by less blood transfusion [b]Inferior primary composite end point for efficacy in MitraClip arm (55% vs. 73% in surgical arm, p = 0.007), driven by more surgical MV repair during follow-up
EVEREST II (high-risk cohort)	Prospective, multicenter, single-arm study	78	Mean age—77 STS mortality score—14% Baseline NYHA III/IV—90% Functional MR—59%	Successful MitraClip implantation in 96% (75/78) with MR reduction achieved in 80% (62/78) Thirty days mortality—7.7% One-year survival rate—76%
TRAMI registry	Multicenter single-arm registry in Germany	486 (177 in prospective and 309 in retrospective)	Mean age—75 STS mortality score—11% Logistic EuroSCORE—23% Baseline NYHA III/IV—93% Functional MR—67%	Acute procedural success rate—94% (with MR reduction into moderate to mild degree) No procedure-related death In-hospital and follow-up mortality (85 days median follow-up duration)—2.5% and 12.5%, respectively
ACCESS EUROPE	Multicenter prospective single-arm registry	567	Mean age—74 Logistic EuroSCORE—23% Baseline NYHA III/IV—85% Functional MR—77%	MitraClip implant rate—99.6% Thirty days mortality—3.4% One-year mortality—17.3% MR ≤ grade 2 at one year—79%

[a] Patient characteristics of EVEREST II trial are of the MitraClip arm.

[b] Freedom from MR >2+, surgical mitral valve repair, and death at 12 months.

[c] Major adverse event at 30 days defined as the composite of death, myocardial infarction, reoperation for failed mitral valve surgery, nonelective cardiovascular surgery for adverse events, stroke, renal failure, deep wound infection, mechanical ventilation for more than 48 h, gastrointestinal complication requiring surgery, new-onset permanent atrial fibrillation, septicemia, and transfusion of two units or more of blood.

Table 40.2 Summary table of core clinical trials

Study	Design	N (MitraClip)
EVEREST I	Feasibility	55
EVEREST II	Roll-in	60
	Single-arm high-risk	78
	Randomized to MitraClip	184
REALISM continued access	Single-arm high-risk, non-high-risk	888
Compassionate/emergency use	Nonrandomized	66
ACCESS Europe Phase I	Commercial registry	567
ACCESS Europe Phase II	Commercial registry	286
COAPT	Randomized to heart failure therapy	17
RESHAPE	Randomized to heart failure therapy	1
ANZ	Single-arm	54
Commericial	Commercial use	8633
Total		10,889

regardless of patient subset and MR etiology. Lastly, durability of the MitraClip beyond 2 years remains uncertain and will need to be confirmed with follow-up studies of previously conducted clinical trials.

Future perspective and conclusions

The MitraClip is a safe and effective alternative approach to surgical MV repair (or replacement) for the treatment of symptomatic severe MR with suitable MV anatomy. This novel device has the potential to effectively improve MR and, therefore, cardiac function and quality of life of the treated patient with minimum invasiveness. Based on results from clinical studies, in current practice, the MitraClip is more suitable for certain patient populations, such as those with a higher surgical risk, older age, cardiac dysfunction, and degenerative MR. In order to evaluate further the efficacy of the MitraClip in high-risk surgical patients with functional MR, a multicenter trial (COAPT) in the United States and RESHAPE in Europe that randomizes this patient population to the MitraClip and conventional medical therapy is currently underway.

References

1. Iung B, Vahanian A. Epidemiology of valvular heart disease in the adult. *Nat Rev Cardiol* 2011;8(3):162–72.
2. Mirabel M, Iung B, Baron G, Messika-Zeitoun D, Detaint D, Vanoverschelde JL et al. What are the characteristics of patients with severe, symptomatic, mitral regurgitation who are denied surgery? *Eur Heart J* 2007;28(11):1358–65.
3. Alfieri O, Maisano F, De Bonis M, Stefano PL, Torracca L, Oppizzi M et al. The double-orifice technique in mitral valve repair: A simple solution for complex problems. *J Thorac Cardiovasc Surg* 2001;122(4):674–81.
4. Vahanian A, Alfieri O, Andreotti F, Antunes MJ, Baron-Esquivias G, Baumgartner H et al. Guidelines on the management of valvular heart disease (version 2012). *Eur Heart J* 2012;33(19):2451–96.
5. Bonow RO, Carabello BA, Chatterjee K, de Leon AC, Jr., Faxon DP, Freed MD et al. 2008 Focused update incorporated into the ACC/AHA 2006 guidelines for the management of patients with valvular heart disease: A report of the American College of Cardiology/American Heart Association Task Force on Practice Guidelines (Writing Committee to Revise the 1998 Guidelines for the Management of Patients With Valvular Heart Disease): endorsed by the Society of Cardiovascular Anesthesiologists, Society for Cardiovascular Angiography and Interventions, and Society of Thoracic Surgeons. *Circulation* 2008;118(15):e523–661.
6. Feldman T, Kar S, Rinaldi M, Fail P, Hermiller J, Smalling R et al. Percutaneous mitral repair with the MitraClip system: Safety and midterm durability in the initial EVEREST (Endovascular Valve Edge-to-Edge REpair Study) cohort. *J Am Coll Cardiol* 2009;54(8):686–94.
7. Feldman T, Foster E, Glower DD, Kar S, Rinaldi MJ, Fail PS et al. Percutaneous repair or surgery for mitral regurgitation. *N Engl J Med* 2011;364(15):1395–406.
8. Luk A, Butany J, Ahn E, Fann JI, St Goar F, Thornton T et al. Mitral repair with the Evalve MitraClip device: Histopathologic findings in the porcine model. *Cardiovasc Pathol* 2009;18(5):279–85.
9. Whitlow PL, Feldman T, Pedersen WR, Lim DS, Kipperman R, Smalling R et al. Acute and 12-month results with catheter-based mitral valve leaflet repair: The EVEREST II (Endovascular Valve Edge-to-Edge Repair) High Risk Study. *J Am Coll Cardiol* 2012;59(2):130–9.
10. Schillinger W, Franzen O, Baldus S, Hausleiter J, Butter C, Schäfer U et al. ACCESS-EUROPE—An observational study of the MitraClip° system in Europe. *ESC Congress* 2012 2012.
11. Baldus S, Schillinger W, Franzen O, Bekeredjian R, Sievert H, Schofer J et al. MitraClip therapy in daily clinical practice: Initial results from the German transcatheter mitral valve interventions (TRAMI) registry. *Eur J Heart Fail* 2012;14(9):1050–5.
12. Siegel RJ, Biner S, Rafique AM, Rinaldi M, Lim S, Fail P et al. The acute hemodynamic effects of MitraClip therapy. *J Am Coll Cardiol* 2011;57(16):1658–65.

41

Mitral valve insufficiency: Other new mitral valve repair techniques

Ted Feldman

Percutaneous therapy for mitral regurgitation (MR) has been defined by leaflet repair with the MitraClip for the last several years.[1] This device has been utilized to treat the largest number of patients among the various catheter therapies for MR. The details of this approach are presented in Chapter 40. The degree to which all of the remaining therapy devices lag behind MitraClip leaflet repair reflects the complexities and challenges of both the treatment approaches and the disease itself.

The substantial challenges for percutaneous treatments for MR are reflected in part by the number of devices that are developing in the field, and also by the number of approaches that have already fallen by the wayside (Table 41.1). Several types of devices are in development. Most of the device approaches mimic or approximate some form of surgical therapy. MitraClip is the only device for direct leaflet repair. Most of the remaining devices are versions of an annuloplasty procedure. Direct and indirect

Table 41.1 Percutaneous mitral repair devices

Ongoing development
    Leaflet repair
    CS annuloplasty
    Direct annuloplasty
    Cerclage
    Mitral spacer
    Chordal replacement
    Valve replacement
Devices that are no longer being developed
    PS3—left atrial reshaping
    Percutaneous transvenous mitral annuloplasty (PTMA)—coronary sinus straightening rods
    Monarc—coronary sinus annuloplasty spring compression
    Recor—radiofrequency annular remodeling
    Coapsys—transventricular chamber and annulus remodeling

annuloplasty devices have been tested. Percutaneous valve replacement has been accomplished in its earliest forms. Several completely novel catheter-based therapies are also under development.

It is instructive to consider some of the devices that have failed and are no longer being developed. Two coronary sinus (CS) devices are no longer under development. This is mainly due to unanticipated mechanical stresses that the CS imposes on implanted devices. Both the Viacor (Viacor, Wilmington, MA, USA) PTMA CS straightening device[2] and the Edwards Monarc[3] (Edwards Life Sciences, Irvine, CA, USA) were troubled by device fracture. These devices were made of nickel–titanium (nitinol) and fracture of the metal occurred from repetitive movement in the CS. It had been assumed that the long history of CS pacing wire implants was a good basis for further development of annuloplasty implants. The annuloplasty devices differ from pacing wires in that they are more rigid. The concept that if a paperclip is bent frequently enough it will ultimately break is the principle behind this problem. For PTMA, device wire fracture led to perforation of the CS and lung.[2] The development of the third CS annuloplasty device, the Cardiac Dimensions Carillon (Cardiac Dimensions, Kirkland, WA, USA), will be described in detail. This device has also had wire fracture, which did not result in complications, and the cause of fracture has ultimately been overcome.

Among the devices remaining under development, annuloplasty approaches have had the largest human experience. The annuloplasty devices can be divided into indirect and direct categories.

Indirect annuloplasty

There is one remaining indirect annuloplasty approach still under development in patients. Indirect annuloplasty via the CS has been developed by Cardiac Dimensions using the Carillon device.[4] The device has a fixed length and is composed of a bridge element with two mirror-image helical anchors at either end (Figure 41.1). The anchors are oversized relative to the venous dimensions to provide stable anchoring. The distal anchor is placed in the distal CS or great cardiac vein, and the proximal anchor close to the CS ostium.

CS access is obtained via internal jugular venous cannulation. A 9 French guide catheter is placed in the CS and angiography is performed. A measuring catheter is used to assess the length of the CS for device size selection (Figure 41.1).

The distal anchor is pushed out of the delivery catheter in the distal CS, and the bridge element is exposed. The guide catheter and device system are pulled up as a unit to shorten the CS, and then the proximal anchor is released in the CS ostium. At this point, assessments are made of the potential for coronary artery compression and the degree of reduction of MR. If efficacy looks adequate, the device is released. If MR reduction is not adequate or if there is coronary compression, the device can be recaptured and removed.

Coronary compression is an important issue for CS devices in general and the Carillon specifically. The CS crosses over the circumflex coronary or a circumflex marginal branch in as many as two-thirds of patients.[5] Thus, there is significant potential for the compression of a coronary artery by a CS device. At least one case of coronary compression with acute infarction has been described with the Monarc device, which is no longer under development. For the Carillon, it is possible to assess the potential for coronary compression at the time of implantation by looking at coronary angiography during the device deployment, before the device is released.[6] There is still considerable learning needed to understand what degree of compression warrants device recapture versus what can be safely left alone. The use of computed tomographic angiography to facilitate patient selection also requires further experience.

The clinical results of CS annuloplasty with the Carillon have recently been reported from the TITAN Trial.[7] Fifty-three patients from seven European centers were included. Inclusion criteria were NYHA class II–IV symptoms with dilated ischemic or nonischemic cardiomyopathy and at least moderate functional MR. The LV ejection fraction had to be less than 40%. The device was implanted in 36/53 and recaptured in 17/53. Transient coronary compromise was the indication for recapture in eight patients and <1 grade MR reduction in nine. It is important to note that coronary arteries were crossed by the implant in 34/53 patients (64%), but coronary compromise led to device recapture in only 8/53 patients (15%).

CS annuloplasty was associated with significant decreases in quantitative measures of MR, including regurgitant volume, effective regurgitant orifice area (EROA), vena contracta, and mitral regurgitant jet area:left atrial area ratio (MRJA/LAA) from baseline up to 12 months. The average reduction from baseline to 12 months ranged up to 50% for both EROA and regurgitant volume. Comparing the implanted cohort with the nonimplanted cohort, there was a significant difference between the two cohorts, with a continued decrease of functional mitral regurgitation (FMR) up to 12 months noted only in the implanted patients. There was also a reduction in LV end-diastolic diameter, end-systolic diameter, and end-diastolic end-systolic volume between baseline and up to 12 months. Reverse remodeling was noted in the implanted group, compared with continued ventricular enlargement in the nonimplanted group. Functional improvements in exercise performance and quality of life (QOL) were apparent by 1 month in the implanted cohort. A significant difference between groups was observed for both the 6 m walk distance and QOL at 1 year.

In summary, devices could be implanted in two-thirds of patients. In the one-third in whom the device was not implanted, the reason for recapture was roughly divided

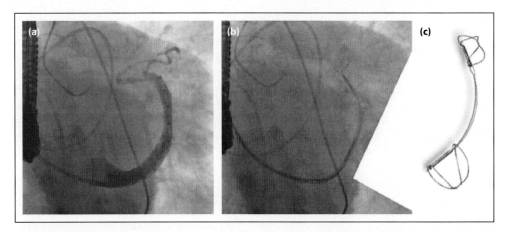

Figure 41.1 The Cardiac Dimensions Carillon device is placed via the coronary sinus. (a) A calibrated catheter in the coronary sinus, allowing for measurement and device length selection. (b) The distal anchor protruding from the tip of a guide catheter. (c) A photograph of the device oriented anatomically as it is seen in (b).

between coronary compromise and insufficient reduction in MR grade. Among implanted patients, there was a continued decrease in measures of MR severity and LV dilatation during the 1 year follow-up, and compared with the nonimplanted patients. QOL and functional capacity measures improved.

The Carillon has received Conformité Européenne (CE) approval and is in commercial use in Europe. Early experience is consistent with the TITAN trial outcomes. One of the surprising experiences has been continued improvement in MR reduction through the first year after device implantation.

Direct annuloplasty

Direct annuloplasty devices have been used only in feasibility studies to date. The Guided Delivery Systems (Santa Clara, CA, USA) Accucinch uses a transventricular retrograde delivery approach (Figure 41.2). A guide catheter with a curve similar to an Extra Back Up (EBU) shape is passed across the aortic valve and the tip placed behind

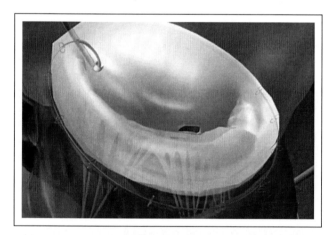

Figure 41.2 **(See color insert.)** The Guided Delivery System Accucinch involves placing anchors in the mitral annulus and subannular left ventricular myocardium via retrograde left ventricular access. A string or tether is used to tension the anchors and diminish the mitral annular circumference.

the anterior mitral leaflet in the subannular space. This is used for a delivery system that places up to a dozen nitinol anchors in the basal myocardium underneath the mitral annulus. A tether is run through the anchors. Cinching of the tether plicates the circumference of the annulus (Figure 41.3). The tether also plicates the myocardium at the base of the left ventricle, thus resulting in some left ventricular remodeling. This is an important feature of the device, since patients with functional MR have either dilatation or distortion of the left ventricle, and annuloplasty by itself does not treat the ventricular disease. The Mitralign (Mitralign, Tewksbury, MA, USA) device uses a similar retrograde approach for the guide catheter.[8] The 14 F guide is used to deliver two pairs of pledgets into the mitral annulus. Each pair is plicated to shorten the annulus (Figure 41.4). For the Mitralign system, radio-frequency wires are used to traverse the annular tissue for pledget placement, with delivery of the cinching force directly into the annulus. A phase I trial with this device is underway in Europe. A third system uses transseptal left atrial access to place a mitral ring directly into the native valve annulus. The Valtech Cardioband (Valtech Cardio, Or Yehuda, Israel) uses screw anchors placed directly into the mitral annulus to anchor an annuloplasty ring.[9] This device most closely replicates surgical annuloplasty, although the current version of the ring does not completely encircle the annulus. While a percutaneous delivery system has been developed, current experience with the device is mostly open surgical.

Yet another method for annuloplasty uses radio-frequency energy to shrink the collagen in the annulus. The QuantumCor (Bothell, WA, USA) system has been used in preclinical models.[10] The appeal of an energy-based method is that no implant is needed and no foreign body is left behind. The delivery of radio-frequency energy is controlled by maximum temperatures, sensed by thermocouples. In a sheep study, variable degrees of acute annular contraction could be achieved. The reduction in antero-posterior distance of the mitral annulus was about 25%. At necropsy in this model, there was no evidence of thrombosis or damage to coronary arteries or cardiac vein. The efficacy of this device in patients remains untested.

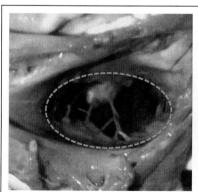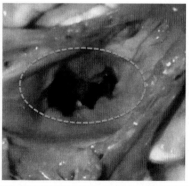

Figure 41.3 **(See color insert.)** In a bench-top ovine model, the left panel shows the mitral orifice before the Guided Delivery System's tether is tightened. The degree of circumferential cinching can be appreciated in the right-hand panel, where the dotted line represents the original mitral orifice.

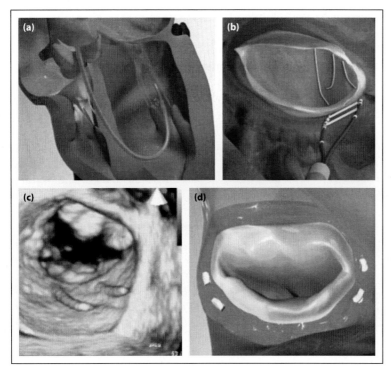

Figure 41.4 (**See color insert.**) The Mitralign system uses retrograde left ventricular access, shown in (a). A guide catheter was placed below the posterior leaflet annular tissue. In (b), radio-frequency wires are seen to traverse the annulus, for delivery of pledgets that are used to cause cinching of the annulus. In (c), a three-dimensional left atrial echocardiographic view shows two wires placed through the annulus. Ultimately, two pairs of wires are used. (d) A schematic of the two pairs of pledgets on either side of the mitral annulus.

LV chamber remodeling with annuloplasty

An approach to treating functional MR by remodeling the LV chamber in conjunction with compressing the mitral annulus has been accomplished using the Coapsys surgical device (Myocor, Minneapolis, MN, USA).[11] The company lost funding and went out of business in 2008, but the device concept and trial results represent an important accomplishment. The device was composed of two epicardial pads, anchored on the anterior and posterior LV surfaces with a tensioning cable passed through the LV cavity to pull the pads together, thus reducing the septal–lateral dimension of the mitral annulus and at the same time diminishing the LV chamber diameter (Figure 41.5).

Experience with the surgical device has shown sustained reductions in MR and LV chamber dimensions for more than 1 year. A percutaneous transpericardial version of the surgical system was created with successful placement in two patients.[12] This proof of concept for successful LV chamber remodeling is an important finding. A great limitation of conventional annuloplasty is that the underlying problem, LV dilatation, is not treated by the annular device. It remains to be seen if this concept will emerge in the form of other devices or systems for chamber remodeling.

Chordal replacement

Surgical repair and replacement of chordae tendineae has been in use for many years, and has become increasingly

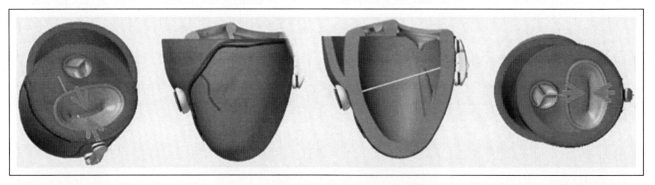

Figure 41.5 (**See color insert.**) The Myocor device uses pads on the anterior and posterior surfaces of the left ventricle, with a cord traversing the left ventricular chamber. This allows for compression of both the left ventricular chamber and the mitral orifice. In a beating-heart surgical approach, this procedure produced similar degrees of reduction in mitral regurgitation compared with surgical annuloplasty, with better survival. (Adapted from Grossi EA et al. *J Am Coll Cardiol* 2010;56(24):1984–93.)

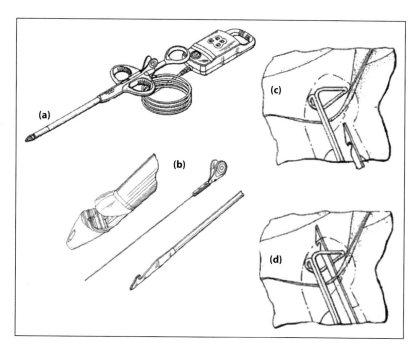

Figure 41.6 The NeoChord system uses a transapical delivery system as shown in (a). The distal end of the delivery catheter in (b) has a sensing mechanism to verify leaflet grasping. (c, d) show the method by which an ePTFE suture is drawn through the leaflet to create a neochord. The neochord is anchored in the apex. (From USPTO website, application number: 12/254,807, publication number: US 2009/0105751 A1.)

successful. Minimally invasive chordal replacement using apical access is under development as an alternative to open chordal replacement, and as a precursor to a percutaneous approach. NeoChord (Eden Prairie, MN, USA)[13] and TransCardiac Therapeutics (Atlanta, GA, USA; makers of MitraFlex) are two companies involved in this effort to design artificial chordae tendineae for direct implantation through the apex of a beating heart, using echo and/or thoracoscopic guidance. The NeoChord system grasps the prolapsed leaflet using the expandable jaws of the device (Figure 41.6). A fiber-optic monitoring device confirms that the leaflet has been adequately captured, and then an expanded polytetrafluoroethylene (ePTFE) suture is deployed and attached to the leaflet. The suture is then pulled through the apex of the heart. The correct length of the ePTFE suture is determined using real-time echocardiographic guidance and observing the improvement in MR in the beating heart in real time. The suture is then secured to the apex of the heart. The surgical system has received CE approval.

Mitral Spacer

A novel concept for diminishing the regurgitant mitral orifice is to place a cylinder in the orifice to occupy the open malcoaptation space. This concept was derived from observations that in some cases after right ventricular pacing leads were placed across a regurgitant tricuspid valve, the pacing wire resulted in decreased regurgitation. The Mitra

Spacer (Cardiosolutions, West Bridgewater, MA, USA) is a saline-contrast balloon anchored to the left ventricular apex (Figure 41.7). It is designed for placement in the left side of the heart by either percutaneous femoral venous

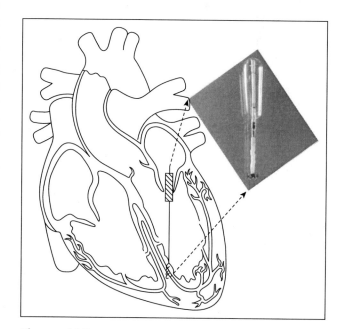

Figure 41.7 The Mitral Spacer concept is illustrated here. The device is anchored in the left ventricular septum or apex, and the spacer "floats" in the mitral orifice to occupy the regurgitant orifice space. (From USPTO website, application number: 12/872,228, publication number: US 2010/0324668 A1.)

and transseptal access or by the surgical transapical route. The device does not directly alter the mitral anatomy, but rather provides a "sealing surface" for the leaflets, with a resultant reduced MR. The spacer balloon works by filling the MR orifice as it straddles the mitral valve with part of the balloon in the ventricle and part of the balloon in the left atrium. There is a valve in the balloon that allows filling to the desired amount to diminish MR. Patients with a Mitral Spacer can still undergo future valve repair or replacement surgery if necessary. The device is in the early stages of development and several patients have undergone temporary implants.

Valve replacement

There has been a parallel path to mitral repair to achieve valve replacement.[14] There are several challenges that make mitral replacement more difficult than transcatheter aortic valve replacement. The native mitral orifice is larger, so the devices must be correspondingly larger profile. The mitral orifice is "D" shaped, so a round prosthesis is a greater challenge. There is not the heavy calcification associated with aortic valve disease to provide an anchoring surface for a mitral device. These factors have combined to make replacement of the mitral valve a much more complex undertaking. At the time of this writing, only a single patient has undergone percutaneous native valve replacement. There has been greater success with using existing aortic valve devices to replace degenerated mitral bioprostheses, or failed prior surgical annuloplasty.[15]

Conclusion

The development of catheter-based approaches for mitral valve repair and replacement has progressed slowly and steadily, and clearly at a less rapid pace than percutaneous aortic valve replacement. This is largely due to the complexity of the mitral valve apparatus anatomically and to the multifactorial nature of the pathophysiology of MR. The success of surgical repair for degenerative MR has set a high bar for any percutaneous method, and thus, percutaneous approaches for degenerative MR have been applied almost entirely to patients who are considered high risk for surgery. For functional MR, progress is being made, and clinical benefits such as reduced rates of rehospitalization are being shown in early studies of catheter-based approaches to reduce MR in patients

with ischemic or cardiomyopathy-related heart failure.[16] The challenge of percutaneous mitral valve replacement is clearly greater than for aortic valve replacement, and great efforts are being invested in developing this therapy as well.

References

1. Feldman T, Foster E, Glower DG et al. Percutaneous repair or surgery for mitral regurgitation. *N Engl J Med* 2011;364:1395–406.
2. Machaalany J, St-Pierre A, Sénéchal M et al. Fatal late migration of viacor percutaneous transvenous mitral annuloplasty device resulting in distal coronary venous perforation. *Can J Cardiol* 2013;29(1):130. e1–4. Epub 2012 May 22.
3. Webb JG, Harnek J, Munt BI et al. Percutaneous transvenous mitral annuloplasty: Initial human experience with device implantation in the coronary sinus. *Circulation* 2006;113:851–5.
4. Maniu CV, Patel JB, Reuter DG et al. Acute and chronic reduction of functional mitral regurgitation in experimental heart failure by percutaneous mitral annuloplasty. *J Am Coll Cardiol* 2004;44:1652–61.
5. Tops LF, Van de Veire NR, Schuijf JD et al. Noninvasive evaluation of coronary sinus anatomy and its relation to the mitral valve annulus: Implications for percutaneous mitral annuloplasty. *Circulation* 2007;115:1426–32.
6. Schofer J, Siminiak T, Haude M et al. Percutaneous mitral annuloplasty for functional mitral regurgitation: Results of the CARILLON mitral annuloplasty device European Union study. *Circulation* 2009;120:326–33.
7. Siminiak T, Wu JC, Haude M et al. Treatment of functional mitral regurgitation by percutaneous annuloplasty—Results of the TITAN Trial. *Eur J Heart Fail* 2012;14(8):931–8.
8. Frerker C, Schäfer U, Schewel D et al. Percutaneous approaches for mitral valve interventions—A real alternative technique for standard cardiac surgery? *Herz* 2009;34(6):444–50.
9. Maisano F, Vanermen H, Seeburger J et al. Direct access transcatheter mitral annuloplasty with a sutureless and adjustable device: Preclinical experience. *Eur J Cardiothorac Surg* 2012;42(3):524–9.
10. Goel R, Witzel T, Dickens D, Takeda PA, Heuser RR. The QuantumCor device for treating mitral regurgitation: An animal study. *Catheter Cardiovasc Interv* 2009;74(1):43–8.
11. Grossi EA, Patel N, Woo YJ et al. RESTOR-MV study group. Outcomes of the RESTOR-MV Trial (randomized evaluation of a surgical treatment for off-pump repair of the mitral valve). *J Am Coll Cardiol* 2010;56(24):1984–93.
12. Pedersen WR, Block P, Leon M et al. iCoapsys mitral valve repair system: Percutaneous implantation in an animal model. *Catheter Cardiovasc Interv* 2008;72(1):125–31.
13. Seeburger J, Leontjev S, Neumuth M et al. Trans-apical beating-heart implantation of neo-chordae to mitral valve leaflets: Results of an acute animal study. *Eur J Cardiothorac Surg* 2012;41(1):173–6; discussion 176.
14. Lutter G, Quaden R, Osaki S et al. Off-pump transapical mitral valve replacement. *Eur J Cardiothorac Surg* 2009;36:124–8.
15. Feldman T. Antegrade approach for percutaneous valve impantation. *Catheter Cardiovasc Intervent* 2012;80:704–5.
16. Whitlow P, Feldman T, Pedersen W et al. The EVEREST II high risk study: Acute and 12 month results with catheter based mitral valve leaflet repair. *J Am Coll Cardiol* 2012;59:130–9.

42

Mitral valve insufficiency: Transcatheter mitral valve implantation

Monique Sandhu, David Gregg, and Daniel H. Steinberg

Introduction

For patients with severe mitral regurgitation, surgical repair or replacement has long been considered the standard of care to improve heart failure and functional status and limit progressive left ventricular dilation and failure. Knowledge about the optimal surgical treatment approach has evolved with the development of new valves and surgical techniques. In general, we have learned that mitral valve repair is preferred over replacement when possible, as this maintains ventricular geometry and mitigates the risks of a prosthetic valve. When necessary, mitral valve replacement is most successful when the subvalvular apparatus is preserved. Treatment of valve disease continues to evolve, and reviewing the lessons of surgical valve treatment is important when considering the benefits and potential challenges to another frontier in mitral valve therapies, transcatheter mitral valve implantation (TMVI). This chapter serves to review the evolution of surgical valve care and outline how this experience pertains to TMVI.

Surgical therapies for mitral regurgitation (repair vs. replacement)

The first mechanical mitral valve replacement was performed in 1960 by Dr. Albert Starr with the "ball-in-cage" Starr–Edwards valve. This surgical replacement was accomplished by complete excision of the mitral valve leaflets, chordae tendinae, and tips of the papillary muscles. While the operation represented a true breakthrough in cardiovascular therapeutics, up to 50% of these patients developed low output cardiac failure despite normal mechanical valve function and perioperative mortality rates approached 37%.[1]

It was hypothesized that the high mortality rate with the Starr–Edwards prosthesis and reductions in left ventricular ejection fraction were directly related to severing the continuity of the mitral annulus and papillary muscles.[2] Initially, the complete excision method was necessary to manage the high-profile Starr–Edwards valve without having interference by retained chordal structures.[3] Not yet recognizing the geometric benefits of chordal preservation, even after the development of new, lower-profile mechanical valve and bioprosthetic valve technology, mitral valve replacements were still performed in this conventional manner until the early 1980s.

Suboptimal outcomes with mitral valve replacement stimulated growing interest in mitral valve repair and preservation of the subvalvular apparatus. Techniques including leaflet plication and mitral orifice narrowing were intuitively attractive but had unreliable outcomes. Carpentier and his associates eventually developed what has come to be known as the "French correction," a series of repairs; the most central to these repairs was the annuloplasty ring as well as the quadrangular resection, chordal shortening, and chordal transection.[4,5]

Mitral valve repair has some very important advantages over replacement. First, the repair itself negates the need for long-term anticoagulation or the risk of prosthetic valve degeneration, decreasing overall morbidity and diminishing the risk of future thromboembolic events. The lack of foreign prosthesis also decreases the subsequent risk of infection.[1] Of equal importance, repair maintains the subvalvular architecture, leading to improvements in left ventricular function, postoperative morbidity and mortality, and sustained long-term outcomes.

Limitations of mitral valve repair

Though associated with better outcomes, the complexity of the mitral valve anatomy inevitably leads to a surgical repair that is more challenging, both intellectually and

Table 42.1	Technical targets for mitral valve repair			
Leaflet repair		**Annulus repair**	**Chord repair**	**Commissure repair**
Posterior leaflet quadrangular resection the "French correction" Carpentier technique "sliding leaflet plasty" Foldover leaflet advancement Alfieri stitch "edge-to-edge repair"		Annuloplasty ring	Reduction of chord height via implantation Artificial PTFE chordae Chordal transfer Chordal shortening	Commissuroplasty

technically, than the conventional replacement. Commonly, a surgical mitral valve repair requires at least one if not multiple surgical techniques (Table 42.1), and this usually includes an annuloplasty ring plus an additional form of repair based on valvular pathology. High-quality repair depends on both valvular pathology and operator experience and expertise. At high-volume centers, repair rates can approach 80–90% with 10-year freedom from reoperation approaching 93%;[6] however, this is not necessarily the norm, and in 2003, of the mitral valve procedures reported in the STS (Society of Thoracic Surgery) database, only 36% of valves considered repairable actually underwent repair.[7]

Another limitation of mitral repair is that not all valves are suitable for repair. The classic techniques for mitral repair are targeted primarily to degenerative valve disease and to a lesser extent rheumatic valve disease. At times, the valvular pathology may preclude a good repair. For example, severe annular calcification may prevent adequate ring implantation and a small mitral valve area may increase the risk of functional mitral stenosis. Additionally, though degenerative mitral valve disease is probably the most common mechanism of severe mitral regurgitation undergoing surgical repair, a growing proportion of patients have severe *functional* mitral regurgitation, often due to ischemic heart disease or dilated cardiomyopathy. In this case, the pathology may relate less to the valve and more to the ventricle, and repair has proven less successful. For instance, McGee et al. reported 585 patients undergoing annuloplasty for function mitral regurgitation. Over 6 months following surgery, 28% of patients developed 3+ or greater mitral regurgitation with left ventricular dysfunction being the primary predictor of late failure.[8]

Chordal-sparing mitral replacement

Armed with the understanding that subavalvular preservation was paramount for optimal LV function and outcomes following mitral regurgitation, lower-profile mechanical and bioprosthetic valves were designed so that the chordal structures would not interfere with valve function. Indeed, comparisons between conventional mitral valve replacement and chordal-sparing mitral valve replacement have

demonstrated improved left ventricular ejection fraction, decreased left ventricular volumes, decreased pulmonary artery pressures, improved long-term survival, and improved overall morbidity and mortality.[9] Although repair is generally considered the preferred modality for surgical correction of mitral regurgitation, a prospective randomized trial of 47 patients undergoing total or partial chordal-sparing mitral valve replacement found complete chordal sparing to be the preferred surgery with improved outcomes in end-systolic and end-diastolic volumes, left ventricular wall stress, return to preoperative ejection fraction, and improved left ventricular mass.[10] As a result, enthusiasm continued to grow for chordal-sparing replacement, particularly when mitral repair would likely be suboptimal. Complete chordal-sparing, however, with current surgical tools is not feasible in all patients such as those with poor anatomic features for repair, ischemic mitral regurgitation, and those at higher surgical risk where the risk of multiple bypass runs to optimize the repair may outweigh the benefits of a quicker, more reliable operation.

Transcatheter mitral valve implantation

As discussed extensively in earlier chapters, percutaneous mitral repair represents an attractive alternative to mitral valve repair in select patients. The primary limitation of any percutaneous repair technique is that each device can enact only a single form of repair. This is an important issue when considering the proportion of surgical repair procedures that employ more than one technique. For instance, with the Alfieri surgical procedure (which serves as the model for the mitral clip procedure), 208 of the initial 260 cases reported by Alfieri et al. had concomitant annular reduction and the lack of an annular reduction surgery was the single largest predictor of reoperation for mitral regurgitation.[11,12] While in no way does this imply that percutaneous repair techniques have no role in cardiovascular therapy, it does suggest that the relative role of each device will be somewhat limited to higher-risk, appropriately selected patients in whom surgical repair is not ideal.

In view of positive outcomes and similar short- and long-term surgical outcomes with chordal-sparing mitral valve replacements, TMVI is a particularly attractive alternative. Moreover, the other major limitation of percutaneous mitral repair is that residual regurgitation cannot be truly expected to match that seen with surgical repair, and even in high-risk patients, considerable debate exists as to whether any residual regurgitation greater than trace–mild is acceptable. In the case of TMVI, the full benefit of a mitral replacement can be achieved without the full risk of cardiac surgery. In particular, TMVI could be especially beneficial in high-risk patients with functional mitral regurgitation. In addition to the elevated operative risk, these patients typically have less reliable repairs.

The development of a percutaneously delivered mitral prosthesis is challenging for multiple reasons. First, the mitral valve is generally larger than the aortic and pulmonary valves, and thus there are challenges in developing a deliverable technology. The delivery of the mitral valve prosthesis is difficult as it is by nature larger than the transcatheter aortic valves that have thus far been developed. Proper positioning and alignment represents a second challenge, and the ideal access route has yet to be determined. Third, the annulus of the mitral valve is saddle-shaped and not necessarily calcified. As a result, anchoring may prove difficult and there is concern for minimizing paravalvular leak. Once the valve is deployed, it is imperative to form a tight seal to minimize the degree of paravalvular leak and thus subsequent hemolysis. Lastly, proximity to the left ventricular outflow tract (LVOT), circumflex, and coronary sinus must be recognized and understood, as obstruction in any of these can be detrimental.[3]

Trials of TMVI

Early attempts at TMVI have focused on the treatment of dysfunction of previously placed surgical bioprosthetic valves, as the prosthetic valve architecture creates a supportive conduit and framework to anchor a percutaneous valve. In these cases, current balloon-expandable valve technology has a logical role. Multiple small series examining transapical mitral valve-in-valve implantations have been reported in Europe. One such study performed in Germany looked at six patients with severe mitral regurgitation of their previously placed bioprosthetic mitral valve who were deemed too high-risk surgical candidates to undergo repeat surgical mitral valve replacement. The patients underwent a mini-left thoracotomy and transapical puncture. An Edwards SAPIEN (Edwards Lifesciences, Irvine, CA, USA) valve was implanted in reverse fashion, overlapping the previously placed bioprosthetic valve using both echocardiographic and fluoroscopic guidance. The patients were followed with serial transthoracic echocardiograms at baseline, prior to discharge, and at 30 days. Five of the six patients survived with improvements in their New York Heart Association (NYHA) class by at least one class and improvement in the

degree of mitral regurgitation. There was a trace paravalvular leak in two of the five survivors.[13]

A number of animal trials are being conducted with different devices designed for treatment of native mitral valve dysfunction. In one such trial, a series of transapical self-expanding stent valves were implanted in 10 pigs. On imaging follow-up (transesophageal echocardiogram and ventriculogram), there was optimal stent positioning/deployment in all of the pigs. All 10 pigs had normal hemodynamics with no significant arrhythmias, no migration, no embolization, and mild paravalvular leak in 3/10 of the animals. There was no significant mitral valve gradient, left ventricular outflow tract gradient, or mitral regurgitation in any of the animals.[14] Similar studies are beginning to show the feasibility of transcutaneous mitral valve implantation of native valve disease in other animal models. TMVI will likely have unique effects on annulus and left ventricular geometry, and it may represent the ultimate valve-sparing procedure, leaving not only the subvalvular apparatus in place but also the native valve.

The CardiAQ (CardiAQ Valve Technologies, Irvine, CA, USA) is the first TMVI system used in man to treat native disease. The prosthesis is delivered via a 30 F venous sheath that then requires a transseptal puncture for antegrade delivery. The valve is mounted on a nitinol frame and is able to anchor itself to the annulus using anchors that come together as the valve is deployed, thereby overcoming part of the aforementioned struggle that a lack of annular calcium and subsequent lack of radial force produce. A wire is used for the transseptal puncture and crosses the mitral valve. The Copenhagen maneuver is performed to ensure that the wire is not caught within the papillary muscle. The tricuspid, porcine valve is loaded on the catheter and is designed for a multistage deployment and controlled release. The valve is self-positioning on the native mitral valve annulus and the entire procedure is performed by an interdisciplinary team. Thus far, the CardiAQ valve is the only transcutaneous mitral valve that has been used in man. It was successfully used for compassionate use on an 86-year-old gentleman with severe mitral regurgitation, and though the patient died, subsequent autopsy showed successful deployment of the mitral valve.[15]

The Neovasc Tiara (Neovasc, Richmond, BC, Canada) valve is currently being designed with a transapical delivery system and plans to also develop a transfemoral delivery system. The platform is very compact and the pericardial tissue valve is mounted on a D-shaped annulus that is designed to match the floor of the left atrium and the mitral annulus, thereby minimizing its ability to cause left ventricular outflow tract obstruction. It has a self-expanding frame that secures itself using an atrial skirt and an anchoring feature on the ventricular side.[16] The team used to deliver the Neovasc Tiara is similar to the CardiAQ and the procedure can be performed in a catheterization lab or a hybrid operating room.

The Endovalve (MicroInterventional Devices, Bethlehem, PA, USA) is delivered via a transapical approach. The Endovalve is combined with an additional Permaseal technology that allows for a sutureless closure of the apical myocardium. The Permaseal device is initially placed at the apex of the left ventricle. It is composed of six anchors that are attached to one another via elastic stays that form an orifice in the middle. The anchors have barbs that separate away from the shaft of the anchor once the Permaseal device has been deployed. The catheter is then advanced through the central orifice into the left ventricle to the level of the mitral valve. The low-profile, bioprosthetic valve is deployed within the annulus of the mitral valve. It has similar soft tissue anchors to the ones seen on the Permaseal device that form a 360° seal around the mitral annulus and attach the prosthetic valve. The catheter is then removed and the elastic stays of the Permaseal rebound, thus achieving hemostasis. The device has been successfully implanted in one sheep thus far and there is preparation for future animal trials.[17]

Future directions

Evolving TMVI technology is promising and may prove to offer results comparable to surgical chordal sparing replacements without the risk of conventional cardiac surgery. In high-risk or inoperable patients, this may represent a true advance. Analogous to transcatheter aortic valve replacement, it is reasonable to expect that as animal studies prove feasibility and potential efficacy, first-in-man trials will lead to small compassionate use series in truly inoperable patients. These will be followed by larger-scale randomized trials evaluating these technologies in patients considered inoperable for traditional repair/replacement procedures.

The ideal valvular pathology, patient risk profiles, specific devices, and timelines for TMVI are yet to be determined. TMVI is likely to eventually have an important role in treating high-risk patients with severe, functional mitral regurgitation, and this population is only likely to increase over the next decade, given an aging population with increasing comorbid disease states. Practically, as with any new technology, the theoretical attractiveness will have to be proven both safe and effective in clinical trials before its ultimate role can be defined.

References

1. Reardon MJ, David TE. Mitral valve replacement with preservation of the subvalvular apparatus. *Curr Opin Cardiol* [Review]. 1999;14(2):104–10.

2. Rao C, Hart J, Chow A, Siannis F, Tsalafouta P, Murtuza B et al. Does preservation of the sub-valvular apparatus during mitral valve replacement affect long-term survival and quality of life? A microsimulation study. *J Cardiothorac Surg* [Comparative Study]. 2008;3:17.

3. Maisano F, La Canna G, Colombo A, Alfieri O. The evolution from surgery to percutaneous mitral valve interventions: The role of the edge-to-edge technique. *J Am Coll Cardiol* [Review]. 2011;58(21):2174–82.

4. Perier P, Clausnizer B, Mistarz K. Carpentier "sliding leaflet" technique for repair of the mitral valve: Early results. *Ann Thorac Surg* 1994;57(2):383–6.

5. Carpentier A, Chauvaud S, Fabiani JN, Deloche A, Relland J, Lessana A et al. Reconstructive surgery of mitral valve incompetence: Ten-year appraisal. *J Thorac Cardiovasc Surg* 1980;79(3):338–48.

6. Sakamoto Y, Hashimoto K, Okuyama H, Ishii S, Hanai M, Inoue T et al. Long-term assessment of mitral valve reconstruction with resection of the leaflets: Triangular and quadrangular resection. *Ann Thorac Surg* [Clinical Trial]. 2005;79(2):475–9.

7. Savage EB, Ferguson TB, Jr., DiSesa VJ. Use of mitral valve repair: Analysis of contemporary United States experience reported to the Society of Thoracic Surgeons National Cardiac Database. *Ann Thorac Surg* 2003;75(3):820–5.

8. McGee EC, Gillinov AM, Blackstone EH, Rajeswaran J, Cohen G, Najam F et al. Recurrent mitral regurgitation after annuloplasty for functional ischemic mitral regurgitation. *J Thorac Cardiovasc Surg* 2004;128(6):916–24.

9. Peter CA, Austin EH, Jones RH. Effect of valve replacement for chronic mitral insufficiency on left ventricular function during rest and exercise. *J Thorac Cardiovasc Surg* [Research Support, U.S. Govt, P.H.S.]. 1981;82(1):127–35.

10. Yun KL, Sintek CF, Miller DC, Pfeffer TA, Kochamba GS, Khonsari S et al. Randomized trial comparing partial versus complete chordal-sparing mitral valve replacement: Effects on left ventricular volume and function. *J Thorac Cardiovasc Surg* [Clinical Trial Comparative Study Randomized Controlled Trial Research Support, Non-U.S. Govt]. 2002;123(4):707–14.

11. Alfieri O, Maisano F, De Bonis M, Stefano PL, Torracca L, Oppizzi M et al. The double-orifice technique in mitral valve repair: A simple solution for complex problems. *J Thorac Cardiovasc Surg* 2001;122(4):674–81.

12. Maisano F, Caldarola A, Blasio A, De Bonis M, La Canna G, Alfieri O. Midterm results of edge-to-edge mitral valve repair without annuloplasty. *J Thorac Cardiovasc Surg* 2003;126(6):1987–97.

13. Seiffert M, Conradi L, Baldus S, Schirmer J, Knap M, Blankenberg S et al. Transcatheter mitral valve-in-valve implantation in patients with degenerated bioprostheses. *J Am Coll Cardiol Cardiovasc Interv* 2012;5(3):341–9.

14. Lozonschi LG. Ed. Progress with transcatheter mitral valve replacement III: Lutter-Lozonschi-Bioprosthesis. Transcatheter Cardiovascular Therapeutics (TCT); 2011; San Francisco, CA.

15. Songaard et al. Featured Lecture: CardiAQ program update: Featuring the world's first successful transcatheter mitral valve implant. Transcatheter Cardiovascular Therapeutics (TCT); 2012; Miami, FL.

16. Banai S, Jolicoeur EM, Schwartz M et al. Tiara: A novel catheter-based mitral valve bioprosthesis: Initial experiments and short-term pre-clinical results. *J Am Coll Cardiol* 2012;60:1430–1.

17. Hermann HC. Ed. Transcatheter mitral valve replacement. Transcatheter Cardiovascular Therapeutics (TCT); 2012; Miami, FL.

43

Tricuspid valve insufficiency: Background and indications for treatment

Alexander Lauten and Hans Reiner Figulla

Introduction

Tricuspid valve insufficiency (TI) is a common condition that is observed in more than 80% of healthy individuals.[1] Isolated mild TI is typically well tolerated and patients may remain asymptomatic for many years without specific treatment. However, as TI is frequently secondary to right ventricular dilatation, it is also commonly associated with late stages of left heart valve, myocardial, or pulmonary disease. In these patients, concomitant moderate or severe TI has a significant impact on functional status and long-term survival. Compared with aortic and mitral valve disease, there is comparatively sparse data from large trials to determine the optimal management strategy for this condition. Surgical therapy is the only established treatment presently available in this difficult patient population. However, in patients with long-standing, symptomatic TI, surgical mortality is high and the decision for surgery is a frequent subject of debate in clinical practice.

Anatomy and function of the tricuspid valve

The tricuspid valve is embedded in the right ventricular inflow tract in the junction between the right atrium (RA) and the right ventricle (RV). The tricuspid annulus (TVA) is a three-dimensional, highly dynamic structure that changes size and shape during the cardiac cycle due to contraction of the surrounding myocardium.[2] It provides a firm and pliable base for the three valve leaflets (anterior, posterior, and septal) and is in continuity with the aortic and mitral annulus. The three leaflets are unequal in size with the anterior leaflet being the largest. Each cusp has a strong central fibrous portion that thins out toward the perimeter where the chordae insert connecting the leaflets to the large anterior, medial, and the often bifid inferior papillary muscle.

Valve function depends on the structural integrity and concerted action of all these components, including the subvalvular apparatus and the RV. Differing preload conditions of the RV alter the geometry of the annulus and the subvalvular apparatus and affect valve function. This is of relevance in patients under anesthesia when the degree of TR is assessed by intraoperative transesophageal echo, which may be significantly reduced compared with preoperative evaluation.[3,4] Several other cardiac structures are in proximity to the TV and are at risk during surgical or catheter-based interventions. The right coronary artery runs along the anterior portion of the TV and can be compromised during surgical repair or replacement. The septal portion of the tricuspid annulus is adjacent to the atrioventricular node, which can be compromised by sutures placed too deeply during TV surgery, producing complete heart block. Several studies have shown that the need for pacemaker implantation after TV surgery is higher than after other valve interventions. In a recent report evaluating the outcome of 416 patients undergoing TV surgery (repair: $n = 310$; replacement: $n = 106$), 7.7% required implantation of a permanent pacemaker postoperatively.[5] This finding is in line with the incidence of early postoperative pacemaker requirement of 5–8% reported in the literature, although an incidence as high as 28% has been reported in one study.[6–8]

Natural history and pathophysiology of tricuspid regurgitation

The prevalence of moderate-to-severe TR in the general US population is estimated at 1.6 million cases.[9] In a retrospective study by Nath et al. investigating the frequency and impact of TR on long-term prognosis in 5223 subjects, moderate or severe TR was observed in 11.8% and 3.8% of all cases, respectively. With increasing severity of TR,

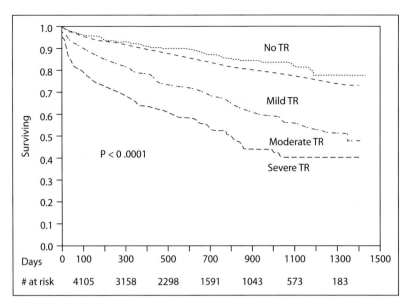

Figure 43.1 Impact of tricuspid regurgitation on long-term survival. Kaplan–Meier survival curves for 5223 consecutive patients with tricuspid regurgitation undergoing transthoracic echocardiography at the Palo Alto Veterans Affairs Health Care System between 1998 and 2002. Survival is significantly worse in patients with moderate and severe TR. (Adapted from Nath J, Foster E, Heidenreich PA. *J Am Coll Cardiol* 2004;43:405–9.)

1-year survival decreased and was reduced to 63.9% in patients with severe TR (Figure 43.1).[10] In the above study, only 64 patients (1.2%) had TR of primary origin resulting from disease processes directly affecting the structure of the valve (primary or organic TR). Primary TR may be caused by infective endocarditis, endomyocardial fibrosis, or the carcinoid syndrome. Carcinoid heart disease is a rare type of valve disease affecting primarily the right-sided heart valves by elevated plasma serotonin levels.[11] Moreover, primary TR occurs in congenital heart disease such as Ebstein's anomaly, and following trauma or leaflet perforation due to pacemaker leads.[10] In the majority of patients, TR is "functional" and therefore not related to primary valve pathology. Functional tricuspid regurgitation (FTR) is frequently observed in the advanced stage of multivalvular heart disease or myocardial disease. Coexisting severe TR is found in approximately 30% of patients with severe mitral regurgitation and represents a subset with a particularly poor long-term follow-up and a high-risk group for surgical intervention.[12] Furthermore, in patients with pulmonary disease, associated pulmonary hypertension increases RV afterload and may eventually lead to FTR.

Because RV stroke volume is partially expelled backwards into the venous system, severe TR causes a rise in mean RA pressure and decrease in cardiac output and RV afterload. At an earlier stage, this decrease in RV afterload may initially actually mask a decreased RV contractility. However, volume overload leads to progressive dilatation of the RV with dysfunction and worsening of TR. The associated rise in RA pressure results in systemic venous congestion that manifests as peripheral edema and hepatic congestion with cirrhose cardiaque. Although the gradual development of severe TR may be tolerated chronically for long periods, the condition eventually leads to RV failure.

Echocardiographic assessment and grading of tricuspid regurgitation

TV function and severity of TR are routinely assessed by transthoracic echocardiography, which also provides important information regarding the etiology of TR by assessing tricuspid leaflet morphology and function as well as RV function and pulmonary artery (PA) pressure (Figure 43.2).

Echocardiographic evaluation should focus on the exclusion of morphologic abnormalities of the tricuspid valve to distinguish between structural and functional TR. In structural TR, specific findings may include vegetations in endocarditis, leaflet retraction, thickening or reduced mobility in rheumatic or carcinoid disease, leaflet prolapsing in myxomatous or posttraumatic disease as well as congenital malformations such as Ebstein's anomaly. The diameter of the TVA measured in the transthoracic four-chamber view is 28 ± 5 mm and significant annular dilation is defined by a diastolic diameter of ≥40 mm.[13] During RV contraction, the annular area decreases by approximately 25–30%, which is essential for leaflet coaptation and competence of the valve.[13–15] In functional TR, a coaptation distance >8 mm has been reported in patients with significant tethering (distance between the tricuspid annular plane and the point of coaptation in midsystole from the apical four-chamber view).[16,17]

Further structural changes of the TV complex associated with the development of FTR may be observed using real-time three-dimensional echocardiography.[18,19] In healthy subjects, the TVA is a nonplanar, elliptical-shaped structure with the posteroseptal portion located most apically. In contrast, the development of FTR is associated

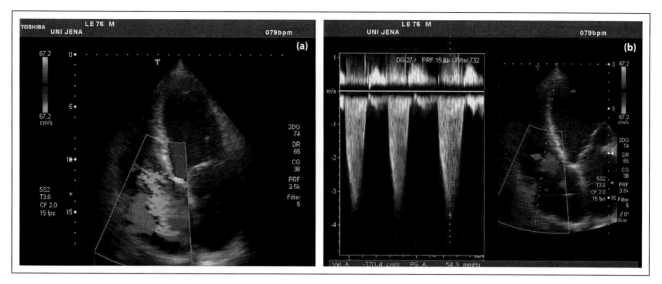

Figure 43.2 (**See color insert.**) Assessment of tricuspid regurgitation and assessment of pulmonary artery pressure. (a) Two-dimensional echocardiography with color-flow Doppler imaging demonstrating severe tricuspid regurgitation with enlargement of the right ventricle and right atrium. (b) Using continuous-wave Doppler and the modified Bernoulli equation, right ventricular and pulmonary artery systolic pressures are indirectly assessed at 55 mmHg.

with flattening of the annulus and an increased annular area primarily due to dilatation of the posterior and lateral segments along the RV free wall (Figure 43.3). This observation is relevant during surgical TV repair, as optimally shaped annuloplasty rings restoring the shape of the TV may favorably affect TV function and RV contractility.

Echocardiographic assessment of TR should also include RV function. Tricuspid annular plane systolic excursion (TAPSE) (<15 mm), tricuspid annulus systolic velocity (<11 cm/s), and RV end-systolic area (>20 cm²) may be used to identify patients with RV dysfunction.[17]

Elevated PA pressure plays a key role in the development and determination of the severity of FTR as it results in dilatation and remodeling of the RV.[20] As a rule, when systolic PA pressure increases beyond 55 mmHg, TR can occur despite anatomically normal tricuspid leaflets, whereas TR occurring with systolic pulmonary artery pressures less than 40 mmHg is likely to reflect a structural abnormality of the valve apparatus.[21]

The presence of intracardiac devices such as defibrillator or pacemaker leads crossing the TV requires careful evaluation of leaflet mobility as these devices may interfere with TV function and cause pacemaker-induced TR. The clinical significance of this entity has been suggested in case reports and small series; however, it is likely more relevant than currently acknowledged. In a recent report by Kim et al. studying the effect of intracardiac devices in 248 patients, the authors observed a worsening of TR by one grade after device implantation in 24.2%.[22] The extraction of existing transvalvular leads is not recommended in patients with TR based on current guidelines due to the adherence of the device to the valve and the subvalvular apparatus and the subsequent risk of injury.[23]

Indications for treatment

Currently, surgical valve repair or replacement is the only established treatment to restore TV function. Over the past

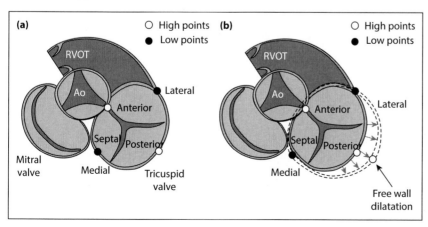

Figure 43.3 Three-dimensional view of the tricuspid valve relative to anatomic structures. (a) Tricuspid valve viewed from the right atrium. (b) Dilatation along the free wall aspect of the tricuspid valve with functional tricuspid regurgitation (dashed lines). Ao, aorta; RVOT, right ventricular outflow tract. (Adapted from Ton-Nu TT. *Circulation* 2006;114:143–9.)

few decades, there have been significant advances in surgical technique resulting in an improvement of early and late outcomes. However, compared with aortic and mitral valve surgery, TV procedures are much less frequently performed and there is a lack of large randomized trials. Therefore, the timing of surgical intervention remains controversial. In general, valve repair is preferable to valve replacement and surgery should be carried out early enough to avoid irreversible RV dysfunction.[17]

As considered by the ACC/AHA guidelines, the decision for TV surgery has to take different factors into account, including the degree and etiology of TR, the severity of symptoms, as well as previous or concomitant cardiac procedures required at the same setting (Table 43.1).

In patients with mild isolated TR, the general practice is to follow TV disease and, if necessary, treat symptoms of volume overload by pharmacologic therapy. Initial treatment is aimed at fluid and sodium restriction. Oral or intravenous diuretics are effective; however, this therapy may further decrease cardiac output and physical capacity. No data are available evaluating the efficacy of pharmacologic therapy in patients with TR.

In patients with moderate or moderate to severe TR, the decision to intervene is more complex. If there is a structural lesion of the valve besides annular dilatation, then surgery is considered beneficial. Otherwise, the decision for TV surgery depends on the surgeon's experience and the overall condition of the patient.

In patients with isolated severe symptomatic TR, surgical intervention should generally be performed (Table 43.1). Although these patients respond well to diuretic therapy, delaying surgery is likely to result in irreversible RV damage, organ failure, and poor results of late surgical intervention.[17]

A common clinical scenario regards the question whether to perform concomitant TV surgery in patients undergoing planned cardiac surgery for left-sided valve lesions. As noted in the 2012 ESC guidelines, correction of TR should be performed at the time of surgical correction of left-sided valve disease in patients with severe TR. It should also be considered in patients with moderate primary TR, as well as in patients with mild or moderate secondary TR and significant dilatation of the annulus (≥40 mm).

The current practice was long influenced by the paradigm that functional TR would improve after treatment of the left-sided valve leasions.[24] Although some evidence actually supports this concept, several studies have demonstrated the persistence or even progression of residual TR in patients after isolated mitral valve surgery.[25–29] TVA dilatation is considered an ongoing process that may progress to severe TR if left untreated and reoperation for recurrent or worsening TR is associated with a significant mortality.[27,30] According to the current guidelines, adjunctive tricuspid repair is clearly recommended in patients with severe TR undergoing mitral valve surgery. If significant TR is ignored, it negatively impacts early postoperative outcomes, functional class, and long-term survival (Figure 43.1).[10,31]

This is further supported by a study performed by Dreyfus et al. The authors visually assessed the tricuspid valve in 311 patients undergoing mitral valve repair. TV annuloplasty was concomitantly performed in those patients whose tricuspid annular diameter was greater than twice the normal size ($n = 148$, ≥70 mm) regardless of the grade of regurgitation. During follow-up, functional NYHA class and TR grade were significantly improved in patients who had undergone annuloplasty.[27] Thus, for patients undergoing planned cardiac surgery, literature sources support performing concomitant TV repair based on dilatation of the TV annulus at an early stage even in the absence of severe TR in order to avoid later deterioration of tricuspid insufficiency.

Table 43.1 2006 ACC/AHA guidelines (2008 focused update) pertaining to the surgical management of tricuspid valve disease/regurgitation

Class I
 Tricuspid valve repair is beneficial for severe TR in patients with MV disease requiring mitral valve surgery. (Level of evidence: B)

Class IIa
 1. Tricuspid valve replacement or annuloplasty is reasonable for severe primary TR when symptomatic. (Level of evidence: C)
 2. Tricuspid valve replacement is reasonable for severe TR secondary to disease/abnormal tricuspid valve leaflets not amenable to annuloplasty or repair. (Level of evidence: C)

Class IIb
 Tricuspid annuloplasty may be considered for less than severe TR in patients undergoing MV surgery when there is pulmonary hypertension or tricuspid annular dilatation. (Level of evidence: C)

Class III
 1. Tricuspid valve replacement or annuloplasty is not indicated in asymptomatic patients with TR whose pulmonary artery systolic pressure is less than 60 mmHg in the presence of a normal mitral valve. (Level of evidence: C)
 2. Tricuspid valve replacement or annuloplasty is not indicated in patients with mild primary TR. (Level of evidence: C)

ACC: American College of Cardiology; AHA: American Heart Association; TR tricuspid regurgitation.

Current techniques for TV surgery

TV repair is the preferred method to correct TR and is associated with better perioperative and long-term outcome than TV replacement.[5,32–35] A repair can be performed in the majority of patients with FTR if the leaflets and the subvalvular apparatus are structurally normal. In such patients, surgical repair focuses on reducing annular size, which can be performed by a number of different options. The efforts to achieve the most durable results have resulted in an ongoing debate as to whether annular plication should be achieved by ring implantation (open or closed) rather than by means of a partial purse-string suture technique ("DeVega technique"). The DeVega technique involves placement of a double row of running sutures around two-thirds of the circumference of the TVA. Annuloplasty rings usually cover the same portion of the TV annulus as the DeVega repair, thus also sparing the area of the conduction system and reducing the risk of heart block. Ring annuloplasty is more durable with a lower incidence of recurrent TR than suture annuloplasty.[30,36–39]

Another less commonly used technique, the edge-to-edge tricuspid valve repair has been suggested as providing an effective adjuvant procedure for severe residual TR following annuloplasty.[40–42] The procedure is analogous to mitral valve repair by leaflet approximation (Alfieri type) and involves anchoring the anterior leaflet to the facing edges of the septal and posterior leaflets of the TV, thus creating a triple orifice. Another technique involves annular bicuspidalization by placing a pledget-supported suture from the anteroposterior to the posteroseptal commissure, thus approximating the anterior and posterior portion of the TVA. It has been reported effective in isolated cases.[43]

Prosthetic TV replacement is reserved for advanced structural valve disease. It carries a higher perioperative failure rate and worse long-term survival compared with valve repair. A recent study followed 42 patients over a 17-year period after isolated or combined (mitral and/or aortic) tricuspid valve replacement. Sixty-nine percent had a bioprosthetic valve; the remainder received a mechanical implant. In-hospital mortality in this report was 26% with right heart failure as the primary cause of death. Ten-year survival was 37%, and 31% were free of major cardiovascular events at 10 years.[44] These findings are in line with those of others.[32,35,45,46] The high failure rate of prosthetic TV replacement is attributed to the change in flow and the distortion of the normally crescent-shaped TV annulus resulting from the rigid frame of the prosthetic valve with negative impact on geometry and contraction dynamics of the RV.[44]

Disclosures

None.

References

1. Singh JP, Evans JC, Levy D et al. Prevalence and clinical determinants of mitral, tricuspid, and aortic regurgitation (the Framingham Heart Study). *Am J Cardiol* 1999;83:897–902.

2. Simon R. Size and motion of the tricuspid annulus. *Circulation* 1983;67:709.

3. De Simone R, Lange R, Iacono A, Hagl S. [Role of transesophageal echocardiography in tricuspid valve repair]. *Cardiologia* 1994;39:87–101.

4. Drexler M, Erbel R, Dahm M, Mohr-Kahaly S, Oelert H, Meyer J. Assessment of successful valve reconstruction by intraoperative transesophageal echocardiography (TEE). *Int J Card Imaging* 1986;2:21–30.

5. Guenther T, Noebauer C, Mazzitelli D, Busch R, Tassani-Prell P, Lange R. Tricuspid valve surgery: A thirty-year assessment of early and late outcome. *Eur J Cardiothorac Surg* 2008;34:402–9.

6. Sung K, Park PW, Park KH et al. Is tricuspid valve replacement a catastrophic operation? *Eur J Cardiothorac Surg* 2009;36:825–9.

7. Jokinen JJ, Turpeinen AK, Pitkanen O, Hippelainen MJ, Hartikainen JE. Pacemaker therapy after tricuspid valve operations: Implications on mortality, morbidity, and quality of life. *Ann Thorac Surg* 2009;87:1806–14.

8. Do QB, Pellerin M, Carrier M et al. Clinical outcome after isolated tricuspid valve replacement: 20-year experience. *Can J Cardiol* 2000;16:489–93.

9. Stuge O, Liddicoat J. Emerging opportunities for cardiac surgeons within structural heart disease. *J Thorac Cardiovasc Surg* 2006;132:1258–61.

10. Nath J, Foster E, Heidenreich PA. Impact of tricuspid regurgitation on long-term survival. *J Am Coll Cardiol* 2004;43:405–9.

11. Moller JE, Connolly HM, Rubin J, Seward JB, Modesto K, Pellikka PA. Factors associated with progression of carcinoid heart disease. *N Engl J Med* 2003;348:1005–15.

12. Koelling TM, Aaronson KD, Cody RJ, Bach DS, Armstrong WF. Prognostic significance of mitral regurgitation and tricuspid regurgitation in patients with left ventricular systolic dysfunction. *Am Heart J* 2002;144:524–9.

13. Lancellotti P, Moura L, Pierard LA et al. European Association of Echocardiography recommendations for the assessment of valvular regurgitation. Part 2: Mitral and tricuspid regurgitation (native valve disease). *Eur J Echocardiogr* 2010;11:307–32.

14. Waller BF, Howard J, Fess S. Pathology of tricuspid valve stenosis and pure tricuspid regurgitation—Part II. *Clin Cardiol* 1995;18:167–74.

15. Waller BF, Howard J, Fess S. Pathology of tricuspid valve stenosis and pure tricuspid regurgitation—Part I. *Clin Cardiol* 1995;18:97–102.

16. Fukuda S, Gillinov AM, McCarthy PM et al. Determinants of recurrent or residual functional tricuspid regurgitation after tricuspid annuloplasty. *Circulation* 2006;114:I582–7.

17. Vahanian A, Alfieri O, Andreotti F et al. Guidelines on the management of valvular heart disease (version 2012). *Eur Heart J* 2012;33:2451–96.

18. Ton-Nu TT, Levine RA, Handschumacher MD et al. Geometric determinants of functional tricuspid regurgitation: Insights from 3-dimensional echocardiography. *Circulation* 2006;114:143–9.

19. Fukuda S, Saracino G, Matsumura Y et al. Three-dimensional geometry of the tricuspid annulus in healthy subjects and in patients with functional tricuspid regurgitation: A real-time, 3-dimensional echocardiographic study. *Circulation* 2006;114:I492–8.

20. Hinderliter AL, Willis PWt, Long WA et al. Frequency and severity of tricuspid regurgitation determined by Doppler echocardiography in primary pulmonary hypertension. *Am J Cardiol* 2003;91:1033–7,A9.

21. Bonow RO, Carabello BA, Chatterjee K et al. 2008 focused update incorporated into the ACC/AHA 2006 guidelines for the management of patients with valvular heart disease: A report of the American College of Cardiology/American Heart Association Task Force on Practice Guidelines (Writing Committee to revise the 1998

guidelines for the management of patients with valvular disease). Endorsed by the Society of Cardiovascular Anesthesiologists, Society for Cardiovascular Angiography and Interventions, and Society of Thoracic Surgeons. *J Am Coll Cardiol* 2008;52:e1–142.

22. Kim JB, Spevack DM, Tunick PA et al. The effect of transvenous pacemaker and implantable cardioverter defibrillator lead placement on tricuspid valve function: An observational study. *J Am Soc Echocardiogr* 2008;21:284–7.

23. Love CJ, Wilkoff BL, Byrd CL et al. Recommendations for extraction of chronically implanted transvenous pacing and defibrillator leads: Indications, facilities, training. North American Society of Pacing and Electrophysiology Lead Extraction Conference Faculty. *Pacing Clin Electrophysiol* 2000;23:544–51.

24. Cohn LH. Tricuspid regurgitation secondary to mitral valve disease: When and how to repair. *J Card Surg* 1994;9:237–41.

25. Hannoush H, Fawzy ME, Stefadouros M, Moursi M, Chaudhary MA, Dunn B. Regression of significant tricuspid regurgitation after mitral balloon valvotomy for severe mitral stenosis. *Am Heart J* 2004;148:865–70.

26. Duran CM, Pomar JL, Colman T, Figueroa A, Revuelta JM, Ubago JL. Is tricuspid valve repair necessary? *J Thorac Cardiovasc Surg* 1980;80:849–60.

27. Dreyfus GD, Corbi PJ, Chan KM, Bahrami T. Secondary tricuspid regurgitation or dilatation: Which should be the criteria for surgical repair? *Ann Thorac Surg* 2005;79:127–32.

28. Tager R, Skudicky D, Mueller U, Essop R, Hammond G, Sareli P. Long-term follow-up of rheumatic patients undergoing left-sided valve replacement with tricuspid annuloplasty—Validity of preoperative echocardiographic criteria in the decision to perform tricuspid annuloplasty. *Am J Cardiol* 1998;81:1013–6.

29. Sadeghi HM, Kimura BJ, Raisinghani A et al. Does lowering pulmonary arterial pressure eliminate severe functional tricuspid regurgitation? Insights from pulmonary thromboendarterectomy. *J Am Coll Cardiol* 2004;44:126–32.

30. McCarthy PM, Bhudia SK, Rajeswaran J et al. Tricuspid valve repair: Durability and risk factors for failure. *J Thorac Cardiovasc Surg* 2004;127:674–85.

31. Bonow RO, Carabello BA, Kanu C et al. ACC/AHA 2006 guidelines for the management of patients with valvular heart disease: A report of the American College of Cardiology/American Heart Association Task Force on Practice Guidelines (writing committee to revise the 1998 Guidelines for the Management of Patients With Valvular Heart Disease): Developed in collaboration with the Society of Cardiovascular Anesthesiologists: Endorsed by the Society for Cardiovascular Angiography and Interventions and the Society of Thoracic Surgeons. *Circulation* 2006;114:e84–231.

32. Chang BC, Lim SH, Yi G et al. Long-term clinical results of tricuspid valve replacement. *Ann Thorac Surg* 2006;81:1317–23, discussion 1323–4.

33. Singh SK, Tang GH, Maganti MD et al. Midterm outcomes of tricuspid valve repair versus replacement for organic tricuspid disease. *Ann Thorac Surg* 2006;82:1735–41.

34. McGrath LB, Gonzalez-Lavin L, Bailey BM, Grunkemeier GL, Fernandez J, Laub GW. Tricuspid valve operations in 530 patients. Twenty-five-year assessment of early and late phase events. *J Thorac Cardiovasc Surg* 1990;99:124–33.

35. Kawano H, Oda T, Fukunaga S et al. Tricuspid valve replacement with the St. Jude Medical valve: 19 years of experience. *Eur J Cardiothorac Surg* 2000;18:565–9.

36. Tang GH, David TE, Singh SK, Maganti MD, Armstrong S, Borger MA. Tricuspid valve repair with an annuloplasty ring results in improved long-term outcomes. *Circulation* 2006;114:I577–81.

37. Peltola T, Lepojarvi M, Ikaheimo M, Karkola P. De Vega's annuloplasty for tricuspid regurgitation. *Ann Chir Gynaecol* 1996;85:40–3.

38. De Paulis R, Bobbio M, Ottino G et al. The De Vega tricuspid annuloplasty. Perioperative mortality and long term follow-up. *J Cardiovasc Surg (Torino)* 1990;31:512–7.

39. Fukuda S, Song JM, Gillinov AM et al. Tricuspid valve tethering predicts residual tricuspid regurgitation after tricuspid annuloplasty. *Circulation* 2005;111:975–9.

40. De Bonis M, Lapenna E, La Canna G et al. A novel technique for correction of severe tricuspid valve regurgitation due to complex lesions. *Eur J Cardiothorac Surg* 2004;25:760–5.

41. Castedo E, Canas A, Cabo RA, Burgos R, Ugarte J. Edge-to-Edge tricuspid repair for redeveloped valve incompetence after DeVega's annuloplasty. *Ann Thorac Surg* 2003;75:605–6.

42. Castedo E, Monguio E, Cabo RA, Ugarte J. Edge-to-edge technique for correction of tricuspid valve regurgitation due to complex lesions. *Eur J Cardiothorac Surg* 2005;27:933–4; author reply 934–5.

43. Deloche A, Guerinon J, Fabiani JN et al. [Anatomical study of rheumatic tricuspid valve diseases: Application to the study of various valvuloplasties]. *Ann Chir Thorac Cardiovasc* 1973;12:343–9.

44. Iscan ZH, Vural KM, Bahar I, Mavioglu L, Saritas A. What to expect after tricuspid valve replacement? Long-term results. *Eur J Cardiothorac Surg* 2007;32:296–300.

45. Filsoufi F, Anyanwu AC, Salzberg SP, Frankel T, Cohn LH, Adams DH. Long-term outcomes of tricuspid valve replacement in the current era. *Ann Thorac Surg* 2005;80:845–50.

46. Carrier M, Hebert Y, Pellerin M et al. Tricuspid valve replacement: An analysis of 25 years of experience at a single center. *Ann Thorac Surg* 2003;75:47–50.

44

Tricuspid valve insufficiency: Melody valve in the tricuspid position

Phillip Roberts

Introduction

Over the last few decades, percutaneous transcatheter valve replacement has moved from being experimental to routine practice in defined patient groups. Transcatheter valve replacement of the arterial valves has led the way with the recognition that suitable landing zones or anchor points enable safe delivery of percutaneous valves.[1] In the case of the pulmonary valve and right ventricle (RV)-to-pulmonary artery (PA) connection, most of the patients will have had previous surgical interventions; however, in the aortic position, the great majority of interventions are in the native calcified aortic valve. To date, animal work on the native atrioventricular connection has not translated to human practice.[2] However, it was inevitable that with the surgical creation of an anchor point in the previously operated atrioventricular valve connection that technically, it would be possible to rehabilitate a previously inserted bioprosthesis by utilizing a valve-in-valve strategy.[3] Early reports of the feasibility of transcatheter bioprosthetic tricuspid valve rehabilitation were initially hybrid and subsequently, percutaneous strategies were introduced using Edwards valves.[3–5]

The first percutaneous tricuspid valve rehabilitation using the Melody valve was performed by Cheatham and Zahn (personal communication) with the first case report and series reported by Roberts et al.[6,7] As with most low-volume procedures, cardiac centers regularly performing arterial valve implants will have a small number of patients who have undergone a percutaneous atrioventricular valve replacement or rehabilitation. Although this has been demonstrated as technically feasible, there is no published data as to the long-term outcome for this patient group and meaningful numbers are only likely to be achieved with a multicenter collaboration.

The debate continues as to whether mechanical or bioprosthetic valves are the best surgical implant for the tricuspid valve position. The low-flow situation in the tricuspid valve compromises mechanical valve function and although bioprosthetic tricuspid valve implants will deteriorate with the passage of time, in addition to the standard benefits with this type of valve, the possibility of valve-in-valve rehabilitation is facilitated.

Thus, there is a small group of patients who will have a surgically positioned bioprosthesis or in exceptional congenital cardiac cases, a surgically created right atrium (RA)–RV connection that will be suitable for percutaneous transcatheter valve rehabilitation. Universal to all of this patient group is the surgically created landing zone or anchor point.

Preparation

Careful review of the original surgical records is essential to confirm the internal device dimensions of the previously surgically inserted tricuspid valve, and with the help of the manufacturer specifications along with optimal preoperative imaging, optimal device choice can be made prior to the procedure. The Medtronic Melody valve is suitable for sizes that are 18–22 mm and currently, the Edwards valves are available in 23, 26, and 29 mm sizes. Both the Melody and Edwards valves are suitable for insertion in the tricuspid position with the final choice dictated by the internal dimensions of the original bioprosthesis.

Catheterization

Given the size of the delivery sheaths and the importance of the patient being still during the procedure, general anesthesia is recommended. Standard percutaneous vessel access strategies are utilized with the use of local anesthesia, heparinization, and antibiotics after access is obtained. As with all percutaneous transvascular cardiac interventions, the presence of surgical backup is prudent. Pre- and posthemodynamic data are obtained. Transoesophageal

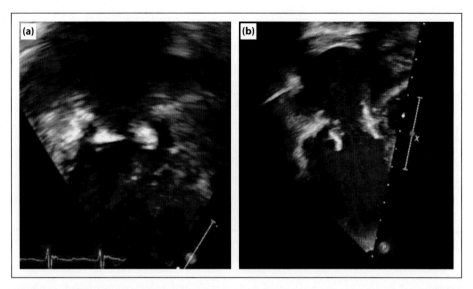

Figure 44.1   Transthoracic echocardiogram, an apical view. (a) shows a severely stenosed bioprosthesis that can be seen to be widely patent on (b) postinsertion of a 22 mm Melody™.

ultrasound is not essential, but its use during the procedure helps to monitor for complications including tamponade, ventricular dysfunction, air embolization, and assessment of the final result postdelivery of the new valve. Some operators use intracardiac echocardiography from the contralateral femoral vein to guide and assess valve deployment and function. Ultrasound-guided vessel access allows assessment of the vessels in a patient group who are likely to have at least one previous procedure where vessel damage may have occurred. Invasive arterial blood pressure monitoring is recommended.

Although it would seem logical that right internal jugular access would give the most direct route to the tricuspid valve,

small case series to date show that delivery is just as feasible from the femoral route. As with all percutaneous transcatheter valve procedures, it is important that there is a stable wire position. It is recommended that an Amplatzer Super Stiff 0.035 inch wire or Lunderquist wire are positioned in the distal pulmonary artery to optimize wire stability. Predilatation is useful in the severely stenosed bioprosthesis and also allows the operator to interrogate and clearly identify the potential points of stenosis within the previously inserted bioprosthesis and to confirm that the appropriate valve size will be selected. In most cases, the originally inserted bioprosthesis will act as an adequate anchor point; however, if there are any concerns, then prestenting to create

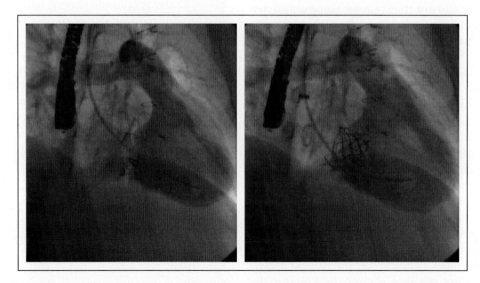

Figure 44.2   Pre- and post-RV angiograms showing that the tricuspid regurgitation has been successfully treated postinsertion of a 22 mm Melody™ valve.

a more secure landing zone[8] is appropriate but at the cost of potentially reducing the final dimension of the yet-to-be-inserted percutaneous valve. The standard inflation techniques as advised by the manufacturer of the valve should be followed. It is important to ensure that the transcatheter valve is appropriately mounted on the balloon in the correct orientation to ensure that catastrophic obstruction to flow does not occur. As the valve is being antegradely inserted, there is not typically a requirement for ventricular pacing to reduce cardiac output. Figures 44.1 and 44.2 are echocardiographic and fluoroscopic images before and after valve implantation, respectively.

Discussion

To date, the technical feasibility of percutaneous rehabilitation of the right-sided atrioventricular (AV) connection has been demonstrated but long-term data as to valve function under the right heart-loading conditions are not yet available. Intuitively, one would expect the valve to work well; however, there are case series reporting rapid degeneration of the newly inserted bioprosthesis. In view of this, adequate preparation of both the patient and his or her family should include the fact that this type of procedure is aimed at reducing the total number of potential bypass procedures for atrioventricular valve replacement that a patient

may require in his or her lifetime. If the connection is of adequate size, it should be technically possible to repeat the procedure if the implanted bioprosthesis deteriorates.

References

1. Bonhoeffer P, Boudjemline Y, Saliba Z et al. Percutaneous replacement of pulmonary valve in a right-ventricle to pulmonary-artery prosthetic conduit with valve dysfunction. *Lancet* 2000;356(9239):1403–5.
2. Boudjemline Y, Agnoletti G, Bonnet D et al. Steps toward the percutaneous replacement of atrioventricular valves: An experimental study. *J Am Coll Cardiol* 2005;46(2):360–5.
3. Webb JG, Wood DA, Ye J, Gurvitch R et al. Transcatheter valve-in-valve implantation for failed bioprosthetic heart valves. *Circulation* 2010;121(16):1848–57.
4. Van Garsse LAFM, ter Bekke RMA, van Ommen VGVA. Percutaneous transcatheter valve-in-valve implantation in stenosed tricuspid valve bioprosthesis. *Circulation* 2011;123(5):e219–21.
5. Weich H, Janson J, van Wyk J et al. Transjugular tricuspid valve-in-valve replacement. *Circulation* 2011;124(5):e157–60.
6. Roberts P, Spina R, Vallely M, Wilson M, Bailey B, Celermajer DS. Percutaneous tricuspid valve replacement for a stenosed bioprosthesis. *Circ Cardiovasc Interv* 2010;3(4):e14–5.
7. Roberts PA, Boudjemline Y, Cheatham JP et al. Percutaneous tricuspid valve replacement in congenital and acquired heart disease. *J Am Coll Cardiol* 2011;58(2):117–22.
8. Kenny D, Hijazi ZM, Walsh KP. Transcatheter tricuspid valve replacement with the Edwards SAPIEN valve. *Catheter Cardiovasc Interv* 2011;78:267–70.

45

Tricuspid valve insufficiency: SAPIEN valve in the tricuspid position

Kiran K. Mallula, Damien Kenny, and Ziyad M. Hijazi

Introduction

With the advent of transcatheter pulmonary and aortic valve replacement, attempts have been ongoing to extend this technology to both atrioventricular valves. Percutaneous tricuspid valve replacement (TVR) was described as early as 2005 by Boudjemline and colleagues in an animal model.[2] They devised a self-fabricated self-expandable stent formed of two disks separated by a tubular part. The ventricular disk was covered by a polytetrafluoroethylene (PTFE) membrane to ensure complete annular sealing, and the atrial disk was left uncovered to prevent occlusion of the coronary sinus. The diameter of the two disks was chosen to be slightly larger than the diameter of the tricuspid annulus to allow for anchoring. Mechanical fixation was ensured by trapping the annulus between the two disks. An 18 mm bovine jugular vein valve was sutured in the tubular part of the device. The device was tested in native tricuspid valves. However, one problem related to the orthotopic position was sufficient fixation of the valve in the highly dynamic tricuspid annulus. The second issue was the fact that tricuspid regurgitation (TR) in humans is usually secondary to the right heart dilation and so it is a challenge to rely on the annular size. Bai et al.[3] described in sheep the use of a self-fabricated stented valve comprising a unidirectional semilunar valve of porcine pericardium that was sutured onto a ring and mounted on a double-edge nitinol stent. PTFE was not used to cover the stent, which enabled the delivery system to be as compact as a 14 F delivery system. Again, the major limitation was that these valved stents were <18 mm diameter whereas pathologic TR in humans results in tricuspid annular dilation up to 30–40 mm. Lauten et al.[4] evaluated the concept of heterotopic TVR via implantation of self-expanding valves in the superior vena cava (SVC) and inferior vena cava (IVC) of sheep. This allowed for sufficient valve fixation and carried low risk to cardiac structures. However, although this reduces the amount of venous regurgitation,

it does not reduce the right ventricular and atrial volume overload. Although stable transcatheter stent–valve delivery is routine across the native aortic valve with calcific aortic stenosis, the remaining locations have largely required prosthetic material to provide support for the stent–valve complex and thus, reported transcatheter TVR to date in humans has been limited to patients with previous TVR.

The first human transcatheter tricuspid valve-in-valve implantation was described by Webb et al.[5] using a transatrial delivery of the Edwards SAPIEN valve (Edwards Lifesciences, Irvine, CA). A right intercostal surgical approach with direct right atrial puncture was used to facilitate coaxial positioning of the SAPIEN valve within the surgical bioprosthesis. Since this time, extended experience with the SAPIEN valve has been limited to case reports.[1,6–13]

This chapter (see Table 45.1) exclusively focuses on the transcatheter implantation of the Edwards SAPIEN valve in the tricuspid position and highlights the procedure in detail, describing the merits and demerits of the system and various approaches that have been utilized.

Indications for percutaneous TVR

There are no current guidelines for transcatheter TVR. However, the common consensus recommendations from the various published case reports and studies[5,7,11,14,15] include patients with a failing bioprosthetic tricuspid valve and the following:

1. Significant right heart failure symptoms
2. Patients at high risk for repeat surgery after primary surgical valve replacements who are candidates for valve-in-valve procedure
3. Patients with multiple comorbidities, including atrial fibrillation, chronic rheumatic heart disease, severe pulmonary hypertension, chronic obstructive pulmonary disease (COPD), renal failure on dialysis, frail, severe RV failure, and morbid obesity

Table 45.1 All case reports of TVR using the SAPIEN valve with patient and perioperative characteristics

Author	Age	Sex	Diagnosis	Prior surgical tricuspid valve	Approach	Presenting	Pacing	Imaging	ESV
Hon (2010)	48	F	Carcinoid	Mosaic 27	Transatrial	No	Yes	TEE	26 XT
Webb (2010)	48	N/A	N/A	Moasia 27	Transatrial	No	Yes	TEE	26
Cerillo (2011)	71	F	N/A	Hancock 27	RIJ	No	Yes	TEE	26
Gewellig (2011)	8	F	Tricuspid failure after transcatheter VSD closure	CE 25	RIJ	No	Yes	TTE	26 XT
Nielsen (2011)	69	M	Endocarditis	CE 27	Transatrial	No	Yes	TEE	26
Calvert (2011)	61	F	RHD	Porcine BP 29	Femoral	No	Yes	TEE	26
Kenny (2011)	20	M	PA with IVS s/p 1.5 repair; endocarditis of TV BP	CE Perimount 27	Femoral	Yes	Yes	N/A	26
Hoendermis (2011)	22	F	Ebsteins anomaly	St Jude Epic 29	Femoral	No	Yes	TEE	26 XT
Van Garsse (2011)	74	F	Partial AV canal s/p repair	CE 25	RIJ	No	Yes	ICE, TEE	23
Cheung (2012)	81	M	TVR; MVR	Mitroflow 27	Transatrial	No	Yes	TEE	26
	77	F	Ebsteins s/p repair;Redo TVR; ASD; and His ablation s/p PM	CE 33	Transatrial	No	Yes	TEE	29 XT
Weich (2011)	38	F	RHD	CE Perimount 31	RIJ	No	No	TEE	XT with inflation to 27
Bentham (2012)	N/A	N/A	Ebstenoid malformation; s/p porcine TV BP	Melody valve 22		No	N/A	TEE	23
Cerillo (2012)	61	F		CE Perimount Plus 29	RIJ	No	Yes	N/A	29 XT

4. Younger female patients intending to avoid anticoagulation and who want to have children
5. Young patients with multiple cardiac surgeries/sternotomies
6. Tricuspid valve stenosis with mean gradient of >5 mmHg

Edwards SAPIEN valve

This consists of bovine pericardial tissue housed in a stainless steel stent with a polyethylene terephthalene skirt. The valve leaflets undergo anticalcification treatment during production in an attempt to maximize longevity. The currently available diameters include 23 and 26 mm valves. A newer version of the valve (SAPIEN XT) on a cobalt–chromium frame features semiclosed leaflets and a smaller crimped profile than the SAPIEN and comes in 20, 23, 26, and 29 mm diameters. The SAPIEN has been extensively used in the aortic position and also in the pulmonic

position and has been shown to be effective, at least in the short term.[16] There have been case reports of its off-label use in the tricuspid position to re-valve a failed bioprosthetic tricuspid valve.[8,9]

Advantages of the SAPIEN valve

1. Large available stent diameter of this valve makes it very suitable to use in the tricuspid position, given the large tricuspid bioprostheses (BP) that are used for TVR.[9]
2. The short length of the stented valve with the 26 mm valve measuring 16 mm ensures that the stent does not significantly protrude into the right ventricle (RV).
3. The delivery system is steerable and useful for navigation around tighter curves.
4. Stent durability is also thought to be a benefit of this system with more than 50,000 SAPIEN valves implanted worldwide without the report of structural failure.

Disadvantages of the SAPIEN valve

1. Large and rigid delivery systems: Technically, the delivery system used with the SAPIEN valve is bulky, and this may be an issue when navigating tortuous curves;[17] however, this should not greatly influence position within the more accessible tricuspid area and smaller delivery systems are becoming available.[9]
2. Owing to the short length of the stented valve, the window for accurate positioning is narrow and prestenting is advised.

Procedure

Preprocedural planning is vital. An appreciation of the size of the surgical bioprosthesis and the extent of the calcification is important to guide decision making regarding prestenting and the size of balloon and stents used. A multidisciplinary team approach is advised with surgical backup available and on standby, particularly in centers with limited experience. The use of advanced preprocedural imaging techniques (CT) is varied and the potential benefits in fine-tuning decision making are as yet unclear.

Imaging

Transesophageal echocardiogram (TEE) (with three-dimensional [3D] reconstruction) is invaluable for determining the size of the tricuspid valve annulus. Usually, this can be best determined in the short-axis view or the four-chamber view, but confirmation of the size should be made from multiple views. It also helps to determine the internal diameter of the surgically placed prosthesis. During deployment of the valve, it is invaluable in the assessment of

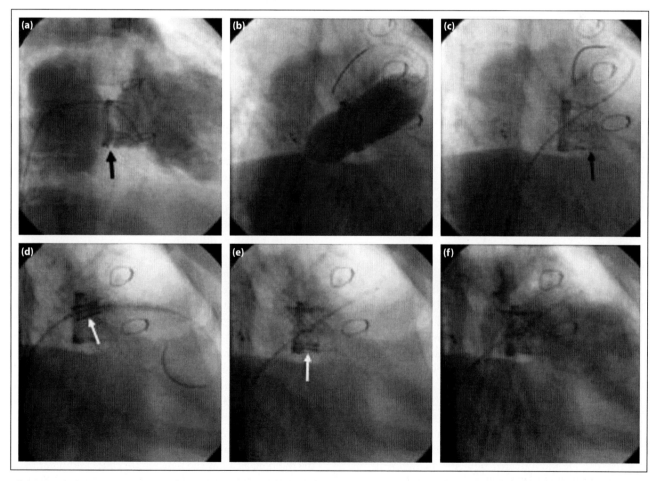

Figure 45.1 Initial right ventricular angiogram demonstrating severe TR with contrast seen filling the entire right atrium. The preexisting bioprosthesis is indicated by the black arrow (b,c). Balloon inflation of the stent with excellent position across the preexisting mounted tricuspid bioprosthesis (black arrow). (d) Positioning the Edwards SAPIEN valve across the preexisting stent for deployment in the tricuspid position (white arrow). (e) The Edwards valve following deployment with excellent position within the existing stent (white arrow). (f) Repeat right ventricular angiogram following stent deployment demonstrates minimal TR and no paravalvar leak. (Adapted from Kenny D, Hijazi ZM, Walsh KP. *Catheter Cardiovasc Interv* 2011;78(2):267–70.)

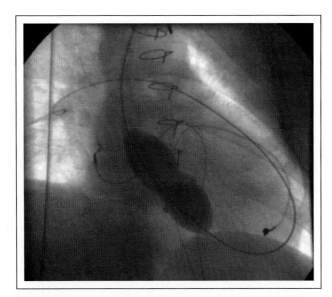

Figure 45.2 A contrast-filled balloon inflated within the bioprosthetic valve was useful in identifying the site and degree of maximum stenosis as well as allowing for predilation. (Adapted from Roberts PA et al. *J Am Coll Cardiol* 2011;58(2):117–22.)

proper coaxial positioning of the valve inside the tricuspid BP, especially in the setting of nonradiopaque tricuspid BPs where the fluoroscopy may not be that helpful. Valves can be deployed without fluoroscopy landmarks. Intracardiac echo can be employed along with or instead of TEE; however, it is vital that the catheter position within the right atrium does not interfere with valve deployment. It may be useful when there is scatter from a previously placed mechanical valve that may render TEE imaging to be inadequate.[11]

Femoral approach

The procedure (see Figure 45.1) can be performed in a monoplane or biplane cardiac catheterization suite under general anesthesia.[1,9,17] Intravenous antibiotics and heparin should be administered as per the unit protocol. Femoral venous access can be obtained with preplacement of two vascular closure devices, as a large delivery sheath will be required. Crossing the tricuspid valve may be tricky and may entail using a long Mullins transseptal sheath (Medtronic Minneapolis, MN) to help orient a smaller catheter such as a balloon wedge pressure catheter (Arrow International, Reading, PA) to cross into the RV.[1] After performing initial hemodynamic assessment, a right ventriculogram may confirm severe TR and a dilated right atrium. Subsequently, a 0.035 inch Lunderquist wire (Cook Medical, Bloomington, IN) or Amplatz Extra Stiff (St Jude Medical, St Paul, MN) or any other stiff wire can be placed in the right pulmonary artery and a long sheath advanced to the right ventricle. The tip of the wire may be shaped into a curve to facilitate contouring within the RV. Balloon sizing of the tricuspid

bioprosthesis with a compliant balloon is optional (Figure 45.2) although it may help to determine the degree of stenosis and the size of the transcatheter heart valve (THV) to be used and also to delineate the landing zone for the intended stent placement based on the level of maximal stenosis and precise positioning of the valved stent.[18] Balloon valvuloplasty may be necessary in the setting of severe stenosis if there is concern regarding the ability to cross the valve with larger delivery systems. However, dilation well below the original annulus size is recommended. Rapid atrial pacing (or left ventricular pacing) may be used to facilitate balloon stability during inflation. Coaxial positioning of the transcatheter valve into the degenerated bioprosthesis is important since the inability to align the valve properly, resulting in an angled, nonparallel position, increases the risk of an unstable valve position, and embolization. This has been the cause of much discussion, with debate regarding optimal wire position to achieve this, with some advocates for a right ventricular apical wire position; however, generally, wire position within the pulmonary artery is advised. Given the short length of the SAPIEN valve, prestenting is preferable and will provide a more stable landing zone;[9] however, many case reports have implanted the valve within the native sewing ring without prestenting (Table 45.1). The choice of balloon size should be based on the extent of the stenosis and the size of the bioprosthetic valve ring. Large-diameter bioprosthetic valves (>30 mm) may not be a contraindication as marked encroachment upon the lumen of these valves may occur with pure stenosis. In mixed valve disease, more caution is advised with larger bioprosthetic rings and balloon sizing in these situations is vital. In general, prestenting to a diameter of 2 mm less than the size of the SAPIEN valve to be used is advised when significant regurgitation is present. The SAPIEN valve is prepared by crimping the valve onto the balloon with a specialized manual crimping tool to achieve symmetrical valve compression over the balloon. The valve must be crimped in a similar orientation when using it in the pulmonary position (reverse orientation of that when used for transfemoral transcatheter aortic valve placement). The access sheath is then upsized to the Edwards hydrophilic sheath and at this stage, the guide wire may be repositioned toward the right ventricular apex. However, caution is advised, as wire perforation of the right ventricle is a concern. When using the Novoflex or Retroflex delivery catheters, full flexion may be required to negotiate the acute curve in the right atrium. This is a significant advantage of the Edwards system. When using the newer SAPIEN XT valve, care has to be taken when pulling the valve onto the balloon, as it has the potential to cause folding or damage to the valve cusps and may lead to residual insufficiency after deployment. The valve is subsequently deployed with or without the use of rapid atrial pacing and a subsequent right ventricular angiogram can demonstrate competency of the THV. In the absence of prestenting, the overlapping of the sewing ring of the bioprosthesis with the valve stent

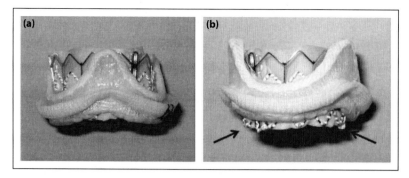

Figure 45.3 (**See color insert.**) Transcatheter valve deployed within a surgical prosthesis (SAPIEN THV and Carpenter–Edwards). (a) Incorrect positioning. The outflows of the surgical prosthesis and THV are superimposed. During balloon deployment, the prosthetic struts may be splayed, allowing the THV to embolize. (b) Correct positioning. The THV overlaps the sewing ring of the surgical prosthesis allowing more secure fixation. (Adapted from Webb JG et al. *Circulation* 2010;121(16):1848–57.)

is crucially important to minimize the embolization (Figure 45.3).[5] Once deployed, full reassessment can be carried out. Hemostasis can be achieved with either a preclosure device or a figure-of-eight suture. Aspirin is generally recommended for at least 6 months.

SVC (transjugular) approach

The jugular venous approach provides an attractive approach to the tricuspid valve with a straighter course than the femoral vein.[8,10–12,19,20] Ultrasound-guided puncture of the right internal jugular vein is advised. A venogram may

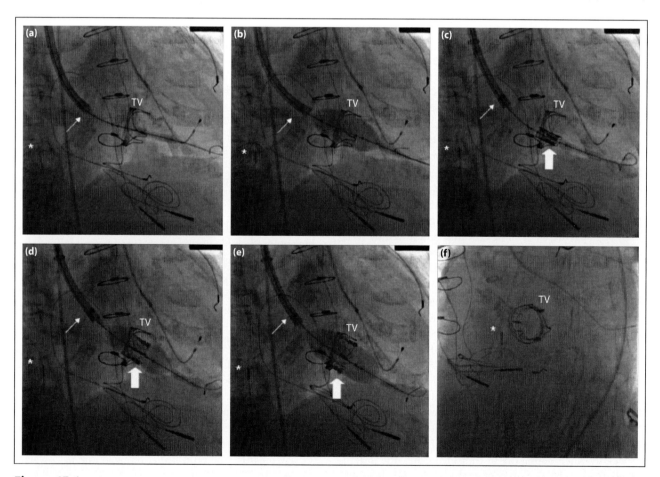

Figure 45.4 Fluoroscopy in transjugular approach with ICE (asterisk) catheter in the RA:[11] (a) Position of guide wire in RV apex with the balloon crossing the tricuspid valve. (b) Balloon valvuloplasty. (c) ESV 23 mm (large arrow) crimped on the balloon, and positioned in the tricuspid valve orifice. (d) Gradual balloon inflation and valve positioning. (e) Totally inflated balloon during valve implantation. (f) Final result of valve-in-valve position. (Adapted from Van Garsse LA, Ter Bekke RM, van Ommen VG. *Circulation* 2011;123(5):e219–21.)

assist in determining the adequacy of size. The right internal jugular vein can also be isolated with a small surgical incision and a purse-string placed. A similar approach as described above is then employed with a stiff wire placed in the pulmonary artery (see Figure 45.4). Over this, the sheath can be upsized to the appropriate delivery sheath size.

One disadvantage of the jugular venous approach especially when the tricuspid bioprosthesis is horizontal to the caval orientation may relate to the fact that the downward pushing force from above may cause prolapse of the bioprosthesis into the IVC.[12] The parallel position of the tricuspid valve to the caval veins can hamper the balloon to cross the heavily calcified tricuspid annulus. The angle of approach to the tricuspid prosthesis may not always be appropriate.[6]

Transatrial approach

This procedure should be performed in a hybrid procedure room with facilities to undergo emergent open-heart surgery.[5–7,13] Under general anesthesia, a double-lumen endotracheal tube is used to isolate the right lung. The patient is positioned in a partial left lateral (45°) position with the right arm hyperextended exposing the right lateral chest wall. Both groins are exposed to facilitate emergency cardiopulmonary bypass. TEE is used to confirm the internal diameter of the dysfunctional valve as described above. Under fluoroscopy, the surface landmark of the midposition of the bioprosthesis is identified in two planes using a radiopaque marker to optimize the incision site. A right anterior minithoractomy can be performed through the fourth intercostal space to expose the right atrium. A circumferential set of purse-string sutures with Teflon pledgets may be placed through the pericardium around the target puncture site to control bleeding. The patient can then be heparinized at a low dose and monitored by serial clotting times with a goal ≥300. Two long spinal needles are pierced into the myocardium for fibrillation. A 6 or 7 F vascular sheath with a dilator is then advanced into the right atrium in the implanting view and a hydrophilic wire can be easily positioned inside the pulmonary trunk. Sometimes, the crossing of the stenotic valve may require the use of a pulmonary flotation catheter due to the acute angle encountered between the chest wall and the plane of the tricuspid valve.[6] The hydrophilic wire can then be replaced by an Amplatz Super Stiff wire and then the Edwards sheath can be exchanged over it. The SAPIEN THV is then positioned carefully under fluoroscopy and echocardiographic guidance. The latter is crucial especially when deploying in translucent BP. The heart is fibrillated for the deployment of the THV and then defibrillated about 10 s after completion. The delivery sheath and wire are removed after confirmation of accurate position and function. Hemostasis is achieved and the chest wall is closed over a pleural drain. The main benefit offered by this approach is the accurate coaxial positioning of the THV within the tricuspid bioprosthesis. However, patients undergoing this procedure are often extremely fragile. Owing to multiple prior operations, they may develop tenacious pleuro–pericardial adhesions and re-entering the chest and dissection of these adhesions carries a significant risk of damaging the lung and cardiac structures leading to pneumothorax, subcutaneous emphysema, and recurrent pleural effusions.[10]

Pacing

Rapid pacing has been described to ensure accurate positioning of balloon-expandable valves. A transvenous lead cannot be placed in the RV as it may be jailed over the bioprosthetic valve when the THV is deployed. The pacing catheter may be introduced into the left ventricle (LV) from a femoral arterial access.[17] Otherwise, a quadripolar electrophysiology (EP) pacing catheter can be placed in the coronary sinus or atrial pacing may be considered if adequate ventricular capture is achievable. An epicardial pacing system will require planning for surgical access.[1] However, it is feasible when a transatrial approach is contemplated since the temporary pacing leads can be placed in the RV myocardium.[7]

Sizing considerations

Prosthetic heart valves are usually described according to their external diameter.[5] However, the relevant diameter is the inner diameter for valve-in-valve implantation. Internal diameter varies by the manufacturer, model, and size. Although manufacturers may report the internal diameter, the nomenclature is far from being standardized and may be misleading. Moreover, calcified, bulky, or torn tissue leaflets, pannus, and variations in valve design have unpredictable implications. Imaging modalities such as CT and 3D echocardiography are useful tools that can be employed preprocedurally to determine the size of the effective annulus. Other preoperative modalities include intracardiac echocardiography (ICE), angiography, and measurement of the annulus by using a sizing balloon.

Complications can include the following:[14]

1. Acute complications related to the procedure include device embolization, residual insufficiency, fatal arrhythmias, and chordal rupture due to the ends of the stented valves.
2. Insufficiency: The possible causes of regurgitation are either insufficient coaptation at lower right ventricular pressures or mild leaflet damage due to "inverted loading."[8]
3. Complete heart block: Owing to the proximity of the conduction system, there is a remote risk of causing acquired heart block.

4. Infective endocarditis has been reported in a patient who underwent Melody valve implantation in the tricuspid position.[14]
5. Paravalvar leaks: They have been reported both in animal studies[2] and in one case in humans.[7] If the stent valve does not adapt completely to the inner ring of the BP, a paravalvar leak may ensue. The development of new stent valves with an exterior cuff is expected to decrease the significance of paravalvar leaks.
6. Early valve failure: This may be related to individual patient factors and propensity to attack the foreign tissue. It may thus be beneficial to include a workup for immunologic and inflammatory markers when this is suspected. However, evidence to recommend this routinely is lacking. One hypothesis may be related to the poor hemodynamics associated with dilated poorly contractile right atria that may result in limited valve leaflet mobility such that the valve fails to open and close satisfactorily with each cardiac cycle. This could result in a rapid deterioration in valve function as the leaflets contract and fibrose.[21]
7. Death: No deaths have been reported so far with this procedure that is in contrast to surgical reports of TVR that carry high mortality rates particularly in smaller patients.[22]

Conclusion

Overall, percutaneous TVR with the Edwards SAPIEN valve is achievable with a high procedural success rate when undertaken by groups experienced with other THVs in the pulmonic and aortic positions. This procedure may reduce the total number of open cardiac bypass procedures that a patient may have to undergo during his or her lifetime and does not appear to prevent the future use of a surgical approach, if it is required. This is a novel procedure that has so far been attempted in very high-risk patients and is done as an off-label use of the currently available THVs for humanitarian reasons. Transcatheter valve implantation in the tricuspid position remains highly experimental and if implanted, these valves require long-term surveillance. Long-term studies assessing the valve function in the tricuspid position in relation to RV systolic and diastolic pressures, ejection fraction, stent fracture, arrhythmia, and exercise capacity are awaited.

References

1. Calvert PA, Himbert D, Brochet E, Radu C, Iung B, Hvass U et al. Transfemoral implantation of an Edwards SAPIEN valve in a tricuspid bioprosthesis without fluoroscopic landmarks. *EuroIntervention* 2012;7(11):1336–9.
2. Boudjemline Y, Agnoletti G, Bonnet D, Behr L, Borenstein N, Sidi D, et al. Steps toward the percutaneous replacement of atrioventricular valves: An experimental study. *J Am Coll Cardiol* 2005;46(2):360–5.
3. Bai Y, Zong GJ, Wang HR, Jiang HB, Wang H, Wu H, et al. An integrated pericardial valved stent special for percutaneous tricuspid implantation: An animal feasibility study. *J Surg Res* 2010;160(2): 215–21.
4. Lauten A, Figulla HR, Willich C, Laube A, Rademacher W, Schubert H, et al. Percutaneous caval stent valve implantation: Investigation of an interventional approach for treatment of tricuspid regurgitation. *Eur Heart J* 2010;31(10):1274–81.
5. Webb JG, Wood DA, Ye J, Gurvitch R, Masson JB, Rodes-Cabau J, et al. Transcatheter valve-in-valve implantation for failed bioprosthetic heart valves. *Circulation* 2010;121(16):1848–57.
6. Hon JK, Cheung A, Ye J, Carere RG, Munt B, Josan K, et al. Transatrial transcatheter tricuspid valve-in-valve implantation of balloon expandable bioprosthesis. *Ann Thorac Surg* 2010;90(5):1696–7.
7. Nielsen HH, Egeblad H, Klaaborg KE, Hjortdal VE, Thuesen L. Transatrial stent–valve implantation in a stenotic tricuspid valve bioprosthesis. *Ann Thorac Surg* 2011;91(5):e74–6.
8. Gewillig M, Dubois C. Percutaneous re-revalvulation of the tricuspid valve. *Catheter Cardiovasc Interv* 2011;77(5):692–5.
9. Kenny D, Hijazi ZM, Walsh KP. Transcatheter tricuspid valve replacement with the Edwards SAPIEN valve. *Catheter Cardiovasc Interv* 2011;78(2):267–70.
10. Cerillo AG, Salizzoni S, Rinaldi M, Glauber M. Tricuspid valve-in-valve implantation: The transjugular approach. *Eur J Cardiothorac Surg* 2012;42(6):1056.
11. Van Garsse LA, Ter Bekke RM, van Ommen VG. Percutaneous transcatheter valve-in-valve implantation in stenosed tricuspid valve bioprosthesis. *Circulation* 2011;123(5):e219–21.
12. Weich H, Janson J, van Wyk J, Herbst P, le Roux P, Doubell A. Transjugular tricuspid valve-in-valve replacement. *Circulation* 2011;124(5):e157–60.
13. Cheung A, Soon JL, Webb JG, Ye J. Transatrial transcatheter tricuspid valve-in-valve technique. *J Card Surg* 2012;27(2):196–8.
14. Roberts PA, Boudjemline Y, Cheatham JP, Eicken A, Ewert P, McElhinney DB, et al. Percutaneous tricuspid valve replacement in congenital and acquired heart disease. *J Am Coll Cardiol* 2011;58(2):117–22.
15. Roberts P, Spina R, Vallely M, Wilson M, Bailey B, Celermajer DS. Percutaneous tricuspid valve replacement for a stenosed bioprosthesis. *Circ Cardiovasc Interv* 2010;3(4):e14–5.
16. Kenny D, Hijazi ZM, Kar S, Rhodes J, Mullen M, Makkar R, et al. Percutaneous implantation of the Edwards SAPIEN transcatheter heart valve for conduit failure in the pulmonary position: Early phase 1 results from an international multicenter clinical trial. *J Am Coll Cardiol* 2011;58(21):2248–56.
17. Hoendermis ES, Douglas YL, van den Heuvel AF. Percutaneous Edwards SAPIEN valve implantation in the tricuspid position: Case report and review of literature. *EuroIntervention* 2012;8(5):628–33.
18. Jux C, Akintuerk H, Schranz D. Two melodies in concert: Transcatheter double-valve replacement. *Catheter Cardiovasc Interv* 2012;80:997–1001.
19. Cerillo AG, Chiaramonti F, Murzi M, Bevilacqua S, Cerone E, Palmieri C, et al. Transcatheter valve in valve implantation for failed mitral and tricuspid bioprosthesis. *Catheter Cardiovasc Interv* 2011;78(7):987–95.
20. Cerillo AG, Berti S, Glauber M. Transjugular tricuspid valve-in-valve implantation: A safe and effective approach. *Ann Thorac Surg* 2011;92(2):777–8.
21. Bentham J, Qureshi S, Eicken A, Gibbs J, Ballard G, Thomson J. Early percutaneous valve failure within bioprosthetic tricuspid tissue valve replacements. *Catheter Cardiovasc Interv* 2013;82:428–35.
22. Bartlett HL, Atkins DL, Burns TL, Engelkes KJ, Powell SJ, Hills CB, et al. Early outcomes of tricuspid valve replacement in young children. *Circulation* 2007;115(3):319–25.

46

Tricuspid valve insufficiency: Percutaneous caval stent valve implantation for treatment of tricuspid insufficiency

Alexander Lauten and Hans Reiner Figulla

Introduction

Recently, transcatheter therapy has expanded the treatment options for patients with heart valve disease. Several interventional concepts have been suggested for the treatment of severe tricuspid regurgitation (TR) and are currently in different developmental stages.[1-4] Transcatheter prosthetic valve implantation into the caval veins is one of these concepts that has been extensively evaluated preclinically and also applied for compassionate treatment in human patients.[5,6] This chapter reviews the pathophysiologic background and current evidence of caval valve implantation and examines the potential role of this approach for interventional treatment of severe TR.

Challenges associated with interventional treatment of native tricuspid valve insufficiency

To date, transcatheter treatment of TR has been performed as compassionate treatment in isolated human cases and is still investigational. No commercial transcatheter device specifically designed for TV disease is available and experimental data on the percutaneous treatment of TV disease are limited.[1,2,7] This is partially due to the fact that transcatheter TV replacement is associated with major challenges related to sufficient fixation of the percutaneous device in the highly dynamic tricuspid annulus as well as the predominantly secondary nature of TV disease. Further, TR has traditionally assumed a lower priority than other valve diseases with less commercial interest in such developments. In contrast, for percutaneous repair of the mitral valve, multiple interventional concepts have been

suggested and several devices are under development, primarily aiming to reproduce the effects of surgical mitral valve repair by annuloplasty or leaflet repair.[8-11]

Compared to the aortic annulus, the TVA offers a greater variability and less resistance for device fixation because of its larger diameter and lower proportion of the fibrous tissue. Size and flexibility of the TV and the surrounding myocardium hamper positioning and long-term fixation of transcatheter devices and there are no adjacent structures to facilitate implantation of such devices.

Percutaneous valve implantation for treatment of insufficiency of the native tricuspid valve

Although percutaneous repair of the TV is conceptually attractive, it remains arguable whether repair concepts can be implemented on the TV with durable long-term results. In the presence of an unmet need for effective treatment of severe TR in nonsurgical patients, transcatheter valve replacement may offer an alternative treatment option. From the interventional perspective, there are two basic principles regarding the percutaneous replacement of the TV depending on the site of valve implantation—an *orthotopic* versus *heterotopic* valve replacement (Figure 46.1).

In *orthotopic* valve replacement, the prosthetic valve is implanted in an anatomically correct position in the TV annulus, thus restoring the functional separation of the RV and right atrium (RA). In 2005, Boudjemline et al. experimentally investigated this approach by means of implanting a double-disk nitinol stent with a semilunar valve into the TVA. Although in this study technical feasibility was demonstrated to some degree in healthy sheep, several difficulties relating to sufficient fixation of the self-expanding valve

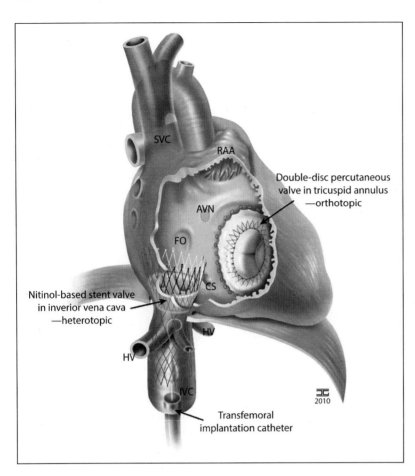

Figure 46.1 (See color insert.) Right atrial view with percutaneous devices suggested for transcatheter TV replacement. Position of self-expanding stent valves in the tricuspid annulus (orthotopic) and in the IVC (heterotopic) in chronic right ventricular pressure overload. Relevant anatomic structures include the coronary sinus ostium (CS), the foramen ovale (FO), and the atrioventricular node (AVN). IVC, inferior vena cava; SVC, superior vena cava; RAA, right atrial appendage.

in the highly dynamic tricuspid annulus were observed.[2] Owing to the anatomic structure and the flexibility of the surrounding myocardium, this site of implantation offers little resistance for orthotopic long-term fixation of stent-based valves with the current technique. Annulus dilatation may reach >70 mm in functional TR and is associated with the loss of anatomical landmarks between RV and RA. A device intended for orthotopic TV replacement would require unique solutions for stent and catheter design as well as tissue valve engineering (e.g., a 70 mm tissue valve would require a leaflet height of >40 mm to avoid prolapsing into the RA). Thus, it is unlikely that the various difficulties associated with the procedure of *orthotopic* valve replacement, will be resolved within the near future.

Orthotopic percutaneous tricuspid valve implantation has, however, been performed as a valve-in-valve-procedure after the failure of surgically implanted bioprosthetic valves or conduits.[12–15] These procedures have been performed in selected cases and a small series using balloon-expandable stent valves was designed for either aortic (Edwards SAPIEN, Edwards Lifescience, Irvine, CA, US) or pulmonary (Melody valve, Medtronic, Minneapolis, MN, US; Figure 46.4b and c) valve implantation. In these reports, percutaneous valve replacement has been performed with a high rate of technical and functional success. Although long-term results are

not yet available, this concept may be considered as a potential treatment option for degenerated bioprosthetic tricuspid valves in selected patients.

An obviously attractive alternative is *heterotopic* tricuspid valve replacement involving implantation of stent valves into the inferior and superior vena cava (SVC). This concept was recently investigated in an experimental study in animals, demonstrating function and hemodynamic effects of the caval valves.[7] After creation of TR via papillary muscle avulsion, self-expanding valves were implanted in the IVC and SVC using a transjugular approach in sheep. In this study, the onset of TR resulted in a significant reduction of cardiac output and a ventricular wave in the IVC. After implantation of both valves, cardiac output and systolic backflow in the caval veins improved significantly (Figure 46.2). Unpublished data demonstrate valve function for a period of up to 6 months after implantation in this model.

After demonstration of feasibility in preclinical studies, this treatment concept was recently performed for the first time for compassionate treatment in a human patient.[5] In this patient, a self-expanding valve was implanted into the IVC at the cavoatrial junction to reduce regurgitant backflow. In this experience, excellent valve function was observed after deployment, resulting in a marked reduction

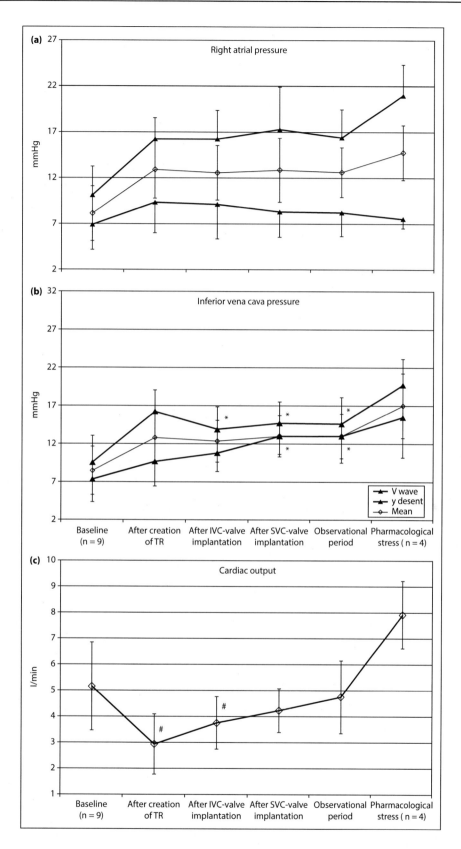

Figure 46.2 Time course of right atrial pressure, IVC pressure, and cardiac output in a chronic sheep model: Creation of TR results in increase of systolic and diastolic RAP (a) and ICVP (b). After implantation of IVC valve, systolic IVCP decreases and diastolic IVCP increases. (c) Cardiac output is decreased with TR and recovers during valve implantation and observational period. * Significantly different from corresponding right atrial pressure ($p < 0.05$); # significantly different from baseline value ($p < 0.05$).

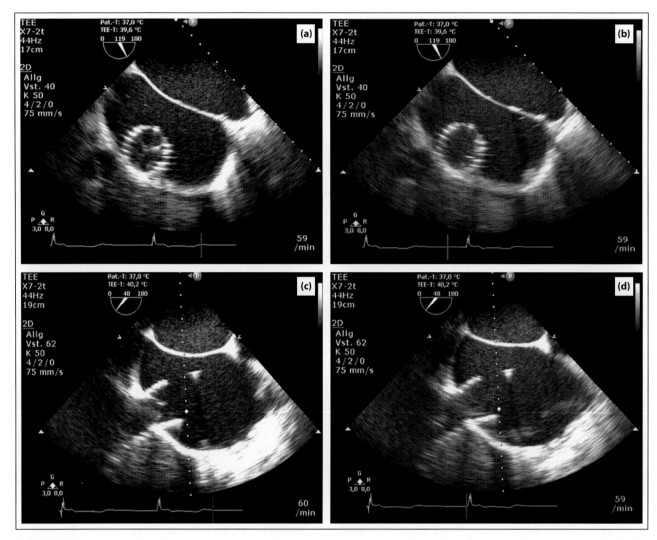

Figure 46.3 Echocardiographic evaluation of prosthetic valve function in a human patient: Systolic closure (a and b) and diastolic opening (c and d) of the pericardial valve is visualized by transesophageal echocardiography after the implantation procedure. Short-axis and long-axis views of the device after deployment. Doppler interrogation confirmed valvular competence and a continuously antegrade blood flow in the IVC and the hepatic veins without flow reversal.

of caval pressure and an abolition of backflow to the IVC (Figures 46.3a–d and 46.4a and b). Early after the procedure, the patient suffered from temporary neck pain and recurring epistaxis, which subsided when anticoagulation with heparin was discontinued and replaced by coumarin. Three weeks after implantation, the patient was discharged to a cardiac rehabilitation program. During follow-up visits, she reported improved physical capacity from NYHA functional class IV to III. Peripheral edema did not recur and ascites resolved partially; however, it remained detectable secondary to hepatic cirrhosis. Sequential echocardiographic exams over a follow-up period of 3 months confirmed continuous excellent device function without paravalvular leakage. However, after 3 months, the patient was readmitted to the hospital due to major intracranial hemorrhage, which she died from within 72 h. Autopsy confirmed correct device position and function. The

stent valve was strongly fixed to the IVC by fibrous covering, making device migration beyond this period highly unlikely (Figure 46.4c).

Compared to the orthotopic approach, the heterotopic procedure benefits from the advantage of a straightforward implantation technique due to the distance to vulnerable cardiac structures. The introduction of foreign material in the RV inflow tract is avoided, permitting a potentially lower risk of injury to ventricular structures and making this an attractive approach to the interventional cardiologist.

However, although caval valve implantation is a rather simple procedure, this approach has important limitations, currently restricting its use to nonsurgical patients with symptomatic TR in the end-stage heart disease. Although venous regurgitation is prevented by heterotopic valves, RV and RA overload persist after valve implantation, resulting

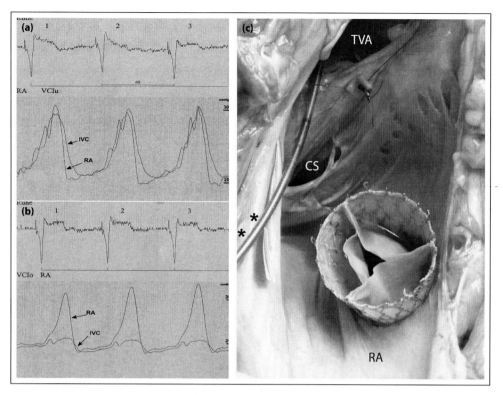

Figure 46.4 **(See color insert.)** First-in-man application of heterotopic tricuspid valve implantation. (a) Severe TR with IVC congestion is present before device implantation. Right heart catheterization confirms a prominent ventricular wave of 30 mmHg in the RA and the IVC. (b) Deployment of a self-expanding valve resulted in the immediate abolition of regurgitation into the IVC and lowered the mean IVC pressure. Excellent device function was documented during follow-up. (c) Macroscopic specimen showing the bioprosthetic valve in the IVC during autopsy 3 months later. Three months after the procedure, the patient died from cerebral ischemia with secondary hemorrhage. TVA, tricuspid annulus; RA, right atrium; CS, coronary sinus. Asterisk: RV pacing lead crossing the TVA.

in ventricularization of the RA with potential deleterious effects on cardiac function and atrial rhythm during long-term follow-up. Further, caval valve implantation addresses the regurgitation of blood only in the caval veins, a condition not found in every patient with severe TR. In this condition, the RA functions as a compliant reservoir by retaining part of the regurgitant volume and thus limiting systolic flow reversal in the caval veins. Therefore, only patients with proven systolic flow reversal in the caval veins and the preserved RV function potentially benefit from this treatment. Furthermore, symptoms of right heart congestion are caused by elevation of mean IVC pressure that may be slightly reduced after caval valve implantation. Current experience shows, however, that due to RV dysfunction and elevation of mean RA pressure, vena cava pressure is not normalized after caval valve implantation but still remains elevated, which also limits the hemodynamic and functional benefit of the procedure.

Summary

For a large number of patients with functional TR in an advanced stage of multivalvular heart disease, a readily available transcatheter approach could offer a treatment alternative. Their number is likely to increase in the future due to the demographic development and the widespread application of interventional therapies for left heart valve disease. Although transcatheter TV replacement is desirable, as it avoids the trauma of conventional surgery, there are numerous challenges regarding sufficient device fixation and function. Heterotopic valve implantation is a technically simple, straightforward interventional technique and has been successfully applied for compassionate treatment in human patients. Hemodynamic improvement has been demonstrated; however, the clinical benefit of the procedure is still unclear and important hemodynamic limitations apply.

Acknowledgment

The authors thank J. Geiling, Institute of Anatomy, Friedrich Schiller University of Jena, for his excellent illustrations. The work is funded by research grants from the Federal Ministry of Education and Research (#01 EZ 0907).

Disclosures

None.

References

1. Bai Y, Zong GJ, Wang HR et al. An integrated pericardial valved stent special for percutaneous tricuspid implantation: An animal feasibility study. *J Surg Res* 2010;160:215–21.
2. Boudjemline Y, Agnoletti G, Bonnet D et al. Steps toward the percutaneous replacement of atrioventricular valves an experimental study. *J Am Coll Cardiol* 2005;46:360–5.
3. Roberts PA, Boudjemline Y, Cheatham JP et al. Percutaneous tricuspid valve replacement in congenital and acquired heart disease. *J Am Coll Cardiol* 2011;58:117–22.
4. Lauten A, Figulla HR, Willich C, Jung C, Krizanic F, Ferrari M. Transcatheter implantation of the tricuspid valve in the inferior vena cava: An experimental study. *J Heart Valve Dis* 2010;19:807–8.
5. Lauten A, Ferrari M, Hekmat K et al. Heterotopic transcatheter tricuspid valve implantation: First-in-man application of a novel approach to tricuspid regurgitation. *Eur Heart J* 2011;32:1207–13.
6. Lauten A, Figulla HR, Willich C et al. Percutaneous caval stent valve implantation: Investigation of an interventional approach for treatment of tricuspid regurgitation. *Eur Heart J* 2010;31:1274–81.
7. Lauten A, Figulla HR, Willich C et al. Heterotopic valve replacement as an interventional approach to tricuspid regurgitation. *J Am Coll Cardiol* 2010;55:499–500.
8. Fedak PW, McCarthy PM, Bonow RO. Evolving concepts and technologies in mitral valve repair. *Circulation* 2008;117:963–74.
9. Masson JB, Webb JG. Percutaneous treatment of mitral regurgitation. *Circ Cardiovasc Interv* 2009;2:140–6.
10. Feldman T, Foster E, Glower DG et al. Percutaneous repair or surgery for mitral regurgitation. *N Engl J Med.* 2011;364(15):1395–1406.
11. Feldman T, Kar S, Rinaldi M et al. Percutaneous mitral repair with the MitraClip system: Safety and midterm durability in the initial EVEREST (endovascular valve edge-to-edge repair study) cohort. *J Am Coll Cardiol* 2009;54:686–94.
12. Van Garsse LA, Ter Bekke RM, van Ommen VG. Percutaneous transcatheter valve-in-valve implantation in stenosed tricuspid valve bioprosthesis. *Circulation* 2011;123:e219–21.
13. Zegdi R, Khabbaz Z, Borenstein N, Fabiani JN. A repositionable valved stent for endovascular treatment of deteriorated bioprostheses. *J Am Coll Cardiol* 2006;48:1365–8.
14. Tanous D, Nadeem SN, Mason X, Colman JM, Benson LN, Horlick EM. Creation of a functional tricuspid valve: Novel use of percutaneously implanted valve in right atrial to right ventricular conduit in a patient with tricuspid atresia. *Int J Cardiol* 2010;144(1):e8–10.
15. Straver B, Wagenaar LJ, Blom NA et al. Percutaneous tricuspid valve implantation in a Fontan patient with congestive heart failure and protein-losing enteropathy. *Circ Cardiovasc Interv* 2011;4:112–3.

Tricuspid valve insufficiency: Catheter closure of paravalvular leaks

Sameer Gafoor, Jennifer Franke, Stefan Bertog, Daniel H. Steinberg, Laura Vaskelyte, Ilona Hofmann, and Horst Sievert

Introduction

Paravalvular leak (PVL) presents with regurgitation and is often a significant problem for patients with bioprosthetic or mechanical heart valves.[1] Often manifesting as heart failure (85% of all presenting symptoms) and hemolysis (13–47% of all presenting symptoms and signs).[2,3] PVL has a prevalence as high as 5–17% of all mechanical valves.[4–6]

The mechanism of leaks is not well understood. The alignment between the sewing ring and annulus may be incomplete because of significant annular calcification. The tissue around valves can weaken as a result of chronic infection. Even the sutures themselves may not allow significant apposition of the valve with the annulus. All these can lead to significant PVL.

How can PVL be treated? Unfortunately, repeat surgery portends a worse prognosis, with mortality rates for the first redo, second redo, or third redo surgery of 13%, 15%, and 35%, respectively.[2] Each repeat operation is less likely to be successful. Therefore, there is ample room for percutaneous approaches.

It is important to select the right patients for PVL closure. Prior to beginning a case, it is important to exclude active infection, valve instability, and/or cardiac thrombus.[5]

Paravalvular leak: Imaging

There are a variety of methods to diagnose PVL—transthoracic echocardiography (TTE), transesophageal echocardiography (TEE), computerized tomography (CT), and magnetic resonance imaging (MRI)—however, none of them are perfect and all come with significant advantages and disadvantages. The important pieces of information to ascertain are valve type, location of leak, size of leak, shape of leak, severity of leak, and number of leaks.

Echocardiography allows the ability to directly compare preprocedural and intraprocedural results. However, echocardiography is prone to artifact from prosthetic shadowing.[7] Aortic PVL can be diagnosed and evaluated often with TTE; mitral PVL often requires TEE (although TTE may be useful for original diagnosis). Three-dimensional (3D) echocardiography adds the ability to determine the path of a leak, which can often take a serpentine course. We perform all our PVL interventions with TEE guidance (often with 3D characterization of leak size and course).

CT and MRI add additional information. Retrospective electrocardiogram (ECG)-gated reconstruction allows diastolic and systolic characterization. Unfortunately, artifacts secondary to calcification or the valve can blur the leak itself, making it difficult to visualize. CT, which has better spatial resolution, requires contrast dye and also involves exposure to more radiation.[8]

Paravalvular leak: Location

A clock face is often used to describe both aortic and PVLs. The three commissures are assigned an hour on the clock face (between left and right coronary sinus as 5 o'clock, between right and noncoronary sinus as 8 o'clock, and noncoronary and left coronary sinus as 11 o'clock). This lexicon helps in communication between the imager and operator and also to monitor leaks pre- and postclosure. Statistically speaking, aortic leaks are most often between 7 and 11 o'clock (46%) and also between 11 and 3 o'clock.[9]

Both clock face and anatomic criteria can be used to describe mitral PVL location. Location is based on the mitral valve annulus using terms such as medial, lateral, anterior, and posterior. The clock face for the mitral valve starts with the 12 o'clock position between the aortic and mitral valve A2, the 3 o'clock position as the posteromedial commissure and interatrial septum, and the 6 o'clock position as the posterior annulus midpoint. According to this system, mitral PVL is found often between 10 and 2 (45%) and between 6 and 7 o'clock (37%).[9]

Paravalvular leak: Sizing

Although the course of the leak may be serpentine, with an orifice that is crescentic or oval in shape, some assumptions can be made about the size of the PVL. Echocardiogram can be used with the vena contracta of the leak as an estimate, although this is not perfect. With the advent of 3D, the leak can be measured in multiple directions. CT and MRI may provide more information if an echocardiogram is unclear. We do not recommend balloon sizing—there is a risk of balloon rupture as a consequence of sharp edges due to annular calcium. Once the leak is measured, this dictates the device, which dictates the delivery system guide or sheath size.

Paravalvular leak: Access

Aortic or medial mitral PVLs can be approached by transfemoral access. We use a 0.035" wire, often a hydrophilic one (e.g., Terumo Glidewire, Terumo Medical Corporation, Somerset, New Jersey) inside a 5 Fr diagnostic catheter (JR4 or MP). The wire crosses the leak and the catheter follows the wire. This wire is substituted for a stiff 0.035" wire (e.g., Amplatzer Extra Stiff wire, from St. Jude Corporation, Minneapolis, MN, USA). The delivery system guide or sheath is then advanced over the stiff wire, the stiff wire is removed, and the device is placed in the correct position. If more support is needed for the catheter or delivery system to cross the leak, a rail can be made (either by transseptal access and snare or by externalizing the wire through transapical access). If the aortomitral curtain is crossed, it is often necessary to protect this from significant stress by covering a bare wire with a catheter at all times.

Sometimes, transseptal access is needed, either for mitral PVL or difficult aortic PVL. Any transseptal system should be used, and this can be performed under transesophageal guidance. We would recommend an inferior and midway between the anterior and posterior position (you cannot state midway between superior and posterior since the short axis shows anterior/posterior relations and the long axis shows the inferior/superior relations) for puncture for most leaks, although it is just as important to make sure that the transseptal puncture is performed safely, as it is to find a specific spot to cross the septum that will allow crossing of the leak.

When a mitral leak cannot be crossed through other methods or if there are mechanical heart valves in both aortic and mitral positions, transapical access can be considered. The transapical access can be achieved either percutaneously or via limited thoracotomy under direct vision.

For the percutaneous transapical approach, in addition to echocardiographic/fluoroscopic visualization to determine the position of the ventricular apex, it is also important to perform concomitant coronary angiography to avoid the coronary arteries. A sheath (often 4 Fr) is delivered and heparin is given. A device is often utilized to close the entry site, for example, Amplatzer PDA occluder (St. Jude Corporation). We save this as the third and last option, as there is an increased risk of complications from tamponade, hemothorax, or puncture of a coronary artery. Follow-up TTE and chest x-ray is highly recommended.

Paravalvular leak: Device selection

There are very limited devices designed specifically for PVL (Amplatzer vascular plug III and Occlutech PVL devices). Other devices designed for other purposes have often been used. The ideal device has the appropriate size and shape for the leak and does not interfere with the valve leaflets. Furthermore, it does not interfere with other vital structures, for example, the coronary ostia in the case of aortic valve or left ventricular outflow tract in the case of mitral valve. Optimally, only one device is needed.

The device size is dependent on measurements from echocardiogram (TEE and 3D whenever possible). Angiography helps in the case of aortic PVL when this can be seen next to the valve. Some may use external catheter size to approximate leak size, but this is also dependent on calcification and tortuosity, which can cause difficulty in a catheter's ability to cross the leak. We follow this general algorithm—for a small cylindrical leak, an Amplatzer vascular plug (AVP) II or PDA occluder may be best. For an oval or crescentic leak, the AVP III is more ideal. If the leak is small or has significant angulation, an AVP IV is better, as it is more flexible.

Putting it all together: Aortic PVL

Retrograde transfemoral approach is the optimal strategy for aortic PVL. TEE is used for imaging, with description of the leak on the clock face as described earlier. Once the leak is crossed with a hydrophilic wire and then a 5 Fr diagnostic catheter (often JR4, MP, or Amplatz-1), this is exchanged over a stiff wire for a delivery system guide catheter or sheath, for example, a Cook shuttle sheath (Cook Corporation, Bloomington, IN, USA). The device is then delivered through this delivery system.

If there is significant tortuosity or difficulty in crossing the leak, more support can be obtained by building a rail. A transseptal rail involves transseptal access with subsequent snaring of the original wire within the left atrium; an apical ventricular rail involves left ventricular puncture and having the wire through the apex. Figures 47.1 and 47.2 demonstrate aortic PVL closure.

Subsequent aortic angiography is often necessary to rule out coronary compression and evaluate the valve for

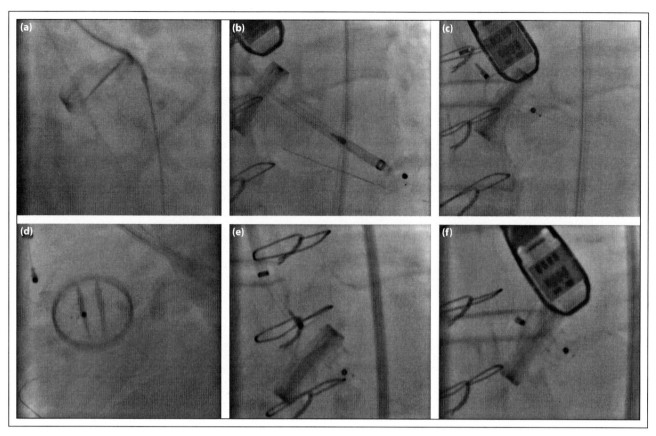

Figure 47.1   Aortic PVL, single device. 74-year-old male with PVL in relation to mechanical aortic valve. The leak is an eccentric leak in the region of the noncoronary cusp and measured 10 × 3 mm on the echocardiogram. Right femoral arterial access was obtained and a 5 Fr sheath was placed. A 5 Fr AL1 guide catheter and Terumo hydrophilic 0.035″ wire were used to cross the leak in a retrograde manner (a). This catheter was exchanged over an Amplatz Extra Stiff wire for a 7 Fr Cook shuttle sheath, which was placed in the left ventricle (b). A 0.014″ Ironman wire was placed as access protection through the PVL into the left ventricle. A 10 mm PDA occluder device was attempted but was unsuccessful in closing the defect (c) and was removed. The 0.014″ wire stayed in place (d). A 4 Fr 125 cm JR4 catheter was placed coaxial inside the shuttle sheath to traverse the PVL over the 0.014″ wire and reestablish the shuttle sheath across the leak (not pictured). Then a 12/3 mm AVP III device was placed across the leak (e). After fluoroscopic and echocardiographic confirmation of minimal leak and good valve function, the device was released (f).

regurgitation. The valve should not have an increased gradient and should have free-moving leaflets. If the device was implanted in the area of the noncoronary cusp, special attention should be given to the anterior mitral valve leaflet.

Putting it all together: Mitral PVL

After evaluating the leak with TEE, the first approach is to try the simplest approach: retrograde transfemoral approach with a 5 Fr IM or JR4 catheter and a hydrophilic 0.035″ guide wire. Once this is across, the wire can be exchanged for a stiff wire and then the delivery system (guide catheter or long sheath). The wire is removed, the device is advanced, and then the device is deployed. By deploying the first disk within the left atrium, it is simpler to visualize on TEE. If there is an issue with support, transseptal access with snare can be used to make a rail.

As stated earlier, it is important to protect the aortomitral continuity with a catheter whenever possible.

When the retrograde transfemoral approach is not successful, an antegrade transseptal approach can have some benefits. It is important to cross posteriorly to avoid the aorta and superiorly to have enough catheter room to reach both medial and lateral leaks. A similar approach with a 0.035″ hydrophilic wire, 5 Fr JR4 or MP catheter, stiff wire exchange, and then exchange for the delivery system (guide catheter or long sheath) is used. If support is still an issue, a transarterial rail is recommended. Another option is to advance the transseptal sheath through the defect. Some centers have used an Agilis system (St. Jude Corporation) if the catheter is not able to reach the defect or if the puncture site was suboptimal. The advantage is that it offers increased steerability; the disadvantage is a larger transseptal puncture and increased cost of the procedure. Figures 47.3 through 47.5 show examples of mitral PVL.

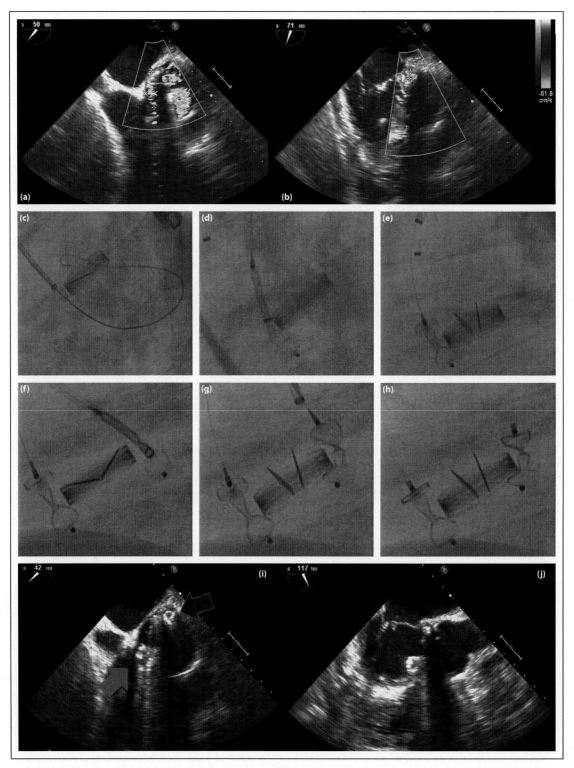

Figure 47.2   (**See color insert.**) Aortic PVL, multiple leaks. After having a mechanical aortic valve in 2008, the patient presented 4 years later with symptoms of heart failure and severe regurgitation. A 5 × 11 mm PVL was noted near the left coronary cusp and 5 × 8 mm PVL was noted in the area of the noncoronary cusp (a and b). A 5 Fr MP catheter and 0.035″ hydrophilic wire was used to cross the leak near the noncoronary cusp. This was then exchanged over an Amplatz ES 0.035″ wire (c) for a 10 Fr Cook shuttle sheath. This was then used to advance an AVP III size 5 × 14 mm device (d), which was then deployed (e). Similar access was obtained through the other femoral artery and a similar technique was used to cross the leak near the left coronary cusp. An AVP III 5 × 14 mm device was also implanted (f through h). Follow-up echocardiographic views at 42° and 117° show the position of the noncoronary cusp (green arrow) and left coronary cusp (red arrow) devices (i and j). Both aortic and mitral valve leaflets moved well on TEE.

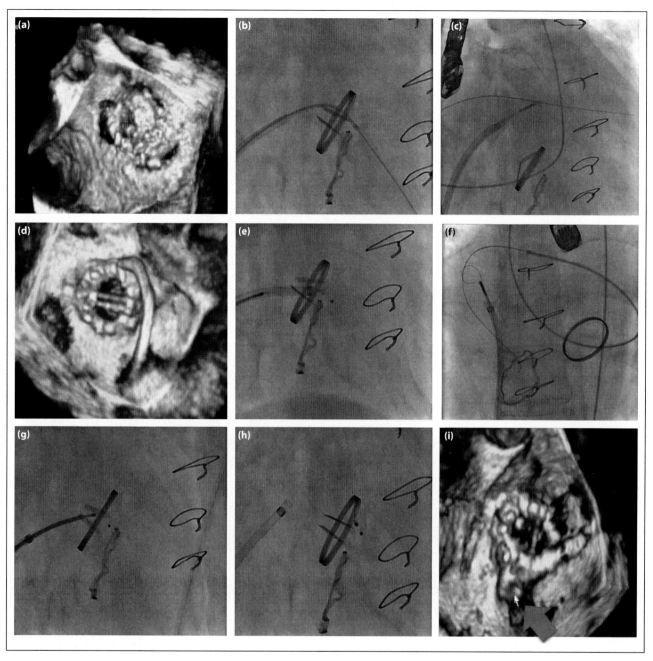

Figure 47.3 (**See color insert.**) Mitral PVL, one device. Several years after placement of a mechanical mitral valve prosthesis and tricuspid ring, the patient developed severe mitral regurgitation with reversal of flow in pulmonary veins. This was due to two paravalvular mitral leaks, one anterolateral (orifice 6 × 15 mm) and one posterior (orifice 10 × 8 mm) (a). The anterolateral leak was close to a section of tissue that interfered with leaflet motion; therefore, a decision was made to only pursue the posterior leak. Rather than approaching the leak retrograde, the decision was made to approach the leak antegrade due to presumed easier access to the posterior leak. After placement of a 5 Fr sheath in the right femoral artery and a 9 Fr sheath in the right femoral vein, transseptal puncture was performed. Antegrade crossing was obtained (wire and diagnostic catheter) but the sheath did not cross (b). Therefore, a 5 Fr JR4 catheter and 0.035″ Terumo wire were introduced through the aorta and the leak was crossed retrograde; the Terumo wire was advanced and snared through a transvenous/transseptal sling in the left atrium and externalized (c and d). This allowed the transseptal 9 Fr sheath to be advanced through the leak. A 10 mm Amplatzer muscular VSD occluder was brought through the leak but caused mitral valve impingement (e). Therefore, this was removed and retrograde access from the aorta and sling in the left atrium was again obtained (f). Next, an Amplatzer 10 mm PDA occluder was placed across the defect (g and h), which did not interfere with mitral leaflet movement. Echocardiography showing final device position is seen (i).

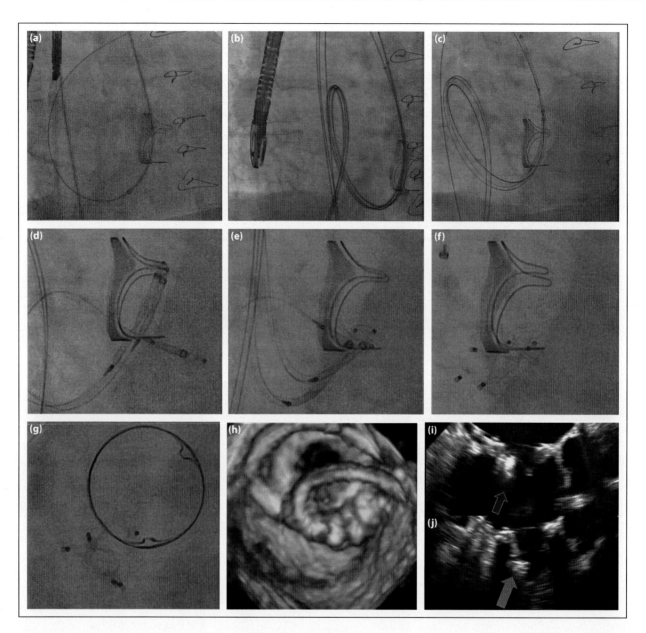

Figure 47.4 **(See color insert.)** Mitral PVL, multiple leaks. Large mitral PVLs. After the patient had placement of a bioprosthetic MVR in 2004, he developed one long PVL that extended over 1/4 of the bioprosthetic valve. A 5 Fr sheath was placed in the right femoral artery. A 5 Fr JR4 catheter and 0.035" Terumo hydrophilic wire were used to cross the leak (a). After femoral venous access with a 6 Fr sheath, transseptal access was obtained. A snare was used to externalize the Terumo wire from the left atrium through the right femoral vein. An Amplatz Extra Stiff wire was used to exchange the transseptal sheath for an 18 Fr sheath. The same wire was used to exchange for an 18 Fr sheath; through this, three Amplatz ES wires were used to exchange this for three 6 Fr Cook shuttle sheaths (b and c). Through these three sheaths, two 12 mm AVP 2 devices and one 10 mm AVP 2 were advanced into the leak (d and e) and deployed (f and g). The position of the devices is also visible on the echocardiogram (h). When deploying mitral PVL devices antegrade, it is important to make sure that the mitral valve leaflets are not affected by the ventricular side of the device (i)—this requires readjustment and redeployment so that the leaflets are not affected (j).

After the device is placed, TEE should show mobile mitral leaflets, open pulmonary veins, and if the leak was anterior, an unobstructed mitral valve. Angiography is insufficient to make this determination. We do not release a device until these requirements are satisfied.

Device success

There are many ways to characterize device success, but the device should treat the problem if it is there to solve—there should be a sizable decrease in regurgitation and

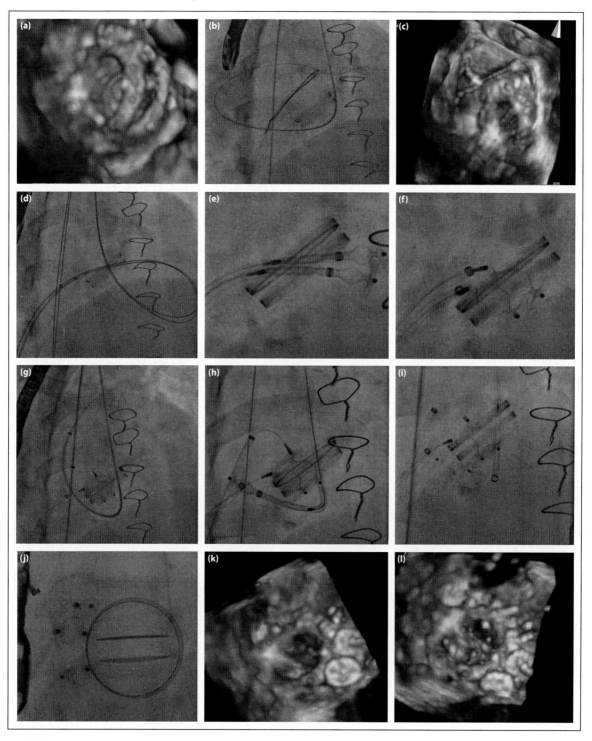

Figure 47.5 **(See color insert.)** Mitral PVL, multiple leaks. The patient presented with severe mitral PVL. He presented with an anteromedial leak from 1 to 4 o'clock (orifice 4 × 19 mm), and by 5 o'clock, presented with a second leak (orifice 4 × 3 mm). The large orifice is seen on the echocardiography (a). A 5 Fr sheath was placed in the right femoral artery. A 5 Fr JR4 catheter and 0.035" hydrophilic wire was advanced across the anteromedial leak. A 6 Fr sheath was placed in the right femoral vein. Transseptal access was obtained and a snare was used to grab and externalize the wire (b and c). An Amplatz ES wire was then used to exchange this transseptal sheath for a 10 Fr sheath. Through this 10 Fr sheath, two Amplatz ES wires were used to exchange for two 6 Fr Cook shuttle sheaths (d). Two AVP II size 10 mm were advanced and deployed (e and f). The leak at 5 o'clock was approached retrograde. The 5 Fr sheath in the right femoral artery was upsized to a 6 Fr sheath. A 5 Fr JR4 catheter and Terumo wire was used to cross the leak (f). A snare was advanced transseptally into the left atrium, used to capture the wire (g), and then externalized. An 8 mm AVP II was advanced (h) and deployed (i and j). The mitral valve leaflets moved normally. The devices are visible on TEE from atrial (k) and ventricular aspect (l).

improvement in symptoms. The patient should have a TTE for aortic leak and TEE for mitral leak at 6 months (or earlier if symptoms persist). If there is hemolysis, the hemoglobin/hematocrit should also be monitored.

Special situations

Multiple leaks

Our paradigm is to close the major leak only at first, so we can identify the offending device if there is significant infection/hemolysis. If multiple devices are placed, one may not be the infectious source and therefore should not be removed. We place multiple devices or close multiple leaks if there is uncertain follow-up or with two equally sized large leaks.

One approach for multiple-device placement is the same-sheath approach (both devices go through the same sheath one after the other). Device one crosses and is deployed. Next, the wire and delivery catheter are used to cross the leak again, and the second device is advanced and deployed. With this method, only one access is needed. However, with this approach, the first device needs to be fully released before the second device can be advanced.

Another method is with new access. Contralateral femoral access and device advancement may be sufficient for aortic PVL (Figure 47.2). In the case of mitral PVL, this requires a transseptal approach and dilating the septal access point to accommodate a larger sheath. The larger sheath should be a sum of the sheaths required for the individual devices (if the two devices need two 6 Fr sheaths, the septum should be crossed with a 12 Fr sheath). Then two (or three wires for three devices) are used to cross the sheath, these wires are exchanged for stiff wires, and the prior large sheath is switched to the multiple-delivery systems. The independent devices are then delivered (see Figures 47.4 and 47.5).

Preserving PVL access with device placement

When the wire crosses the leak only with great difficulty (e.g., tortuous anatomy and/or suboptimal transseptal catheter position), it is also possible to preserve PVL access during device placement with a 0.014″ coronary wire (Figure 47.1). This allows the ability to preserve access—which is crucial if the device must be removed because it is not the correct size or causes leaflet compromise. However, this carries with it the risk that the wire will not be retrievable after the device is released.

Complications

Complications occur and must be avoided when possible. These include valve interference (3.5–5%), stroke,

endocarditis, postprocedural hemolysis, device erosion, emergent cardiac surgery (0.7–2%), and death (1.4–2%). One study showed major adverse events at 30 days (death, myocardial infarction, stroke, major bleeding, and emergency surgery) of 8.7%. Embolized devices from the aortic position are often large and go to the iliac bifurcation and can be removed percutaneously; those from the mitral position may get caught at the left ventricular outflow tract and may require surgery.

Long-term survival

As mentioned before, there should be a sizable decrease in regurgitation and improvement in symptoms. The patient should have a TTE for aortic leak and TEE for mitral leak at 6 months (or earlier if symptoms). If there is hemolysis, the hemoglobin/hematocrit should also be monitored.

Technical success rate is reported as between 77% and 86%, and clinical improvement is between 67% and 77%. A study by Ruiz et al. reported long-term survival at 6, 12, and 18 months as 91.9%, 89.2%, and 86.5%, respectively. Sorajja et al.[10] found 1–2-year survival after PVL closure of 70–75% with an estimated 3-year survival of 64.3%.

References

1. Vongpatanasin W, Hillis LD, Lange RA. Prosthetic heart valves. *N Engl J Med* 1996;335:407–16.
2. Genoni M, Franzen D, Vogt P et al. Paravalvular leakage after mitral valve replacement: Improved long-term survival with aggressive surgery? *Eur J Cardiothorac Surg* 2000;17:14–9.
3. De Cicco G, Russo C, Moreo A et al. Mitral valve periprosthetic leakage: Anatomical observations in 135 patients from a multicentre study. *Eur J Cardiothorac Surg* 2006;30:887–91.
4. Rallidis LS, Moyssakis IE, Ikonomidis I, Nihoyannopoulos P. Natural history of early aortic paraprosthetic regurgitation: A five-year follow-up. *Am Heart J* 1999;138:351–7.
5. Pate GE, Al Zubaidi A, Chandavimol M, Thompson CR, Munt BI, Webb JG. Percutaneous closure of prosthetic paravalvular leaks: Case series and review. *Catheter Cardiovasc Interv* 2006;68:528–33.
6. Davila-Roman VG, Waggoner AD, Kennard ED et al. Prevalence and severity of paravalvular regurgitation in the artificial valve endocarditis reduction trial (AVERT) echocardiography study. *J Am Coll Cardiol* 2004;44:1467–72.
7. Zoghbi WA. New recommendations for evaluation of prosthetic valves with echocardiography and Doppler ultrasound. *Methodist Debakey Cardiovasc J* 2010;6:20–6.
8. Ruiz CE, Jelnin V, Kronzon I et al. Clinical outcomes in patients undergoing percutaneous closure of periprosthetic paravalvular leaks. *J Am Coll Cardiol* 2011;58:2210–7.
9. Krishnaswamy A, Kapadia SR, Tuzcu EM. Percutaneous paravalvular leak closure—Imaging, techniques and outcomes. *Circ J* 2013;77:19–27.
10. Sorajja P, Cabalka AK, Hagler DJ et al. Percutaneous repair of paravalvular prosthetic regurgitation: Acute and 30-day outcomes in 115 patients. *Circ Cardiovasc Interv* 2011;4(4):314–21.

Tricuspid valve insufficiency: Catheter closure of perforated sinus of Valsalva

Prafulla Kerkar and Joseph DeGiovanni

Introduction

The three outpouchings of the proximal ascending aorta above the hinge points of the aortic valve leaflets and from which the two coronary arteries arise were described by the Italian anatomist Antonio Valsalva and these now bear his name.[1] Congenital weakness, infection, or trauma to the wall of these outpouchings or sinuses results in a windsock-shaped aneurysm, first described by Hope in 1939 and later by Thurman in 1940.[2] Some of these aneurysms perforate or rupture into a cardiac chamber (often the right ventricle [RV] or right atrium [RA] but less commonly into the left atrium, left ventricle, or pulmonary artery) causing a large shunt. Rarely, they rupture into the pericardium, when it is invariably fatal. The majority (around 95%) rupture into the RV or the RA, presumably because of their proximity to the aorta and also due to the lower pressure in these chambers. Aneurysms most commonly originate from the right coronary sinus (70–90%), less commonly from the noncoronary sinus (10–20%), and rarely from the left sinus (<5%).[3]

Rupture of an aneurysm of the sinus of Valsalva (RASV) may present with clinically impressive symptoms or even catastrophic collapse, but some 20% are asymptomatic.[2] Only a third present with chest pain or severe dyspnea, and the rest usually develop breathlessness gradually. Unruptured aneurysms are largely asymptomatic but can cause chest pain from coronary artery compression, heart block with syncope through dissection of the ventricular septum, obstruction to the right or left ventricular outflow tract (RVOT/LVOT), tricuspid regurgitation (TR) through prolapse across the valve, or aortic regurgitation (AR) caused by distortion of the aortic valve leaflets.

The mechanism of the aneurysm formation and subsequent rupture is a congenital weakness of the elastic tissue in the media between the attachment of the aortic valve leaflets and the aorta. Acquired RASV can result following surgery to the aortic valve, coronary intervention, or infection, although the substrate may already coexist.

There is a higher prevalence in the East compared to Western countries and, in the Oriental population, it is more commonly associated with a ventricular septal defect (VSD), in some series up to 50%; the latter is often doubly committed or juxta-arterial and the rupture is from the right sinus to the RV.[4] Around 25% may have AR. The mean age of presentation is in the third decade of life but can occur in children as well as octogenarians. RASV is 4 times more common in males.[2]

Presentation

Symptoms, when present, include pain in the chest but may also involve the back and abdomen, breathlessness, syncope, stroke, or death. Various types of heart murmurs may be audible but typically, a continuous murmur is present and this may be accompanied by a thrill. Features of heart failure eventually occur. In severe cases, circulatory collapse and multiorgan failure result from a huge drop in cardiac output and with a very low aortic diastolic pressure.

Not uncommonly, rupture occurs during physical or emotional stress, including pregnancy. Rarely, an episode of infective endocarditis may be the precipitating factor.[2] There is no way of predicting which unruptured ones are likely to burst and this makes it difficult to decide whether to proactively repair these or even whether to repair them if heart surgery is being carried out for another pathology. If RASV is left unrepaired, the majority die within 1 year although there are reported cases that have survived a few decades after rupture.

Investigations

Electrocardiogram

This may be normal but may show ischemia if there is coronary compression or coronary steal. There may be variable degrees of atrio-ventricular block. Eventually, biventricular hypertrophy occurs but not in the acute phase.

Chest radiography

At presentation, the heart size may be normal but with increased pulmonary congestion. Eventually, cardiomegaly sets in but the aortic root is not dilated. This modality is of limited value.

Echocardiogram/Doppler

Cross-sectional echocardiography often provides the diagnosis including details of the sinus involved, the chamber where the aneurysm exits, and its size, but also shows associated lesions, such as VSD, AR, RVOT, and LVOT obstruction, TR, or effusion. Additional detail may be obtained with transoesophageal echocardiography (TOE) including three-dimensional (3D) imaging that is very helpful for guiding device closure of RASV (Figures 48.1 and 48.2, Videos 48.1 through 48.7). In addition, this provides vital information about RV and LV size and function and their progress over time.

Angiography

Catheterization is nowadays carried out during an interventional procedure to close the RASV and not simply for diagnosis. This provides details about the size, shape, position, and exit point of the RASV and these are essential in deciding which type and size of device to choose as well as the site for optimal placement.

Computerized tomography/cardiac magnetic resonance (CMR)

Increasingly, these are carried out in non-urgent settings when there is a suspicion of RASV and, although not essential, the imaging detail helps to prepare a strategy for closure.[3]

Indications for intervention

RASV often causes a large and acute shunt that produces symptoms. These can be managed with medical antifailure treatment initially. There is often a period of clinical improvement as the pulmonary vascular resistance rises and the ventricles adapt to the hemodynamics. But eventually, heart failure occurs, which may lead to death often within 1 year; *all RASV should, therefore, be closed*. Medical treatment consists of diuretics, vasodilators, and inotropes.

The first reported surgical repair was in 1956 from the Mayo Clinic.[2] The techniques have evolved over the years and the acute and long-term results of surgery are excellent

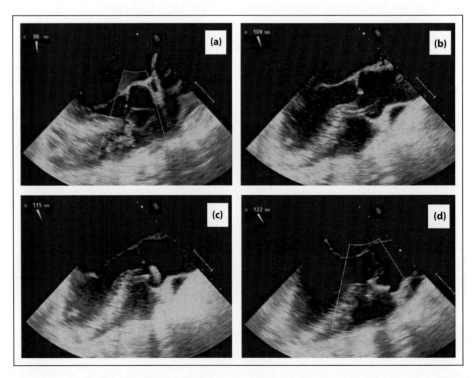

Figure 48.1 (**See color insert.**) Intraprocedural TOE in the long-axis view showing (a) perforated aneurysm of the right coronary sinus draining into the RVOT with turbulent color flow across. (b) Following CC with ADO, there is complete closure with no color flow across. (c) The delivery sheath can be seen crossing the defect from the RVOT into the ascending aorta. (d) The aortic disk with its attached delivery cable passing through the sheath being pulled to block the aortic end of the defect.

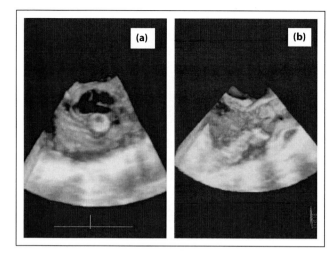

Figure 48.2 (See color insert.) Transoesophageal 3D acquisition in the short-axis (a) and long-axis (b) views following CC of RASV from RCC to RVOT showing the deployed ADO *en face* and in profile.

with hospital mortality of <5% in the largest-reported series.[2] Surgery is still an option when there are associated lesions (not amenable to catheter repair) but for isolated RASV, catheter closure (CC) is the current practice. The Mayo Clinic experience reports a 95% survival after 20 years of surgical repair.[5] Recurrence is very rare when patch repair is used. Factors that contribute to late mortality include aortic valve replacement or bacterial endocarditis.

CC of RASV has become safe and feasible and it is the treatment of choice when there are no associated lesions that require surgery. The procedure should be carried out at the earliest opportunity once the patient is stable but occasionally, it has to be done in the acute phase[6] when exceptional support is required, such as ventilation and inotropes, or if there is target organ damage, such as progressive renal/liver failure. About 70% of patients with RASV are potentially eligible for CC.[7]

There are no reports of CC of unruptured aneurysms and if this is considered in the future, it is likely to be limited to some of the asymptomatic group.

Catheter intervention

General

The procedure may be carried out under conscious sedation or general anesthesia. The latter is preferred if TOE is used and this is recommended as it provides vital guidance during device deployment, particularly when combined with 3D imaging; moreover, TOE is very helpful to assess the degree of AR during device deployment and prior to release.

The procedure is usually carried out through the femoral vessels. The commoner approach is to access both

femoral vessels to create an arteriovenous (AV) loop although some can be simply closed from the arterial side. Intravenous heparin 100 units per kilogram is administered and antibiotics are given according to the local policy of the department.

Equipment

- Pigtail for aortogram
- Judkins right coronary catheter to cross the aneurysm
- Angled glide wire (Terumo, Japan) exchange length
- Amplatz gooseneck snare kit (ev3 Europe, Paris, France) or Entrio snare™ (Bard, Murray Hill, NJ)
- Noodle wire (St. Jude Medical, Golden Valley, MN) for AV loop (optional)
- Delivery sheath to deploy the device, for example, Mullins/Flexor sheaths (Cook Cardiology, Bloomington, IN) or TorqVue (St. Jude Medical)
- Occlusion devices: Nitinol-based plugs; the commonest used is the Amplatzer duct occluder (ADO)[6–9] (St. Jude Medical) but other devices based on a nitinol mesh, such as Amplatzer septal occluder[10] or muscular VSD device[11] (St. Jude Medical) have been used successfully. Rarely, Gianturco coils (Cook) may be used for small defects[12]

Procedure

Once the catheters are inserted and the patient heparinized, hemodynamic evaluation is carried out that may include measurement of the aortic and pulmonary artery pressures—the former will show a wide pulse pressure with a low diastolic and the latter may be elevated to a variable degree. In addition, a saturation run will estimate the severity of the shunt; however, the decision to close an RASV is not dependent on the shunt size and all of them should be considered for closure.

Angiography may be carried out in the biplane although a single plane may suffice. The aortic sinus where the aneurysm arises from is usually known in advance from noninvasive imaging. If the right sinus is involved, a 30° right anterior oblique (RAO) and 30° left anterior oblique (LAO) projections are helpful (Figures 48.3a and b), and if the noncoronary sinus is involved, an LAO 30° with cranial 30° (Figure 48.4) gives a clear image of the fistula and its relationship to the aortic valve and the right coronary artery. Customized angiographic views may be necessary. If the shunt size is large and there is superimposition of structures, it may not be possible to get all the details of the RASV, in which case, a selective angiogram within the aneurysm may help. Owing to the high-flow aortic runoff, a rapid high-volume injection is preferred for better opacification.

Sizing of the RASV and of the device is generally done with a combination of angiography and TOE. Although balloon sizing may be carried out, this is not usually required.

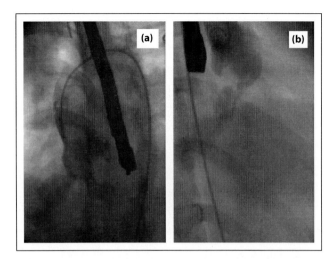

Figure 48.3   Aortic root angiogram in LAO (a) and RAO (b) projections showing RASV arising from the right sinus and emptying into the RA.

If the ADO is used, the size of the device should be 2–4 mm larger than the landing zone, which is usually at the aortic end of the RASV. Unnecessary oversizing must be avoided in view of the close proximity of the aortic valve, the conduction system, and the right coronary artery. However, at times, due to flimsy margins, oversizing to 4 mm becomes necessary. If a muscular VSD device is used, the size should be equal to the landing zone, as these devices have a bigger rim than the ADO.

During CC, the Judkins right coronary catheter usually enters the RASV easily, often ending in the exit chamber but if this is not feasible, the use of a Terumo wire facilitates crossing the fistula. Most large RASVs are recommended to be closed from the venous side, although retrograde arterial closure is feasible but not with the ADO.

When a device is delivered from the venous side, once the fistula has been crossed from the aorta, an AV loop is created (using a snare to grab the exchange length noodle wire [Figure 48.4c] to exteriorize it from the femoral vein). A delivery sheath is introduced over the noodle wire in the femoral vein, crossing the fistula from the right side and parking the sheath in the ascending aorta. For this approach, the ADO (St. Jude Medical) or a similar design is the commonest device used and this is ideally suited to repair the aneurysm and close the shunt. The small distal rim of the ADO allows closure of the os of the aneurysm at the aortic end with very little likelihood of interference with the aortic valve or the right coronary artery (Figure 48.4). If done from the arterial approach, the device used has to be a VSD device (St. Jude Medical) or a similar device made from a nitinol mesh. A vascular plug may be considered in some cases although this may not be as stable.

Irrespective of the approach and device used, positioning is guided by fluoroscopy as well as TOE (Figure 48.1, Videos 48.1 through 48.4). The latter is of immense importance to control for occurrence of any AR and limits the use of contrast. Recently, we have performed successful CC of RASV under TOE guidance in a critically ill patient with anuria on

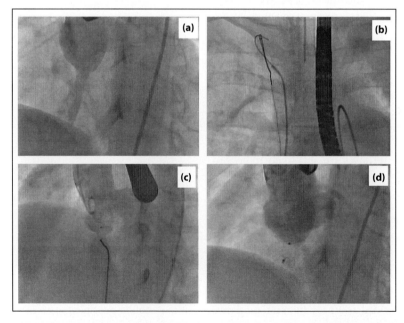

Figure 48.4   (a) Aortic root angiogram in LAO cranial projection showing RASV from noncoronary sinus to RA. (b) Following deployment and release of ADO, aortogram confirms good position of the device with no AR. (c) After crossing the defect with a Judkins right catheter, fluoroscopy shows snaring of the noodle wire positioned in the superior vena cava for creation of the AV loop. (d) ADO deployed at the os of the aneurysm with some waist indicating adequate size of the device; angiogram confirms the optimal position and absence of any significant AR prior to release.

dialysis *without using any contrast* (as yet unpublished). Test contrast injections carried out through the delivery sheath and/or through a pigtail in the aorta also help in optimal placement of the device (Figure 48.4d). Once the device is in place and stable without occurrence of any new significant AR or conduction defects, it can be released according to the type of attachment of the device, for example, unscrewed with St. Jude Medical devices. After release, the result is checked on TOE including 3D imaging (Figures 48.1b and 48.2, Videos 48.2, 48.5 through 48.7) and angiography (Figure 48.4b) and final hemodynamics are measured.

Postprocedure management

An electrocardiogram (ECG) and echocardiogram are carried out prior to discharge, which usually takes place 48–72 h after the procedure. Apart from confirming the position of the device, it is important to check for a residual shunt and AR.

Antiplatelet medication, such as aspirin, is usually prescribed for 6 months. Some prefer to add clopidogrel for 6 weeks.[7] During follow-up, it is important to make sure that there is no hemolysis due to residual shunting. Minimizing risks of endocarditis, including good dental care and appropriate prophylaxis when necessary should be practiced. Surveillance for aortic valve function remains important.

Midterm follow-up up to 5 years so far appears excellent following CC of RASV[7] and this approach is therefore the treatment of choice.

Indications for surgery

Surgery carries very good immediate and long-term results, but nowadays it is restricted to the following situations:

- Patients who have an associated VSD especially when juxta-arterial
- Significant AR where an aortic valve resuspension or aortic valve replacement is needed
- Failure of CC due to a large perforation, or prolonged/severe hemolysis after device placement

Complications

- *Generic:* These include infection, pulse loss, thromboembolic events, and internal bleeding
- *Specific:* These include device migration, hemolysis, encroachment of aortic valve leaflets, and mild AR may occur even without leaflet entrapment, due to after-load mismatch, that is, a sudden increase in the afterload following disconnection of the low-resistance pulmonary circuit. Rarely, AV conduction disturbances[13] and right coronary compromise [14] may occur

Results

CC of RASV was first reported by Cullen et al. in 1994, in a patient with a recurrent RASV, 10 years after the previous surgical repair using the Rashkind umbrella.[15] Since then, in recent times, there have been several case reports, interesting case presentations at interventional meetings, and a small series of cases of CC of RASV using the popular and effective Amplatzer or Amplatzer-like devices.[6–11,13,14] The first series of eight patients was reported by Arora et al.[9] In 2010, Kerkar et al.[7] published the largest series of 20 patients with a success rate of 90% (18 of 20), using the ADO. Patients with coexisting VSD or significant AR requiring surgery, large RASV with aortic end >12 mm, RASV with multiple rupture sites, and those with any suspicion or evidence of infective endocarditis were excluded. However, two patients in this series had associated defects (coarctation of aorta in one and ostium secundum ASD in the other[16]) that were corrected by the catheter technique. Acute complications encountered were residual shunting in five patients (small in four, moderate with self-abating hemolysis in one) and trivial procedure-related AR in four patients. On a median follow-up of 24 months (range 1–60 months), the residual shunting disappeared in three out of five and procedure-related AR vanished in two out of four. There was no AR progression, recurrence, or infective endocarditis or device embolization.

Conclusion

CC of RASV is an established, first-choice procedure often closed with nitinol-based plug devices, such as the ADO from St. Jude Medical. The results are excellent and these persist during follow-up. Surgery is indicated for specific situations, such as a very large perforation not suitable for transcatheter closure or associated lesions that require surgical repair.

All RASV should be closed. The contentious issue is whether the unruptured RASVs should be proactively occluded but there is no evidence to support that this is beneficial, at least from a hemodynamics point of view but they have been known to be a source of systemic emboli.

The techniques have been established and the commonest device used is the ADO or devices with similar shape delivered from the femoral vein.

Acknowledgments

The authors wish to acknowledge Dr. Phatarpekar AU and Dr. Patil RS, for their great help in the preparation of the manuscript.

References

1. Valsalva AM. *Arteriae Magnae Sinus*. In: Morgagni JB. Ed. *Opera*. Venice: Pitteri. p. 1740:1–129.

2. Kirklin JW, Barratt-Boyes BG. Congenital sinus of Valsalva aneurysm and aortico-left ventricular tunnel. In: Kouchoukos NT, Blackstone EH, Hanley FL, Kirklin JK. Eds. *Cardiac Surgery*. 4th ed. Philadelphia, PA: Elsevier Saunders, 2013. pp. 1326–41.

3. Hoey ET, Kanagasingam A, Sivananthan MU. Sinus of Valsalva aneurysms: Assessment with cardiovascular MRI. *Am J Roentgenol* 2010;194:W495–504.

4. Chu SH, Hung CR, How SS et al. Ruptured aneurysms of the sinus of Valsalva in Oriental patients. *J Thorac Cardiovasc Surg* 1990; 99:288–98.

5. Van Son JA, Danielson GK, Schaff HV et al. Long-term outcome of surgical repair of ruptured sinus of Valsalva aneurysm. *Circulation* 1994;90:II20.

6. Kerkar P, Suvarna T, Burkule N et al. Transcatheter closure of ruptured sinus of Valsalva aneurysm using the Amplatzer duct occluder in a critically ill post-CABG patient. *J Invasive Cardiol* 2007;19:E169–71.

7. Kerkar PG, Lanjewar CP, Mishra N et al. Transcatheter closure of ruptured sinus of Valsalva aneurysm using the Amplatzer duct occlude: Immediate results and mid-term follow-up. *Eur Heart J* 2010;31:2881–7.

8. Fedson S, Jolly N, Lang RM et al. Percutaneous closure of ruptured sinus of Valsalva aneurysm using the Amplatzer duct occluder. *Catheter Cardiovasc Interv* 2003;58:406–11.

9. Arora R, Trehan V, Rangashetty UM et al. Transcatheter closure of ruptured sinus of Valsalva aneurysm. *J Interv Cardiol* 2004;17:53–8.

10. Abidin N, Clarke B, Khattar RS. Percutaneous closure of ruptured sinus of Valsalva aneurysm using an Amplatzer occluder device. *Heart* 2005;91(2):244.

11. Schaeffler R, Sarikouch S, Peuster M. Transcatheter closure of ruptured sinus of Valsalva aneurysm (RSVA) after aortic valve replacement using the Amplatzer muscular VSD occluder. *Clin Res Cardiol* 2007;96:904–6.

12. Rao PS, Bromberg BI, Jureidini SB et al. Transcatheter occlusion of ruptured sinus of Valsalva aneurysm: Innovative use of available technology. *Catheter Cardiovasc Interv* 2003;58:130–4.

13. Karlekar SM, Bhalghat P, Kerkar PG. Complete heart block following transcatheter closure of ruptured sinus of Valsalva aneurysm. *J Invasive Cardiol* 2012;24:E314–17.

14. Lihua G, Daxin Z, Feng Z et al. Percutaneous device closure of ruptured sinus of Valsalva aneurysm: A preliminary experience. *J Invasive Cardiol* 2013;25(10):492–6.

15. Cullen S, Sommerville J, Redington A. Transcatheter closure of a ruptured aneurysm of the sinus of Valsalva. *Brit Heart J* 1994;71:479–80.

16. Mehta N, Mishra N, Kerkar P. Percutaneous closure of a ruptured sinus of Valsalva aneurysm and atrial septal defect. *J Invasive Cardiol* 2010;22:E82–5.

49

Atrial septal defect: Background and indications for ASD closure

John L. Bass

Definition

An atrial septal defect (ASD) is a congenital hole in the atrial septum. It is one of the commoner forms of congenital heart disease, occurring in 5–10% of children with cardiac malformations at birth. In adulthood, it accounts for 25–30% of newly diagnosed congenital heart defects. Normally, the foramen ovale provides a communication between the atria prior to birth. This is necessary to allow blood to fill the left side of the heart when pulmonary blood flow is minimal. A flap of tissue covers this opening after birth when the ductus arteriosus closes and the right ventricular output is directed only into the pulmonary arteries. With an ASD, the communication remains, allowing blood to mix between the atria.

Physiology

The direction and amount of blood flowing through an isolated ASD depends on the size of the communication and the diastolic properties of the right and left ventricles. With a large ASD, the pressures in both atria are essentially equal and flow depends on the ease with which each ventricle fills. Both ventricles pump to the systemic circulation *in utero*, and their volume and thickness, and thus their compliance, are similar. The pressure required to fill the right and left ventricles is similar immediately after birth. At this point, there may be relatively little flow through an ASD.

Pulmonary vascular resistance dramatically falls with the first breath. There is a further, slower but continuous fall in pulmonary vascular resistance over the next few months of life. Right ventricular myocardial thickness decreases as a result of the decreased resistance and pressure, and right ventricular compliance increases. The right ventricle is gradually able to accept more blood than the left ventricle at the same diastolic pressure. Thus, the left-to-right shunt through an ASD increases with increasing right ventricular compliance. Small defects may be pressure restrictive and limit flow beyond ventricular compliance.

Diagnosis

The left-to-right shunt through the ASD produces increased flow through the right side of the heart with increased flow across the tricuspid and pulmonary valves. This produces flow murmurs across these valves—a systolic ejection murmur at the upper left sternal border from the pulmonary valve, and a diastolic murmur at the lower sternal border from the tricuspid valve. The larger end-diastolic volume prolongs ejection from the right ventricle, and splitting of the second heart sound widens from delayed closure of the pulmonary valve. The normal respiratory variation in splitting of the second heart sound is lost as left-to-right shunting through the ASD decreases with increased systemic venous return during inspiration, and splitting becomes "fixed." The ASD shunt produces right atrial and right ventricular enlargement that is seen on echocardiography (Figure 49.1), and can produce a precordial bulge. The amount of blood flow to the lungs is increased. A chest roentgenogram shows cardiomegaly with increased pulmonary vascular markings, but no left atrial enlargement as it is "decompressed" across the ASD. Electrocardiograms may show right axis deviation, right atrial enlargement, and a right ventricular volume overload pattern.

The clinical findings of an ASD mirror those of the gradual increase in the left-to-right shunt. At birth, there is relatively little flow through the ASD, and there are no clinical findings. The murmur of increased flow across the pulmonary valve usually appears during the first year of life, followed later by widening of the second heart sound and subsequently a tricuspid flow murmur. The classical auscultation findings may not be apparent until at least 2–3 years of age. The murmurs are subtle, and sometimes

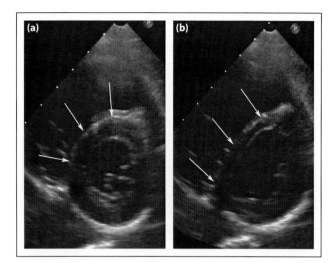

Figure 49.1　Parasternal short-axis echocardiographic images from a patient with a large ASD. The contour of the ventricular septum (arrows) is rounded in the systole (a) as left ventricular pressure exceeds that of the right ventricle. During diastole (b), the contour of the ventricular septum (arrows) is flattened as the mitral and tricuspid valves are open, and the diastolic pressures in the right and left ventricles are equalized through the large ASD.

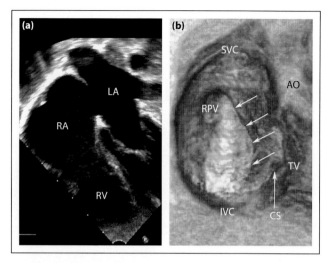

Figure 49.2　(a) Two-dimensional echocardiogram recorded from an apical four-chamber view. The right atrium (RA) and right ventricle (RV) are enlarged. Between the RA and the left atrium (LA), there is "dropout" of echoes from a large secundum ASD. (b) Three-dimensional tissue imaging of a secundum ASD from a cardiac computed tomographic angiogram. (Courtesy of Charles Shepard, MD, University of Minnesota, Minneapolis, MN.) A rim of atrial septum extends superiorly and anteriorly (arrows) with no rim posteriorly or inferiorly by the inferior vena cava (IVC). AO = aorta, CS = coronary sinus, RPV = right pulmonary vein, SVC = superior vena cava, TV = tricuspid valve.

incomplete, and the clinical diagnosis of an ASD may be delayed into later childhood and adult life.

The diagnosis of an ASD is suspected from the clinical findings, and evidence of a large left-to-right shunt is seen on the chest roentgenogram. The gold standard for making the diagnosis is observation of the defect on echocardiography (Figure 49.2). Transthoracic imaging is usually sufficient in children, but a poor echocardiographic window may necessitate transesophageal imaging in larger patients and adults. Other imaging modalities such as computed tomography and magnetic resonance imaging may also be used to document the presence of a defect in the atrial tissue (Figure 49.2). Before two-dimensional echocardiographic imaging was developed, many patients with an ASD were sent for surgical repair based on classical clinical, roentgenographic, and electrocardiographic findings. Device closure of an ASD requires a complete evaluation of ASD anatomy and pulmonary and systemic venous return with details of size and location of the defect and elucidation of associated abnormalities.

Effects

The deleterious effects of having an ASD are related to the increased flow through the pulmonary vasculature, and the enlargement of right-sided cardiac chambers. An isolated large ASD may increase pulmonary blood flow from 2 to 4 times normal. The lungs are able to accommodate this increased flow by dilating vessels and recruiting the available pulmonary circulation, and pulmonary artery (PA) pressure is usually normal in children with a large

ASD. Over decades, however, there is vasoconstriction with increased arteriolar muscle, and eventually permanent intimal changes with fixed elevation in pulmonary vascular resistance may develop. Pulmonary hypertension does not usually appear until beyond the second decade of life.

Children with trisomy-21 have an accelerated pulmonary vascular response to increased pulmonary blood flow with an ASD, and may develop permanent pulmonary vascular changes in the first few years of life. Children with pulmonary disease (e.g., lung disease of prematurity) are affected more by the increased pulmonary blood flow than normal children. This may be manifested as frequent respiratory infections or delayed weaning from respiratory support.

Most children with ASDs seem normal to their parents, are active, and participate in sports. Their growth and development are usually normal. However, most families note an increase in activity tolerance after closure of the defect. So, the symptoms of dealing with the left-to-right shunt are real but not noticeable. It has been shown that closure of "small" left-to-right shunts (>1.5:1) in young adults improves exercise tolerance as measured by stress test.

Rarely, children with an ASD may develop symptoms during the first year of life with frequent respiratory infections and failure to thrive. These children's ASDs are not anatomically different from older children with large ASDs who have seemed normal. It is not clear why this defect affects a few children more significantly, although the possibility of abnormally decreased left ventricular compliance has been raised. Long-standing increased pulmonary blood flow and right-sided cardiac enlargement in adults with large ASDs often produces more symptoms of exercise intolerance.

Chronic enlargement of the right atrium and ventricle can lead to fibrosis, and arrhythmias are common in adults with ASDs. When surgical closure was performed under the age of 15, no atrial fibrillation or flutter was seen on Holter monitor at 15-year follow-up. This same group had a 6% incidence of atrial tachyarrhythmias 26 years after surgery, although 26% complained of palpitations.[1] At least half of the patients with an untreated ASD over 45 years of age have chronic or intermittent atrial fibrillation. Atrial arrhythmias persisted in 60% of the patients repaired over age 40, with new atrial flutter or fibrillation in 12% of the patients.[2] This may form the substrate for a thrombus in the left atrial appendage with the risk of systemic embolus.

Indications for closure

Closure of an ASD should be performed before developing permanent damage to the pulmonary vasculature from increased pulmonary blood flow, or myocardial fibrosis with arrhythmias from right atrial enlargement. The trick, then, is early identification of patients with an ASD at risk for these complications.

The size of a left-to-right shunt (expressed as a ratio of pulmonary-to-systemic blood flow [Qp:Qs]) that damages the pulmonary vasculature is generally accepted to be 2:1. The gold standard of calculating this ratio is by cardiac catheterization. The calculation depends on acquiring the oxygen saturation in the pulmonary veins and arteries (PV, PA) and the systemic arterial and "mixed" systemic venous saturations (SA, MV). The equation solves to (SA–MV saturations)/(PV–PA saturations). An ASD presents significant challenges for this measurement. Since the left-to-right shunt occurs at the atrial level, there is no mixing chamber for the venous return from the superior and inferior venae cavae. Maneuvers to solve this include assuming the contribution of the superior and inferior caval veins (50:50 in infants and 40:60 in older patients), or simply using the superior vena caval saturation. The case for the latter choice is strengthened by variable inferior caval saturations caused by streaming of renal and hepatic flows. When PV and arterial saturations are close, significant error can result from the narrow arteriovenous oxygen difference in the denominator, inflating the calculated size of the shunt. At best, the shunt size calculated at cardiac catheterization must be considered as an approximation because of the assumptions involved.

The minimum size of a left-to-right shunt requiring intervention is not clear. A poll of 205 pediatric cardiologists was obtained in 1971.[3] When the shunt was larger than 1.5:1, 70% of respondents recommended closure, and 96% recommended closure when the Qp:Qs was at least 2:1. In general, shunts between 1.5:1 and 2:1 are closed when accompanied by typical clinical findings, cardiomegaly with increased pulmonary vascular markings on the chest roentgenogram, or right-sided cardiac enlargement on the echocardiogram.

Patients with right atrial enlargement are at risk for developing fibrosis and atrial arrhythmias. This risk increases with increasing age. Closure of an ASD in a patient with right atrial enlargement and no other explanation should be performed electively but should not be delayed. Once fibrosis has developed, atrial arrhythmias may persist after closure, although decreased right atrial size after eliminating the shunt may decrease the frequency or severity of the arrhythmia.

Timing

Elective closure of an isolated ASD is usually performed between 2 and 5 years of age, the time when clinical findings usually become typical. Closure of the ASD in children with trisomy-21 should occur in the first year of life because of the risk of early pulmonary vascular disease. Children with failure to thrive, recurrent respiratory infections, or with chronic respiratory conditions who are not improving may need closure in the first few months of life, and their respiratory status may be significantly improved.

Closure of an ASD in adults deserves special comment. Early reports of the natural history of ASD suggested high percentages of exercise intolerance, cyanosis, and death (25% by age 27, 50% by age 36, and 75% by age 60). As echocardiography has become available to make the diagnosis of an ASD in patients with fewer symptoms, it is clear that these data are too pessimistic. Surgical closure over the age of 40 years does not improve mortality compared to medical treatment.[4] However, paradoxical emboli, arrhythmias, heart failure, and quality of life (NYHA class) were improved. Adults with smaller shunts (1.2–2:1) had as much improvement in VO$_2$ max and decrease in RV size as patients with larger shunts (>2:1).[5] When the diagnosis of a large ASD is established in adult life, closure should be performed when the diagnosis is made.

Contraindications

Device closure of an ASD depends on the defect being entirely surrounded with rims of tissue—a secundum ASD (Figure 49.3). In about 20% of patients, the ASD may be in a different location. Primum ASDs have atrioventricular valve tissue forming the inferior rim of the defect (Figure 49.3) and are not amenable to device closure. Sinus venosus defects at the superior or inferior vena cava also lack rims for a device to capture, and the superior defects are often associated with partial anomalous pulmonary

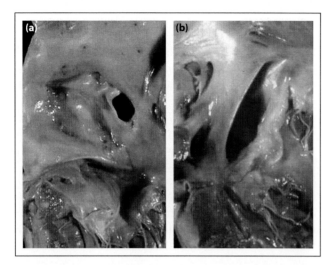

Figure 49.3 (a) Pathologic specimen of a secundum ASD. The defect is entirely surrounded by rims of atrial tissue, good anatomy for device closure. (b) Pathologic specimen of a primum ASD. The inferior margin of the defect is composed of the atrioventricular valve, and device closure of this defect is impossible. (Courtesy of Jesse E. Edwards Registry of Cardiovascular Disease, St. Paul, Minneapolis, MN.)

venous connection. Defects in the wall of the coronary sinus are rare and may be accompanied by a defect in the atrial septum where the coronary sinus ostium would be expected. These nonsecundum ASDs are not amenable to device closure.

Elevated pulmonary vascular resistance (>5 WU) and pulmonary hypertension (PA pressure more than 50–70 mmHg) may be considered as contraindications to closure.

Summary

Closure of large ASDs that result in right-sided cardiac enlargement and classical clinical findings should be electively performed at 2–3 years of age to minimize the risk of later arrhythmias and prevent increased pulmonary vascular resistance. Earlier closure may be indicated for symptoms of congestive heart failure or when associated with significant pulmonary parenchymal disease. When the defect is detected later in life, closure will result in improved morbidity, even beyond the age of 40 years.

The best course for patients who have smaller ASDs is less clear. But the inaccuracies of oximetry for measuring shunt size with an ASD, and demonstrated improvement in right-sided enlargement and exercise tolerance in adults with shunts as small as 1.2:1, suggest that consideration should be given to closing even these smaller defects.

References

1. Roos-Hesselink JW, Meijboom RJ, Spitaels SEC et al. Excellent survival and low incidence of arrhythmias, stroke and heart failure long-term after surgical ASD closure at young age. A prospective follow-up study of 21–33 years. *Eur Heart J* 2003;2003:190–7.
2. Gatzoulis MA, Freeman MA, Siu SC et al. Atrial arrhythmia after surgical closure of atrial septal defects in adults. *N Engl J Med* 1999;340:839–46.
3. Moss AJ, Siassi B. The small atrial septal defect—Operate or procrastinate? *J Pediatr* 1971;79:854–7.
4. Attie F, Rosas M, Granados N et al. Surgical treatment for secundum atrial septal defect in patients ≥40 years old. A randomized clinical trial. *J Am Coll Cardiol* 2001;38:2035–42.
5. Brochu M-C, Baril J-F, Core A et al. Improvement in exercise capacity in asymptomatic and mildly symptomatic adults after atrial septal defect percutaneous closure. *Circulation* 2002;106:1821–6.

50

Atrial septal defect: Amplatzer-type ASD occluders

Mustafa Al-Qbandi, Qi-Ling Cao, and Ziyad M. Hijazi

Introduction

Most secundum types of atrial septal defects (ASD) are amenable for transcatheter closure. The Amplatzer septal occluder (ASO) is a unique device that combines the advantage of being a double-disk device with a self-centering mechanism.[1] It is the first and only device to ever receive full approval in 2001 for clinical use from the United States Food and Drug Administration (FDA). Since its initial human use in 1995,[2] it is now the most commonly used device worldwide to close the ASD. Yet, increasing in popularity is another device of similar shape, but with different technology, called the Occlutech Figulla occlude, first introduced in 2003 (Occlutech AB, Helsingborg, Sweden). The Flex II, the third-generation Occlutech occluder has a very flexible technology that allows it to adjust and fit a wide variety of geometries. We will first give a detailed description of the original Amplatzer device followed by features of the ASD Occlutech device that are different from the Amplatzer device.

Amplatzer device

The ASO device (St. Jude Medical, Plymouth, MN, USA) is a self-expandable double-disk device made of a nitinol wire mesh (Figure 50.1).[1-3] The ASO device is constructed from a 0.004–0.0075 inch nitinol (55% nickel; 45% titanium) wire mesh that is tightly woven into two flat disks. There

is a 3–4 mm connecting waist between the two disks, corresponding to the thickness of the atrial septum. Nitinol has superelastic properties with shape memory. This allows the device to be stretched into an almost linear configuration and placed inside a small sheath for delivery and then reforms to its original configuration within the heart when not constrained by the sheath. The device size is determined by the diameter of its waist and is constructed in various sizes ranging from 4–40 mm (1 mm increments up to 20 mm; 2 mm increments from size 20 up to the largest device currently available at 40 mm). The two flat disks extend radially beyond the central waist to provide secure anchorage. Patients with secundum ASD usually have L–R shunt. Therefore, the left atrium (LA) disk is larger than the right atrium (RA) disk. For devices 4–10 mm in size, the LA disk is 12 mm and the RA disk is 8 mm larger than the waist. However, for devices larger than 11 mm and up to 32 mm in size, the LA disk is 14 mm and the RA disk is 10 mm larger than the connecting waist. For devices 34 mm and larger, the LA disk is 16 mm larger than the waist and the RA disk is 10 mm larger than the waist. Both disks are angled slightly toward each other to ensure firm contact of the disks to the atrial septum. There is a total of three Dacron polyester patches sewn securely with polyester thread into each disk and the connecting waist to increase the thrombogenicity of the device. A stainless steel sleeve with a female thread is laser welded to the RA disk. This sleeve is used to screw the delivery cable to the device.

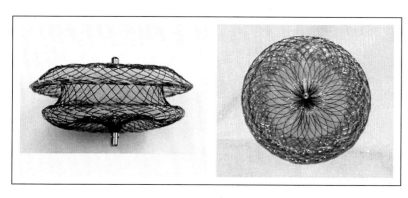

Figure 50.1 The Amplatzer septal occluder (ASO) consists of three components: Left, side view showing a left atrial disk on top, a connecting waist, and a right atrial disk. Polyester fabric fills these three components. Right, *en face* view of the left atrial disk.

For device deployment, we recommend using a 6 Fr delivery system for devices <10 mm in diameter; a 7 Fr delivery system for 10–15 mm devices; a 8 Fr sheath for 16–20 mm devices; a 9 Fr sheath for 22–28 mm devices; a 10 Fr sheath for 30–34 mm devices; a 12 Fr sheath for the 36 and 38 mm device, and a 14 Fr sheath for the 40 mm device. The 40 mm device is not available in the United States.

Amplatzer delivery system

The delivery system is supplied sterilized and separate from the device. It contains all the equipment needed to facilitate device deployment. It consists of

Delivery sheath of specified French size and length and appropriate dilator
Loading device, used to collapse the device and introduce it into the delivery sheath
Delivery cable (ID = 0.081"): The device is screwed onto its distal end and it allows for loading, placement, and retrieval of the device. Recently, the manufacturer has introduced a new delivery system (TorqVue® FX delivery system) with a cable that has an inner core; pulling back the core wire makes the angle flexible between the device and cable.
Plastic pin vice: This facilitates unscrewing of the delivery cable from the device during device deployment.
Touhy–Borst adapter with a side arm for the sheath, to act as a one-way stop-bleed valve

All delivery sheaths have a 45° angled tip. The 6 Fr sheath has a length of 60 cm, the 7 Fr is available in lengths of 60 and 80 cm, and the 8, 9, 10, and 12 Fr sheaths are all 80 cm in length.

Optional but recommended equipment

Amplatzer sizing balloon

The Amplatzer sizing balloon is a double-lumen balloon catheter with a 7 Fr shaft size. The balloon is made from nylon and is very compliant, making it ideal for sizing secundum ASD by flow occlusion and preventing overstretching of the defect. The balloon catheter is angled at 45° and there are radiopaque markers (positioned inside the balloon for calibration at 2, 5, and 10 mm). The balloon catheters are available in three sizes: 18, 24, and 34 mm.

NuMED sizing balloons

An alternative to the above balloon is the NuMED sizing balloon (NuMED Hopkinton, NY, USA) that is available in sizes 20 mm × 3 cm, 25 mm × 3 cm, 30 mm × 3–5 cm, and 40 mm × 3–5 cm. There are radiopaque markers for calibration inside the balloon at 10–15 mm. The shaft size is 8 Fr.

Amplatzer Super Stiff exchange guide wire—0.035 inch

It is used to advance the delivery sheath and dilator into the left upper pulmonary vein.

Occlutech ASD device

The Occlutech Figulla Flex ASD device (Occlutech AB, Helsingborg, Sweden) is technically similar to the Amplatzer device.[4] It is a double-disk device made of a self-expanding nitinol wire mesh fully recapturable and repositionable before release.

The Occlutech surface technology was developed in order to obtain the highest possible biocompatibility of the implant. A special oxidation process that creates a layer of titanium oxide gives the Occlutech occluders their characteristic golden color (Figure 50.2).

The patented braiding system allows Occlutech to manufacture its occluders without mounting any clamp or hub. The connector is shaped from laser-welded biocompatible nitinol only, using no other metals. The amount of material implanted in this area is reduced over 70% by utilizing a proprietary welding process to form a ball specifically designed for compatibility with the delivery system (cable). In addition to reducing the amount of material implanted and giving a less traumatic tip, this gives several additional advantages. Most importantly, by not locking the strands at the distal part into a rigid structure, the occluders remain more flexible providing

- Superior adaptation to the septal tissue upon implantation
- Superior adaptation to challenging anatomy
- Sizing flexibility reducing the number of sizes needed in stock
- Softer rims

In order to achieve an optimal acute outcome and minimize any residual shunt when closing an ASD, it is important not to undersize.[5-8] The Occlutech Figulla Flex II range of occluders has been designed to allow flexibility when matching the size of the occluder to the defect. Each device size covers up to approximately 3 mm. Figulla Flex II ASD Occluder sizes are 4, 5, 6, 7.5, 9, 10.5, 12, 13.5, 15, and 16.5 mm. From 18 to 40 mm, the range is 18, 21, 24, 27, 30, 33, 36, 39, and 40 mm. The Figulla Flex Uni is used for multifenestrated ASDs and its sizes range from 17/17, 24/24, 28.5/28.5, 33/33, and 40/40 mm.

The device–cable connection (see Figure 50.2) is not a screw but a ball-and-socket mechanism. When the device is connected to the cable, the occluder can be angled some 50° without any major drag on the device. This supports placement under difficult conditions, especially in defects with deficient rims and where the angle of the desired placement is different from the angle of delivery system. In addition, the

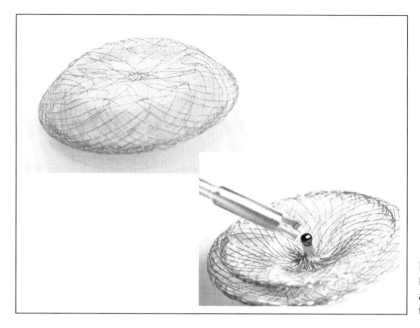

Figure 50.2 **(See color insert.)** The Occlutech Figulla Flex II device: Note the difference in the attachment mechanism. Occlutech has the ball in the right atrial disk.

actual tip of the delivery system or the cable can be shaped to the desired angle suiting any implantation technique. Occlutech's specially developed "Kinza" technology allows the preimplantation shaping of the tip. Once the device is in place, the cable is disconnected from the device by a release mechanism of forceps (unlike Amplatzer's screw mechanism). The forceps release has a lock mechanism that needs to be unscrewed (if secured initially—an optional feature).

The unique, flexible braiding allows the implant to adapt to the shape of the defect and effectively close it. Since the waist of the Occlutech occluders is substantially softer than any other device, the implant adapts to the defect without causing unnecessary pressure. The soft waist, coupled with the flexible disks, reduces any risk of erosion.

The sheath: The unique Occlutech braiding technology has allowed Occlutech to reduce the required size of the delivery sheath by 1–3 Fr sizes. On average, the required diameter has been reduced by 20%, an important feature, especially in small children. The sheath is the Mullins type and consists of a smooth outer layer and a low-friction inner layer reinforced with metal braiding. The braid improves the strength of the sheath and provides radiopacity. The sheath has a proximal female connector for connection to the dilator or to the loader. The sheath accepts Occlutech stiff guide wire 0.035 260 J-3 mm. The range of the sheath is 7–12 Fr. There are two 8 Fr sizing balloons, 25 and 35 mm.

Patient selection

The indication for ASD closure using the ASO is the secundum-type ASD demonstrated by echocardiography with (1) symptomatic patients or hemodynamically significant shunt (Qp/Qs >1.5 or evidence of right ventricular

enlargement as evidenced by echocardiography; we usually do not depend on the Qp/Qs ratio to determine the importance of the shunt, but rather on the size of the right ventricle); or (2) patients with small atrial defect and a history of paradoxical embolization resulting in a stroke, transient ischemic attack, or peripheral embolism. Contraindications for the use of the ASO include (1) patients with an associated anomalous pulmonary venous drainage requiring surgery, (2) patients with sinus venosus defects, (3) patients with primum ASD, (4) a deficient rim (<5 mm) from the ASD to the superior or inferior vena cava, right upper or lower pulmonary vein, coronary sinus, mitral or tricuspid valve (outside the United States, a deficient anterior rim toward the aorta is not a contraindication for the ASO; however, in the United States, as of January 2012, the manufacturer deemed a deficient anterior rim to be a contraindication to use the ASO in such patients), (5) associated other cardiac anomalies requiring surgical repair, (6) pulmonary vascular resistance of greater than 8 Woods units, (7) sepsis, or (8) contraindication to antiplatelet therapy.

Precatheterization evaluation

Echocardiographic assessment of the type, size, and number of ASDs is of paramount importance for planning the device closure.[9] Transesophageal echocardiography (TEE) can provide superior anatomical detail of the defect and the surrounding structures. Figure 50.3 details the TEE views that need to be obtained in order to assess suitability for device closure. Transthoracic echocardiography (TTE) is usually sufficient for children with good imaging windows. It is essential to assess if there is associated anomalous pulmonary venous drainage and to assess the adequacy of all rims. If the septum has more than one hole, the bigger hole is

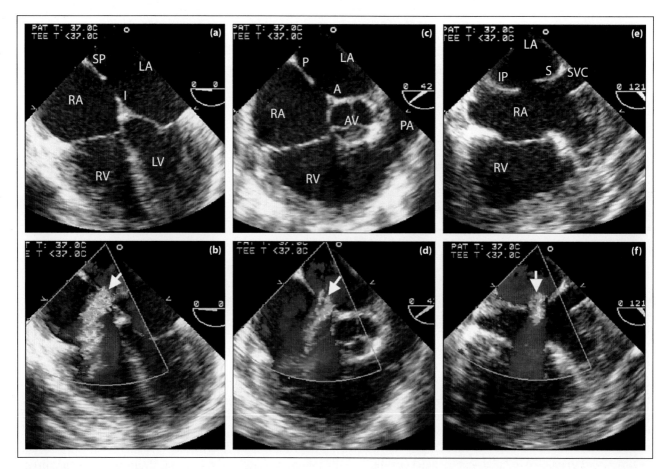

Figure 50.3 (**See color insert.**) Transesophageal echocardiographic images in a patient with secundum atrial septal defect demonstrating the essential views for selection of patients to undergo device closure using the Amplatzer or the Occlutech devices. Top images are without and bottom images same views with color Doppler. (a,b) Four-chamber view (0° omni plane) showing the defect with left-to-right shunt (arrow), the inferior anterior rim (I), and the superior-posterior rim (SP). (c,d) Classic short-axis view at about 40° demonstrating the defect (arrow); the anterior rim (A) and the posterior rim (P). (e,f) Bicaval view at about 120° demonstrating the superior rim (S) and the inferior rim (IP) and the defect (arrow). LA: left atrium; RA: right atrium; RV: right ventricle; SVC: superior vena cava; IVC: inferior vena cava; LV: left ventricle; PA: pulmonary artery.

usually located in the superoanterior septum, while the smaller hole is located in the inferoposterior septum. Three-dimensional echocardiography may provide a better defect morphology and structural relationships. Nevertheless, the accuracy of its reconstructed images is heavily dependent on the technical expertise of the echocardiographer. Forty-eight hours prior to the procedure, patients are asked to take aspirin 3–5 mg/kg per day.

Transcatheter closure of secundum ASD: Step-by-step technique

Materials and equipment

Single- or biplane cardiac catheterization laboratory: We prefer to work with a single-plane fluoroscopy system; this allows larger room for the echo machine and for anesthesia if needed.

TEE or intracardiac echocardiography (ICE): We prefer the ICE technology using the AcuNAV catheter (Acuson, a Siemens Company).

The full range of device sizes, delivery, and exchange (rescue) systems must be readily available in the room:

Sizing balloon catheters: Different sizes should be available.

A multipurpose catheter to engage the defect and the left upper pulmonary vein.

Suprastiff exchange length wire, we prefer the 0.035-inch Amplatzer suprastiff exchange length guide wire with a 1 cm floppy tip, but any extra-stiff J-tipped wire may be used.

Personnel

Interventional cardiologist appropriately proctored to perform device closure

Cardiologist—noninvasive to facilitate TEE or ICE

Anesthesiologist—if procedure is performed under TEE guidance

Nurse certified to administer conscious sedation if performed under ICE guidance

Catheterization laboratory technicians

Procedure

The right femoral vein is accessed using a 7–8 Fr short sheath. An arterial monitoring line can be inserted in the right femoral artery, especially if the patient's condition is marginal or if the procedure is performed under TEE and general endotracheal anesthesia. If the femoral venous route is not available, we advocate the transhepatic approach. A subclavian or internal jugular venous are very difficult approaches for maneuvering the device deployment, especially with large defects. We administer heparin to achieve activated clotting time (ACT) >200 s at the time of device deployment. Antibiotic coverage for the procedure is recommended. We usually use cefazolin 1 g intravenously. The first dose is given at the time of the procedure and two subsequent doses are given 6–8 h apart.

Routine right heart catheterization should be performed in all cases to ensure presence of normal pulmonary vascular resistance. The left-to-right shunt can also be calculated.

Echocardiographic assessment of the secundum ASD should be performed simultaneously either by TEE or ICE (Figure 50.4). A comprehensive study should be performed looking at all aspects of the ASD anatomy (location, size, presence of additional defects, and adequacy of the various rims).

The important rims to look for are

Superior/SVC rim: This is best achieved using the bicaval view.

Anterior-superior/aortic rim: This is the least important rim. Often, many patients lack this rim. This is best seen in the short-axis view.

Inferior/IVC and coronary sinus rim: This is an important rim to have. Best seen in the bicaval view.

Posterior rim: This can be seen best in the short-axis view at the aortic valve level.

How to cross the ASD. Select a multipurpose catheter; the MP A2 catheter has the ideal angle. Place the catheter at the IVC/RA junction. The IVC angle should guide the catheter to the ASD; keep a clockwise torque on the catheter while advancing it toward the septum (posterior). If unsuccessful, place the catheter in the SVC and slowly pull the catheter into the RA and keep a clockwise posterior torque to orient the catheter along the atrial septum until it crosses the defect. TEE/ICE can be very useful to guide the catheter across difficult defects.

Right upper pulmonary vein angiogram. It can be useful to perform an angiogram in the right upper pulmonary vein (Figure 50.5) in the hepatoclavicular projection (35° LAO/35° cranial). This delineates the anatomy, shape, and length of the septum. This may become handy when the device is deployed but not released, the operator can position the I/I in the same view of the angiogram and compare the position of the device with that obtained during the deployment (Figure 50.5).

Defect sizing. Position the MP A2 catheter in the left upper pulmonary vein. Prepare the appropriate sizing balloon according to the manufacturer's guidelines. We prefer to use the 34-mm balloon since it is longer and during balloon inflation it sits nicely across the defect. Pass an extra-stiff floppy/J-tipped 0.035 inch exchange length guide wire (Amplatzer Super Stiff wire). This gives the best support within the atrium for the balloon, especially in large defects. Remove the MP A2 catheter and the femoral sheath. We advance the sizing balloon catheter over the wire directly without a venous sheath. Most sizing balloons require 8–10 Fr sheaths. The balloon catheter is advanced over the wire and placed across the defect under both fluoroscopic and echocardiographic guidance. The balloon is then inflated with diluted contrast until the left-to-right shunt ceases as observed by color-flow Doppler TEE/ICE (stop-flow technique). The best ECHO view for measurement is to observe the balloon in its long axis (Figure 50.4). In this view, the indentation made by the ASD margins can be visualized and a precise measurement made.

Fluoroscopic measurement. Angulate the x-ray tube so the beam is perpendicular to the balloon. This can be difficult but the various calibration markers can help. Ensure that the markers are separated and discrete. Measure the balloon diameter at the site of the indentation as per the diagnostic function of the laboratory (Figures 50.4 and 50.5). If a discrepancy exists between the echocardiographic and the fluoroscopic measurements, we have found that the echocardiographic measurement is usually more accurate.

Once the size is determined, deflate the balloon and pull it back into the IVC, leaving the wire in the left upper pulmonary vein.

This is a good time to recheck the ACT and give the first dose of antibiotics.

Device selection. If the defect has adequate rims (>5 mm), we usually select a device 0–2 mm larger than the balloon-stretched diameter. However, if the superior/anterior rim is deficient (less than 5–7 mm), we select a device 2–4 mm larger than the balloon-stretched diameter. Lately, we have been closing ASDs without balloon sizing. Our choice for the device size depends on the echocardiographic

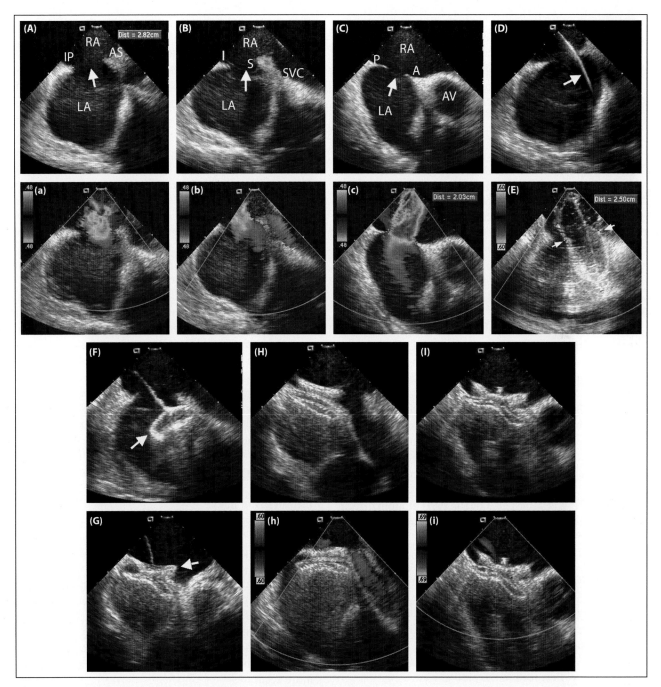

Figure 50.4 **(See color insert.)** Intracardiac echocardiographic images in a 59-year-old patient with a secundum atrial septal defect measuring 28 mm demonstrating the various steps of closure. (A and a) Septal view without and with color Doppler showing the defect (arrow) with left-to-right shunt, the anterior/superior (AS) rim, and the inferior/posterior rim (IP). (B and b) Bicaval view (long-axis view) without and with color Doppler showing the superior rim (S) and inferior rim (I). (C and c) Short-axis view without and with color Doppler showing the defect with left-to-right shunt (arrow), the anterior rim (A), and the posterior rim (P). (d) Septal view showing wire passage (arrow) through the defect. (e) Similar view as (d), during stop-flow technique of balloon sizing. RA: right atrium; LA: left atrium; SVC: superior vena cava; AV: aortic valve. (f) Deployment of the left atrial disk (arrow) of a 28-mm Amplatzer septal occluder. (g) Deployment of the right disk of the device (arrow). (H and h) Bicaval view without and with color Doppler after the device has been released showing good device position and no residual shunt and unobstructed SVC flow. (I and i) Short-axis view after the device has been released, again showing good device position and no residual shunt.

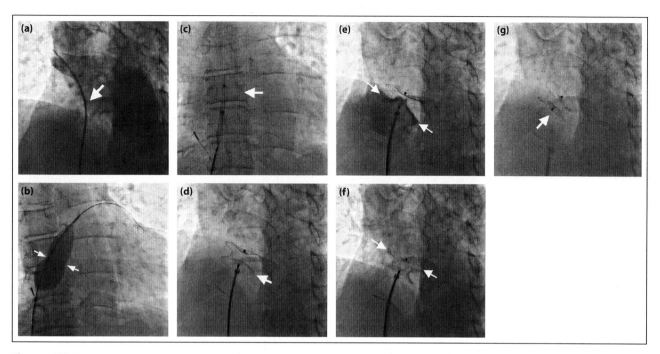

Figure 50.5 Cine fluoroscopic images demonstrating the steps of closure in the same patient as Figure 50.4. (a) Angiography in the right upper pulmonary vein in the hepatoclavicular projection demonstrating a secundum-type ASD (arrows). (b) Cine image straight frontal demonstrating the sizing balloon with a waist (arrows), indicating the stretched diameter or stop-flow diameter. (c) Left atrial disk (arrow) has been deployed in the left atrium (straight frontal). (d) Deployment of the right atrial disk (arrow) in same view as image (a). (e) Angiogram in the right atrium via side arm of delivery sheath demonstrating good device position (the RA disk opacifies) (arrows) indicating it is all in the RA, and the LA disk does not opacify. (f) Pulmonary levophase of the previous angiogram showing that the LA disk opacifies (arrows), indicating it is in the LA, and the RA disk does not opacify, indicating it is in the right atrium. (g) Final cine image of the device after release showing good device position. Compare this image with image (a). This indicates the device to be in good position.

measurements of the defect by color Doppler (ICE). We choose a device about 20% larger than the two-dimensional size by color Doppler in children. Once the device size is selected, open the appropriate-sized delivery system. Flush the sheath and dilator. The proper size delivery sheath is advanced over the guide wire to the left upper pulmonary vein (Figures 50.4 and 50.5). Both dilator and wire are removed, keeping the tip of the sheath inside the left upper pulmonary vein. Extreme care must be exercised not to allow passage of air inside the delivery sheath. An alternative technique to minimize an air embolism is passage of the sheath with the dilator over the wire until the inferior vena cava, then the dilator is removed and the sheath is advanced over the wire into the left atrium while continuously flushing the side arm of the sheath. The device is then screwed to the tip of the delivery cable, immersed under normal saline and drawn into the loader underwater seal to expel air bubbles out of the system. A Y-connector is applied to the proximal end of the loader to allow flushing with saline. The loader containing the device is attached to the proximal hub of the delivery sheath. The cable with the ASO device is advanced to the distal tip of the sheath, taking care not to rotate the cable while advancing it in the long sheath to prevent premature unscrewing of the device. Both cable and delivery sheath are pulled back as one unit to the middle of the left atrium. The position of the sheath can be verified using fluoroscopy or TEE/ICE.

The LA disk is deployed first under fluoroscopic and or echocardiographic guidance (Figures 50.4 and 50.5). Caution should be taken not to interfere with the left atrial appendage.

Part of the connecting waist should be deployed in the left atrium, very close (about 2–4 mm) to the atrial septum (the mechanism of ASD closure using the ASO or the Occlutech is stenting of the defect). While applying constant pulling of the entire assembly and withdrawing the delivery sheath off the cable, the connecting waist and the right atrial disk are deployed in the ASD itself and in the RA, respectively (Figures 50.4 and 50.5). Proper device position can be verified using different techniques: (1) Fluoroscopy in the same projection as that of the angiogram. A good device position is evident by the presence of two disks that are parallel to each other and separated from each other by the atrial septum (Figure 50.5). In the same view, the operator can perform the Minnesota wiggle (the cable is pushed gently forward and pulled backward). A stable device position manifests by the lack of movement of the device in either direction. (2) TEE/ICE: The echocardiographer should make sure that one disk is in each chamber. The long-axis view should be sufficient to evaluate the superior and inferior parts of the septum and the short-axis view for the anterior and posterior parts of the disk (Figure 50.4). It is of paramount importance to document the device position using two orthogonal views! One view only is not good enough to determine good device position! (3) The last method to verify device position can be achieved by angiography. This is done with the camera in the same projection as the first angiogram to profile the septum and device using either the side arm of the delivery sheath or via a separate angiographic catheter inserted in the sheath used for ICE, or via a separate puncture site. Good device position manifests by opacification of the right atrial disk alone when the contrast is in the right atrium and opacification of the left atrial disk alone on pulmonary levophase (Figure 50.5).

If device position is not certain or is questionable after all these maneuvers, the device can be recaptured entirely or partly and repositioned following similar steps. Once the device position is verified, the device is released by a counterclockwise rotation of the delivery cable using a pin vise. There is often a notable change in the angle of the device as it is released from the slight tension of the delivery cable and it self-centers within the ASD and aligns with the interatrial septum. To assess the result of closure, repeat TEE/ICE with color Doppler and angiography (optional) in the four-chamber projection in the RA with pulmonary levophase (Figure 50.4). Patients receive a dose of an appropriate antibiotic (commonly cephazolin at 1 g) during the catheterization procedure and two further doses at 8-h intervals. Once the procedure is completed, recheck the ACT and if appropriate, remove the sheath and achieve hemostasis. If ACT is above 250 s, we have been reversing the effect of heparin by using protamine sulfate. Patients are also asked to observe endocarditis prophylaxis when necessary for 6 months after the procedure, as well as aspirin 81–325 mg orally once daily for 6 months. In adult patients, we add 75 mg clopidogrel daily for 2–3 months. Full activity including competitive sports is usually allowed after 4 weeks of implantation. Magnetic resonance imaging (if required) can be done any time after implantation.

Postprocedure monitoring. It is very important to have the patients recover overnight in a telemetry ward. Some patients may experience an increase in atrial ectopic beats. Rarely, some patients may have sustained atrial tachycardias. Resume aspirin therapy 81–325 mg per day after the procedure and continue it for 6 months. As mentioned above, we have been adding clopidogrel 75 mg for adult patients for a total of 2–3 months. We have noticed that adding clopidogrel minimizes postprocedure headaches.

The following day, an ECG, a CXR (PA and lateral), and a TTE with color Doppler should be performed to assess device position and presence of residual shunt. The chest radiograph is optional.

Patients are followed up after 1–3 months, then at 6 months, and then yearly thereafter. During these follow-up visits, an ECG and a TTE are performed. If the device position is good with no residual shunt at the 2 year follow-up, subsequent, follow-up can be done every 3–5 years. We recommend not discharging these patients from care. Rare cases of erosions have been reported after 9 years from closure using the ASO.

Infective endocarditis prophylaxis is discontinued after 6 months if the closure is complete.

Results

The initial human use of ASO in 30 patients showed a complete closure rate of 80% at 24-h follow-up.[2] At that time, the result was very encouraging compared to all other contemporary devices. With the improvement of device and deployment techniques, the results became more and more promising. The United States FDA approved the ASO in December 2001. The data presented to the FDA for the approval revealed that the procedure success rate was 97.6% (413/423). The complete closure rate at 1 day, 6 month, and 12 month follow-up was 96.7% (404/418), 97.2% (376/387), and 98.5% (326/331), respectively. Major adverse events occurred in only 7 (1.6%) out of 442 patients, including device embolization in 4, cardiac arrhythmia requiring major treatment in 2, and delivery system failure in 1. Minor adverse events occurred in 27 (6.1%) out of 442 of patients, including cardiac arrhythmia with minor treatment in 15 (3.4%), thrombus formation in 3 (0.7%), headache in 2, allergic reaction in 2, delivery system failure in 2, device embolization with percutaneous removal in 1, extremity tingling in 1, and urinary tract disturbance in 1.

Complications/problems encountered during ASD closure

1. *Device embolization/migration:* This complication is rare (about 1%) and usually occurs in patients with a large ASD and deficient rims. Most of these embolizations do not cause acute hemodynamic collapse. The device can be snared and retrieved percutaneously; however, a larger sheath (+2 Fr) than the one used for delivery may be needed to remove the device. The presence of a cardiovascular surgeon in house is essential when closing ASDs with devices.

2. *Arrhythmia:* The study with an ambulatory electrocardiographic monitoring showed that supraventricular ectopy was noted in 26 (63%) out of 41 patients immediately after the device closure, including 9 patients

(23%) with nonsustained supraventricular tachycardia.[10] Changes in atrioventricular (AV) conduction occurred in 3 patients (7%). A complete AV block is a potential risk, but rare (<1%). Suda et al. reported that 10 out of 162 (6.2%) patients presented with a new onset ($n = 9$) or aggravation of a preexisting ($n = 1$) AV block.[11] Three of them occurred during the procedure, 7 patients were first noted 1–7 days later. All AV blocks (first degree in 4, second degree in 4, and third degree in 2) resolved or improved spontaneously, with no recurrence at midterm follow-up.

3. *Cardiac erosion or perforation:* Amin et al. reported that the ASO might cause cardiac erosion in 0.1% of patients, which all occurred at the dome of the atria, near the aortic root.[12] The risks for erosions may be seen in patients with deficient aortic rim and/or superior rim or the use of oversized ASO. Divekar et al. reported similar findings that ASO-associated cardiac perforations uniquely involve the anterosuperior atrial walls and adjacent aorta.[13] Most (66.6%) of the cardiac perforations occurred after a patient's discharge. One cardiac perforation occurred 3 years after device closure. The above findings imply that high-risk patients need closer follow-up. Our protocol to diagnose erosions includes performing an echocardiogram the following day. If there is a new pericardial effusion or an increasing one, we repeat the echocardiogram after 12 h and reassess. If the effusion is stable, then we discharge the patient and bring him or her back after 3 days for a repeat echocardiogram. In May 2012, the United States FDA held a panel to review ASD device closure complications. The panel discussed all potential complications with emphasis on erosions. For more details, the reader is referred to an article written by Diab et al.[14]

4. *Cobra head formation:* The left disk maintains a high profile when deployed, mimicking a cobra head. This can occur if the left disk is opened in the pulmonary vein or the left atrial appendage, or if the left atrium is too small to accommodate the device size. It can also occur if the device is defective or if the device has been loaded with unusual strain on the device. If this occurs, check the site of deployment; if appropriate, recapture the device, remove it, and inspect it. If the "cobra head" forms outside the body, use a different device. If the disk forms normally, try deploying the device again. Do not release a device that has a "cobra head" appearance to the left disk.

5. *Recapture of the device:* To afford the smallest sheath size for device delivery, its wall thickness is small with a resultant decrease in sheath strength. To recapture a device prior to its release, the operator should hold the sheath at the groin with his/her left hand and with his/her right hand pull the delivery cable forcefully inside the sheath. If the sheath is damaged/kinked (accordion effect), use the exchange (rescue) system to change the damaged sheath. First, extend the length of the cable by screwing the tip of the rescue cable to the proximal end of the cable attached to the device, then remove the sheath. Or, if the sheath is 9 or 12 Fr, introduce the dilator of the rescue system over the cable inside that sheath until it reaches a few centimeters from the tip of the sheath. These dilators will significantly strengthen/stiffen the sheath allowing the operator to pull back the cable with the dilator as one unit inside the sheath. Then the operator can decide what to do next (change the entire sheath system or the device).

6. Release of the device with a prominent Eustachian valve: To avoid the possibility of cable entrapment during release, advance the sheath to the hub of the right disk. Then release the cable and immediately draw back inside the sheath before the position of the sheath is changed.

General remarks

1. *ASO versus surgical closure of ASD:* A multicenter, non-randomized concurrent study was performed in 442 patients with ASO closure and 154 patients with surgical closure from March 1998 to March 2000, which showed that the early, primary, and secondary efficacy success rates were not statistically different between the two groups.[15] However, the complication rate was lower and the length of hospital stay was shorter for device closure than for surgical closure. Kim et al. reported that ASO closure not only had equal effectiveness but also cost less compared to surgical closure (11,541 versus 21,780 U.S. dollars).[16]

2. *Echocardiographic guidance:* TEE has been successfully used for guiding transcatheter closure of ASD.[17–20] However, TEE requires general anesthesia. ICE, using an AcuNav catheter, (Siemens Medical, Iselin, NJ, USA) can eliminate the need for general anesthesia and has been proven effective to guide the device closure of ASD with less fluoroscopy and procedure time compared to TEE.[20–25]

3. *Multiple ASDs:* A multiple ASD closure is more challenging than a single ASD. If the septum has more than one hole, the bigger hole is usually located in the superoanterior septum, while the smaller hole is located in the inferoposterior septum. Because the LA disk is 12–16 mm larger than the waist and the stenting of the larger defect may squeeze the smaller defect, the two close defects may be closed with one device.[26] For two defects with wide separation (>7 mm), two devices are required to achieve successful closure. Rarely, three devices are needed to close three defects. Cao et al. reported 22 patients with more than one ASD who were successfully closed with more than one device.[27] The smaller device is usually deployed first, but not released until the larger device is positioned across the defect. If the stability of both devices is confirmed, the devices are

released sequentially, starting with the smaller device. Chun et al. described a case of multiple atrial septal defects that were "consolidated" into a single defect using blade atrial septostomy for successful closure with single ASO,[28] we do not advocate this technique.

4. *Large ASD*[29]: To date, ASO is suitable for a large ASD up to 40 mm in diameter. However, a large defect, especially associated with deficient rims, is still challenging. In such circumstances, oftentimes, when deploying the LA disk, the disk becomes perpendicular to the atrial septum, resulting in prolapse into the right atrium. There are several techniques that can be used to overcome such difficulties in aligning the LA disk to be parallel to the atrial septum that will result in a successful procedure.[30]

a. *Hausdorf sheath* (Cook, Bloomington, IN, USA) is a specially designed long sheath with two curves at its end.[31] The two posterior curves help align the left disk parallel to the septum. This sheath is available in sizes 8–12 Fr. Under fluoroscopic and echocardiographic guidance, if the initial deployment of the left disk is not ideal, counterclockwise rotation of the sheath until the side arm of the sheath is parallel to the ground and closer to the operator (when this is achieved, the tip of the sheath points posterior) will orientate the tip posterior and further deployment of the left disk will be parallel to the septum.

b. *Right upper pulmonary vein technique:* This technique is only recommended in larger patients. Carefully, position the delivery sheath in the right upper pulmonary vein; advance the device to the tip of the sheath, then partially deploy the left disk in the right upper pulmonary vein;[32–34] quickly retract the sheath to deploy the remainder of the left disk; this will result in the disk jumping from that location to be parallel to the atrial septum. Quick and successive deployment of the connecting waist and the right disk is carried out before the sheath may change its position or prior to the left disk prolapsing through the defect to the RA.

c. *Left upper pulmonary vein technique:* This technique can be used in children as well as in adults. Carefully position the delivery sheath in the left upper pulmonary vein. Advance the device to the tip of the sheath and start deploying the left disk inside the vein. Continue deployment of the waist and right disk to create an American football appearance within the vein.[33] As the sheath reaches the RA, the left disk disengages from the pulmonary vein and the disk jumps to be parallel to the atrial septum. Continuous retraction of the sheath over the cable with pulling of the entire assembly toward the RA will result in parallel alignment of the left disk to the septum.

d. *Dilator-assisted technique:* After deployment of the left disk, a long dilator (usually of the delivery sheath being used) is advanced into the LA by an assistant from the contralateral femoral vein to hold the superior anterior part of the left disk and prevent it from prolapsing into the RA, while the operator continues to deploy the waist and right disk in their respective locations.[31] Once the right disk is deployed in the RA, the assistant withdraws the dilator back to the RA.

e. *Balloon-assisted technique:* Dalvi et al. reported the balloon-assisted technique to facilitate device closure of large ASDs and to prevent prolapsing of the left disk into the RA.[35] In essence, it is similar in concept to the dilator technique. During device deployment, they used a balloon catheter to support the left disk of the ASO, preventing its prolapse into the RA.

f. *Right coronary Judkins guide catheter technique:* This technique is used only if the device size is less than 16 mm. Position an 8 Fr delivery sheath in the LA. Then preload the device inside the 8 Fr Judkins coronary guide catheter (inner lumen is 0.098"). Advance the entire assembly (device/cable/guide catheter) inside the delivery sheath until the catheter reaches the tip of the sheath. Bring the sheath back to the inferior vena cava, keeping the coronary catheter in the LA. Owing to the curve of the catheter, once the left disk is deployed in the LA, a counterclockwise rotation of the guide will result in alignment of the left disk to be parallel to the septum. Continue deployment of the waist and right disk in their respective locations. We found this technique to be of use in small children.

All these techniques have been used successfully to align the LA disk parallel to the atrial septum. Owing to these difficulties, the manufacturer of the Amplatzer device designed a new delivery sheath (TorqVue FX delivery system) where there is a hard-core wire inside a flexible cable. Once the device is pushed to the tip of the sheath, the stiffer core wire is pulled back to the IVC while the flexible thin cable is attached to the device. This allows positioning of the device without much tension on the disks, thus preventing prolapse of the left disk to the right atrium.

References

1. Hamdan MA, Cao QL, Hijazi ZM. Amplatzer septal occluder. In: Rao PS, Kern MJ, editors. In *Catheter Based Devices for the Treatment of Non-Coronary Cardiovascular Disease in Adults and Children.* Philadelphia: Williams and Wilkins; 2003, p. 51–9.
2. Masura J, Gavora P, Formanek A, Hijazi ZM. Transcatheter closure of secundum atrial septal defects using the new self-centering Amplatzer septal occluder: Initial human experience. *Catheter Cardiovasc Diagn* 1997;42:388–93.

3. Omeish A, Hijazi ZM. Transcatheter closure of atrial septal defects in children and adults using the Amplatzer Septal Occluder. *J Interv Cardiol* 2001;14:37–44.

4. Pac A, Polat TB, Cetin I, Oflaz MB, Balli S. Figulla ASD occluder versus Amplatzer Septal Occluder: A comparative study on validation of a novel device for percutaneous closure of atrial septal defects. *J Interv Cardiol* 2009;22:489–95.

5. Aytemir K, Oto A, Ozkutlu S et al. Early-mid term follow-up results of percutaneous closure of the interatrial septal defects with occlutech figulla devices: A single center experience. *J Interv Cardiol* 2012;25:375–81.

6. Demir B, Tureli HO, Kutlu G, Karakaya O. Percutaneous closure of a postoperative residual atrial septal defect with the Occlutech Figulla Occluder device. *Turk Kardiyol Dern Ars* 2012;40:55–8.

7. Krizanic F, Sievert H, Pfeiffer D et al. The Occlutech Figulla PFO and ASD occluder: A new nitinol wire mesh device for closure of atrial septal defects. *J Invasive Cardiol* 2010;22:182–7.

8. Ilkay E, Kacmaz F, Ozeke O et al. The efficiency and safety of percutaneous closure of secundum atrial septal defects with the Occlutech Figulla Occluder: Initial clinical experience. *Turk Kardiyol Dern Ars* 2010;38:189–93.

9. Harper RW, Mottram PM, McGaw DJ. Closure of secundum atrial septal defects with the Amplatzer septal occluder device: techniques and problems. *Catheter Cardiovasc Interv* 2002;57:508–24.

10. Hill SL, Berul CI, Patel HT et al. Early ECG abnormalities associated with transcatheter closure of atrial septal defects using the Amplatzer septal occluder. *J Interv Card Electrophysiol* 2000;4:469–74.

11. Suda K, Raboisson MJ, Piette E, Dahdah NS, Miro J. Reversible atrioventricular block associated with closure of atrial septal defects using the Amplatzer device. *J Am Coll Cardiol* 2004;43:1677–82.

12. Amin Z, Hijazi ZM, Bass JL, Cheatham JP, Hellenbrand WE, Kleinman CS. Erosion of Amplatzer septal occluder device after closure of secundum atrial septal defects: Review of registry of complications and recommendations to minimize future risk. *Catheter Cardiovasc Interv* 2004;63:496–502.

13. Divekar A, Gaamangwe T, Shaikh N, Raabe M, Ducas J. Cardiac perforation after device closure of atrial septal defects with the Amplatzer septal occluder. *J Am Coll Cardiol* 2005;45:1213–8.

14. Diab K, Kenny D, Hijazi, ZM. Erosions, erosions and erosions! Device closure of atrial septal defects. How safe is safe? *Cathet Cardiovasc Interven* 2012;80:168–74.

15. Du ZD, Hijazi ZM, Kleinman CS, Silverman NH, Larntz K. Comparison between transcatheter and surgical closure of secundum atrial septal defect in children and adults: results of a multicenter nonrandomized trial. *J Am Coll Cardiol* 2002;39:1836–44.

16. Kim JJ, Hijazi ZM. Clinical outcomes and costs of Amplatzer transcatheter closure as compared with surgical closure of ostium secundum atrial septal defects. *Med Sci Monit* 2002;8:CR787–91.

17. Hijazi ZM, Cao Q, Patel HT, Rhodes J, Hanlon KM. Transesophageal echocardiographic results of catheter closure of atrial septal defect in children and adults using the Amplatzer device. *Am J Cardiol* 2000;85:1387–90.

18. Mazic U, Gavora P, Masura J. The role of transesophageal echocardiography in transcatheter closure of secundum atrial septal defects by the Amplatzer septal occluder. *Am Heart J* 2001;142:482–8.

19. Figueroa MI, Balaguru D, McClure C, Kline CH, Radtke WA, Shirali GS. Experience with use of multiplane transesophageal echocardiography to guide closure of atrial septal defects using the amplatzer device. *Pediatr Cardiol* 2002;23:430–6.

20. Latiff HA, Samion H, Kandhavel G, Aziz BA, Alwi M. The value of transesophageal echocardiography in transcatheter closure of atrial septal defects in the oval fossa using the Amplatzer septal occluder. *Cardiol Young* 2001;11:201–4.

21. Hijazi Z, Wang Z, Cao Q, Koenig P, Waight D, Lang R. Transcatheter closure of atrial septal defects and patent foramen ovale under intracardiac echocardiographic guidance: Feasibility and comparison with transesophageal echocardiography. *Catheter Cardiovasc Interv* 2001;52:194–9.

22. Koenig P, Cao QL, Heitschmidt M, Waight DJ, Hijazi ZM. Role of intracardiac echocardiographic guidance in transcatheter closure of atrial septal defects and patent foramen ovale using the Amplatzer device. *J Interv Cardiol* 2003;16:51–62.

23. Koenig PR, Abdulla RI, Cao QL, Hijazi ZM. Use of intracardiac echocardiography to guide catheter closure of atrial communications. *Echocardiography* 2003;20:781–7.

24. Alboliras ET, Hijazi ZM. Comparison of costs of intracardiac echocardiography and transesophageal echocardiography in monitoring percutaneous device closure of atrial septal defect in children and adults. *Am J Cardiol* 2004;94:690–2.

25. Bartel T, Konorza T, Arjumand J, et al. Intracardiac echocardiography is superior to conventional monitoring for guiding device closure of interatrial communications. *Circulation* 2003;107:795–7.

26. Roman KS, Jones A, Keeton BR, Salmon AP. Different techniques for closure of multiple interatrial communications with the Amplatzer septal occluder. *J Interv Cardiol* 2002;15:393–7.

27. Cao Q, Radtke W, Berger F, Zhu W, Hijazi ZM. Transcatheter closure of multiple atrial septal defects. Initial results and value of two- and three-dimensional transoesophageal echocardiography. *Eur Heart J* 2000;21:941–7.

28. Chun TU, Gruenstein DH, Cripe LH, Beekman RH, III. Blade consolidation of multiple atrial septal defects: A novel approach to transcatheter closure. *Pediatr Cardiol* 2004;25:671–4.

29. Hijazi ZM, Ted F, Mustafa A, Horst S. *Transcatheter Closure of ASD's and PFO's: A Comperhensive Assessment*, 1st ed. Minneapolis, Minnesota: Cardiotext; 2010.

30. Fu YC, Hijazi ZM. The Amplatzer septal occluder, a transcatheter device for atrial septal defect closure. *Expert Rev Med Devices* 2008;5:25–31.

31. Wahab HA, Bairam AR, Cao QL, Hijazi ZM. Novel technique to prevent prolapse of the Amplatzer septal occluder through large atrial septal defect. *Catheter Cardiovasc Interv* 2003;60:543–5.

32. Berger F, Ewert P, Abdul-Khaliq H, Nurnberg JH, Lange PE. Percutaneous closure of large atrial septal defects with the Amplatzer Septal Occluder: Technical overkill or recommendable alternative treatment? *J Interv Cardiol* 2001; 14: 63–7.

33. Varma C, Benson LN, Silversides C et al. Outcomes and alternative techniques for device closure of the large secundum atrial septal defect. *Catheter Cardiovasc Interv* 2004;61:131–9.

34. Kannan BR, Francis E, Sivakumar K, Anil SR, Kumar RK. Transcatheter closure of very large (> or =25 mm) atrial septal defects using the Amplatzer septal occluder. *Catheter Cardiovasc Interv* 2003;59:522–7.

35. Dalvi BV, Pinto RJ, Gupta A. New technique for device closure of large atrial septal defects. *Catheter Cardiovasc Interv* 2005;64:102–7.

51

The Figulla-Occlutech device

Carlos A. C. Pedra, Simone R. F. Fontes Pedra, Rodrigo N. Costa, and Marcelo S. Ribeiro

Introduction

The Figulla-Occlutech occluder was introduced in Europe in 2003 and since then over 20,000 implants for atrial septal defect (ASD) and patent foramen ovale (PFO) closure have been performed worldwide according to the company track records. However, this device is not available in Canada, the United States, Japan, and China at the time of this writing.

Device

The Figulla-Occlutech ASD occluders (Occlutech, Jena, Germany) are individually braided using very thin (40–150 µm or 0.00157–0.00590 inches) and numerous strands of nitinol (80 in total). All strands end proximally requiring no clamp on the left disk (Figure 51.1a and b). This results in a smaller amount of uncovered metallic material

in the left atrium (LA). Also, the absence of a clamp on the left disk minimizes the risks of inadvertent trauma to the cardiac structures in the LA when deploying the device. Enhanced flexibility results from a single weld on the right side and the thinner and more numerous strands of nitinol. These strands are covered by a biocompatible titanium oxide layer, which gives the Figulla-Occlutech occluder its typical golden appearance.

The newer Flex generations (second and third) of the Figulla-Occlutech ASD occluders do not have any threaded hub or clamp to provide a screwing attachment to the delivery cable. By utilizing a combined laser/plasma welding process to form a rounded pin (the connecting ball) at the center portion of the right atrial (RA) disk (Figure 51.1c), the amount of metallic material utilized in this area was further reduced by over 70%. This connecting ball was specifically designed for compatibility with the newer delivery

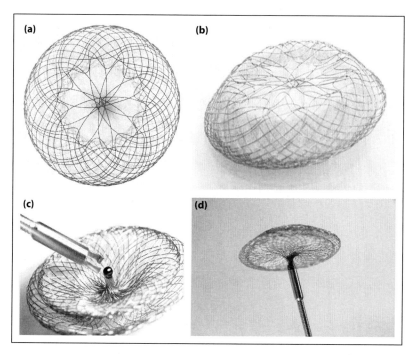

Figure 51.1 The Figulla-Occlutech ASD occluder. (a) *En face* view of the LA disk. Note the unique braiding pattern and the lack of a distal clamp resulting in less amount of exposed metal. (b) An angled view of the LA disk, which is larger than the RA disk. (c) The RA disk has a central welded ball to connect with the jaw of the bioptome-like delivery cable. (d) The connecting ball is pulled into the distal pod of the delivery cable.

Table 51.1 Sizes of the Figulla-Occlutech devices and their components

Type	Ø Waist (mm)	Ø LA Disk (mm)	Ø RA Disk (mm)
29 ASD 04	4.0	11.0	9.0
29 ASD 05	5.0	14.0	11.0
29 ASD 06	6.0	16.5	12.5
29 ASD 07	7.5	18	14
29 ASD 09	9	20.5	16.5
29 ASD 10	10.5	22	18
29 ASD 12	12.0	27	23
29 ASD 15	15.0	30	26
29 ASD 18	18.0	33	29
29 ASD 21	21.0	36	32
29 ASD 24	24.0	39	35
29 ASD 27	27.0	42	38
29 ASD 30	30.0	45	41
29 ASD 33	33.0	48	43
29 ASD 36	36.0	52	46
29 ASD 39	39.0	54	49
29 ASD 40	40.0	55	50

system through a coupling mechanism (Figure 51.1c and d). In the latest generation (third) of the device, also called Figulla Flex II, the ultimate profile of the stretched/collapsed device was substantially reduced by 1–3 Fr due to a unique design in which the left disk has a different braiding pattern than the proximal disk (Figure 51.1a and b). This also contributed to the reduction of metal on the left disk.

The device size is determined by the diameter of its waist, which is 2.5–3.5 mm long. The Figulla-Occlutech occluders are available in the following sizes: 4, 5, 7.5, 9, 10.5, 12, 13.5, 15, 16.5, 18, 21, 24, 27, 30, 33, 36, 39, and 40 mm (Table 51.1). The 4, 5, 13.5, and 16.5 mm may not be available in some countries. The number of sizes needed in inventory can be reduced due to the 3 mm increments for devices larger than 12 mm. The LA disk is 7–16 mm and the RA disk is 5–11 mm larger than the waist (Table 51.1).

The company has also developed a device that was specifically designed for closing multifenestrated ASDs: the Figulla® Flex UNI. In this design, both disks have the same diameter and are connected by a thin waist (Figure 51.2a and b). It is available in five sizes corresponding to the diameter of both disks: 17, 24, 28.5, 33, and 40 mm.

Delivery system

In its first generation, the Occlutech ASD occluders were connected to the delivery cable through a male–female screwing mechanism. The delivery system has undergone substantial improvement after the launching of the Figulla Flex I and II, the second and third generations of the device. In the latest system, the flexible metallic delivery cable is somewhat similar to a bioptome. There is a two-part handle equipped with a rotational safety locking system at the proximal (operator) extremity and a coupling pod at the distal end. The operator (or an assistant) exposes the coupling jaw out of the distal pod of the delivery cable by moving both parts of the handle away from each other. For this maneuver, some gentle force should be applied to overcome the resistance provided by a coil that separates both parts. The jaw is then connected to the central ball of the device (Figure 51.1c). The tension on both parts of the handle is released so that the exteriorized jaw can pull the ball into the pod (Figure 51.1d), establishing the connection between the device and the delivery cable. This connection is secured and locked by rotating the safety knob on the handle. Before final device release, the system allows a tilted angle of 45–50° without any tension on the implant (Figure 51.3). This pivoting mechanism minimizes the amount of tension between the RA disk and the delivery cable, which avoids possible undesirable "jumps" of the cable upon final release. In addition to the optimized angulation between the delivery system and the implant, the actual tip of the delivery system can be shaped to any desired angle. The attachment system is safe and avoids any risk of inadvertent release during handling. It also allows complete retraction of the device into the sheath if necessary, giving full retrievability/recapturability capabilities to the system.

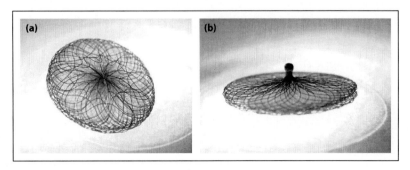

Figure 51.2 The Figulla® Flex UNI. (a, b) Different views of the Figulla Flex UNI showing two flat disks of the same size.

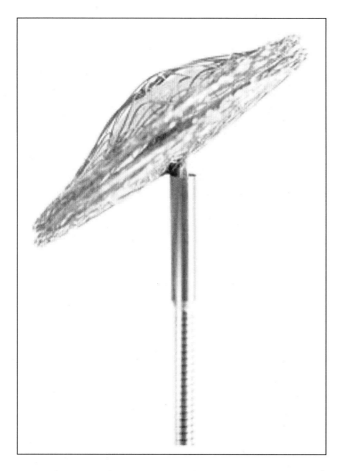

Figure 51.3 The connection of the Figulla occluder to the delivery cable. The pivoting system allows for a 45–50° angle between the device and the delivery cable.

Once an adequate device position is achieved within the atrial septum, the occluder is released from the delivery system. First, the locking system on the handle is unlocked by rotating the red safety knob counterclockwise. The coupling jaw is then exteriorized by maneuvering both parts of the handle, which releases the connecting ball of the device from the delivery cable. The delivery cable is finally brought back into the sheath. If the device is not immediately released after the coupling jaw is exteriorized, it may be necessary to rotate the delivery cable slightly to allow for complete uncoupling.

Additional equipment

Sizing balloons

Either the NuMED (NuMED, Hopkinton, NY, USA) or the new Occlutech sizing balloons can be employed. The latter is available in two sizes (diameter/length): 25 mm/45 mm (filling volume: 25 mL; maximum filling volume: 35 mL; maximum diameter: 27 mm) and 35 mm/50 mm (fill-ing volume: 60 mL; maximum filling volume: 90 mL;

Table 51.2 Device size and sheath compatibility for the Figulla and Figulla Flex I

Type	Recommended sheath size	Required flex-pusher
29 ASD 06	7 Fr	50FP100 (dark blue)
29 ASD 07	7 Fr	50FP100 (dark blue)
29 ASD 09	7 Fr	50FP100 (dark blue)
29 ASD 10	7 Fr	50FP100 (dark blue)
29 ASD 12	10 Fr	50FP120 (dark green)
29 ASD 15	10 Fr	50FP130 (orange)
29 ASD 18	12 Fr	50FP130 (orange)
29 ASD 21	12 Fr	50FP140 (black)
29 ASD 24	12 Fr	50FP150 (pink)
29 ASD 27	14 Fr	50FP160 (white)
29 ASD 30	14 Fr	50FP170 (yellow)
29 ASD 33	14 Fr	50FP180 (light blue)
29 ASD 36	14 Fr	50FP180 (light blue)
29 ASD 39	14 Fr	50FP180 (light blue)
29 ASD 40	14 Fr	50FP180 (light blue)

maximum diameter: 40 mm). The shaft is 8 Fr and 70 cm long. The balloons run over 0.035 inch guide wires. There are two radiopaque markers inside the balloon at 5 mm intervals.

Delivery sheaths

We have used the long blue Mullins-type sheath from Cook (Cook, Bloomington, IN, USA) to deliver the first and second generation of Figulla-Occlutech occluders (Table 51.2). Recently, Occlutech has introduced a new delivery set consisting of a braided delivery sheath with a dilator, a hemostatic valve (a Touhy–Borst adapter), and a transparent loader. The sheath has a 45° distal curve and is 80 cm long. Its profile is 7–12 Fr with 1 Fr increments. The dilator has a 0.035 inch guide wire compatibility. For the new Figulla Flex II, the required diameter of the sheath has been reduced by 1–3 Fr (Table 51.3), which is of para-mount importance for use in small children. Compatibility between device size and sheath profile should be checked before their use (Tables 51.2 and 51.3).

Patient selection

The indications and contraindications for transcatheter ASD closure have been discussed in the designated chap-ter. Of note, we have not considered a deficient anterior rim as a contraindication for ASD closure with any type of device, especially acknowledging that 40–50% of all ASDs have some deficiency of this rim. In our experience, ASDs not suitable for transcatheter closure include too

Table 51.3 Device size and sheath compatibility for the Figulla Flex II

Type	Recommended sheath size	Required flex-pusher
29 ASD 04	7 Fr	50FP100 (dark blue)
29 ASD 05	7 Fr	50FP100 (dark blue)
29 ASD 06	7 Fr	50FP100 (dark blue)
29 ASD 07	7 Fr	50FP100 (dark blue)
29 ASD 09	7 Fr	51FP100 or 52FP100 (light blue)
29 ASD 10	7 Fr	51FP100 or 52FP100 (light blue)
29 ASD 12	9 Fr	51FP120 or 52FP120 (yellow)
29 ASD 15	9 Fr	51FP120 or 52FP120 (yellow)
29 ASD 18	9 Fr	51FP120 or 52FP120 (yellow)
29 ASD 21	11 Fr	51FP150 or 52FP150 (purple)
29 ASD 24	11 Fr	51FP150 or 52FP150 (purple)
29 ASD 27	12 Fr	51FP160 or 52FP160 (blue)
29 ASD 30	12 Fr	51FP160 or 52FP160 (blue)
29 ASD 33	12 Fr	51FP160 or 52FP160 (blue)
29 ASD 36	12 Fr	51FP160 or 52FP160 (blue)
29 ASD 39	12 Fr	51FP160 or 52FP160 (blue)
29 ASD 40	12 Fr	51FP160 or 52FP160 (blue)

large defects (over 35–40 mm in adults); too large an ASD in relation to the size of the patient, especially in small (10–15 kg) children in whom a large device may impair proper functioning of AV valves, pulmonary veins, and coronary sinus; and ASDs with more than one deficient rim, especially contralateral rims. We believe that the use of real-time 3D transesophageal echocardiography (TEE) is the best tool to provide a thorough assessment of the anatomy of the atrial septum in challenging cases, especially with regard to the adequacy of the surrounding rims of the defect (Figure 51.4).

Precatheterization evaluation

In our experience, children with adequate echo windows are properly screened using transthoracic echocardiography (TTE). Adolescents and adults are better screened using TEE, especially with 3D capabilities. Patients are started on aspirin (3–5 mg/kg per day; max: 200 mg) a couple of days before the procedure. Older patients (>40–50 years) should be checked for left ventricular diastolic dysfunction and started on diuretics and vasodilators a couple of days before the procedure.

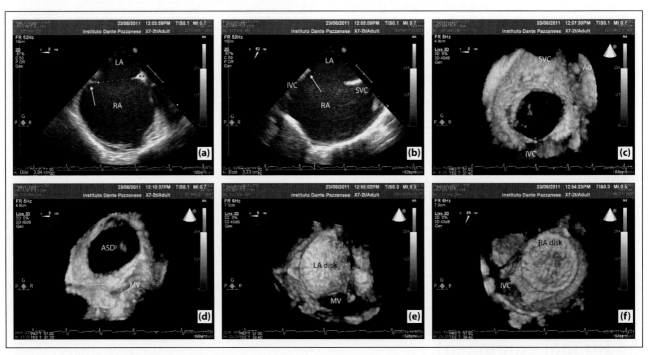

Figure 51.4 (**See color insert.**) A large ASD closed with a 39 mm Figulla ASD device. (a) On short-axis view on 2D TEE, the ASD measured 30–31 mm. The anterior rim (asterisks) and the posterior rim (arrow) are of good size. LA: left atrium. RA: right atrium. (b) On long-axis (bicaval) view on 2D TEE, the ASD measured 32 mm. The posteroinferior rim (arrow) is somewhat deficient. SVC: superior vena cava. IVC: inferior vena cava. (c) 3D TEE. RA view. The use of 3D TEE allowed for a better delineation of the large ASD and the adequate surrounding rims. IVC: inferior vena cava. SVC: superior vena cava. Ao: aorta. (d) 3D TEE. LA view. There is sufficient amount of tissue separating the mitral valve (MV) and the ASD, which defined the adequacy of the posteroinferior rim. (e) 3D TEE after device release. LA view. Note the LA disk is well apposed to the atrial septum distant from the mitral valve (MV). The disk is flat with no metallic clamp. There is no space between the disk and the surrounding rims. (f) 3D TEE after device release. RA view. Note the RA disk is well positioned within the atrial septum with no space between it and the surrounding rims.

Device implantation technique

The procedure is performed under general anesthesia if monitored by TEE or under sedation if guided by intracardiac echocardiography (ICE). The implantation technique is similar to the ones that have been used for other ASO-type occluders. However, some technical aspects specific to the implantation of the Figulla-Occlutech occluders or related to the way we perform such procedures merit discussion. We believe that balloon sizing (or balloon interrogation) of the defect is mandatory in the following scenarios: defects associated with a floppy or an aneurismal posterior septum; a large anterior defect associated with (a) smaller posteroinferior defect(s) when the use of a single device is contemplated to close all defects; two distant (>7–8 mm) defects requiring the use of two different devices; and defects that might be too large for the size of the patient, especially in young children. In patients with a single defect surrounded by a reasonably thick septum, we have not yet balloon-sized the defect. We simply take into account the largest measurement using several echo views and use a device that is 15–30% larger than the largest diameter. This same guideline is applied for very large defects (>30 mm) (Figure 51.4). As such, we estimate that in about 30–50% of the patients, the stretched diameter is not performed anymore. When it is performed, a Figulla occluder that is 0–2 mm larger than the stretched diameter is selected for implantation. We have slightly oversized the device (2–4 mm larger than the stretched diameter) in cases with deficient rims, especially the retroaortic. Although this may be a risk factor for erosion using the ASO, this has not been an issue as yet with the more flexible Figulla-Occlutech device.

The more standard technique for device implantation includes opening the LA disk followed by the waist by slowly retracting the sheath and pushing the cable (two-hand technique). Sometimes, especially with larger devices, the LA disk of the Figulla occluder does not reconfigure entirely, retaining a globe appearance. The lack of the distal clamp may partially explain this observation. If this happens, the entire system should be carefully pushed against the roof of the LA to help to flatten the left disk. The lack of a distal clamp and less metallic material on the LA disk of the Figulla device minimizes possible damage to the roof of the LA. After the whole system is pulled back toward the atrial septum, allowing the waist to stent the defect, the RA disk is deployed in the RA. Meticulous echocardiographic assessment of all steps described above guides the operator through the procedure. If the device is in a proper position as determined by echocardiography, it is released following the above-mentioned steps. We usually do not perform a wiggle to ensure device stability within the atrial septum. We find this not only unnecessary but also hazardous since it may dislodge the device from a proper location and/or damage intracardiac structures with risk of erosion. If device position is uncertain or inappropriate on echo, the device should be entirely or partly recaptured and repositioned. After the device is released, full echocardiographic assessment is repeated.

The most common problem encountered during device implantation is LA disk prolapse through the anterior portion of the defect behind the aorta, especially in very large defects with clockwise rotation of the cardiac mass due to an enlarged right ventricle. Although there have been a number of techniques described to deal with this problem when using an ASO, it is our impression that device prolapse occurs less frequently with the Figulla-Occlutech occluder. This may be due to the enhanced flexibility of the Figulla device, which results in a better alignment with the plane of the atrial septum after the LA disk and the connecting waist have been fully exteriorized. If the LA disk still prolapses through the defect, a simple maneuver to overcome this technical difficulty is to rotate the delivery sheath clockwise, keeping it in a parallel fashion in relation to the spine in the posteroanterior view on fluoroscopy.

Multiple ASD closure is more challenging and technically demanding. The techniques to tackle those defects with the Figulla-Occlutech devices are similar to the ones employed for other nitinol devices (Figure 51.5).

Postprocedure follow-up

These measures are common to all nitinol ASD devices and are no different for the Figulla occluder. Of note, we perform serial echocardiograms the following day and at the 1, 6, and 12 month visits. Follow-up visits should be scheduled every 2–5 years thereafter. Aspirin is maintained for 6 months. Standard guidelines for endocarditis prophylaxis should be applied.

Results

From April 2008 to December 2012, we have performed 100 procedures of transcatheter ASD closure using the first and second generation of the Occlutech-Figulla occluders. A preliminary experience has been published before.[1] Because of the higher profile of the sheaths required for implantation of the first and second generation, we avoided their use in smaller children. As such, the median age and weight at implantation was 24 years (3–82 years) and 55 kg (14–92), respectively. Sixty-three patients were female. Fifteen patients had multiple defects that were closed with a single device implanted in the larger hole. Three patients required two devices to close two distant defects (Figure 51.5). Three patients had a multifenestrated septum that required closure using a Figulla PFO occluder (the UNI Flex occluder was not available at the time of the procedure). In four patients, a custom-made fenestrated device was used due to left diastolic dysfunction in three elderly patients and

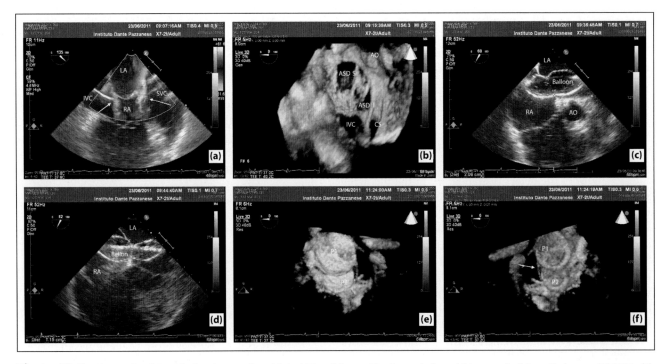

Figure 51.5 (**See color insert**.) The closure of multiple ASDs with two Figulla occluders. (a) Long-axis (bicaval) view on 2D TEE with color-flow mapping showing two ASDs (arrows) separated by a 15 mm tongue of tissue. The superior defect (near the superior vena cava—SVC) measured 15 mm and the inferior defect (near the inferior vena cava—IVC) measured 8 mm. (b) 3D TEE, RA view. The use of 3D TEE allowed for a better appreciation of the underlying anatomy. Both defects are delineated at best and the distance to the surrounding structures such as the coronary sinus (CS), aorta (Ao), and inferior vena cava (IVC) are unequivocally displayed. ASD S: superior ASD. ASD I: inferior ASD. (c) Balloon interrogation of the superior defect. The stretched diameter measured 20 mm. (d) Balloon interrogation of the inferior defect. The stretched diameter measured 11.5 mm. (e) 3D TEE. LA view. A 21 mm device was implanted in the superior defect (P1) and a 12 mm device in the inferior ASD (P2). There is some overlap of both occluders with a pinpoint residual defect (arrow) between them. There was complete closure within 6 months after endothelialization of the devices. (f) 3D TEE. RA view. The immediate residual defect (arrow) is again delineated at best between the overlapping occluders.

due to a smaller right ventricular size in a child with pulmonary atresia and intact interventricular septum who was previously submitted to RF-assisted pulmonary dilation and pulmonary artery stenting (Figure 51.6). Seventy-five procedures were performed using the first-generation device, while the Figulla Flex was used in the remainder. Median size of the defect was 19 mm (6–38) (excluding the multifenestrated ASDs) and the median stretched diameter was 23 mm (10–40 mm). Median device size was 24 mm (9–40). In 34 patients, balloon sizing of the defect was not performed. Successful implantation was achieved in all patients. In one patient, there was thrombus formation within the sheath that resolved with judicious aspiration and proper anticoagulation. There was one device (12 mm) embolization to the descending aorta. The device was retrieved using a snare followed by successful closure of the defect using a larger (18 mm) device. One patient with a very large defect (33 × 36 mm) in whom a 40-mm device was implanted had a remaining small residual leak (2 mm) at the posteroinferior aspect (near the inferior vena cava) of the atrial septum

(Figure 51.7). Another patient with multiple defects had a remaining 2 mm uncovered posteroinferior defect after implantation of two devices. The remainder had complete closure of the defect. No patient experienced significant arrhythmias or had erosions. We have not seen any cobra formation during deployment. Interestingly, the fenestrations remained patent in two patients who had 6 months of follow-up.

This encouraging experience is in line with the information drawn from observational studies encountered in the still limited literature available.[2–6]

Complications with the Figulla occluder

Some possible complications specific to the Figulla-Occlutech occluders merit consideration. When this device embolizes, it may be more difficult to snare and retrieve it since it has a single weld on the RA disk. On

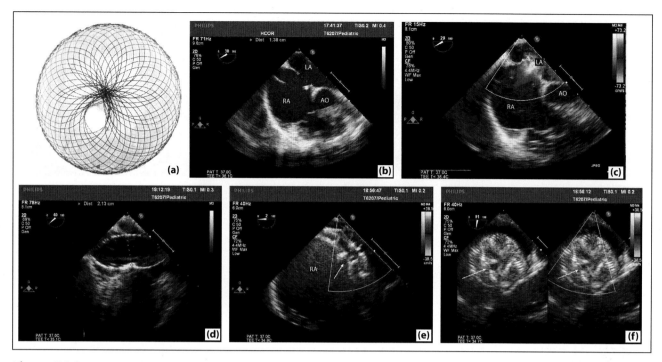

Figure 51.6 **(See color insert.)** Use of a fenestrated Figulla ASD occluder. A 4-year-old female patient (15 kg) previously submitted to radio-frequency-assisted pulmonary valve dilatation, left pulmonary artery stenting, and Blalock–Taussig–Thomas shunt occlusion. Right ventricular size was smaller (tricuspid valve Z value of –2.5) and there was predominantly right-to-left shunt through a 14 mm ASD. The stretched diameter was 21 mm. There was no hemodynamic compromise after test occlusion of the ASD. A 21 mm fenestrated Figulla Flex device was implanted at first but it was too large for the size of the child. It was replaced by an 18 mm fenestrated occluder, which was implanted uneventfully through a transhepatic approach. Systemic oxygen saturation increased from low 80s to low 90s. (a) Picture of the custom-made fenestrated device. The size of the fenestration varies with the size of the device (4–8 mm). In this patient, the fenestration was 4 mm. (b) Short-axis view on 2D TEE showing the 14 mm ASD. (c) Right-to-left shunting demonstrated by color-flow mapping on short-axis view on 2D TEE. (d) Sizing balloon across the ASD. The stretched diameter was 21 mm. (e) An 18 mm device in place on short-axis view on 2D TEE. The fenestration (arrow) can be seen in the more anterior aspect of the device allowing some right-to-left shunt on color-flow mapping (red color). (f) An *en face* view of the LA disk was obtained on TEE. The fenestration (arrow) is nicely displayed on 2D view (left) and with color-flow mapping (right).

the other hand, due to its enhanced flexibility, it may be easier to drag it through a vessel in a partially collapsed form. Although the lack of reports of cardiac erosion or perforation after the use of the Figulla-Oclutech occluder is encouraging, this must be interpreted with caution. If the estimated incidence of erosion of 0.1% as published by Amin et al. after the use of the ASO was observed with the Figulla occluder, we would expect at least 20 cases out of 20,000 implants performed worldwide (according to the company track record). This has not been observed and might be due to a variety of reasons. The denominator may be overestimated since the company tracks shipped devices and not necessarily implanted ones. It is possible that this complication might be underreported in the literature. However, this is unlikely since it is usually symptomatic and can be catastrophic. On the other hand, it may have been possible that operators implanting the Figulla device have learned with previously accumulated experience with the ASO and have avoided the

use of oversized devices in high-risk situations, eventually decreasing the rate of erosions. Finally, the Figulla occluder may be less traumatic to the anterosuperior atrial wall and adjacent aorta due to its enhanced flexibility. With such a low estimate of the incidence of erosions, only a very large number of patients (maybe those specifically at risk) followed for a long period of time will determine the real incidence of this severe complication.

Conclusions

Transcatheter closure of ASDs using the Figulla-Occlutech occluder is operator friendly, safe, and effective. The device performs as well as the ASO in a wide range of scenarios in older children, adolescents, and adults. The reduction in the profile of the required sheaths for implantation achieved in the third and latest generation of the device will likely expand its use for smaller children.

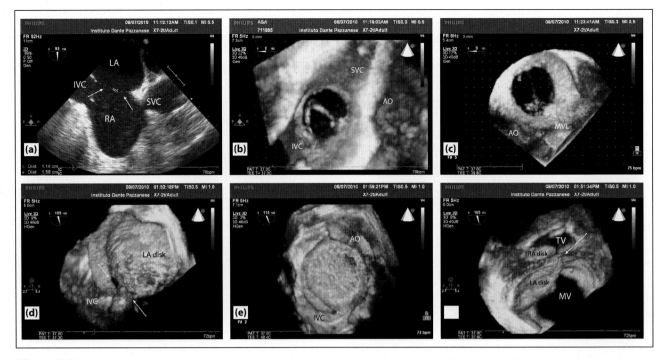

Figure 51.7 **(See color insert**.) The closure of multiple ASDs with a single large device. (a) Long-axis (bicaval) view on 2D TEE showing two defects (arrows) separated by a flimsy tongue of tissue. RA: right atrium. LA: left atrium. SVC: superior vena cava. IVC: inferior vena cava. (b) 3D TEE. RA view. The two defects and the tissue strand between them are better appreciated using 3D technology. IVC: inferior vena cava. SVC: superior vena cava. AO: aorta. (c) 3D TEE. LA view. The defect is profiled from the LA side. AO: aorta. MVL: mitral valve anterior leaflet. A decision was made to place the device in the superior defect. (d) 3D TEE. LA view after device deployment before release. There is a half-moon residual defect (arrows) in the posteroinferior aspect of the atrial septum due to the tension of the delivery cable. IVC: inferior vena cava. (e) 3D TEE. LA view after device release. There was a significant decrease in the size of the residual defect (arrow) after the occluder was released from the delivery cable. (f) 3D TEE. LA view after device release. The superior portion of the atrial septum (arrow) is nicely seen in between the two disks. MV: mitral valve. TV: tricuspid valve.

Acknowledgment

The authors would like to thank Mr Hakan Akpinar from Occlutech for providing pictures of the devices and some specific technical information.

References

1. Pedra CAC, Pedra SF, Costa RN, Braga SLN, Esteves CA, Fontes VF. Initial experience with percutaneous occlusion of the ostium secundum atrial septal defect with the Figulla device. *Rev Bras Cardiol Inv* 2010;18(1):81–8.

2. Halabi A, Hijazi ZM. A new device to close secundum atrial septal defects: First clinical use to close multiple defects in a child. *Catheter Cardiovasc Interv* 2008;71:853–6.

3. Krizanic F, Sievert H, Pfeiffer D, Konorza T, Ferrari M, Hijazi Z, et al. The Occlutech Figulla PFO and ASD occluder: A new nitinol wire mesh device for closure of atrial septal defects. *J Invasive Cardiol* 2010;22(4):182–7.

4. Cansel M, Pekdemir H, Yağmur J, Tasolar H, Ermis N, Kurtoglu E, et al. Early single clinical experience with the new Figulla ASD occluder for transcatheter closure of atrial septal defect in adults. *Arch Cardiovasc Dis* 2011;104(3):155–60.

5. Van Den Branden BJ, Post MC, Plokker HW, Ten Berg JM, Suttorp MJ. Percutaneous atrial shunt closure using the novel Occlutech Figulla device: 6-Month efficacy and safety. *J Interv Cardiol* 2011;24(3):264–70.

6. Aytemir K, Oto A, Ozkutlu S, Kaya EB, Canpolat U, Yorgun H, et al. Early-midterm follow-up results of percutaneous closure of the interatrial septal defects with occlutech figulla devices: A single center experience. *J Interv Cardiol* 2012;25(4):375–81.

52

The Cera Lifetech device

Worakan Promphan

Introduction

Nickel–titanium alloy (nitinol) is widely used as a substrate for the double-disk device. However, *in vivo* nickel release is still a matter of potential contribution to allergic reaction or carcinogenicity even though there have been no consensus reports on how much nickel level might affect human health. To reduce these possible risks and to improve biocompatibility, Lifetech Scientific Corporation (Shenzhen, China) has developed a closure device made of nitinol coated with bioceramic titanium nitride (TiN), the Cera™ ASD Occluder. This type of coating technology prevents nickel leaching and may promote rapid tissue endothelialization after implantation (Figure 52.1).[1] This device received approval for clinical use for the European Union in 2009.

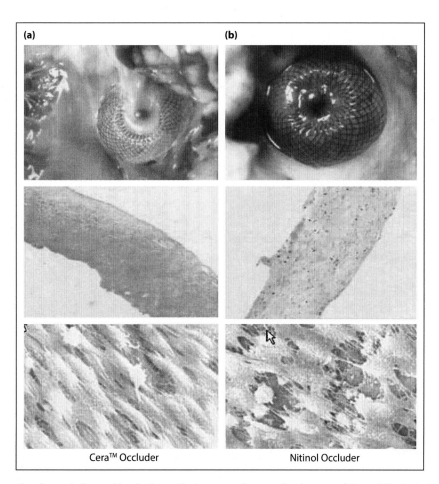

Figure 52.1 **(See color insert.)** Gross, histologic, and electron microscopic pictures of Cera ASD Occluder compared with the untreated nitinol device in an animal model 3 months after implantation.

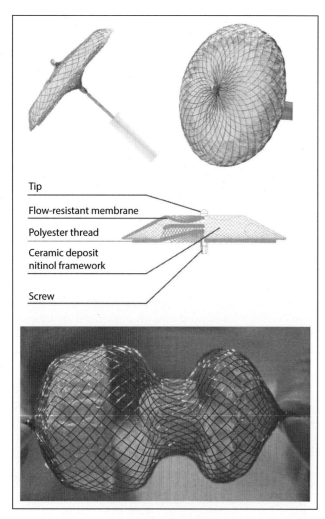

Tip

Flow-resistant membrane

Polyester thread

Ceramic deposit
nitinol framework

Screw

Figure 52.2 The Cera ASD Occluder.

The device

The Cera ASD Occluder (Figures 52.2 and 52.3) is a self-expandable double-disk device made of a treated nitinol wire mesh that is shaped into two flat disks with a connecting waist similar to Amplatzer™ Septal Occluder (ASO) (St. Jude Medical, St. Paul, MN, USA). A porous polyethylene terephthalate (PET) membrane is sewn to the left and right atrial disks and the connecting waist to promote thrombogenicity after implantation. The device size is determined by its waist diameter, ranging from 6 to 42 mm (2 mm increments) with a connecting waist length of 4 mm. The right atrial disk diameter is larger than its waist, that is 8 mm for the waist diameter <12 and 10 mm for the waist 12–42 mm. The left disk is 4 mm larger than the right disk for the waist that is <32 mm, whereas it is 6 mm larger for the 34–42-mm devices. The device connects to the delivery cable by a screw mechanism. In 2013, Lifetech Company is planning to launch a second generation of the Cera ASD Occluder, the CeraFlex™ ASD Occluder (Figure 52.4). This new-generation device will provide more angulation with less tension of the delivery cable to the attached device, which may simplify procedural steps.

The delivery system

The delivery system for Cera ASD Occluder is supplied separately in a sterile package.

Delivery sheath: Two types of delivery sheath are available, a conventional SFA SteerEase™ Introducer and a Fustar™ Steerable Introducer (Figure 52.5). Both

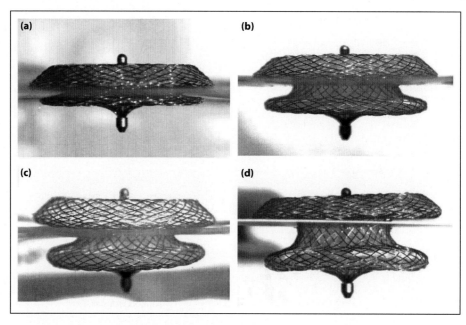

Figure 52.3 The Cera ASD Occluder 26 mm implanted in different diameters of the sizing plate. (a) 26 × 26 mm diameter, (b) 22 × 22 mm diameter, (c) 20 × 20 mm diameter, and (d) 18 × 22 mm diameter.

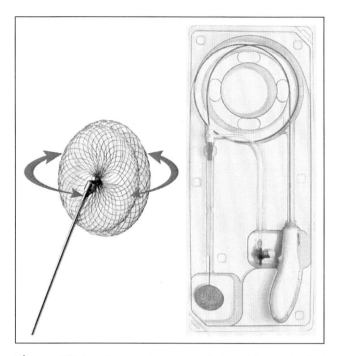

Figure 52.4   The CeraFlex ASD Occluder with a preloaded delivery system.

of them are kink-resistant sheaths with a hemostatic valve to prevent blood reflux and air embolism. There is a radiopaque marker band at the distal end for easy location and accurate positioning. The SFA SteerEase is an 80-cm-long and 45° angled tip sheath with the size ranging from 7 (for 6–8 mm device) to 14 Fr (for 32–42 mm device). The Fustar is a steerable sheath that has an ability to adjust the angle and direction of the tip end from 0° to 160°. The sizes range from 5 to 14 Fr, with the length of the deflectable end 30 and 50 mm (12 and 14 Fr sheaths are available only for the 50 mm deflectable length with angulation ability of 0–90°). The Fustar™ Steerable sheath is available in three different lengths: 55, 70, and 90 cm.

Loader: A short sheath with a hemostatic valve is used to collapse and introduce the device into the delivery sheath.

Delivery cable: There are two sizes of the cable (5 and 6 Fr) to screw onto the device for loading, placement, and retrieval.

Patient selection

As with the Amplatzer disk device, patient selection is one of the most important steps for transcatheter ASD closure. The indications and contraindications for implanting the

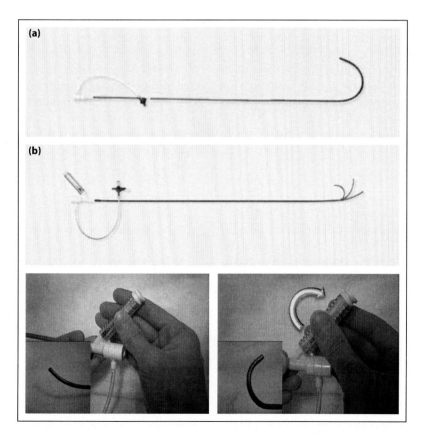

Figure 52.5   The Lifetech delivery sheaths. (a) SFA SteerEase Introducer and (b) Fustar Steerable Introducer.

Cera Septal Occluder are similar to ASO. Patients must be thoroughly assessed for position/dimension/number of the defect(s), supporting rims, septal floppiness/malalignment, associated lesions (such as anomalous pulmonary venous returns or mitral valve disorders), degree/direction of atrial shunt, and estimated pulmonary arterial pressure (by velocity of tricuspid regurgitation or pulmonic regurgitation jets). Transthoracic echocardiography (TTE) and/or transesophageal echocardiography (TEE) are important tools for ASD evaluation in pre-, peri-, and postprocedural stages. Although TEE can provide superior anatomical details of the defect and surrounding structure, TTE is usually sufficient for children, with a good image window.

Implantation procedure

The procedure can be performed under local or general anesthesia with TTE, TEE, or intracardiac echocardiogram (ICE) guidance depending on the patient's condition and institutional preference. Venous access is routinely performed at the right or left femoral vein. Arterial access is usually not required unless continuous arterial blood pressure monitoring or assessment of shunt volume for calculation by Fick method is indicated. As for other devices, heparin 100 U/kg is routinely and intravenously administered to maintain activated clotting time (ACT) >200 s at the time of device deployment. Evaluation of pulmonary arterial pressure and pulmonary vascular resistance is mandatory in all ASD cases prior to closure. Comprehensive echocardiographic evaluation should be reperformed. If ASD is suitable for closure, the procedure can proceed by crossing the atrial septum with a multipurpose catheter into the left upper pulmonary vein. Then, a stiff exchange length 0.035 guide wire is positioned in the left upper pulmonary vein and the catheter is removed. If the defect needs to be evaluated by balloon sizing, the catheter with a compliant balloon is subsequently advanced over the wire and placed across the defect using fluoroscopic (at 30–45° left anterior oblique projection) and echocardiographic guidance. The balloon is inflated with diluted contrast using the stop-flow technique and then the diameter is measured in the balloon's long-axis view.

With all adequate rims and without septal floppiness, the device size should be 2–3 mm greater than the largest diameter measured by a two-dimensional echocardiogram (2DE) or increasing 0–2 mm from the stop-flow diameter of balloon sizing. With deficient anterior–superior (aortic) rim and/or floppy posterior septum, increasing 4–6 mm from a 2DE largest diameter is usually required to ensure device stability. However, implanting an oversized device in the absence or deficiency of an aortic rim may potentiate the risk of erosion. Once a suitable device is selected, prepare the proper size of the delivery system. Advance the sheath over the guide wire to the left upper pulmonary vein. Be careful while manipulating a large sheath into the pulmonary vein since it may injure the vessel, causing perforation or rupture. Then remove the dilator and wire, leaving the tip of the sheath in the left atrium or inside the left upper pulmonary vein. Open the sheath's stopcock to allow blood to bleed back and then reflush the sheath to ensure that there is no air bubble inside the system. Prepare the proper device by screwing to the tip of the delivery cable and withdrawing into the loader underwater seal while continuously flushing with saline to expel air bubbles out of the system. Introduce the loader into the diaphragm of the sheath and begin deployment steps as with ASO.

Several techniques have been described to facilitate device placement.[2] The Lifetech Company has developed the new implantation technique by using the Fustar Steerable sheath (Figure 52.5). By rotating the side-arm knob clockwise, the sheath's tip will angulate, allowing the left disk to stay perpendicular to the atrial septum. This technique is suitable for patients with deficient aortic/posterior rim or with septal malalignment. A steerable sheath is also beneficial when catheter advancement is carried out from an unusual route (such as the internal jugular vein).

Similar to ASO implantation, echocardiography (Figure 52.6) is the key for procedural success. To ensure a stable position of the device, echocardiographic evaluation (TTE, TEE, or ICE) in different angles must be comprehensively performed before release. This assessment includes checking the position/configuration of the device, looking for residual leak(s)/additional hole(s)/disturbance of the device to adjacent structures and pericardial effusion. Once a favorable device position is demonstrated, the device is then released in a counterclockwise rotation of the delivery cable using a pin vise (Figure 52.7).

Commencing cefazolin (100 mg/kg/day in children or 1 g/dose in adults) is usually recommended during the procedure and 2–4 further doses are recommended at 6 h intervals. Endocarditis prophylaxis is indicated when necessary for 6 months after the procedure. Aspirin in the antiplatelet dose is given orally once daily for 6 months. The patient with a large device may require double antiplatelet therapy for the first month after the procedure. Prior to discharge, TTE and ECG should be evaluated. Full activity is usually allowed after 4 weeks of implantation.

Results

A multicenter clinical trial was conducted in 11 Chinese Heart Centers to evaluate safety and efficacy of the Cera

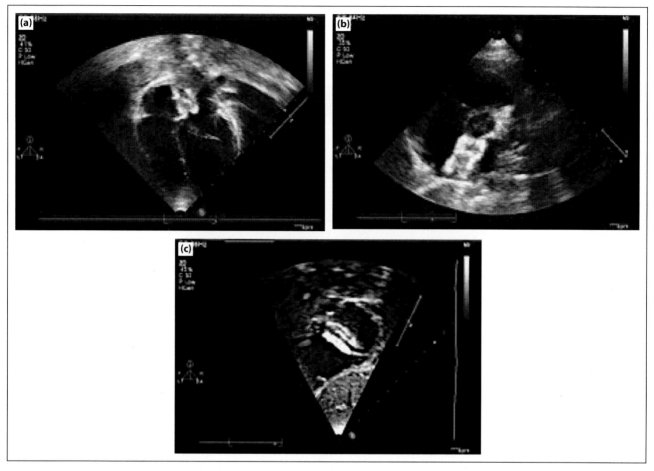

Figure 52.6 Transthoracic echocardiographic pictures of postimplanted Cera ASD Occluder with different views. (a) Apical four-chamber view, (b) parasternal short-axis view, and (c) subcostal view.

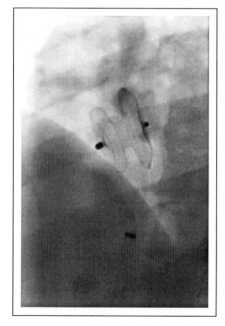

Figure 52.7 Fluoroscopic picture of the postimplanted Cera ASD Occluder in LAO projection.

Occluder in October 2011 (personal communication, Lifetech Company). Seventy-eight ASDs were enrolled in the Cera ASD Occluder group. These data showed that Cera devices were safely implanted in most cases even though one patient needed surgical removal of an embolized occluder and ASD repair within 24 h. Within the median follow-up time of 31 months, there was no recorded case of erosion, endocarditis, or death. One patient had a transient nodal block that was completely recovered at 3-month follow-up. Three cases had trivial to small residual shunts at 6-month follow-up.

Conclusion

The Cera ASD Occluder is a double-disk device with TiN/Ti bioceramic coating. It can reduce *in vivo* nickel release[1] and may prevent adverse outcomes from nickel allergy. As of 2012, more than 3000 Cera ASD Occluders have been successfully implanted in more than 22 countries worldwide. Although initial information has shown a safe and effective result for clinical use, further study is necessary to determine the long-term outcome in a larger population of patients.

References

1.   Zhang DY, Zhang ZW, Zi ZJ, Zhang Y, Zeng W, Chu PK. Fabrication of graded TiN coatings on nitinol occluders and effects on *in vivo* nickel release. *Bio-Med Mater Eng* 2008;18:387–93.

2.   Amin Z, Hijazi ZM, Bass JL, Cheatham JP, Hellenbrand W, Kleinman C. Erosion of Amplatzer septal occluder device after closure of atrial septal defects: Review of registry of complications and recommendations to minimize future risk. *Catheter Cardiovasc Interv* 2004;63:496–502.

53

ASD-R PFM device

Miguel A. Granja, Alejandro Peirone, Jesus Damsky Barbosa, Alexandra Heath, and Luis Trentacoste

Introduction

Percutaneous closure has evolved as the treatment of choice for the majority of ostium secundum-type atrial septal defects. The overall safety and effectiveness of the interventional procedure has compared favorably with surgical repair.[1-3] Long-term clinical outcomes have been excellent: good quality of life, functional class improvement, and ventricular remodeling have been the rule after the procedure.[4] For over three decades, there has been a great enthusiasm to develop the ideal device for ASD closure. An effort to design such an occlusion device began in 2002 in La Paz, Bolivia, with Dr. Franz Freudenthal, who started with animal experience leading to human experience and finally came up with the idea of the "pfm family of devices" that includes the Nit-Occlud® ASD-R, Nit-Occlud® PFO, and Nit-Occlud® PDA-R devices (pfm-medical, Cologne, Germany).[5]

The device

The Nit-Occlud ASD-R is a double-umbrella, self-expandable, self-centering, and premounted device knitted from a single nitinol wire without any soldering or protruding clamps or screws on either side of the occlusor. It consists of two circular retaining disks made of nitinol wire mesh linked together by a short connecting waist (Figure 53.1). Although the device characteristics, such as the nitinol framework, loading maneuver, delivery technique, and deployment are similar to other self-expandable devices, the ASD-R has a distinct design based on two aspects:

- "Reverse configuration" (Figure 53.2) (Video 53.1) of a single-layer left atrial disk that is completely covered by a polyester membrane sutured to the borders, minimizing the amount of metal on the left atrial side with the potential of promoting faster endothelialization as well

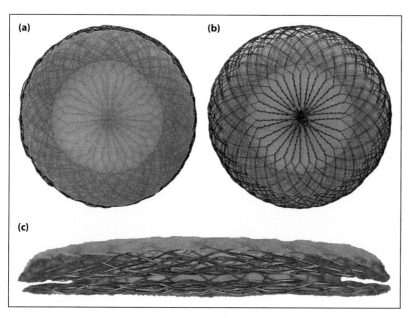

Figure 53.1 (a) Frontal view of the left atrial disk, which is completely covered by a polyester membrane. (b) View of the right atrial disk. (c) Lateral view of the device showing the disks linked by a short connecting waist. (With permission from pfmmedical, Cologne, AG.)

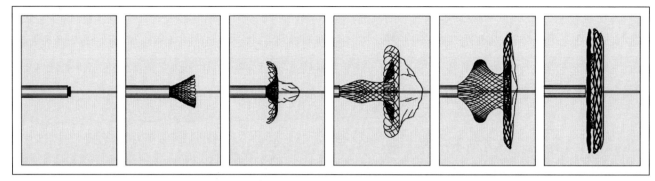

Figure 53.2 Schematic representation of the "reverse" configuration of the left atrial disk. (With permission from pfmmedical, Cologne, AG.)

as reducing the incidence of thrombosis. This peculiar configuration of the left atrial disk tightly fixes the implant to the left atrial aspect of the interatrial septum, offering a secure anchoring mechanism and minimizing the risk of "pulling-through" during implantation or inadvertent embolization after release. Careful reverse distal disk opening is devised to prevent any left atrial wall injury, especially avoiding opening the device inside the left atrial appendage. Nevertheless, in special circumstances when opening the device is required in either the left or the right pulmonary veins, it can be safely accomplished with partial deployment within the vein itself, reaching a complete final reconfiguration once the device is pulled into the left atrial body (Figure 53.3) (Video 53.2). Two platinum markers are applied to the wire ends of the left atrial disk for radiological guidance during implantation. Both disks are made of the same diameter. To improve its closure rate, a polyester membrane is also sewn onto the right atrial disk.

• A "snare-like" release mechanism (Figure 53.4) includes a central "locking wire" that crosses the device entirely (Figure 53.5) and a "pusher" with a distal wire noose ("eyelet"). The locking wire is attached to the right atrial

side of the implant by four accessory wires connected to the pusher, which is covered by a "catheter" that allows adequate flushing possibilities for the system to avoid air embolism and clot formation. For release, a distal "security seal" is removed and the "locking wire" is retracted, disengaging the noose and freeing the implant (Figure 53.6) (Video 53.3).

The Nit-Occlud ASD-R is available in 12 different sizes ranging from 8 to 30 mm in stent diameter with 2 mm increments. They require 8–14 Fr Nit-Occlud long tip-braided sheaths (pfmmedical) for delivery.

Device selection is dictated by a combination of measurements by transesophageal/intracardiac echocardiography and the stretched diameter using balloon sizing following the "stop-flow" technique. The recommended diameter of the selected device should be the same size or up to 2 mm larger than the defect. However, oversizing is not relatively forgiving with this device, resulting in an excessive bulging of the RA disk showing a suboptimal final configuration. If the selected device size is correct, the final appearance even before release shows an occlusor with a very low profile splayed over the interatrial septum

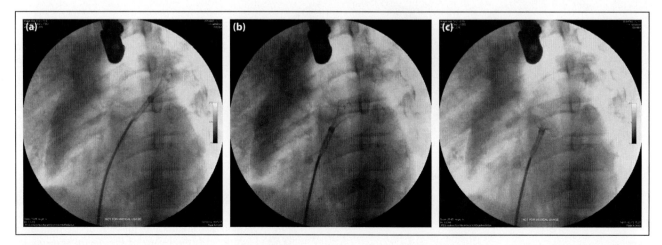

Figure 53.3 The left atrial disk is deployed in the left upper pulmonary vein (a), subsequently retrieved into the left atrium (b), and finally completely configured outside the pulmonary vein (c).

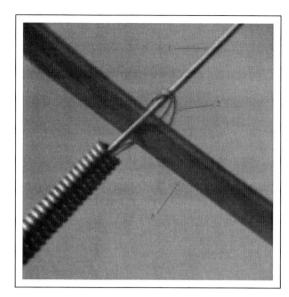

Figure 53.4 The release mechanism. The device (3) is connected to the pusher via the retaining wire (2). A locking wire (1) fixes this connection. (With permission of pfmmedical, Cologne, AG).

(Figure 53.7). To obtain its lowest profile, it is important to finish a gentle "pull and push" maneuver (Minnesota wiggle), pushing the right disk until it adopts a "concave shape" (Figure 53.8) usually accompanied by a "click" sensation on the operator's hands (Video 53.4).

The implantation technique is similar to that of other double-disk, self-expandable devices. The occluder is retrievable, easy to position with a simple and tension-free release mechanism that allows for recapturing and

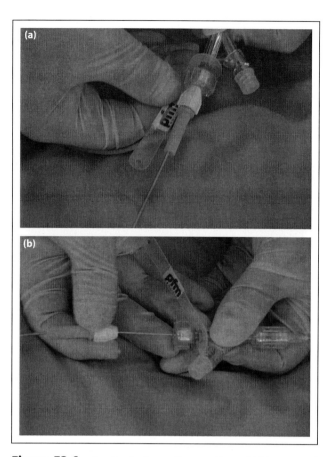

Figure 53.6 For final release, the security seal (a) is removed and the locking wire (b) is retracted. (With permission from Cardiotext Publishing.)

repositioning several times before release. During implantation, visualization on echocardiography and fluoroscopy is optimal (Figures 53.9 and 53.10).

Experiences and outcomes

The first human implantation was performed by Dr. Alexandra Heath and coworkers at Kardiocentrum in La Paz, Bolivia, in 2007 (personal communication). This group, between May 2007 and February 2011, implanted the device in 53 patients. Four attempts were unsuccessful due to the identification of either a large defect or insufficient rims. The mean age at intervention was 17.8 years (3–67), mean weight was 35.5 kg (13–75), and mean Qp/Qs was 1.9 (1.1–4.0). Taken into consideration that the majority of patients lived at high altitude (more than 2500 m over the sea level), the mean systolic pulmonary artery pressure was 36 mm Hg (26–68). The mean ASD diameter after balloon sizing using the "stop-flow technique" was 16.3 mm (5.4–26 mm) and the mean implanted device size (connecting waist) was 19.3 mm (8–28 mm).

Complete defect closure was achieved immediately in 71.4% of patients, increasing to 91.7% after 24 h, 93.7% after

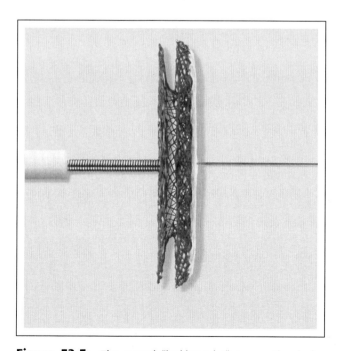

Figure 53.5 The central "locking wire" crosses the device entirely. (With permission from pfmmedical, Cologne, AG.)

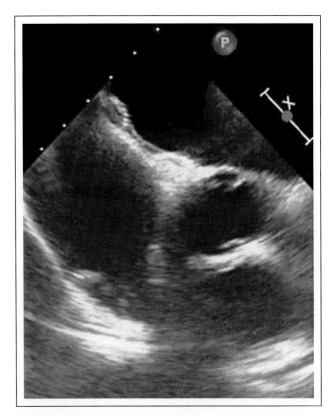

Figure 53.7 Final TEE long-axis view shows the device profile after implantation.

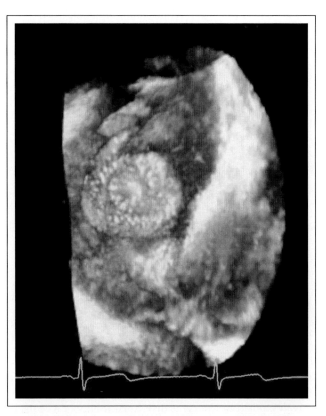

Figure 53.9 (**See color insert.**) Left atrial 3D TEE view showing the left atrial disk in position covering the defect completely.

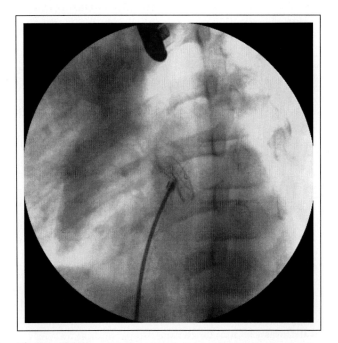

Figure 53.8 Angiographic view of the device showing the "concave shape" of the right atrial disk before release.

1 month, and 100% at 6 month evaluation. Clinical examination, electrocardiogram (ECG), and transthoracic echocardiography at 24 hours, 7 days, 3, 6, 12 months, and then yearly were performed during follow-up. One patient suffered device embolization immediately after release (presumably due to a rip of a very thin rim) and was referred for surgical device retrieval and ASD patch closure with an uneventful recovery.

During a mean follow-up time of 9.1 months (6–39 months), no other device-related complications were detected.

In Argentina, the use of the device began under the humanitarian law in 2009 and was implanted in six patients by one of the authors (MAG). Later, the device was officially approved for clinical use by ANMAT (local medical devices approval authority) in September 2011 and the data presented in this chapter are a combined experience from the four Argentine authors.

From October 2011 to September 2012, 73 patients (48 female) were evaluated and fulfilled inclusion criteria to undergo an attempt of transcatheter closure of an ostium secundum-type ASD using the Nit-Occlud ASD-R device that was selected by the interventional cardiologist as an alternative to the standard use of other available devices. All interventions were performed under general

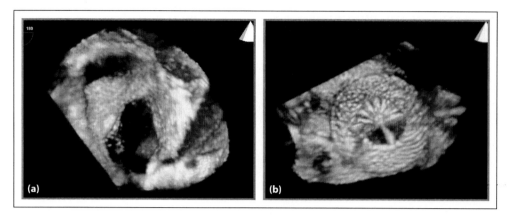

Figure 53.10 **(See color insert.)** (a) A large ostium secundum-type ASD is visualized on 3D TEE from the RA side. (b) A Nit-Occlud ASD-R device, which is still attached to the delivery system, has been implanted and shows an adequate device position. (Courtesy of Simone Fontes Pedra.)

anesthesia using transesophageal echocardiography guidance. After the procedure, the patients were prescribed aspirin (5–10 mg/kg, maximum 100 mg) once daily for 6 months.

Five patients showed an accessory small ASD located in close proximity to the larger ASD, and a multifenestrated ASD was observed in four additional patients.

The median age was 15.1 years (4–60) and median weight was 37.7 kg (12–81). The mean ASD diameters were 13.7 (7–20), 14.8 (7–22), and 15.5 mm (9–24) measured by transthoracic echocardiography, transesophageal echocardiography, and balloon sizing, respectively. In eight patients, balloon sizing was not performed, and the anatomy of the defect was considered adequate for closure avoiding this technique.

The mean device size utilized was 17.5 mm (10–26 mm) (size of the connecting waist). In four patients presenting a multifenestrated ASD, a Nit-Occlud PFO device® (Figure 53.11) was implanted (20 and 26 mm devices). The median pulmonary artery mean pressure obtained in these cases was 20.2 ± 4.53 mmHg (13–34 mmHg) and the mean Qp/Qs ratio was 1.82 ± 0.35 (1.5–2.6). The implantation success rate was 97.2%.

In a 5-year-old female patient with a large defect, the device was not released and was consequently retrieved due to the immediate appearance of an intermittent atrioventricular block that completely recovered after retrieval of the device. In one patient, immediate embolization occurred after a presumable membrane rip of a multifenestrated septum using a 14 mm ASD-R device that was recovered using a "snare and wire technique" through a 14 F sheath from the descending aorta (Figure 53.12). The defect was finally occluded during the same procedure implanting a 26 mm PFO device. Additionally, in one patient, a small thrombus located at the tip of the sheath was detected on transesophageal echocardiography before device delivery. Consequently, the thrombus was aspirated, anticoagulation was reinforced, and the procedure continued without complications.

All closures were achieved from a femoral vein access using 8–14-F-long Mullins sheaths (Nit-Occlud® sheaths were unavailable in Argentina at that time). The median

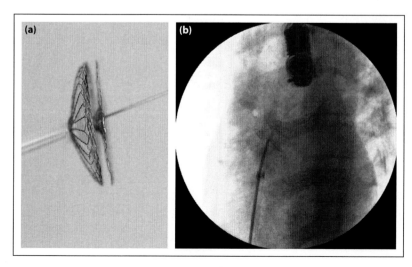

Figure 53.11 (a) Nit-Occlud PFO device. (b) Angiographic view of a Nit-Occlud PFO device implanted in a multifenestrated ASD.

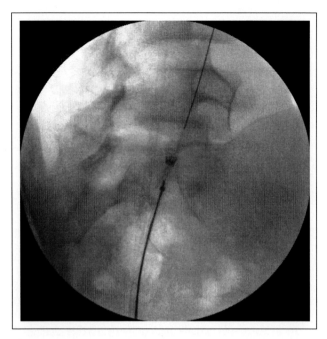

Figure 53.12 An embolized Nit-Occlud ASD-R 14 device is retrieved from the descending aorta using a snare and a 14-F-long sheath advanced through the femoral artery.

fluoroscopy time was 9.7 min (7–38 min). The mean follow-up time was 7.9 months (1–36) and evaluated by transthoracic echocardiography with color Doppler at 3 months from implantation, 70/72 patients (97.2%) showed complete closure. The remaining two patients had a small persistent antero-superior leak. Pre- and postprocedure (at 24 h) ECGs and a Holter monitor performed at 3 months after intervention, showed no significant conduction or rhythm changes. There were no other major or minor complications detected.

Conclusions

Following an initial learning curve gaining experience implanting the Nit-Occlud ASD-R device, the authors have drawn some preliminary conclusions: it is a user-friendly, low profile, and very flexible system with a high closure rate,

no RA–LA pin, less metal in the LA disk, a simple release mechanism, and eco-friendly. On the other hand, the erosion rate is still unknown, mainly due to a limited follow-up time and the fact that the total number of implanted cases require larger delivery sheaths for implantation and the device is not available for closure of very large ASDs (maximum stretched diameter for closure 28–30 mm).

Although experience in recovering the device after embolization is limited, it seems to be no different than other available devices.

A larger number of patients and longer follow-up time are required to assess its ultimate clinical performance.

Acknowledgments

To Mr Frank Thiel from pfmmedical AG, for his collaboration in preparing the device figures.

To Mrs Carol Syverson from Cardiotext Publishing, for obtaining permission to use images previously published.

To Mr Fernando Lopez and Mr Gustavo Ronderos from pfmmedical, Argentina, for their help in collecting the pictures utilized to prepare the figures.

References

1. Du Z, Hijazi Z, Kleinman C, Silverman N, Larntz K. Comparison between transcatheter and surgical closure of secundum atrial septal defect in children and adults: Results of a multicenter non-randomized trial. *J Am Coll Cardiol* 2002;39:1836–44.

2. Visconti K, Bichell D, Jonas R, Newburger J, Bellinger D. Development outcome after surgical versus interventional closure of secundum atrial septal defect in children. *Circulation* 1999;100:145–50.

3. Butera G, Biondi-Zoccai G, Sangiorgi G, Abella R, Giamberti A, Bussadori C et al. Percutaneous versus surgical closure of secundum atrial septal defects: A systematic review and meta-analysis of currently available clinical evidence. *EuroIntervention* 2011;7:377–85.

4. Peirone A, Contreras A, Ferrero A, da Costa RN, Pedra SF, Pedra CA. Immediate and short-term outcomes after percutaneous atrial septal defect closure using the new Nit-Occlud ASD-R device. *Catheter Cardiovasc Interv*. 2014 Feb 12.

5. Granja M, Freudenthal F. The PFM device for ASD closure. In: Hijazi Z, Feldman T, Abdullah Al-Qbandi MH, Sievert H. Eds. *Transcatheter Closure of ASDs and PFOs*. Minneapolis, MN: Cardiotext Publishing, 2010. pp. 423–9.

54

Cocoon device

Worakan Promphan

Introduction

The self-expandable nitinol-containing atrial septal defect (ASD) device has been widely used worldwide and has been acknowledged for its excellent outcome.[1,2] However, there was concern about nickel leaching after implantation. Cocoon™ Septal Occluder (CSO) (Vascular Innovation, Bangkok, Thailand) has been developed to reduce this possible unfavorable consequence. By a process called plasma deposition, ultrathin layers of platinum atoms are deposited on the surface of nitinol wires. With this concept, without changing the properties of the nitinol material, nano-coating of platinum on the CSO can prevent nickel release following implantation.[3] In 2010, CSO along with its accessories was approved for use in the European Union.

The device and loading system

Although the structure of the CSO appears similar to the Amplatzer™ Septal Occluder, ASO (St. Jude Medical, St. Paul, MN, USA), the CSO was braided from platinum-coated nitinol wires and filled with three circular polypropylene sheaths to enhance thrombogenicity (Figures 54.1 through 54.3). The size of the device is indicated as the diameter of the central connecting waist. The minimum device diameter is 8 mm while the maximum diameter is 40 mm (2 mm increments). The connecting waist length is 3 mm for a device diameter of 8–10 mm and 4 mm for a device diameter of 12–40 mm. The right atrial disk diameter is larger than its waist, which is 10 mm. The left disk is 2 mm larger than the right disk for a device size of 8–10 mm, 4 mm larger for a device of 12–32 mm, and 6 mm larger for a device of 34–40 mm.

The delivery system consists of a loading tube, a stopcock, a braided delivery sheath, and a delivery cable. The delivery sheath is an 80-cm-long and 90° angled tip sheath with the size ranging from 8 (for 8–14 mm device) to 14 Fr (for 30–40 mm device). The device connects to the delivery cable by a screw mechanism.

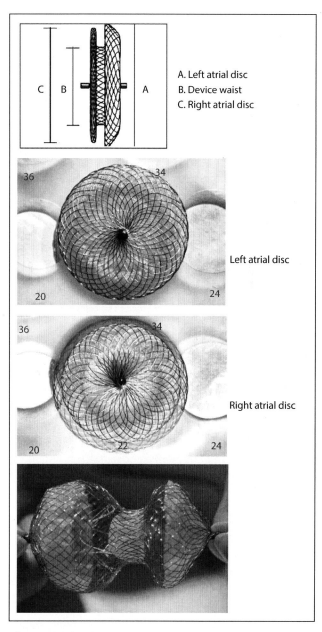

A. Left atrial disc
B. Device waist
C. Right atrial disc

Left atrial disc

Right atrial disc

Figure 54.1 The CSO.

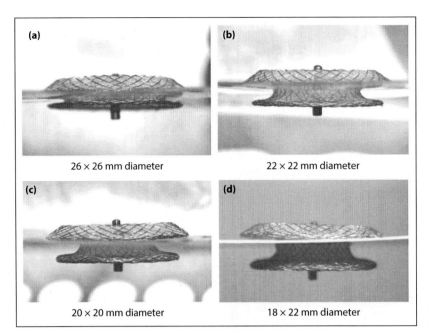

(a) 26 × 26 mm diameter

(b) 22 × 22 mm diameter

(c) 20 × 20 mm diameter

(d) 18 × 22 mm diameter

Figure 54.2   The CSO 26 mm implanted in different diameters of the sizing plate.

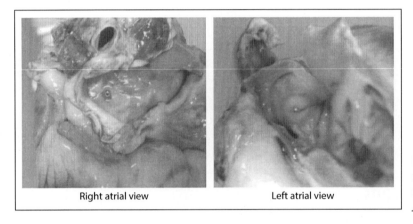

Right atrial view

Left atrial view

Figure 54.3   (**See color insert.**) Gross specimens of CSO 6 weeks after implantation in swine model. (From Lertsapcharoen P et al. *Indian Heart J* 2006;58:315–20.)

Patient selection

The indications and contraindications for using the CSO are identical to those for the ASO. Generally speaking, patients with ostium secundum ASD are eligible for CSO implantation when they have significant left-to-right shunt (Qp/Qs > 1.5, an evidence of right ventricular volume overload) and have sufficient septal rims (deficient retro-aortic rim is usually feasible with caution concerning early or late erosion). However, patients with irreversible pulmonary arterial hypertension or with anomalous pulmonary venous returns might not benefit from transcatheter ASD closure. Therefore, comprehensive anatomical and physiological evaluations are the most important keys to success for device implantation. In children, transthoracic echocardiography (TTE) can provide sufficient details of the defect and surrounding structures, while transesophageal echocardiography (TEE) usually allows superior information in adults or children with poor imaging windows. The intracardiac echocardiogram (ICE) is reserved for periprocedural evaluation in some institutions.

Implantation procedure

The procedural steps are similar to ASO implantations that can be performed under local or general anesthesia (depending on the patient's condition and operator's preference). The echocardiogram (TTE, TEE, or ICE) is the most reliable guiding tool for the whole procedure. The right or left femoral vein is the routine route of access. Arterial access is usually not necessary except: (1) if the patient requires coronary artery assessment/intervention, (2) if the patient needs continuous arterial blood pressure monitoring, and (3) an assessment of shunt volume for calculation by Fick method is required. Intravenous administration of heparin 50–100 U/kg is indicated to

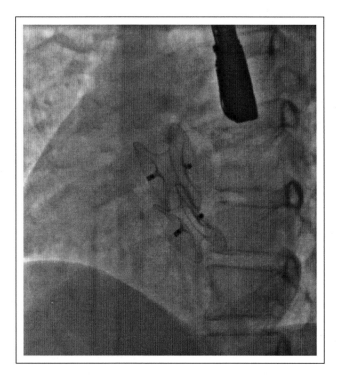

Figure 54.4 Fluoroscopic picture of postimplanted double CSOs in LAO projection.

maintain activated clotting time (ACT) >200 s at the time of device deployment. The defect can be nicely crossed and placed at the left upper pulmonary vein by a multipurpose catheter. Then, the catheter is removed over an exchange length stiff guide wire. Balloon sizing can be done (if necessary) over this wire. Once the suitable device is chosen, advance the appropriate-sized delivery sheath over the wire and leave the tip of the sheath in the left atrium or into the proximal left pulmonary vein. Allow the blood to bleed back by lowering the sheath below the level of the heart. Once back bleed is verified, flush the sheath with an adequate amount of saline.

The properly sized device is attached to the delivery cable by screwing it on and withdrawing it into the loader underwater. The loader should be continuously flushed during this step. Push the loader against the sheath until a "click" sound is audible. By echocardiographic and fluoroscopic guidance, open the left disk in the mid-left atrium once the device is at the tip of the sheath. Pull back the whole system as one unit to approximate the left disk to the atrial septum. The waist and the right disk are then released by withdrawing the sheath over the cable. The device position and configuration are rechecked by echocardiography and fluoroscopy. Once a favorable device position is demonstrated, it is released via a counterclockwise rotation of the cable using a pin vise (Figures 54.4 through 54.6).

Intravenous administration of cefazolin is usually indicated during and a day after the procedure. Aspirin in an antiplatelet dose is given orally once daily for at least 6 months. Some patients with a large device implant may require additional clopidogrel during the first month after the procedure. Prior to discharge, routine TTE and ECG should be performed in all cases. Full activity is usually allowed 4 weeks after implantation.

Results

The initial human use of CSO in 29 patients showed complete closure within 1 month after implantation without device-related complications in 1 year follow-up.[3] As of

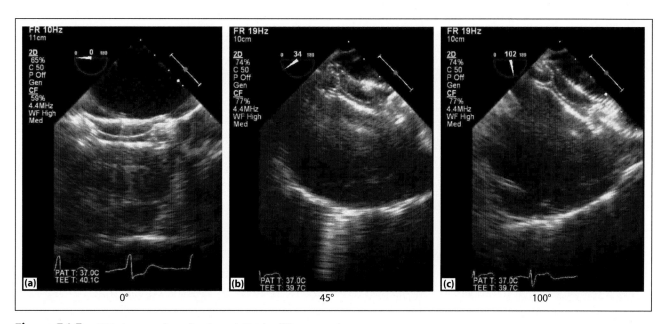

Figure 54.5 TEE pictures of postimplanted CSO in different angles.

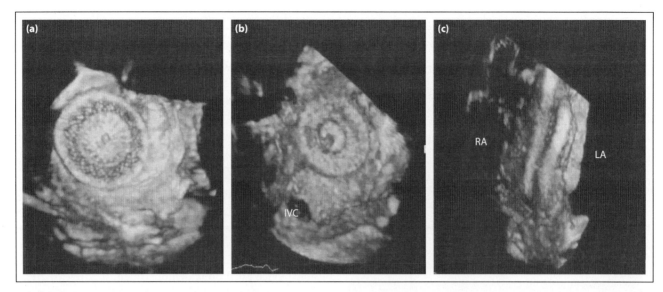

Figure 54.6 **(See color insert.)** Three-dimensional TEE pictures of postimplanted CSO in different views. (a) Left atrial aspect, (b) right atrial aspect, and (c) interatrial.

July 2012, more than 4000 CSO have been successfully implanted in eight Asian and six European countries. The retrospective evaluation from five institutions in India (presented in CSI 2012 by Dr. Ravi Narayan, Bangalore, India) showed successful CSO implantation in 360 cases. Five cases had immediate embolization (3.3%). At 1 year follow-up, there was no late embolization, thrombus, or residual shunt. In Thailand, three different brands of ASD devices are available: ASO, CSO, and Occlutech™ Septal Occluder (OSO). We reviewed 148 adults treated by these three different brands in regard to safety and efficacy (Tables 54.1 and 54.2). The mean follow-up time was 31.3, 21.8, and 19.4 months in the ASO, CSO, and OSO groups, respectively. Residual shunt on the first day after implantation was approximately 40% in each group, which completely disappeared 1 month later in all cases. We experienced

device embolization in three cases (one in each group). Two patients had massive pericardial effusion (one in ASO, one in CSO) requiring surgical treatment. One patient of the CSO group who previously had atrial fibrillation developed stroke a month after implantation. There was no mortality in any of the groups. With this review, we concluded that all three brands demonstrated favorable outcomes with fewer complications in the midterm period. (The study will be presented at the PICS & AICS meeting to be held in January 2013 in Miami.)

Conclusion

By closure of the secundum ASD by a platinum-coated disk device, the CSO can prevent nickel release with favorable

Table 54.1 Baseline demographic and procedural data of different brands of ASD device

	ASO (n = 60)	CSO (n = 52)	OSO (n = 36)
Mean age (year)	39.5 ± 16.4	40.9 ± 13.4	43.4 ± 14.4
Sex (M:F)	9:51	18:34	8:28
Mean PAP (mmHg)	18.2 ± 5.0	33.9 ± 4.3	21.9 ± 7.9
Rhythm			
NSR	60	48	36
AF	2	4	3
Deficient aortic rim (%)	33.3	36.5	44.4
ASD diameter in the major axis from TEE (mm)	21.9 ± 12.9	23.5 ± 4.3	19.1 ± 3.6
Diameter of the implanted device (mm)	28.5 ± 6.6	27.6 ± 7.8	24.1 ± 3.5
Size difference (mm)	5.2 ± 2.6	5.3 ± 2.8	4.9 ± 1.3

ASO, Amplatzer Septal Occluder; CSO, Cocoon Septal Occluder; OSO, Occlutech Septal Occluder; PAP, pulmonary arterial pressure; NSR, normal sinus rhythm; AF, atrial flutter/fibrillation; ASD, atrial septal defect; TEE; transesophageal echocardiogram.

Table 54.2 Follow-up information of different brands of device

	ASO (n = 60)	CSO (n = 52)	OSO (n = 36)
Follow-up duration (months)	31.3 ± 14.9	21.8 ± 10.3	19.4 ± 8.5
Residual shunt (%)			
24 h	41.7	42.1	42.9
1–3 months	0	0	0
12 months	0	0	0
Complications			
Immediate embolization (within 24 h after implantation)	1	1	1
Late embolization	0	0	0
Immediate postprocedural pericardial effusion	0	0	0
Immediate postprocedural pericardial effusion	1	1	0
Erosion	0	0	0
Stroke	0	1	0

ASO, Amplatzer Septal Occluder; CSO, Cocoon Septal Occluder; OSO, Occlutech Septal Occluder.

midterm outcomes. However, comprehensive assessment for long-term efficacy and possible complications (i.e., erosion, thromboembolism, and late arrhythmia) are notably necessary.

References

1. Kefer J, Sluysmans T, Hermans C et al. Percutaneous transcatheter closure of interatrial septal defect in adults: Procedural outcome and long-term results. *Catheter Cardiovasc Interv* 2012;79:322–30.

2. Kutty S, Hazemm AA, Brown K et al. Long-term (5- to 20-year) outcomes after transcatheter or surgical treatment of hemodynamically significant isolated secundum atrial septal defect. *Am J Cardiol* 2012;109:1348–52.

3. Lertsapcharoen P, Khongphatthanayothin A, Srimanachota S et al. Self-expanding platinum-coated nitinol devices for transcatheter closure of atrial septal defect: Prevention of nickel release. *J Invasive Cardiol* 2008;20:279–83.

4. Lertsapcharoen P, Khongphatthanayothin A, La-orkhun V et al. Self-expanding nanoplatinum-coated nitinol devices for atrial septal defect and patent ductus arteriosus closure: A swine model. *Indian Heart J* 2006;58:315–20.

55

Starway device

Ting-Liang Liu and Wei Gao

Device introduction

Atrial septal defect (ASD) is a common congenital heart disease. The Starway Cardi-O-Fix ASD occluder is a self-expandable, double-disk implantable device made from a nitinol wire mesh, similar to the Amplatzer septal occluder (St. Jude Medical, USA). The two disks are linked together by a short connecting waist corresponding to the size of the ASD. In order to increase its closing ability, the disks and the waist are filled with polyester fabric membranes (Figure 55.1). It is specifically designed for the occlusion of ASD. These occluders are available in sizes from 4 to ~44 mm and can be delivered through 6 F to ~14 F delivery sheaths depending on the required size of the device (Table 55.1). This type of ASD device has been widely used for transcatheter closure of secundum ASD.

Patient selection

Starway Cardi-O-Fix ASD occluders can be used in patients with secundum ASDs. Patients who have echocardiographic evidence of a secundum ASD with a diameter ≤36 mm and a distance of ≥5 mm from the margins of the defect to the coronary sinus, mitral valves, and right upper pulmonary vein will be the candidates.

ASD device implantation

Before device implantation, echocardiography is performed to evaluate the ASD size, location, margin, and relation with adjacent cardiac structures. Patients are monitored by transthoracic echocardiography (TTE), transesophagus echocardiography (TEE), or intracardiac echography (ICE). After sheath placement, heparin is given at 100 IU/kg to keep the activated clotting time above 200 s. A standard right heart catheterization is performed following puncture of the femoral vein. If a sizing balloon catheter is used, the device size chosen is usually the same or one size larger (1–2 mm bigger) than the stretched diameter. Although ICE or TEE can provide optimal images, both methods are relatively inconvenient or fairly expensive. Many patients or pediatric heart centers cannot afford the expense of purchasing and maintaining these systems, especially in developing countries. And in most pediatric patients, both TTE and TEE have proven to be reliable for the assessment of the defect rims and play an important role in guiding the device deployment. In recent years, we have performed the closure of ASDs in more than 500 patients successfully under TTE guidance. According to our experience, the device size chosen is usually 3–4 mm larger than the maximal diameter of the defect measured

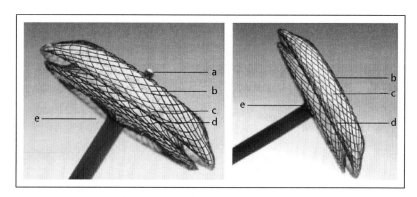

Figure 55.1 Starway Cardi-O-Fix ASD occluder. (a) Distal wire ring, (b) left atrial disk metal mesh, (c) fluid-resistance membrane, (d) right atrial disk, and (e) proximal wire ring and nut.

ASD device size	Recommended delivery system
4–13 mm	6 F
14–18 mm	7 F
19–22 mm	8 F
24–28 mm	9 F
30–32 mm	10 F
34–44 mm	12 F

Table 55.1 Recommended delivery system for Starway ASD device

by TTE if the maximal defect is less than 20 mm, and if the defect is more than 20 mm, the device size selected is generally 4–6 mm larger than the maximal diameter. The selected device is screwed onto the delivery cable by a screw at the end of the device and compressed into a loader. Then the device is advanced through a sheath without rotation. Under x-ray and/or echocardiographic guidance, the left atrial disk is deployed in the left atrium. The ASD device is deployed by withdrawing the sheath over the delivery cable to expand the right atrial disk. When the device position is confirmed, the device is released from the delivery system (Figure 55.2). Final assessment is conducted by echocardiography to confirm the device location and residual shunting. Routinely, patients receive a dose of an appropriate antibiotic (commonly cefazolin at 20 mg/kg) during the catheterization procedure and two further doses at 8 h intervals, as well as aspirin (5 mg/kg/day) for 6 months. Standard bacterial endocarditis prophylaxis is recommended for 6 months or until complete closure.[1–3]

Results

Starway Cardi-O-Fix ASD occluders have been introduced in over 200 medical centers in China and are exported to over 20 countries. Between 2002 and 2013, transcatheter closure with Starway ASD devices was performed in 25,456 patients. The immediate procedure success rate was 99% with good closure effects. The technical success rate was 99.8%. The ages of patients ranged from 2 to ~81 years and the mean age was 27.4 years. The male-to-female ratio was 1:1.5. The selected ASD device sizes were 4~44 mm. The most frequently used device sizes were 22~32 mm. The delivery systems used ranged from 6F to ~14 F depending on the required size of the device. The procedure time

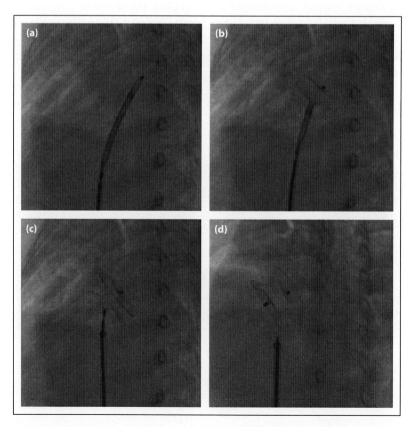

Figure 55.2 Transcatheter closure steps by fluoroscopy. (a) Delivery sheath with the collapsed device in the left atrium. (b) Deployment of the left atrial disk of the device. (c) The device fully deployed (both disks) but not released yet. (d) Device released across the defect.

ranged from 25 to ~60 min. The exposure time ranged from 2 to ~10 min.[4,5]

Complications

Complications may occur during transcatheter closure of ASD, such as air embolism, thrombosis, arrhythmia, device dislodgement, cardiac tamponade, and so on.

The total rate of complications during transcatheter closure of ASD using Starway ASD occluder devices since 2002 is less than 5% (in 25,456 patients).

The major complications included five deaths (the causes of death were cardiac tamponade, larger occluder displacement that got stuck at the cardiac valve, etc.), and 17 complications of cardiac tamponade. The residual shunts observed were less than 0.5%. Twenty-four cases of short-period migraine and two cases of transient ST-segment elevation were observed.[6]

Discussion

Transcatheter closure is now widely accepted as the preferred choice for treating secundum ASD. There is a similar rate of closure success comparing the transcatheter closure with surgical treatment; nevertheless, transcatheter closure not only presents a low complication rate and short hospital stay but also avoids surgical scarring and postoperative pain. There are a number of significant factors that are crucial to prevent complications and to achieve a high closure rate, such as the selection of suitable patients based on a sufficient rim, the selection of the correct size of device depending on the accurate assessment of the stretched diameter of the ASD, and echocardiography guidance to ensure the device position.

Device displacement and device embolism are early complications that may require emergent surgical treatment. Cardiac arrhythmias are also a known complication that may be controlled medically or recover spontaneously, but some arrhythmias may require cardioversion. Arrhythmias often occur during the operation as well as in the short period after the operation, but in some cases, they could remain long-term risks after ASD closure.

Conclusion

The Starway Cardi-O-Fix ASD occluder is specifically designed for the occlusion of ASD. It has a high closure rate and low risk of complication. The Starway Cardi-O-Fix ASD occluder has been registered in China SFDA since 2002 and has had CE certification since 2007. The Cardi-O-Fix ASD occluder is safe and effective in the clinical environment.

Acknowledgments

We wish to thank Dr. Zheng Zeng (Starway Med, Beijing, China), Dr. Wei Huang, and Ms Lin-Lin Jiang for collecting data and statistical analysis. We would also like to thank the technical, echocardiography, and nursing staff in the Department of Cardiology at the Shanghai Children's Medical Center for their hard work.

References

1. Masura J, Gavora P, Formanek A et al. Transcatheter closure of secundum atrial septal defects using the new self-centering amplatzer septal occluder: Initial human experience. *Catheter Cardiovasc Diagn* 1997;42:388–93.
2. Hijazi ZM, Cao Q, Patel HT et al. Transesophageal echocardiographic results of catheter closure of atrial septal defect in children and adults using the Amplatzer device. *Am J Cardiol* 2000;85:1387–90.
3. Fu YC, Cao QL, Hijazi ZM. Closure of secundum atrial septal defect using the Amplatzer Septal Occluder. In Sievert H, Qureshi SA, Wilson N, Hijazi ZM. Eds. *Percutaneous Interventions for Congenital Heart Disease*. London: Informa Healthcare, 2007. pp. 265–75.
4. Xie DM, Liu ZL, Liao YL et al. Clinical analysis of transcatheter closure of atrial septal defect using device made in China. *Gan Nan Yi Xue Yuan Xue Bao*. 2010;30:375–6 (Chinese).
5. Dai ZX, Guo YX, Fang CM et al. Comparison of three domestic-made ASD occluder device in the closure of atrial septal defects. *Chin Heart J* 2005;17:263–4 (Chinese).
6. Wang X, Hu DY, Sun Q et al. Transient ST-segment-elevation during transcatheter closure of atrial septal defect (ASD) with ASD occlude made in China: A report of two cases. *Chin Heart J* 2008;20:752–9.

56

Atrial septal defect: Cardia ASD occluder

Emanuela de Cillis, Tommaso Acquaviva, and Alessandro Santo Bortone

Introduction

Atrial septal defect (ASD) is the cardiac congenital anomaly most frequently found in adults, affecting 8% of the adult population with congenital heart disease, with a slight predominance in women (3:2). It is classified based on the anatomical location and relationship with adjacent anatomical structures. Typically, the indication to the closure of ostium secundum ASD is defined by hemodynamic parameters.[1] Data from the surgical literature suggest that the correction of an ASD should be considered in patients in whom the Qp/Qs ratio is equal to or >1.5. The treatment is recommended in patients with echocardiographic evidence of right ventricular dilatation and/or cardiac failure and may be considered in patients with pulmonary hypertension. Paradoxical embolism may also be considered as an indication for closure. From a clinical point of view, patients generally complain of effort dyspnea. Rarely, there is an evidence of right heart failure. It is rather rare to observe a neurological cryptogenic event in the presence of ASD, given that the flow is from left to right. In patients with secundum ASD, it is common to observe the presence of incomplete right bundle branch block on an electrocardiogram.

Often, there is a moderate dilatation of the right ventricle. Prolonged left-to-right shunting and excessive pulmonary blood flow may lead to pulmonary hypertension that may proceed to Eisenmenger's syndrome, and right heart failure. Percutaneous closure of secundum ASDs has been performed for many years both in the adult and pediatric population. The first attempt of percutaneous correction of ASD was performed in 1974 by King and Mills. Since then, technology has improved over time and numerous devices are currently commercially available.

A principal determinant of success in percutaneous closure of ASD is the choice of an appropriate device, as the actual effectiveness of each particular type of occluder is likely to depend on the differing atrial septal morphology encountered. Among the commercially available occluder devices, the last generation of Atriasept occluder device (Cardia, Eagan, MN, USA), shows additional novel improvements in safety and performance. The aim of this chapter is to describe the main technical and procedural characteristics of these devices intended for ASD closure in terms of safety and efficacy, anatomical assessment utilizing intracardiac echocardiography and fluoroscopy, and eventual clinical outcome on the basis of the authors' experience and recent literature data.

Device description and technical solution implemented over time to improve the Cardia performance

The Cardia occluder was born as a device for PFO closure. Indeed, the first generation (PFO-STAR) was a double umbrella with a four-arm frame made from two crossing wire struts of solid nitinol with titanium endcaps. The right and left atrial sails were made from 2-mm-thick square pieces of PVA (Ivalon/polyvinyl alcohol) foam. The endcaps acted like an area for suturing PVA to the frame and softened the tips of the strut wires. There was a 2 mm centered cylinder separating the sails.

In the second generation (Cardia-STAR), the frame was strengthened by using seven strands of nitinol in each strut wire.

The third generation (Cardia PFO) was characterized by enhancing the strut wires with 19 strands of nitinol, the sails becoming hexagonal instead of square. The PVA sail material was placed on the outer surface of the left atrial arms of the device, thereby reducing the possibility of thrombus formation.

In the fourth generation (Intrasept), the center element consists of multijoined titanium struts, permitting each sail to articulate independently from the other in three dimensions. This allows optimal conformation to the septal anatomy and reduces the degree of fatigue on the device and surrounding structures. This device was indicated for small

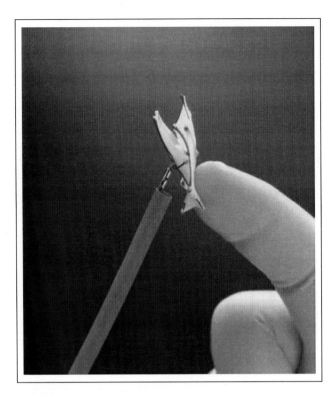

Figure 56.1   Intrasept device (fourth generation) in which the center element is realized in multijoined titanium, permitting each sail to articulate independently from the other in 3D dimension.

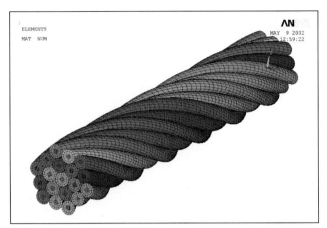

Figure 56.2   (**See color insert.**) 19-strand NiTi wires woven in petal shape.

ASDs but due to the lack of a self-centering mechanism, it was not ideal for medium or large ASDs (Figure 56.1).

In the fifth generation (Atriasept I), the addition of a different diameter-centering ring of PVA makes this device ideal for the treatment of both PFO and ASD. Moreover, the centering sail articulation was improved and device loading and retrieving were greatly simplified. The strut wires were reduced to 13 strands.

Finally, in the sixth version (Atriasept II), the right atrial struts and endcaps have been replaced with a rounded wire sail similar to the left sail without any pointed edges, thus improving the safety profile of the device. The stranded-wire struts are 19-strand nitinol wires woven and constituted in petal shapes that maximize fatigue resistance while maintaining an appropriate tension (Figure 56.2). Atriasept II is a double-rounded occluder in which the right atrial struts and endcaps have been completely replaced with a second rounded sail. This new design has no pointed arms or rough saw blade-style edges and presents a fully smooth and rounded profile, thus improving and maximizing safety. The dual-articulating sails along with the patented self-centering mechanism allows for easy deployment of the device as well as a super low profile within the atria. The complete Atriasept system consists of three components: the device, the delivery forceps, and the introducer. The device is fully retrievable in the sense that it can be regrasped

with the delivery forceps at the grasping knob, withdrawn into the delivery catheter, and removed (Figure 56.3). The Atriasept ASD double-round device shows centering mechanisms sized from 6 to 34 mm with the outside diameter disks (14/7 mm per side) larger than the centering mechanism. The sheath profile varies from 9 to 13 F in size (Figure 56.4). The device is composed of four materials: nitinol struts with titanium caps on each end, titanium centerposts, polyvinyl alcohol 8PVA (IvalonVR foam sails), and polypropylene sutures. The frame of the device is constructed from two titanium centerposts and three sets of stranded nitinol wires (Figure 56.5). The delivery forceps are flexible and have non-sharpened jaws, which serve to hold and/or release the device

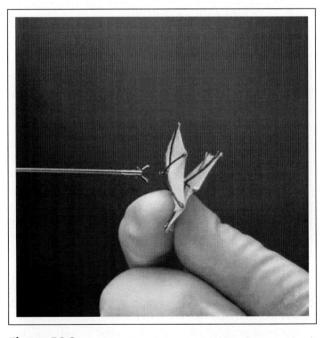

Figure 56.3   The device is fully retrievable in the sense that it can be regrasped with the delivery forceps at the grasping knob, withdrawn into the delivery catheter, and removed.

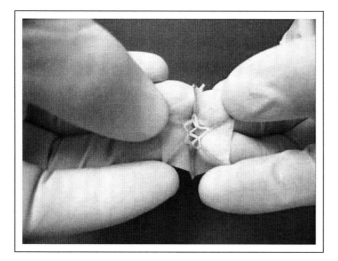

Figure 56.4   Atriasept ASD double-round device shows sizes-centering mechanisms.

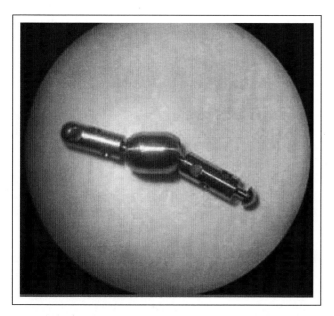

Figure 56.5   Titanium centerpost allows articulation of each sail.

at the grasping knob. The handle of the delivery forceps provides a locking mechanism that prevents detachment of the device, allowing a controlled release only when ready (Figure 56.6). Very recently, the company has produced a new ASD-dedicated device that presents additional improvements, including an innovative design with the left sail that is very flat, an increased radial force, new caliber dimensions for a Mullins sheath (9 Fr for ASD up to 18 mm), and a new self-centering mechanism better suited to eliminating the possibility of residual shunting. Additionally, transseptal puncture is feasible with this design (Figures 56.7 and 56.8).

Procedural aspects of Atriasept ASD closure

In most centers, the procedure is performed via the right femoral venous route, using transesophageal echocardiography monitoring under general anesthesia. Increasingly, intracardiac echocardiography (ICE) monitoring is also employed, which has some advantages over transesophageal echocardiography (TEE).[2,3] In our laboratory, all ASD closure procedures were performed using ICE (AcuNav 8 Fr, Acuson Siemens) guidance under local anesthesia with mild conscious sedation. Bilateral venous access was gained and two introducer sheaths (8 and 9 F) were placed respectively in the right and left common femoral vein. The 8 F sheath allows the introduction of 10 MHz ICE probe (AcuNav; Siemens Medical Solutions, Malvern, PA), which guarantees direct visualization of the atrial chambers and the atrioventricular valves. During percutaneous ASD closure, the images were typically obtained from the right atrium. The positioning of deflectable and directional catheters at the center of the right atrial cavity, with a right and posterior inclination of the transducer, provides an excellent imaging of the septum and surrounding structures. ICE images were acquired with a scan of 90° originating from the right atrium where the transducer is positioned. The marker located on the operator side has been positioned on the left side of the field of view (Figure 56.9).

Once the probe has been advanced into the right atrium at the level of the interatrial septum, a multipurpose 6 Fr

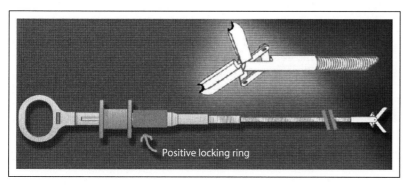

Positive locking ring

Figure 56.6   The delivery forceps are flexible with nonsharpened jaws, which serve to hold and/or release the device at the grasping knob. The handle of the delivery forceps provides a locking mechanism that prevents detachment of the device, allowing a controlled release only when ready.

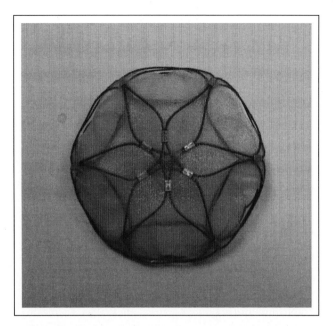

Figure 56.7 New ASD-dedicated device with an innovative design and the left sail very flat.

catheter is inserted into the right atrium to cross the defect and a 260 cm super-stiff exchange guide is advanced in the left atrium and preferably into the superior left pulmonary vein. The maximum static diameter of the defect can be measured with the aid of ICE and/or with balloon sizing. The dimensions of tissue margins surrounding the ASD are important to increase the chance of procedural success. A rim equal to or greater than 5 mm is generally considered adequate. The dimensions of the superior and inferior rims are of particular importance for the success of the procedure, although in small series, there has been effective closure even in the presence of deficient margins.[4]

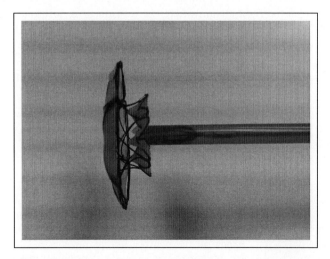

Figure 56.8 New ASD-dedicated device with an improvement of self-centering mechanism.

Typically, the diameter of the ASD obtained from the stretching effect of balloon measurement is >30% compared with the basal diameter, although thanks to the high resolution of ICE, the risk of overestimation is reduced. Therefore, it is possible to base the choice of device size on the ICE measurement without using the sizing balloon. Otherwise, a sizing balloon is inflated with a mixture of contrast media and saline in a ratio of 1:4 and at this point, the central part of the balloon is visible both to fluoroscopy and the ICE, thanks to the predefined calibration markers (Figure 56.10). Generally, in the same way, as classical devices are used to close ASD, the choice of the Atriasept device size is larger than the "stretched" diameter by 1–4 mm.

Because of the range of device diameter, the size of the Mullins introducer catheter may range from 9 to 13 F. Once you choose the most appropriately sized introducer, the femoral sheath is replaced with a long and curved Mullins sheath (80 cm) that needs to be placed in the pulmonary vein and the dilator retracted along the stiff guide wire (Figure 56.11). It is important to carefully purge the introducer sheath to avoid air embolus. At this point, the Atriasept device is inserted into the Mullins sheath. It is common to feel a slight resistance during initial insertion of the loaded device into the introducer. Using fluoroscopy, the delivery forceps and the device secured at the grasping knob is advanced inside the introducer sheath. When the device has reached the tip of the introducer, the whole system is withdrawn at the upper portion of the left atrium. During this maneuver, the introducer is withdrawn slowly while holding the cable release, and the left atrial sail opens (Figure 56.12).

Under both fluoroscopic and ICE guidance, the whole system is pulled back until the left atrial sail is well supported on the left side of the interatrial septum. Finally, the introducer is further retracted to allow opening of the right atrial sail (Figure 56.13). At this point, the device should be well positioned with both sails well secured on each side of the septum (Figure 56.14). Stability can be assessed by intracardiac ultrasound Doppler visualization of the defect from both sides of the device. It is also possible to inject contrast medium or saline solution in the introducer to display the right atrium and highlight any residual shunt through the ASD, with the occluder device well positioned across the defect and held in place by the delivery forceps. If no or only minimal residual shunting is detected, the device is released by opening the delivery forceps (Figure 56.15). It is essential to keep light traction during forceps opening until the device is released. Once the device is released, the position of the device and the disappearance of the shunt by color Doppler is assessed using the ICE transducer. Clearly, it is important to ensure that the atrioventricular valves are not encroached upon by the device. A small residual shunt through the device is not infrequent immediately after the release while severe residual shunts indicate a malposition of the device or the presence of a second defect. When the end result is judged satisfactory, both venous introducer sheaths are removed.

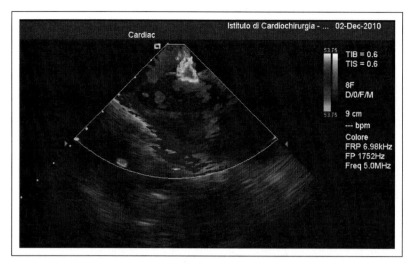

Figure 56.9 (**See color insert.**) ICE with left-to-right ultrasound Doppler visualization of an ostium secundum ASD.

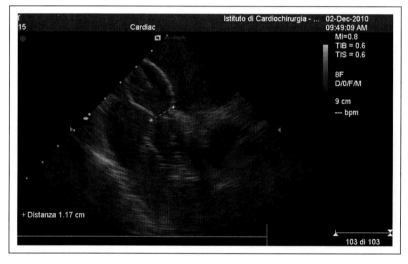

Figure 56.10   Sizing balloon is inflated with a mixture of contrast media and saline and the central part of the balloon is visible at the ICE and provides the sizing diameter. In this patient, the stretched diameter was 11 mm and we choose a 12 mm Atriasept occluder device.

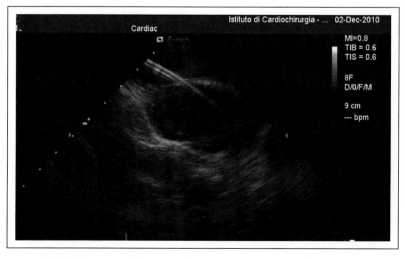

Figure 56.11   Mullins sheath (80 cm) was positioned across the defect and then the stiff guide wire was withdrawn from the left superior pulmonary vein.

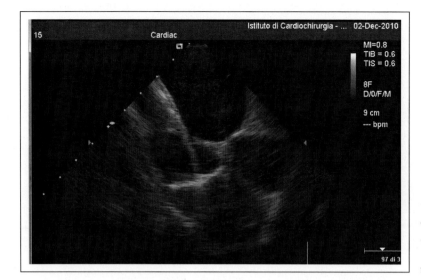

Figure 56.12 When the device has reached the tip of the introducer, the whole system is withdrawn at the upper portion of the left atrium. During this maneuver, the introducer is withdrawn slowly and the left atrial sail opens.

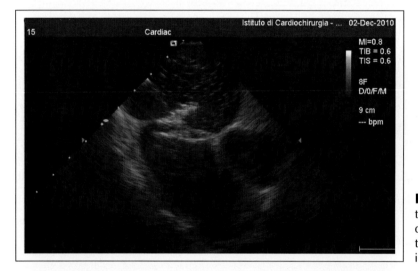

Figure 56.13 The system is pulled back jointly together until the left atrial sail is well supported on the left side of the interatrial septum and only the introducer is further retracted to allow opening of the right atrial sail.

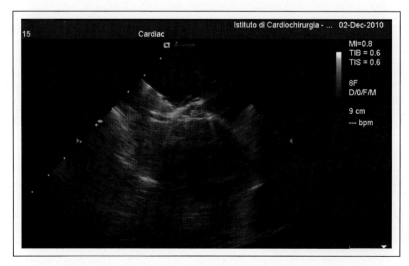

Figure 56.14 The device is well positioned with both sails well secured from each side of the septum.

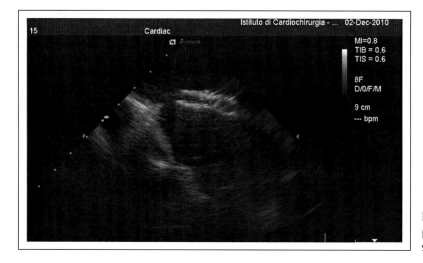

Figure 56.15 The device has been released, perfectly conforming to the anatomy of the septum.

Implantation of an ASD closure device potentially carries complications.[5] Dislocation and embolization of the device are well-known complications of ASD closure. There are "operator-dependent" errors and procedural errors, among which the most common are the incomplete grasping of the device to the delivery forceps, inappropriate choice of the type of device, or underestimation of the device's size, malposition, and early release. Taking into account that the current literature data mainly refer to the Atriasept occluder experience in small- and medium-sized ASDs, in the presence of large defects, it is generally believed that the devices of larger dimensions are prone to a higher incidence of embolization due to the inadequacy of one of the rims of the defect, which does not allow an optimal sealing of the device. In addition, several reports demonstrated that larger devices (or undersized) were found to be more susceptible to malposition and dislocation or embolization. The retrieval techniques of the Atriasept may be more challenging than devices classically used for the ASD closure (such as the Amplatzer septal occluder), but in all cases, a "goose-neck" snare and the use of a large-bore venous or arterial sheath is required.[6]

The development of new devices for percutaneous closure of secundum ASD has significantly increased the number of procedures in the cathlab for adult patients. The growing expertise in the use of these devices is increasing over time and they are currently employed in many centers as an alternative to surgical correction. The short- and medium-term results have been very positive.[7]

During the Atriasept closure procedure, the quality of the images obtained with ICE is shown to be similar if not higher than that of transesophageal ultrasound, allowing the acquisition of new and more accurate diagnostic information. In particular, the images captured on anatomical details of ASD, the adequacy of rims, and relations with the surrounding cardiac structures are excellent as well as the echogenicity of the device.

Our experience suggests that percutaneous closure of ASD with the Cardia Atriasept device, appears safe and beneficial in patients with secundum ASD. A principal determinant of procedural success is the choice of an appropriate device for the specific defect morphology encountered, and the effectiveness of the commercially available occluder devices is likely to depend on differing anatomy. The Atriasept device, due in part to its high flexibility, easy loading, and extremely low profile, showed excellent performance in differing anatomical configurations of interatrial septum, making them particularly suitable for small and medium ASDs and also for larger defects. Current experience shows that in comparison to the extensive use of more established devices (Amplatzer PFO occluder, etc.), a reasonably comparable outcome was obtained with the use of the Atriasept.

References

1. King TD, Mills NL. Nonoperative closure of atrial septal defect. *Surgery* 1974;75:383.
2. Boccalandro F, Baptista E, Muench A et al. Comparison of intracardiac echocardiography versus transesophageal echocardiography guidance for percutaneous transcatheter closure of atrial septal defect. *Am J Cardiol* 2004;93(4):437.
3. Koenig PR, Abdulla RI, Cao QL et al. Use of intracardiac echocardiography to guide catheter closure of atrial communications. *Echocardiography* 2003;20(8):781.
4. Du ZD, Koenig P, Cao QL et al. Comparison of transcatheter closure of secundum atrial septal defect using the Amplatzer septal occlude associated with deficient versus sufficient rims. *Am J Cardiol* 2002;90(8):865.
5. Chessa M, Carminati M, Butera G et al. Early and late complications associated with transcatheter occlusion of secundum atrial septal defects using the Amplatzer device. *J Am Coll Cardiol* 2002;39:1061.
6. De cillis E, Chessa M, Acquaviva T et al. How to retrieve the so-called "unretrievable" Amplatzer device: Tips and tricks. *Minerva Cardioangiol* 2010;58(3):421–2.
7. Steiger Stolt V, Chessa M, Aubry P et al. Closure of ostium secundum atrial septum defect with the Atriasept occluder: Early European experience. *Catheter Cardiovasc Interv* 2010;75:1091–95.

57

Atrial septal defect: Complications of device closure of ASDs

Jeremy Asnes and William E. Hellenbrand

Introduction

Major complications related to transcatheter closure of secundum atrial septal defects (ASDs) and patent foramen ovale (PFO) appear to be rare. However, most published studies of transcatheter ASD and PFO closure include a variety of devices, delivery systems, and techniques, thus limiting the ability to accurately quantify the risks associated with individual devices. Furthermore, single-device studies have generally included small numbers of subjects and, thus, the power of these studies to detect potentially important events is limited. Lack of a uniform classification scheme for procedural complications across studies and reports further hampers our ability to draw broadly generalizable conclusions regarding the safety of percutaneous closure. With these limitations in mind, this chapter will review several of the most commonly encountered complications of percutaneous ASD and PFO closure.

Reported complications of transcatheter ASD and PFO closures are listed in Table 57.1. Complications can be considered in terms of their severity as well as in terms of their temporal relationship to the implant procedure. Multicenter and single-center studies of transcatheter ASD and PFO closures demonstrate major complication rates of 0.2–5.9% and minor complication rates of 3.4–27.7%.[1–3] This compares favorably with recently published surgical ASD closure data.[4] A nonrandomized multicenter trial comparing the Amplatzer Septal Occluder (ASO) to surgical closure showed percutaneous closure with the ASO to have lower major and total complication rates when compared with surgery (1.6% vs. 5.4%, $p = 0.03$ and 7.2% vs. 24%, $p < 0.001$).[3,4] Similarly, the Gore HELEX Multicenter Pivotal Study found device closure with the Gore HELEX device to have a higher rate of clinical success—a composite evaluation of safety and efficacy 12 months postprocedure—compared with surgical closure (91.7% vs. 83.7%; $p < 0.001$).[1]

Table 57.1 Complications of device closure

Procedural complications	Postprocedural complications
• Air embolism	• Aortic insufficiency
• Arrhythmia	• Arrhythmia
• Atrial tachycardia	• Atrial tachycardia
• Heart block	• Heart block
• AV valve impingement	• Device component fracture
• Cardiac perforation	• Erosion
• Coronary compression	• Embolization
• Embolization	• Endocarditis
• Esophageal injury (TEE)	• Migraine
• Pulmonary edema	• Thrombosis/ thromboembolism
• Septal injury	
• Thrombosis/ thromboembolism	
• Vascular injury	

The majority of complications occur during the implant procedure. However, it has become clear over the past decade that complications—particularly erosion, arrhythmia, and thromboembolism—although rare, may occur long after device implant. Thus, an appropriate frequency and duration for routine postprocedure surveillance has yet to be defined.

Procedural complications

Procedural complications associated with transcatheter ASD closure (i.e., those occurring during device implant) are listed in Table 57.1. Procedural risk can be effectively mitigated with close attention to atrial anatomy, technique, and anticoagulation.

Large-diameter, long, hemostatic sheaths are required for closure of ASD and PFO. These sheaths increase the risk for vascular injury, air emboli, and cardiac perforation. Positioning delivery sheaths across the atrial septum often requires placement of a guide wire in a pulmonary vein. Incorrect guide wire position has resulted in LA free wall and LA appendage perforation. Catheter, guide wire, sheath, and dilator perforation of the pulmonary vein have been reported in conjunction with ASD closure procedures. When required, the authors generally prefer the left upper pulmonary vein for distal guide wire position. An appropriately positioned guide wire will appear outside of the heart border and will cross the left bronchus air column on a straight anteroposterior fluoroscopic image. The use of a relatively flexible guiding catheter and confirmation of catheter position prior to guide wire placement will help avoid perforation through the LA appendage or free wall. Echocardiography (intracardiac echocardiogram [ICE] or transesophageal echocardiography [TEE]) can be used to confirm wire position prior to sheath positioning. The use of a J-tip guide wire with at least a 3-cm floppy tip also reduces the risk of pulmonary vein trauma.

Long hemostatic sheaths positioned in the LA create significant risk for systemic air embolization. Withdrawal of dilators from long sheaths can result in air entrainment and subsequent embolization. Several techniques for safe and effective de-airing have been described. In one such method, the dilator is withdrawn, leaving the guide wire in place while the sheath tip is kept at the inferior vena cava right atrial junction. The sheath is then carefully flushed paying attention to avoid air entrainment through the hemostatic valve system. Inadvertently introduced air bubbles will flow across the tricuspid valve and out to the PAs instead of the Ao. Once purged, the sheath is advanced over the guide wire to the LA (without the dilator). Alternatively, the sheath and dilator can be advanced to the pulmonary vein orifice as a unit. Leaving the guide wire in place, the dilator is then slowly withdrawn. The guide wire helps to keep the sheath centered in the pulmonary vein and prevents the sheath tip from abutting the atrial wall. This allows free flow of LA blood through the sheath, purging the sheath as the dilator is withdrawn. Finally, one can advance the sheath and dilator to the proximal pulmonary vein as a unit. The dilator can then be "unlocked" from the sheath and the sheath advances over the dilator until the tips of the sheath and dilator are aligned within the pulmonary vein. The guide wire can then be slowly withdrawn and a large volume flush syringe attached to the dilator. Gentle negative pressure on the syringe should result in evacuation of any air in the dilator lumen and easy return of blood. If blood is not easily returned, then the sheath and dilator should be pulled back as a unit into the LA while continuous gentle negative pressure is applied

until blood return is achieved. Once free blood return is achieved, the dilator can be slowly withdrawn while continuously infusing saline from the syringe. This will avoid vacuum formation and entrainment of air.

Extra caution must be taken when patients have obstructive breathing patterns. The negative intrathoracic pressure generated under these conditions can draw air into the heart through the long sheath. Proximal sheath and catheter hubs should be kept well below atrial level during all the maneuvers described above and should never be left open to air.

The placement of large sheaths, guidewires, and inherently thrombogenic devices within the LA creates risk for thromboembolic events during percutaneous ASD closure. Thrombi attached to device-delivery components are occasionally identified by echocardiography during closure procedures. These thrombi can easily migrate to the pulmonary or systemic circulations. These events can be avoided with appropriate dosing and vigilant monitoring of anticoagulation, frequent flushing of long sheaths, and, in cases requiring multiple deployment attempts, "washing" of the device and delivery components in fresh saline—especially if potential thrombi are identified echocardiographically. The authors recommend systemic heparinization with a goal activated clotting time (ACT) of 225–250 s. ACTs should be checked every 20–30 min during the procedure and should be at or above the goal prior to entry into the LA. Protamine should never be used after device closure.

Patients should be treated with aspirin for 3 days prior to the procedure. Antiplatelet medications should be continued for a minimum of 6 months after implant. As published data indicate increased risk of device-related thrombus in older patients, we recommend the use of a second antiplatelet agent (i.e., clopidogrel) in addition to aspirin for the initial 3 months after implant in patients older than 18 years. Reports also suggest that device endothelialization may be inhibited in some circumstances such as with the use of antiproliferative medications or in the setting of arteriovenous (AV) valve insufficiency directed at device components. Such circumstances may require prolonged antiplatelet treatment although there is insufficient data to define the appropriate criteria.

Arrhythmia

Atrial tachyarrhythmias are among the most commonly reported complications associated with device closure. There does not appear to be an association between device type and arrhythmia risk; however, there is increased risk with ASD versus PFO closure. Arrhythmia is rare in young patients undergoing closure. Intraprocedural atrial fibrillation and flutter are often self-limited or easily extinguished with catheter manipulation. However, intraprocedural or immediate postprocedural cardioversion is occasionally required. In the authors' experience, as well as in published case reports, periprocedural direct current (DC) cardioversion has resulted in device embolization.[5] There are theoretical advantages to atrial overdrive pacing and chemical cardioversion due to the lack of skeletal muscle activation. Regardless, cardioversion should not be delayed, as there is increased potential for thrombus formation on the device in the setting of a disorganized atrial rhythm. Therapeutic levels of anticoagulation should be maintained until sinus rhythm is restored.

Varying degrees of heart block, including third degree, have been reported with device closure of atrial communications. This complication is likely related to stretching of the atrial myocardium and/or device encroachment on the AV node. A preprocedure electrocardiogram (ECG) should be obtained on all patients. The baseline PR interval and rhythm should also be noted immediately prior to device placement. Prior to device release, the rhythm and PR interval should be carefully evaluated. Moderate PR prolongation has been reported to occur in up to 5% of patients and is most commonly noted on postprocedural electrocardiography. In the absence of progressive prolongation and higher degrees of block, such patients can be followed closely with serial ECGs and/or Holter monitoring. Most patients will have return of normal conduction after a month or so. If the PR interval is prolonged beyond the upper limits of normal or higher degrees of AV block are noted, the device should be withdrawn or removed surgically. In most reports, normal conduction will return with device withdrawal. In many reports, device withdrawal in the cath lab was followed by subsequent successful closure with a smaller device. Obviously, this can only be achieved if the initial device was oversized.

Ventricular arrhythmias—nonsustained ventricular tachycardia and/or premature ventricular contractions—may indicate device embolization to or through a ventricle. These may be transient with subsequent ejection of the device to the aorta or pulmonary artery. The authors recommend in-hospital observation for a minimum of 12–18 h following device implantation. Continuous rhythm monitoring during this time may allow for early recognition of device embolization.

Postprocedural tachyarrhythmias

In the authors' experience, nonsustained atrial tachyarrhythmias are the most common postprocedural rhythm abnormality. Although rare in children, palpitations are frequently reported in adult patients. Occasionally, there is enough arrhythmia burden and/or sufficient symptomatology to warrant a brief course of β-blockade to suppress ectopy. In the vast majority of cases, ectopy subsides and β-blockade can be withdrawn after 6–12 weeks.

Postprocedural atrial fibrillation and/or flutter have been reported in up to 14% of cases with 8–12% being new onset.[6,7] Other tachyarrhythmias—AVNRT, WPW—have been reported as well although the substrate for these is obviously not device related. Postprocedural tachyarrhythmias are more common in older patients. Since preexisting arrhythmia increases the risk for postprocedure rhythm abnormalities, patients with arrhythmia symptoms prior to device implant should undergo formal rhythm assessment. Preexisting arrhythmia may require treatment before device implantation. Ablation procedure-related access to the left atrium via transseptal puncture can be complicated in patients following device closure.

Stagnation of the atrial blood pool associated with atrial arrhythmias may increase the risk of thromboembolic events in patients with newly implanted (<6 months) devices due to incomplete endothelialization. Therefore, careful echocardiographic evaluation for thrombus on or near the device is required prior to chemical or DC cardioversion.

Embolization

Device embolization has been reported with all commonly used closure devices. In a large, US community-based multicenter study of the ASO, embolization was the most commonly reported major complication with an incidence of 0.7%.[8] Other studies show ASO embolization rates of 0.55–1.7%.[3,5,9] In the Gore HELEX Multicenter Pivotal Study, the embolization rate was 1.7%.[1] Embolization occurs most often at the time of implant and the overwhelming majority of events occur within 24 h of the implant procedure. However, late embolization, days to weeks after implant, has been infrequently reported.

Implanters must be familiar with risk factors for embolization, avoidance strategies, and retrieval techniques. While percutaneous device retrieval is often successful, surgical intervention is sometimes required. Therefore, device implantation should only be performed in settings where cardiothoracic surgical services are available.

Most embolizations result in movement of the device to either the right or left atrium. However, devices may migrate to the ventricle, the aorta, or the branch pulmonary arteries. An important obstruction of ventricular inflow or outflow has only rarely been reported.

Embolization events have been associated with Valsalva (emesis, cough), vigorous TEE probe manipulation, DC cardioversion, and cardiopulmonary resuscitation. As the vast majority of events occur within 24 hours of device implantation, it is recommended that patients remain in hospital for 18–24 hours after implant and that a transthoracic echocardiogram must be performed prior to discharge. There are reports of late embolization events identified weeks after implant, but these are rare. In one such case, embolization was felt to be related to contact sports participation 72 hours after implant.[3] Thus, restriction from contact sports participation for 4–6 weeks after device implant may be warranted.

Device undersizing and septal rim deficiency, particularly of the IVC rim, are the most common causes of device embolization. Additionally, a thin, mobile septum primum or septal aneurysm increases the risk for device instability.

Gross device misalignment with prolapse of the device is generally identified easily and can be rectified with complete or partial device recapture and repositioning. More difficult to identify are the subtle errors in device positioning. Careful echocardiographic assessment of rim capture prior to final device release is essential to avoid embolization. Septal rim must be visualized between the left and right atrial device components in multiple imaging planes prior to release. The inferior rim is typically the most difficult to assess. The combination of a device-related artifact, thinness of the septum, proximity of device components, and delivery system-related distortion in this location makes visualization of the septum between the left and right device components particularly challenging. While ICE imaging may be superior to TEE for visualization of this region, trans-gastric sagittal TEE imaging planes can be helpful when ICE is not available. For the ASO and Gore HELEX Septal Occluder (GHSO) devices, gentle traction or forward tension on the delivery system can help to slightly separate the left and right components, allowing identification of the rim tissue within the device. For the ASO, this must be done with the delivery sheath pulled back from the device. Significant force during this maneuver can dislodge a well-seated device.

Color-flow Doppler imaging can aid in confirming rim capture. Residual shunt despite apposition of the left and right atrial device components frequently indicates failure to capture the septal tissue. It is common to see a leak at the anterior superior or aortic rim prior to release due to device distortion by the delivery system. An inferior leak is uncommon. Residual shunt can also be seen if an additional, potentially unrecognized defect is present at the margin of the device. Fluoroscopically, separation of the inferior device components usually indicates rim capture though this can be subtle. Gantry angulation is usually required to obtain an imaging angle perpendicular to the plane of the device.

All device-delivery systems distort the attached device and septum to some degree prior to final release. Newer delivery system designs such as the St. Jude Amplatzer TorqVue FX system have helped to minimize distortion by providing a more flexible coupling mechanism between the delivery system and device. However, the implanter must anticipate conformational changes and their impact on device alignment and stability prior to release. The delivery system should be positioned such that the least amount of torque is applied to the device at the time of release. When significant torque is present, the release will result in dramatic shifts that may dislodge the device position.

Embolizations occur even in the setting of appropriate rim capture. Therefore, the operator must be familiar with device-retrieval techniques. Furthermore, the catheterization laboratory must be stocked with appropriate retrieval equipment including snare catheters, a variety of shaped catheters that will accommodate snares, bioptomes, and 12–18 F long sheaths.

Understanding device construction and mechanics is critical to successful retrieval. For example, the ASO can only be retrieved if the screw hub on the RA disk can be snared. This may necessitate manipulation of the device within a cardiac chamber, a pulmonary artery, or the aorta such that the RA screw hub is facing the retrieval catheter. Controlling device position with an atraumatic guide wire or bioptome can be helpful in this regard. A wire can generally be passed through the device once it is in a good position for capture. The nitinol wire frame can also be grabbed with a bioptome to stabilize or manipulate its position. The bioptome will not allow for grabbing the screw hub itself. Once the screw hub is appropriately exposed, a gooseneck snare can be positioned around the base of the hub. There is a small ridge between the nitinol wires and the hub that allows purchase. Difficulty is often encountered when attempting to pull the snared hub into a sheath as the hub tends to align perpendicular to the orifice of the sheath. For this reason, it is helpful to use a sheath that is a minimum of 2 Fr sizes greater than the recommended delivery sheath. Additionally, the sheath tip can be beveled if a sheath without a wire braid is used. This increases the cross-sectional area of the sheath orifice and eases hub entry. A beveled sheath should always be introduced and advanced with a dilator to avoid vessel injury from the cut edge of the sheath. Linear splitting of beveled sheaths by retrieval snares and catheters has been described. This can allow for entrapment of cardiac and vascular structures and can impede device retrieval. Therefore, care must be taken to identify the position of the beveled tip and its relationship to the device on fluoroscopy. It can also be helpful to retract the device from the opposite side using a bioptome while simultaneously pulling the snared RA hub into the retrieval sheath. This elongates the device and can help center the hub. Finally, a series of coaxial sheaths can be used such that the retrieval sheath is itself deployed through a larger, shorter sheath, thus allowing the inner sheath and snared device to be pulled into the larger sheath.

The GHSO device has a cord attached to the right atrial islet that allows the operator to retrieve an embolized or malpositioned device even after the lock loop has been set. The operator must secure the cord and then retract the device using the delivery system. A "popping" or "unzipping" will be felt as the lock loop opens and closes, allowing the RA and center islets and the Gore-Tex material to pull off the loop. Care must be taken to ensure that there is enough distance between the introducer sheath and the lock loop to allow the lock loop to open. If the sheath is too close to the lock loop, it will prevent the loop from opening and the operator will feel the resistance. If additional force is applied to overcome the resistance, the retrieval cord will break. If the retrieval cord has already been withdrawn or the breaks the GHSO device can be snared or grabbed with a bioptome and retrieved, though this is significantly more difficult. As with retrieval of the ASO, misalignment of GHSO device components—islets and lock loop—with the retrieval sheath can make retrieval difficult. Thus, large coaxial sheaths can significantly aid in retrieval.

Devices that have embolized to the PA or Ao should not be pulled retrograde acrs the semilunar valves. Devices in the PA should be retrieved through a long sheath positioned across the pulmonary valve. Devices in the Ao should be retrieved through a retrograde arterial sheath.

Similarly, devices in either the left or right ventricle should not be forcefully pulled across the mitral or tricuspid valve but should be retrieved in the ventricle or associated great artery. Stiff sheaths, dilators, and devices must be manipulated with caution. Fatal ventricular perforation during attempted device retrieval has been reported. Retrieval from the great arteries is generally easier than from within a cardiac chamber.

During any attempted retrieval, the operator must remember to provide adequate anticoagulation to avoid the formation of thromboemboli on the device or retrieval equipment. Retrieval efforts often add significantly to the procedure time and so anticoagulation must be monitored and adjusted as needed.

There are situations in which retrieval should not be attempted. Retrieval of devices entangled in the chordal apparatus of the mitral or tricuspid valve may result in significant valve damage. If the device cannot be easily freed, the patient should be referred for surgery rather than risk the need for AV valve repair or replacement. Other situations may arise in which the device size or peculiarities of the device position prevent safe retrieval. When retrieval is not possible, if the device construction permits, it is often helpful to position an atraumatic guide wire through the device to "pin" the device in place. This prevents more distal movement of the device and allows the surgeon to quickly locate and control it. The wire can be removed once the device is under surgical control. This technique is valuable regardless of the device's position.

Erosion

Erosion of closure devices through the atrial wall has been well described in multiple case reports and case series. While rare, these events are of particular concern because they remain unpredictable and potentially lethal. Despite significant effort on the part of the industry, academia, and regulatory agencies, the etiology and risk factors for device erosion remain difficult to study due to inconsistent reporting of both device implants and erosion events. Furthermore, when reported, event reports vary greatly in the amount and quality of clinical information including pre- and postprocedural imaging, making identification of commonalities across events difficult.

Erosion events have been reported with several devices including Atriasept, Blockaid, Starflex, SolySafe, ASO, Amplatzer PFO Occluder, and Amplatzer Cribriform Occluder (ACO) in both on-label and off-label applications.

The ASO, ACO, and GHSO, the only approved ASD closure devices in the United States, are the most studied in terms of erosion. In 2012, the US Food and Drug Administration (FDA) Circulatory System Devices Advisory Panel reviewed all available data on adverse events related to on-label use of the ASO and GHSO for closure of secundum ASDs. Data were drawn from manufacturer databases, clinical studies, literature review, and the FDA's Manufacturer and User Facility Device Experience database. Cases were reconciled to avoid duplication.

No GHSO erosions were identified. A total of 202 potential ASO erosions were identified worldwide (Table 57.2). Of the 202 potential cases, 97 were confirmed as erosion events. The remaining 105 cases of pericardial effusion were not due to erosion but were trivial postprocedural erosions that resolved spontaneously.

Cardiac erosion sites are presented in Table 57.3. Left atrial erosions predominated, likely due to the larger diameter of the LA disk. Aortic root injury and/or perforation were noted

Table 57.2   ASO-related erosion data

Source	Potential erosions ($n = 202$)	Confirmed—not erosion events ($n = 105$)	Confirmed erosions ($n = 97$)
Literature	44	28	16
Field event report	122	46	76
PAS investigator query	10	7	3
PAS	26	24	2

PAS = Postapproval study.

Table 57.3   Site of ASO erosion

Site of erosion ($n = 97$)	Total/with Ao involvement
Left atrium	47 (48.4%)/28 + Ao
Right atrium	26 (26.8%)/22 + Ao
Right and left atria	9 (13.4%)
Unknown	15 (15.5%)

Ao = Aortic.

in 52% of the cases, including 16 cases of aortic–atrial fistula formation. Cardiac tamponade due to hemopericardium was present in 68 cases (70%) at the time of presentation.

The time from implant to erosion varied considerably. While the majority of pediatric erosions (57%) occurred <72 h after implant, only 35% of adult erosions occurred within that time period. Nearly 90% of all erosions occurred within 1 year of implant. However, erosion of the ASO has been reported more than 8 years after implant.[11] While not included in the FDA review, on-label and off-label ACO erosion has been reported. In one case, ACO erosion was associated with isometric exertion 5 years after implant.

Erosion was fatal in eight of the 97 confirmed cases (8.2%). There were no fatalities in patients <15 years of age. All fatal erosions occurred within 16 months of implant. In each of the eight fatal erosions, there was either device oversizing, anterior–superior rim deficiency, or both. For the purposes of the panel analysis, device oversizing was defined as *an implanted device diameter >150% of the largest native (not balloon sized) ASD diameter as measured by echocardiography in any view.* Aortic rim deficiency was defined as *anterior–superior rim length <5 mm in more than one consecutive imaging plane or absence of the aortic rim altogether.*

While the etiology of ASO erosion remains ill defined, some conclusions can be drawn from the available data. All but two of the 97 erosion cases involved device oversizing, anterior–superior rim deficiency, or both. Furthermore, all pediatric erosions and 84% of adult erosions involved anterior–superior rim deficiency. Thus, it is reasonable to conclude that device oversizing and aortic rim deficiency independently, and in combination, increase erosion risk.

Device size may also independently increase erosion risk, as 75% of erosion cases involved devices larger than 18 mm. This may be explained in part by differences in device construction. While devices <18 mm are formed from a 0.004 inch nitinol wire, devices of 18 mm and larger are formed from a 0.006 inch wire and devices of 26 mm and larger are formed from a 0.0075 inch wire. As wire thickness and resulting device stiffness increases mechanical device–tissue interactions, it may be more conducive to tissue erosion.

Lack of accurate implant data limits the ability to accurately determine the true incidence of ASO erosion and erosion-related mortality. While known, the number of devices shipped overestimates ASD implants. Device registration has been voluntary; thus the number of registered devices underestimates the true number of implants due to underregistration. Furthermore, not all registered devices have been implanted for on-label indications. Finally, erosion events are underreported. With these limitations in mind, using a combination of returned device registration cards and product shipment totals, it has been estimated that the overall ASO erosion rate is 0.04–0.17% or 0.4–1.7 erosions/1000 implants. The incidence of erosion-related mortality is 0.004–0.015% or roughly 1–2 fatalities/10,000

implants. When counseling our prospective patients, we inform them that the risk of erosion is 0.15–0.2% and that approximately one in 10 erosion events are fatal. This mortality risk favorably compares with the current-era surgical mortality (0.13–0.36%).[4,12] However, important caveats must be kept in mind when comparing these mortality figures. Surgical mortality is reported as either discharge or 30-day mortality and so does not include deaths outside of these reporting windows. On the other hand, erosion mortality data are event driven and have no specified reporting window. While nonerosion mortality is exceedingly rare, erosion mortality figures do not represent all device implant-related mortality and, thus, underrepresent the overall procedural mortality to a small degree.

Implanters must be familiar with these data to appropriately inform patients and families regarding the risks of device closure. Furthermore, implanters must be cognizant of appropriate ASD-sizing techniques and rim assessment. Real-time echocardiography and stop-flow sizing utilizing an ultra-compliant balloon should be performed in all cases to avoid device oversizing. In patients with aortic rim deficiency, consideration should be given to the use of the GHSO or to surgical closure.

Pulmonary edema

Transcatheter ASD closure in patients with left ventricular diastolic dysfunction—most commonly patients >60 years of age—can result in acute pulmonary edema and the need for emergent intubation and anticongestive therapy.[13] In this setting, the atrial left-to-right shunt unloads the left heart and may mask the diastolic dysfunction. Elimination of the atrial "pop-off" causes a sudden increase in LV preload, a rise in LA pressure, and the development of acute pulmonary edema. Therefore, in patients at risk for diastolic dysfunction, temporary balloon occlusion of the ASD with simultaneous measurement of LV end-diastolic pressure or pulmonary capillary wedge pressure should be performed. If LV end-diastolic pressures increases to >25 mmHg or increases by more than 10 mmHg, consideration should be given to the institution of a preconditioning regimen prior to ASD closure.

Thromboembolism

While the risk of device thrombosis is low thromboembolism, both intraprocedural and postprocedural, has been well described.[14,15] As noted above, all patients without a specific contraindication should receive aspirin for 3 days prior to device implant. Animal models have demonstrated complete device endothelialization at 3 months; however, late device thrombosis, while rare, has been reported. We recommend the use of a second antiplatelet agent (i.e., clopidogrel) in addition to aspirin for the initial 3 months after implant in patients older than 18 years. Reports suggest that device endothelialization may be inhibited in some circumstances such as with the use of antiproliferative medications or in the setting of AV valve insufficiency directed at device components.[16,17] Such circumstances may require prolonged antiplatelet treatment, although there is insufficient data to define the appropriate criteria. Any unexplained thromboembolic event following ASD device closure should prompt careful echocardiographic evaluation of the device.

References

1. Jones TK, Latson LA, Zahn E, Fleishman CE, Jacobson J, Vincent R et al. Results of the U.S. multicenter pivotal study of the Helex septal occluder for percutaneous closure of secundum atrial septal defects. *J Am Coll Cardiol* Jun 5 2007;49(22):2215–21.

2. Fiarresga A, De Sousa L, Martins JD, Ramos R, Paramés F, Freitas I et al. Percutaneous closure of atrial septal defects: A decade of experience at a reference center. *Rev Port Cardiol* May 2010;29(5):767–80.

3. Du ZD, Hijazi ZM, Kleinman CS, Silverman NH, Larntz K, Amplatzer Investigators. Comparison between transcatheter and surgical closure of secundum atrial septal defect in children and adults: Results of a multicenter nonrandomized trial. *J Am Coll Cardiol* Jun 5 2002;39(11):1836–44.

4. DiBardino DJ, McElhinney DB, Kaza AK, Mayer JE. Analysis of the U.S. Food and Drug Administration Manufacturer and User Facility Device Experience database for adverse events involving Amplatzer septal occluder devices and comparison with the Society of Thoracic Surgery congenital cardiac surgery database. *J Thorac Cardiovasc Surg* Jun 2009;137(6):1334–41.

5. Chessa M, Carminati M, Butera G, Bini RM, Drago M, Rosti L et al. Early and late complications associated with transcatheter occlusion of secundum atrial septal defect. *J Am Coll Cardiol* Mar 20 2002;39(6):1061–5.

6. Sadiq M, Kazmi T, Rehman AU, Latif F, Hyder N, Qureshi SA. Device closure of atrial septal defect: Medium-term outcome with special reference to complications. *Cardiol Young* Jul 11 2011;22(01):71–8.

7. Spies C, Khandelwal A, Timmermanns I, Schräder R. Incidence of atrial fibrillation following transcatheter closure of atrial septal defects in adults. *Am J Cardiol* Oct 1 2008;102(7):902–6.

8. Everett AD, Jennings J, Sibinga E, Owada C, Lim DS, Cheatham J et al. Community use of the Amplatzer atrial septal defect occluder: Results of the multicenter MAGIC atrial septal defect study. *Pediatr Cardiol* Apr 2009;30(3):240–7.

9. Levi DS, Moore JW. Embolization and retrieval of the Amplatzer septal occluder. *Catheter Cardiovasc Interv* Apr 2004;61(4):543–7.

10. Poommipanit P, Levi D, Shenoda M, Tobis J. Percutaneous retrieval of the locked Helex septal occluder. *Catheter Cardiovasc Interv* May 1 2011;77(6):892–900.

11. Roberts WT, Parmar J, Rajathurai T. Very late erosion of Amplatzer septal occluder device presenting as pericardial pain and effusion 8 years after placement. *Catheter Cardiovasc Interv* 2013;82:E592–4.

12. Sarris GE, Kirvassilis G, Zavaropoulos P, Belli E, Berggren H, Carrel T et al. Surgery for complications of trans-catheter closure of atrial septal defects: A multi-institutional study from the European Congenital Heart Surgeons Association. *Eur J Cardiothorac Surg* Jun 2010;37(6):1285–90.

13. Schubert S, Peters B, Abdul-Khaliq H, Nagdyman N, Lange PE, Ewert P. Left ventricular conditioning in the elderly patient to prevent congestive heart failure after transcatheter closure of atrial septal defect. *Catheter Cardiovasc Interv* Mar 2005;64(3):333–7.

14. Krumsdorf U, Ostermayer S, Billinger K, Trepels T, Zadan E, Horvath K et al. Incidence and clinical course of thrombus formation on atrial septal defect and patient foramen ovale closure devices in 1000 consecutive patients. *J Am Coll Cardiol* Jan 21 2004;43(2):302–9.

15. Taaffe M, Fischer E, Baranowski A, Majunke N, Heinisch C, Leetz M et al. Comparison of three patent foramen ovale closure devices in a randomized trial (Amplatzer versus CardioSEAL–STARflex versus Helex occluder). *Am J Cardiol* May 1 2008;101(9):1353–8.

16. Astroulakis Z, El-Gamel A, Hill JM. Failed endothelialisation of a percutaneous atrial septal defect closure device. *Heart* 2008; 94(5):580.

17. Zaidi AN, Cheatham JP, Galantowicz M, Astor T, Kovalchin JP. Late thrombus formation on the Helex septal occluder after double-lung transplant. *J Heart Lung Transplant* Jul 2010;29(7):814–6.

58

Patent foramen ovale closure: Background, indications for closure, and clinical trial results

Daniel H. Steinberg, Stefan Bertog, and Horst Sievert

Introduction

As an essential component of intrauterine circulation, the foramen ovale is a tunnel bound by the superior septum secundum on the right atrial side and inferior septum primum on the left atrial side.[1] It allows oxygenated blood to flow from the inferior vena cava and right atrium into the left atrium and systemic circulation. Shortly after birth, pulmonary resistance decreases, left atrial pressure increases, and the foramen ovale physiologically closes. It usually fuses over the ensuing 2 years; however, in up to 30% of the population, it may remain patent.[2] A patent foramen ovale (PFO) is often of no clinical consequence, but it has been implicated in multiple disease processes including migraine headaches and cryptogenic stroke. Percutaneous device closure has been proposed to prevent recurrent events in patients with PFO. This chapter is dedicated to the background, indications, and clinical trial results of PFO closure.

Background

Physiologically, a PFO is a communication between the right and left atrium. As left atrial pressure is usually higher than right atrial pressure, this communication is typically inconsequential. However, when right atrial pressure increases, such as during exercise, coughing, or a physiologic Valsalva maneuver, shunting of blood or other substances may occur from the right atrium into the left atrium and the systemic circulation.

PFO has been implicated in multiple processes including decompression sickness,[3] platypnea–orthodeoxia syndrome,[4] migraine headaches,[5] and cryptogenic stroke.[6] The underlying mechanism is the passage of material across the PFO and into the systemic circulation. From an incidence/prevalence standpoint, the primary academic, clinical, and industry interests have focused on cryptogenic stroke and migraine headaches.

Cryptogenic stroke and PFO

Stroke is one of the most important causes of morbidity and mortality both in the United States and Europe. Of over 700,000 strokes in the United States, 87% were presumed ischemic in nature, and of these, 40% occurred with no known cause, leaving 140,000 "cryptogenic" strokes per year.[7,8] While PFO is not associated with increased morbidity in the general population, patients with cryptogenic stroke have increased prevalence of PFO compared with those with a documented cause of stroke.[9–12] This association is particularly prominent in patients with increased right–left shunting, including those with larger PFO and coexisting atrial septal aneurysm.[1,13,14]

For patients with cryptogenic stroke and PFO, secondary prevention is multifactorial. Primary therapy often involves antiplatelet or anticoagulation therapy. Importantly, however, prospective, randomized data favoring a particular therapy do not exist. In the PFO in cryptogenic stroke study (PICCS) trial, of all patients with cryptogenic stroke and PFO enrolled, 17.9% of patients treated with aspirin had an event (stroke or death) over 2 years compared with 9.5% of patients treated with anticoagulation. This difference was not significant, as the total number of patients in either group and the number of events was too small to allow any conclusions regarding the efficacy of either agent.[15]

Migraine headaches and PFO

Occurring in approximately 17% of females and 6% of males, migraine headaches are characterized by unilateral, dull, and deep-throbbing crescendo headaches with slow but complete relief. Often, an "aura" consisting of vague visual, sensory, or gustatory symptoms may precede the headache by up to 60 min. With a median frequency of 1–5 episodes per month, migraine headaches are associated with significant disability and economic burden.[16–19]

Multiple reports demonstrate increased right–left shunting in patients with migraine headaches, particularly those with aura. The exact mechanism is unknown, but it is presumed that microemboli or vasoactive substances typically inactivated in the lungs enter the systemic circulation in an active form and lead to an aura.[20] In one study, Anzola and colleagues[21] examined 113 migraine patients with aura, 53 migraine patients without aura, and 25 healthy controls by transcranial Doppler and found right–left shunting in 48% of those with aura, 23% of those without aura, and 20% of healthy controls ($p < 0.001$ across groups).

Medical therapy for migraine headaches aims at acute treatment with pain medications and preventive management to decrease the frequency and intensity of recurrent events. Preventative medications include β-blockers, calcium channel blockers, tricyclic antidepressants, and serotonin antagonists. Relative to placebo, these strategies can result in 30–50% improvements in migraine symptoms, but curative therapy is rare.[22]

PFO closure

Although not without controversy, the fundamental indication for PFO closure is prevention of recurrent events. As medical therapy for secondary prevention of stroke or migraine is often suboptimal, and no medical therapy has been systemically studied in prospective, randomized trials, the possibility that a device implant may provide safe and effective closure of the PFO and prevent recurrent stroke or migraine is intuitively attractive. The extent to which intuition translates into actuality is a matter of considerable debate.

Cryptogenic stroke

As noted above, stroke is a leading cause of morbidity and mortality, and its occurrence leads to mental and physical disability and psychological stress, particularly regarding the possibility of a recurrent event. There is little argument that *any* modifiable risk factor should be addressed to reduce the risk of recurrent stroke, and in patients with cryptogenic stroke, PFO may be the only potentially modifiable risk factor. Therefore, as a safe and effective means to prevent further right–left shunting, PFO closure in patients with cryptogenic stroke appears both reasonable and appropriate.

The controversy lies in the fact that these associations are mostly circumstantial. Although there is a reasonable association between PFO and cryptogenic stroke, PFO is found incidentally in a significant proportion of the general population, many of these patients never develop stroke, and much of the evidence associating the two comes from case control as opposed to population-based studies.[12] Next, a right–left shunt cannot definitively be proven as the underlying etiology of many cryptogenic strokes, and many patients with stroke and PFO have additional risk factors for stroke. Additionally, in medically managed patients with cryptogenic stroke due to PFO, the recurrence rate is only about 2% per year.[15] Finally, although PFO closure is safe, it is neither risk free nor 100% effective as PFO closure has been associated with device embolization, erosion, thrombus formation, atrial arrhythmias, and residual shunting.[23]

Migraine headaches

The case with migraines is also uncertain. The initial association of PFO and migraine headaches was incidentally noted in a study of PFO closure for decompression sickness. In this study, of 37 patients who also had migraine headaches, 19 (45%) reported cessation of their headaches following PFO closure. Mechanistically, the correlation of PFO and migraine is interesting, particularly given the correlation of larger right–left shunts with migraine and stroke.[24] However, as with cryptogenic stroke, the association between PFO and migraine is more circumstantial than definitive.

Clinical trial results

The literature contains many case series and registries supporting the feasibility, efficacy, safety, and results of PFO closure with various devices (Figure 58.1), each to be discussed in separate chapters. Though some of these devices are approved and in use, significant controversy exists throughout the world. The roots of this controversy are looming questions regarding PFO as a true risk factor for stroke or migraine and the relative lack of prospective, randomized clinical evidence supporting PFO closure versus medical therapy.

Cryptogenic stroke

In 2007, a Food and Drug Administration (FDA) panel concluded that there was insufficient evidence to recommend for or against PFO closure in patients with cryptogenic stroke and PFO, and they strongly recommended enhanced efforts to enroll patients in randomized trials to demonstrate the role of PFO closure.[25] At the time, the primary evidence supporting PFO closure was a single-center study of 308 nonrandomized patients with cryptogenic stroke and PFO who underwent PFO closure ($n = 150$) or treatment with medical therapy ($n = 158$).[26] In this study, patients undergoing PFO closure had larger right–left shunts, and more prior events. At 4 year follow-up, there was a nonsignificant trend toward a reduction in strokes or transient ischemic attacks (TIAs) in patients who underwent closure compared with those treated with medical therapy (7.8% vs. 22.2%, respectively, $p = 0.08$).[26]

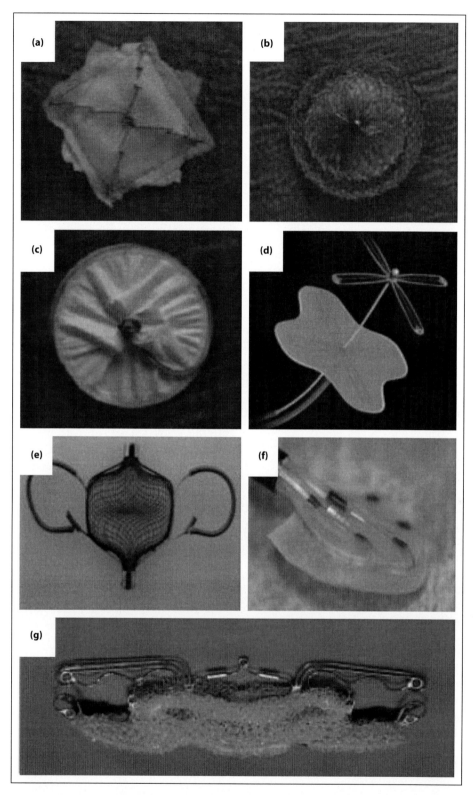

Figure 58.1   PFO devices. (a) NMT septal occluder (NMT Medical, MA, USA). (b) Amplatzer PFO occluder (AGA Medical, MN, USA). (c) HELEX septal occluder (WL Gore and Associates, AZ, USA). (d) Premere (St. Jude, MN, USA). (e) SeptRx (Secant Medical, PA, USA). (f) PFx (Cierra, CA, USA). (g) Coherex Flatstent (Salt Lake City, UT, USA).

More recent studies

In patients with cryptogenic stroke and PFO, the CLOSURE 1 (evaluation of the STARFlex septal closure system in patients with a stroke or TIA due to the possible passage of a clot of unknown origin through a PFO) represents the first large-scale, prospective, randomized trial evaluating PFO closure versus medical therapy.[27] Investigators randomized 909 patients with cryptogenic stroke or TIA and a PFO to device closure with the STARFlex (NMT Medical, Boston, MA) system ($n = 447$) or medical therapy ($n = 462$) consisting of warfarin (target INR 2.0–3.0), aspirin 325 mg, or a combination of aspirin 81 mg and warfarin to target International Normalized Ratio (INR). The choice of medical therapy was left to the investigators' discretion. By intention to treat analysis, there was no significant difference between groups in the primary combined endpoint of death, recurrent stroke, or TIA (5.5% closure, 6.8% medical, and $p = 0.37$) at 2 year follow-up.[27] Additionally, there were no differences in any of the individual endpoints, and there were no differences based on the type of analysis (intention to treat vs. per protocol) performed. Though CLOSURE 1 is a negative trial, controversy exists regarding whether these results reflect this particular device or PFO closure in general. Indeed, only 87% of cases were successful (lower than that seen in other studies), and complication rates were seemingly higher as well.[27]

More recently, a meta-analysis of 52 single-arm, seven nonrandomized comparative trials, and CLOSURE-1 was performed by Kitsios and colleagues.[28] Forty-nine of these studies included 7013 patients who underwent PFO closure, and 17 of these studies included 1903 patients treated with medical therapy. They concluded that recurrent stroke rates were 0.36 (0.24–0.56) in patients who underwent closure versus 2.53 (1.91–3.35) in patients treated medically ($p < 0.01$). Regarding medical therapy, anticoagulation appeared superior to antiplatelet therapy with rates of 1.27 (0.44–3.64) for anticoagulation compared with 3.17 (1.94–5.18) for antiplatelet therapy.[28]

At the 2012 Transcatheter Cardiovascular Therapeutics conference, two highly anticipated trials were presented. The randomized evaluation of recurrent stroke comparing PFO to established current standard-of-care treatment (RESPECT) trial evaluated 980 patients with cryptogenic stroke and PFO in the United States and Canada. Patients were randomized to medical therapy or PFO with the Amplatzer PFO device (St. Jude Medical, Minneapolis, MN).[29] Medical therapy included aspirin alone, warfarin alone, aspirin, or clopidogrel with dypyradimole and aspirin and clopidogrel. The primary endpoint was ischemic events over 2 year follow-up, and the event rate was lower in patients undergoing device closure (1.6%) than in the medical therapy arm (3.0%). This 46.6% relative reduction translates into an absolute reduction of 1.4% and a number needed to treat of 71.5, and it was not significant in the intention-to-treat analysis. However, in both the per-protocol and as-treated analyses, the benefit was more pronounced and statistically significant (Table 58.1).

Not surprisingly, the results of the RESPECT trial are subject to controversy when coupled with nuances in statistical design and scientific method. While it is difficult to ignore relative stroke reduction ranging from 46.6% to 72.7% in patients undergoing PFO closure, the low stroke rate in the medical therapy arm is also reassuring, the absolute magnitude of benefit is not quite as robust, and the overall adverse event rate between the two groups did not differ (23.0% closure vs. 21.6% medical, $p = NS$). Importantly, there were no instances of device thrombosis or erosion.[29]

The second randomized trial presented was the percutaneous treatment of foramen ovale versus medical treatment in patients with cryptogenic embolism (PC) trial.[30] In this study, 414 patients with stroke or TIA due to paradoxical thromboembolism were randomized to PFO closure with the Amplatzer PFO device ($n = 210$) or medical therapy ($n = 214$). The primary endpoint was a composite of death, stroke, TIA, or peripheral embolism over a mean of 4.5 years. Patients undergoing PFO closure had a 34% relative risk reduction in the primary endpoint (HR 0.63, 95% CI 0.24–1.62, and $p = 0.34$). As this difference was not significant, the authors concluded that PFO closure did not reduce recurrent events in patients with stroke due to paradoxical embolism. Of note, the lower than expected 4% event rate in the medical therapy arm raises the possibility that this study was underpowered to detect a difference between treatment arms.[30]

In aggregate, the above studies suggest that PFO closure is both safe and effective for secondary prevention of cryptogenic stroke. The low event rates seen in the single-center registries are reproduced in the randomized studies utilizing the Amplatzer device. Also evident, medical therapy in

Analysis	Description	Relative risk reduction (%)	p-value
Intent to treat	Patients counted based on how they are randomized, not on how they are treated	50.8	0.083
Per protocol	Patients counted by whether the protocol was followed	63.4	0.03
As treated	Patients counted by how they were treated	72.7	0.007

Table 58.1 Results of the RESPECT trial by analysis performed

the modern era results in favorable outcomes with event rates lower than expected in all three randomized studies. The GORE HELEX septal occluder for PFO closure in stroke patients (REDUCE) is another randomized trial that will shed further light on the subject.

Migraine Headaches

While numerous small series demonstrate improvements in migraine symptoms with PFO closure, only one prospective, randomized trial is published. The Migraine Intervention with STARFlex Trial (MIST) evaluated 432 eligible migraine-with-aura patients. Of these, 163 had transesophageal echocardiographic evidence of moderate–large shunts and 147 were randomized to PFO closure or a sham procedure with a primary endpoint of complete migraine cessation. There was no difference between groups in the primary endpoint, but, excluding two outliers, there was significant reduction in migraine frequency in the patients undergoing closure.[31]

Not surprisingly, controversies surrounding this trial include device selection and study design. The issues with device selection reflect those of CLOSURE 1, specifically, whether the STARFlex device is an appropriate measure of PFO closure safety and efficacy. Regarding the study design, many question the primary endpoint of complete migraine cessation. Given the debate regarding a truly "causal" role of PFO with migraine, and the largely retrospective evidence base suggesting improvement in migraine with aura following PFO closure, it is hoped that the prospective randomized investigation to evaluate incidence of headache reduction in subjects with migraine and PFO using the Amplatzer PFO occluder to medical management (PREMIUM) study will answer this question.

Conclusions

While PFO closure is largely considered safe and effective, questions remain regarding the pathophysiologic or causative role that PFO plays in various disease processes, particularly cryptogenic stroke and migraine headaches. Although several devices are approved for throughout the world, none of them definitively reduce recurrent events compared with medical therapy. Considering recently published and presented trials, it is unlikely that this will change anytime soon. For patients with recurrent events despite medical therapy, many agree that PFO closure is a reasonable option. However, for patients with a single cryptogenic stroke and PFO who have not been medically treated, the definitive role for PFO closure remains controversial and requires further study to fully define.

On another note, though not statistically significant, the RESPECT trial results can also be viewed favorably.

As medical therapy is imperfect, committing a patient to this without discussing PFO closure seems as premature as recommending first-line PFO closure. Perhaps, the best solution is consideration of individual patient factors, the likelihood of recurrent events, and the risks versus benefits of closure. Balanced patient discussion, a push for clinical trial enrollment, and thoughtful data interpretation will hopefully lead to more definitive data and improved long-term outcomes.

References

1. Meier B, Lock JE. Contemporary management of patent foramen ovale. *Circulation* 2003;107(1):5–9.
2. Hagen PT, Scholz DG, Edwards WD. Incidence and size of patent foramen ovale during the first 10 decades of life: An autopsy study of 965 normal hearts. *Mayo Clin Proc* 1984;59(1):17–20.
3. Knauth M, Ries S, Pohimann S, Kerby T, Forsting M, Daffertshofer M et al. Cohort study of multiple brain lesions in sport divers: Role of a patent foramen ovale. *BMJ* (Clinical Research ed.) 1997;314(7082):701–5.
4. Waight DJ, Cao QL, Hijazi ZM. Closure of patent foramen ovale in patients with orthodeoxia-platypnea using the Amplatzer devices. *Catheter Cardiovasc Interv* 2000;50(2):195–8.
5. Wilmshurst PT, Nightingale S, Walsh KP, Morrison WL. Effect on migraine of closure of cardiac right-to-left shunts to prevent recurrence of decompression illness or stroke or for haemodynamic reasons. *Lancet* 2000;356(9242):1648–51.
6. Webster MW, Chancellor AM, Smith HJ, Swift DL, Sharpe DN, Bass NM et al. Patent foramen ovale in young stroke patients. *Lancet* 1988;2(8601):11–2.
7. Sacco RL, Ellenberg JH, Mohr JP, Tatemichi TK, Hier DB, Price TR et al. Infarcts of undetermined cause: The NINCDS Stroke Data Bank. *Ann Neurol* 1989;25(4):382–90.
8. Rosamond W, Flegal K, Friday G, Furie K, Go A, Greenlund K et al. Heart disease and stroke statistics—2007 update: A report from the American Heart Association Statistics Committee and Stroke Statistics Subcommittee. *Circulation* 2007;115(5):e69–171.
9. Lechat P, Mas JL, Lascault G, Loron P, Theard M, Klimczac M et al. Prevalence of patent foramen ovale in patients with stroke. *N Engl J Med* 1988;318(18):1148–52.
10. Meissner I, Khandheria BK, Heit JA, Petty GW, Sheps SG, Schwartz GL et al. Patent foramen ovale: Innocent or guilty? Evidence from a prospective population-based study. *J Am Coll Cardiol* 2006;47(2):440–5.
11. Di Tullio MR, Sacco RL, Sciacca RR, Jin Z, Homma S. Patent foramen ovale and the risk of ischemic stroke in a multiethnic population. *J Am Coll Cardiol* 2007;49(7):797–802.
12. Davis D, Gregson J, Willeit P, Stephan B, Al-Shahi Salman R, Brayne C. Patent foramen ovale, ischemic stroke and migraine: Systematic review and stratified meta-analysis of association studies. *Neuroepidemiology* 2012;40(1):56–67.
13. Steiner MM, Di Tullio MR, Rundek T, Gan R, Chen X, Liguori C et al. Patent foramen ovale size and embolic brain imaging findings among patients with ischemic stroke. *Stroke* 1998;29(5):944–8.
14. De Castro S, Cartoni D, Fiorelli M, Rasura M, Anzini A, Zanette EM et al. Morphological and functional characteristics of patent foramen ovale and their embolic implications. *Stroke* 2000;31(10):2407–13.
15. Homma S, Sacco RL, Di Tullio MR, Sciacca RR, Mohr JP. Effect of medical treatment in stroke patients with patent foramen ovale: Patent foramen ovale in cryptogenic stroke study. *Circulation* 2002;105(22):2625–31.

16. Boureau F, Joubert JM, Lasserre V, Prum B, Delecoeuillerie G. Double-blind comparison of an acetaminophen 400 mg—Codeine 25 mg combination versus aspirin 1000 mg and placebo in acute migraine attack. *Cephalalgia* 1994;14(2):156–61.

17. Stewart WF, Shechter A, Rasmussen BK. Migraine prevalence. A review of population-based studies. *Neurology* 1994;44(6 Suppl 4):S17–23.

18. Silberstein SD. Migraine. *Lancet* 2004;363(9406):381–91.

19. Lipton RB, Hamelsky SW, Stewart WF. Epidemiology and impact of headache. In: Silberstein SD, Lipton RB, Dalessio DJ. Eds. *Wolff's Headache and Other Head Pain*. New York: Oxford University Press, 2001. pp. 85–107.

20. Schwerzmann M, Nedeltchev K, Meier B. Patent foramen ovale closure: A new therapy for migraine. *Catheter Cardiovasc Interv* 2007;69(2):277–84.

21. Anzola GP, Magoni M, Guindani M, Rozzini L, Dalla Volta G. Potential source of cerebral embolism in migraine with aura: A transcranial Doppler study. *Neurology* 1999;52(8):1622–5.

22. Ramadan NM, Schultz LL, Gilkey SJ. Migraine prophylactic drugs: Proof of efficacy, utilization and cost. *Cephalalgia* 1997;17(2):73–80.

23. Tobis J, Shenoda M. Percutaneous treatment of patent foramen ovale and atrial septal defects. *J Am Coll Cardiol* 2012;60(18):1722–32. Epub 10/09/2012.

24. Anzola GP, Morandi E, Casilli F, Onorato E. Different degrees of right-to-left shunting predict migraine and stroke: Data from 420 patients. *Neurology* 2006;66(5):765–7.

25. Slottow TL, Steinberg DH, Waksman R. Overview of the 2007 Food and Drug Administration circulatory system devices panel meeting on patent foramen ovale closure devices. *Circulation* 2007;116(6):677–82.

26. Windecker S, Wahl A, Nedeltchev K, Arnold M, Schwerzmann M, Seiler C et al. Comparison of medical treatment with percutaneous closure of patent foramen ovale in patients with cryptogenic stroke. *J Am Coll Cardiol* 2004;44(4):750–8.

27. Furlan AJ, Reisman M, Massaro J, Mauri L, Adams H, Albers GW et al. Closure or medical therapy for cryptogenic stroke with patent foramen ovale. *N Engl J Med* 2012;366(11):991–9. Epub 03/16/2012.

28. Kitsios GD, Dahabreh IJ, Abu Dabrh AM, Thaler DE, Kent DM. Patent foramen ovale closure and medical treatments for secondary stroke prevention: A systematic review of observational and randomized evidence. *Stroke* 2012;43:422–31.

29. Carroll JD, Saver JL, Thaler D, Smalling RW, Berry S, MacDonald LA et al. Eds. Randomized evaluation of recurrent stroke comparing PFO closure to established current standard of care treatment. *Transcatheter Cardiovascular Therepeutics*. Miami, FL: Boca Raton, 2012.

30. Meier B, Kalesan B, Khattab AA, Hildick-Smith D, Dudek D, Andersen G et al. Eds. Percutaneous closure of foramen ovale versus medical treatment in patients with cryptogenic embolism. The PC trial. *Transcatheter Cardiovascular Therapeutics*. Miami, FL: Boca Raton, 2012.

31. Dowson A, Mullen MJ, Peatfield R, Muir K, Khan AA, Wells C et al. Migraine Intervention with STARFlex Technology (MIST) trial: A prospective, multicenter, double-blind, sham-controlled trial to evaluate the effectiveness of patent foramen ovale closure with STARFlex septal repair implant to resolve refractory migraine headache. *Circulation* 2008;117(11):1397–404.

59

Patent foramen ovale closure: Amplatzer-type PFO occluders

Bernhard Meier and Fabien Praz

Introduction

The Amplatzer patent foramen ovale (PFO) occluder (St. Jude Medical, Plymouth, MN, USA) is derived from the Amplatzer atrial septal defect occluder. It consists of two flat self-expendable retention disks interconnected by a short, thin, and flexible waist. The disks are formed by 0.005 inch nitinol wire and filled with polyester fabric (Dacron). The currently available sizes are shown in Figure 59.1.

The world's first Amplatzer PFO occluder was implanted on September 10, 1997 (by this author in the presence of Kurt Amplatz). Owing to the remarkable device

performance and the ease of implantation, complete closure rate, and safety with the lowest incidence of embolization and thrombus formation,[1,2] it has since dominated all other techniques to close PFOs.

Technique of Amplatzer PFO occluder implantation

The main steps are summarized in Table 59.1. Some centers prefer to use echocardiographic guidance or size the PFO with a balloon. The most recent roughly 2000 PFO closures

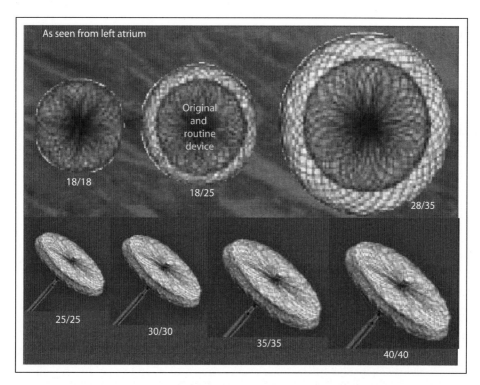

Figure 59.1 Amplatzer PFO occluders. Top row: original devices. Bottom row: cribriform devices with twin disks. The disk diameters are indicated in millimeters (left-sided disk first). Minimal required sheath size 8 French for the first 4 devices from the left, 9 French for the remainder, and 10 French for the device at the bottom right (1 French = 0.3 mm).

Table 59.1   Technique with Amplatzer PFO occluder
• Preintervention work-up preferably with TEE
• ≤1 night at hospital
• Local anesthesia
• No echocardiographic guidance
• Access: right femoral vein
• 0.035 inch ordinary (normal-length or exchange-length) guide wire
• Multipurpose or Judkins right coronary catheter to cannulate PFO unless guide wire alone passes easily
• No balloon sizing
• 9 French sheath accommodates most occluders
• Right atrial contrast injections (LAO cranial)
• Antibiotics (0–3 doses)
• Acetylsalicylic acid 100 mg (5 months) and clopidogrel 75 mg (1 month)
• Prophylaxis against endocarditis (for 2–6 months)

LAO = left anterior oblique; PFO = patent foramen ovale; TEE = transesophageal echocardiography.

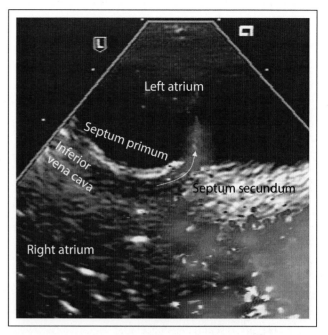

Figure 59.2   Transesophageal echocardiogram performed for suspicion of paradoxical stroke through a PFO, immediately after a prolonged Valsalva maneuver. The gray flame with the curved arrow indicates a temporary right-to-left shunt through the PFO.

at our center have been performed without these measures. In none of the rare problems encountered was it deemed that periprocedural echocardiography or balloon sizing would have been of help. Stripping the procedure to the bare essentials has allowed us to curb cost and reduce the procedure time to less than 30 min with only a short duration of fluoroscopy use.[3] This technique is being adopted by an increasing number of centers worldwide.

Echocardiographic properties relevant for PFO closure

The PFO can be passed with very few exceptions when it has unequivocally been demonstrated in a transesophageal echocardiogram at the preintervention work-up. Figure 59.2 shows the rare instance with a demonstrable color Doppler right-to-left shunt. Figures 59.3 through 59.5 show a PFO with transesophageal echocardiography, pointing out some of the salient features. False-negative diagnosis by transesophageal echocardiography may occur when the wrong echocardiographic plane was used for assessment, or with insufficient contrast medium (aerated saline, Hemaccel, Echovist, Levovist, etc.) concentration, absent or inadequate Valsalva maneuver, or poor coordination between Valsalva maneuver and contrast medium injection. The Valsalva maneuver should be maintained for at least 20 s. This results in reduced filling of the entire heart. At the release time of the Valsalva maneuver, the venous blood pooled in the lower body rushes back to the right atrium. This results in the right atrium being well filled, while the left atrium remains temporarily underfilled. The physiological situation will be reestablished a few seconds later, when the blood has circulated through the lungs. Hence, the bubbles typically pass the PFO only for a few heartbeats. This makes it even more important

to be ready in the optimal echocardiographic plane to catch and document the bubble passage. This plane is typically found somewhere with a 60°–90° flexing of the multiplanar probe.

Although the maximum PFO gaps can often be measured (Figure 59.5), they are of little value for PFO closure with the Amplatzer technique. First, PFO may be a slit of more than 20 mm length and the gap between the lips forming the valve-like PFO is smaller toward the edges of the slit. Second, when inserting a device to close a PFO, the septum primum will be pulled toward the septum secundum by the left atrial device before deploying the right atrial device. This can be compared with sticking a folded umbrella through a door that is ajar. When opening it on the other side of the door, and trying to pull the umbrella back through the door, the door will be pulled shut. It is irrelevant how far it can maximally be opened.

The presence and extent of a hypermobile septum primum (atrial septal aneurysm) (Figure 59.6), a Chiari network (Figure 59.7), or a Eustachian valve (Figures 59.8 and 59.9) can be nicely demonstrated by transesophageal echocardiography. Again they are not important for the Amplatzer technique, notwithstanding a few exceptions discussed below.

Occasionally, it is possible to diagnose a PFO quite reliably with transthoracic echocardiography. However, while the diagnosis of a floppy septum primum (atrial septal aneurysm) is quite easy by transthoracic echocardiography, PFOs are more difficult to document (Figure 59.10).

The less-invasive alternative, of transcranial Doppler ultrasound, can also be used for an accurate diagnosis of

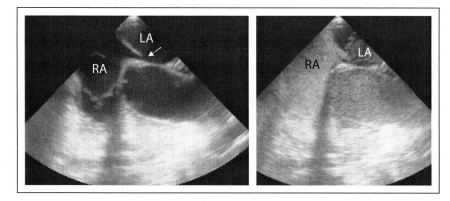

Figure 59.3 Transesophageal echocardiogram performed for demonstration of a PFO. Left: High suspicion of a PFO (arrow). Right: The PFO is ultimately proved by a bubble transit after a Valsalva maneuver. LA = left atrium; RA = right atrium.

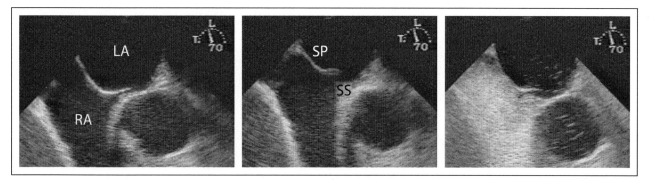

Figure 59.4 Transesophageal echocardiogram performed for demonstration of a PFO. Left: During the Valsalva maneuver, the septum primum is usually deviated toward the right atrium (RA). The picture indicates that a possible PFO will be of the tunnel type. Center: After releasing the Valsalva maneuver, the mobile septum primum (SP) moves away from the triangular wedge-like septum secundum (SS). This is highly suggestive of a PFO. Right: The arrival of contrast bubbles immediately after the release of the Valsalva maneuver and their passage through the PFO tunnel into the left atrium (LA) unequivocally document the PFO and reconfirm its tunnel shape.

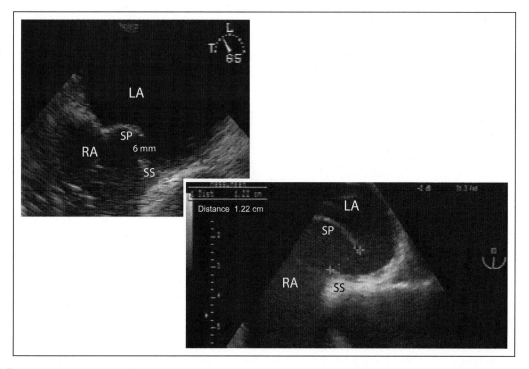

Figure 59.5 Attempts to echocardiographically size the maximum gap of PFOs after a proper Valsalva maneuver. The 6 mm and 1.22 cm distances between the edges of the septum primum (SP) and the septum secundum (SS) are not relevant for the technique or choice of device with Amplatzer PFO occluders. LA = left atrium; RA = right atrium.

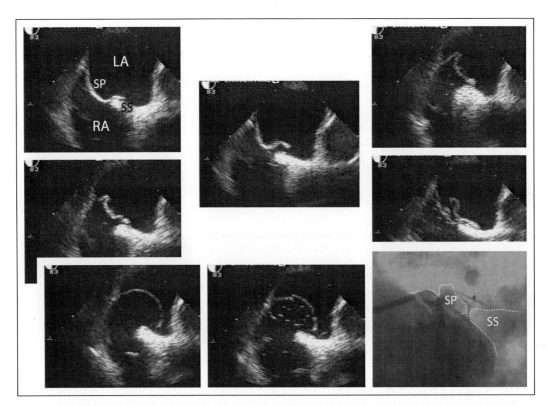

Figure 59.6 Atrial septal aneurysm, an expression of a redundant septum primum (SP), in different positions. While the position at the bottom left strongly suggests a PFO, its proof needs the visualizations of bubbles passing through the gap (bottom center). The insert at the bottom right shows a right atrial contrast injection during fluoroscopy, in this case after positioning a 35 mm Amplatzer PFO occluder in the projection used for the echocardiographic pictures. While the device sits tight on the tongue-like septum secundum (SS), the curtain-like SP is still undulating between the caudal disk halves (dotted lines). LA = left atrium; RA = right atrium.

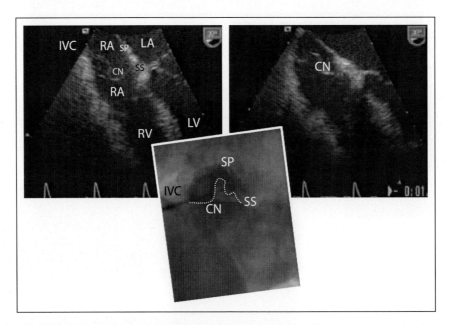

Figure 59.7 Transesophageal echocardiogram showing a Chiari network (CN). It is seen spanning the right atrium (RA) from the inferior vena cava (IVC) to the septum secundum (SS). It must not be confused with a mobile septum primum (SP), that is, an atrial septal aneurysm. In this patient, the SP is clearly distinguishable from the CN and immobile. The lower insert shows a right atrial contrast injection during fluoroscopy in the patient after implanting a 25 mm Amplatzer PFO occluder in the PFO using the same projection. Again it is important not to mix up the CN with the SP, which would lead to the misdiagnosis of erroneous placement of the caudal part of the device in the left atrium. LA = left atrium; LV = left ventricle, RV = right ventricle.

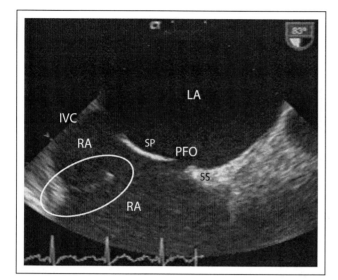

Figure 59.8 Transesophageal echocardiogram showing a Eustachian valve (circle) protruding from the lateral orifice of the inferior vena cava (IVC) toward the PFO or in this case a small ASD, because the septum primum (SP) falls short of reaching the septum secundum (SS). In contrast to the Chiari network, the Eustachian valve only partially traverses the right atrium (RA).

a right-to-left shunt, when screening for a PFO. It has been shown to have sensitivity comparable to transesophageal echocardiography in detecting and quantifying right-to-left shunts. An important disadvantage is the lack of anatomic information.

Implantation procedure

Different protocols exist for percutaneous Amplatzer PFO closures. The one used at our center (Table 59.1) has stood the test of time in more than 2000 implantations. It allows to accomplish the procedure in less than 30 min, with the patient returning to full physical activities a few hours later.[3]

The right femoral vein is punctured through a small skin incision and a regular 0.035 inch J-tip guide wire is advanced through the needle up to the right atrium. In about one-third of cases, it will pass the PFO easily, as the PFO is situated directly opposite the exit of the inferior vena cava into the right atrium. In the remainder of the cases, a multipurpose or right Judkins catheter is advanced directly through the skin without an introducer. With the catheter tip below the hepatic vein and pointing medially, the guide wire is advanced toward the atrial septum. This will cross the PFO in another one-third of the patients. Should that fail, the PFO is looked for usually in a frontal projection by sliding along the interatrial septum with the tip of the catheter pointing from 8 to 2 o'clock and torquing it in both directions, as soon as the tip gets caught in the region of the fossa ovalis. Occasionally, a straight guide wire or even a steerable coronary guide wire is required to negotiate the PFO. Other special technical details for crossing the PFO are discussed later. After the PFO is crossed, 5000 units of heparin are given. The guide wire in the left atrium allows the deployment sheath to be advanced into the left atrium. To make a place for it, the multipurpose catheter (if one had been used) is withdrawn into the inferior vena cava, but not

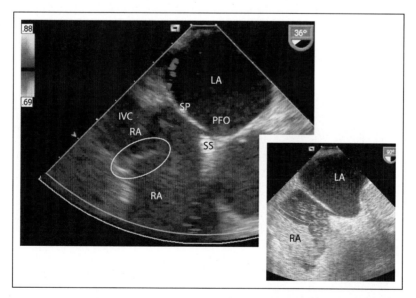

Figure 59.9 Transesophageal echocardiogram showing a Eustachian valve (circle) similar to the one in Figure 59.8 in the presence of a PFO. There is a spontaneous left-to-right shunt through the PFO (Doppler flow signal). The flow from the inferior vena cava (IVC) through the right atrium (RA) covering the Eustachian valve is shown by Doppler flow signals. The insert in the bottom right corner shows the situation during a bubble test with the Eustachian valve (outlined by a dotted line) separating the almost bubble-free inflow from the inferior vena cava from the bubble-laden blood coming from the superior vena cava (lower part of the right atrium). Some of the bubbles still manage to cross the PFO. It is understandable that in the presence of a Eustachian valve, a bubble study through the arm may be falsely negative and fail to diagnose a PFO. LA = left atrium; SP = septum primum; SS = septum secundum.

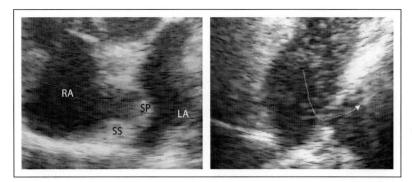

Figure 59.10 Transthoracic echocardiogram in an apical four-chamber view showing an atrial septal aneurysm (left) and a train of bubbles crossing the septum after Valsalva (dotted arrow, right). LA = left atrium; RA = right atrium; SP = septum primum; SS = septum secundum.

yet removed from the groin to prevent venous oozing while the Amplatzer PFO occluder is prepared.

A 9 French Amplatzer introducer set is opened. Although smaller devices require only an 8 French sheath, using a 9 French sheath allows free device selection. A larger PFO occluder may become necessary if the standard 25 mm occluder, with its 18 mm left-sided disk, is pulled through the PFO without having exerted exaggerated traction during an attempt to place it at the septum (Figure 59.11). Reasons to use a larger Amplatzer PFO occluder without first attempting a 25 mm device are the presence of a huge atrial septal aneurysm representing a risk of device embolization (Figure 59.6), an extremely long tunnel with the possibility of running out of material on the right disk of a 25 mm device before reaching the right atrium at the end of the tunnel (Figures 59.12 and 59.13), a particularly thick and triangular, lipomatous septum secundum, or rarely, in a case with a large aortic root protruding close to the fossa ovalis, the risk of aortic erosion by the disk rims (Figure 59.14).

The pusher cable is screwed into the central female screw of the right atrial disk of the Amplatzer PFO occluder. To make sure that it will unscrew properly at the time of release, the screw is completely tightened down, but then unscrewed half a turn. This typically produces an audible click, the first millimeter of unscrewing is the toughest in an analogy to automobile wheel nuts. The device is then pulled backward into the short loader sheath in a water bowl, then pushed out and retracted only once to eliminate air bubbles. Repeating this procedure may result in a doughnut shape of the right disk. The tip of the device is left protruding out of the loader a few millimeters, to avoid airspace between the loader tip and the tip of the device.

Once the device is loaded and ready, the catheter possibly used to pass the PFO is pulled out of the femoral vein. If a short 0.035 inch guide wire is being used, a liquid-filled syringe is attached to the end of the catheter at the time the wire disappears at its hub, while the tip of the catheter has not yet come out of the patient. With a powerful injection, the wire is kept across the interatrial septum, while completely withdrawing the catheter further until the tip is out. Sometimes, just swirling the catheter while retracting it suffices to avoid pulling the guide wire along. Such maneuvers are not necessary with a long guide wire. However, a long guide wire is more cumbersome throughout the remainder of the procedure. The bleeding ensuing after removal of the multipurpose catheter is scrutinized

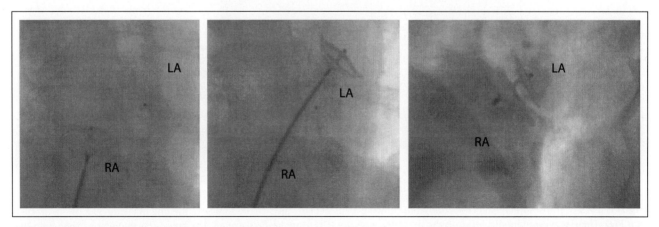

Figure 59.11 Hypermobile septum primum (atrial septal aneurysm) preventing anchorage of a 25 mm Amplatzer PFO occluder, which is dislocated into the right atrium (RA, left panel) or the left atrium (LA, center panel) at three consecutive deployment attempts. Substituting a 35 mm Amplatzer occluder solves the problem (right panel). The incorrect positions of the device are recognized by two criteria: (1) Parallel position of the disk with no space in between (well shown in center panel) and (2) free movability of the device away from the region of the interatrial septum.

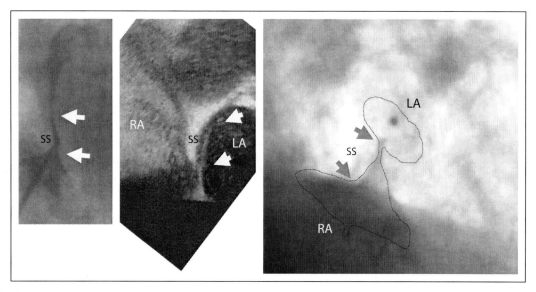

Figure 59.12   A long PFO tunnel (ends marked by arrows, left and center panel) requiring a 35 mm device (right panel). The angiographic (left and right panel) and the echocardiographic (center panel) pictures are aligned in a similar projection for easier understanding. LA = left atrium; RA = right atrium; SS = septum secundum.

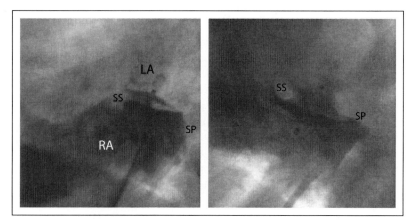

Figure 59.13   Incorrect position of a 25 mm Amplatzer PFO occluder (left panel). The septum secundum cannot be properly engaged because the septum primum (SP) yields easily, allowing the device to shift away from the septum secundum (SS). This is overcome by a 35 mm Amplatzer PFO occluder, in spite of continued significant indentation of the septum primum by the delivery catheter. LA = left atrium; RA = right atrium.

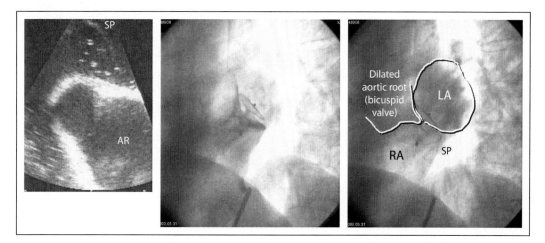

Figure 59.14   Implantation of a 35 mm Amplatzer PFO occluder (rather than a 25 mm) in a patient with a dilated aortic root because of a bicuspid valve. It was deemed that a larger device would embrace the aortic root rather than indenting it with its sharp rim, thereby decreasing the risk of erosion. The transesophageal echocardiographic picture on the left shows the dilated aortic root (AR), the mobile septum primum (SP), and bubbles passing through the PFO. The angiographic picture in a left anterior oblique projection is shown with and without labels. LA = left atrium, RA = right atrium.

for the absence of arterial blood. If arterial bleeding is seen, then this indicates that the puncture has been carried out traversing an artery to access the vein. In that case, a new puncture should be performed before introducing the 9 French sheath, to avoid an arteriovenous fistula.

The introducer sheath is advanced over the guide wire. While entering the groin, the end of the guide wire is moved in a to-and-fro fashion to avoid kinking of the guide wire at the tip of the sheath crossing the tissue and the wall of the vein. Once the tip of the sheath is within the vein, progress is easy and the wiggling of the guide wire maneuver can be stopped. Some operators prefer a stiff guide wire; however, the straight path of the PFO closure does not necessitate this.

The tip of the dilator in the sheath is stopped proximal to the end of the guide wire in the left atrium and the introducer sheath itself is advanced while keeping the dilator still. Once it has reached a position in the middle of the left atrium, the dilator and the guide wire are withdrawn, keeping the hub of the sheath below the level of the heart to avoid air being sucked into the sheath. The hub of the sheath is closed with a finger as soon as the obturator and the wire have been removed completely. When back bleeding from the sheath is copious, the sheath is flushed with a syringe of saline.

It has been recommended to leave the sheath tip in the right atrium, when removing the dilator and advance it only into the left atrium after it has been flushed. This may reduce the risk of air embolism into the left atrium. On the other hand, the mismatch between the small guide wire upon which the large bore sheath has to be advanced through the PFO occasionally precludes the advancement, as the rim may catch the edge of the septum secundum. Since air embolism has virtually been eliminated by using a sheath without a side port for the initial part of the procedure outlined above, this precaution appears to be no longer warranted.

Keeping the hub below the level of the heart—usually lateral to the right thigh—the short loader sheath with the device stretched out in it and protruding a few millimeters, is connected to the sheath placed in the left atrium, making sure that there is backflow from the sheath at the moment of attachment of the loader. The device is then advanced without fluoroscopy until half of the pusher cable has entered the sheath, after which fluoroscopy should be used.

A left anterior oblique cranial projection is ideal to position the device across the septum. In this projection, first, the left disk is pushed completely out of the sheath and the sheath and pusher cable are pulled back as a unit under fluoroscopic control. As soon as the left disk reaches the PFO and the septum, it will pull the valve closed and change the position of the disk to one that is parallel to the interatrial septum (Figure 59.15). Maintaining tension on the pusher cable, the sheath is withdrawn further until the right-sided disk is opened. Relaxing both the sheath and the cable, the right-sided disk will adapt itself to the right side of the interatrial

septum. The fluoroscopy angle is adjusted to profile the two disks perpendicularly as two parallel lines. These should form a V-shape open to the top left (Figures 59.14 and 59.15). This proves that the septum secundum is between the disks. Before releasing the device by unscrewing it counterclockwise, a small injection of contrast medium into the right atrium is performed (Figure 59.15). For this, the Y-connector (part of the delivery set) is inserted on the pusher cable and connected to the sheath. The sheath is then flushed. Initially, arterial blood remaining in the sheath from the left atrium will be aspirated followed by dark blood from the right atrium. The contrast medium injection will ascertain the correct position of the device (Figure 59.15), which then can be released. For documentation, an additional injection through the sheath may be performed, after readjusting the x-ray plane to see the device again in a perpendicular fashion, in case it has changed its angle at release (Figure 59.16).

The sheath is then removed and light manual pressure is maintained on the femoral vein. This may also be carried out by the patient. After keeping the groin still for about 1 hour, the patient can usually get out of bed, briefly again pressing on the groin, to prevent bleeding from the punctured vein due to the weight of the blood column from head to groin in the erect position. After that, the patient should be able to perform any type of physical activity, including driving, unless significant sedation or tranquilizer drugs have been administered.

During or before the intervention, an oral or intravenous antibiotic is administered, which may be repeated a few hours later and again the next morning, if the patient is still an inpatient. Acetylsalicylic acid (100 mg per day) and clopidogrel (75 mg per day) are prescribed starting on the day of the intervention for 5 and 1 months, respectively. The patient is instructed to observe the usual prophylaxis against endocarditis, at least for a couple of months. All medications can usually be stopped once an echocardiogram, preferably transesophageal, has proved a tight seal of the device, without any sign of thrombosis at least 4 months after the intervention.

Important points to check before releasing the device

A proof of correct positioning of the device, before its release from the pusher cable, is of paramount importance. While some centers deem transesophageal or intracardiac echocardiography necessary, we have defined a number of angiographic features that appear equally reliable and are easier to obtain. The most important one is the so-called Pacman sign,[4] explained in Figures 59.17 through 59.24. The angiographic examples convincingly demonstrate that the quality of the transesophageal echocardiographic demonstration of correct position (Figure 59.24) can be matched by angiography.

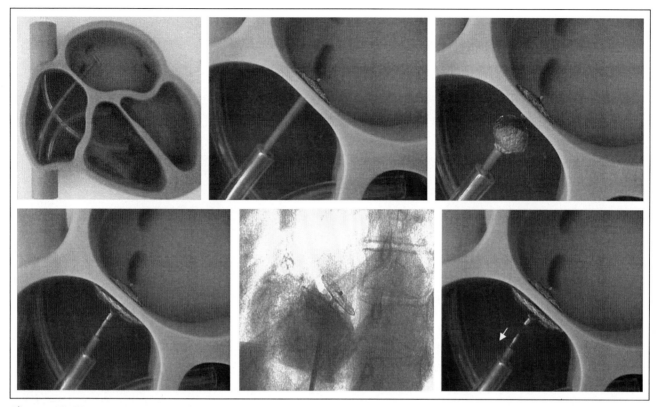

Figure 59.15 Steps for implantation of a 25-mm Amplatzer PFO occluder from top left to bottom right. After placing an 8 French introducer centrally in the left atrium, the left-sided disk (diameter 18 mm) is deployed (top left) and the introducer and device are pulled back as a unit until stopped by the septum (top center). While keeping traction on the pusher cable, the right-sided disk is opened (top right). Relaxing the introducer and the pusher cable allows the right-sided disk to adapt to the septum (bottom left). Before releasing the device, an injection of at least 10 mL of contrast medium through the introducer in a projection delineating the device as two parallel disks, usually left anterior oblique with cranial tilt, is used to ascertain the correct position of the device (bottom center). Finally the device is released by unscrewing it from the pusher cable (arrow, bottom right).

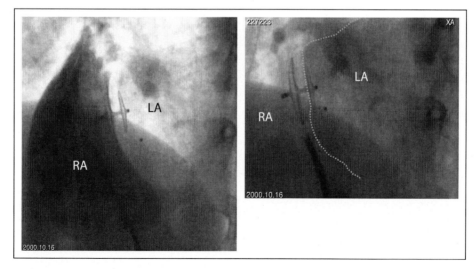

Figure 59.16 Angiographic documentation of Amplatzer PFO occlusion by injections of contrast medium through the introducer in a left anterior oblique projection with cranial angulation. The right atrium (RA) is clearly delineated (left panel). After the contrast has passed through the lungs (levophase), the left atrial border is also visible (right panel, dotted line) albeit more faintly. LA = left atrium.

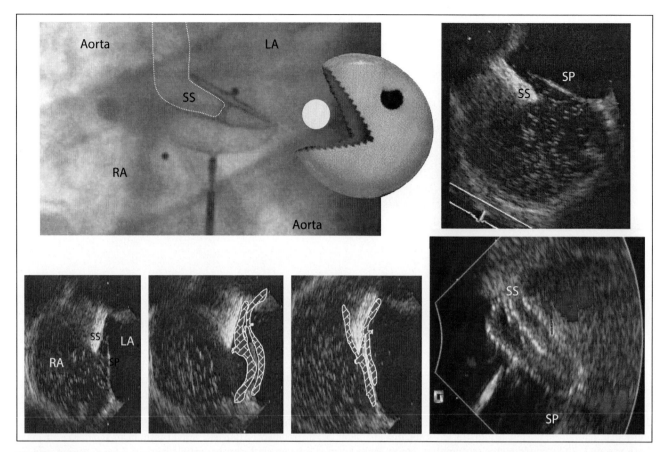

Figure 59.17   Pacman sign for correct placement of PFO occluder. The top left panel shows a 25 mm Amplatzer PFO occluder placed correctly. Even without dye injection, the V-shape of the two disks can be appreciated. Separation of left side of the disk is caused by the muscular septum secundum (dotted outline) while the paper-thin septum primum to the right does not separate the two disks. The right panels show the transesophageal echocardiographic picture in an analogous projection without (top) and with (bottom) the device. The bottom left panels show the echocardiographic situation in the projection used angiographically with an incorrect (center) and correct (right) superimposed Amplatzer PFO occluder. LA = left atrium; RA = right atrium; SP = septum primum; SS = septum secundum.

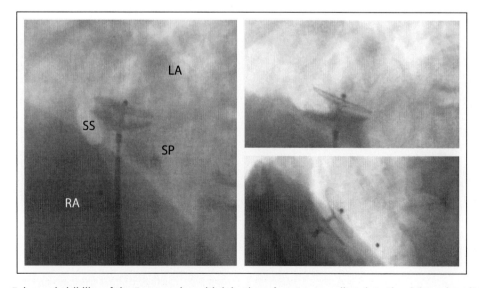

Figure 59.18   Enhanced visibility of the Pacman sign with injection of contrast medium into the right atrium (RA). The uvula-like septum secundum (SS) is clearly delineated by the contrast medium. On the left, it is not between the two disks of this 18-mm Amplatzer PFO occluder. The right disk had to be withdrawn into the introducer and again released with more tension to obtain the correct position (right) before (top) and after (bottom) release. LA = left atrium; SP = septum primum.

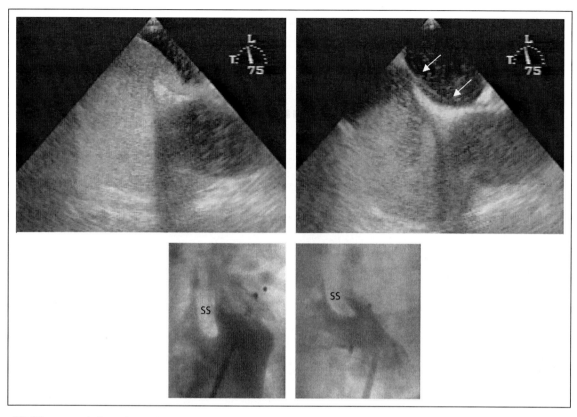

Figure 59.19   Tunnel-shaped PFO demanding particular attention to the Pacman sign. Top panels: Transesophageal echocardiography with bubble test. The right panel exhibits the length of the tunnel (arrows). A first attempt with a 25 mm Amplatzer PFO occluder resulted in a negative Pacman sign (bottom left). This could be corrected by withdrawal and redeployment of the right disk (right panel).

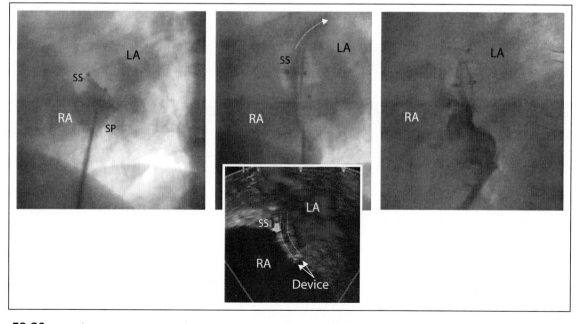

Figure 59.20   Amplatzer 18 mm PFO occluder erroneously released without a reliable Pacman sign. Left panel: the right atrial disk of the device is merely indenting rather than straddling the septum secundum (SS). After release from the pusher cable, the right atrial disk slips into the PFO tunnel, resulting in a significant residual shunt (center panel, arrow). The device should have been replaced for a 25 mm PFO occluder to safely embrace the septum secundum before release. The residual shunt was still present at the 6 month follow-up transesophageal echocardiogram (bottom insert). At that time it was remedied with the implantation of a second Amplatzer PFO occluder (right panel). LA = left atrium; RA = right atrium; SP = septum primum.

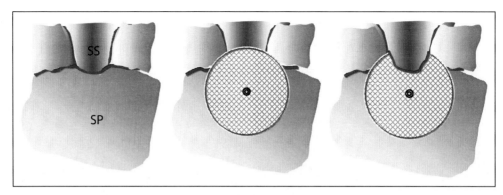

Figure 59.21   Artist's rendering of the Pacman sign, as seen from right atrium in Figures 59.17 through 59.20. The tongue-like septum secundum (SS) encompasses only a small segment of the upper septum (left). The correct position of the Amplatzer occluder is depicted in the center and the incorrect position in the right panel. Although there is no real risk of complete embolization of the device, the incorrect position harbors a high propensity of a residual shunt (Figure 59.20).

Complications and follow-up examinations after Amplatzer PFO occlusion

It is recommendable to perform a transesophageal echocardiogram at 4–6 months after the device implantation (Figure 59.25).

Although the rapidity of endocardial coverage of the device may vary, animal studies and examinations of devices, removed at different time periods after implantation, proved that coating with fibrinogen occurs within the first hours and endocardialization is complete at the latest at 4 months (Figure 59.26).

Thrombotic problems with the Amplatzer occluders are rare. This constitutes one of the significant advantages of this device over other devices.[1] In our personal experience, with over 2000 Amplatzer occluders and routine 6 month follow-up transesophageal echocardiography, three cases with thrombus on the device were found (Figure 59.27). In two cases, the thrombus resolved after vitamin K antagonist oral anticoagulation for 3–6 months. The third patient

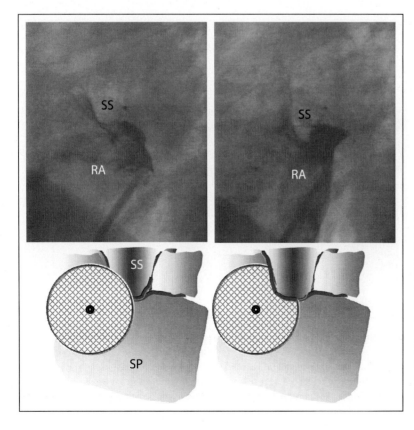

Figure 59.22   Situation with a partially prolapsing Amplatzer PFO occluder at the septum secundum (SS). An eccentric placement of the device is visible by a contrast medium injection into the right atrium (RA, top panels). At first, a correct sandwich position of the septum secundum between the two disks appears. However, during washout of the dye, a lateral prolapse of the septum secundum beyond the right atrial disk becomes apparent. The situation is schematically explained (bottom panel) with the potential risk of partial prolapse of the right atrial disk into the left atrium like the case in Figure 59.20 (bottom right). SP = septum primum.

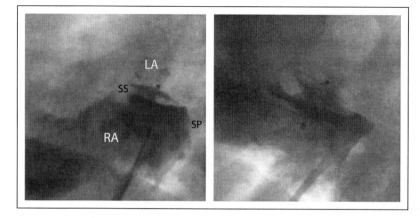

Figure 59.23   Rare occasion, in which a 25 mm Amplatzer PFO occluder is too small to produce a positive Pacman sign (left, septum secundum [SS]) and cannot be straddled between the disks. This is remedied by replacing it with a 35 mm Amplatzer PFO occluder (right). LA = left atrium; RA = right atrium; SP = septum primum.

was orally anticoagulated for a year but the findings of the thrombus persisted. The patient has been followed conservatively for over 10 years with no clinical events. Late thrombus formation, several years after implantation, has been reported only in a few cases worldwide with different devices, including one case after PFO closure using an Amplatzer septal occluder (8 mm).

Erosion of the superior atrial wall, left or right, into the pericardium or into the aorta, has been described with most devices, including the Amplatzer PFO occluder. Its incidence is estimated to range between 0.01% and 0.03%.[5] Debate is ongoing whether the risk of such a complication depends on the size of the device. It is likely that a device, not in contact with the aorta, will be less prone for erosion as the main mechanism is rubbing against the pulsating aorta. On the other hand, a small device may have a higher risk of incomplete closure of the PFO, although it may not always be necessary to cover the entire width of

the mouth of the PFO, as closing one half of a valve should prevent the other half from opening. A large device might embrace the aorta rather than poking it with its sharp edge and, therefore, may also have less propensity for erosion. The complete occlusion rate may be jeopardized, because of failure of a large device to hug the interatrial septum. The advantages or disadvantages of small or large devices are explained in Figure 59.28. A reasonable compromise is to use the 25-mm Amplatzer PFO occluder for the routine case. It is fairly reliable in establishing a positive Pacman sign during implantation; it has a low, albeit not zero, risk of eroding the aorta and a high potential for complete or sufficient coverage of the PFO mouth, with >90% complete and permanent closure of the PFO.

In our experience, residual shunts occur in about 8% of the patients, requiring implantation of a second device in about 3%. Importantly, the incidence of residual shunts is strongly device-dependent, reaching up to 30% with some

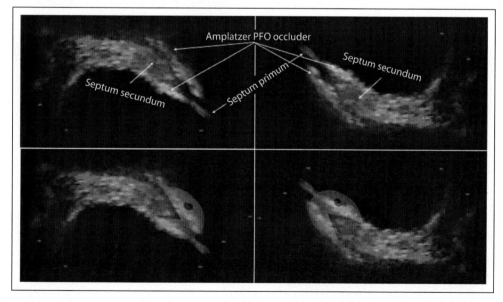

Figure 59.24   **(See color insert.)** Left: Demonstration of a positive Pacman sign by transesophageal echocardiography in the projection usually seen during fluoroscopy. The bottom panel explains where the name "Pacman sign" derives from. Right: The same situation seen in the projection typical for transesophageal echocardiography.

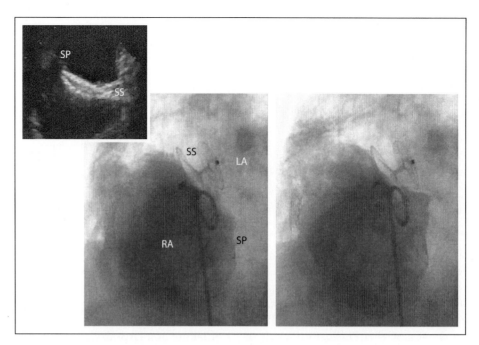

Figure 59.25 Transesophageal echocardiography (left top) and right atrial angiography (right bottom) examination at 6 month follow-up after successful and complete PFO closure with a 25 mm Amplatzer PFO occluder. The left angiographic picture is taken during and the right after a prolonged Valsalva maneuver. While the septum secundum (SS) remains immobile, the thin and flaccid septum primum (SP, atrial septal aneurysm) is pushed toward the right atrium (RA) during and freely prolapses into the left atrium (LA) after the Valsalva maneuver.

of the other devices. Several mechanisms have been considered to explain incomplete closure, with the most common one being an inadequate large device placed eccentrically (Figures 59.21, 59.22, 59.28, and 59.29). Other predictors of residual shunt have been discussed, including the presence of an atrial septal aneurysm or a Eustachian valve, large defects, and device size >30 mm.[3] The options for remedy are limited to implantation of a second device allowing complete closure in nearly all the patients (Figure 59.29).

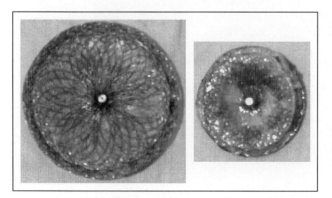

Figure 59.26 Endothelialization depicted on the example of two Amplatzer atrial septal defect occluders (same material as PFO occluders) removed at different times (seen from right atrial view). On the left is a 34 mm device removed 5 h after implantation. It already shows homogeneous coverage with fibrin. On the right is a 24 mm device removed at 4 months. It shows complete coverage with a glistening new endocardium.

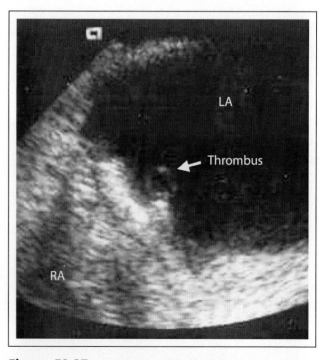

Figure 59.27 Drop-like mobile but organized thrombus attached to the left-sided nipple of an Amplatzer 25 mm PFO occluder at a 6 month follow-up transesophageal echocardiogram. The right atrium (RA) is filled with bubbles and proving the tightness of the occlusion, as no bubbles transit into left atrium (LA).

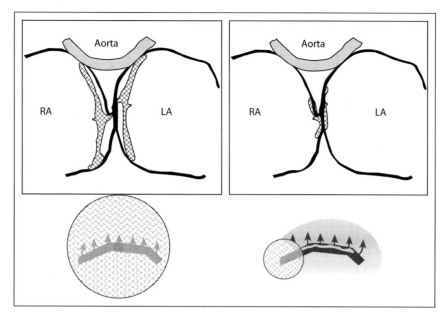

Figure 59.28 Depiction of advantages and disadvantages of large and small PFO occluder devices. Left: The large device will fairly reliably cover the entire PFO mouth (bottom). However, it will not be hugging the septum in a snug fashion and it has the potential of eroding the atrial wall, while rubbing against the aorta. Right: A small device will conform perfectly to the septum and be devoid of the risk of eroding the atrial wall. However, it may only cover part of the PFO mouth (bottom), particularly when placed eccentrically, which cannot be avoided by fluoroscopy or by transesophageal echocardiography during implantation.

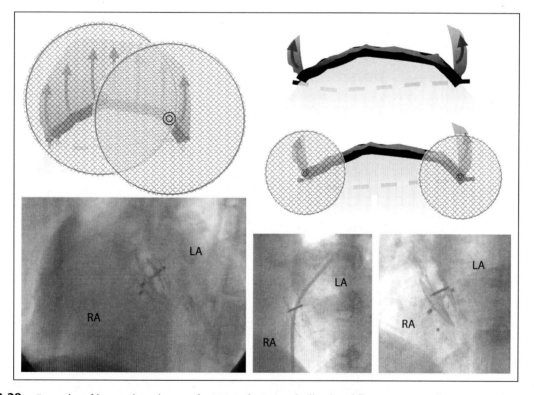

Figure 59.29 Examples of incomplete closure of a PFO. Left: Eccentrically placed first 25 mm Amplatzer PFO occluder is too small to cover the entire width of the PFO. The PFO can be completely closed by implantation of a second occluder. Right top: Most of the PFO is fused except for the two edges of the mouth. This is best treated by two small devices being implanted separately (right center). The bottom left panel shows the aspect of two 25 mm Amplatzer PFO occluders side by side with the contour of the right atrium (RA) delineated by contrast medium. The bottom right panels show the implantation of a 25 mm Amplatzer PFO occluder to correct a leaky PFO-Star occluder implanted several months earlier (left: introducer across the septum through the PFO-Star occluder, right: Amplatzer PFO occluder straddling the PFO-Star occluder). The left atrium (LA) is faintly outlined by contrast medium.

Another important concern is new-onset atrial fibrillation following PFO closure, because it has the potential to provoke cerebral events. Its incidence has been reported from 7–15%, but this was similar to that in patients with a stroke of non-PFO etiology. The presence of a device or its size has not been identified as a predictor or producer of atrial fibrillation, although it may well be.[6]

Patients with a known nickel allergy can develop transient chest pain and pericardial effusion, probably due to excessive inflammatory response. This has rarely led to surgical device explantation.[5]

Use of the Amplatzer atrial septal defect occluder for PFO closure

In some patients, the septum primum does not reach the septum secundum, thereby resulting in a secundum atrial septal defect. If the gap is just a few millimeters by transesophageal echocardiography, we generally use a PFO device. Gaps >10 mm may be better treated with balloon sizing and an appropriate-sized atrial septal defect device. The concept of opening the PFO to a maximum and then closing it with an appropriate-sized atrial septal defect device will be free of the risk of eccentric placement and incomplete coverage as may happen with PFO occluders. However, in longish PFO tunnels, it will deploy rather awkwardly (Figure 59.30).

Pitfalls of Amplatzer PFO occluder implantation

A high-quality transesophageal echocardiogram may alert the operators to most of the potential pitfalls before the

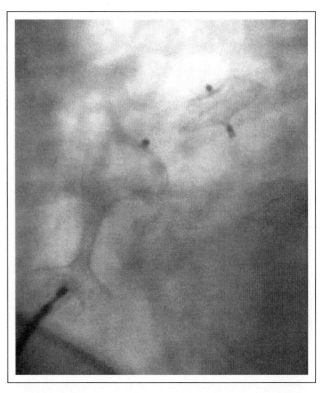

Figure 59.30   Poor choice of device. A 15 mm Amplatzer atrial septal defect occluder was used to close a funnel-shaped PFO. While it occluded the PFO, the left atrial disk remained distorted. A 10 mm Amplatzer atrial septal defect occluder had been previously placed in the left atrial appendage to avoid anticoagulation in this 70-year-old patient with atrial fibrillation and a history of coumadin necrosis. The 15 mm Amplatzer atrial septal defect occluder device had been found to be too large for the left atrial appendage and was afterward employed for the PFO closure for availability.

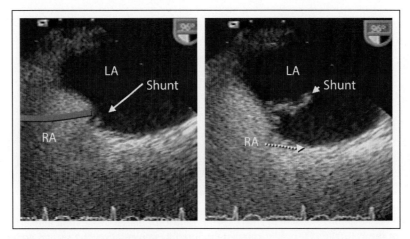

Figure 59.31   Impossibility to cannulate a PFO suspected from clearly demonstrated bubbles crossing on transesophageal echocardiography. The left panel shows a bubble about to cross close to the junction of the septum secundum with the septum primum, which is aneurysmal (left side). The right panel shows more bubbles appearing in the left atrium, but this time their point of transit is less clear. It was impossible to cannulate the suspected hole because the catheter (superimposed in the left panel) wound up in the aneurysmatic pouch when looking for the hole and the actual foramen ovale canal (dotted arrow) proved tight.

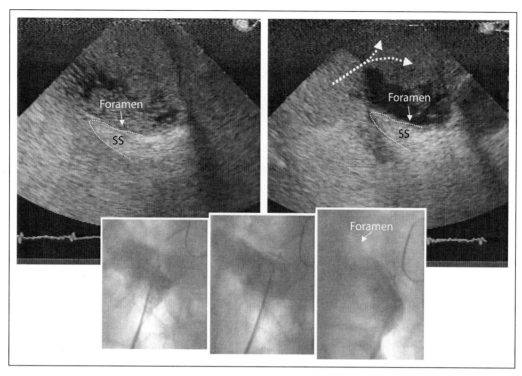

Figure 59.32 In a case similar to the one in Figure 59.31, the transesophageal bubble passage looked straightforward. However, when checking for the initial bubble transit, it clearly indicated that the passage was through a small hole in the redundant septum primum (dotted arrows) rather than through the foramen, which was tight. The small atrial septal defect in the aneurysmal septum primum could be cannulated and a 25 mm Amplatzer PFO occluder was inserted. The completely parallel position of the two disks (negative Pacman sign) in addition to the fact that the device appeared to be in the right atrium rather than at the level of the septum (bottom left) were explained by the fact, that the hole was not the PFO but a small atrial septal defect in a redundant septal aneurysm. Pushing the device toward the left atrium proved that it was indeed at the level of the septum (bottom center). The final position showed it in the middle of the septum primum at a clear distance from the foramen (bottom right). The half circle in the top right corner of the bottom panels is a Carpentier–Edwards ring after mitral valve reconstruction. SS = septum secundum.

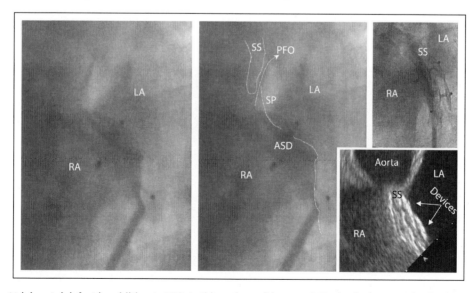

Figure 59.33 Atrial septal defect in addition to PFO. In this patient with a true PFO, the device was mistakenly placed in an unrecognized small ASD (left). The anatomy is outlined in the center panel, showing that the PFO remains open. The situation can be suspected, diagnosed, and corrected without the need of echocardiography on the basis of the parallel position of the two disks and the residual shunt to the left of the implanted device. A second 25 mm Amplatzer PFO occluder implanted through the PFO corrected the problem (right top). An 8 month follow-up transesophageal echocardiogram shows the two PFO occluders, one in the atrial septal defect and the other in the PFO, and documents complete closure of both holes (right bottom).

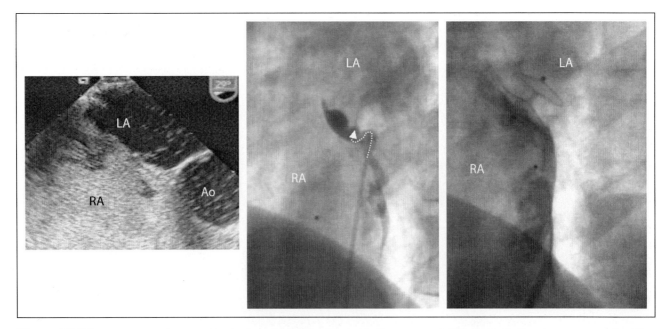

Figure 59.34   Bubble transit suggestive, but not diagnostic of a PFO (left). Because of difficulty in finding the passage, a dye injection into the foramen was carried out, revealing a pinhole leaving the canal perpendicularly (probably in a corner of the foramen) (center). Passage could be negotiated with a Judkins right coronary catheter (center) and the foramen was closed with a 25 mm Amplatzer PFO occluder (right). AO = aorta; LA = left atrium; RA = right atrium.

procedure. Figure 59.19 shows the case of a particularly long tunnel that required an increased pull, while deploying the right-sided disk to create the Pacman sign. Such a situation may give rise to selecting a 35 mm Amplatzer PFO occluder from the beginning (Figure 59.12).

On the other hand, even a high-quality transesophageal echocardiogram may be misleading. Unless the bubble passage through the gaping PFO was clearly demonstrated, difficulties or failures to cannulate may occur. Figures 59.31 through 59.34 demonstrate such examples.

Figure 59.35 depicts a case, in whom a persistent left superior vena cava was mistaken for a large atrial septal defect at transesophageal echocardiography, performed because of a cryptogenic stroke. The diagnosis was

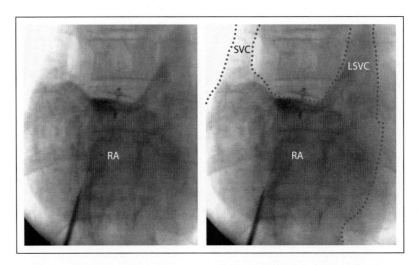

Figure 59.35   A 61-year-old woman with cardiomegaly on x-ray and a cryptogenic stroke. Transthoracic echocardiography misdiagnosed a persistent left superior vena cava (LSVC) as a 2 cm atrial septal defect. The atrial septal defect was deemed the culprit for paradoxical embolism. A bubble study was not done due to the mistakenly assumed left-to-right shunt, which in fact was the venous inflow into the right atrium (RA). During attempted closure of the presumed atrial septal defect, the LSVC was recognized in addition to the normal superior vena cava (SVC). To account for the cryptogenic stroke, a PFO was looked for, found, and occluded with a 25 mm Amplatzer PFO occluder. It assumed a horizontal position due to the anomalous anatomy.

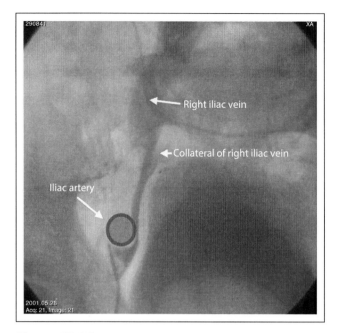

Figure 59.36 Thrombosed right iliac vein. The PFO could be occluded by accessing the right iliac vein through a collateral. The access was further complicated by the fact that the collateral circled around a tortuous iliac artery.

angiographically modified during the planned atrial septal defect closure. Incidentally, a PFO was found and it was successfully closed.

As with all procedures requiring venous access to the heart, local venous anomalies or thromboses may cause

difficulties for the interventional cardiologist (Figure 59.36). Cannulation and closure of the PFO is easiest from the right femoral vein. However, it can also be accomplished from the left femoral vein or a vein of the upper half of the body.

If it is impossible to unscrew the pusher cable from the device because the device rotates in unison with the cable, the introducer should be pushed firmly against the device, perhaps even invaginating a part of the right atrial disk, while unscrewing the pusher cable. This increases friction and tends to keep the device from rotating (Figure 59.37). If this maneuver fails, the device will have to be removed and unscrewed outside the body the first quarter turn and then reinserted.

In the rare case of premature release of the device during deployment or embolization subsequently, Amplatzer devices are best retrieved by a Dotter basket, a gooseneck snare, a wire loop, or biopsy forceps (Figure 59.38) and brought into an easily accessible place, where an attempt should be made to either capture the female plug on the right atrial disk with a catheter, reinsert the screw of the pusher cable, or capture the female plug at its neck with a biotome or a gooseneck snare. The latter grip may still not allow the device to be retrieved back into an introducer, as the female screw may approach obliquely at the entrance of the introducer. Cutting off the tip of the introducer obliquely enlarges the entry. In some cases, it may only be possible to retract the device to the femoral vein (or artery) from where it will have to be removed with a surgical cutdown.

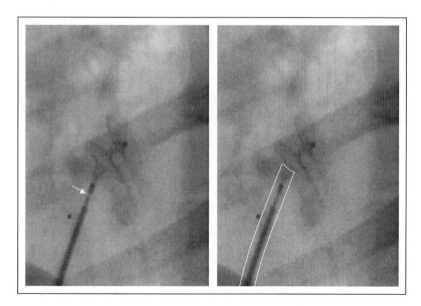

Figure 59.37 Difficulty in deploying an 18 mm Amplatzer PFO occluder, because the device keeps rotating in concert with the pusher cable when the operator trying to unscrew it. By pulling part of the right disk back into the sheath (outlined in the right panel), the device could be immobilized and deployment was successful. This problem occurs more often with small devices (less friction against the tissue) and can be prevented by releasing the device half a turn before inserting it into the sheath or before exiting the sheath. On the other hand, before advancing an Amplatzer device out of the sheath, it should always be ascertained, that the pusher is not already halfway unscrewed, as in this picture showing the thin screw appearing between the female screw of the device and the solid part of the pusher cable (arrow in left panel).

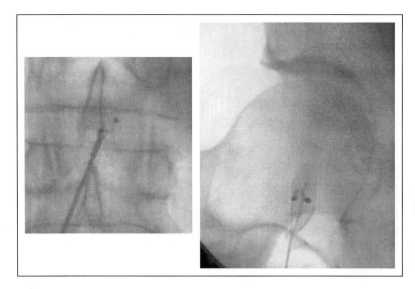

Figure 59.38 Attempt to grab an embolized Amplatzer occluder by its female plug with a bioptome (left) in the descending aorta. As the grip was not strong enough to pull it back into an sheath, the device was caught between the disks with a wire loop and pulled into the femoral artery (right) from where it was removed with a cutdown.

Incidental angiographic diagnoses of PFO

In patients needing cardiac catheterization for another reason, in particular, right heart catheterization patients in whom the suspicion of a PFO arises without prior diagnostic transesophageal echocardiogram, for example, during percutaneous coronary intervention (PCI) for acute myocardial infarction; (Figures 59.39 and 59.40), or patients either refusing transesophageal echocardiography or yielding a questionable finding, the PFO can easily be sought for, documented (Figures 59.39 and 59.40), or excluded (Figure 59.41) by direct angiography.

Occasionally, angiography may have to be used to correct an erroneous diagnosis of a PFO by echocardiography (Figure 59.41). Such echocardiographic errors are due

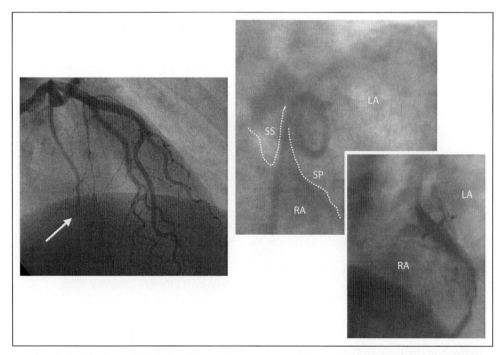

Figure 59.39 Acute myocardial infarction in a 34-year-old woman with no risk factors. The infarction was caused by an embolic occlusion of a small left circumflex coronary artery (left panel, arrow). The patient underwent emergency catheterization at 2 am. The most likely reason for such a situation is a PFO. It was looked for, found, and documented with a pigtail catheter straddling it (center panel). It took about 5 min to occlude it with a 25 mm Amplatzer PFO occluder. The PFO closure prolonged the procedure by less than 30 min. LA = left atrium; RA = right atrium; SP = septum primum; SS = septum secundum.

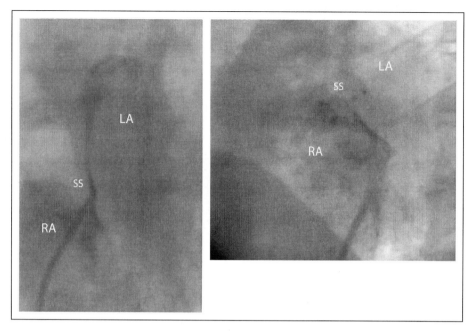

Figure 59.40   Documentation and impromptu closure of PFO suspected in a 53-year-old man referred for emergency coronary angioplasty because of an acute myocardial infarction showing an embolic occlusion of a coronary artery without atherosclerosis, which raised the suspicion of a PFO. The PFO was looked for, found, and closed during the same emergency catheterization session. The documentation occurred with a multipurpose catheter (left panel) depicting a tunnel PFO when injecting with the tip leaning against the septum secundum (SS). A 25 mm Amplatzer PFO occluder was implanted (right panel). LA = left atrium; RA = right atrium.

to overinterpretation of bubbles appearing late in the left atrium, shunts or normal connections in the pulmonary circulation, or shunts in other places of the interatrial septum (Figures 59.31 and 59.32). In particular, the appearance of exclusively small bubbles in the left atrium after more than four heartbeats does not indicate the presence of a PFO.

General remarks

Several observational studies and meta-analyses have established the superiority of percutaneous PFO closure over medical treatment. The results of two randomized trials performed with the Amplatzer PFO closure device have become available and confirm the trend toward

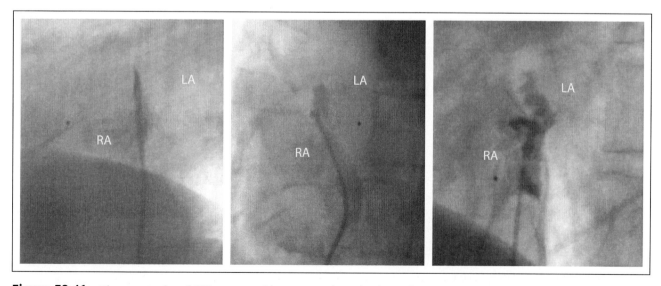

Figure 59.41   Three examples of PFOs suspected by transesophageal echocardiography, but not present. A dye injection into the fossa ovalis depicts the tunnel of the PFO with no exit into the left atrium in all three cases (left: left anterior oblique projection; center and right: frontal projection). LA = left atrium, RA = right atrium.

superiority. The RESPECT trial was a prospective randomized multicenter event-driven trial involving 69 centers in the United States.[7] Although the primary analysis (intention to treat cohort) was not statistically significant, secondary analysis (e.g., as per protocol or as treated cohort) clearly supports a better outcome for the closure group. A stroke risk reduction of 47–73% was observed in the analyses. Another multicenter randomized trial, the PC trial,[8] has corroborated these findings, showing a relative stroke risk reduction of 80% after percutaneous PFO closure, which did not reach statistical significance, probably due to lack of power.

To occlude a PFO with an Amplatzer PFO occluder is currently the easiest therapeutic catheter intervention known to adult cardiologists. This will help in coping with the possibly increasing number of patients who may be referred for PFO closure. Theoretically, 25% of the population could undergo the procedure if a PFO were to be considered a hazard ominous enough to warrant primary prevention with implantation of a device in the heart.[4]

References

1. Krumsdorf U, Ostermayer S, Billinger K, Trepels T, Zadan E, Horvath K et al. Incidence and clinical course of thrombus formation on atrial septal defect and patient foramen ovale closure devices in 1000 consecutive patients. *J Am Coll Cardiol* 2004;43(2):302–9.
2. Taaffe M, Fischer E, Baranowski A, Majunke N, Heinisch C, Leetz M et al. Comparison of three patent foramen ovale closure devices in a randomized trial (Amplatzer versus CardioSEAL-STARflex versus Helex occluder). *Am J Cardiol* 2008;101(9):1353–8.
3. Wahl A, Tai T, Praz F, Schwerzmann M, Seiler C, Nedeltchev K et al. Late results after percutaneous closure of patent foramen ovale for secondary prevention of paradoxical embolism using the Amplatzer PFO occluder without intraprocedural echocardiography: Effect of device size. *J Am Coll Cardiol Cardiovasc Interv* 2009;2(2):116–23.
4. Wahl A, Meier B. Patent foramen ovale and ventricular septal defect closure. *Heart* 2009;95(1):70–82.
5. Verma SK, Tobis JM. Explantation of patent foramen ovale closure devices: A multicenter survey. *J Am Coll Cardiol Cardiovasc Interv* 2011;4(5): 579–5.
6. Burow A, Schwerzmann M, Wallmann D, Tanner H, Sakata T, Windecker S et al. Atrial fibrillation following device closure of patent foramen ovale. *Cardiology* 2008;111(1):47–50.
7. Carroll JD, Saver JL, Thaler DE, Smalling RW, Berry S et al. Randomized evaluation of recurrent stroke comparing PFO closure to established current standard of care treatment (RESPECT). *N Engl J Med* 2013;368(12):1092–100.
8. Meier B, Kalesan B, Mattle HP, Khattab AA, Hildick-Smith D et al. Percutaneous closure of patent foramen ovale versus medical treatment in patients with cryptogenic embolism (PC Trial). *N Engl J Med* 2013;368(12):1083–91.

60

Disorders of the atrial septum: Closure with HELEX or Gore septal occluder

Matt Daniels and Neil Wilson

Incomplete development or failure of fusion of the two components of the atrial septum (the septum primum and septum secundum) leads to a direct communication—an atrial septal defect (ASD), or a patent foramen ovale (PFO)—a flap-like communication. This group of anatomical lesions is common (~one-third of the adult population) and generally benign. This is not always the case and, therefore, a clinical need exists to deliver safe and effective closure in cases of large defects associated with hemodynamically significant intracardiac shunts or following events of suspected paradoxical embolism. In the case of paradoxical embolism, patients with this pathology are often young, and come for treatment to mitigate lifetime risks that are low in absolute terms (~1–2%/year), but high in relative terms (80 times higher than age-matched controls). Device treatment in this group has a chance of being efficacious if the potential harm of intervention is significantly less than the attributable risk of the lesion itself.

Although percutaneous approaches have greatly reduced the need for open surgical repair, it is important to acknowledge the role surgery still has: to treat very large and complex defects of the atrial septum and to rescue embolized devices when percutaneous retrieval fails. It is also important to consider the evolution of percutaneous devices in the context of the early surgical experiences of closure via direct suture, or patch interposition. Various patch materials have been used ranging from autologous pericardium to synthetic polymers. Among the synthetic materials, expanded polytetrafluoroethylene (ePTFE or GOREtex, WL Gore and Associates, Flagstaff, AZ, USA) has demonstrated desirable properties such as reduced thrombogenicity and rapid endothelialization when compared with alternatives such as collagen-coated or Dacron-sealed materials.

In the 1990s, the progression of minimally invasive percutaneous strategies—which come with a smaller attendant risk and morbidity compared with open repair—redefined the standard of care[1] and inspired the development of percutaneous delivery systems that are able to deploy and

retain Gore-Tex within the beating adult heart to template endothelialization and, thus, exclude structural defects from the circulation. Initial *in vitro* and *in vivo* feasibility and biocompatibility studies[2] in large animals led to first-in-man use in 1999.[3] Three iterations of the device have been used clinically: the first two are known as the Gore HELEX, and the more recent arrival has been rebranded the Gore septal occluder (GSO). Importantly, the theoretical advantages of this family of devices extend beyond the properties of the synthetic patch because of a minimal metal scaffold design enabling these devices to maintain a low profile, and an atraumatic contour compared with other retrievable percutaneous devices that may be used to treat the same lesion.

We will now discuss the HELEX and GSO in turn, highlighting important differences in design, implantation procedure, and outcome measures of safety and efficacy, which are more readily available for the HELEX device as the first-in-man GSO use[4] was relatively recent and only available for use in Europe since June 2011.

HELEX device

The HELEX device is a retrievable non-self-centering double-disk device consisting of a single 0.012 inch nitinol wire, wound as two opposing spirals, on which is bonded a curtain of hydrophilic ePTFE. When the device is advanced from the control catheter, it forms two identical-size planar parallel disks, which sandwich the septal tissue (Figure 60.1). Ring markers on the wire frame demarcate the external limit of the right and left disks and the common internal boundary to aid fluoroscopy-guided delivery. It is supplied in a 9 F integral delivery system in sizes from 15 to 35 mm, in 5 mm increments. The delivery system itself is made of an outer delivery catheter, an inner control catheter (for deployment or withdrawal), and a central mandrel used to deploy the locking mechanism

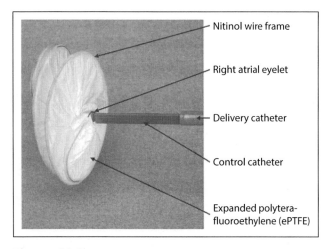

Nitinol wire frame

Right atrial eyelet

Delivery catheter

Control catheter

Expanded polytera-fluoroethylene (ePTFE)

Figure 60.1 The HELEX septal occluder. (From WL Gore & Associates, Flagstaff, AZ, USA.)

(Figure 60.2). A safety cord is attached to the tip of the control catheter and looped through the right atrial eyelet of the device back into the control catheter lumen to enable retrieval even after deployment and locking. The individual components are manipulated by a series of maneuvers of the Y-arm hub of the distal catheter (Figure 60.3), commonly referred to as the "push, pinch, pull" technique.

Adjustments to the winding pattern of the disks and to the delivery system were early iterative developments of the HELEX to aid implantation. Echocardiographic device visualization was enhanced by the use of hydrophilic ePTFE supporting the needs of multimodality imaging during structural intervention.

Sizing and anatomical compatibility

Anatomical assessment of intra-atrial communications in the context of the surrounding atrial tissue is undoubtedly important, and particularly so for the HELEX device. As a non-self-centering device, it is particularly useful in the

setting of a fenestrated intra-atrial septum as one device may cover many adjacent lesions. A trade-off for this versatility is the requirement to accurately size the diameter of the defect and to follow a manufacturer's recommend device to defect sizing ratio of at least 1.6:1, which sets an upper limit of defect diameter at ~20 mm for the range of devices available. In practical terms, the less mathematically onerous ratio of 2:1 is acceptable in adult patients, but in small children, the absolute size of the atria can limit device reconfiguration and preclude the use of all sizes available. There are no absolute guides to help in this setting and the adage that you can only use smaller devices in small children remains true. Our experience has taught us to reconsider any strategy to use a >30 mm device in a child <25 kg.

The device has been widely used in a range of clinical settings[5-10] but a recurring theme in case reports and live case discussions is that in addition to large defects precluded by the sizing rule, the HELEX device may not lock appropriately in PFO anatomy with a relatively long fixed tunnel length in excess of 10 mm. This is because the device absolutely requires the integrity of the locking mechanism, which runs through all three eyelets. Long tunnel anatomy prevents the right and left disks coming to rest without tension. Lengthening the distance between the left and right disks extends the length the locking loop must capture beyond its engineered range, and may result in a "missed eyelet capture."

Procedure

PFO/ASD closure represents the largest volume of activity in most structural intervention programs. Since the last edition of this book, we have adopted a number of changes to our practice to try and further minimize potential complications and maximize echocardiographic assessment of anatomical and physiological parameters, which we believe will be important for retrospective analysis of patient selection and outcome. More than 95% of the cases in our center are outpatient "day case" procedures performed with intracardiac echocardiography and limited

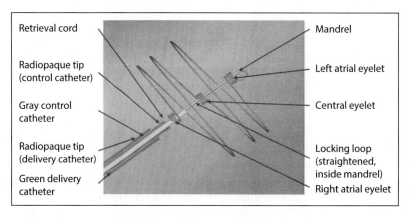

Retrieval cord

Radiopaque tip (control catheter)

Gray control catheter

Radiopaque tip (delivery catheter)

Green delivery catheter

Mandrel

Left atrial eyelet

Central eyelet

Locking loop (straightened, inside mandrel)

Right atrial eyelet

Figure 60.2 A HELEX septal occluder schematic.

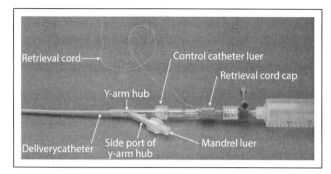

Figure 60.3 The HELEX septal occluder delivery system.

sedation with short-acting benzodiazepine drugs. Our average procedure time is in the region of 36 min, radiation doses are less 250 μGm^2, and a total fluoroscopy time typically less than 2 min.

Femoral venous access is obtained with two high-frequency ultrasound-guided punctures to the same common femoral vein if the patient weighs >50 kg, and to left and right veins if the patient weighs less. A 35-cm-long 9 F sheath with a hemostatic valve is inserted over a long 0.035 inch guide wire at the distal puncture site. This will be used for the 8 F ICE (intracardiac echocardiogram) catheter and taking the distal position means that once positioned, the ICE catheter hub can rest between the patient's legs, reducing inadvertent movements that can occur with the various catheter manipulations required for device deployment. We use a long sheath for the ICE catheter as it is not positioned with a guide wire and, therefore, it can be difficult to appreciate that the catheter has entered a pelvic vein until discomfort, and potentially venous trauma, has been caused to the patient. The long sheath, which is inserted over a wire, allows delivery to the distal inferior vena cava in most patients.

A second short 12 F (Cook) sheath with a hemostatic valve is inserted at the proximal puncture site. The 0.035 guide wire is positioned through this sheath to the right atrium to ensure IVC continuity, prior to positioning of the ICE catheter within the right atrium. Anatomical assessment of relevant septal anatomy (unstretched dimension, number of defects, and margins in the case of ASD; Eustachian ridge, Chiari network, and septal mobility in the case of PFO) and physiology (color Doppler flow for ASD; color Doppler plus superior vena cava (SVC) and IVC agitated saline contrast injections for PFO) is then performed.

If the ASD appears to be suitable for percutaneous closure, the patient is anticoagulated with weight-adjusted unfractionated heparin (100 IU/kg) before the lesion is crossed. In the case of a suspected PFO, the sensitivity and specificity of the screening echocardiogram (transthoracic echocardiography [TTE] or transesophageal echocardiography [TOE]) is approximately 90%; therefore, up to 10% of cases presenting for invasive assessment may be expected to be false positives and may not have a demonstrable intracardiac defect. Accordingly, we do not give heparin until

we have supportive data from agitated saline or fluoroscopic contrast injection that a defect is present, to minimize adverse outcomes at the site of vascular puncture, or cardiac trauma following probing of the fossa ovalis.

Typically, we use a 6 F end-hole diagnostic catheter to engage and cross an atrial defect, as this allows the use of the shorter (180 cm) stiff wire required for balloon interrogation and device positioning. The alternative multipurpose catheter (MPAII) requires a longer (260 cm) wire with technical/logistical implications in the cath lab where a usable table length is little more than 2 m. In cases of extreme septal mobility, or where the septal aneurysm billows into the right atrium and the septal defect is superiorly placed, it can be technically impossible to engage it with either of these catheters and in this situation we typically use a Judkins Right 4 catheter. With the catheter in the left atrium, it is directed to the left upper pulmonary vein, sometimes with the help of the 0.035 inch guide wire. The experience from left atrial appendage closure suggests that it would be prudent to avoid catheter manipulation in this friable structure, which sits in plane with the target left-sided pulmonary veins.

We manually deform the soft end of a heavy-duty guide wire (e.g., Amplatzer Super Stiff wire) and prolapse the curved tip into the left upper pulmonary vein through the deaired catheter. Having removed the diagnostic catheter used to access the pulmonary vein, we advance a sizing balloon (typically a PTS sizing balloon 20, 25, 30, 40 mm; Numed Hopkinton NY/BBraun Interventional Systems, Bethlehem PA, USA). Gentle balloon inflation reveals the maximum size of the PFO or ASD. We prefer to measure in a 30–45° LAO fluoroscopic projection. We employ the "stop-flow" method for ASDs based on the intracardiac echo color Doppler observations. A device is then chosen based on the size of the defect in the context of adjacent anatomy, in particular morphology and thickness of the secundum septum. The contribution of ICE during defect sizing is mainly to exclude the presence of other defects, to assess adjacent cardiac structures, and to guide the extent of balloon inflation. Accurate sizing may be difficult by ICE alone, as correct probe orientation to provide perfect alignment with the equator of the balloon's waist, while confidently visualizing both sides of the balloon can be hampered by metal artifacts from the wire and competition for space in the right atrium from the inflated balloon. For this reason, we rely on the fluoroscopic measurement, calibrated against the 1 cm markers on the balloon catheter.

Once selected, the device is loaded into the flushed delivery catheter in the small "water bath" provided in the packaging by pulling the gray control catheter, and is flushed further with saline until all air has been expelled. Loading should be performed with the occluder and the distal portion of the delivery catheter submerged in heparinized saline solution, with a heparin flush attached to the red retrieval cord cap. When flushing is complete, the gray control catheter with the attached syringe is withdrawn until only 3 cm of the device is outside the delivery catheter. This will cause the mandrel to bend slightly. At this time, the mandrel luer lock is loosened and the occluder is completely withdrawn into the delivery catheter by pulling the gray control catheter. The mandrel will exit the side port of the Y-hub and protrude by 3–4 cm. The red cap is reattached to secure the safety cord. Once loaded, the delivery catheter is advanced from the groin into the heart using the stiff wire through the distal monorail guide wire port on the catheter, which will accommodate wires up to 0.035 inches. Deployment can begin with the distal portion of the catheter in the mid left atrium using a series of "push, pinch, pull" maneuvers detailed below. Fluoroscopic intermediates are shown in Figure 60.4. Figure 60.5 shows the appearance of the device on transesophageal echo after full deployment and release.

The left atrial disk is deployed under fluoroscopic and echo guidance by repeating the following steps. Fixing the delivery catheter, the gray control catheter is advanced in the left atrium until the tan mandrel luer stops against the side port of the Y-hub. The tip of the control catheter should not touch the atrial wall. If space in the left atrium is inadequate, the control catheter should be advanced in smaller steps. Fixing the delivery and the control catheter, the mandrel is pulled back approximately 2 cm. Thus, the left atrial disk is gradually configured. The above steps are repeated until the central eyelet of the occluder exits the delivery catheter, indicating that the left atrial disk is completely deployed. This is then pulled into contact with the atrial septum, easily visible on echocardiography. To ensure it is closely opposed to the atrial septum, the tan mandrel may be slightly withdrawn.

To constitute the right atrial disk, the gray control catheter is fixed while the delivery catheter is pulled back gently until the mandrel luer lock touches the side port of the Y-arm hub. The mandrel luer is tightened. The right atrial disk is now exposed by simply fixing the delivery catheter and advancing the control catheter until it stops at the Y-arm hub, where the control catheter luer lock is then tightened. The position and configuration of the disks should be controlled by both echocardiography and fluoroscopy. Both disks should be flat and close-fitting to the atrial septum, with atrial septal tissue in between them.

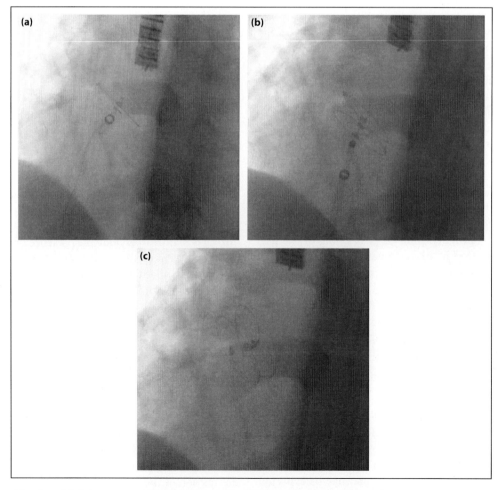

Figure 60.4   (a) Left atrial disk at septum; (b) both disks applied either side of the septum prior to locking; (c) postdevice locking and removal of delivery catheter.

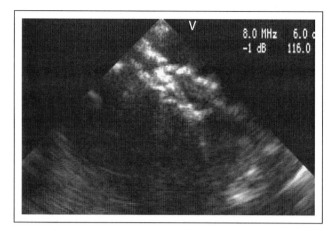

Figure 60.5 A TOE image of the device in place at the end of the procedure.

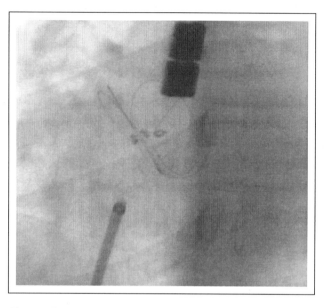

Figure 60.6 Left and right atrial disks appear splayed as they sit astride the aorta in this anterior–superior situated ASD.

If the position is not satisfactory at this point of the procedure, the HELEX occluder may be repositioned before locking the device (see below). When the device appears well positioned, the red retrieval cord cap is removed and the mandrel luer lock is loosened. The locking mechanism is activated by sharply pulling the mandrel a distance of 4–5 cm coaxially while fixing the delivery catheter in place. If the device position is not acceptable after this step, the occluder may be removed as it is still loosely attached to the control catheter via the retrieval cord (see below).

When a good device position has been achieved, the delivery system as a whole is removed from the patient. The retrieval cord will move through the control catheter hub and through the right atrial eyelet of the occluder, thereby releasing it completely.

A special note is needed for the ASD sited antero–superior close to the aorta and where there is a deficient rim: by necessity, the left and right aspects of the device have to sit astride the aorta. In this instance, there is a certain amount of "splaying" of the device, evident under fluoroscopy. This must not be interpreted as an abnormal configuration. TOE will demonstrate the disks astride the aorta and effective closure. An understanding of the anatomy of such defects bears this out. Figure 60.6 demonstrates a device astride the aorta producing effective closure.

Repositioning of the device is an option if it is considered suboptimal. This is only possible prior to engaging the locking mechanism. If the occluder is already locked and its position is not acceptable, it has to be recaptured using the retrieval suture, and cannot be reused (see below). To begin the retrieval process, the red retrieval cord cap and the mandrel luer need to be tightened first. Gently pulling back the gray control catheter, the device is completely withdrawn into the delivery catheter as it was during the initial loading procedure (see above). The delivery catheter is then repositioned within the left atrium and the device is redeployed following the above-mentioned steps. If increased force is necessary

during repositioning, parts of the HELEX system may be damaged or kinked. In this case, we recommend completely removing the HELEX system and using a new device.

Recapture of the occluder may be necessary if its position is not acceptable after lock release or if repositioning is not possible without applying increased force. The mandrel luer lock must be open. With the red retrieval cord cap removed, the retrieval cord is gently withdrawn, leaving some 5 cm or so distance between it and the right atrial eyelet of the device. Now, the red retrieval cord cap is firmly reattached and the control catheter is withdrawn, causing the device to return into the delivery catheter in its linear form. This step should be performed with caution to avoid interference of the device eyelets with the tip of the delivery sheath, which may lead to breakage of the retrieval cord. If complete withdrawal of the device into the delivery catheter would require excessive force, the control catheter and the delivery catheter may be withdrawn together with parts of the device remaining out of the delivery catheter. In this case, it might be necessary to remove the whole system together with the introducer sheath.

Complications and management

In the case of an *embolization* or malposition of the occluder after the retrieval cord has been removed, the device can be snared at any point of its frame using a loop snare. A long sheath of at least 10 F should be positioned near the occluder, allowing for complete retraction of the device. If parts of the device remain outside the long sheath, the device, snare, and sheath have to be removed as a whole.

In a small percentage of patients treated with the HELEX device, a wire frame fracture has been observed. Frame fractures usually do not require any action as they do not affect the function of the device and the metal frame is encased in a curtain of ePTFE. Should there be concern about encroachment or viability of a fractured device on vital structures of the heart, surgical removal should be considered.

Follow-up and medication

After a HELEX device implantation, our practice is to recommend aspirin monotherapy in antiplatelet dosage unless there has been a clear history of recent migraine (present in up to two-thirds of cryptogenic stroke patients) in which case clopidogrel is added for 3–4 months to try and prevent the rebound migraine phenomenon that was reported following device closure.[11]

The duration of antiplatelet therapy depends on the indication for closure. For ASDs in the context of intracardiac shunts, 6 months should be sufficient to protect the patient from on-device thrombus formation during the endothelialization process, which is complete in 3 months in experimental animals. In the case of a paradoxical embolism, it may be prudent to continue antiplatelet therapy indefinitely, as this would be the standard practice if intervention was not considered. This is particularly true in the case of a stroke, where effective secondary prevention has been demonstrated for oral antiplatelet regimes.

Endocarditis prophylaxis is recommended for 6 months.

The role, timing, and nature of follow-up and postprocedure imaging are uncertain. Our standard practice was to see patients at 3 months, and perform transthoracic echocardiography at that visit, with a Doppler assessment to assess residual shunting and document the final device position. This approach may not detect small shunts and device-associated thrombi when compared with a more invasive imaging approach, such as transesophageal echocardiography. However, in a retrospective analysis of almost 300 patients treated with PFO closure using the HELEX device in our center, we have only identified two definite strokes supported by neuroimaging among eight patients with a neurological event postprocedure. The average follow-up time was 30 months. None of these events occurred during the 3-month follow-up period. Thus, with a low event rate postclosure it appears that the main role of the follow-up is to exclude late device migration rather than preempt future events.

Published outcomes

Currently, there is no published formal trial data for the HELEX device. REDUCE,[12] a phase III prospective randomized control trial of the HELEX and GSO device versus standard medical therapy in imaging-proven cryptogenic strokes, continues to enroll patients in North America and Europe and aims to complete enrollment shortly and, therefore, complete the trial in 2018, if all patients are followed for the upper 5-year provision of the trial.

In a meta-analysis of >15,000 patients initially reported in various case series of PFO closure following cryptogenic stroke,[13] HELEX device use accounted for the smallest proportion (8.9% of cases) where device use was established. However, in these patients, recurrent stroke, atrial arrhythmia, surgical intervention, and device thrombus rates were the lowest of the five major devices used, which appears to be encouraging.

Clearly, it is impossible to accurately compare the relative absolute merits of devices in this setting due to reporting and publication bias. Moreover caution must be exercised in the face of these data, which have an order of magnitude difference in outcomes that would be expected to be uniform across all devices, and are in disagreement with data obtained in randomized trials (e.g., bleeding complications—0.2% for Starflex in this analysis vs. 2.6% in the device arm of the randomized Closure 1 trial).

The other point this analysis overlooks is the difficulty some operators have encountered trying to use the HELEX device; in particular, the delivery mechanism being relatively complex and the device itself being physically light when compared with the alternatives. As a result, malposition/deployment events are more likely to be encountered, particularly during the learning curve. The implication here is that HELEX usage may have been limited to a subset of more simple lesions that may have a natural history different from more complex lesions suited to more rigid devices.

Be that as it may, in centers that have persevered with this device,[14] early closure rates do appear to be lower[15] than the more rigid devices, which to a degree impose cardiac anatomy to the device, rather than the device conforming to the septal anatomy. The extent to which this may influence clinical outcomes remains unclear and it may be relevant to note that to date no HELEX device erosions have been reported.

In an attempt to improve the HELEX concept of a flexible ePTFE predominant device, and in particular to simplify the practicalities of delivery and improve early closure rates while maintaining the safety and biocompatibility record, WL Gore and Associates have developed the GSO[16] with first-in-man use in 2011.[4]

Gore septal occluder

This remains a non-self-centering double-disk device supplied on an integral delivery system based on an ePTFE curtain encasing a nitinol frame held together by a locking loop running from the left to the right atrial disks. The GSO has five wires covered by a hydrophilic ePTFE film, such that when deployed two disks of equal size form in a five-petal arrangement (Figure 60.7). To enhance fluoroscopic visualization, a platinum core has been introduced to the nitinol frame. The delivery handle incorporates the

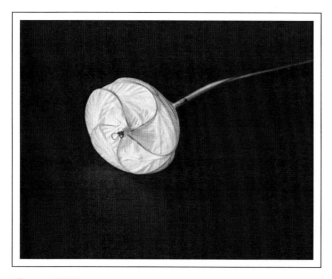

Figure 60.7   The Gore septal occluder.

deployment mechanism of the HELEX into a much simplified slider with a side port for de-airing (Figure 60.8). The device is available in 15 mm to 30 mm sizes in 5 mm intervals. All devices have the same delivery catheter dimensions. The sizing ratio of ~2:1 is still recommended.

Procedure

Vascular access, echocardiographic assessment, anticoagulation, and balloon interrogation of the septum are identical to the HELEX procedure details given above. We tend to oversize the device if a long tunnel or thick secundum septum is seen, as the device still requires the locking mechanism to remain intact. We will also perhaps extend the 2:1 ratio in the event of an ASD with a deficient aortic rim.

Once the device size is determined, the packaging is opened, revealing the device and delivery system configured in packaging, which is designed with a reservoir to facilitate flushing and loading. The reservoir is filled with heparinized saline, before the operator turns attention to the handle and removes the packaging insert, liberates the flush port (to which we normally attach a three-way tap), mobilizes the safety cord away from the delivery mechanism, and checks the integrity of the luer lock in the delivery catheter, which if loose can allow the device to lock prematurely while being deployed.

A 10 mL heparinized saline flush activates the lubricious hydrophilic coating inside the delivery mechanism. The slider is then moved distally navigating the chicane engineered in the handle; this brings the right and left disks into the delivery catheter sequentially. The device and delivery catheter are then completely de-aerated by two to three slow injections of 20 mL heparinized saline into the flush port. The delivery catheter is advanced through the venous sheath into the heart using the distal guide wire port on the catheter along the prepositioned guide wire in the left pulmonary vein. Once the catheter is in the left atrium, the wire is removed. Further de-aerating is not required.

To begin deployment, the ideal position for the end of the delivery catheter is the center of the left atrium (Figure 60.9a), as this will accommodate the device as it emerges in a straight and relatively rigid form initially. Sometimes, it may not be possible to deploy in this position, for example, when a PFO tunnel directs the catheter obliquely toward the top of the left atrium, or when the left atrium is too small to accommodate the advancing tip of the device. In these cases, we recommend the use of an "uncovering" technique where the left disk is advanced while the delivery catheter is withdrawn as this prevents device protrusion from the luminal position of the catheter and, thus, minimizes the risk of cardiac perforation.

Left disk deployment is monitored with echo and fluoroscopy, and controlled by movement of the red slider in the opposite direction to that which loaded it into the delivery catheter. In our experience, we find that complete deployment and compaction of the left disk often requires the right disk to partially be advanced in the left atrium. The right disk is then drawn back into the delivery system, using the slider, bringing the left disk back to the tip of the delivery catheter. The whole delivery system is then drawn slowly backward until resistance is felt as the left disk encounters the left side of the atrial septum. At this point, we often see that the right atrial disk begins to emerge, which is the cue to complete movement of the slider in order to deliver the right disk (Figure 60.9b). If necessary, both disks can be recaptured and repositioned by reversal of this process and gentle torquing of the delivery catheter.

Prior to locking the device, it is important to bring the septum and device into a neutral position, as the tendency is to have too much tension on the right side by the process described above. Locking the device is performed by firmly

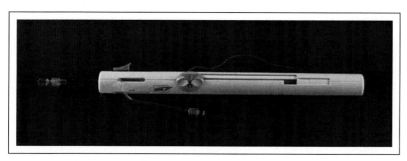

Figure 60.8   The delivery handle for the Gore septal occluder.

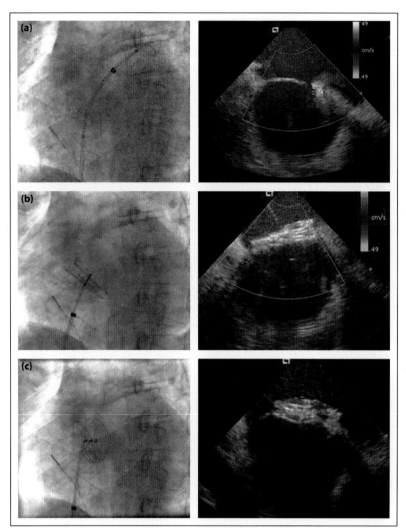

Figure 60.9 (See color insert.) Fluoroscopic and intracardiac echo images of the key steps in deployment of the Gore septal occluder in a secundum ASD. (a) With the delivery catheter in the left atrium, the device is advanced configuring the left disk first. (b) The device is then drawn back to the septum, and the right disk deployed. (c) The device is then locked and released using the delivery handle. It is normal to see the device realign as it is liberated from the delivery catheter.

holding the distal end of the delivery handle with the right hand, and with the left hand against that resistance, sliding the release mechanism (Figure 60.9c). In contrast to the importance of direct visualization of the locking mechanism in the HELEX device, which could be difficult in larger patients, additional wires present in the GSO give rise to an obvious appearance in the event of the locking mechanism failure (Figure 60.10).

At this point, the safety cord remains intact, so if the device appears satisfactory, it can be removed by lifting the red toggle on the slider and with gentle traction away from the patient in the plane of the heart. The cable is 3 m long, and it is normal to feel a loss of resistance at about 1.5 m as the cord emerges from the device. If too much resistance is felt, we would encourage operators to look at the relative position of the right disk and delivery catheter. Normally locking the device separates the two, but sometimes if the delivery handle is pushed during this maneuver, the two can sit closely opposed, which hampers removal of the safety cord. With the device liberated, the delivery system can be removed from the patient.

If there is concern about the device because of failure of the locking mechanism, malposition, or embolization after it has been locked, the device can be recaptured using the safety cord. This first action is to unscrew the luer lock on the delivery catheter, advancing the distal catheter toward the device and retracting the right disk with the slider. The catheter is then moved into the left atrium and the remainder of the device recaptured, before the whole system is withdrawn.

We routinely repeat IVC agitated saline injections from the 12 F venous sheath to confirm device efficacy by comparison to the predevice IVC injection. Complete closure is anticipated in >90% of patients even when we incorporate simultaneous transcranial Doppler assessment to detect small shunts with greater sensitivity.

Follow-up and management

We continue to use the same recommendations for antiplatelet therapy and endocarditis prophylaxis as for the HELEX device described above.

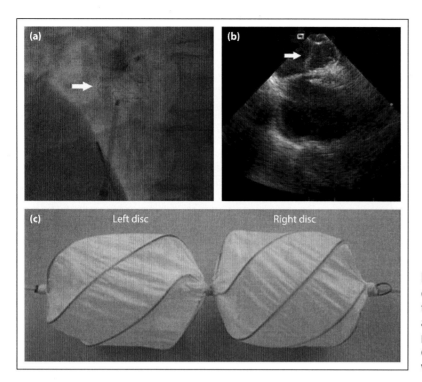

Figure 60.10   Fluoroscopic (a) and intracardiac (b) images of a 20 mm device in a PFO where the right disk failed to retain its configuration after locking and release. The arrows indicate the position of unconstrained appearance of the right disk. (c) Appearance of the Gore septal occluder without the central locking mechanism.

Our first 100 implants were followed up at 30 days (clinical assessment, ECG, transthoracic echo) and 90 days (clinical assessment, ECG, agitated saline transthoracic echo), but as we failed to demonstrate device migration, thrombus, or large residual shunt in this population, we have now adopted a less intensive assessment of patients at 50–90 days (clinical, ECG, transthoracic echo) and plan to reserve repeat bubble testing for patients with unusual anatomical appearance at TTE, divers treated to prevent decompression sickness, or patients with a suspected second event (although we have not had any patients in this group yet).

Arrhythmia

Early in our use of this device, a number (5–10%) of patients reported an awareness of abnormal heart rhythm that appeared maximal in intensity/frequency in the 14–21 day postclosure interval. A number of these individuals, who were concerned in particular by the unusual timing of the symptoms, were able to obtain ECGs during the arrhythmia episode largely identifying benign forms of atrial arrhythmia (principally atrial ectopy). One patient had atrial fibrillation, which was managed with anticoagulation and rate-control therapy. Overall, this phenomenon seems to be short-lived and at 30 days the subjective sensation, and objective ECG proof, had resolved.

Based on this experience, we now tell patients that they may expect some arrhythmia in the 2–3 week postclosure interval, which we assume reflects a more vigorous endothelialization process accounting for the apparent increase in early closure rates. We advise patients to seek attention

if the associated symptoms are sustained or compromising. However, since we have begun to offer this advice there has been a clear reduction in self-initiated event reporting.

Published outcomes

The GSO has been approved for use in the REDUCE trial, so as for the HELEX device, some randomized control trial data may become available in the 2015–2018 period.

As for all new devices, long-term follow-up data are not yet available, but to date there have been approximately 3000 implants of the GSO worldwide with publications of relatively small series (largest $n = 229$).[17] These have documented commendable safety and efficacy with a high incidence of complete closure with an absence of serious complications in both ASD[18,19] and PFO case series, which compare favorably with more established devices.[17,20,21] The versatility of the device has been demonstrated in closing multiple fenestrations of the atrial septum with implantation of interlocking devices,[22] closure of long tunnel PFO, and closure of fenestrated Fontan circulation.[23]

Overall

We are of the impression that the changes to the delivery mechanism make the GSO much easier to use and implant than the HELEX. The new device configuration makes identification of failures of the locking mechanism more obvious, but also much less common, and the range of anatomy that can be closed now includes longer tunnels and extremely mobile septa.[16] Early complete closure rates appear improved; >90% with the GSO compared with 60% with the HELEX. These apparent mechanical advantages according to early case series have not been associated with adverse events. However, like all medical devices used in young patients, long-term data are required to make judgments on harm and efficacy.

References

1. Webb G, Gatzoulis M. Atrial septal defects in the adult recent progress and overview. *Circulation* 2006;114:1645–53.
2. Zahn EM, Wilson N, Cutright W, Latson LA. Development and testing of the Helex septal occluder, a new expanded polytetrafluoroethylene atrial septal defect occlusion system. *Circulation* 2001;104(6):711–6.
3. Latson LA, Zahn EM, Wilson N. Helex septal occluder for closure of atrial septal defects. *Curr Interv Cardiol Rep* 2000;2(3):268–73.
4. Søndergaard L, Loh PH, Franzen O, Ihlemann N, Vejlstrup N. The first clinical experience with the new GORE° septal occluder (GSO). *EuroIntervention* 2013;9(8):959–63.
5. Pedra CA, Pedra SR, Esteves CA et al. Transcatheter closure of secundum atrial septal defects with complex anatomy. *J Invasive Cardiol* 2004;16(3):117–22.
6. Dobrolet NC, Iskowitz S, Lopez L et al. Sequential implantation of two Helex septal occluder devices in a patient with complex atrial septal anatomy. *Catheter Cardiovasc Interv* 2001;2:242–6.
7. Krumsdorf U, Keppeler P, Horvath K et al. Catheter closure of atrial septal defects and patent foramen ovale in patients with an atrial septal aneurysm using different devices. *J Interven Cardiol* 2001;1:49–55.
8. Sievert H, Horvath K, Zadan E et al. Patent foramen ovale closure in patients with transient ischemia attack/stroke. *J Interven Cardiol* 2001;2:261–6.
9. Onorato E, Melzi G, Casilli F et al. Patent foramen ovale with paradoxical embolism: Mid-term results of catheter closure in 256 patients. *J Interven Cardiol* 2003;1:43–50.
10. Peuster M, Beerbaum P. A novel implantation technique for closure of an atypical fenestration connecting the right atrial appendage to an extracardiac conduit by use of a 15 mm Helex device in a patient with a total cavopulmonary connection. *Z Kardiol* 2004;10:818–23.
11. Bhindi R, Ruparelia N, Newton J, Testa L, Ormerod OJ Acute worsening in migraine symptoms following PFO closure: A matter of fact? *Int J Cardiol* Oct 8 2010;144(2):299–300.
12. http://www.strokecenter.org/trials/clinicalstudies/gore-helex-septal-occluder-gore-septal-occluder-for-patent-foramen-ovale-pfo-closure-in-stroke-patients-the-gore-reduce-clinical-study.
13. Agarwal et al. Meta-analysis of transcatheter closure versus medical therapy for patent foramen ovale in prevention of recurrent neurological events after presumed paradoxical embolism. *JACC Int* 2012;7:777–89.
14. Heinisch C, Bertog S, Wunderlich N, Majunke N, Baranowski A, Leetz M, et al. Percutaneous closure of the patent foramen ovale using the HELEX® Septal Occluder: Acute and long-term results in 405 patients. *EuroIntervention* 2012;8(6):717–23.
15. Taaffe M, Fischer E, Baranowski A, et al. Comparison of three patent foramen ovale closure devices in a randomized trial (Amplatzer versus CardioSEAL/STARflex versus Helex occluder). *Am J Cardiol* 2008;101(9):1353–8.
16. MacDonald ST, Daniels MJ, Ormerod OJ. Initial use of the new GORE° septal occluder in patent foramen ovale closure: Implantation and preliminary results. *Catheter Cardiovasc Interv* 2013;81(4):660–5.
17. Thomson JD, et al. Patent foramen ovale closure with the gore septal occluder: Initial UK Experience. *Catheter Cardiovasc Interv* 2014;83(3):467–73.
18. Smith B, Thomson J, Crossland D, Spence MS, Morgan GJ. UK multicenter experience using the gore septal occluder (GSOTM) for atrial septal defect closure in children and adults. *Catheter Cardiovasc Interv* 2014;83:581–6.
19. Nyboe C, Hjortdal VE, Nielsen-Kudsk JE. First experiences with the GORE® Septal Occluder in children and adults with atrial septal defects. *Catheter Cardiovasc Interv* 2013 Feb 13. doi:10.1002/ccd.24851.
20. Musto C, Cifarelli A, Fiorilli R, De Felice F, Parma A, Nazzaro MS, et al. Comparison between the new gore septal and amplatzer devices for transcatheter closure of patent foramen ovale. *Circ J* 2013;77(12):2922–7.
21. Freixa X, Ibrahim R, Chan J, Garceau P, Dore A, Marcotte F, et al. Initial clinical experience with the GORE septal occluder for the treatment of atrial septal defects and patent foramen ovale. *EuroIntervention* 2013;9(5):629–35. doi: 10.4244/EIJV9I5A100.
22. Lockhart CJ, Magee AG. Closure of multiple fenestrations in an aneurismal atrial septum using overlapping GORE HELEX septal occluders. *Catheter Cardiovasc Interv* 2012;79(7):1176–7.
23. Lockhart CJ, Johnston NG, Spence MS Experience using the new GORE Septal Occluder at the margins. *Catheter Cardiovasc Interv* 2013;81(7):1244–8.

61

Patent foramen ovale closure: Premere septal occluder

Franziska Buescheck and Horst Sievert

Introduction

Premere™ PFO closure system

The Premere PFO Closure System (St. Jude Medical, Maple Grove, MN, USA) is a percutaneous, transcatheter self-explanding, dual-anchor arm occlusion device that is specifically designed to accommodate PFO with its special anatomy. It is available in diameters of 20 and 25 mm. It received CE mark in January 2005.

The anchors are made of nickel–titanium alloy (nitinol). The left anchor arm has an open architecture, a low profile, and a small surface area to discourage thrombus formation and reduce the potential for atrial tissue erosion. Only the right anchor is enveloped between two layers of knitted polyester (PET) fabric. The arms are designed with a low profile and a low surface area to minimize exposure to thrombogenic surfaces and to assist in rapid endothelialization. A flexible PET-braided tether runs through the center of the anchor and holds the two anchors together. The distance between the two arms is adjustable by the implanting physician; thus, the Premere can accommodate variable PFO tunnel lengths. The anchors are locked together after delivery before the tether is cut. A schematic drawing of the implant portion of the Premere PFO closure device with the delivery system is depicted in Figures 61.1 and 61.2.

Each anchor consists of four radiating clover-leaf-like arms as shown in Figure 61.3. A radiopaque outer marker rivet is placed at the ends of each arm. At the center of the anchor, a radiopaque left side hub is permanently fixed to the left anchor and the tether.

The right atrial anchor is similar to the left atrial anchor. It has also a right-side hub marker that is longer than that of the left anchor and has a flange to allow for retrieval if needed.

In addition, the nitinol anchor is enclosed within a sealed pouch made of PET (Figure 61.3). The right atrial anchor rides freely on the tether in both directions for ease of advancement and retrieval.

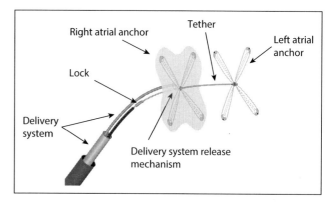

Figure 61.1 Isometric view of the implant assembly of the Premere PFO Closure System.

The tether consists of a braided white PET suture-like material. The tether termination engages with the left-side hub marker of the left atrial anchor. Near the proximal end of the tether is a marker. It denotes the position to move the tether retention clip after deployment of the left anchor. On the proximal side of the right atrial anchor, the tether is trimmed after placement of the anchors and lock.

The tether lock is made of nitinol tubing with six tabs that are placed on two circumferential planes. The tether

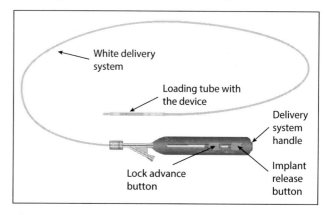

Figure 61.2 Premere delivery system.

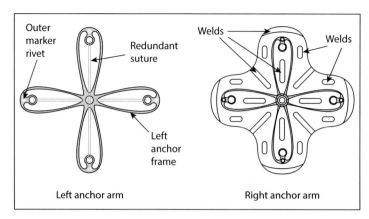

Figure 61.3 Left and right anchor arm frame.

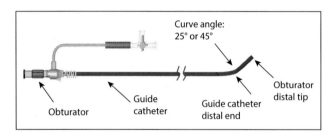

Figure 61.4 Guide catheter and obturator.

runs through the center of the lock. The tabs are designed to dig into the tether so that it is movable only in one direction. The lock can be advanced distally but the tabs prevent it from moving proximally. For visibility, the tether lock is encased within the lock marker.

The tether cutter system is advanced over the tether through the tether guide lumen after the delivery catheter system is removed. The cutter shaft is stationary and bonded to the cutter hub. The cutter hub is rotated clockwise. As the cutter shaft advances forward, it rotates and cuts the tether.

The guide catheter is available in two distal curve shapes to provide a better accommodation to the different anatomies of the patients. The two curves of the guide catheter are

- 25° radius of curvature
- 45° radius of curvature

Except for the radius of curvature of the distal tip, the two guide catheters are identical. Each guide catheter consists of an obturator, a proximal hub with a standard side arm for flushing.

An obturator is supplied with the guide catheter. The obturator has a guide wire lumen and a tapered distal end. The schematic of the guide catheter is shown in Figure 61.4.

Implantation

Attach a 20 cm³ syringe with heparinized saline to the luer fitting on the blue Premere delivery sheath. Evacuate air

from the delivery sheath, the Premere dilatator/obturator, and the delivery system.

- Place a short 9 F sheath and a multipurpose catheter into the left upper pulmonary vein.
- After the PFO measurements, exchange the 9 F sheath of the 11 F introducer sheath and load the dilator/obturator into the Premere delivery sheath.
- Advance the delivery sheath and dilator/obturator along the guide wire into the right atrium, through the PFO into the left atrium.
- Remove the guide wire and ensure that the tip of the delivery sheath is in the mid-left atrium.
- Keep the dilator/obturator hub below atrial level and ensure that blood is flowing freely out of the hub. Slowly remove the dilator/obturator as you maintain a constant column of blood out of the proximal end of the dilator/obturator.
- Open the stopcock on the delivery sheath and allow blood to flow out. Gently tap on the hub of the delivery sheath to remove any trapped air into the hub so that the air exits through the stopcock.
- Flush the delivery sheath with heparinized saline and close the stopcock.
- Fill a 20 cm³ syringe with heparinized saline and attach it to the luer fitting on the Premere PFO Closure System.
- While taking care to keep the loading tube in a generally horizontal orientation, maintain pressure on the 20 cm³ syringe. Observe saline exiting the distal end of the loading tube.
- Advance the loading tube into the hub until its shoulder fits correctly against the hub of the delivery sheath.
- Transfer the implant assembly into the delivery sheath by slowly advancing the Premere PFO Closure System at least 5 cm into the delivery sheath. Withdraw the loading tube from the delivery sheath until it is adjacent to the proximal hub of the delivery catheter of the delivery system. Remove the 20 cm³ syringe from the Premere PFO Closure System and verify the position of the delivery sheath in the mid-left atrium.

- Under fluoroscopy guidance, advance the Premere Implant through the delivery sheath until the implant is near the distal tip of the delivery sheath.
- Deploy the left atrial anchor by slowly advancing the delivery system until the radiopaque markers on the tips of the left atrial anchor arms expand (Figures 61.5 and 61.6).

It is critical to ensure that the right anchor does not exit the delivery sheath as you advance the left anchor. If the right atrial anchor is inadvertently deployed, see the "Retrieval" section.

- Once the left anchor is deployed, place your hand on the mark located on the tether of the Premere PFO Closure System. The tether is used to maintain the tactile feel of the septum and to direct device placement.
- Apply slight tension to the tether to maintain the orientation of the left atrial anchor perpendicular to the end of the delivery sheath. Slowly retract both the delivery sheath and the tether until you have seated the left anchor securely against the septal wall.
- Lightly ground the tether with your hand.
- With your other hand, continue to retract the delivery sheath into the mid-right atrium. As you retract the

delivery sheath, the delivery system will slide back over the fixed tether (Figure 61.7).
- Verify under fluoroscopy the position of the delivery sheath in the right atrium. While maintaining slight tension on the tether, slowly advance the right atrial anchor out of the delivery sheath by advancing the delivery system. Continue to advance the right anchor until it is seated against the septal wall of the right atrium.
- If necessary, the right anchor can be repositioned by retracting and subsequently readvancing the delivery system (Figure 61.8).

Care should be taken to ensure that the right atrial anchor is not advanced into the PFO track. Ensure that the anchor arms are not constrained or prolapsed into the PFO tunnel (Figure 61.9).

- Loosen the Touhy–Borst on the Premere delivery system. Maintain tension on the tether and advance the inner delivery catheter. This movement will advance the lock mechanism. This procedure should be done under fluoroscopic guidance. Continue advancing the lock mechanism until the radiopaque marker on the lock mechanism is adjacent to the radiopaque marker of the right atrial anchor.

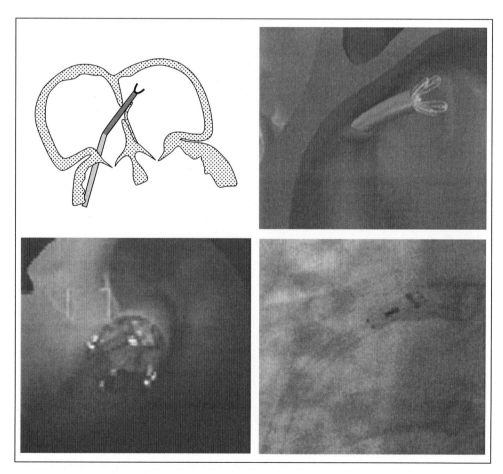

Figure 61.5   The outer delivery catheter pushes the LAA into the left atrium.

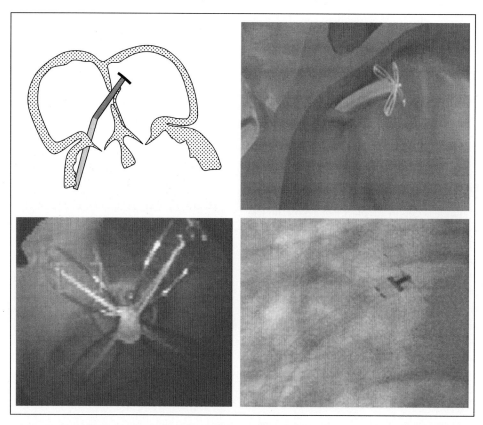

Figure 61.6   The LAA is released from the guide catheter allowing it to unfold.

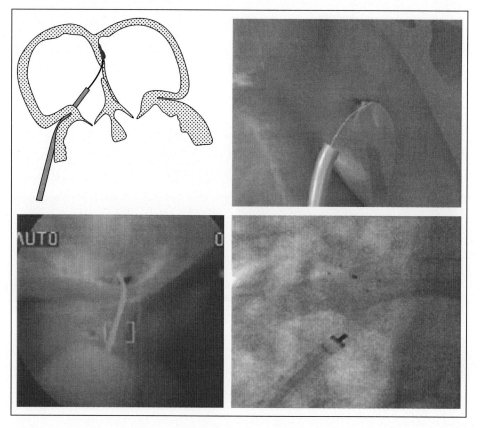

Figure 61.7   The guide catheter is withdrawn into the right atrium while the LAA is holding the PFO flap against the interatrial septal wall.

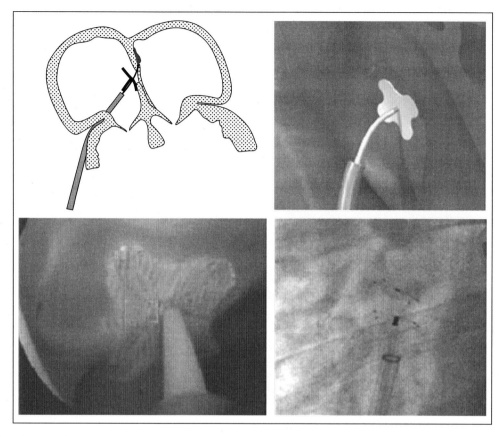

Figure 61.8   The delivery catheter system pushes the RAA against the interatrial septum.

- Retract the Premere delivery system just into the tip of guide catheter.
- Pull on the tether to ensure that the implant is securely in place. Observe this under fluoroscopy. Depress and hold the tether retention clip button and slide it proximally off the tether.
- Slide the Premere delivery system proximally off the tether.
- Introduce the proximal end of the tether into the distal end of the cutter. Advance the tether until it exits the cutter. Slight rotation of the tether may be required to advance it through the proximal opening of the cutter.
- Maintain tension on the tether and advance the cutter into the proximal end of the guide catheter. While maintaining tension on the tether, advance the cutter until the radiopaque marker on the cutter is adjacent to the radiopaque marker on the lock mechanism. Observe this under fluoroscopy.
- While maintaining tension on the tether, rotate the cutter wheel clockwise until the tether has been cut. This will be observed by a change in tension on the tether and typically by a change in position of the radiopaque marker of the cutter relative to the radiopaque marker on the lock mechanism.
- Rotate the cutter wheel counterclockwise to its original position and then remove the cutter and the cut tether together out of the guide catheter (Figures 61.10 through 61.12).

System retrieval

In the event that the implant needs to be removed (prior to advancing the lock), the following steps should be followed:

Prior to withdrawing the guide from left atrium to right atrium:

- Align the guide catheter coaxially with the left atrial anchor and pull on the tether. The left anchor will prolapse into the distal end of the guide catheter.

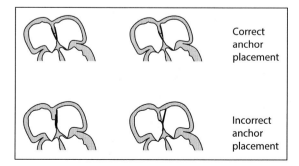

Correct anchor placement

Incorrect anchor placement

Figure 61.9   Illustration for correct and incorrect placement.

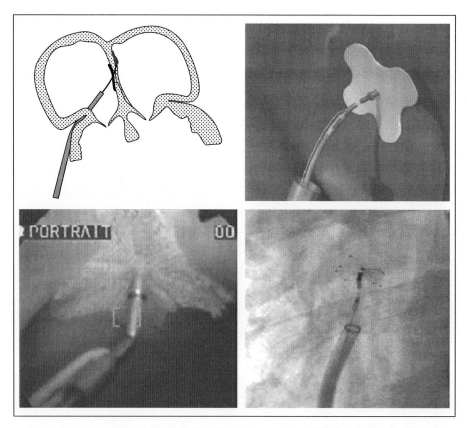

Figure 61.10   The delivery catheter system is withdrawn from the guide catheter and the tether cutter system guided to the implant side by the tether.

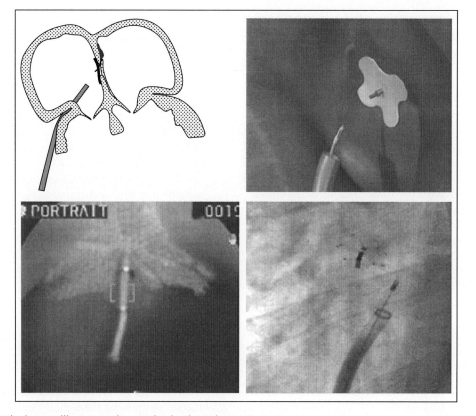

Figure 61.11   The images illustrate tether cutting by the tether cutter system.

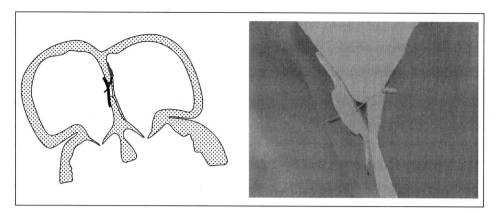

Figure 61.12   PFO closed by the implant assembly.

- Reinsert the implant-loading tube into the hemostasis valve on the hub of the Premere guide catheter.
- Care should be taken to ensure that the tip of the guide catheter is unobstructed and not in contact with the tissue. Slowly remove the Premere system from the guide catheter.

Prior to advancing the lock:

- Remove the tether retention clip off the proximal end of the tether.
- Unscrew the Y-adapter, releasing the inner delivery catheter from the outer delivery catheter.
- Slide the inner delivery catheter off the tether and out of the outer delivery catheter.
- Load a 10-mm-diameter snare over the hub and loading tube at the proximal end of the outer delivery catheter.
- Advance the snare through the hemostasis valve on the guide catheter and down to the distal end of the delivery system.
- The radiopaque marker on the hub of the right atrial anchor should be adjacent to the radiopaque shaft of the delivery system.
- While maintaining the position of the right atrial anchor and the delivery system, advance the snare onto the hub of the right atrial anchor. The radiopaque wire of the snare should be clearly visible over the radiopaque hub of the right atrial anchor.
- Actuate the snare mechanism until it is very firmly down on the hub of the right atrial anchor.
- Align the guide catheter coaxially with the right atrial anchor and withdraw the snare and delivery system. The right anchor will prolapse into the distal end of the guide catheter.
- Advance the Premere guide catheter back through the PFO track.
- Align the guide catheter coaxially with the left atrial anchor and pull on the tether. The left anchor will prolapse into the distal end of the guide catheter.
- Reinsert the implant-loading tube into the hemostasis valve in the hub of the Premere guide catheter.

Premere retrieval basket

The Premere retrieval basket consists of a funnel-shaped mesh of braided, nitinol wire that is mechanically crimped to a stainless-steel shaft.

It is indicated for use in extracting a Premere PFO Closure System implant that has been deployed incorrectly. The retrieval basket is only required in the event that both the right and left atrial anchors have been inadvertently placed in the same atrium.

Procedure

- Attach a 20 cm^3 syringe filled with heparinized saline solution to the luer fitting on the carrier tube. Flush the carrier tube and the retrieval basket.
- To use the retrieval basket, the Premere Closure System delivery catheter must be removed and the tether must not have been cut. Insert the tether into the eye of the tether-threading tool.
- Holding the free end of the tether, retract the tether-threading tool through the retrieval basket and loading tube until the tether-threading tool and tether exit the opposite side of the loading tube. Release the tether and remove and discard the tether-threading tool.
- Apply tension to the proximal end of the tether and insert the loading tube into the delivery sheath.
- Advance the retrieval basket into the delivery sheath and slide the loading tube out of the delivery sheath.
- Advance the retrieval basket to the distal tip of the delivery sheath and expand into the atrium.
- The retrieval basket should be observed with fluoroscopy and ultrasound when advancing to the desired location.
- Pull the implant assembly into the basket with the tether until it is completely seated at the bottom of the funnel-shaped basket.
- Pull both the tether and shaft of the basket together until the implant is withdrawn into the delivery sheath and completely removed.

The CLOSEUP trial was conducted to determine the safety of placement and effectiveness of the Premere device in closure of patent foramen ovale.[1] It showed that the Premere device was safely implanted in all (n = 67) cases and provided complete closure of the PFO in 87% of the cases at 6 months. Closure rate was clearly related to the device size. The 20 mm device had a better closure rate than the 15 mm device that was only available initially. There was no serious device-related adverse event either during device implantation or during follow-up. One patient had two episodes of atrial fibrillation that had resolved by 4 months postimplant. One patient reported transient left arm weakness. He did not seek medical attention at the time and no work-up was performed. This patient had no evidence of device thrombus formation at any evaluation and the PFO was found to be closed on echo/bubble study. No thrombus was seen at follow-up in the CLOSEUP trial.

Stanczak et al. reported a series of 263 patients who underwent PFO closure with the Premere device. Implantation success was 99.6%, complete closure occurred in 93% and the 30-day adverse event rate was 5.4%. At 30 days, atrial fibrillation was reported in 6 patients and at longer term follow-up (19 months), 3.5% of patients had a stroke or transient ischemic attack. Thrombus formation was found in only one patient (0.4%).[2]

These data as well as the data from the CLOSEUP trial indicate that closure of PFO can be successfully and safely completed.

References

1. Buescheck F, Sievert H, Kleber F, Tiefenbacher C, Krumsdorf U, Windecker S, Uhleman F, Wahr DW. Patent foramen ovale using the Premere device: The results of the CLOSEUP trial. *J Interven Cardiol* 2006;19:328–33.
2. Stanczak LJ, Bertog SC, Wunderlich N, Franke J, Sievert H. PFO closure with the Premere PFO closure device: Acute results and follow-up of 263 patients. *Eurointervention* 2012;8(3):345–51.

62

Patent foramen ovale closure: PFM PFO occluder

Tina Edwards-Lehr, Jennifer Franke, Stefan Bertog, Kristina Renkhoff, and Horst Sievert

Introduction

The Nit-Occlud® PFO is a new patent foramen ovale closure device developed by PFM Medical AG (Figures 62.1 and 62.2). It belongs to the "Nit-Occlud family" along with an atrial septal defect (ASD) and patent ductus arteriosus closure device. All these devices carry a typical feature—they are constructed of a single nitinol wire mesh (Figure 62.2) and do not have protruding clamps. As the wire mesh is solely composed of nitinol, the device is flexible and can adapt well to the septal wall. The Nit-Occlud PFO consists of a double-layer right atrial disk and a single-layer left atrial disk, reducing the amount of material by half in the left atrium to lower the thromboembolic risk. An integrated polyester membrane on the right atrial disk and a polyester membrane facing the left atrium are intended to accelerate endothelialization. The Nit-Occlud PFO is available in the following diameters: 20, 26, and 30 mm. It received CE mark in July 2010.

Implantation

The Nit-Occlud PFO system consists of the occluder and its delivery system with a disposable handle. Standard methods are used for vascular access and for the preparation of the system. The device comes premounted on a 9 or 10 F implantation catheter, and is easy to position and deploy. The distance between the PFO and the aortic root and between the PFO and the junction of the superior vena cava is measured in transesophageal echocardiography to select the correct occluder size. For the 20 and 26 mm Nit-Occlud PFO, a 9 F Nit-Occlud Implantation Sheath is recommended, and for the 30 mm Nit-Occlud PFO, a 10 F Nit-Occlud Implantation Sheath is recommended. After flushing of the transportation sheath through the side access of the Y-connector with heparinized saline solution, the Nit-Occlud PFO is loaded into the transportation sheath and flushed with saline solution once

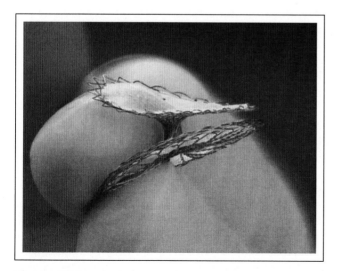

Figure 62.1   Nit-Occlud PFO. (Courtesy of PFM Medical AG.)

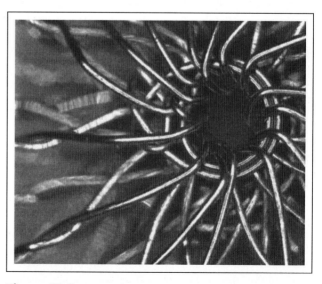

Figure 62.2   Nit-Occlud PFO is knitted out of a single nitinol wire. (Courtesy of PFM Medical AG.)

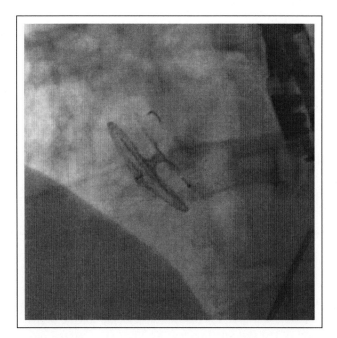

Figure 62.3   Final position of Nit-Occlud PFO as seen in fluoroscopy.

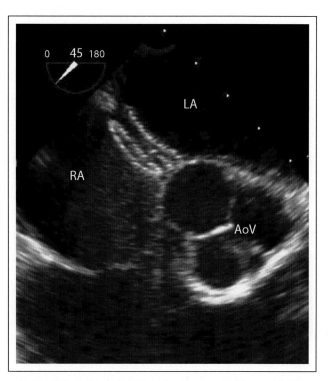

Figure 62.4   Final position of Nit-Occlud PFO as seen during transesophageal echocardiography. RA = right atrium, LA = left atrium, AoV = aortic valve.

again to prevent air embolism. Thereafter, the transportation sheath is connected to the Nit-Occlud Implantation Sheath via the luer connection. The Nit-Occlud PFO is pushed to the distal end of the implantation sheath using the delivery system. The implantation technique of the Nit-Occlud PFO is similar to that of the other commonly used closure devices. To assure optimal position, the device can be repositioned, withdrawn into the implantation sheath, or removed, as long as the release mechanism is not triggered yet. The umbrella is released from the delivery system by turning the hand wheel on the disposable handle clockwise. The final position of the Nit-Occlud PFO is shown under fluoroscopy (Figure 62.3) and in transesophageal echocardiography (Figure 62.4). In the event of embolization, the occluder can be retrieved using a lasso or a biopsy forceps technique.

Clinical trial

Between August 2009 and June 2010, 63 patients were included in a prospective, noncomparative, and single-center clinical investigation titled "Procedural Success and Safety of the Nit-Occlud PFO Closure Device and Its Application System" in Frankfurt, Germany, to assess the effectiveness, safety, and practicability of implantation of the Nit-Occlud PFO. Encouraging preliminary results were presented in July 2010, showing successful

implantation in 62 of 63 patients (98.4%).[1] In one patient, the device was successfully implanted, but could not be released from the delivery system. It was retrieved into the delivery system and a 25-mm Amplatzer® PFO Occluder was implanted successfully. All patients participated in the 6 week follow-up with transesophageal echocardiography, which revealed no residual shunt during Valsalva maneuver in 49.2% (31/63) of the patients and a severe residual shunt in 17.5% (11/63) of the patients. The device was stable in all patients, but dislocated into the PFO tunnel in two patients (3.1%). No thromboembolic events, thrombus formation, or arrhythmias were detected during the 6 week follow-up. Although not part of the protocol, longer-term follow-up was performed at the investigating center for the majority of patients. Fifty of 63 patients (79.4%) underwent 6 month follow-up with transesophageal echocardiography showing no residual shunt during Valsalva maneuver in 70% of the patients and a severe residual shunt in 2% of the patients.[2] A transient ischemic attack occurred in two (4%) patients without the presence of any residual shunt. One patient experienced an episode of atrial fibrillation that lasted for 5 h. Forty patients participated in a 1 year follow-up. Of these patients, complete closure was seen in 83% (33/40).

No moderate or severe shunt was detected in any patient. Two patients experienced a transient ischemic attack and one patient had a stroke due to vertebral artery dissection. In all three patients, there was no residual shunt during transesophageal echocardiography. No intracardiac thrombi, device embolization, or arrhythmias occurred at 1-year follow-up.

References

1. Renkhoff K, Joy S, Lehr T et al. New PFO devices: PFM Medical Device. Presented at Congenital and Structural Interventions, Frankfurt, Germany, July 8–11, 2010.
2. Momberger J, Renkhoff K, Joy S et al. Follow-up on PFM Medical Device. Presented at Congenital and Structural Interventions, Frankfurt, Germany, June 23–25, 2011.

63

Patent foramen ovale closure: CoherexFlatStent occluder

Ilona Hofmann, Stefan Bertog, and Horst Sievert

CoherexFlatStent EF PFO closure system

The CoherexFlatStent EF PFO Closure System™ (Coherex Medical, Salt Lake City, Utah) consists of a self-expanding, multicellular, planar nitinol device, and a rapid exchange delivery catheter (Figures 63.1 and 63.2). It has been CE marked and is commercially available in the European Union, Canada, Australia, and New Zealand.

The CoherexFlatStent EF device is the second generation of the CoherexFlatStent Closure System and contains an additional layer of polyurethane foam in comparison to the first generation (the acronym stands for enhanced foam). It is an in-tunnel PFO device that mechanically closes the PFO within the tunnel. As a result, the surface area of the device exposed to left and right atrium is significantly reduced, and the anatomy of the septum is preserved. These features potentially reduce the risk of device-associated thrombus formation, erosion, and arrhythmias. The

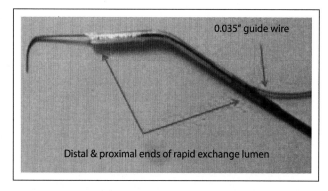

Figure 63.2 Rapid exchange system (distal and proximal ends of rapid exchange lumen).

device consists of a 51-μm-thick nitinol frame covered with polyurethane foam. The polyurethane foam stimulates tissue growth inside the tunnel. The device has anchors reaching out of the PFO tunnel and attaching to the walls of the left and right atrium (Figure 63.1). The micro-tines on the device provide additional stability of the implant within the tunnel. Tantalum markers along the framework facilitate visualization during implant placement. The system is available in two sizes, 13 and 19 mm. The 13 mm device is used for balloon-sized PFO diameters <8 mm and the 19 mm device is used for balloon-sized PFO diameters >8 mm and <12 mm.

The delivery system is a multilumen catheter designed for use with a 0.035" guide wire and has a 9.5 cm rapid exchange rail. The delivery system has a distal end (RX Lumen), in which the device is compressed for release within the PFO and a proximal end, which consists of a stationary handle, lock button, deployment slide, and release knob (Figure 63.3). The device is connected to three tethers with the proximal end of delivery by deployment slide (Figure 63.4). Activation of the release knob releases the device from the delivery system.

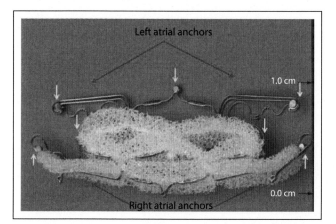

Figure 63.1 CoherexFlatStent device. (Courtesy of Coherex Medical). Yellow arrows show radiopaque markers.

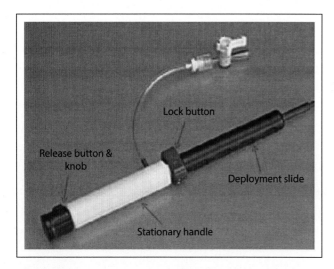

Figure 63.3   Single-operator delivery system handle.

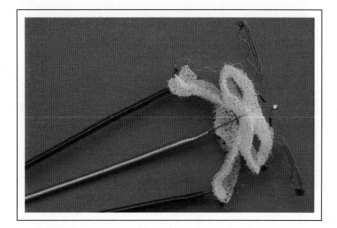

Figure 63.4   Three tether attachments.

Deployment of the FlatStent EF device

The delivery catheter, including the RX Lumen, is flushed, so that the guide wire (0.035″ or 0.038″) can be inserted into the RX Lumen. The device is immersed in saline for 3 s and loaded into the delivery system. A 12 F sheath is placed in the femoral vein and the PFO crossed using the guide wire, the distal tip of which is placed in a pulmonary vein. Following balloon sizing of the PFO and device size selection, the tip of the delivery catheter is advanced over the guide wire into the left atrium. The distal anchors are unsheathed and gently retracted to engage the tunnel (Figure 63.5). The body of the device is expanded within the tunnel, drawing the septum primum and the septum secundum into contact. Proximal anchors are released adjacent to the right side of the interatrial septum (Figure 63.6). After confirming the correct and stable position, the guide wire is removed and the device can be released from the delivery system by activating the release knob (Figure 63.7). It can be resheathed and repositioned until final detachment (Figure 63.8).

Follow-up and medication

After PFO closure, patients receive clopidogrel 75 mg once daily for 1 month and acetylsalicylic acid 100 mg once daily for 3 months. Antimicrobial endocarditis prophylaxis is recommended for 6 months.

Transesophageal echocardiography should be performed for the detection of residual shunt, thrombi, and assessment of device position 1 and 6 months after the procedure.

Who is suitable for CoherexFlatStent EF device?

- Simple PFO with no atrial septal aneurysm (ASA) (type I tunnel)
- PFO with interatrial septal aneurysm (type II tunnel) and adequate functional tunnel length for an in-tunnel device

What does "adequate functional tunnel length" mean? The PFO functional tunnel length is defined as the overlap of the septum primum and septum secundum where the septum primum remains parallel to the septum secundum

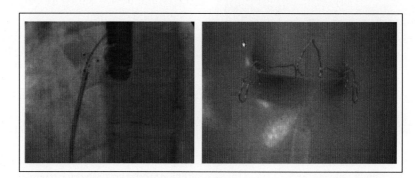

Figure 63.5   (**See color insert.**) Distal anchors open into the left atrium.

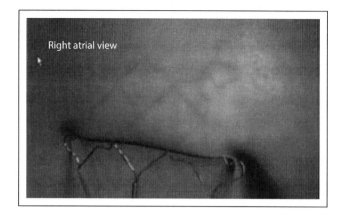

Figure 63.6 (**See color insert.**) Proximal anchors open into the right atrium.

during all phases of the heart cycle. Such parallel overlap of at least 4 mm is essential for stable implantation of this in-tunnel device (Figures 63.9 and 63.10). Furthermore, the distance between the septum secundum and primum in this tunnel should be <8 mm because too large a gap may increase the risk of a residual shunt.

Who is not suitable for CoherexFlatStent EF device?

- PFO with an interatrial septal aneurysm and inadequate functional tunnel length (type III tunnel) (Figure 63.11).

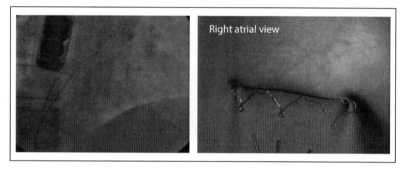

Figure 63.7 (**See color insert.**) CoherexFlatStent EF detached.

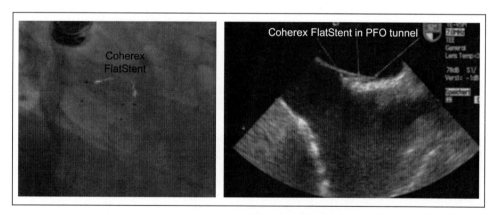

Figure 63.8 CoherexFlatStent EF under fluoroscopy and bicaval view TEE after release.

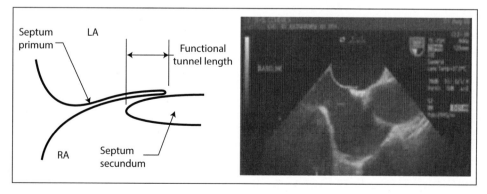

Figure 63.9 Simple PFO with no ASA (type I tunnel).

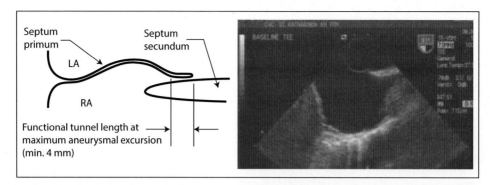

Figure 63.10   PFO with aneurysm and adequate tunnel length for in-tunnel device (type II tunnel).

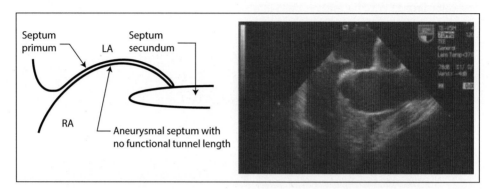

Figure 63.11   PFO with aneurysm and inadequate tunnel length for in-tunnel device (type III tunnel).

Clinical studies and results

The results from the Coherex-EU Study were published in 2014.[1] In this prospective, nonrandomized, multicenter study, device implantation was successful in 100% successful. The clinically effective closure rate during 6 month follow-up was 88%. Device embolization occurred in four cases. In these cases, in addition to the PFO, an interatrial septal aneurysm was present with an insufficient (<4 mm) tunnel length (type III). All devices were retrieved percutaneously. No thrombus, erosion, arrhythmia, or device-induced valvular incompetence was reported during 6 month follow-up.

Conclusion

The CoherexFlatStent EF device is an in-tunnel device. As a result, the exposed surface area is significantly reduced. This may reduce the risk of device-induced complications, particularly thrombus formation, erosion, and arrhythmias. Sufficient functional tunnel length (>4 mm) is essential for safe implantation of this device and can be easily assessed by transesophageal echocardiography or intracardiac echocardiographic imaging. The FlatStent EF PFO Closure System is easy to use and may be suitable for most PFO patients.

Reference

1. Sievert H, Wunderlich N, Reiffenstein I et al. Initial clinical experience with the Coherex FlatStent and FlatStent EF PFO closure system for in-tunnel PFO closure: Results of the Coherex-EU study. *Catheter Cardiovasc Interv* 2014;83(7):1135–43.

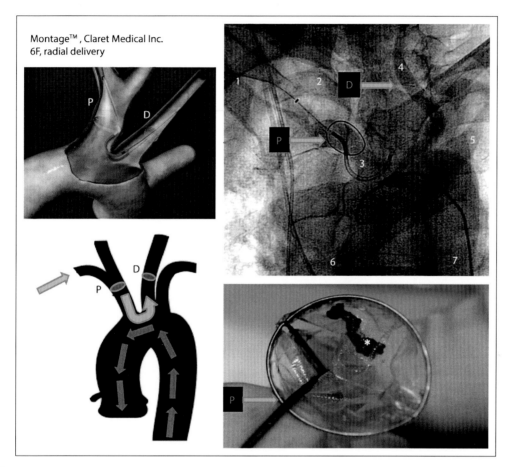

Figure 29.5 Montage—Distal embolic protection device. Embolic protection devices are developed to prevent transcatheter aortic valve implantation (TAVI)-related embolism into the brain supplying vessels. The Montage dual-filter embolic protection device is delivered over a 0.014" guide wire from a left-radial approach (6 F). The proximal filter (P) is placed within the innominate artery; the distal filter (D) is to be delivered into the left common carotid artery (blue arrows indicate the delivery route of the protection device [blue circles], the pathway of a transfemoral valve delivery is indicated with gray arrows). This system allows retrieval of embolic debris (asterisk, "*"). 1—Right subclavian artery, 2—right common carotid artery, 3—common brachiocephalic trunk/anonymous artery, 4—left common carotid artery, 5—left subclavian artery, 6—ascending aorta, 7—descending aorta. (Reproduced from Claret Medical, Inc. With permission.)

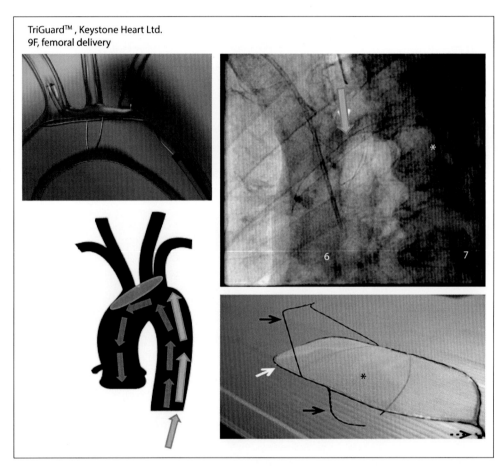

Figure 29.6 TriGuard—Distal embolic protection device. The Keystone TriGuard embolic protection device is delivered from a femoral approach (9 F) and deployed in the aortic arch. The deflection shield allows coverage of the ostia of the arch vessels (blue arrows indicate the delivery route of the protection device [blue circle], the pathway of a transfemoral valve delivery is indicated with gray arrows). The nitinol frame (white arrow) holds a nitinol mesh (white asterisk) which is kept in place by upper and lower stabilizers (black arrows), to achieve maximal coverage of the aortic trifurcation throughout the intervention. 6—Ascending aorta, 7—descending aorta. (Reproduced from Europa Digital & Publishing. With permission.)

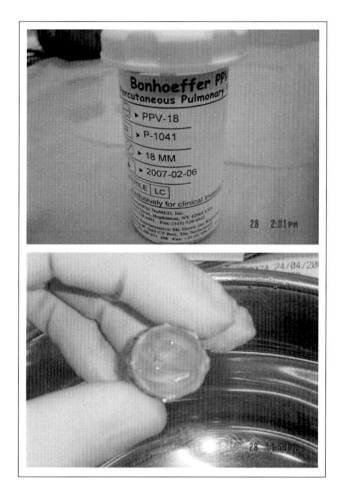

Figure 34.1 Bonhoeffer PPV.

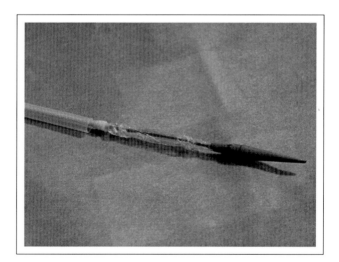

Figure 34.2 Delivery system with BIB balloon and outer sheath.

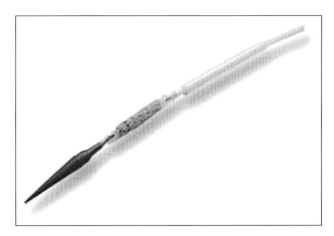

Figure 34.3 Appropriate loading of the PPV on the BIB balloon of the delivery system.

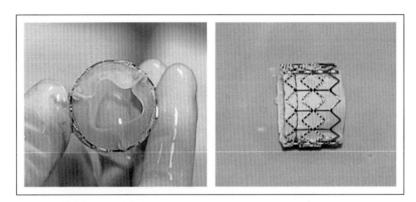

Figure 35.1 The Edwards SAPIEN transcatheter heart valve. The valve (shown *en face* on the left and from the side on the right) is available in 23 mm or 26 mm diameter. It consists of three bovine pericardial cusps mounted into a stainless-steel, balloon-expandable stent.

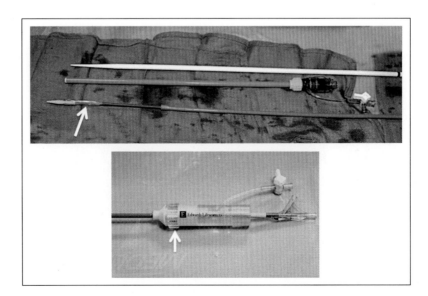

Figure 35.2 The delivery system that includes the 35-cm-long delivery sheath and dilator and the RetroFlex delivery catheter that has a tapered steerable tip (shown in the top panel), which facilitates valve crossing; white arrow indicates the location of the valve on the catheter. The handle of the Retroflex catheter (shown in the bottom panel) has a nob (arrow) to steer the tip of the catheter.

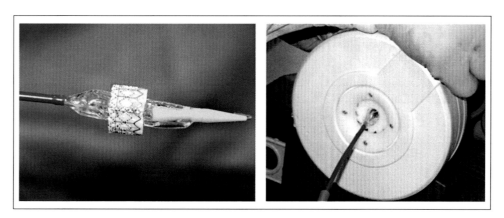

Figure 35.4 Left: The valve is positioned on the delivery balloon, green suture line lined up away from the yellow tip. Right: Valve being crimped using the crimping tool.

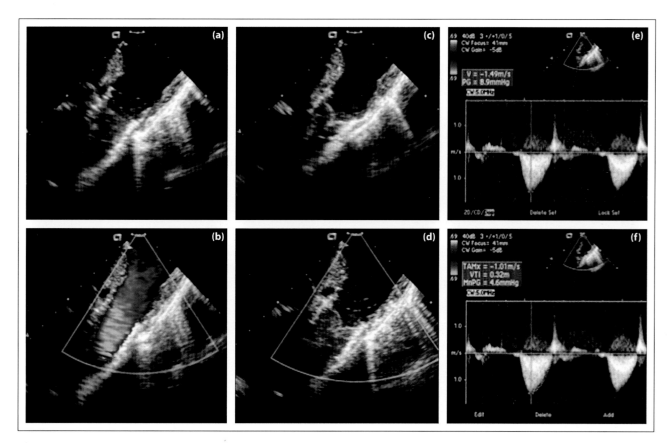

Figure 35.5 Intracardiac echocardiography. (a) After prestenting the RVOT, (b) color Doppler demonstrates free pulmonic insufficiency. (c) After deployment of Edwards SAPIEN valve, (d) color Doppler demonstrates trivial pulmonic insufficiency. (e) Continuous-wave Doppler across the RVOT at baseline showing significant gradient. (f) Continuous-wave Doppler across the RVOT following valve implantation showing reduction in gradient.

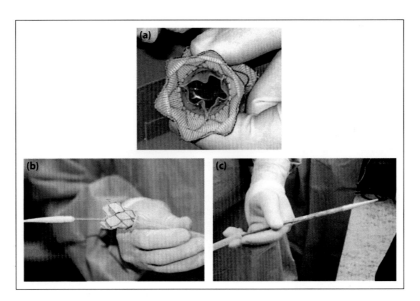

Figure 36.5 A new Medtronic self-expanding valve, currently in development, is being designed for native RVOTs. (a) Demonstration of the short-axis view of the valve. (b) Loading the valve into the delivery system. (c) The valve fully loaded and ready for delivery.

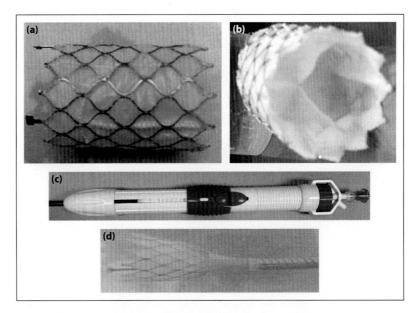

Figure 36.6 Series of images outlining the Lifetech self-expanding pulmonary valve system. (a) Demonstration of the long-axis view of the expanded valve. (b) Demonstration of the short-axis view of the outflow end of the valve with the three tissue leaflets seen clearly. (c) The delivery system allows for rapid or slow deployment with (d) a superelastic reinforced end to allow flaring and recovery after over two-thirds of the device is deployed.

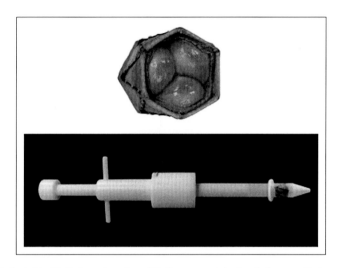

Figure 36.8 The No-React Injectable BioPulmonic valve with the perventricular delivery catheter seen in the bottom panel.

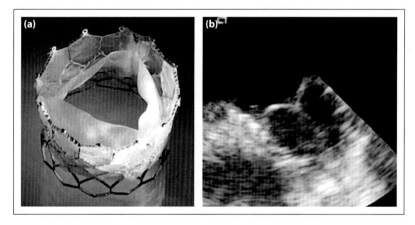

Figure 36.9 (a) The Colibri valve. (b) Intracardiac echocardiographic image of the valve following deployment in the RVOT in a canine model.

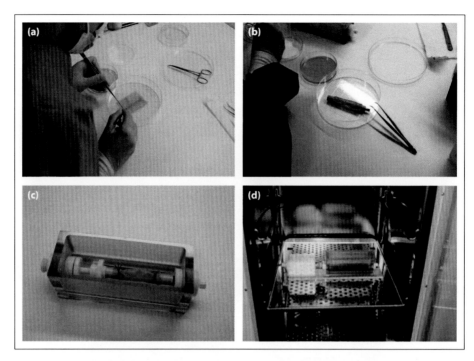

Figure 36.10 Series of images outlining the development of a core-matric scaffold for seeding of stem cells and the ultimate development of a tissue-engineered scaffold. Human cord blood stem cell-derived smooth muscle cells were seeded onto a core scaffold and incubated for 2 days before the assembly of the conduit. (a) Sewing the two pieces of scaffold together as a cylinder. (b) The core column is sheathed in tissue-engineered conduit, before being installed on the bioreactor. (c) Tissue-engineered conduit, installed and fixed in the bioreactor. (d) Tissue-engineered conduit incubating in the bioreactor at 37°C incubator.

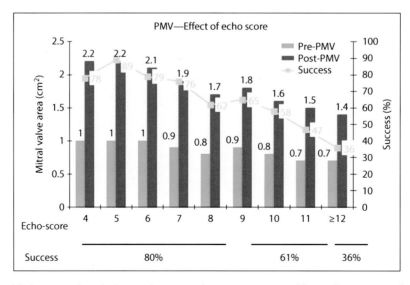

Figure 37.5 Relationship between the echo score, the pre- and post-PMV MVA, and immediate success after PMV.

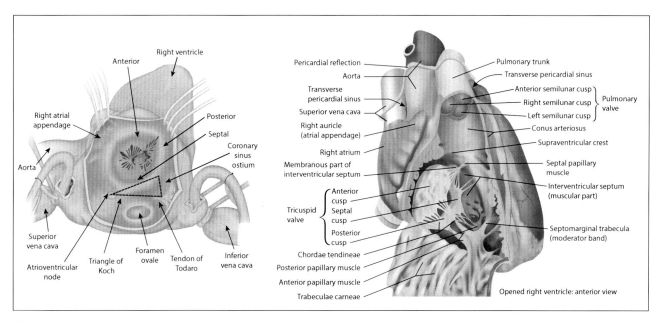

Figure 38.1 Anatomy of TV and subvalvular apparatus. (From Gray H, Standring S. Eds. *Gray's Anatomy: The Anatomical Basis of Clinical Practice*. 39th ed. Edinburgh, UK: Churchill Livingstone Elsevier, 2005. pp. 1003–4.)

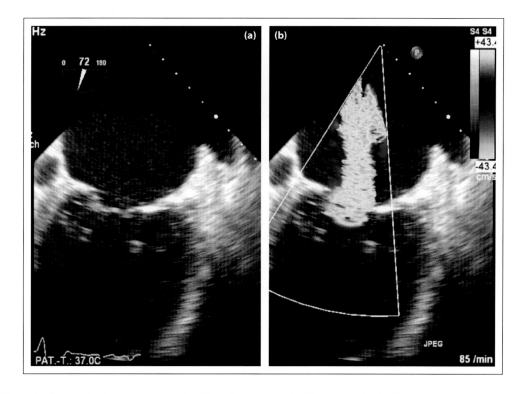

Figure 39.1 Mitral regurgitation, type I: annulus dilatation. As seen in (a), the annulus is dilated, leading to the central wide color flow pattern seen in (b).

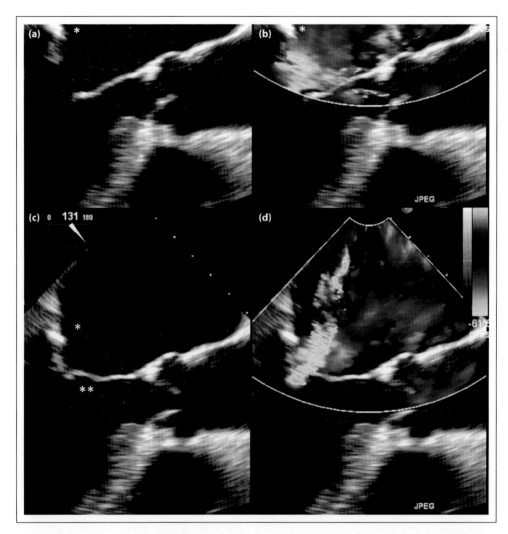

Figure 39.3 Mitral regurgitation, type III: restrictive leaflets. The posterior leaflet in diastole is seen without color in (a) and with color in (b), marked by the single asterisk. (c) The patient in systole, where the posterior leaflet has not moved due to restriction (single asterisk). Of note, the anterior leaflet has risen to meet the posterior leaflet (double asterisk), but there is still significant regurgitation (d).

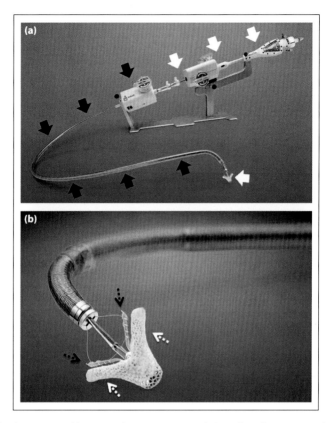

Figure 40.1 The MitraClip device system. (a) Two main components of the MitraClip system. Black arrows indicate the steerable guide catheter and white arrows the clip delivery system that is advanced through the steerable guide catheter. (b) The MitraClip attached on the tip of the clip delivery catheter has two arms (white broken arrows) and two grippers (black broken arrows).

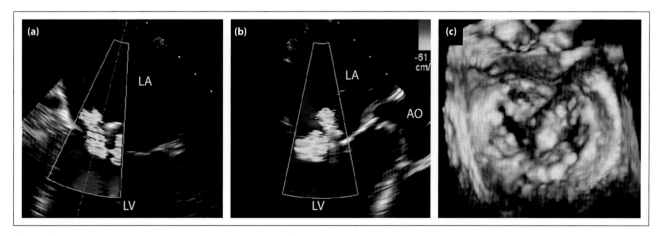

Figure 40.4 The direction of the clip shaft is optimized by the manipulation of the steerable guide catheter and clip delivery system. Following the opening of the MitraClip in the left atrium, under a intercommissural two-chamber view, the clip shaft is directed to divide the regurgitation jet (a). The direction of the clip shaft is adjusted so that the shaft is perpendicular to the mitral annulus both in intercommissural two-chamber (a) and LVOT view (b). On determination of clip shaft trajectory, it is rotated to position the clip arm perpendicular to the commissure. Three-dimensional reconstruction of TEE image facilitates this maneuver (c).

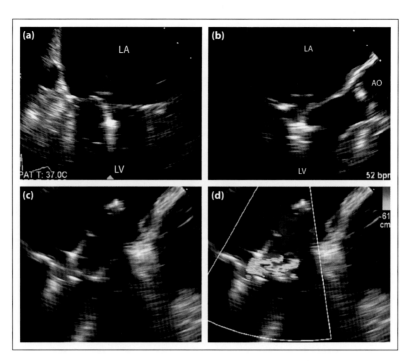

Figure 40.5 The clip delivery system is slowly advanced into the left ventricle with real-time TEE guidance using an intercommissural two-chamber (a) and LVOT view (b). On final confirmation of the clip arm position, the clip delivery system is slowly pulled back immediately under the mitral valve leaflet to grasp. The LVOT view is the standard view, as this allows slight adjustment of clip arm in anterior–posterior direction (c). Using color Doppler, the clip arm is completely closed to confirm the reduction of regurgitation jet (d).

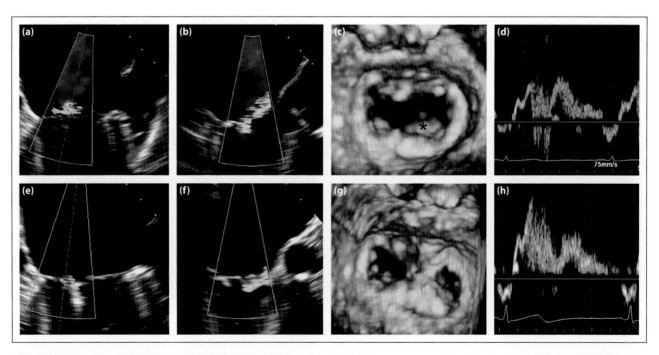

Figure 40.6 A case of successful repair with the MitraClip in a patient with mitral regurgitation due to flail posterior leaflet. Baseline TEE showed significant eccentric mitral regurgitation (a and b) due to frail P2 posterior leaflet (asterisk in c). A Doppler of a pulmonary vein showed systolic flow reversal (d). Following deployment of the mitral clip, successful improvement of MR was observed (e and f). Three-dimensional reconstruction of the TEE image showed successful deployment of the MitraClip at the target portion of mitral valve (g) and systolic flow reversal of pulmonary vein also improved (h).

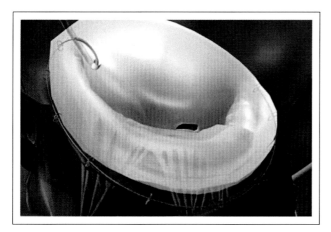

Figure 41.2 The Guided Delivery System Accucinch involves placing anchors in the mitral annulus and subannular left ventricular myocardium via retrograde left ventricular access. A string or tether is used to tension the anchors and diminish the mitral annular circumference.

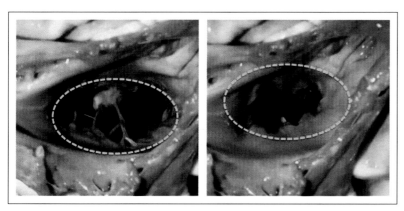

Figure 41.3 In a bench-top ovine model, the left panel shows the mitral orifice before the Guided Delivery System's tether is tightened. The degree of circumferential cinching can be appreciated in the right-hand panel, where the dotted line represents the original mitral orifice.

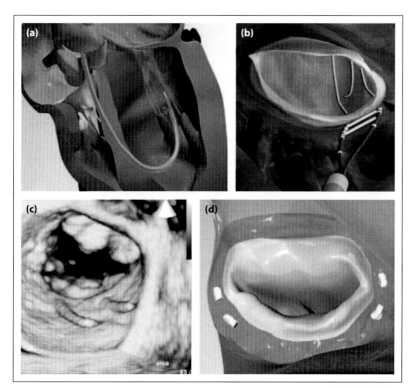

Figure 41.4 The Mitralign system uses retrograde left ventricular access, shown in (a). A guide catheter was placed below the posterior leaflet annular tissue. In (b), radio-frequency wires are seen to traverse the annulus, for delivery of pledgets that are used to cause cinching of the annulus. In (c), a three-dimensional left atrial echocardiographic view shows two wires placed through the annulus. Ultimately, two pairs of wires are used. (d) A schematic of the two pairs of pledgets on either side of the mitral annulus.

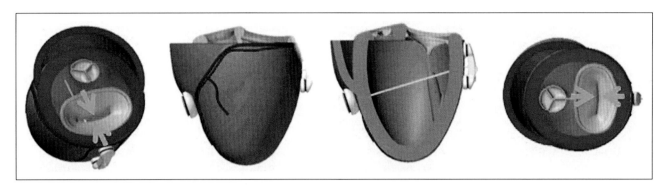

Figure 41.5 The Myocor device uses pads on the anterior and posterior surfaces of the left ventricle, with a cord traversing the left ventricular chamber. This allows for compression of both the left ventricular chamber and the mitral orifice. In a beating-heart surgical approach, this procedure produced similar degrees of reduction in mitral regurgitation compared with surgical annuloplasty, with better survival. (Adapted from Grossi EA et al. *J Am Coll Cardiol* 2010;56(24):1984–93.)

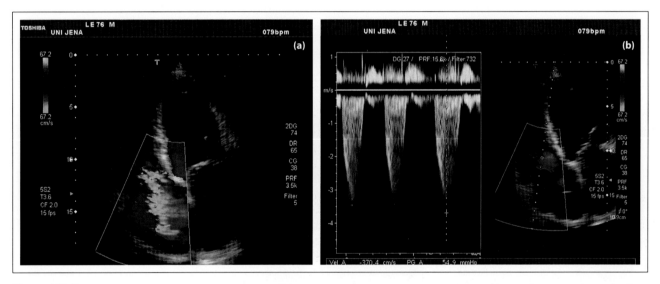

Figure 43.2 Assessment of tricuspid regurgitation and assessment of pulmonary artery pressure. (a) Two-dimensional echocardiography with color-flow Doppler imaging demonstrating severe tricuspid regurgitation with enlargement of the right ventricle and right atrium. (b) Using continuous-wave Doppler and the modified Bernoulli equation, right ventricular and pulmonary artery systolic pressures are indirectly assessed at 55 mmHg.

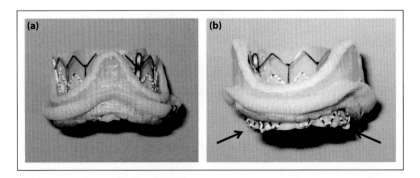

Figure 45.3 Transcatheter valve deployed within a surgical prosthesis (SAPIEN THV and Carpenter–Edwards). (a) Incorrect positioning. The outflows of the surgical prosthesis and THV are superimposed. During balloon deployment, the prosthetic struts may be splayed, allowing the THV to embolize. (b) Correct positioning. The THV overlaps the sewing ring of the surgical prosthesis allowing more secure fixation. (Adapted from Webb JG et al. *Circulation* 2010;121(16):1848–57.)

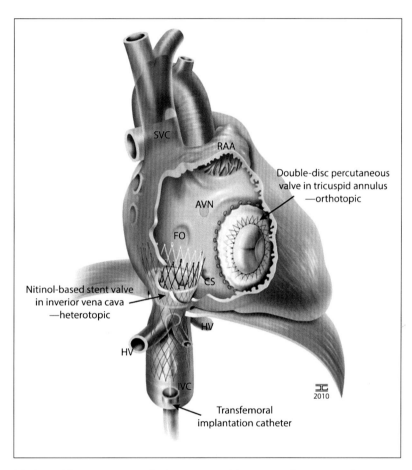

Figure 46.1 Right atrial view with percutaneous devices suggested for transcatheter TV replacement. Position of self-expanding stent valves in the tricuspid annulus (orthotopic) and in the IVC (heterotopic) in chronic right ventricular pressure overload. Relevant anatomic structures include the coronary sinus ostium (CS), the foramen ovale (FO), and the atrioventricular node (AVN). IVC, inferior vena cava; SVC, superior vena cava; RAA, right atrial appendage.

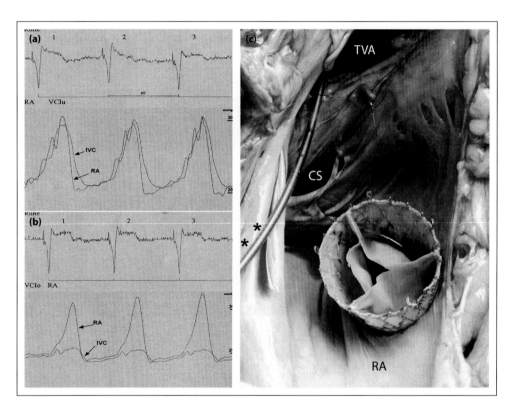

Figure 46.4 First-in-man application of heterotopic tricuspid valve implantation. (a) Severe TR with IVC congestion is present before device implantation. Right heart catheterization confirms a prominent ventricular wave of 30 mmHg in the RA and the IVC. (b) Deployment of a self-expanding valve resulted in the immediate abolition of regurgitation into the IVC and lowered the mean IVC pressure. Excellent device function was documented during follow-up. (c) Macroscopic specimen showing the bioprosthetic valve in the IVC during autopsy 3 months later. Three months after the procedure, the patient died from cerebral ischemia with secondary hemorrhage. TVA, tricuspid annulus; RA, right atrium; CS, coronary sinus. Asterisk: RV pacing lead crossing the TVA.

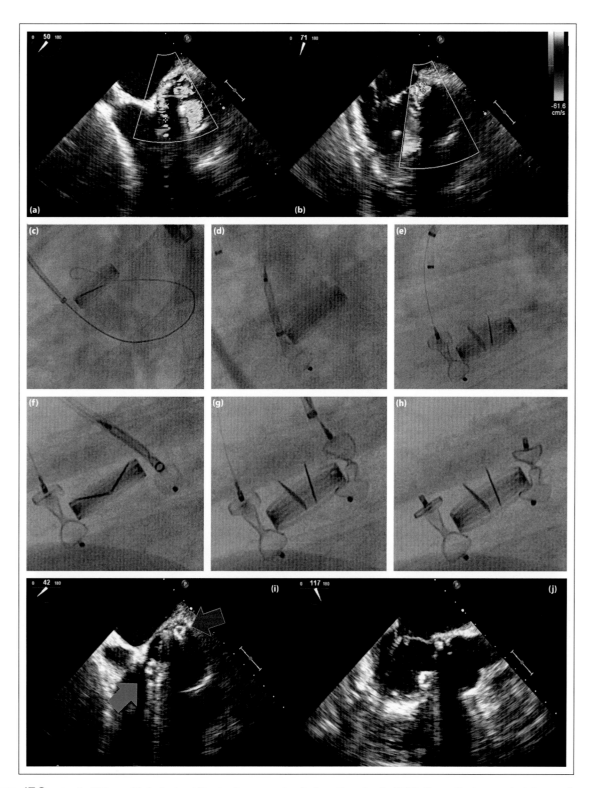

Figure 47.2 Aortic PVL, multiple leaks. After having a mechanical aortic valve in 2008, the patient presented 4 years later with symptoms of heart failure and severe regurgitation. A 5 × 11 mm PVL was noted near the left coronary cusp and 5 × 8 mm PVL was noted in the area of the noncoronary cusp (a and b). A 5 Fr MP catheter and 0.035" hydrophilic wire was used to cross the leak near the noncoronary cusp. This was then exchanged over an Amplatz ES 0.035" wire (c) for a 10 Fr Cook shuttle sheath. This was then used to advance an AVP III size 5 × 14 mm device (d), which was then deployed (e). Similar access was obtained through the other femoral artery and a similar technique was used to cross the leak near the left coronary cusp. An AVP III 5 × 14 mm device was also implanted (f through h). Follow-up echocardiographic views at 42° and 117° show the position of the noncoronary cusp (green arrow) and left coronary cusp (red arrow) devices (i and j). Both aortic and mitral valve leaflets moved well on TEE.

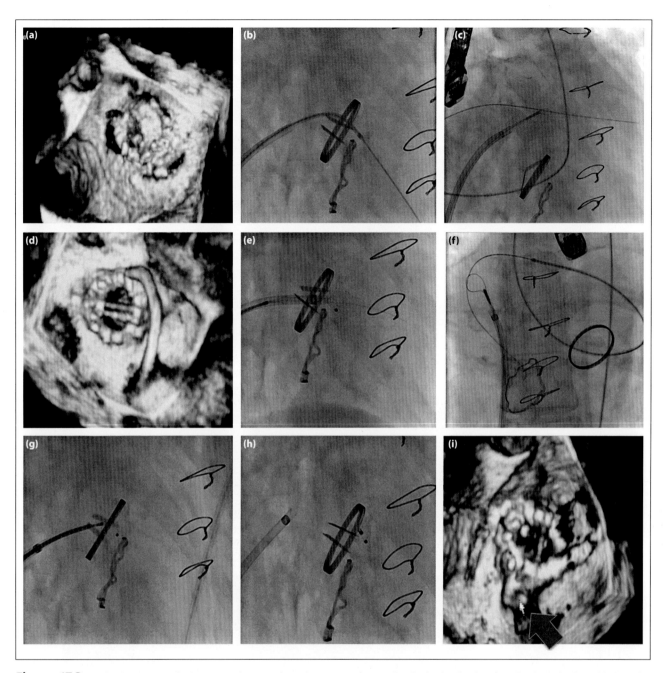

Figure 47.3 Mitral PVL, one device. Several years after placement of a mechanical mitral valve prosthesis and tricuspid ring, the patient developed severe mitral regurgitation with reversal of flow in pulmonary veins. This was due to two paravalvular mitral leaks, one anterolateral (orifice 6 × 15 mm) and one posterior (orifice 10 × 8 mm) (a). The anterolateral leak was close to a section of tissue that interfered with leaflet motion; therefore, a decision was made to only pursue the posterior leak. Rather than approaching the leak retrograde, the decision was made to approach the leak antegrade due to presumed easier access to the posterior leak. After placement of a 5 Fr sheath in the right femoral artery and a 9 Fr sheath in the right femoral vein, transseptal puncture was performed. Antegrade crossing was obtained (wire and diagnostic catheter) but the sheath did not cross (b). Therefore, a 5 Fr JR4 catheter and 0.035″ Terumo wire were introduced through the aorta and the leak was crossed retrograde; the Terumo wire was advanced and snared through a transvenous/transseptal sling in the left atrium and externalized (c and d). This allowed the transseptal 9 Fr sheath to be advanced through the leak. A 10 mm Amplatzer muscular VSD occluder was brought through the leak but caused mitral valve impingement (e). Therefore, this was removed and retrograde access from the aorta and sling in the left atrium was again obtained (f). Next, an Amplatzer 10 mm PDA occluder was placed across the defect (g and h), which did not interfere with mitral leaflet movement. Echocardiography showing final device position is seen (i).

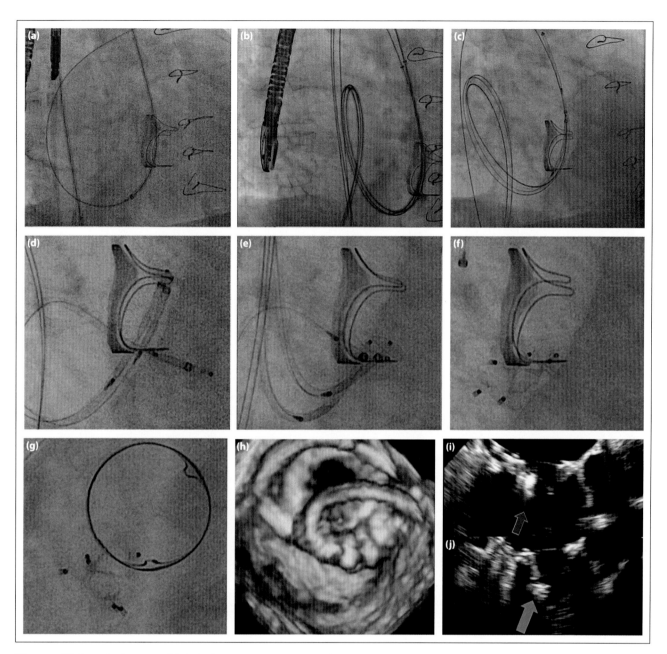

Figure 47.4 Mitral PVL, multiple leaks. Large mitral PVLs. After the patient had placement of a bioprosthetic MVR in 2004, he developed one long PVL that extended over 1/4 of the bioprosthetic valve. A 5 Fr sheath was placed in the right femoral artery. A 5 Fr JR4 catheter and 0.035" Terumo hydrophilic wire were used to cross the leak (a). After femoral venous access with a 6 Fr sheath, transseptal access was obtained. A snare was used to externalize the Terumo wire from the left atrium through the right femoral vein. An Amplatz Extra Stiff wire was used to exchange the transseptal sheath for an 18 Fr sheath. The same wire was used to exchange for an 18 Fr sheath; through this, three Amplatz ES wires were used to exchange this for three 6 Fr Cook shuttle sheaths (b and c). Through these three sheaths, two 12 mm AVP 2 devices and one 10 mm AVP 2 were advanced into the leak (d and e) and deployed (f and g). The position of the devices is also visible on the echocardiogram (h). When deploying mitral PVL devices antegrade, it is important to make sure that the mitral valve leaflets are not affected by the ventricular side of the device (i)—this requires readjustment and redeployment so that the leaflets are not affected (j).

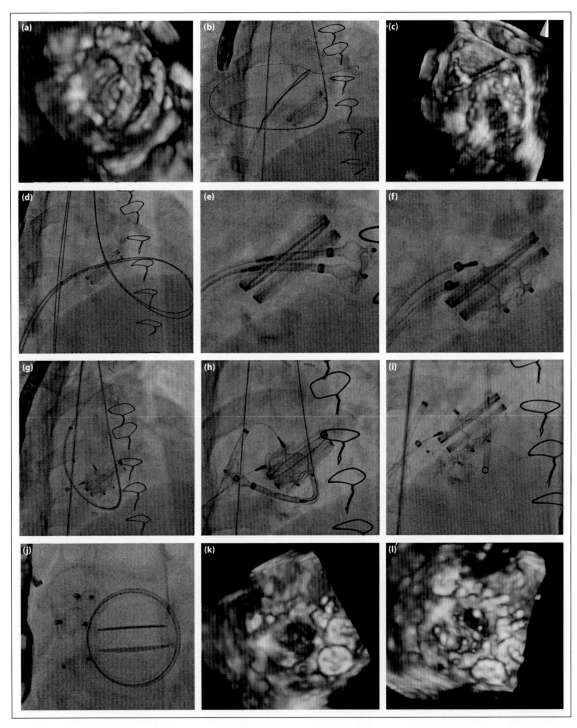

Figure 47.5 Mitral PVL, multiple leaks. The patient presented with severe mitral PVL. He presented with an anteromedial leak from 1 to 4 o'clock (orifice 4 × 19 mm), and by 5 o'clock, presented with a second leak (orifice 4 × 3 mm). The large orifice is seen on the echocardiography (a). A 5 Fr sheath was placed in the right femoral artery. A 5 Fr JR4 catheter and 0.035″ hydrophilic wire was advanced across the anteromedial leak. A 6 Fr sheath was placed in the right femoral vein. Transseptal access was obtained and a snare was used to grab and externalize the wire (b and c). An Amplatz ES wire was then used to exchange this transseptal sheath for a 10 Fr sheath. Through this 10 Fr sheath, two Amplatz ES wires were used to exchange for two 6 Fr Cook shuttle sheaths (d). Two AVP II size 10 mm were advanced and deployed (e and f). The leak at 5 o'clock was approached retrograde. The 5 Fr sheath in the right femoral artery was upsized to a 6 Fr sheath. A 5 Fr JR4 catheter and Terumo wire was used to cross the leak (f). A snare was advanced transseptally into the left atrium, used to capture the wire (g), and then externalized. An 8 mm AVP II was advanced (h) and deployed (i and j). The mitral valve leaflets moved normally. The devices are visible on TEE from atrial (k) and ventricular aspect (l).

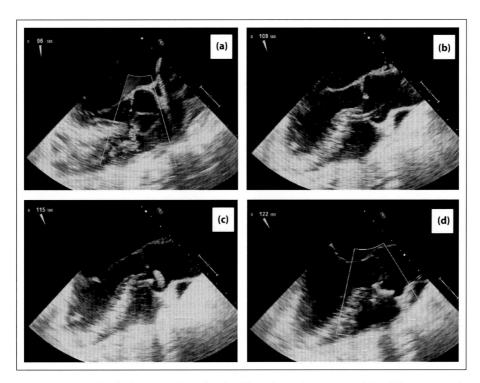

Figure 48.1 Intraprocedural TOE in the long-axis view showing (a) perforated aneurysm of the right coronary sinus draining into the RVOT with turbulent color flow across. (b) Following CC with ADO, there is complete closure with no color flow across. (c) The delivery sheath can be seen crossing the defect from the RVOT into the ascending aorta. (d) The aortic disk with its attached delivery cable passing through the sheath being pulled to block the aortic end of the defect.

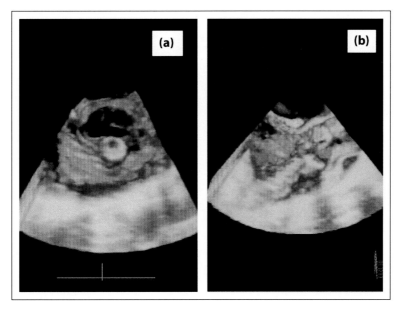

Figure 48.2 Transoesophageal 3D acquisition in the short-axis (a) and long-axis (b) views following CC of RASV from RCC to RVOT showing the deployed ADO *en face* and in profile.

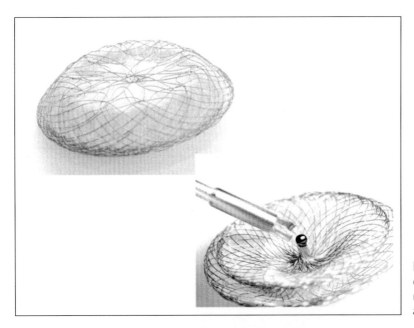

Figure 50.2 The Occlutech Figulla Flex II device: Note the difference in the attachment mechanism. Occlutech has the ball in the right atrial disk.

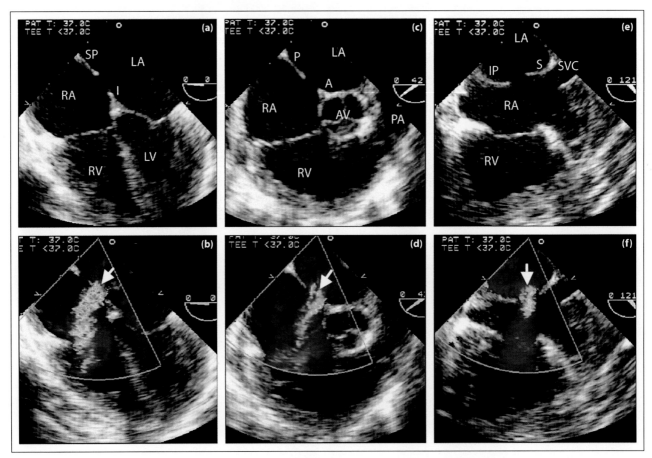

Figure 50.3 Transesophageal echocardiographic images in a patient with secundum atrial septal defect demonstrating the essential views for selection of patients to undergo device closure using the Amplatzer or the Occlutech devices. Top images are without and bottom images same views with color Doppler. (a,b) Four-chamber view (0° omni plane) showing the defect with left-to-right shunt (arrow), the inferior anterior rim (I), and the superior-posterior rim (SP). (c,d) Classic short-axis view at about 40° demonstrating the defect (arrow); the anterior rim (A) and the posterior rim (P). (e,f) Bicaval view at about 120° demonstrating the superior rim (S) and the inferior rim (IP) and the defect (arrow). LA: left atrium; RA: right atrium; RV: right ventricle; SVC: superior vena cava; IVC: inferior vena cava; LV: left ventricle; PA: pulmonary artery.

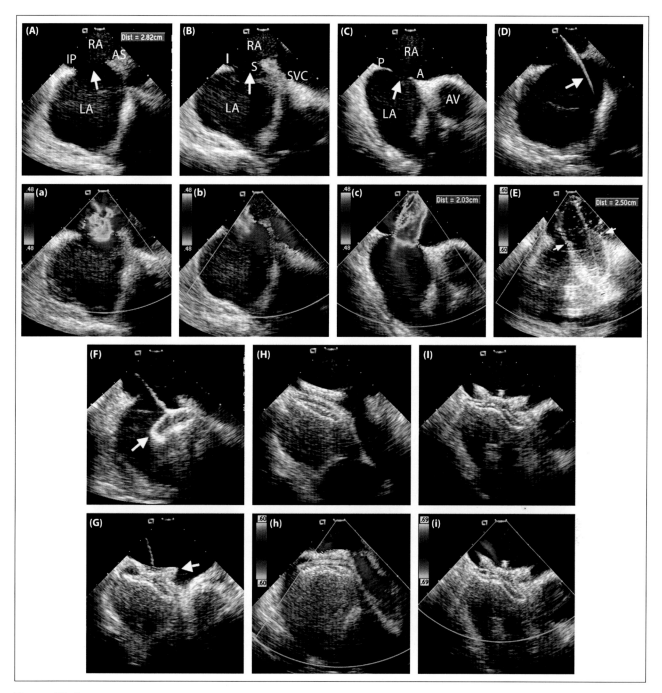

Figure 50.4 Intracardiac echocardiographic images in a 59-year-old patient with a secundum atrial septal defect measuring 28 mm demonstrating the various steps of closure. (A and a) Septal view without and with color Doppler showing the defect (arrow) with left-to-right shunt, the anterior/superior (AS) rim, and the inferior/posterior rim (IP). (B and b) Bicaval view (long-axis view) without and with color Doppler showing the superior rim (S) and inferior rim (I). (C and c) Short-axis view without and with color Doppler showing the defect with left-to-right shunt (arrow), the anterior rim (A), and the posterior rim (P). (d) Septal view showing wire passage (arrow) through the defect. (e) Similar view as (d), during stop-flow technique of balloon sizing. RA: right atrium; LA: left atrium; SVC: superior vena cava; AV: aortic valve. (f) Deployment of the left atrial disk (arrow) of a 28-mm Amplatzer septal occluder. (g) Deployment of the right disk of the device (arrow). (H and h) Bicaval view without and with color Doppler after the device has been released showing good device position and no residual shunt and unobstructed SVC flow. (I and i) Short-axis view after the device has been released, again showing good device position and no residual shunt.

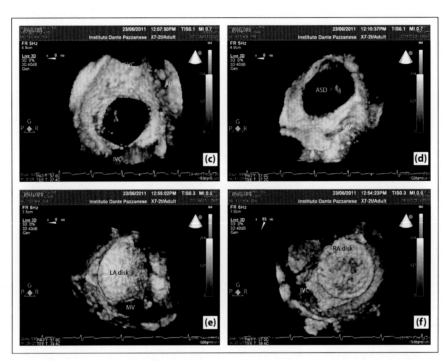

Figure 51.4 A large ASD closed with a 39 mm Figulla ASD device. (c) 3D TEE. RA view. The use of 3D TEE allowed for a better delineation of the large ASD and the adequate surrounding rims. IVC: inferior vena cava. SVC: superior vena cava. Ao: aorta. (d) 3D TEE. LA view. There is sufficient amount of tissue separating the mitral valve (MV) and the ASD, which defined the adequacy of the posteroinferior rim. (e) 3D TEE after device release. LA view. Note the LA disk is well apposed to the atrial septum distant from the mitral valve (MV). The disk is flat with no metallic clamp. There is no space between the disk and the surrounding rims. (f) 3D TEE after device release. RA view. Note the RA disk is well positioned within the atrial septum with no space between it and the surrounding rims.

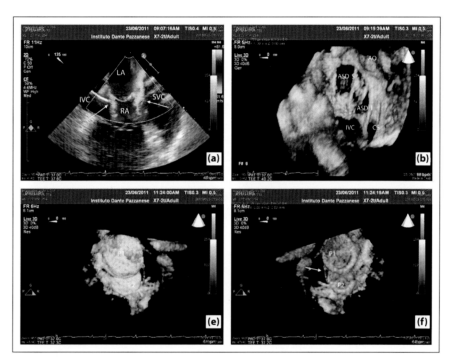

Figure 51.5 The closure of multiple ASDs with two Figulla occluders. (a) Long-axis (bicaval) view on 2D TEE with color-flow mapping showing two ASDs (arrows) separated by a 15 mm tongue of tissue. The superior defect (near the superior vena cava—SVC) measured 15 mm and the inferior defect (near the inferior vena cava—IVC) measured 8 mm. (b) 3D TEE, RA view. The use of 3D TEE allowed for a better appreciation of the underlying anatomy. Both defects are delineated at best and the distance to the surrounding structures such as the coronary sinus (CS), aorta (Ao), and inferior vena cava (IVC) are unequivocally displayed. ASD S: superior ASD. ASD I: inferior ASD. (e) 3D TEE. LA view. A 21 mm device was implanted in the superior defect (P1) and a 12 mm device in the inferior ASD (P2). There is some overlap of both occluders with a pinpoint residual defect (arrow) between them. There was complete closure within 6 months after endothelialization of the devices. (f) 3D TEE. RA view. The immediate residual defect (arrow) is again delineated at best between the overlapping occluders.

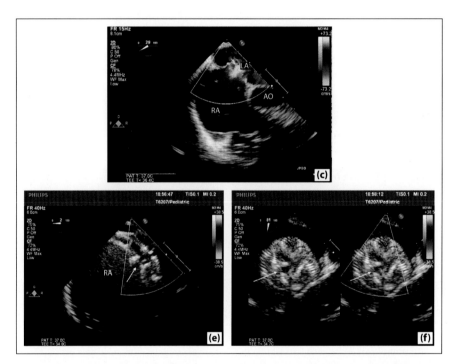

Figure 51.6 Use of a fenestrated Figulla ASD occluder. A 4-year-old female patient (15 kg) previously submitted to radio-frequency-assisted pulmonary valve dilatation, left pulmonary artery stenting, and Blalock–Taussig–Thomas shunt occlusion. Right ventricular size was smaller (tricuspid valve Z value of −2.5) and there was predominantly right-to-left shunt through a 14 mm ASD. The stretched diameter was 21 mm. There was no hemodynamic compromise after test occlusion of the ASD. A 21 mm fenestrated Figulla Flex device was implanted at first but it was too large for the size of the child. It was replaced by an 18 mm fenestrated occluder, which was implanted uneventfully through a transhepatic approach. Systemic oxygen saturation increased from low 80s to low 90s. (c) Right-to-left shunting demonstrated by color-flow mapping on short-axis view on 2D TEE. (e) An 18-mm device in place on short-axis view on 2D TEE. The fenestration (arrow) can be seen in the more anterior aspect of the device allowing some right-to-left shunt on color-flow mapping (red color). (f) An *en face* view of the LA disk was obtained on TEE. The fenestration (arrow) is nicely displayed on 2D view (left) and with color-flow mapping (right).

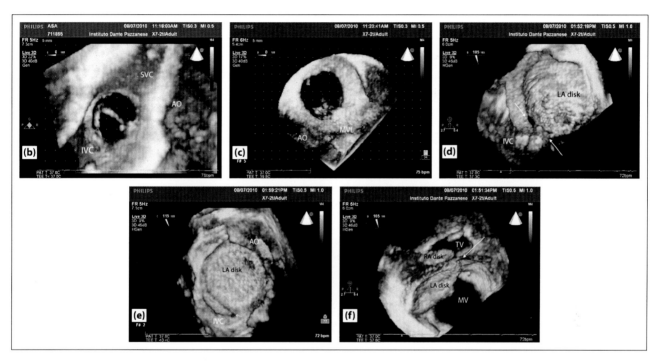

Figure 51.7 The closure of multiple ASDs with a single large device. (b) 3D TEE. RA view. The two defects and the tissue strand between them are better appreciated using 3D technology. IVC: inferior vena cava. SVC: superior vena cava. AO: aorta. (c) 3D TEE. LA view. The defect is profiled from the LA side. AO: aorta. MVL: mitral valve anterior leaflet. A decision was made to place the device in the superior defect. (d) 3D TEE. LA view after device deployment before release. There is a half-moon residual defect (arrows) in the posteroinferior aspect of the atrial septum due to the tension of the delivery cable. IVC: inferior vena cava. (e) 3D TEE. LA view after device release. There was a significant decrease in the size of the residual defect (arrow) after the occluder was released from the delivery cable. (f) 3D TEE. LA view after device release. The superior portion of the atrial septum (arrow) is nicely seen in between the two disks. MV: mitral valve. TV: tricuspid valve.

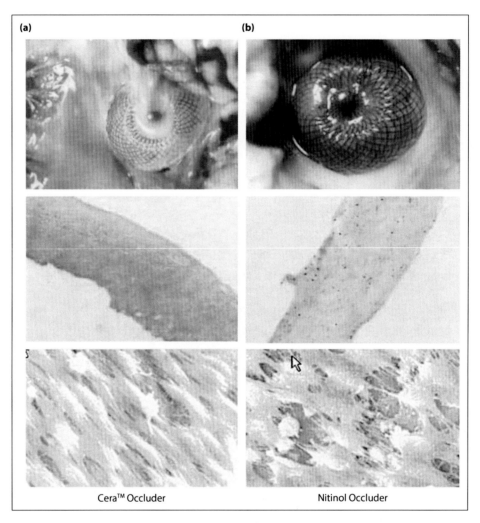

(a) **(b)**

Cera™ Occluder | Nitinol Occluder

Figure 52.1 Gross, histologic, and electron microscopic pictures of Cera ASD Occluder compared with the untreated nitinol device in an animal model 3 months after implantation.

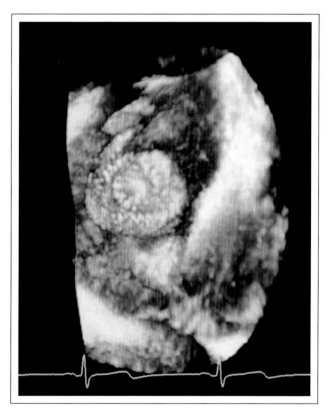

Figure 53.9   Left atrial 3D TEE view showing the left atrial disk in position covering the defect completely.

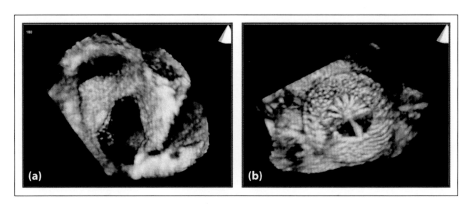

Figure 53.10 (a) A large ostium secundum-type ASD is visualized on 3D TEE from the RA side. (b) A Nit-Occlud ASD-R device, which is still attached to the delivery system, has been implanted and shows an adequate device position. (Courtesy of Simone Fontes Pedra.)

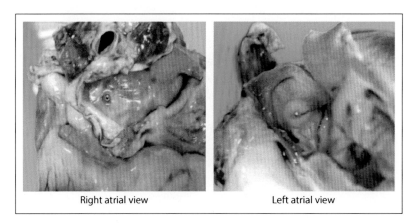

Right atrial view   Left atrial view

Figure 54.3 Gross specimens of CSO 6 weeks after implantation in swine model. (From Lertsapcharoen P et al. *Indian Heart J* 2006;58:315–20.)

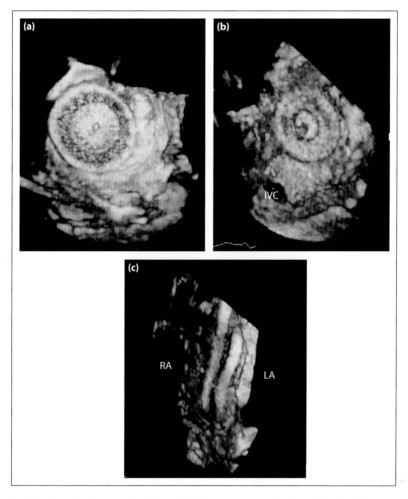

Figure 54.6 Three-dimensional TEE pictures of postimplanted CSO in different views. (a) Left atrial aspect, (b) right atrial aspect, and (c) interatrial.

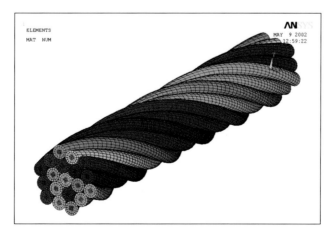

Figure 56.2 19-strand NiTi wires woven in petal shape.

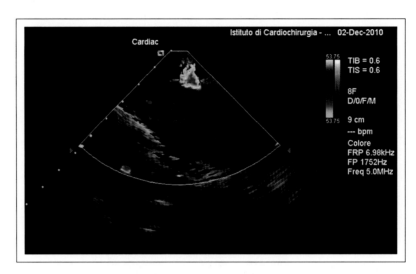

Figure 56.9 ICE with left-to-right ultrasound Doppler visualization of an ostium secundum ASD.

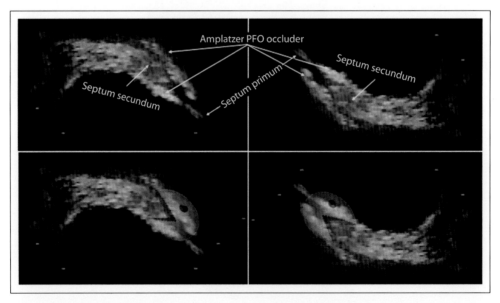

Figure 59.24 Left: Demonstration of a positive Pacman sign by transesophageal echocardiography in the projection usually seen during fluoroscopy. The bottom panel explains where the name "Pacman sign" derives from. Right: The same situation seen in the projection typical for transesophageal echocardiography.

64

Patent foramen ovale closure: SeptRx occluder

Katharina Malsch, Jennifer Franke, Stefan Bertog, and Horst Sievert

Introduction

The SeptRx IPO™ (IntraPocket Occluder) PFO closure system (SeptRx, Fremont, CA, USA) is one of the newer generation closure systems for PFOs. It is an in-tunnel closure system exclusively designed for PFOs. It cannot be used for atrial septal defect (ASD) or ventricular septal defect (VSD) closures. The PFO is closed by using stretching and a natural adhesion response to bring the septum primum and secundum together. In contrast to umbrella and double-umbrella devices, it does not rely on endothelialization for closure. The low profile and limited exposure of foreign material to the circulation may minimize the risk of atrial arrhythmias and thrombus formation. A first-in-man implantation was performed in 2006.

Device

The device (Figure 64.1) consists of a flexible nitinol frame, a braided nitinol mesh in the middle of the frame, and four anchors that secure the device between the septum primum and secundum and prevent embolism. Tantalum radiopaque markers optimize device visualization during fluoroscopy and deployment. The device has been designed to adapt to a wide range of PFOs. This is achieved by the flexibility of the frame and anchors, allowing accommodation to various tunnel lengths and interatrial septal morphologies. On the left atrial side, the anchors are long and curled and suspended around the septum primum. On the right atrial side, the anchors have an angled design to secure the device on the septum secundum. Permanent closure is stimulated by the body's natural adhesion response. The SeptRx IPO (IntraPocket Occluder) PFO Closure System is available in two sizes and is designed to fit defect lengths of 4–20 mm and flat widths of 4–19 mm (Table 64.1).

Delivery system

An over-the-wire delivery system facilitates SeptRx IPO PFO closure system implantation. The device is preloaded onto the stainless steel delivery system (Figure 64.2) and connected by two positive paddle locks. These paddle locks secure the device and can be opened for delivery by a thumbscrew release mechanism.

Procedure

A careful PFO anatomy assessment before device implantation including balloon sizing under fluoroscopy and/or other imaging techniques such as transesophageal echocardiography (TEE), 3D TEE, or intracardiac echocardiography (ICE) is essential.[1–3] The PFO tunnel diameter

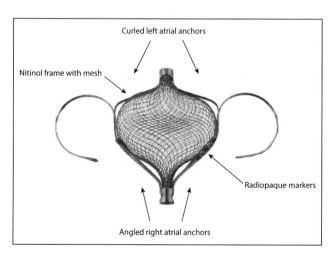

Figure 64.1 SeptRx IPO (IntraPocket Occluder) PFO closure system.

Table 64.1	Device selection sizes		
PFO length (mm)	PFO flat width (mm)	PFO diameter (mm)	SeptRx IPO PFO closure system
4–20	4–14	2.5–9	14
4–20	4–19	2.5–12.5	19

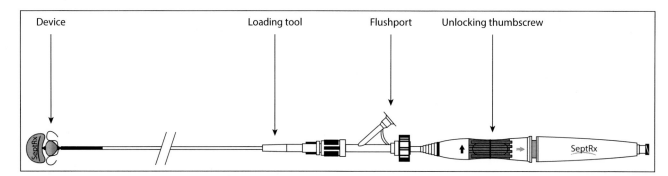

Figure 64.2   Delivery system.

is measured by balloon sizing. The flat width and tunnel length are measured by TEE or ICE. The flat width is the width of the tunnel if septum primum and septum secundum are in a neutral position to each other. These values determine the device size. Flat width is typically approximately 1.5 times the balloon diameter.

Table 64.1 shows the available sizes of the device in connection with length, flat width, and diameter of the PFO.

After crossing of the PFO, defect sizing, and choice of the correct device size, a 9 Fr sheath is advanced over a 0.035 inch guide wire into the left atrium. Before loading the SeptRx device onto the delivery system, it is flushed thoroughly through the hub with a saline-filled syringe and pulled into a loading tool. Special attention should be paid to the right and left atrial anchors to avoid entanglement within the nitinol mesh. Subsequently, the device is loaded into the delivery sheath and advanced until the left atrial anchors emerge in the left atrium. The delivery system and sheath are pulled back until these anchors engage the left atrial edge of the PFO (Figure 64.3). For orientation, fluoroscopy imaging is useful: To assure a correct device position, during fluoroscopy imaging, the radiopaque markers should be on the right side of the device (Figure 64.4). This step is important because, otherwise, the right atrial anchors cannot be secured by the septum secundum. Afterward, the device is deployed within the tunnel by further pulling back the sheath while maintaining device position. During this maneuver, the right atrial anchors should engage the limbus in the right atrium (Figure 64.5). For this step, it is essential to ensure that the right atrial anchors are outside the tunnel. Otherwise, only the left atrial anchors secure the device at the septum primum. In fluoroscopic assessment, the right atrial anchors should deflect downward. The SeptRx delivery system can be pulled and pushed to ensure that the device is correctly positioned in the PFO. A final check using different imaging modalities should be performed before releasing the device to ensure

- That the three radiopaque markers are on the right side of the device
- That the right atrial anchors are outside of the tunnel
- That the device is relaxed within the tunnel and does not become straight

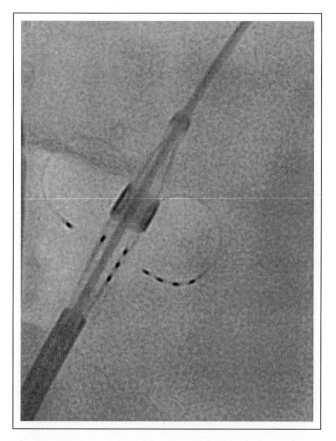

Figure 64.3   Fluoroscopic image during left atrial anchor release and correct orientation of radiopaque markers.

- That the anchors are not disengaged from the septum primum and secundum

If the device is not satisfactorily positioned in the PFO, it can be recaptured and the deployment can be repeated.

Once the device position is satisfactory, the implant is released by exposing the paddle locks by turning a simple mechanism on the handle of the delivery system. Unlocking of the delivery system is indicated by the covered orange indicator strip. After turning the rotating nut in the direction of the black arrow, the delivery system is disconnected from the device (Figure 64.6). The last step

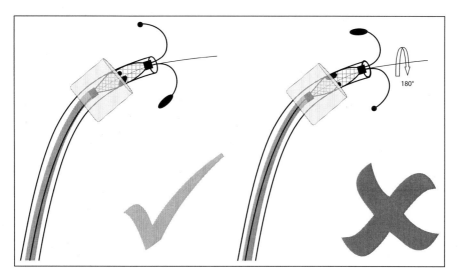

Figure 64.4   Correct/incorrect device orientation.

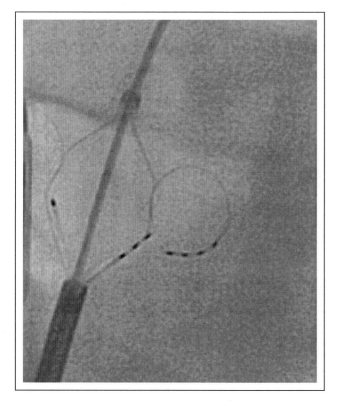

Figure 64.5   Fluoroscopic image during right atrial anchor release.

is to remove the delivery system, the guide wire, and the sheath from the patient (Figure 64.7).[5]

Clinical experience

A pilot, nonrandomized, single-center, open-label, non-comparative, and prospective interventional clinical investigation of the SeptRx IPO (IntraPocket Occluder)

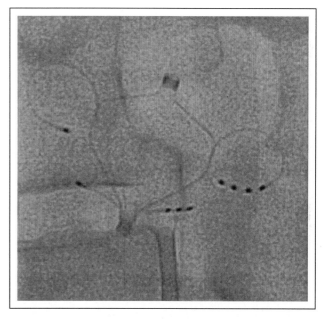

Figure 64.6   Fluoroscopic image: Device release.

PFO closure system was conducted between July 2006 and May 2007 in Frankfurt, Germany. The aim was a safety and efficacy evaluation. Thirteen patients were enrolled. PFO closure with the SeptRx device was successfully performed in 11 patients. Owing to the patients' PFO anatomy, implantation of the SeptRx device was not possible in two of the 13 patients. Follow-up after 30 days including history and physical examination, electrocardiography, transcranial Doppler studies, and TEE with bubble contrast demonstrated complete closure in six of the 11 patients. Four patients had a minimal (5–10 bubbles) and one patient had a moderate (10–30 bubbles) shunt. At 180 days post-procedure, complete closure occurred in all patients.[4] In June 2011, the InterSEPT In-Tunnel SeptRx European

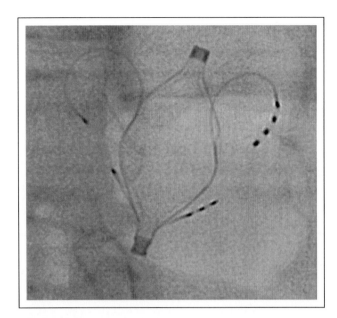

Figure 64.7 Fluoroscopic image after removal of delivery system, guide wire, and sheath.

PFO Trial: A prospective, multicenter study to evaluate the safety and performance of the SeptRx IPO PFO closure system was initiated at the CardioVascular Center, Frankfurt, Germany, and Institut Cardiovasculaire Paris Sud, Massy, France, and is ongoing. As of this writing, 47 patients have been enrolled. The follow-ups are scheduled after 1, 3, 6, and 12 months (Figure 64.8).

References

1. Vigna C, Marchese N, Zanchetta M et al. Echocardiographic guidance of percutaneous patent foramen ovale closure: Head-to-head comparison of transesophageal versus rotational intracardiac echocardiography. *Echocardiography* 2012;29(9):1103–10.
2. Seca L, Cação R, Silva J et al. Intracardiac echocardiography imaging for device closure of atrial septal defects—A single-center experience. *Rev Port Cardiol* 2012;31(6):407–12.
3. Parizkova B, Webb ST. Perioperative transoesophageal echocardiography. *J Perioper Pract* 2011;21(9):318–24.

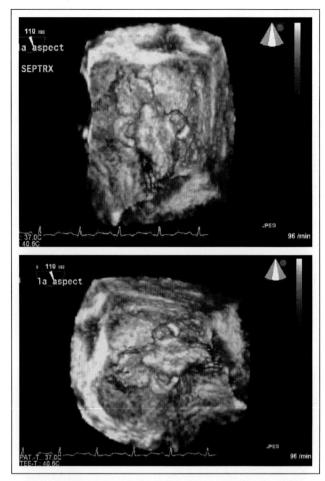

Figure 64.8 **(See color insert.)** 3D TEE image: Long-axis view, view from the left atrium to the interatrial septum 3 months after implantation.

4. Zimmermann WJ, Heinisch C, Majunke N et al. Patent foramen ovale closure with the SeptRx device initial experience with the first "In-Tunnel" device. *J Am Coll Cardiol Cardiovasc Interv* 2010;3(9):963–7.
5. Tang B. The SeptRx™ Intrapocket PFO Occluder (IPO). Presented at the *Congenital and Structural Interventions*, Frankfurt, Germany, July 8–11, 2010.

65

Patent foramen ovale closure: Suture-based PFO closure

Anthony Nobles

Suture-based PFO closure

Closure of patent foramen ovale (PFO) is performed in patients at risk of stroke and/or migraine. The two treatment options for closure of PFO are occlusion large metal-framed "umbrella" devices that are placed in both the left and right atria, and surgical suture closure in an open-surgical on-pump procedure. The less invasive occlusion method can be percutaneously performed by an interventionist in the catheter laboratory. The more invasive approach is "open surgical," which requires a cardiac surgeon to place a suture into the PFO structure and close the tunnel. In Europe, the most common approach is the percutaneous one. In the United States, the occluders are not Food and Drug Administration (FDA) approved, leaving only the surgical solution. The success of these procedures are well documented, as are their respective risks and complications. Therefore, there is a need for the development of a technology that is not a "device" and that can equal or improve on the results of open surgical closure through a percutaneous cardiology-based procedure. This led to the development of the suture-based PFO closure system, NobleStitch™. This system delivers a surgical-based suture to the PFO to acutely close the tunnel without leaving a device in either the right or left atrium. The system is a fully integrated "throw-and-catch" system that delivers a polypropylene suture to the PFO through a 12 F catheter system. The NobleStitch includes a pretied polypropylene knot, which is delivered over the 3-0 suture. Excess suture is then cut by using the integrated cutter leaving only the suture and knot.

NobleStitch PFO suture-based closure system

The NobleStitch system consists of three parts. The first is the catheter to deliver the secundum septum suture. The second is the catheter to deliver the primum septum suture. The third is the knot delivery catheter (Figure 65.1).

The 12 F catheter system has a 75 cm working length. The suture-carrying arm of each of the secundum and primum catheters is uniquely shaped to couple to the anatomy, allowing the needle to take a surgical tissue bite. The knot is of radiopaque polypropylene, which allows visual confirmation of the knot location and its proper placement.

Suture placement

The procedure is performed through a transfemoral venous puncture. A 14 F straight sheath is placed in the right atrium (which never passes through the PFO, thus reducing the risk of sheath-borne air emboli). A 0.030" guide wire is placed through the PFO into the left atrium. A 0.018" guide wire is then placed in the superior vena cava (SVC). This two-wire system, which acts like a "Y" in the road, assures proper secundum positioning. The two wires are loaded into the distal tip of the secundum catheter and advanced under fluoroscopic guidance to the right atrium. At approximately 45–50° left anterior oblique (LAO) projection, the orientation should, in most cases, provide adequate visualization. With the distal tip of the secundum

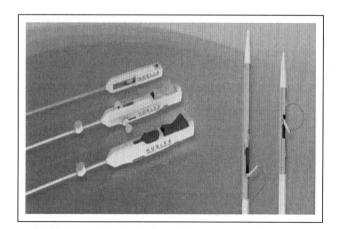

Figure 65.1 The NobleStitch PFO closure system.

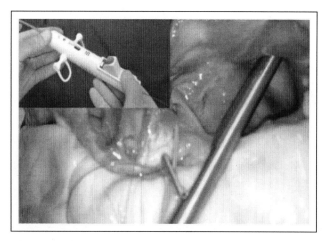

Figure 65.2 (**See color insert.**) The NobleStitch secundum suture-carrying arm being opened in the right atrium with distal tip in the SVC.

catheter in the SVC, the device is activated by opening the suture-carrying arm (Figure 65.2) and advancing it forward, which will place it against the secundum septum.

A small dye injection is used to verify proper positioning (Figure 65.3). The needle is advanced through the secundum septum (Figure 65.4), then picks up the suture; the arm is then closed and the catheter withdrawn.

The 0.018″ guide wire is removed and the primum catheter is advanced over the 0.030″ guide wire through the PFO, allowing the suture-carrying arm to be opened in the left atrium (Figure 65.5). It is then withdrawn until it contacts the septum primum. A small dye injection is used to verify proper catheter positioning. The needle then picks up the suture and the arm is closed and the primum catheter and 0.030″ wire are withdrawn.

The two ends of the withdrawn sutures are tied together and the remaining end of the secundum suture is pulled until the knot is removed and the suture is automatically formed into an "S" configuration through the PFO (Figure 65.6). The

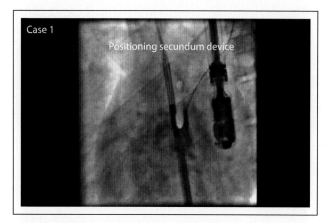

Figure 65.3 The NobleStitch secundum catheter visualized under fluoroscopy to verify final positioning prior to needle deployment.

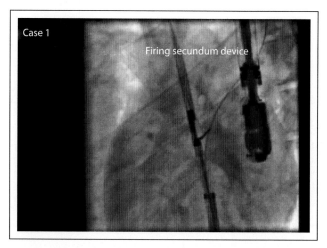

Figure 65.4 The needle passing through the secundum septum retrieving the suture.

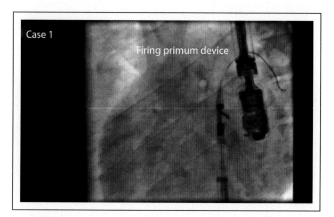

Figure 65.5 The primum septum catheter engaged with the primum.

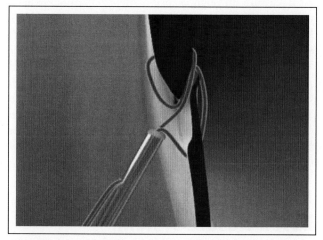

Figure 65.6 (**See color insert.**) The NobleStitch KwiKnot over the 3-0 polypropylene suture forming the "S"-shaped suture that will pull the primum septum into the tunnel forming a "valve-like" effect, closing the tunnel, and eliminating right-to-left shunting.

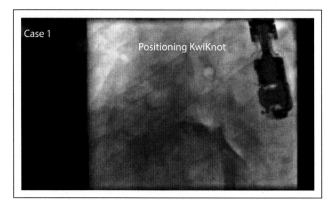

Figure 65.7   Positioning the KwiKnot and verifying closure prior to engaging the polypropylene knot.

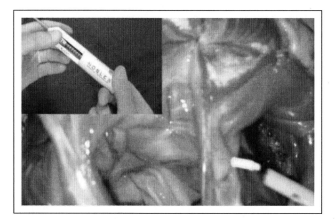

Figure 65.8   (See color insert.) The KwiKnot deploying the polypropylene suture knot in the right atrium.

"S" configuration pulls the soft floppy edge of the PFO into the tunnel, creating a valve-like effect, as the suture is tightened. This substantially reduces the chance for a potential residual shunt compared with the open surgical approach of tunnel suturing. The pretied knot is advanced over the suture, which is visualized under fluoroscopy (Figure 65.7).

The knot is then deployed tightly against the septum and cut (Figure 65.8) leaving only the polypropylene knot in the right atrium and nothing in the left atrium. The septum primum is pulled inside the tunnel and forms a "one-way valve" that stops "left-to-right" flow. The results are

confirmed by completion angiogram and are compared with the preprocedural angiogram (Figure 65.9) showing the effect of the suture in a large PFO tunnel.

Benefits of percutaneous suture-based PFO closure

The benefits of the percutaneous approach versus on-pump open cardiovascular surgical intervention are well documented. These include lower morbidity and mortality and a reduction of other complications associated with the surgical approach. There are additional benefits in using NobleStitch versus an open- surgical suture:

Potential complications/ benefits	Percutaneous NobleStitch suturing	Open surgical suturing
Open thoracic surgical complications and risks	No	Yes
Real-time feedback on a beating heart	Yes	No
Single suture	Yes	No
Residual shunt	Low	Yes
Shunt confirmation	Yes	No

The benefits of the NobleStitch over the "Umbrella Device" implants are potentially significant.

Potential complications/ benefits	NobleStitch	Umbrella device
Migration	No	Yes
Erosion	No	Yes
Perforation	No	Yes
Nickel allergy	No	Yes
Anticoagulation therapy	No	Yes
Inhibits future transseptal procedures	No	Yes
Residual shunt	Low	Yes
Embolic stroke from device	No	Yes

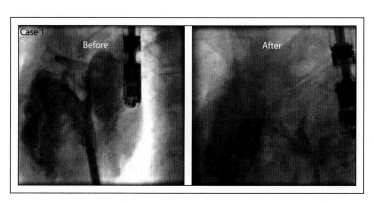

Figure 65.9   The PFO tunnel before and after closure showing the polypropylene knot and closure of the shunt.

The effects of trial data on PFO closure and the rationale for suture-based closure

There is a great deal of discussion on whether PFO closure for stroke or migraine provides clinical benefits over medical therapy. Recent trials, including RESPECT,[*] PC, and "The Effect of Patent Foramen Ovale Closure on Visual Aura without Headache or Typical Aura with Migraine Headache"[†] by Jonathan Tobis, MD, have demonstrated positive results using closure versus medical therapy with proper patient selection. However, the "nonbelievers" continue to argue that the risk of placing a large permanent implant device outweighs the benefit over medical therapy. This is where the NobleStitch "no-device" suture approach may provide the solution. The NobleStitch device can be used on most PFO patients without the known adverse effects that would normally be associated with an "umbrella device." Therefore, there is little rationale not to suture closed a PFO in cases of potential stroke or migraine. Although there have not been large randomized trails using the NobleStitch, the clinical studies performed have supported these benefits.

Summary

Suture-based closure using the NobleStitch system is safe and effective in closing PFO. This approach reduces or eliminates the significant risks associated with "umbrella device closure" technique. Suture-based closure using the NobleStitch system provides a potentially better long-term result compared with open surgical closure. The system is simple to use and can be performed with fluoroscopic guidance. The use of the NobleStitch suture-based closure may provide the solution for PFO closure as the gold standard for stroke and migraine.

---

[*] RESPECT, Randomized evaluation of recurrent stroke comparing PFO closure to established current standard-of-care treatment. John D. Carroll, MD, Jeffrey L. Saver, MD, 2012—TCT.

[†] The effect of PFO closure on visual aura without headache or typical aura with migraine headache. Hamidreza Khessali, MD, M. Khalid Mojadidi, MD, Rubine Gevorgyan, MD, Ralph Levinson, MD, Jonathan Tobis, MD, JACC—Vol. 5, No. 6, 2012.

66

Patent foramen ovale closure: Other new PFO closure techniques

Ilona Hofmann, Stefan Bertog, and Horst Sievert

The current concepts of transcatheter closure of patent foramen ovale (PFO) rely on the placement of a permanent implant device. Most of these devices are accompanied by excellent closure rates and some have been tested in randomized trials with good clinical results. However, the presence of an intracardiac foreign body poses several potential problems: atrial fibrillation, thrombus formation, device fracture, embolization, and erosion. Hence, under ideal circumstances, a concept that leaves little or no foreign material behind while providing reliable closure with no or few procedural complications would be desirable. The ideal device would be no device!

Nondevice closure

The first transcatheter technique for PFO closure without an implantable device was the PFx™ Closure System (Cierra, Redwood City, CA, USA). It was a percutaneous system that emitted monopolar radio-frequency (RF) energy to close the PFO by welding the septum primum and secundum together. The underlying principle was an increase in tissue temperature in the PFO tunnel, leading to denaturation of collagen and other proteins followed by cooling. The result was a tissue bond between the septum secundum and primum. The PFx Closure System consisted of a catheter with a metal electrode at the distal end and an elastomeric distal housing covering the electrode (Figure 66.1a) and an RF generator with impedance monitoring and automatic shutoff (Figure 66.1b). The PFx catheter was delivered into the right atrium, and the left atrium was not entered, thereby reducing the risk of thromboembolism. A clinical trial was performed between 2005 and 2007. One hundred and thirty patients underwent RF application for PFO closure. Although feasibility could be demonstrated, the 6-month closure rate was low (55%), particularly for larger defects. However, a closure rate of 72% was achieved in patients whose balloon-sized defect was <8 mm in diameter[1] and the secondary closure rate (closure after a second

RF application) was 63%.[2] The company discontinued this technology in 2009.

Similarly, the CoAptus Closure System Device (CoAptus Medical Corporation, Redmond, WA, USA) used RF energy to coapt the septum secundum and primum mechanically. The device (energy source) was removed after completion of the procedure leaving nothing behind. Animal trials had been performed with promising results but the company was shut down for financial reasons (Figure 66.2).

The Terumo (Terumo Medical Corporation, Somerset, NJ, USA) PFO closure system is the first device using bipolar RF energy. The device catheter is delivered into the right atrium, but in contradistinction to the PFx Closure System, the left atrium is entered. Initial animal results demonstrated feasibility and safety. Further clinical studies are pending.

Suture-based techniques

Percutaneous suture closure emulates the surgical procedure and leaves behind only minimal foreign material (the suture). The NobleStitch EL PFO closure system (Nobles

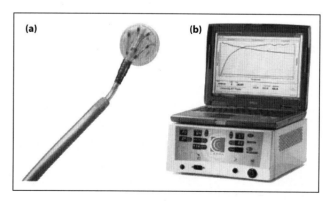

Figure 66.1 **(See color insert.)** PFx Closure System. (a) Radio-frequency electrode, (b) radio-frequency generator. (Courtesy of Cierra, Redwood City, CA, USA.)

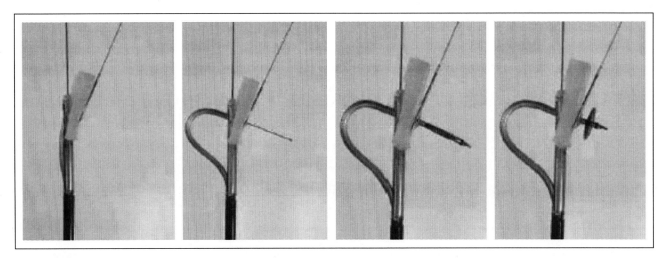

Figure 66.2 CoAptus. (Courtesy of CoAptus Medical Corporation, Redmond, WA, USA.)

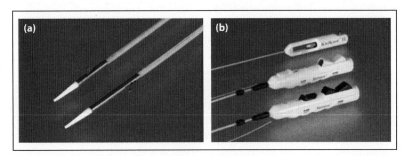

Figure 66.3 The NobleStitch (a) and the KwiKnot (b). (Courtesy of Nobles Medical Technology, Fountain Valley, CA, USA.)

Medical Technology, Fountain Valley, CA, USA) is a catheter- and suture-based system. It has been CE marked and is commercially available in Germany and the United Kingdom.

The system includes the NobleStitch (Figure 66.3a) and the KwiKnot (Figure 66.3b). The NobleStitch consists of needles and arms, the working length is 90 cm, and it is available in 6, 8, and 12 Fr. Fourteen French venous access is required. A single 4-0 polypropylene suture is placed through the septum secundum and primum, thereby closing the PFO tunnel with a single suture. The sutures are then tied together using the proprietary KwiKnot with an integrated suture cutter (Figure 66.4). The NobleStitch can be used for a PFO with sufficient tunnel length. It cannot be used for a PFO with short tunnels and atrial septal defects (ASDs).

Bioabsorbable devices

Bioabsorbable occluders are similar to the aforementioned concepts in that no permanent foreign material is left behind. The BioSTAR device (NMT Medical, Boston, MA, USA) was a modification of the STARFlex (NMT Medical) consisting of a metal framework and a totally bioabsorbable matrix (Figure 66.5). It had been CE marked and was available in sizes of 23, 28, and 33 mm. In the BEST (BioSTAR evaluation study),[3] successful device

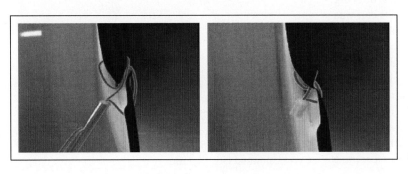

Figure 66.4 **(See color insert.)** NobleStitch suture-mediated PFO closure.

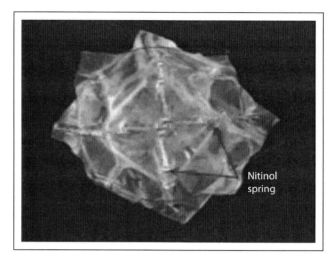

Figure 66.5 The BioSTAR device. (Courtesy of NMT Medical, Boston, MA, USA.)

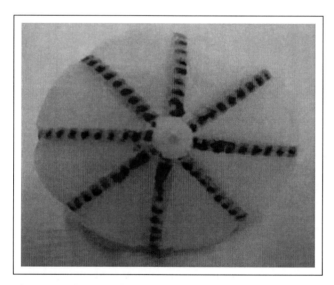

Figure 66.6 The BioTREK device. (Courtesy of NMT Medical, Boston, MA, USA.)

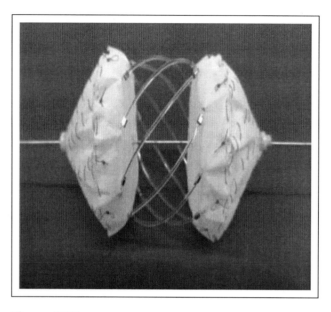

Figure 66.7 The CARAG biodegradable Occluder (Courtesy of CARAG-Swiss engineering.)

entirely bioabsorbable. The novel bioabsorbable polymer (P4HB) is a noninflammatory natural metabolite.

Other biodegradable devices are being developed. The CARAG biodegradable Septal Occluder is based on the original Solysafe design, the metal frame of which is replaced by a proprietary polylactic coglycolic acid (PLGA) biodegradable compound (Figure 66.7). The device is the first biodegradable framework device successfully used in chronic animal trials, demonstrating excellent short- and intermediate-term endothelial response. At the time of this writing, this device is undergoing preclinical testing.

References

1. Sievert H, Ruygrok P, Salkeld M et al. Transcatheter closure of patent foramen ovale with radiofrequency: Acute and intermediate term results in 144 patients. *Catheter Cardiovasc Interv* 2009;73:368–73.
2. Sievert H, Fischer E, Heinisch C, Majunke N, Roemer A, Wunderlich N. Transcatheter closure of patent foramen ovale without an implant: Initial clinical experience. *Circulation* 2007;116:1701–6.
3. Mullen MJ, Hildick-Smith D, De Giovanni JV et al. BioSTAR evaluation study (BEST): A prospective, multicenter, phase I clinical trial to evaluate the feasibility, efficacy, and safety of the BioSTAR bioabsorbable septal repair implant for the closure of atrial-level shunts. *Circulation* 2006;114:1962–7.
4. Van den Branden BJ, Post MC, Jaarsma W, ten Berg JM, Suttorp MJ. New bioabsorbable septal repair implant for percutaneous closure of a patent foramen ovale: Short-term results of a single-centre experience. *Catheter Cardiovasc Interv* 2009;74:286–90.
5. Van den Branden BJ, Luermans JG, Post MC, Plokker HW, Ten Berg JM, Suttorp MJ. The BioSTAR(r) device versus the CardioSEAL(r) device in patent foramen ovale closure: Comparison of mid-term efficacy and safety. *EuroIntervention* 2010;6:498–504.
6. Van den Branden BJ, Post MC, Plokker HW, ten Berg JM, Suttorp MJ. Patent foramen ovale closure using a bioabsorbable closure device: Safety and efficacy at 6-month follow-up. *J Am Coll Cardiol Cardiovasc Interv* 2010;3:968–73.

implantation was achieved in 98%. The closure rate at 6 months was reported at 96%. In contrast, Van den Branden et al.[4] report a closure rate of only 55% at 1 month and 71% and 76% at 6 months, respectively.[5,6] It is conceivable that postprocedure, double-antiplatelet agent administration (aspirin and clopidogrel) had a negative effect on the closure rate. When platelets are activated as a result of endothelial damage during PFO closure, stimulation of smooth muscle cell proliferation and migration may contribute to the synthesis of the connective tissue and closure. Aspirin and clopidogrel therapy could inhibit the formation of neo-endothelium and natural healing induced by the bioabsorbable device and, thereby, closure. The BioTREK device (Figure 66.6) was designed to be 100% reabsorbable. The device consists of circular patches and eight ribs that are

67

Patent foramen ovale closure: Complications of device closure of PFOs

Lutz Buellesfeld and Stephan Windecker

Interventional device closure of patent foramen ovale (PFO) is one of the safest procedures in invasive cardiology. After establishing the diagnosis and exclusion of the accompanying atrial septal defects, the procedure is straightforward in experienced hands, when performed under local anesthesia with fluoroscopic guidance requiring an 8–12 F venous access. The low risk and simplicity of PFO closure led to the widespread utilization of this technique during the past two decades and has been considered as a potent therapeutic approach to eliminate the risk for recurrent paradoxical embolism. All the currently available devices are fully repositionable and retrievable, resulting in a high level of reproducibility and success of the intervention.

The vast majority of clinical experience in PFO closure is based on observational studies, whereas the results of randomized clinical trials were reported only recently.[1] The evidence on safety issues among patients undergoing PFO device closure is available from two meta-analyses, the first published in 2006, including 11 studies with 1970 patients,[2] the second published in 2012, with inclusion of 39 studies and 8185 patients,[3] as well as the randomized CLOSURE, RESPECT, and PC trials.[4–6] Both meta-analyses summarizing the experience with different PFO occluders are limited by differences in registry design, including a lack of uniform endpoint definitions and incomplete monitoring, while the three randomized clinical trials comparing PFO closure with medical treatment enrolled patients prospectively with appropriate adverse event monitoring and event adjudication.

The evidence published so far is mainly related to the Amplatzer PFO occluder, followed by the CardioSeal and Starflex occluders (both are from NMT Medical, Boston, MA), the latter two are no longer commercially available, as well as the HELEX device (Gore Medical, Flagstaff, AZ). The relevant differences between the devices, whenever apparent, are highlighted in the chapter.

Timing of complications

As related to the occurrence of adverse events, three different time periods need to be considered in patients undergoing PFO closure:

- The procedural phase
- The postprocedural period until full device endothelialization ensues, which is achieved within the first 1–3 months
- The subsequent "late" phase

Procedure-related events, which will be discussed in detail below, may occur during the procedural phase, as shown in Table 67.1, whereas some events, such as device thrombosis and atrial arrhythmias, also manifest themselves later.

Specific adverse events

The overall rate of device-related complications among patients undergoing PFO closure is low, with approximately 4.1 complications per 100 patient years.[3] These adverse events are related to the device as well as to the various procedural steps during the intervention. The most important complications and their frequency are summarized in Table 67.2.

Atrial arrhythmias

Atrial arrhythmias may occur in approximately 3.9% of patients.[3] They range from simple premature atrial beats to atrial fibrillation (1.2%, 95% confidence interval 0.7–1.7) and, rarely, atrial flutter (0.1%, 0–0.2) may occur during the procedure as well as during the follow-up period. The mechanism is local irritation either by the manipulation in the atria during device implantation, or by the implanted device itself with an acute and/or delayed inflammation.

Table 67.1 Overview of type and timing of potential adverse events related to PFO closure

Adverse events	Procedural	Postprocedure to complete endothelialization	Late
Atrial arrhythmias	X	X	X
Bleeding complications	X		
Thrombus	X	X	
Air embolism	X		
Embolization/malposition	X	X	
Effusion/tamponade	X		
Infection	X	X	

Table 67.2 Frequency of device-related adverse events in patients undergoing PFO closure

Adverse events	Rate (%)	95% CI
Atrial arrhythmias	3.9	2.7–6.1
Bleeding complications	1.7	1.1–2.4
Thrombus	0.6	0.3–0.9
Air embolism	0.6	0.2–1.0
Embolization/malposition	0.4	0.2–0.7
Effusion/tamponade	0.3	0–0.6
Infection	0.1	0–0.8

Source: Reported by Agarwal S et al. *J Am Coll Cardiol Cardiovasc Interv* 2012;5(7):777–89.

There appears to be a link to the device design, as shown in the meta-analysis by Agarwal et al.[3] with an incidence of atrial arrhythmias of 1.8% observed with the Amplatzer, 10.2% with the Starflex, and 0.1% with the HELEX occluder. These observations have been indirectly corroborated in the randomized clinical trials with a periprocedural incidence of atrial fibrillation of 5.7% with the Starflex device in CLOSURE I[5] compared with 3.0% and 2.9% with the Amplatzer occluder in the RESPECT and PC trials, respectively. Of note, these events may also be coincidental, given the natural incidence of spontaneous or non-procedure-related atrial arrhythmias in this population.

Access site complications

PFO device closure with established techniques requires venous access, typically established by femoral vein puncture, or alternatively jugular, subclavian, or brachial access. As with all invasive techniques, access site complications may occur, particularly in the case of inadequate hemostasis. The overall rate of access site complications in patients undergoing PFO closure may be up to 1.7% (1.1–2.4), including minor (0.8%, 0.3–1.3) and major hematomas (0.1%, 0–0.2), arteriovenous fistulas (0.2%, 0–0.5), and pseudoaneurysms (0.6%, 0.1–1.2).[3] Complications are related to access vessel size and anticoagulation regimen,

but not to the device design itself. Major vascular access site complications were observed in 3.2% of patients in CLOSURE I and 0.8% of patients in the RESPECT trial.

Thrombus

All established PFO devices have a metal frame of variable size, whose exposure to blood may induce platelet aggregation, activation of the coagulation cascade, and subsequent thrombus formation. Newer generations of devices attempt to address this issue by minimizing the amount of metal and foreign body material. Thrombi on the device surface have been observed in 0.6% of patients, ranging from 0% to 0.1% with the Amplatzer, 0.1–1% with the HELEX, and up to 7–10.2% with the Starflex device.[3,5,7] Thrombus formation may occur on both the left and right atrial side of the device (Figure 67.1) and usually becomes apparent during the postprocedural phase until full device endothelialization has occurred. Besides thrombus formation on the device surface, thrombus may also form in the delivery catheter or on the wire surface used during the procedure, which may accidentally be injected, in case of inadequate device and delivery catheter preparation, flushing, and insufficient anticoagulation. To avoid procedural thrombus formation on both the catheters and the device, patients typically receive a bolus of unfractionated

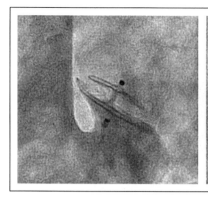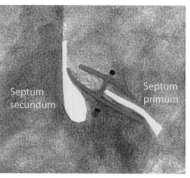

Figure 67.1 (See color insert.) Misplaced Amplatzer PFO occluder. The device is anchored in the PFO tunnel, but does not grasp the septum secundum due to a malpositioned right atrial disk at the antero-superior aspect. Potential consequences include device embolization and an increased risk for a significant residual shunt.

heparin followed by the empiric use of acetylsalicylic acid 75–100 mg once daily for up to 6 months and clopidogrel 75 mg once daily for 1–6 months.

Air embolism

Air embolism is a feared complication whenever the arterial circulation is involved. A rate of 0.6% (0.2–1.0) has been reported among patients undergoing PFO closure.[3] Air embolism is usually clinically silent (most frequently temporary inferior ST-segment elevation due to embolism into the right coronary artery), but may cause symptomatic cerebral or cardiac ischemic symptoms of various degrees. Meticulous evacuation of air from all catheters and devices followed by careful catheter manipulation with attention to maintain the end of the catheter below the right atrial level whenever the catheter is open to air, effectively eliminates the risk of air embolism.

Device embolization and malposition

Device embolization or malposition is reported in 0.4% of cases[3] with a notable learning curve. Complete device embolization is avoidable, when using adequate techniques. Figure 67.2 shows the example of a malpositioned Amplatzer device placed, in which the two disks grasp the septum primum but fail to embrace the septum secundum. Therefore, the device is accidentally seated in the PFO tunnel, which is stable in this particular case, but may result in some residual shunting.

To avoid device embolization or malposition, a thorough evaluation of the atrial septal anatomy should be performed prior to the procedure using transthoracic and transesophageal echocardiography, to determine the size of the defect, the presence of associated atrial septal defects, as well as the presence and size of an atrial septal aneurysm. Particularly, hypermobile and protruding septal aneurysms may influence proper device size selection, as it may obscure the true defect size and prevent stable device anchoring. If identified beforehand, selection of a suitable device can overcome these issues.

Implantation strategies involving periprocedural transesophageal or intracardiac echocardiography are helpful for less-experienced operators to confirm a good device placement, but angiographic delineation of the septum and atrial anatomy using contrast injections may be adequate to achieve a successful result. Moreover, echocardiographic techniques may complicate the procedure by prolonging the procedure time, requiring deep sedation or endotracheal intubation in case of transesophageal echocardiography, and demanding additional human resources. The advantage of reducing the device size as much as possible to minimize the risk of thrombus formation may increase the risk of embolization and malposition.

Pericardial effusion or tamponade

The periprocedural development of pericardial effusions or tamponade is exceedingly rare with a device-independent incidence of approximately 0.3%.[3] Traumatic catheter manipulation or attempts to cannulate the PFO with hydrophilic guide wires may rarely lead to injury of the right atrial wall that can result in pericardial effusions. Significant damage, which results in symptomatic cardiac tamponade, should be suspected whenever a patient becomes hemodynamically unstable during or after PFO closure and must be treated by means of immediate pericardiocentesis and reversal of anticoagulation. Usually, drainage of the effusion suffices with spontaneous closure of the defect subsequently.

Infection

PFO device closure is an invasive procedure to close an intracardiac defect and requires insertion of a foreign body, all of which are risk factors for local and systemic infections if not properly performed under sterile conditions. Nevertheless, the incidence of infections is very low (0.1%), likely due to the very short procedure time and the reduced exposure to infectious agents.[3] As a routine measure, one dose of antibiotics is usually administered in the catheterization laboratory or immediately before the procedure, followed by one or two more doses over the next 12 h, although the use of antibiotics is not supported by any evidence.

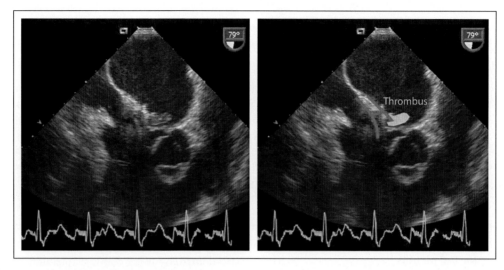

Figure 67.2   **(See color insert.)** Thrombus on the left atrial disk 3 weeks after implantation of an Amplatzer PFO occluder, successfully treated with temporary anticoagulation for 6 months.

Major adverse events

All the above-mentioned procedure-related events could theoretically result in a major adverse event such as death, stroke, or myocardial infarction. However, adverse events are exceedingly rare during interventional PFO closure. Moreover, if they do occur, most of them resolve spontaneously without major sequelae. Wöhrle and colleagues[2] have reported the absence of mortality, stroke, or myocardial infarction (0%) in a systematic review of almost 2000 procedures. This observation has been corroborated in the most recent randomized trials (Table 67.3).

Other events

Residual shunt

The presence of a residual shunt does not represent a complication in the sense of a harmful event, but rather results in failure to provide complete abolition of a right-to-left shunt with the attendant risk of paradoxical embolism. The risk of residual shunts is device related and time dependent.

The overall rate is approximately 12% at 12 months, ranging from 25% after the procedure to 6% beyond 12 months.[3] In addition, the risk of residual shunts ranges from as low as 6% with the Amplatzer PFO occluder to more than 20% with the HELEX device. Shunts may be of different size and are therefore of different clinical importance. Therapeutic options include careful clinical observation, intensified anticoagulation, repeated device closure with implantation of a second device, or surgical device explantation and direction of patch defect closure.

Reintervention

An interventional approach to implant a second device may be required in patients with significant residual shunts and recurrent thromboembolic events. These procedures can be performed with a high rate of success and low complication rates as with the initial procedure. However, when there is a significant residual shunt, which cannot be addressed by a second percutaneous approach, or the presence of a large and mobile thrombi or local infection, a surgical intervention may be indicated. The overall rate of

Table 67.3   Procedural incidence of major adverse events among patients undergoing interventional PFO closure, observed in a meta-analysis including 11 observational registries as well as randomized trials

	Procedural events	
Major adverse events	Woehrle J, meta-analysis (2006) $n = 1970$	RESPECT trial (2012) $n = 499$
Death	0	0
Stroke	0	0
Myocardial infarction	0	n.a.

surgical explantation of PFO devices is approximately 0.3% as recently reported by Verma et al.[8] The primary reasons for surgical explantation of devices were residual shunts (0.09%) and thrombus formation (0.03%). Of note, nonspecific chest pain was the leading cause for device explantation in 0.1% of cases, although the responsible mechanism causing this symptom remains elusive.

References

1. Kitsios GD, Dahabreh IJ, Abu Dabrh AM, Thaler DE, Kent DM. Patent foramen ovale closure and medical treatments for secondary stroke prevention: A systematic review of observational and randomized evidence. *Stroke* 2012;43(2):422–31.

2. Wöhrle J. Closure of patent foramen ovale after cryptogenic stroke. *Lancet* 2006;368(9533):350–2.

3. Agarwal S, Bajaj NS, Kumbhani DJ, Tuzcu EM, Kapadia SR. Meta-analysis of transcatheter closure versus medical therapy for patent foramen ovale in prevention of recurrent neurological events after presumed paradoxical embolism. *J Am Coll Cardiol Cardiovasc Interv* 2012;5(7):777–89.

4. Carroll J. *Randomized Evaluation of Recurrent Stroke Comparing PFO Closure to Established Current Standard of Care Treatment (RESPECT Trial).* Miami, FL: TCT; 2012.

5. Furlan AJ, Reisman M, Massaro J, Mauri L, Adams H, Albers GW et al. CLOSURE I investigators. Closure or medical therapy for cryptogenic stroke with patent foramen ovale. *N Engl J Med* 2012;366(11):991–9.

6. Windecker S. *The PC Trial: A Prospective, Randomized Trial of PFO Closure vs. Medical Therapy in Patients with Cryptogenic Embolism.* Miami, FL: TCT, 2012.

7. Krumsdorf U, Ostermayer S, Billinger K, Trepels T, Zadan E, Horvath K et al. Incidence and clinical course of thrombus formation on atrial septal defect and patient foramen ovale closure devices in 1,000 consecutive patients. *J Am Coll Cardiol* 2004;43(2):302–9.

8. Verma S, Tobis JM. Explantation of patent foramen ovale closure devices: A multicenter survey. *J Am Coll Cardiol Cardiovasc Interv* 2011;4(5):579–85.

68

Ventricular septal defect closure: Background, indications for closure, and clinical trial results

Shakeel A. Qureshi and Sebastian Goreczny

Introduction

Ventricular septal defect (VSD) is the commonest of all significant congenital heart defects and when occurring as an isolated lesion, VSDs account for about 20% of all defects, with the incidence increasing up to 40% in case of multiple congenital heart defects.[1]. Perimembranous VSDs are the most frequent (70%), followed by muscular (15–20%), subarterial (in up to 5%), and finally multiple swiss cheese VSDs. The doubly committed subarterial VSD is more common in the Asian and Far East population and muscular and multiple VSDs are less common in this population.[2,3]

VSDs may decrease in size spontaneously and close, cause congestive cardiac failure in infancy, or progress to pulmonary vascular disease.[4–6] In one study, VSDs closed spontaneously in 71% of patients, with the oldest patient being 19 years of age.[6] An increased rate of spontaneous closure has been reported in muscular VSDs.[7]

For over 50 years, surgical patch closure through a sternotomy with cardiopulmonary bypass has been performed with a low operative mortality and postoperative morbidity. With careful selection, early surgery, and improved perioperative care, currently, most patients experience normal quality of life when compared with age-matched controls.[8–10] However, the possible complications and the incidence of mortality and morbidity is likely to increase in patients with multiple defects, associated lesions, or with reoperation.[11,12] Atrioventricular block (AVB) has been reported in up to 8% of patients, although in the modern era, the incidence is <1%, reoperation due to significant residual leak in up to 6%, or for indications other than residual leak in up to 2%.[13,14] Furthermore, patient discomfort, sternotomy, scar, postpericardiotomy syndrome, arrhythmias, infections, or neurological complications add to the limitations of this treatment.[10] In addition, behavioral and school performance difficulties as well as long-term impairment of developmental and neurocognitive functions can occur with cardiopulmonary bypass surgery.[10,15]

Interventional closure of VSDs has been performed for over two decades with varying results. This approach has several advantages, such as avoidance of a sternotomy and cardiopulmonary bypass, causing less pain, no scar, and a shorter hospital stay. For selected defects, muscular or residual postsurgical, interventional closure is as effective as surgery, but with lower incidence of complications. In addition, in many centers and in many countries, percutaneous interventional treatment may be considered to be less expensive than the standard surgical approach and so potentially expands the population that may be offered the treatment.[16] The disadvantages include the need for x-ray radiation and contrast injection; however, with constantly improving imaging techniques such as three-dimensional (3D) echocardiography, 3D rotational angiography and magnetic resonance imaging (MRI), and their associated road mapping, the need for these may be reduced in the future.

Surgical treatment remains the gold standard for the treatment of VSDs. Interventional closure has been performed as an alternative in many types of VSDs. In the recent past, percutaneous treatment of the commonest type of VSDs, that is, perimembranous, has brought both hope with high rate of early success and disappointment with late complete heart block, bringing this treatment into question and indeed, it was abandoned by many.[17] In the meantime, new devices have been developed and introduced and further experience with the traditional devices has been gained.

Historical perspective

Percutaneous VSD closure was initially described by Lock et al.[18] In this study, seven defects, including congenital, postinfarct, and residual after surgery, were closed in six patients, who were considered as unsuitable candidates for surgery. For closure, the defects were approached and crossed from the left ventricle, an arteriovenous guide wire circuit was established, and a Rashkind double umbrella was used to occlude the defects. Apart from one device, which embolized immediately after release, the remaining devices stayed in place and resulted in reduction of the shunt or complete closure. This preliminary report proved that transcatheter VSD closure was feasible and soon gave way for the next generation of devices to be used.

Bridges et al.[19] reported on 12 patients who underwent percutaneous closure of 21 defects—19 muscular, and two residual defects after surgery. Six of the patients presented with associated complex heart lesions and the remaining patients had undergone prior pulmonary artery banding. The Clamshell umbrella device (NMT) was implanted successfully in all the defects, with no major early as well as late complications. Although residual flow was noticed in 10 of 12 patients, the mean pulmonary-to-systemic flow ratio measured during subsequent cardiac surgery was 1.1, indicating insignificant left-to-right shunt.

Sideris et al.[20] described experience with the Buttoned device in 18 patients with perimembranous[15] and muscular[3] VSDs. Transcatheter closure of 25 defects was attempted, but in seven, the device could not be introduced to the defect or was pulled through the defect prior to its release. In two out of the 18 initially successfully treated patients, a change of the device position from its original position was noticed, resulting in mild aortic regurgitation in one and recurrence of the shunt in the second patient. Both required surgical removal of the device with subsequent VSD closure. During the follow-up, 13 of 16 patients showed complete occlusion, with a trivial residual shunt in the remaining three patients.

Although the initial results looked promising, both the devices used for closure of VSDs and their closure rates were suboptimal. The devices in the first decade had been originally designed for closing patent arterial ducts or atrial septal defects.[21,22] They required large sheaths for delivery as well as complex implantation techniques with limited or no possibility to recapture, reposition, or redeploy the devices. Interference with atrioventricular or aortic valves and a high incidence of hemodynamically significant residual shunts added to their limitations.[18,19]

Modern era

The modern era of percutaneous interventional VSD closure started with the Amplatzer Muscular VSD Occluder, the first device specifically designed for closing muscular VSDs. The device is made of two flat, round disks with waist length corresponding to the thickness of the muscular septum, Dacron patches sewn into the disks to increase closure rate, have a low profile requiring a small delivery sheath, a wide range of sizes, and retrievability, allowing device

repositioning. These characteristics distinguished this type of device from the other devices and contributed to their success. It was introduced into the market in the late 1990s with first human implantations reported by Thanopoulos et al. and Hijazi et al.[23,24] Thanopoulos et al. described successful device implantation in all six patients, ranging in age from 3 to 10 years, with residual shunt noted in one patient. Apart from transient complete left bundle branch block in two patients, no other complications were observed.[23] Hijazi et al. reported their initial experience in eight patients, ranging in age from 2 to 10 years, with mid-muscular VSDs in four, anterior in two, apical in one, and posterior in one. The device was successfully implanted in all cases with trivial residual shunt in six patients, which disappeared in five patients within 24 hours and in one patient at 6-month follow-up. Transient junctional rhythm occurred in one patient with no other complications immediately or during follow-up.[24]

Indications

The hemodynamic significance of a VSD depends on the size of the defect and the ratio of pulmonary and systemic flows and resistances. Although most muscular and a few perimembranous VSDs close spontaneously in the first months of life, patients can present with several clinical scenarios. In large unrestrictive VSDs, young infants may become breathless with failure to thrive within the first few weeks of life. For this group of infants, VSD closure is recommended within the first 3–6 months of life. They are also too small in weight for percutaneous interventional closure as the introduction of standard delivery systems and long sheaths through tortuous routes may cause hemodynamic instability. Furthermore, these infants have large defects, which require a large device, which could interfere with the surrounding structures. For such patients, a hybrid approach with perventricular access can overcome some of the mentioned limitations; however, this group of patients is usually referred for surgery.[25–27]

For asymptomatic patients with volume-overloaded left heart but without pulmonary hypertension, closure of the VSD may be recommended with the aim of avoiding late left ventricular dysfunction related to sustained dilatation. This group of patients is typically most suitable for transcatheter closure, as their VSDs are relatively small.[28–30]

Closure of VSDs in patients with concomitant aortic valve prolapse or regurgitation remains controversial. Most of these patients with the presence of even trivial aortic regurgitation are referred for surgery in many centers. Although for most devices used for percutaneous closure of VSD, the presence of aortic regurgitation is a contraindication; however, the PFM coil (pfm medical ag, Koln, Germany) occluder has been used in this setting with encouraging results.[29,30]

The commonly accepted indications for transcatheter VSD closure include:

- Clinical signs and symptoms:
  - Congestive heart failure
  - Failure to thrive
  - Recurrent respiratory tract infections
  - Shock or respiratory failure
- Hemodynamically significant shunt (Qp:Qs > 1.5) measured by
  - Echocardiography
  - MRI
  - Cardiac catheterization
- Evidence of left-side chamber by
  - Echocardiography
  - MRI
- History of previous infective endocarditis

Contraindications

The most frequently accepted contraindications for transcatheter VSD closure include:

- Weight
  - <5 kg—For the Amplatzer Muscular VSD Occluder and the Nit-Occlud VSD occluder
  - <8 kg—For the Amplatzer Membranous VSD
- Pulmonary vascular disease >7 U/m²
- Sepsis
- Contraindications for antiplatelet therapy
- Distance from the edge of the VSD to the semilunar valves:
  - <2 mm—For the Amplatzer Membranous VSD Occluder
  - <4 mm—For the Nit-Occlud VSD
- Defects associated with other cardiac lesions requiring surgery
  - Some muscular VSDs may be difficult to access surgically and then may be closed with a device via a hybrid right ventricular approach
- Size of the VSD is bigger than the available maximum device size

Preprocedural evaluation

Cross-sectional echocardiography is the mainstay of diagnostic techniques and also provides crucial information for the proper planning of the intervention. Echocardiography can provide information on the number, the location, the size, and relationship of the VSDs to the tricuspid, aortic, and pulmonary valves as well as the degree of aortic and tricuspid regurgitation. In addition, 3D echocardiography is becoming widely available and may provide additional assessment of unusually located

defects and thus enables better understanding of the spatial relationships. Occasionally, in patients with poor diagnostic windows, transesophageal echocardiography (TOE) is required.

The short-axis view at the semilunar valve level is optimal for delineation of the location of the VSD. In this view, perimembranous defects are seen between 7 and 12 o'clock and subarterial defects are seen between 12 and 1 o'clock. The left parasternal long-axis view usually best demonstrates perimembranous VSDs.

The parasternal short-axis view at the level of the mitral valve may be used to visualize membranous VSD. Inlet VSDs appear between 7 and 9 o'clock, midmuscular VSDs appear between 9 and 12 o'clock, and anterior defects appear between 12 and 1 o'clock. The parasternal long-axis view with a tilt toward the pulmonary valve may demonstrate anterior VSDs and the four-chamber view at the level of the atrioventricular valves demonstrated apical, mid-muscular, and inlet defects. Further angulations of the transducer to a five-chamber view may help to visualize subaortic and anterior VSDs.

Technique

Regardless of the type of the VSD and the intended device choice, there are several common steps during each percutaneous VSD closure. After angiographic visualization of the defect from a left ventricular angiogram, the VSD is crossed from the left ventricular side and the guide wire is exteriorized so that an arteriovenous circuit is established. A long delivery sheath is introduced from the venous side over the guide wire circuit across the defect and a device is implanted. Final angiography is performed to assess residual leak and aortic valve competence.

- Anesthesia: Most of these procedures are done under general anesthesia, although sedation can be used.
- Imaging: TOE guidance for device closure is important although in single muscular VSDs, fluoroscopy with transthoracic echocardiography (TTE) monitoring can be performed.
- Vascular access: Both arterial and venous access is required. Usually, 4–5 Fr sheath is placed in the femoral artery and 6–8 Fr sheaths are placed in the femoral vein, when perimembranous or high anterior muscular VSDs are being closed or the internal jugular vein for apical or midmuscular VSDs. Alternatively, in small patients, who may develop significant hemodynamic instability when an arteriovenous circuit is established and a long stiff sheath is placed across the tricuspid valve, a direct hybrid approach can be utilized. In older children in whom similar difficulties are encountered, the VSD may be approached retrogradely from the femoral artery.

- Anticoagulation: Once vascular access has been obtained, intravenous heparin is given to maintain an activated clotting time (ACT) between 200 and 250 s. In case of prolonged procedures, ACT should be regularly monitored and additional doses of heparin should be given as required. Some operators prefer to start aspirin a day prior to the intervention.
- Hemodynamic study: Routine right and left heart catheterization is performed to estimate the degree of shunt, measure the pulmonary artery pressure, and pulmonary vascular resistance.
- Angiography: Left ventriculography is performed to visualize the defect(s) and the distance from the aortic valve. The best projection varies depending on the location of the defect. For perimembranous and anterior muscular defects, 60° left anterior oblique (LAO)/20° cranial is suitable and for the midmuscular, apical, and posterior lesions, the 35° LAO/35° cranial projection are typically the best ones. Alternatively, the posterior septum may be visualized in a 40° LAO projection and the anterior apical septum may be visualized in a left lateral projection.
- Crossing the VSD: The right ventricular trabeculations may make crossing the VSD from the venous side more difficult and if the defect is crossed antegradely, there is a greater likelihood of the sheath becoming entangled in the trabeculations. Therefore, in most cases, the VSD is best approached from the left ventricular side. A 4 or 5 Fr end-hole catheter, such as Judkins right coronary, Cobra, a cutoff Pigtail, or Judkins left coronary, are combined with a long floppy exchange length guide wire, such as Terumo or Noodle wire, to cross the VSD. Alternatively, a flow-directed balloon-tipped end-hole catheter can be advanced and looped in the apex of the left ventricle. With the balloon inflated, both the catheter and a curved guide wire are manipulated to engage the balloon into the VSD. Then while partially deflating the balloon, the guide wire is advanced into the right ventricle and further in to either the pulmonary artery or the right atrium.[23,24,31–33]
- Arteriovenous guide wire loop: Gooseneck snare and catheter (Microvena) of 10–15 mm diameter for children and 20–25 mm for adults, is advanced from the venous access into the pulmonary artery and is used to exteriorize the guide wire to establish an arteriovenous loop.
- Introduction of a long sheath: With the arteriovenous guide wire circuit kept taut, an appropriate-sized delivery sheath is advanced from the vein across the defect and into the ascending aorta. This should be performed with a kissing catheter technique, in which the sheath and dilator assembly are pushed from the venous approach while in contact with an end-hole catheter placed from the arterial side, and both are pulled simultaneously. Locking the loop with arterial forceps attached to the

wire just proximal to the end-hole catheter and also the long sheath makes this maneuver easier.
- The device: Once the device size is chosen, based on echocardiographic and angiographic measurements, the device is loaded in a saline bath to remove air bubbles and is then introduced into the sheath.

Complications

These may occur immediately or late during follow-up.[17,28,30] Immediate complications include

1. Embolization
2. Rhythm disturbances
3. Residual shunt
4. Hemolysis
5. Thromboembolism
6. Endocarditis

Late complications include development of complete heart block, when a perimembranous VSD has been closed.[17,30,34,35]

Clinical trials

No formal randomized clinical trials have been performed to compare device closure with surgery. All the reports are case based, occasionally prospective, but usually retrospective and descriptive studies or registries, which highlight the results and complications.[16,17,20,22,24,30,36–42] These then form the basis for decision making when dealing with individual patients. Furthermore, the population of patients, who are suitable for device closure, are mostly different in age and weight from those who usually undergo surgery and therefore, no meaningful scientific comparison can be made between the two techniques. In particular, extrapolation from the results to highlight superiority or inferiority of a technique needs to be avoided. Some of the selected studies of catheter closure of VSDs are summarized in Tables 68.1 and 68.2. These are not comprehensive tables but some details of these are shown in these tables.

Although it seems reasonable to recommend device closure for muscular and apical VSDs as well as residual defects after the previous surgery, these form a small proportion of patients. It is much more difficult to make unreserved recommendation for closing perimembranous VSDs. Conflicting results have been reported. The European registry raised concerns about the development of late complete heart block in those patients who had perimembranous VSD closed with devices.[17] In most centers in the Western world, device closure for perimembranous VSDs was abandoned. Alternative devices have been developed or some of the original devices have been

Table 68.1 Data from selected studies of catheter closure of VSDs

Year of publication	Author	Number of patients	Age range (years)	Type of VSD	Device type	Procedural success	Complications
1988	Lock et al.[18]	Six with seven VSDs	0.7–82	Post-MI, congenital Postoperative	Rashkind double umbrella	6/7	1—Embolization of device Deaths—All in post-MI patients
1991	Bridges et al.[19]	12 with 21 VSDs	0.8–20.4	Congenital in all muscular 19, postoperative 2	Clamshell septal umbrella	12/12	1—Hemothorax 1—Tricuspid regurgitation by device
1997	Sideris et al.[20]	25	4–35	PMVSD 15 Muscular 3	Buttoned device	18/25	1—Mild AR 1—Recurrence of shunt
1998	Janorkar et al.[21]	16 with 25 VSDs	0.1–4	Mid or anterior muscular 11, apical 14	Rashkind double umbrella	22/25	2—Deaths or major complications
1999	Kalra et al.[22]	30	5.5–33	PMVSD in 28 Muscular in two	Rashkind double-umbrella coil in one	26	1—Coil embolization

VSD = ventricular septal defect, MI = myocardial infarction, PMVSD = perimembranous ventricular septal defect, AR = aortic regurgitation, CHB = complete heart block, AV block = atrioventricular block, TR = tricuspid regurgitation.

Table 68.2 Data from other selected studies of catheter closure of VSDs

Year of publication	Author	Number of points	Age range (years)	Type of VSD	Device type	Procedural success	Complications
1999	Thanopoulos et al.[23]	6	3–10	Muscular	Amplatzer VSD occluder	6	2—Transient left bundle branch block
2000	Hijazi et al.[24]	8	2–10	Muscular	Amplatzer VSD occluder	8	1—Transient junctional rhythm
2002	Chessa et al.[28]	32	0.1–86	Muscular (20 congenital, 12 post-MI)	Amplatzer VSD occluder	30	1—Death from tamponade, 1—Device malposition; 2—Hemolysis
2003	Bass et al.[31]	27	1.25–32	PMVSD	Amplatzer PMVSD occluder	25	None
2003	Arora et al.[43]	137	3–33	PMVSD in 91 Muscular in 46	Amplatzer VSD occluder in 107 Rashkind umbrella in 29	130	2—Complete heart block 2—Tricuspid valve complications
2004	Knauth et al.[44]	170	0.3–73	Congenital 92 Postoperative 78	CardioSEAL/Starflex devices	168	39—Adverse events related to device
2006	Fu et al.[36]	35	1.2–54.4	PMVSD	Amplatzer PMVSD occluder	32	1—CHB 1—Tricuspid valve damage 1—Bleeding
2007	Thanopoulos et al.[45]	54	0.3–13	PMVSD	Amplatzer PMVSD occluder	49/54	5—Early (one with 2:1 AV block); 1—Late CHB
2007	Lim et al.[46]	55	0.02–65	Muscular	CardioSEAL	50	8
2007	Butera et al.[47]	104	0.6–63	PMVSD	Amplatzer PMVSD occluder Muscular VSD occluder	100	13—Early (six had CHB, four early, and two late)
2008	Qin et al.[48]	412	3–65	PMVSD	Modified double-disk device	398	6—had CHB (transient) 3—Embolized devices
2009	Kenny et al.[49]	25	1.8–32.8	PMVSD	Amplatzer PMVSD occluder Muscular VSD occluder	23	2—Had AR
2010	Yang et al.[42]	848	2–73	PMVSD	PMVSD	832	9—Major with CHB in two
2010	Zuo et al.[41]	301	Mean = 9.8	PMVSD	Amplatzer PMVSD occluder	294	11—With AR 16—With TR 18—CHB (15 early, three late)
2012	Zhou et al.[35]	348		PMVSD	Shanghai PMVSD occluder	339	1—Embolized 1—Cardiac tamponade 1—CHB (late)
2012	Wang et al.[39]	525	Mean 5.6	PMVSD	Symmetric PMVSD occluder	502	3—Major (valve related) 1—CHB (transient)
2013	Lee et al.[38]	21	3–42	PMVSD	ADO	21	1—Residual leak needing surgery

VSD = ventricular septal defect, MI = myocardial infarction, PMVSD = perimembranous ventricular septal defect, AR = aortic regurgitation, CHB = complete heart block, AV block = atrioventricular block, TR = tricuspid regurgitation.

modified, resulting in possible gradual reintroduction of this procedure.[50,51] With the recently modified Amplatzer Membranous VSD Occluder 2, the median 1 year follow-up of 19 patients, ranging in age between 1.4 and 62 years, and ranging in weight from 9.3 to 96 kg, has shown no cases of heart block.[51] Although the study population and the follow-up are short, this study does show a difference in age and weight compared with the surgical cases, which tend to be younger and smaller. Apart from softer waists on this and some of the other devices, devices such as the Amplatzer Duct Occluder (ADO) have also been used to close perimembranous VSDs.[32,33,38] It is thought that these devices are less rigid, in particular, the ADO I, as they do not have two disks with a waist between them and so impart less radial force on the septum. Other devices, with asymmetric disks as well as symmetric disks, but with a more flexible waist, are being used in clinical studies, but it remains to be seen whether there is truly a much lower incidence of complete heart block.[34,39–40,52] Furthermore, for smaller children, who may be considered for device closure, hybrid perventricular therapy overcomes many of the technical problems encountered and the risks with the procedure.[25–27,53,54]

The future developments should take into account the concerns about metal devices, their rigidity, and the incidence of complications such as complete heart block. Although softer devices are being developed and used clinically, biodegradable devices will become more important in the future.[55] Indeed, such a device has undergone experimental study already and so, future developments in this field will be exciting.

References

1. Hoffman JIE, Rudolph AM. The natural history of ventricular septal defects in infancy. *Am J Cardiol* 1965;16:634–53.
2. Momma K, Toyama K, Takao A, Ando M, Nakazawa M, Hirosawa K et al. Natural history of subarterial infundibular ventricular septal defect. *Am Heart J* 1984;108:1312–17.
3. Momma K, Ando M, Matsukova R, Soo K. Interruption of the aortic arch associated with deletion of chromosome 22q11 is associated with a subarterial and doubly committed ventricular septal defect in Japanese patients. *Cardiol Young* 1999;9:463–7.
4. Moe DG, Guntheroth WG. Spontaneous closure of uncomplicated ventricular septal defect. *Am J Cardiol* 1987;60:674–8.
5. Alpert BS, Cook DH, Varghese PC et al. Spontaneous closure of small ventricular septal defects: Ten year follow-up. *Pediatrics* 1979;63:204–6.
6. Krovetz IJ. Spontaneous closure of ventricular septal defect. *Am J Cardiol* 1998;81:100–1.
7. Mehta AV, Chidambaram B. Ventricular septal defect in the first year of life. *Am J Cardiol* 1992;70:364–6.
8. Perrault H, Drblik SP, Montigny M et al. Comparison of cardiovascular adjustments to exercise in adolescents 8 to 15 years of age after correction of tetralogy of Fallot, ventricular septal defect or atrial septal defect. *Am J Cardiol* 1989;64:213–7.
9. Klitsie LM, Kuipers IM, Roest AAW et al. Disparity in right vs. left ventricular recovery during follow-up after ventricular septal defect correction in children. *Eur J Cardiothorac Surg* 2013;44:269–74.
10. Meijboom F, Szatmari A, Utens E et al. Long-term follow-up after surgical closure of ventricular septal defect in infancy and childhood. *J Am Coll Cardiol* 1994;24:1358–64.
11. Kitagawa T, Durham III LA, Mosca RS, Bove EL. Techniques and results in the management of multiple ventricular septal defects. *J Thorac Cardiovasc Surg* 1998;115:848–56.
12. Seddio F, Reddy VM, McElhinney DB, Tworetzky W, Silverman NH, Hanley FL. Multiple ventricular septal defects: How and when should they be repaired? *J Thorac Cardiovasc Surg* 1999;117:134–9; discussion 39–40.
13. Andersen HØ, deLeval MR, Tsang VT, Elliott MJ, Anderson RH, Cook AC. Is complete heart block after surgical closure of ventricular septum defects still an issue? *Ann Thorac Surg* 2006;82:948–56.
14. Tucker EM, Pyles LA, Bass JL, Moller JH. Permanent pacemaker for atrioventricular conduction block after operative repair of perimembranous ventricular septal defect. *J Am Coll Cardiol* 2007;50:1196–200.
15. Roos-Hesselink JW, Meijboom FJ, Spitaels SEC et al. Outcome of patients after surgical closure of ventricular septal defect at young age: Longitudinal follow-up of 22–34 years. *Eur Heart J* 2004;25:1057–62.
16. Liu S, Chen F, Ding X, Zhao Z, Ke W, Yan Y et al. Comparison of results and economic analysis of surgical and transcat heteroclosure of perimembranous ventricular septal defect. *Eur J Cardiothorac Surg* 2012;42:e157–62.
17. Carminati M, Butera G, Chessa M et al. Transcatheter closure of congenital ventricular septal defects: Results of the European Registry. *Eur Heart J* 2007;28:2361–8.
18. Lock JE, Block PC, McKay RG, Baim DS, Keane JF. Transcatheter closure of ventricular septal defects. *Circulation* 1988;78:361–8.
19. Bridges ND, Perry SB, Keane JF, Goldstein SA, Mandell V, Mayes JE et al. Preoperative transcatheter closure of congenital muscular ventricular septal defects. *N Engl J Med* 1991; 324:1312–17.
20. Sideris EB, Walsh KP, Haddad JL, Chen CR, Ren SG, Kulkarni H. Occlusion of congenital ventricular septal defects by the buttoned device. "Buttoned Device" Clinical Trials International Register. *Heart* 1997;77:276–9.
21. Janorkar S, Goh T, Wilkinson J. Transcatheter closure of ventricular septal defects using the Rashkind device: Initial experience. *Catheter Cardiovasc Interv* 1999;46:43–8.
22. Kalra GS, Verma PK, Dhall A, Singh S, Arora R. Transcatheter device closure of ventricular septal defects: Immediate results and intermediate-term follow-up. *Am Heart J* 1999;138:339–44.
23. Thanopoulos BD, Tsaousis GS, Konstadopoulou GN, Zarayelyan AG. Transcatheter closure of muscular ventricular septal defects with the Amplatzer ventricular septal defect occluder: Initial clinical applications in children. *J Am Coll Cardiol* 1999;33:1395–9.
24. Hijazi ZM, Hakim F, Al Fadley F, Abdelhamid J, Cao QL. Transcatheter closure of single muscular ventricular septal defects using the Amplatzer muscular VSD occluder: Initial results and technical considerations. *Catheter Cardiovasc Interv* 2000;49:167–72.
25. Amin Z, Danford DA, Lof J, Duncan KF, Froemming S. Intraoperative device closure of perimembranous ventricular septal defects without cardiopulmonary bypass: Preliminary results with the perventricular technique. *J Thorac Cardiovasc Surg* 2004;127:234–41.
26. Bacha EA, Cao QL, Starr JP, Waight D, Ebeid MR, Hijazi ZM. Perventricular device closure of muscular ventricular septal defects on the beating heart: Technique and results. *J Thorac Cardiovasc Surg* 2003;126:1718–23.
27. Bacha EA, Cao QL, Galantowicz ME, Cheatham JP, Fleishman CE, Weinstein SW et al. Multicenter experience with perventricular device closure of muscular ventricular septal defects. *Pediatr Cardiol* 2005;26:169–75.
28. Chessa M, Carminati M, Cao QL et al. Transcatheter closure of congenital and acquired muscular ventricular septal defects using the Amplatzer device. *J Invasive Cardiol* 2002;14:322–7.
29. Michel-Behnke I, Le TP, Waldecker B, Akintuerk H, Valeske K, Schranz D. Percutaneous closure of congenital and acquired

ventricular septal defects—Considerations on selection of the occlusion device. *J Interv Cardiol* 2005;18:89–99.

30. Chungsomprasong P, Durongpisitkul K, Vijarnsorn C, Soongswang J, Lê TP. The results of transcatheter closure of VSD using Amplatzer® device and Nit Occlud® Lê coil. *Catheter Cardiovasc Interv* 2011;78:1032–40.

31. Bass JL, Kalra GS, Arora R, Gavora P, Thanopoulos BD, Torres W et al. Initial human experience with the Amplatzer perimembranous ventricular septal occluder device. *Catheter Cardiovasc Interv* 2003; 58:238–45.

32. Koneti NR, Verma S, Bakhru S, Vadlamudi K, Kathare P, Penumatsa RR et al. Transcatheter trans-septal antegrade closure of muscular ventricular septal defects in young children. *Catheter Cardiovasc Interv* 2013;82:E500–6.

33. Koneti NR, Sreeram N, Penumatsa RR, Arramraj SK, Karunakar V, Trieschmann U. Transcatheter retrograde closure of perimembranous ventricular septal defects in children with the Amplatzer duct occluder II device. *J Am Coll Cardiol* 2012;60:2421–2.

34. Yang R, Kong XQ, Sheng YH et al. Risk factors and outcomes of postprocedure heart blocks after transcatheter device closure of perimembranous ventricular septal defect. *J Am Coll Cardiol Cardiovasc Interv* 2012;5(4):422–7.

35. Zhou D, Pan W, Guan L, Ge J. Transcatheter closure of perimembranous and intracristal ventricular septal defects with the SHSMA occluder. *Catheter Cardiovasc Interv* 2012;79:666–74.

36. Fu YC, Bass J, Amin Z et al. Transcatheter closure of perimembranous ventricular septal defects using the new Amplatzer membranous VSD occluder: Results of the U.S. phase I trial. *J Am Coll Cardiol* 2006;47:319–25.

37. Holzer RJ, Balzer D, Amin Z, Ruiz CE, Feinstein J, Bass J et al. Transcatheter closure of postinfarction ventricular septal defects using the new Amplatzer muscular VSD occluder: Results of a U.S. registry. *Catheter Cardiovasc Interv* 2004;61:196–201.

38. Lee SM, Song JY, Choi JY et al. Transcatheter closure of perimembranous ventricular septal defect using Amplatzer ductal occluder. *Catheter Cardiovasc Interv* 2013;82:1141–6.

39. Wang L, Cao S, Li J et al. Transcatheter closure of congenital perimembranous ventricular septal defect in children using symmetric occluders: An 8-year multi-institutional experience. *Ann Thorac Surg* 2012;94:592–8.

40. Yang R, Sheng Y, Cao K et al. Transcatheter closure of perimembranous ventricular septal defect in children: Safety and efficiency with symmetric and asymmetric occluders. *Catheter Cardiovasc Interv* 2011;77:84–90.

41. Zuo J, Xie J, Yi W, Yang J, Zhang J, Li J et al. Results of transcatheter closure of perimembranous ventricular septal defect. *Am J Cardiol* 2010;106:1034–7.

42. Yang J, Yang L, Wan Y et al. Transcatheter device closure of perimembranous ventricular septal defects: Mid-term outcomes. *Eur Heart J* 2010;31:2238–45.

43. Arora R, Trehan V, Kumar A, Kalra GS, Nigam M. Transcatheter closure of congenital ventricular septal defects. Experience with various devices. *J Interven Cardiol* 2003;16:83–91.

44. Knauth AL, Lock JE, Perry SB, McElhinney DB, Gauvreau K, Landzberg MJ et al. Transcatheter device closure of congenital and post-operative residual ventricular septal defect. *Circulation* 2004;110:501–7.

45. Thanopoulos BV, Rigby ML, Karanasios E et al. Transcatheter closure of perimembranous ventricular septal defects in infants and children using the Amplatzer perimembranous ventricular septal defect occluder. *Am J Cardiol* 2007;99:984–9.

46. Lim DS, Forbes TJ, Rothman A, Lock JE, Landzberg MJ. Transcatheter closure of high-risk muscular ventricular septal defects with the CardioSEAL occluder: Initial report from the CardioSEAL VSD registry. *Catheter Cardiovasc Interv* 2007;70:740–4.

47. Butera G, Carminati M, Chessa M, Piazza L, Micheletti A, Negura DG et al. Transcatheter closure of perimembranous ventricular septal defects: Early and long-term results. *J Am Coll Cardiol* 2007;50:1189–95.

48. Qin Y, Chen J, Zhao X, Liao D, Mu R, Wang S et al. Transcatheter closure of perimembranous ventricular septal defect using a modified double-disk occluder. *Am J Cardiol* 2008;101:1781–6.

49. Kenny D, Morgan G, Bajwa A, Farrow C, Parry A, Caputo M et al. Evolution of transcatheter closure of perimembranous ventricular septal defects in a single centre. *Catheter Cardiovasc Interv* 2009;73:568–75.

50. Velasco-Sanchez D, Tzikas A, Ibrahim R, Miró J. Transcatheter closure of perimembranous ventricular septal defects: Initial human experience with the Amplatzer® membranous™ VSD occluder 2. *Catheter Cardiovasc Interv* 2013;82:474–9.

51. Tzikas A, Ibrahim R, Velasco-Sanchez D et al. Transcatheter closure of perimembranous ventricular septal defect with the Amplatzer® membranous VSD occluder 2: Initial world experience and one-year follow-up. *Catheter Cardiovasc Interv* 2014;83(4):571–80.

52. Jin Y, Han B, Zhang J, Zhuang J, Yan J, Wang Y. Post implant complications with transcatheter closure of congenital perimembranous ventricular septal defects: A single-center, longitudinal study from 2002 to 2011. *Catheter Cardiovasc Interv* 2013;81:666–73.

53. Gan C, Lin K, An Q, Tang H, Song H, Lui RC et al. Perventricular device closure of muscular ventricular septal defects on beating hearts: Initial experience in eight children. *J Thorac Cardiovasc Surg* 2009;137:929–33.

54. Gan C, An Q, Lin K, Tang H, Lui RC, Tao K et al. Perventricular device closure of ventricular septal defects: Six months results in 30 young children. *Ann Thorac Surg* 2008;86:142–6.

55. Huang XM, Zhu YF, Cao J et al. Development and preclinical evaluation of a biodegradable ventricular septal defect occluder. *Catheter Cardiovasc Interv* 2013;81:324–30.

69

Ventricular septal defect closure: Closure of congenital muscular VSD using the Amplatzer-type muscular VSD occluders

Noa Holoshitz, Qi-Ling Cao, and Ziyad M. Hijazi

Introduction

Ventricular septal defect (VSD) is the most common congenital heart disease accounting for approximately 20% of all congenital defects.[1] About 10–15% of VSDs are muscular, located entirely within the muscular portion of the septum. The most common location is apical, followed by the mid- and anterior septum. Occasionally, the defects are multiple (swiss cheese VSDs). Acquired muscular VSDs are very rare and may result from postmyocardial infarction or traumatic injury to the chest.[1] Because muscular VSDs are frequently hidden within the coarse right ventricular (RV) trabeculations, they are difficult to localize through the standard surgical approach via the right atrium. Various surgical approaches have been proposed, but surgery still poses a remarkable challenge and carries certain morbidity and mortality.[1]

Since 1987, the Rashkind and buttoned devices have been used to close muscular VSDs. However, these devices were originally designed for closure of patent ductus arteriosus and atrial septal defects, respectively.[2–4] There were multiple major drawbacks with these devices, including a large delivery sheath (11 Fr), complex implantation techniques, and the inability to reposition the device after deployment. In addition, there was the possibility of interference with the mitral, tricuspid, or aortic valves and the rate of significant residual shunt was as high as 25–60%. The Amplatzer muscular VSD occluder is the only device that is specifically designed for the muscular VSD. Since its initial human use in 1998,[5,6] it has become the most popular and effective device to close muscular VSDs worldwide.

Device

The Amplatzer muscular VSD occluder (St. Jude Medical, Plymouth, MN, USA) is currently the only available device approved by the Food and Drug Administration (FDA) for closure of muscular VSDs. The CardioSeal device had similar US FDA approval; however, the manufacturer ceased to exist. The Amplatzer muscular VSD device is a self-expandable double-disk device made of a nitinol wire mesh (Figure 69.1).[7–10] The thickness of the wire is 0.004–0.005 inches. The connecting waist is 7 mm long and the left and right ventricle disks are 8 mm larger than the waist. Three Dacron polyester patches are sewn securely with polyester thread into the two disks and the waist of the device to enhance thrombosis and to achieve higher closure rates. The RV disk has a stainless-steel sleeve

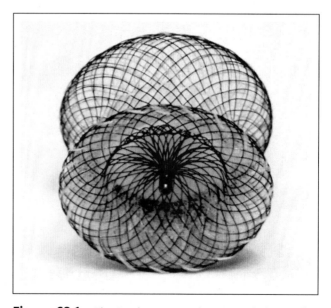

Figure 69.1 The Amplatzer muscular VSD occluder consists of three components: an LV disk, a connecting waist, and an RV disk. The connecting waist is 7 mm long and the two disks are 8 mm larger than the waist. Polyester fabric is present in both disks and the connecting waist.

with a female thread used to screw the delivery cable to the device. The device size corresponds to the diameter of the waist and is available in sizes ranging from 4 to 18 mm in 2 mm increments. The delivery sheath required for deployment of these devices varies from 6 to 9 Fr (6 French sheath for the 4–6 mm devices, 7 French sheath for the 8–10 mm devices, 8 French sheath for the 12–14 mm devices, and a 9 French sheath for the 16–18 mm devices). The mechanism of closure involves stenting of the VSD by the device and subsequent thrombus formation within the device with eventual complete neoendothelialization.

The Amplatzer postinfarction muscular VSD occluder is slightly different from the Amplatzer muscular VSD occluder.[8–11] The connecting waist is longer (10 mm) and the two disks are bigger (10 mm larger than the waist). The device is available in sizes ranging from 16 to 24 mm in 2 mm increments, that are delivered through 8–12 Fr sheaths. It is currently only available through the FDA for emergency or compassionate use in the United States. Refer Chapter 72.

Patient selection

The complete indications for closure of VSDs as outlined by the 2008 ACC/AHA guidelines for adults with congenital heart disease are listed in Table 69.1.[12] Contraindications

---

Table 69.1   Guidelines for VSD closure

Class I:
1. Surgeons with training and expertise in CHD should perform VSD closure operations. (*Level of Evidence: C*)
2. Closure of a VSD is indicated when there is a Qp/Qs (pulmonary-to-systemic blood flow ratio) of 2.0 or more and clinical evidence of LV volume overload. (*Level of Evidence: B*)
3. Closure of a VSD is indicated when the patient has a history of infective endocarditis. (*Level of Evidence: C*)

Class IIa:
1. Closure of a VSD is reasonable when net left-to-right shunting is present at a Qp/Qs greater than 1.5 with pulmonary artery pressure less than two-thirds of systemic pressure and PVR less than two-thirds of systemic vascular resistance. (*Level of Evidence: B*)
2. Closure of a VSD is reasonable when net left-to-right shunting is present at a Qp/Qs greater than 1.5 in the presence of LV systolic or diastolic failure. (*Level of Evidence: B*)

Class IIb:
1. Device closure of a muscular VSD may be considered, especially if the VSD is remote from the tricuspid valve and the aorta, if the VSD is associated with severe left-sided heart chamber enlargement, or if there is PAH. (*Level of Evidence: C*)

Class III:
1. VSD closure is not recommended in patients with severe irreversible PAH. (*Level of Evidence: B*)

---

include (1) distance of less than 4 mm between the VSD and the aortic, pulmonary, mitral, and tricuspid valves, (2) pulmonary vascular resistance of greater than 8 Woods units, (3) sepsis, or (4) contraindication to antiplatelet therapy. For patients weighing more than 5 kg, the percutaneous transcatheter approach is safe and effective and has low morbidity and mortality. However, for smaller patients (less than 5 kg) or patients with other associated cardiac defects requiring concommitant surgical repair, the perventricular approach may be preferred.

Precatheterization evaluation

In order to plan the interventional approach, echocardiographic assessment of the size, number, and location of the VSDs is of paramount importance.[1] The parasternal long-axis view demonstrates anterior VSDs. The short-axis view near the tips of the mitral valve is important in delineating the location of the muscular VSD. In this view, anterior defects appear between 12 and 1 o'clock; midmuscular defects appear between 9 and 12 o'clock, and inlet defects appear between 7 and 9 o'clock. The four-chamber view at the level of the atrioventricular valves demonstrates apical, midmuscular, and inlet defects. If the transducer is angled more anterior to the "five-chamber view," subaortic and anterior VSDs are also delineated.

Device implantation technique

Percutaneous protocol

1. The procedure is preferably performed under general endotracheal anesthesia with continuous transesophageal echocardiographic (TEE) guidance (Figure 69.2).[1,6–10] However, for single muscular VSD, the procedure can be done safely and effectively under fluoroscopic guidance with transthoracic echocardiographic monitoring.
2. Access is obtained in the femoral artery and the femoral vein. If the VSD is midmuscular, posterior, or apical septum, the right internal jugular vein is also accessed. If the VSD is anterior, femoral vein delivery is preferred.
3. Heparin is administered to maintain an activated clotting time (ACT) greater than 200 s at the time of device placement. We monitor the ACT every 30 min after the initial dose.
4. Routine right and left heart catheterization is performed to assess the degree of shunting and to evaluate the pulmonary vascular resistance.
5. Left ventriculography is performed to rule out any additional defects and to create a road map to aid in accessing the defect from the left ventricular side. This is done in a single plane at a 35° left anterior oblique

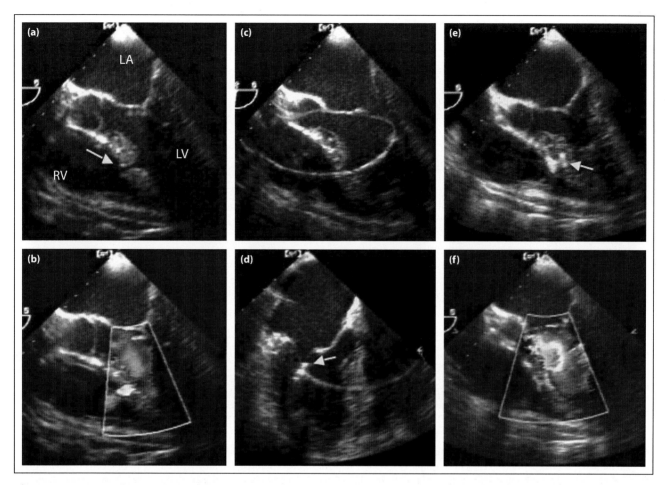

Figure 69.2   (See color insert.) Transesophageal echocardiographic images in modified four-chamber views in a 31-year-old male patient with a 5 mm anterior muscular VSD and left-to-right shunt. (a) View demonstrating the VSD (arrow). LV: left ventricle; RV: right ventricle; LA: left atrium. (b) Similar view to (a) with color Doppler demonstrating the shunt. (c) View demonstrating the arteriovenous wire loop (from the aorta, left ventricle, VSD, right ventricle, and out the jugular vein). (d) Deployment of the LV disk of a 6 mm Amplatzer muscular VSD device in mid-LV cavity (arrow). (e) The device has been released (arrow) in the ventricular septum. Note for an adult, the connecting waist is not long enough, but it achieves closure. (f) Final image with color Doppler demonstrating good device position and no residual shunt.

(LAO)/35° cranial view to profile the muscular septum. For anterior muscular VSDs and perimembranous VSDs, the 60° LAO/15–20° cranial angulation best profiles the VSD.

6. The appropriate device size is chosen to be 1–2 mm larger than the VSD size as measured by TEE or left ventriculography at end-diastole.

7. A 4 or 5 Fr curved end-hole catheter (Judkins right coronary, or Cobra) is used to cross the VSD from the left ventricle (LV) into either the branch pulmonary artery or the superior vena cava with a 0.035 inch Glidewire (Terumo Medical Corporation, Somerset, NJ, USA). When using the Glidewire in a small child, extreme care has to be exercised because perforating the ventricular septum with the wire is not a rare phenomenon! If the VSD is anterior, we cut the tip of a Judkins left coronary catheter and use it to orientate the tip to the defect. On rare occasions, if the VSD cannot be crossed using the Judkins right coronary catheter, we float an end-hole balloon wedge catheter and advance it to the LV cavity until it prolapses back into the ascending aorta. With the balloon inflated, the catheter has the tendency to cross the defect. At this time, advance a wire through the catheter and follow it to the right side of heart. We usually do not like to cross the VSD from the RV side due to the tendency of the sheath to become entangled in the trabeculations.

8. The next step is to snare the wire and exteriorize it from a vein (jugular or femoral). This is done using a gooseneck snare catheter (ev3, Plymouth, MN, USA) with an appropriate loop diameter (for adults, we use 20–25 mm, and for children, 10–15 mm). This

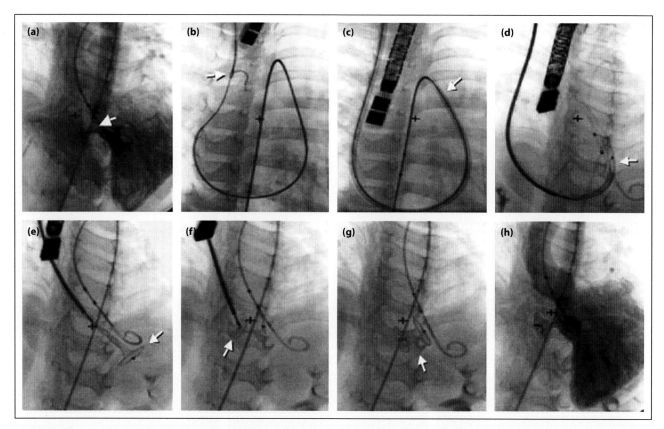

Figure 69.3   (a) Left ventriculography in the left four-chamber view demonstrating an 8 mm muscular VSD (arrow) in a 3.6-year-old boy. (b) Cine image demonstrating the snaring of the wire from the right internal jugular vein (arrow). (c) Cine image demonstrating the delivery sheath over the wire (arteriovenous loop). The sheath tip is in the ascending aorta (arrow). (d) Cine fluoroscopy during passage of a 10 mm Amplatzer muscular VSD device inside the sheath (arrow). (e) Cine fluoroscopy during deployment of the left ventricle disk (arrow) in mid-LV cavity. (f) Cine fluoroscopy during deployment of the RV disk (arrow) on the right ventricle side of the VSD. (g) Cine fluoroscopy after the device (arrow) has been released. (h) Left ventriculography after the device has been released demonstrating good position and no residual shunt.

establishes an arteriovenous loop to provide stability and support for device delivery. Figure 69.3 demonstrates an arteriovenous loop snared through the jugular vein.

9. Over this wire, an appropriate-size delivery sheath is advanced from the vein (jugular or femoral) until the tip of the sheath is in the ascending aorta (Figure 69.3c). We like to keep the position of the sheath in the ascending aorta until the device reaches the tip of the sheath. After removal of the dilator from the sheath, kinking can be a problem. To overcome this problem, we suggest keeping an 0.018 inch Terumo Glidewire inside the sheath, snared from the arterial end to keep constant tension and to facilitate passage of the device inside the sheath, or to use a kink-resistant sheath such as the Arrow-Flex (Teleflex, Research Triangle Park, NC, USA) or the Torq Vu from the device manufacturer.

10. The device is loaded under blood/saline seal in the usual fashion and attached to the delivery sheath. The device is advanced to the tip of the sheath while fluoroscoping and looking for any evidence of air in the system.

11. We usually deploy part of the LV disk at the tip of the sheath before we start bringing the sheath back to the LV cavity. This is done mostly for the anterior VSD where the sheath may jump back to the RV even with slow withdrawal. Once the sheath is in the mid-LV cavity, the remainder of the LV disk is deployed. This can be easily visualized by echocardiography and it is imperative to insure that the disk is not entangled in the mitral valve apparatus. Should this be the case, the device is recaptured or the entire assembly is pushed back inside the LV to release the anterior mitral valve leaflet.

12. The entire device assembly is withdrawn back to the septum with further retraction of the sheath to expand the waist inside the septum (Figure 69.3e).

13. After a good device position is ensured by echocardiography and left ventriculography, the sheath is retracted to expand the RV disk (Figure 69.3f).

14. After echocardiography and left ventriculography confirm the device position is good, the device is released by counterclockwise rotation of the cable using the pin

vise. Once the device is released (Figure 69.3g), the cable should be brought inside the sheath immediately to prevent any injury from the sharp end of the cable.

15. Repeat echocardiography (Figure 69.2f) and left ventriculography (Figure 69.3h) are performed to assess the final result in terms of closure and residual shunt and to assess the function of the tricuspid, mitral, and aortic valve. If there are further defects (multiple or swiss cheese), the same process is repeated.

16. At the end of the procedure, the ACT is checked and if it is below 250 s, the sheaths are removed and hemostasis is achieved. If ACT is >250 s, protamine sulfate can be given to reverse the heparin effect.

17. The patient stays in the hospital overnight for postdevice observation and is usually discharged home the following day.

Perventricular protocol

Indications include (1) small infants (<5 kg) precluding safe percutaneous closure, (2) patients with poor vascular access, or (3) muscular VSD associated with other defects requiring open surgical repair.[11,13,14]

1. The procedure is performed under general endotracheal anesthesia with continuous TEE guidance in the operating room or in the hybrid catherization laboratory. Figure 69.4 demonstrates the steps of closure.

2. After the chest and pericardium are opened by a cardiovascular surgeon, a good location for the puncture of the RV free wall is assessed by echocardiography, which should be away from any papillary muscles and perpendicular to the defect.

3. A 5-0 polypropylene purse-string suture is placed at the chosen location.

4. An 18 gauge needle is introduced through the chosen location into the RV cavity, pointing toward the VSD.

5. A 0.035 inch short Glidewire is passed through the needle and VSD into the LV. The needle is then taken out, leaving the wire in position.

6. Over the wire, the proper-size short sheath with its dilator is advanced to the LV cavity. Then the dilator is taken out. Extreme care is exercised while advancing the sheath over the wire. The dilator is sharp and could injure the LV wall if one is not careful. Once the sheath is inside the LV cavity, de-aeration should take place to prevent any air embolism.

7. The proper-size Amplatzer muscular VSD device is screwed to the delivery cable and loaded inside a sheath smaller than the one through the defect.

8. The device is then advanced inside the delivery sheath under TEE guidance until the LV disk is deployed.

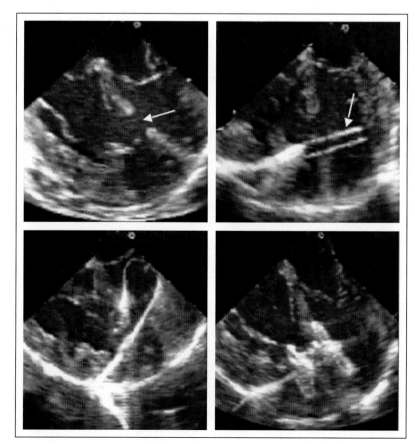

Figure 69.4 Transesophageal echocardiographic images in a 4-month-old baby with large (7–8 mm) anterior muscular VSD who underwent closure of the VSD using the perventricular approach. Top left: Four-chamber view demonstrating the VSD (arrow). Bottom left: Passage of a 0.035" guide wire from the right ventricle free wall to the VSD to the LV cavity. Top right: The tip of a 7 Fr delivery sheath (arrow) in mid-LV cavity. Note the device is in the proximal part of the sheath being advanced to the tip. Bottom right: A 10-mm Amplatzer muscular VSD device has been deployed, but not released yet. This demonstrates good device position.

9. The whole cable/sheath assembly is retracted toward the septum until tension is felt and the device is aligned with the septum by echocardiography.
10. Further retraction of the sheath deploys the connecting waist and the RV disk.
11. After echocardiography confirms good device position, the device is released by counterclockwise rotation of the cable using the pin vise.

On rare occasions, if the VSD cannot be crossed from the RV free wall puncture, one can cross in the retrograde fashion percutaneously (as described above). The wire is advanced via the VSD to the branch pulmonary artery. Then the surgeon advances a short sheath from a puncture in the RV free wall to the main pulmonary artery. Under fluoroscopic guidance, a snare is introduced inside this sheath to the pulmonary artery. The wire that was placed in the pulmonary artery via the VSD is then snared and exteriorized out through the RV free wall. Over this wire, advance the sheath with its dilator until the tip is in the mid-LV cavity. Once this step is achieved, remove the wire and dilator and the remaining steps are followed as described above.

Follow-up

The follow-up protocol includes physical examination, electrocardiography, echocardiography, and chest radiography the following day and at 1 and 6 months (transthoracic echocardiography) after the procedure. Patients are routinely maintained on aspirin 81 mg (3–5 mg/kg for small children) daily or equivalent antiplatelet therapy for 6 months. Patients are instructed to receive infective endocarditis prophylaxis when needed until complete closure is documented at the 6-month follow-up visit.

Possible complications

1. *Device embolization/migration*: This complication is rare, especially if the procedure is performed by an experienced operator and under cautious echocardiographic monitoring. The device can migrate to the LV, aorta, RV, or pulmonary artery. The device can be snared and retrieved percutaneously; however, a larger sheath may be needed. The presence of a cardiovascular surgeon in house is essential for device closure of muscular VSD. Different size and type sheaths and snares should be available on the premises to manage such a complication. Device embolization is not a common complication. In the European registry of transcatheter closure of 430 VSDs (119 were muscular), there were only 5 device embolizations.[15] Furthermore, in a study from the same group out of 40 adult patients with transcatheter closure of a muscular VSD, there were no device emolizations reported.[16] In the US registry of muscular defects, out of 77 muscular VSDs closed percutaneously, there were only 2 device embolizations.[7]

2. *Arrhythmia*: Ventricular arrhythmia may be encountered during catheter manipulations and device deployment, which is usually benign and transient. Conduction disturbances can be seen and complete heart block is rare. On occasions, a Lidocaine drip is initiated to manage ventricular arrhythmias. The anesthesiologist managing such patients should be well versed in managing such arrhythmias. A recent study showed a 10% rate of permanent conduction abnormalities and a 7% rate of transient conduction abnormalities (such as right bundle branch block or left anterior fascicular block) following transcatheter muscular VSD closure with the Amplatzer device.[17] There was one incident of transient second-degree type II block that was resolved and there were no incidents of complete heart block.

3. *Air embolization*: A meticulous technique of catheter and wire exchanges can minimize this complication. It is important to let the sheath bleed back freely once it has entered the left-sided circulation.

4. *Hemolysis*: This complication is rare and usually associated with residual shunting. The authors preferably pre-soak the device with the patient's own blood for about 15–20 min; we believe this technique can reduce residual shunt and improve immediate complete closure.

5. *Valvular regurgitation*: Tricuspid, mitral, or aortic regurgitation may occur due to the impingement of the device on the valvular apparatus or subaortic septum. Therefore, echocardiographic assessment of the valvular regurgitation prior to closure and prior to device release is extremely important. If the device does appear to be entangled in the subvalvular apparatus, we have been successful in recapturing the device and repositioning it.

6. *Pericardial effusion*: This is very rare complication that may result from catheter irritation or minute wire perforation during the procedure. To our knowledge, there have been no cases of tamponade or delayed pericardial effusion after 24 h.

Results
Congenital muscular VSD

A US registry involving 14 tertiary referral centers conducted a prospective, nonrandomized study of device closure of congenital muscular VSDs using the Amplatzer muscular VSD occluder.[7] A total of 83 procedures (percutaneous closure in 77 and perventricular closure in 6) were performed in 75 patients (median age: 1.4 years, range: 0.1–54.1 years). The median size of the VSD was 7 mm (range

3–16 mm) and in 34 of 78 (43.6%) procedures, patients had multiple VSDs (range 2–7). The device was implanted successfully in 72 of 83 (86.7%) procedures. In 17 of 83 (20.5%) procedures, multiple devices were implanted (range 2–3). Procedure-related major complications occurred in 8 of 75 (10.7%) patients, including cerebrovascular accident in 3, death in 2, device embolization in 2, and cardiac perforation in 1. Complete closure rate was 47.2% (34/72), 69.6% (32/46), and 92.3% (24/26) at 24 hour, 6 month, and 12 month follow-up.

The European VSD registry data was published in 2007 by Carminati et al. They reported results on 430 patients with congenital VSDs (119 were muscular); the median age at closure was 8. The median VSD size was 7 mm (3–22 mm), and the device was implanted successfully in 95% of patients. Complications included five device embolizations (1.6%), aortic regurgitation in 14 cases (3.2%), and tricuspid regurgitation in 27 cases (6.3%). There were minor rhythm disturbances in 10 patients (2.3%). Out of the muscular VSD patients there were three cases of transient heart block and one case of complete heart block requiring PPM (0.8%). Complete closure was achieved in 40% of the patients at the time of procedure, 65% at discharge, and 83% at their 3 month follow-up. Longer follow-up was not available. In three cases (0.7%), the residual shunt was severe, requiring additional surgery.[15]

Bacha et al. reported the multicenter experience with perventricular device closure of muscular VSDs in 12 patients (median age of 8.5 months, range 14 days to 4.3 years; median weight of 7 kg, range 3–20 kg).[13] At a median follow-up of 12 months, all patients were asymptomatic and only 2 patients had mild residual shunts. No complications were encountered. More recently, a German multicenter retrospective study of the hybrid technique in 26 patients from 11 centers was published. The procedure was successful in 23 of the 26 patients. During mean follow-up of 1.4 years, a residual shunt that was more than trivial was observed in only one patient.[18]

Percutaneous muscular VSD closure is also proven to be safe when performed in the adult population. Two adult series (median age 34 and 37.9) showed the procedure to have close to 100% success rate with only minor complications.[16,19] There were no procedural deaths or device embolizations reported in these series. In the first series with 40 patients, only 12 had muscular VSDs. The complications reported included a pseudoaneurysm requiring surgery, brachial plexus injury, which resolved following the procedure, and 4 patients had transient arrhythmias.[16] In the second series of 28 patients, only 8 patients had muscular defects. They reported a total of three complications, including one small groin hematoma, nonsustained ventricular tachycardia, and entanglement of the device in the mitral valve apparatus causing severe mitral regurgitation, which resolved when the device was recaptured and repositioned.[19]

The authors' own personal experience with swiss cheese VSD includes many patients who received up to nine devices to close multiple defects and achieved good results.

In summary, the Amplatzer muscular VSD occluder has been shown to be safe and effective in the percutaneous closure of muscular VSDs in the hands of experienced operators. It is currently the only available approved device in the United States for closure of muscular VSDs. Its design makes it easy to use and reposition if necessary. The rate of procedure-related complications such as embolization, arrhythmias, and vascular issues are very low. The low rate of morbidity associated with the procedure makes it an attractive option for most patients.

References

1. Hijazi ZM. Device closure of ventricular septal defects. *Catheter Cardiovasc Interv* 2003;60:107–14.
2. Lock JE, Block PC, McKay RG, Baim DS, Keane JF. Transcatheter closure of ventricular septal defects. *Circulation* 1988;78:361–8.
3. Sideris EB, Walsh KP, Haddad JL, Chen CR, Ren SG, Kulkarni H. Occlusion of congenital ventricular septal defects by the buttoned device. "Buttoned device" Clinical Trials International Register. *Heart* 1997;77:276–9.
4. Kalra GS, Verma PK, Dhall A, Singh S, Arora R. Transcatheter device closure of ventricular septal defects: Immediate results and intermediate-term follow-up. *Am Heart J* 1999;138:339–44.
5. Thanopoulos BD, Tsaousis GS, Konstadopoulou GN, Zarayelyan AG. Transcatheter closure of muscular ventricular septal defects with the amplatzer ventricular septal defect occluder: Initial clinical applications in children. *J Am Coll Cardiol* 1999;33:1395–9.
6. Hijazi ZM, Hakim F, Al-Fadley F, Abdelhamid J, Cao QL. Transcatheter closure of single muscular ventricular septal defects using the amplatzer muscular VSD occluder: Initial results and technical considerations. *Catheter Cardiovasc Interv* 2000;49:167–72.
7. Holzer R, Balzer D, Cao QL, Lock K, Hijazi ZM. Amplatzer muscular ventricular septal defect investigators. Device closure of muscular ventricular septal defects using the Amplatzer muscular ventricular septal defect occluder: Immediate and mid-term results of a U.S. registry. *J Am Coll Cardiol* 2004;43:1257–63.
8. Waight DJ, Cao QL, Hijazi ZM. Amplatzer muscular ventricular septal defect occluder. In: Rao PS, Kern MJ. Eds. *Catheter Based Devices for the Treatment of Non-coronary Cardiovascular Disease in Adults and Children*. Philadelphia: Williams and Wilkins, 2003. pp. 245–51.
9. Chessa M, Carminati M, Cao QL et al. Transcatheter closure of congenital and acquired muscular ventricular septal defects using the Amplatzer device. *J Invasive Cardiol* 2002;14:322–7.
10. Holzer R, Balzer D, Amin Z et al. Transcatheter closure of postinfarction ventricular septal defects using the new Amplatzer muscular VSD occluder: Results of a U.S. Registry. *Catheter Cardiovasc Interv* 2004;61:196–201.
11. Bacha EA, Cao QL, Starr JP, Waight D, Ebeid MR, Hijazi ZM. Perventricular device closure of muscular ventricular septal defects on the beating heart: Technique and results. *J Thorac Cardiovasc Surg* 2003;126:1718–23.
12. Warnes CA, Williams RB, Bashore TM et al. ACC/AHA 2008 Guidelines for the management of adults with congenital heart disease: A report of the American College of Cardiology/American Heart Association task force on practice guidelines. *Circulation* 2008;118:714.
13. Bacha EA, Cao QL, Galantowicz ME, Cheatham JP, Fleishman CE, Weinstein SW et al. Multicenter experience with perventricular

device closure of muscular ventricular septal defects. *Pediatr Cardiol* 2005;26:169–75.

14. Amin Z, Cao QL, Hijazi ZM. Closure of muscular ventricular septal defects: Transcatheter and hybrid techniques. *Catheter Cardiovasc Interv* 2008;72:102–11.

15. Carminati M, Butera G, Chessa M et al. Investigators of the European VSD Registry: Transcatheter closure of congenital ventricular septal defects: Results of the European Registry. *Eur Heart J* 2007;28:2361.

16. Chessa M, Butera G, Negura D et al. Transcatheter closure of ventricular septal defects in adult: Mid-term results and complications. *Int J Card* 2009;133(1):70–3.

17. Robinson JDC, Zimmerman FJ, De Loera O, Heitschmidt M, Hijazi ZM. Cardiac conduction disturbances seen after transcatheter device closure of muscular ventricular septal defects with the amplatzer occluder. *Am J Cardiol* 2006;97:558–60.

18. Michel-Behnke I, Ewert P, Koch A et al. Device closure of ventricular septal defects by hybrid procedures: A multicenter retrospective study. *Catheter Cardiovasc Interv* 2011;77:242.

19. Al-Kashkari A, Balan P, Kavinsky CJ et al. Percutaneous device closure of congenital and iatrogenic ventricular septal defects in adult patients. *Catheter Cardiovasc Interv* 2011;77:260.

70

Ventricular septal defect closure: Closure of perimembranous VSD using Amplatzer-type occluders

Ting-Liang Liu and Wei Gao

Introduction

The atrial septal defect (ASD) is a common congenital heart disease. With the development of cardiac catheterization, transcatheter closure of secundum ASD with the Amplatzer septal occluder (ASO) has become a widespread alternative procedure to surgical repair. Because of the unique design, easy handling, and high complete closure rates, the ASO device has been the one most widely used for catheter closure of secundum ASD.

Device

The ASO device (St. Jude Medical, Plymouth, MN, USA) is a self-centering and self-expandable double-disk device made from a 0.004–0.0075-inch nitinol (55% nickel, 45% titanium) wire mesh (Figure 70.1). Nitinol has superelastic properties with shape memory, so that the device can be stretched into an almost linear configuration and compressed inside a small sheath for delivery and then re-formed to its original configuration when not constrained. There is either a 3-mm or 4-mm connecting waist between two circular flat disks depending on the size of the ASO device. The conjoined waist is designed to completely fill and conform to the rims of the atrial defect. The diameter of the waist represents the device size. Both the disks and the waist are filled with polyester fiber to prevent blood flow and promote closure of the defect. The ASO is available in sizes from 4 to 40 mm, with 1-mm increments from 4 to 20 mm and then in 2-mm increments up to the current largest device of 40 mm. The left atrial disk is slightly larger than the right atrial disk because of the higher left atrial pressure. For devices 4–10 mm, the left disk is 12 mm and the right one is 8 mm larger than the connecting waist. And for devices 11–32 mm, the left disk is 14 mm and the right one is 10 mm larger than the waist. However, for devices larger than 32 mm, the left atrial disk is 16 mm larger than the waist. The device is delivered through long sheaths. A 6 F to 12 F delivery sheath is used depending on the required size of the device.[1-3]

The Amplatzer multifenestrated septal occluder (Cribriform occluder) with a small central waist and equal-sized disks is designed for use in patients with fenestrated atrial septal defects and can be used when an aneurysm of the interatrial septum is present.[4] The narrow waist is placed through one of the central holes in the septal wall, with the disks covering the surrounding holes. This device is available in sizes 18, 25, 30, and 35 mm (disk diameter). An 8 F delivery system is suggested for devices 18, 25, and 30 mm, and a 9 F sheath for the 35-mm Cribriform occluder.

Patient selection

Theoretically, ASO devices can be used in patients with secundum ASD if there is an adequate rim of tissue of more than 5 mm from the margins of the defect to mitral valves, superior and inferior vena cava, right pulmonary vein, and coronary sinus. The aortic rim was not included because the device sat astride the aorta in cases of aortic rim deficiency, and the aorta became a part of the aortic rim.[2,3] But in a recent review of erosion cases by St. Jude Medical (SJM), aortic rim deficiency was present in 88% of the cases in which erosion occurred. In this sense, appropriate assessment of the aortic rim of the secundum ASD should be done before closure.[5]

The Amplatzer Cribriform occluder is a percutaneous ASD closure device intended for the closure of multifenestrated defect. In those candidates, the distance from the central defect to the aortic root or vena cava orifice should be greater than the "radius" of selected device (that means greater than 9, 12.5, 15, and 17.5 mm, respectively).

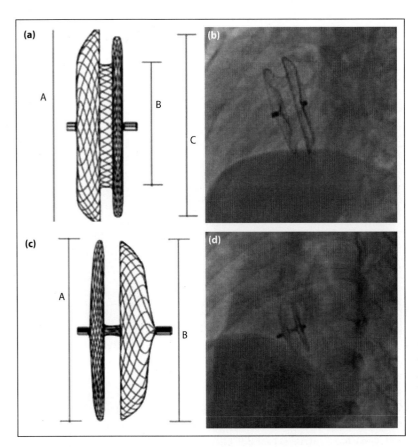

Figure 70.1 The Amplatzer atrial septal defect occluder device (ASO) and the Amplatzer Cribriform occluder (ACO). (a) Schematic picture of ASO. The left atrial disk (A), right atrial disk (C), and the waist part (B) are shown. (b) ASO after release. (c) Schematic picture of ACO, showing the left atrial disk (A) and the right atrial disk (B); (d) ACO after release.

Device implantation technique

Before catheterization, echocardiography is done to evaluate the ASD number, size, location, margin, and relation with adjacent cardiac structures. All patients are continuously monitored by transthoracic echocardiography (TTE), transesophageal echocardiography (TEE), or intracardiac echocardiography (ICE). After sheath placement, heparin is given at 100 IU/kg to keep the activated clotting time above 200 s. A routine right catheterization is performed. If a sizing balloon catheter is used, the device size chosen is usually the same or one size larger (1–2 mm bigger) than the stretched diameter (Figures 70.2 and 70.3). Although ICE or TEE can provide optimal images, both methods are relatively inconvenient or fairly expensive. Many patients or pediatric heart centers cannot afford the high expenses of purchasing and maintaining these systems, especially in the developing countries. And in most pediatric patients, both TTE and TEE have proven to be reliable for assessment of the defect rims and play an important role in guiding device deployment. In recent years, we have performed the closure of ASDs in more than 500 patients successfully under TTE guidance only. According to our experiences, the device size chosen is usually 3–4 mm larger than the maximal diameter of the defect measured by TTE if the maximal defect is less than

20 mm, and if the defect is more than 20 mm, the device size selected is generally 4–6 mm larger than the maximal diameter. The selected device is screwed onto the delivery cable by a central screw at the end of the device until it stops turning. Then it is compressed into a loader by pulling on the delivery cable. The devices are advanced through long sheaths without rotation. Under echocardiographic and/or fluoroscopic guidance, the left atrial disk is deployed in the left atrium first. Then the ASO device is fully deployed by drawing the sheath over the delivery cable to expand the right atrial disk (Figure 70.4). Before releasing the device, the cable is pushed forward and backward to verify the stability of the device (the "Minnesota wiggle").[2] Once the device position is verified, it is released from the delivery system. Final assessment is performed by echocardiography to verify the device location and any residual shunting.

Routinely, the patients receive a dose of an appropriate antibiotic (commonly cefazolin at 20 mg/kg) during the catheterization procedure and two further doses at 8 h intervals, as well as aspirin (5 mg/kg/day) for 6 months. Standard bacterial endocarditis prophylaxis is recommended for 6 months or until complete closure. TTE is done 24 h after the procedure to ensure suitable deployment of the device. Thereafter, follow-up TTE is performed at 1, 6, and 12 months, and then yearly after implantation.

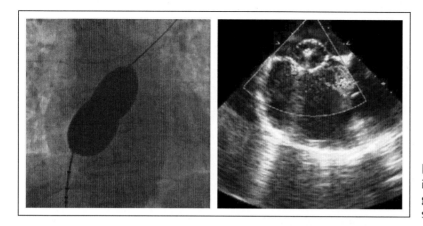

Figure 70.2 (**See color insert.**) Balloon sizing of the defect by fluoroscopy/transesophageal echocardiography (TEE) for measuring the stretched diameter of the atrial septal defect.

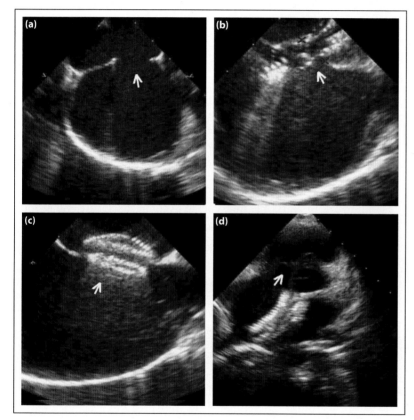

Figure 70.3 Transcatheter closure steps by transesophageal echocardiography (TEE). (a) TEE images in bicaval view, demonstrating left-to-right shunt. (b) Balloon sizing of the defect for measuring the stretched diameter of the defect. (c) The ASO device is deployed across the defect. (d) TEE images immediately after deployment of the ASO device, demonstrating good device position.

Results

Since the introduction of the ASO device, there have been many studies to evaluate the results in different centers. It was reported that procedure success rate ranged from 89.7% to 99.1%. Complete closure immediately ranged from 81.4% to 85.9%. However, at 24 h follow-up, complete closure increased to 94.2% of patients. The closure rate occurred in up to 97.0% at 6 months and 98.2% at 1 year follow-up.[2,3,6–12]

Between January 2001 and September 2011, a total of 683 patients were considered for transcatheter closure with the ASO device in our study. Device closure was successful in 672 patients (98.4%). The clinical data of the patients are listed in Table 70.1. The median size of the defect as measured by TTE/TEE was 11.4 mm (range: 3–31 mm, 155 TEE cases and 528 TTE cases). In 127 cases using the sizing balloon catheter, the median stretched diameter of the defect was 16.7 mm (range: 13–30 mm), and there were 34 patients with multiple ASDs. A total of 677 devices were successfully implanted in 672 patients, the median size of the device was 17.6 mm (range: 6–36 mm). For the patients with multifenestrated defect, Cribriform devices were implanted in 18 patients 12 patients had only 1 ASO device

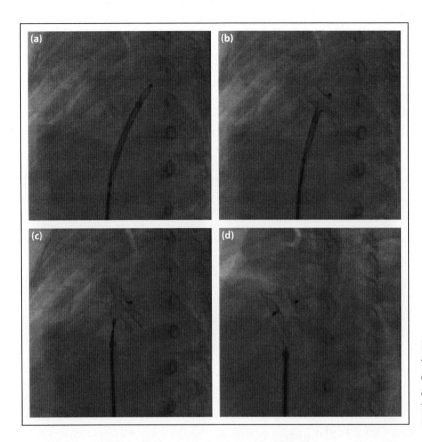

Figure 70.4 Transcatheter closure steps by fluoroscopy. (a) Delivery sheath with the collapsed device in the left atrium. (b) Deployment of the left atrial disk of the ASO device. (c) The ASO device is fully deployed (both disks) but not released yet. (d) Device is released across the defect.

Table 70.1   Characteristics of patients and procedures

	All patients ($n = 672$)
Age (year)	5.8 ± 3.6 (0.9–17.5)
Sex (F/M)	283/389
Weight (kg)	17.5 ± 10.7 (8–67)
Pulmonary-to-systemic flow ratio	2.1 ± 0.8 (1.3–4.0)
Average PAP (mmHg)	27 ± 12.6 (14–45)
Size of ASD with TTE/TEE (mm)	11.4 ± 5.3 (3–31)
Stretched diameter with SBC (mm)[a]	16.7 ± 8.9 (13–30)
Size of the device (mm)	17.6 ± 5.1 (6–36)
Fluoroscopy time (min)	3.6 ± 1.7 (2.1–10.9)
Procedure time (min)	35 ± 8.9 (15–75)

[a] Only 127 patients using SBC.
Note: Data expressed as mean ± SD (range) or number of patients.
PAP, pulmonary artery pressure; ASD, atrial septal defect; TTE, transthoracic echocardiography; TEE, transesophageal echocardiography; SBC, sizing balloon catheter.

implanted, respectively, 3 patients required 2 ASO devices for each one, and 1 patient received 3 devices for closure of multiple defects.

The median fluoroscopy time was 3.6 min (range, 2.1–10.9 min), and the median total procedure time was 35 min (range, 15–75 min). The follow-up time ranged from 1 to 10 years. The time course of complete closure and residual shunt disappearance after device implantation is given in Table 70.2.

Complications

Reported complications encountered during catheter closure of ASD using the ASO device were rare. Some reported complications[6–12] are listed in Table 70.3.

In our series of 672 patients, 1 major and 29 minor complications were observed (Table 70.4). One patient experienced device displacement. This 12-year-old boy with 6-mm tunnel-like ASD measured by TTE received an 8-mm ASO device for the closure, and device embolization was found in the 1 month follow-up. The device was retrieved from the descending aorta in the catheterization laboratory and a 12-mm device was implanted with successful closure of the defect. Minor complications included transient arrhythmia, residual leakage, transient pericardial effusion, and migraine. Transient arrhythmia was observed in 16 patients, including atrial premature beats, ventricular premature beats, and first-degree atrioventricular block, which recovered spontaneously within 6 months without any medical treatment. Pericardial effusion was observed in five patients in the 1 month follow-up, which was mild, and all recovered by 3 months later without further treatment. Trivial residual shunt was observed

Table 70.2 Time course of complete closure and residual shunt disappearance after ASO implantation in all 672 patients in the study

Follow-up	C (%)	TS (%)	SS	MS	LS
Immediate	98.5	1.5	0	0	0
24 h	99.1	0.9	0	0	0
1 month	99.3	0.7	0	0	0
6 months	99.3	0.7	0	0	0
1–5 years	99.3	0.7	0	0	0
5–10 years	99.3	0.7	0	0	0

C, complete closure; TS, trivial residual shunt (color jet width <1 mm); SS, small residual shunt (color jet width 1–2 mm); MS, moderate residual shunt (color jet width 2–4 mm); LS, large residual shunt (color jet width >4 mm).

Table 70.3 Complications encountered during device closure of ASD using the ASO device

Author	n^a	Age (year)	D (mm)	Device (mm)	CX (%)	Type of CX
Kaya	117	2–65	6–30	5–36	2 (1.7%)	1 Device displacement
						1 Supraventricular tachycardia
Berger	200	0.8–77.7	4–28	4–28	1 (0.5%)	1 Device displacement
Kim	560	1.1–75	8–38	9–39	24 (4.3%)	1 Device embolization
						1 Device displacement
						4 Migraine
						5 Transient arrhythmia
						13 Hematoma
Masura	151	11.9 ± 11.6	15.9 ± 4.8	16.1 ± 5.3	0	No significant complications
Majunke	650	18–90	3.1–43	7–40	55 (8.5%)	6 Device embolization
						2 Hemopericardium
						1 Cardiac tamponade
						1 Thrombosis
						1 Ischemic stroke
						1 Peripheral embolism
						4 Heart failure
						3 Transient ischemic attack
						7 Pericardial effusion
						29 Cardial arrhythmia
Ueda	208	8.3 ± 3.8	15 ± 4.2	15 ± 4.3	17 (8.1%)	1 Device embolization
						16 Migraine
Wang	243	2.1–76	5.2–37	8–40	8 (3.3%)	2 Device embolization
						6 Cardiac arrhythmia

[a] Number of patients in series.

D, diameter of defect; CX, complications.

in 10 patients after closure immediately after closure, in 6 patients at 24-hour follow-up, and disappeared in 5 out of 10 patients with trivial residual shunt 1 month later. Three patients experienced mild migraine headaches. During the follow-up period, no further complications such as device displacement, device embolization, cardiac perforation, and cardiac arrhythmia were observed.

Discussion

Transcatheter closure is now widely accepted as the preferred choice for treating secundum ASD. There is a similar rate of closure success comparing the transcatheter closure with surgical treatment; nevertheless, transcatheter closure not only presents a low complication rate and short

Table 70.4 Complications encountered during closure ASD using the ASO

Major complications	n (%)
Device displacement	1 (0.15%)
Device erosion	0
Severe arrhythmias	0
Cardiac perforation	0
Cardiac tamponade	0
Thrombosis	0
Death	0
Minor complications	
Transient arrhythmia	16 (2.4%)
Transient pericardial effusion	5 (0.7%)
Residual leakage	5 (0.7%)
Infective endocarditis	0
Aortic regurgitation	0
Blood transfusion	0
Migraine	3 (0.4%)

hospital stay but also avoids a surgical scar and postoperative pain.[13] There are a number of significant factors that are crucial to prevent complications and to achieve a high closure rate, such as the selection of suitable patients based on a sufficient rim, the selection of the correct size of device dependent on accurate assessment of the stretched diameter of the ASD, and echocardiography guidance to ensure the device position.

Device displacement and device embolization are well-known early complications, which may require emergency surgical retrieval in some cases. Exceptionally, several authors reported delayed embolization of the device even 4 years after implantations.[14,15] The worst of the complications after transcatheter closure of ASD with the Amplatzer device is atrial wall erosion, also called "perforation." Most of the erosions occur in the anterior-superior region of the atrial wall, an area that corresponds to the aortic and superior rim on echocardiography. So the aortic rim of the defect should be taken into consideration.[5]

Most arrhythmias are well controlled medically or recover spontaneously, but some arrhythmias may require cardioversion. Arrhythmias often occur during the procedure and in the short postprocedure period; however, arrhythmias could remain long-term risks after ASD closure. The patients who were older at the time of ASD, especially if the patient had preexisting arrhythmia, had more arrhythmic events.[16,17] No new onset of arrhythmias was detected during follow-up in the present study.

It is also reported that some patients experienced migraine headaches during follow-up.[11] In our study, migraine headaches occurred in three patients. However, there is no confirmed evidence about the relationship between migraine headaches and ASD closure with the ASO.

Both early and long-term follow-ups demonstrate that ASD closure using ASO is safe and effective. The present study also demonstrates an excellent outcome of ASD closure using ASO during a follow-up period up to 10 years.

Conclusion

The ASO device has a distinctive design that combines features such as high complete closure rates and ease of implantation and ability to retrieve, reposition, or recapture the device before release. The short-, intermediate-, and long-term follow-ups have demonstrated high procedural success and low complication rates. In conclusion, transcatheter occlusion of secundum ASD with the ASO device is safe and effective.

Acknowledgments

We wish to thank Dr. Wei Huang and Ms Lin-Lin Jiang for collecting data and statistical analysis. We would also like to thank the technical, echocardiography, and nursing staff in the Department of Cardiology at the Shanghai Children's Medical Center for their hard work.

References

1. Masura J, Gavora P, Formanek A et al. Transcatheter closure of secundum atrial septal defects using the new self-centering Amplatzer septal occluder: Initial human experience. *Cathet Cardiovasc Diagn* 1997;42:388–93.
2. Hijazi ZM, Cao Q, Patel HT et al. Transesophageal echocardiographic results of catheter closure of atrial septal defect in children and adults using the Amplatzer device. *Am J Cardiol* 2000;85:1387–90.
3. Fu YC, Cao QL, Hijazi ZM. Closure of secundum atrial septal defect using the Amplatzer Septal Occluder. In: Sievert H, Qureshi SA, Wilson N, Hijazi ZM. Eds. *Percutaneous Interventions for Congenital Heart Disease.* London: Informa Healthcare, 2007. pp. 265–75.
4. Silvestry FE, Naseer N, Wiegers SE et al. Percutaneous transcatheter closure of patent foramen ovale with the Amplatzer Cribriform septal occluder. *Catheter Cardiovasc Interv* 2008;71:383–7.
5. Mallula K, Amin Z. Recent changes in instructions for use for the Amplatzer atrial septal defect occluder: How to incorporate these changes while using transesophageal echocardiography or intracardiac echocardiography? *Pediatr Cardiol* 2012;33:995–1000.
6. Kaya MG, Baykan A, Dogan A et al. Intermediate-term effects of transcatheter secundum atrial septal defect closure on cardiac remodeling in children and adults. *Pediatr Cardiol* 2010;31:474–82.
7. Berger F, Ewert P, Björnstad PG et al. Transcatheter closure as standard treatment for most interatrial defects: Experience in 200 patients treated with the Amplatzer Septal Occluder. *Cardiol Young* 1999;9:468–73.
8. Kim NK, Park SJ, Shin JI et al. Eight-French intracardiac echocardiography: Safe and effective guidance for transcatheter closure in atrial septal defects. *Circ J* 2012;76:2119–23.
9. Masura J, Gavora P, Podnar T et al. Long-term outcome of transcatheter secundum-type atrial septal defect closure using Amplatzer Septal Occluders. *J Am Coll Cardiol* 2005;45:505–7.
10. Majunke N, Bialkowski J, Wilson N et al. Closure of atrial septal defect with the Amplatzer Septal Occluder I adults. *Am J Cardiol* 2009;103:550–4.

11. Ueda H, Yanagi S, Nakamura H et al. Device closure of atrial septal defect: Immediate and mid-term results. *Circ J* 2012;76:1229–34.

12. Wang JK, Tsai SK, Lin SM et al. Transcatheter closure of atrial septal defect without balloon sizing. *Catheter Cardiovasc Interv* 2008;71:214–21.

13. Bialkowski J, Karwot B, Szkutnik M et al. Closure of atrial septal defects in children: Surgery versus Amplatzer device implantation. *Tex Heart Inst J* 2004;31:220–3.

14. Dhaliwal RS, Singh H, Swami N et al. Removal of displaced and impacted ASD device after 4 years. *Thorac Cardiovasc Surg* 2009;57:233–5.

15. Mashman WE, King SB, Jacobs WC et al. Two cases of late embolization of Amplatzer septal occluder devices to the pulmonary artery following closure of secundum atrial septal defects. *Catheter Cardiovasc Interv* 2005;65:588–92.

16. Kutty S, Hazeem AA, Brown K et al. Long-term (5- to 20-year) outcomes after transcatheter or surgical treatment of hemodynamically significant isolated secundum atrial septal defect. *Am J Cardiol* 2012;109:1348–52.

17. Knepp MD, Rocchini AP, Lloyd TR et al. Long-term follow up of secundum atrial septal defect closure with the Amplatzer septal occluder. *Congenit Heart Dis* 2010;5:32–7.

71

Ventricular septal defect closure: Closure of perimembranous VSD using PFM coil

Trong-Phi Le

Introduction

Ventricular septal defect (VSD) is the most common congenital or acquired heart defect. Surgical closure of VSD, which used to be the gold standard for closing VSDs, carries inherent risks associated with cardiopulmonary bypass. In addition, serious postoperative arrhythmias have arisen and in approximately 1% of cases, complete atrioventricular (AV) block requiring implantation of a pacemaker has occurred.[1]

Transcatheter closure of VSD as an alternative to surgery was first reported in the late 1980s[2] and has gained increasing acceptance in the medical community due to a comparable success rate and low risk of complications.

Today, various devices are available for transcatheter closure of a wide range of muscular and perimembranous defects in children and adults. The most commonly used devices are disk occluders such as Amplatzer VSD devices (St. Jude Medical, St. Paul, MN, USA)[3–9] or Amplatzer-like devices.[10–12] However, occlusion devices with high radial and clamping force may cause injury to the aortic valve and, due to their rigid structure, might not adapt correctly to the anatomic structure of the defect.[13–15] Incorrectly configured devices can cause pressure on the surrounding tissue and, as a consequence, result in serious rhythm disturbances such as AV block.[16–20]

These complications can be avoided by using devices made of highly flexible material such as nitinol coils, which adapt to the shape of a wide range of VSD sizes and morphologies.[15] A softer and more flexible delivery system ensures a less traumatic implantation procedure compared with other occlusion devices.

The NitOcclud Lê VSD coil (PFM, Cologne, Germany) is designed as a reinforced double-disk device for percutaneous transcatheter occlusion of both perimembranous and muscular VSDs. Owing to technical limitations in manufacturing, only VSDs smaller than 8 mm in diameter can be closed with NitOcclud coils. The application of transcatheter coils, however, demands highly experienced and skilled operators.

This chapter describes the PFM NitOcclud Lê VSD coil, its implantation procedure, and the management of potential complications, and summarizes preclinical and clinical experience with the device.

Device and delivery system

The NitOcclud Lê VSD device consists of conical-shaped disks made of nitinol, a biocompatible, nickel–titanium alloy with excellent shape memory. The NitOcclud device is composed of a 0.25 mm nitinol wire with tightly spaced primary windings around a straight core wire and secondary coil loops. The result is a flexible, straight-tension spring with an internal diameter of 0.25 mm and an external diameter of 0.96 mm. The stiffness of the distal primary windings is reinforced by the insertion of a 0.04 mm flat wire, with reduced thickness toward the proximal end. The spring is wound around a fixture with a cone mold and shock heated to form permanent secondary coil loops, resulting in two disks with a small, 2 mm connecting waist.

The proximal right ventricular disk has a smaller diameter and is more flexible compared with the distal left ventricular disk. Polyester fibers are added to the left ventricular disk of the device. These fibers are placed between the tightly spaced primary coil loops.

The NitOcclud VSD coil is built asymmetrically, forming a cone-in-cone shape by reverse position of the proximal disk. After positioning the coil in the defect, the two disks are closely opposed to the septum. A special mechanism is located at the proximal end for the attachment to the core wire of the implantation system (Figure 71.1a and b).

The NitOcclud VSD coil is premounted straight on a flexible 5 or 6 Fr delivery catheter 105 cm in length, which is connected to a disposable handle for detachment. Once correctly positioned, the device can be detached by

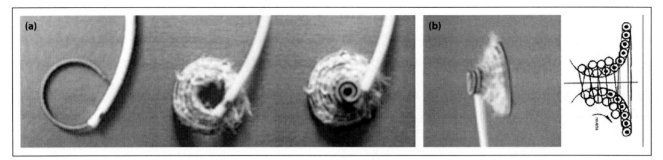

Figure 71.1   (a) The left ventricular disc is covered by dacron fibers except the fist distal coil loop. (b) The distal coil loops are reinforced and the proximal loops are reversed.

withdrawing the core wire (detachment force 12–15 N) under fluoroscopy control (Figure 71.2).

A hemostatic Y-connector is attached to the proximal end of the delivery catheter to allow flushing of the system. The delivery wire is marked in two locations. When the first marker reaches the Y-connector, the coil will be almost fully deployed on the left ventricular side of the defect. Only the last two proximal loops remain within the delivery catheter. They will deploy onto the right ventricular side, once the second marker has reached the Y-connector.

NitOcclud Lê VSD devices are available with a distal loop diameter of 8, 10, 12, 14, and 16 mm (measuring the largest diameter of the left ventricular disk) making the implant suitable for various sizes and shapes of perimembranous and muscular VSDs <8 mm in diameter.

Angiography

Before closure of the VSD, the location and size of the VSD needs to be determined by left ventriculography in the long axial oblique projection. It may be necessary to repeat the

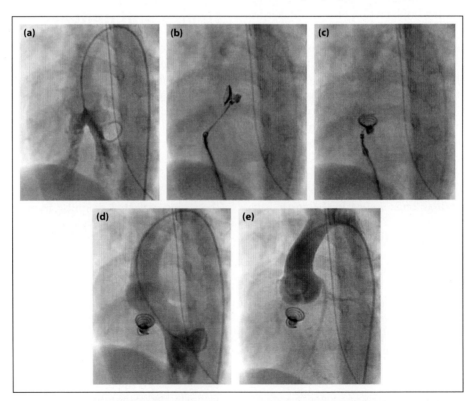

Figure 71.2   (a) Angiogram of the LV in LAO projection. The VSD has a large aneurysm and almost no rims on the aortic annulus. (b) The coil configured in the ascending aorta. There are only two proximal coil loops remaining in the implantation catheter. (c) After passing through the aortic valve, the configured coil adapts itself into the aneurysm of the VSD. The tip of the implantation catheter is now located on the right ventricular side of the interventricular septum. The tip of the long sheath remains close to the septum. (d) Angiogram of the LV following coil release. The coil is lying nicely compressed in the VSD aneurysm. (e) Angiogram of the ascending aorta following coil release. One can recognize the close relationship between the coil and the aortic valve.

injections from different angles to obtain a full profile of the defect (left anterior oblique 30–60°, cranial 20–30°). Owing to the pressure difference and left-to-right shunts, VSDs are shaped conically. In addition, perimembranous VSDs may have aneurysmal septal rims of various sizes and shapes or may have more than one opening into the right ventricle, thus compromising the correct estimation of its size.

The larger diameter of the defect can mostly be seen from the left ventricular side, whereas the effective diameter is measured from the right ventricular side. If the right heart is seen significantly well on the left ventricular angiogram, the size of the VSD might be underestimated when measured with echocardiography, since the echocardiogram would only reveal the smaller diameter. In these cases, balloons are recommended to measure the exact size of the defect. The largest dimension of the VSD at the opening into the right ventricle should be recorded.

Caution should be exerted during the entire procedure because severe arrhythmias can be provoked. The insertion and maneuvering of catheters and guide wires can cause injury to the right coronary artery or the aortic and tricuspid valves.

Standard baseline hemodynamic data should be recorded before the implantation.

Device selection

The coil should have a distal diameter of at least double the size of the effective diameter of the VSD measured on the right ventricular side and be approximately 1–2 mm larger than the VSD diameter from its left ventricular opening.

In case of complex-shaped VSDs with aneurysm of the septum, only the left ventricular diameter of the aneurysm should be used to determine the size of the coil to be used. In such cases, a rim along the aortic valve is not required and the coil should fit into the aneurysmal sac, without the coil protruding into the left ventricular outflow tract.

Patient selection

Hemodynamically stable patients weighing more than 10 kg with muscular or perimembranous VSDs and a diameter of <8 mm are eligible for implantation of the NitOcclud VSD coil. In case of perimembranous VSD, the distance between the cranial rim of the VSD to the aortic valve should be more than 3 mm. However, a rim to the aortic valve is not necessary if the VSD has a well-developed aneurysm.

Concomitant medication

The implantation procedure is performed under general anesthesia or deep conscious sedation. Before implantation of a device, patients should receive full heparinization with a bolus dose of 100 IU/kg. To maintain an activated clotting time (ACT) between 200 and 250 s during the procedure,

repeat dose of heparin is necessary, in case the procedure is prolonged. For the prevention of bacterial endocarditis, administration of antibiotics is recommended. We propose a dosage regime of one dose of cephalosporin (30–50 mg/kg) given intravenously shortly before the intervention and two additional doses of intravenous cephalosporin given 8 and 16 h after the procedure. After the intervention, the patients should receive intravenous heparin over 24 h (200 IU/kg).

Implantation procedure and management of potential problems

Transcatheter closure of VSDs involves complex intracardiac maneuvers with various guide wires, sheaths, catheters, snares, and devices. As always, the best protection against complications is patience and care. This requires close monitoring of the patient during the intervention, proper selection of materials, a cool head, a careful hand, and the willingness to abandon the procedure in unsafe situations.

For the occlusion of muscular VSDs, an arteriovenous (AV) loop is not obligatory because the defect can be reached from the right ventricle via the jugular venous access. If the defect cannot be accessed from the right ventricle, a guide wire circuit is needed.

For the initial crossing of a perimembranous VSD and the placement of the delivery catheter or sheath from the right to the left ventricle from venous access, a through-and-through guide wire circuit is recommended.

The femoral artery is accessed with a 4 or 5 Fr sheath. A 6 or 7 Fr sheath should be used for the venous access.

The VSD is crossed with a 4 Fr Judkins right coronary catheter (Cordis Corporation, Miami, FL, USA), or an Amplatzer right coronary catheter and a J-curved 0.035-inch Terumo 260-cm-long exchange guide wire (Terumo Medical Corporation, Somerset, NJ). The guide wire for the creation of an AV loop should have an appropriate length and a stable distal end.

The pulmonary artery can be entered initially by using a 6 Fr end-hole balloon catheter (Arrow, Reading, PA, USA) to allow the delivery sheath to pass the tricuspid valve without interference with its chordae. The lumen should be large enough to accommodate a snare of up to 15 mm. The Terumo guide wire should be positioned in the pulmonary artery and have a slightly cranial orientation when crossing the VSD, to avoid interfering with the moderator band or the tricuspid valves. The procedure of crossing the VSD and establishing the guide wire circuit should be performed as carefully as possible—there should not be any impediments setting up the AV circuit. In patients with perimembranous VSDs, the position of the aortic valve should be highlighted immediately before the coil is deployed, either by angiography or by placement of a catheter.

The AV guide wire circuit is formed by snaring the Terumo exchange guide wire in the pulmonary artery and pulling it out of the femoral venous access. The snare should be opened in the main pulmonary artery before further advancing the exchange guide wire. No loops should be present in the right ventricle or atrium during this process. The presence of these loops could be an indication that the moderator band or the tricuspid valve apparatus is affected, which can lead to interference or entanglement later on in the process. In this case, repeating the steps to catch the guide wire is advised.

The tip of the arterial catheter is brought down to the upper part of the inferior vena cava after crossing the VSD with the guide wire. The sheath and its dilator are introduced through the femoral vein until both the tips of the dilator and the arterial catheter meet ("kiss") in the inferior vena cava.

The guide wire is pulled on both sides of the system to tighten the AV loop. Then it should be secured at the hub of the catheter and the long sheath with a surgical clamp.

The operators should carefully pull on the arterial catheter and push on the venous sheath to move the sheath from the femoral vein to the ascending aorta across the defect. After the sheath has reached the ascending aorta, the arterial catheter can be replaced over the guide wire by a pigtail catheter. The guide wire circuit is broken by removing the dilator of the long sheath and the guide wire. The pigtail catheter should be pulled back in the descending aorta to prevent interference with the coil during coil exposure.

Before inserting the coil-delivering catheter, the long sheath should be aspirated and flushed to remove any thrombi and prevent any inadvertent embolism.

Before delivering the coil, we recommend pushing the coil delivery catheter 1 cm out of the tip of the long sheath. Otherwise, during the pullback maneuver of the delivery system from the left to the right ventricle, the tension of the rigid sheath could result in a pulling through of the configured coil. All loops except the last two are deployed in the ascending aorta. The tip of the delivery catheter should be kept apart from the tip of the long sheath when pulling the coil back into the left ventricle. Both the delivery catheter and the long sheath are carefully pulled back across the aortic valve and positioned in the left ventricular outflow tract. Once the coil is pulled back into the defect, it should adapt to the shape of the defect. The sheath and the delivery catheter should be moved slightly backward during this process, to prevent the coil pulling through the defect. After the loops are well positioned in the VSD, the remaining two proximal coil loops should be positioned on the right ventricular side of the defect by slowly retracting the catheter from the left into the right ventricle, while the two remaining loops are exposed (Figure 71.2a–e). Prior to releasing the coil, the function of the tricuspid valve must be confirmed using echocardiography; otherwise, an entanglement between the proximal coils and the supporting structures of the valve cannot be completely ruled out.

In muscular VSDs, the tips of the delivery catheter and the long sheath should be in close proximity to the ventricular septum (Figure 71.3a–c) to prevent the loops from interfering with the mitral valve apparatus. It is essential to ensure that the coil does not interfere with the mitral

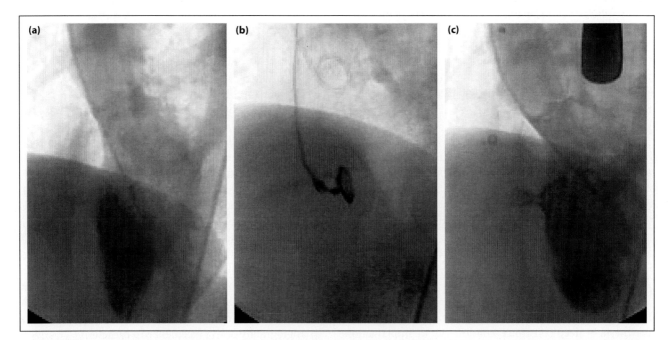

Figure 71.3 (a) Funnel-shaped midmuscular VSD. (b) The coil firmly configured on the interventricular septum to prevent interference with the supporting structures of the mitral valve. (c) Angiogram of the LV following coil release showing the entire coil in the defect without protrusion into the LV cavity.

valve apparatus during deployment of the proximal loops. This can be performed by keeping the tip of the long sheath close to the VSD entrance from the right ventricular side. It is strongly recommended that the position of the configured coil must be checked by echocardiography. After correct positioning of the coil, the same steps are performed as for membranous VSDs.

If too many loops are delivered on the right ventricular side, these loops may interfere with the tricuspid valve apparatus and cause residual shunts. In this case, the coil should be pulled back into the delivery catheter, while the delivery catheter is advanced across the VSD into the left ventricular outflow tract. A new attempt at coil insertion can then be made.

If the delivery catheter cannot be moved into the left ventricular outflow tract, retrieval of the coil via the catheter is necessary. If it is not possible to pull the entire coil back into the delivery catheter, it should be retracted together with the delivery catheter into the long sheath.

The likelihood of the coil becoming entangled in the aortic valve is relatively high if the diameter of the coil is larger than 70% of the diameter of the ascending aorta. Configuration of only four distal loops in the ascending aorta and positioning the remaining loops in the left ventricular outflow tract may minimize the risk in such cases. Another practical option is to place the tip of the long sheath in the left ventricular outflow tract. This ensures positioning of the coil as close to the septum as possible.

If the coil becomes entangled in the aortic valve, it is important to advance the tip of the long sheath to the left ventricular side, thus ensuring the easy passage of the delivery catheter to disentangle the coil from the aortic valve.

In this case, two different situations could develop: either the delivery catheter with the coil is pushed back into the ascending aorta and a new attempt can be started to move the coil from the ascending aorta to the left ventricle, or alternatively, the delivery catheter could fall or tip into the left ventricle. In this case, the operator can still carefully maneuver the coil into the defect.

If the coil needs to be retrieved, we recommend retracting the delivery catheter together with the configured coil into the long sheath. Once the coil is within the lumen of the long sheath, it is straightened in a favorable way and can be retrieved more easily.

If the coil is resisting retrieval, the tip of the catheter may not capture it. The coil can then be retrieved by releasing the snag with careful movements of the catheter. If too much force is exerted, the coil might deploy and release too early.

In some cases, the delivery catheter needs to be completely withdrawn and the sheath needs to be repositioned. In this case, a new approach should be considered as well as a different device size.

Even after the coil is completely opened but has not taken its expected shape, it can still be repositioned by completely retrieving it into the catheter. This must be done in close proximity to the ventricular septum. A new attempt of moving the sheath into the defect can then be made, and the same coil can be repositioned correctly. If the delivery catheter cannot readvance on its own, the coil should be retracted into the catheter and the sheath, which can then be repositioned and the procedure restarted.

Retrieval of prematurely detached coils

In case of early release of the coil from the delivery system before it is correctly positioned, the stiff distal loops will hold it in position; so, there is a low risk of embolization into the right ventricle. The VSD should be recrossed in a retrograde manner and a new guide wire circuit should be established. A long sheath should be positioned close to the proximal end of the coil, and a snare catheter should be advanced inside the long sheath, guided by the guide wire circuit. The coil can then be snared from its right ventricular end and withdrawn into the long sheath. To avoid interference with the tricuspid valve apparatus, the coil should not be placed too deep into the right ventricle.

Another way of dealing with an incorrectly positioned coil is to snare the coil at its distal end and retract it into the descending aorta. It can then be retrieved with a larger arterial long sheath. Otherwise, a guide wire circuit can be established from the contralateral femoral artery, with a similar technique to that described in the previous paragraph. The coil can then be retrieved transvenously with a snare.

Implantation of multiple PFM (products for the medicine) VSD coils. In some large perimembranous VSDs with multiple perforations, the use of multiple coils may be necessary to achieve effective closure (Figure 71.4a and b). In such cases, the first implanted coil should be kept attached, until the subsequent coils are deployed. The deployed coils should then be released together.

Closure of doubly committed VSD. Although initially designed for the closure of perimembranous or muscular VSD only, the PFM VSD coil can be used in some doubly committed VSD (DCVSD) as well. However, the echocardiographically measured defect size should not be larger than 5 mm. Preexisting aortic regurgitation (AR) either remains unchanged or decreases in the first patient group.[21]

A DCVSD is best viewed using lateral fluoroscopy. In many cases, it can be accessed from the right ventricle using an internal jugular venous catheter approach. The size of the shunt observed by echocardiography does not always correspond to the size of the VSD, as a prolapsed aortic valve leaflet often hangs into the defect, partially covering it. Therefore, it is strongly advised that the defect size must be measured using angiography after crossing the defect with the long sheath. The left ventricular disk will be positioned directly under the right coronary cusp

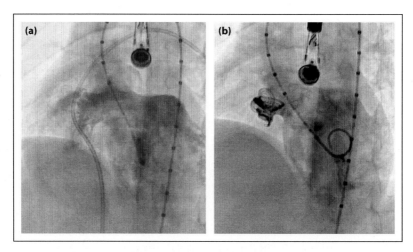

Figure 71.4 (a) Angiogram of the LV with a multiperforated aneurysmal VSD. (b) Angiogram of the LV following the simultaneous implantation of two coils. Both coils remain fully embedded in the large aneurysm.

of the aortic valve, and as a result, it will appear more mobile than the coils placed in perimembranous or muscular VSDs (Figure 71.5a–c).

Other procedural complications

Embolization of the coil into the pulmonary arteries has been reported as a potential late complication of transcatheter closure of VSDs.[22] Usually, this event does not lead to hemodynamic instability.

In cases of embolization, a large long sheath should be inserted into the pulmonary artery. The coil can be caught at the proximal end with a 10–15 mm snare. It should be captured into the long sheath in the pulmonary artery to prevent the loops from interfering with the tricuspid valve apparatus during withdrawal.

Owing to its fibers, the NitOcclud coil can cause hemolysis, especially in the presence of significant residual shunts. In case of a significant decrease in hemoglobin, which does not resolve spontaneously, surgical removal of the device might become necessary.

Postprocedure follow-up

The patient should be transferred into the recovery unit for routine clinical postprocedure observation. Within 12 h of implantation, an electrocardiogram (ECG) and transthoracic echocardiogram should be performed. The patient should not be discharged home any earlier than the next day.

For the following 6 months, the patient should take aspirin (2–3 mg/kg a day, maximum 100 mg/day) and avoid physical exertion for at least 1 month. Prophylaxis

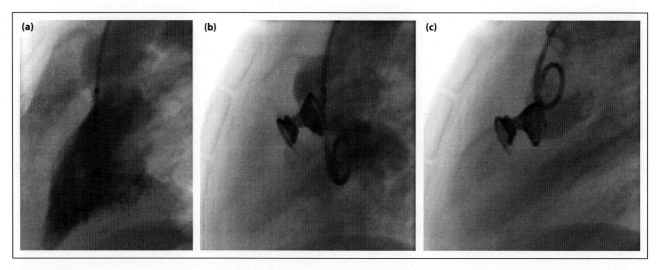

Figure 71.5 (a) DCVSDs can be best demonstrated in lateral projection. The right coronary cusp is partially prolapsed. (b) Angiogram of the LV following coil release. The coil lies directly underneath the right coronary cusp. (c) Angiogram of the ascending aorta following coil release. The coil is in contact with the prolapsed portion of the right coronary cusp.

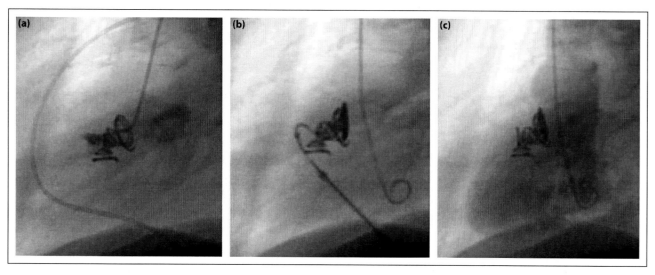

Figure 71.6   (a) Residual shunt after implantation of the first coil. Only 50% of the coil loops are located on the LV side and too many coil loops (four loops) are deployed in the RV. Hand injection into the funnel of the coil using a Judkins right catheter. (b) The second coil is already deployed inside the funnel of the first coil (coil in coil). The last proximal loop of the second coil is placed on the right ventricular side. (c) Complete occlusion after coil-in-coil procedure.

of endocarditis with antibiotics should be pursued for 6 months or until complete occlusion is confirmed. Follow-up evaluation with physical examination, 12-lead ECG, and transthoracic echocardiography should be scheduled after 1 week, 1 month, 6 months, and annually thereafter.

Typically, residual shunts may be closed completely with the implantation of a second coil. The second procedure is recommended after 3–6 months and tends to be easier than the first, since the first coil can act as a guide for the second coil placement in the correct position. There is almost no risk of displacing the first coil during the second procedure. The second coil should be implanted into the funnel of the first coil (Figure 71.6a–c). With subsequent implantations, the closure rate can theoretically approach 100%. After deployment of the second coil, the patient should be reassessed in the same way as after the first procedure.

Preclinical and clinical experience with the PFM NitOcclud coil

Prior to implantation in humans, the NitOcclud VSD device was evaluated in animals with subaortic VSDs.[23] The coil was successfully implanted in 9 of 12 animals (body weight 15–65 kg) with VSD diameters ranging from 4 to 10 mm. In three cases, implantation was abandoned: death occurred in two animals as a result of complete heart block during the procedure, and one animal had a defect that was too large for closure with the available devices. In

five cases, complete closure was successfully achieved at the first attempt, and in four cases, a second implantation was needed. At the last control, five animals had complete closure, and four still had a small ($n = 2$) or moderate ($n = 2$) residual shunt.

At follow-up, no significant arrhythmias or insufficiency of the aortic and tricuspid valves was recorded. Coil embolization occurred in one animal after 3 months, and coil fracture was detected in another animal 6 months after implantation. Histopathological evaluation confirmed biocompatibility similar to other VSD devices.[24]

The first experience in humans was reported in 2005, when a prototype of the NitOcclud coil was implanted in five adult patients, aged 36–60 years, with defect sizes of <5 mm.[23] Three patients had subaortic VSDs, and two patients had muscular VSDs. The procedure was successfully performed in four of the five patients and abandoned in one patient due to unsatisfactory device configuration. No complications were reported during the procedure, and no significant arrhythmias or insufficiency of the aortic and tricuspid valves occurred. Complete occlusion was achieved in two patients with perimembranous VSD and in one with a muscular VSD. A small residual shunt persisted in one patient after device implantation.

As of 2008, 126 VSD closures have been performed with the NitOcclud Lê VSD coil, with only one reported case of embolization.[17] Hemolysis was a very rare complication and occurred in four cases. In only one of these cases was surgical removal of the device necessary after a significant drop in hemoglobin. The other cases resolved spontaneously within 5 days.[22]

A retrospective study reviewed the clinical data of 33 patients, who successfully received the NitOcclud Lê

VSD coil, at a single center in Thailand.[21] The incidence of small residual shunts was 18.2% immediately after the procedure and 15.2% after 6 months. No moderate or large residual shunts, device embolization, or hemolysis were reported in these patients. 39.4% of the patients had trivial-to-mild AR within a day after implantation and no patient had moderate AR. At follow-up, 33% of the patients had trivial-to-mild AR and no patient had moderate AR. One case of third-degree atrioventricular block (AVB) was reported 4 days after implantation. The patient was treated with steroids and the AVB resolved after 5 days.

In an international survey, data from VSDs that were closed using the PFM VSD coil were collected from 12 countries for a total of 448 patients in 27 centers. Implantations were technically feasible in 94% of the patients. The longest follow-up period was 6.5 years. There were no serious complications and there was no mortality or major morbidity. In particular, there were no cases of AV block or other arrhythmias requiring therapy. The defect was occluded successfully in 92% of cases. In approximately 7% of cases, mechanical hemolysis occurred. Of these, 75% were self-limiting. Mechanical hemolysis following coil implantation is usually associated with a residual shunt. In a few cases, in which the hemolysis could not be controlled, the shunt was either closed with a second coil or the patient was referred to a surgical explanation of the coils.

Conclusion

The application of the PFM VSD coil calls for both a high degree of experience in interventional techniques and manual dexterity. With the PFM VSD coil, restrictive perimembranous and muscular VSDs, with diameters of up to 8 mm, can be closed safely and effectively. This makes the PFM VSD coil a valuable alternative to other methods, such as surgical closure or transcatheter closure with Amplatzer occluders or other occluders. There is one aspect in which the PFM coil is superior to the other methods. This is the total freedom from serious arrhythmia such as complete AV block. This is most likely due to the three-dimensional flexibility provided by the coils. The coils conform to the previously existing anatomy of the defect. They do not cause a "stenting" effect, freeing the myocardium to continue its complex movement patterns. The NitOcclud Lê VSD coil is a safe and effective device for transcatheter closure of muscular and perimembranous VSDs of various sizes (<8 mm) and shapes, with or without aneurysms in adults and children.

To summarize, interventional closure of a VSD utilizing the PFM coil has an important role in the management of these defects.

References

1. Andersen HØ, deLeval MR, Tsang VT, Elliott MJ, Anderson RH, Cook AC. Is complete heart block after surgical closure of ventricular septum defects still an issue? *Ann Thorac Surg* 2006;82(3):948–56.
2. Lock JE, Block PC, McKay RG et al. Transcatheter closure of ventricular septal defects. *Circulation* 1988;78(2):361–8.
3. Hijazi ZM, Hakim F, Haweleh AA et al. Catheter closure of perimembranous ventricular septal defects using the new Amplatzer membranous VSD occluder: Initial clinical experience. *Catheter Cardiovasc Interv* 2002;56:508–15.
4. Holzer RJ, de Giovanni J, Walsh K et al. Transcatheter closure of perimembranous ventricular septal defects using the Amplatzer membranous VSD occluder: Immediate and midterm results of an international registry. *Catheter Cardiovasc Interv* 2006;68:620–8.
5. Carminati M, Butera G, Chessa M et al. Transcatheter closure of congenital ventricular septal defects: Results of the European Registry. *Eur Heart J* 2007;28:2361–68.
6. Holzer RJ, Balzer D, Cao QL, Lock K, Hijazi ZM. Device closure of muscular ventricular septal defects using the Amplatzer muscular ventricular septal occluder: Immediate and mid-term results of a U.S. registry. *J Am Coll Cardiol* 2004;43:1257–63.
7. Butera G, Carminati M, Chessa M et al. Transcatheter closure of perimembranous ventricular septal defects—Early and long-term results. *J Am Coll Cardial* 2007;50:1189–95.
8. Quek SC, Tai BC, Khin LW et al. Transcatheter closure of ventricular septal defect using Amplatzer device: A meta-analysis. *Catheter Cardiovasc Interv* 2011;78:1 (S169).
9. Fu YC. Transcatheter device closure of muscular ventricular septal defect. *Pediatr Neonatol* 2011;52:3–4.
10. Li X, Li L, Wang X et al. Clinical analysis of transcatheter closure of perimembranous ventricular septal defects with occluders made in China. *Chin Med J* 2011;124(14):2117–22.
11. Mingbiao G, Xiaohua Y, Xianxian Z et al. Transcatheter device closure of infracristal ventricular septal defect. *Am J Cardiol* 2011;107:110–3.
12. Quansheng X, Silin P, Qi A et al. Minimally invasive perventricular device closure of perimembranous ventricular septal defect without cardiopulmonary bypass: Multicenter experience and mid-term follow-up. *J Thorac Cardiovasc Surg* 2010;139:1409–15.
13. Sideris EB, Walsh KP, Haddad JL et al. Occlusion of congenital ventricular septal defects by the buttoned device. *Heart* 1997;77:276–9.
14. Janorkar S, Goh T, Wilkinson J. Transcatheter closure of ventricular septal defects using the Rashkind device: Initial experience. *Catheter Cardiovasc Interv* 1999;46(1):43–8.
15. Vogel M, Rigby ML, Shore D. Perforation of the right aortic valve cusp: Complication of ventricular septal defect closure with a modified Rashkind umbrella. *Ped Cardiol* 1996;17:416–8.
16. Zhou T, Shen XQ, Zhou SH et al. Complications associated with transcatheter closure of perimembranous ventricular septal defects. *Catheter Cardiovasc Interv* 2008;71:559–63.
17. Predescu D, Chaturvedi RR, Friedberg MK et al. Complete heart block associated with device closure of perimembranous ventricular septal defects. *J Thorac Cardiovasc Surg* 2008;136:1223–8.
18. Masura J, Gao W, Gavora P et al. Percutaneous closure of perimembranous ventricular septal defects with the eccentric Amplatzer device: Multicenter follow-up study. *Pediatr Cardiol* 2005;26:216–9.
19. Yip WC, Zimmerman F, Hijazi ZM et al. Heart block and empirical therapy after transcatheter closure of perimembranous ventricular septal defect. *Catheter Cardiovasc Interv* 2005;66:436–41.
20. Walsh MA, Bialkowski J, Szkutnik M et al. Atrioventricular block after transcatheter closure of perimembranous ventricular septal defects. *Heart* 2006; 92:1295–7.

21. Chungsomprasong P, Durongpisitkul K, Vijarnsorn C et al. The results of transcatheter closure of VSD using Amplatzer° Device and Nit Occlud° Lê Coil. *Catheter Cardiovasc Interv* 2011;78:1032–40.

22. Lê TP, Kozlik-Feldmann R, Sievert H et al. Potential complications of transcatheter closure of ventricular septal defect using the PFM NitOcclud VSD coil. In: Hijazi Z, Feldman T, Cheatham J, Sievert H. Eds. *Complications during Percutaneous Interventions for Congenital and Structural Heart Disease*. London: Taylor & Francis; 2009. pp. 171–4.

23. Lê TP, Vaessen P, Freudenthal F et al. Transcatheter closure of sub-aortic ventricular septal defect (VSD) using a nickel–titanium spiral coil (NitOcclud): Animal study and initial clinical results. *Prog Pediatr Cardiol* 2001;14:83–8.

24. Sigler M, Handt S, Seghaye MC et al. Evaluation of *in vivo* biocompatibility of different devices for interventional closure of the patent ductus arteriosus in an animal model. *Heart* 2000;83:570–3.

72

Ventricular septal defect closure: Postmyocardial and postsurgery VSDs

Kevin P. Walsh and Carla Canniffe

Postmyocardial infarction ventricular septal defects

The incidence of postmyocardial infarction ventricular septal defects (PMIVSDs) was estimated to be between 0.2% and 0.34% in the era of thrombolysis.[1] There are few data available on the incidence in the current setting of primary coronary intervention. Those patients who develop PMIVSDs following acute coronary syndrome (ACS) tend to be older, female, and have a history of hypertension compared with those who do not develop ventricular septal defects following ACS. Angiographically, they tend to demonstrate complete occlusion or Thrombolysis in Myocardial Infarction Study (TIMI) grade 0 or 1 flow of the culprit vessel. The left anterior descending artery has been found to be the culprit artery in the majority of PMIVSD cases, and the absence of significant collateral flow also appears to be an important factor.[1]

The current ESC guidelines recommend urgent surgical repair; however, they acknowledge that there is still no consensus on the optimal timing of surgical repair and on the potential role of percutaneous closure as an alternative to surgical intervention.[2] The 2012 AHA/ACC guidelines recommend emergency surgical repair whether or not there is hemodynamic compromise. They recognize a potential role for percutaneous closure, but emphasize that prospective trials are needed to clarify which patients may benefit from this technique compared with a surgical repair.[3]

PMIVSDs are not discrete holes but rather rupture in a necrotic area or aneurysm of the myocardium.[4] These defects are therefore more akin to a tear (Figure 72.1) with the potential for further expansion, and can be very large or multiple.

Many cardiothoracic surgeons recommend repair after a delay of 3–4 weeks, to allow the development of scar tissue in the surrounding myocardium, which provides a more favorable site for the anchoring of suture and patch material. This approach undoubtedly produces better

results for those who undergo treatment but not necessarily for the patients who may have died or become inoperable in the intervening time. The GUSTO-1 trial reported a 30-day mortality of 74% for those who developed VSDs, compared with 7% in those without this complication. Furthermore, in the patients surgically treated in the trial, 30-day mortality was 47% versus 94% for those who were treated medically.[1] Despite improved surgical techniques, dehiscence of a patch remains relatively common and early mortality postrepair is still reported to be over 40% in some series.[5,6]

Advances in transcatheter closure techniques and devices mean a less invasive approach is a viable alternative for this group of patients. In this chapter, we discuss criteria for patient selection, the technique of device closure, and the clinical outcomes of PMIVSD transcatheter closure reported in the recent literature.

A residual/recurrent VSD postsurgical repair occurs in about 11–35% of the survivors for acute PMIVSD, depending

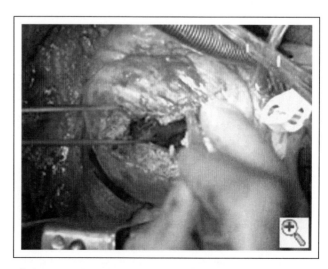

Figure 72.1 Ruptured interventricular septum. A ragged perforation (forceps holding it open) seen at the time of surgical repair.

on the surgical technique used.[5,7] Mortality associated with a second surgical procedure to repair a recurrent PMIVSD has been reported to be as high as 31%.[8] Patients with residual or recurrent defects are clearly natural survivors both from the MI and the surgical repair of the VSD. Furthermore, the tissue surrounding the VSD is likely to be firm and relatively static in size. This group of patients does well with device closure, which avoids the need for a redo open-heart procedure.

While other devices such as the Lock Clamshell device[9,10] have been used to close postinfarct VSDs, this chapter deals with the Amplatzer occluders.[11–16]

Patient selection

Patients are selected for the procedure on the basis of clinical condition, imaging, and institutional experience. Institutions without experience in device occlusion technology are likely to opt for surgical management. Patients with residual or recurrent defects are "natural survivors," have defects with established firm margins, and make ideal cases for a transcatheter approach. Patients in the early acute phase are much more difficult to select for either surgery or device closure. One group reviewed five recent studies (2004–2009) and proposed that those with simple, small-to-moderate-sized (<15 mm) PMIVSDs could be initially treated with a closure device in the subacute setting, whereas those with larger defects measuring ≥15 mm should be referred for immediate surgical repair.[17]

Preprocedure imaging with either transthoracic or/and transesophageal echocardiography (TOE) will help establish whether the defect is amenable to transcatheter closure. Imaging should establish that there is a suitable rim >4 mm for the anchoring of a device, that basal VSDs are >4 mm distance from mitral, tricuspid, and/or aortic valve apparatus, and that the VSD is <3 cm in size. Those with intracardiac thrombus should be referred for surgical management.

If visualization of the defect is suboptimal with either transthoracic echocardiography (TTE) or TOE, then

cardiac magnetic resonance (MRI) or computed tomography (CT) imaging should be considered. The ability of CT or MRI to produce an *en face* view of the septal rupture may help to direct patients toward surgery, if the defect is too large for effective device closure.

We should probably exclude those patients for device closure, who are moribund despite an intra-aortic balloon pump (IABP) and inotropes and also those in whom the defect is too large. Early surgery should be considered for acutely presenting large defects, where surgery with stabilization on cardiopulmonary bypass and infarct exclusion may currently offer better results. This may change if devices with larger diameters and a less porous structure, along with better delivery systems become available.

Patients who are hemodynamically stable at the time of referral and/or who can be stabilized with an IABP, who have a moderate-sized defect (<2 cm), and have a defect that is anatomically amenable to transcatheter closure are good candidates for device closure. Stenting of the infarct-related artery at the time of IABP insertion is considered by some to be helpful.

Technique of transcatheter device closure

Equipment

Devices. Amplatzer ASD devices and congenital muscular VSD devices have been used for PMIVSD patients; however, these devices may not conform well to the thicker interventricular septum in adults and thereby permit significant residual shunting. A specific Amplatzer PMIVSD device has been developed to deal with this issue. This device is similar to the congenital muscular VSD device with a shape like a drum with rims made from a 0.005″ nitinol self-expanding wire mesh and the disks and waist are filled with polyester patches sewn on with polyester thread. The PMIVSD has a longer waist of 10 mm (Figure 72.2a) compared with 7 mm in the MVSD device (Figure 72.2b). The PMIVSD device is available with waist diameters from 16 to

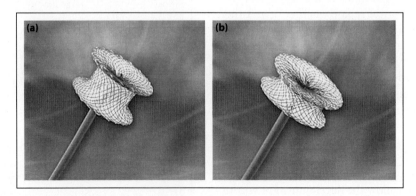

Figure 72.2 Amplatzer muscular ventricular septal defect (VSD) occluders. The device has three components: a left ventricular disk, a connecting waist, and a right ventricular disk. The postinfarct muscular VSD occluder (a) has a 10-mm-long waist compared with 7 mm for the congenital muscular VSD device (b).

Table 72.1   Amplatzer postinfarct muscular VSD occluder

Code	Waist diameter (mm)	RV disk (mm)	LV disc (mm)	Waist length (mm)	Sheath size (Fr)
9-VSDMUSC-PI-016	16	22	24	10	9
9-VSDMUSC-PI-018	18	24	26	10	9
9-VSDMUSC-PI-020	20	26	28	10	10
9-VSDMUSC-PI-022	22	28	30	10	10
9-VSDMUSC-PI-024	24	30	32	10	10

24 mm in 2 mm increments and can be delivered through 9–10 Fr long sheaths (Table 72.1). However, the largest size currently available (24 mm) is too small for some of the defects encountered, particularly if a degree of further expansion of the defect is to be allowed for. The porosity of the device is also of concern as significant residual shunting can continue for a number of weeks after implantation. In addition to a hemodynamic burden, hemolysis through the device may occur, which will compromise an already severely ill patient. Preclotting the device in 20 mL of the patient's unheparinized blood may help to diminish significant early shunting.

Sheaths. Sheath kinking can prevent delivery of the device and often necessitates having to recreate the arterio-venous guide wire circuit (Figure 72.3). Leaving a 0.014" or 0.018" guide wire through the sheath after the dilator and AV wire loop has been withdrawn may help to avoid kinking (Figure 72.4). If the sheath develops a kink as the device is being advanced, then simply withdrawing the sheath while the device is advanced may be enough to get the device through the kinked area.

Braided sheaths may also prevent kinking but the Arrowflex sheath has a polyurethane inner coating, which creates tremendous frictional resistance to the passage of the nitinol device. This can be overcome by back loading the device into the usual St. Jude Medical long delivery sheath and advancing the entire unit inside an Arrowflex sheath 2 Fr sizes larger. The standard Cook sheaths with radiopaque marker bands, although not braided, kink much less frequently than the standard St. Jude Medical sheaths. A 12 Fr Cook sheath can be used to deliver a 24 mm PMIVSD device back loaded in a 10 Fr St. Jude Medical long sheath. Cook also manufactures Flexor sheaths, which are braided and have a Teflon inner lining that permits easy advancement of the device. The new St. Jude Medical-braided sheaths for perimembranous devices are not large enough to deliver the PMIVSD device but can be used to deliver a congenital muscular VSD device.

Catheters and Wires. The usual diagnostic coronary catheters are sufficient. A 7 F monitoring (balloon lumen and guide wire lumen) Swan–Ganz catheter that has a 0.035 guide wire lumen (Model 111F7 Edwards) is worth keeping

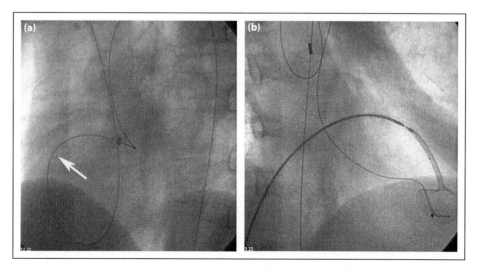

Figure 72.3   Sheath kinking. The long sheath has been introduced from the right internal jugular vein over an arterio-venous (A-V) guide wire loop in a patient with an acute postinfarct VSD (a). The arrow points to the kink on the sheath that developed after removal of the long dilator from the delivery sheath. Recrossing the VSD and snaring out the femoral vein has produced a much gentler angle on the sheath and avoided kinking of the sheath (b) in this patient with an anterior VSD.

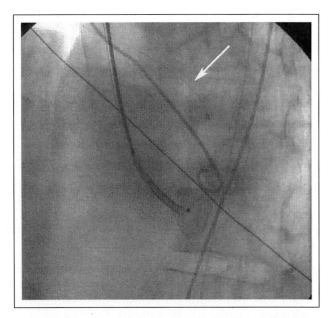

Figure 72.4 Sheath reinforcement. A 0.014 inch coronary guide wire (arrow) has been passed into the long sheath and the device loaded and passed alongside it and opened in the left ventricle.

in stock. Also a 400-cm-long Terumo guide wire (Model NV-GA35403M) may avoid running out of guide wire length during the introduction of the long sheath over the A-V guide wire loop.

Extras. It is advisable to be prepared for any possible complications. We suggest ensuring that all equipment is readily available, and preferably prepared. This includes large sheaths, gooseneck snares and retrieval baskets, as well as temporary pacemaker equipment.

Imaging. TTE or TOE should be performed during the procedure. Transgastric views can be particularly useful for delineating the defect (Figure 72.5); however, TOE imaging usually requires general anesthesia, which patients in cardiogenic shock may tolerate poorly. It is important to visualize the maximum LV, septal, and right ventricular (RV) orifices of the intended defect and to see the guide wire crossing these (Figure 72.6). Otherwise, particularly in patients with multiple defects, the device may end up in an adjacent unimportant defect, which in addition to producing significant residual shunting may impede a second device from completely closing the important defect. TOE does not always provide good images of very apical defects and it may be better to use transthoracic imaging. Three-dimensional echocardiography is being increasingly used during these procedures. As both interventionalists and imaging specialists become more familiar with the technique, it is likely to add value to the procedure by ensuring a better match and alignment of the device(s) in the defect(s).

Angiography allows for a crude assessment of the amount of shunting of contrast before and after device

implantation. It can be the sole imaging modality for patients with single defects, particularly if the defect is well profiled.

Technique

Arterio-Venous Guide wire Circuit. The most common method used has been to cross the defect from the left ventricle and create an arterio-venous guide wire circuit. The left ventricle can be entered through the aortic (retrograde arterial) or mitral valves (transseptal). A right coronary or balloon-wedge catheter is used to cross the defect, often with the aid of a torque wire (Terumo or Storq) (Figure 72.7a). A 6 Fr JR4 and exchange length-angled Terumo guide wire is usually the initial catheter/wire combination chosen. The wire will often be directed to the pulmonary artery from where it can be snared (Figure 72.7b) and pulled out of the jugular or femoral vein. We usually use an Amplatzer 25-mm-diameter gooseneck snare (Microvena). The guide wire course that allows the straightest introduction of the long sheath is chosen. This is usually the jugular vein but may be the femoral vein for anterior defects. It is helpful to use a wedge balloon catheter (7 Fr monitoring [nonthermodilution] Swan–Ganz catheter, Edwards) from the jugular vein to enter the pulmonary artery and pass an exchange wire to introduce the snare catheter, to avoid looping the wire around a chord or papillary muscle of the tricuspid valve, when the guide wire circuit is created. St. Jude Medical-exchange rope wire can be very helpful, as it is very unlikely to kink. The defect can then be balloon sized over the wire (Figure 72.7c), which also ensures that the guide wire is not trapped around the tricuspid valve chordae. The appropriate long sheath (9 Fr for 16 and 18 mm PMIVSD devices, 10 Fr for 20–24 mm PMIVSD devices) and dilator are then introduced over the guide wire (Figure 72.7d). When the tip of the dilator meets the tip of the arterial catheter, the long sheath and arterial catheter are advanced and withdrawn, respectively, using a "kissing" technique. The dilator usually passes into the left ventricle without too much difficulty. The sheath often requires some encouragement by either holding the guide wire circuit taut or, often more usefully, just pushing the sheath over the dilator. It is a mistake to "over-introduce" the long sheath into the left ventricle, as the sheath will buckle when the dilator and wire are removed. After removal of the dilator and de-airing of the long sheath, the guide wire is partly withdrawn via the artery to about the level of the tricuspid valve. The sheath is then clamped, with rubber shods or an artery clamp over the gauze, and the device is introduced and passed down to the level of the guide wire and then advanced while the guide wire is withdrawn. Once the device is at the tip of the sheath, the echocardiogram is checked to ensure that the device does not open inside the mitral tension apparatus. The deployment is monitored mainly on echocardiography

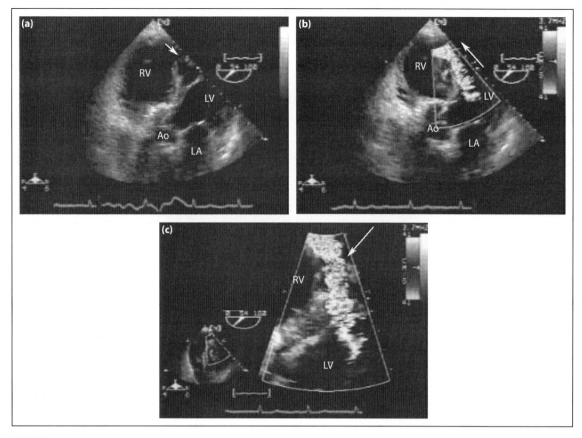

Figure 72.5 Transesophageal echocardiographic (TEE) images of an acute postinfarct VSD. The transgastric view (a) shows the ragged margins of the ruptured (arrow) septum. Color-flow mapping shows (b) a high velocity flow exiting the tunnel such as VSD (arrows) (c). RV, right ventricle; LV, left ventricle; LA, left atrium; Ao, aorta.

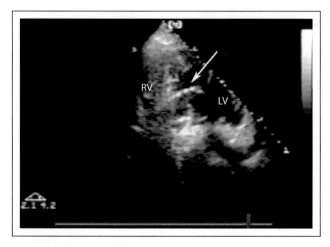

Figure 72.6 TTE image of guide wire passage through a postinfarct VSD. The arrow shows a Terumo guide wire crossing an acute postinfarct VSD from right to left (arrow). Transthoracic imaging confirmed that the wire had passed through the major orifices of the VSD. The right ventricular approach was used in this particular patient to introduce a 24 mm post-MI VSD device without the need for an AV guide wire loop. LA, left atrium; LV, left ventricle; RV; right ventricle.

(Figure 72.7e and f). The RV disk may need time to fully configure. If the lips of the device are tilted into the defect, then the sheath can be advanced back over the device to recapture it and redeploy it. Echocardiography (Figure 72.7g) and angiography are then used to check its final position prior to release. After release of the device, any residual shunting should be through the device; however, at this stage, it may become apparent that there are other significant defects that require further devices. It is usually better to go on and implant the additional devices during the same session.

RV Approach. The technique of using a retrograde arterial approach to cross the defect, create an arterio-venous guide wire loop, and then introduce the delivery sheath transvenously is cumbersome. To simplify the technique, we have sometimes adopted the approach of crossing the maximum RV orifice of the defect with a catheter (right coronary, multipurpose) and/or Terumo guide wire, usually introduced from the right internal jugular vein (Figure 72.8a and b). The guide wire is then directed out through the aortic valve, followed by the catheter and the guide

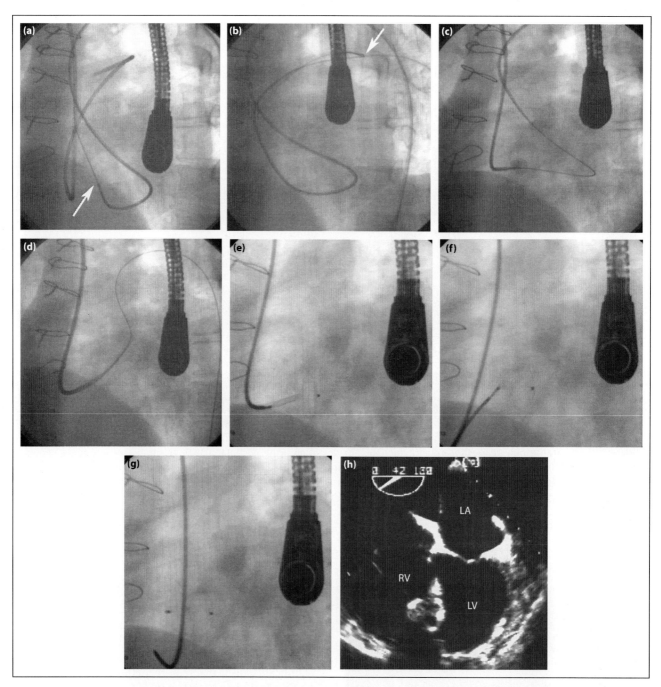

Figure 72.7 Transcatheter closure of a residual postinfarct VSD. The defect is crossed via the retrograde arterial approach (a). Using an El-Gamal catheter, a torque wire (arrow) has been directed from the left ventricle through the VSD and into the right ventricular outflow tract. The exchange length guide wire is then snared out (arrow) from the pulmonary artery using an Amplatz gooseneck snare (b). A 7-F monitoring Swan–Ganz catheter has been passed over the A-V guide wire loop and dye used to inflate the balloon to size the defect (c). The long delivery sheath is then passed from the right internal jugular vein over the A-V guide wire loop into the left ventricle (d). The left ventricular disk (e) followed by the right ventricular disk (f) is deployed and then the device is unscrewed from the delivery cable (g). Transesophageal echo shows the device to be well seated on the ventricular septum (h). LA, left atrium; LV, left ventricle; RV; right ventricle.

wire is passed down the descending aorta or into the subclavian artery. The Terumo wire is exchanged for a normal Teflon-coated J-tipped guide wire. A long sheath and dilator are then hand curved to match the guide wire curve and passed over the guide wire into the left ventricle. Device introduction and deployment then proceed as before. If the long sheath should fall back or kink, then an 8 F right coronary guide catheter inside the long sheath can be used to recross the VSD from the RV and pass the sheath back into the LV for a further attempt.

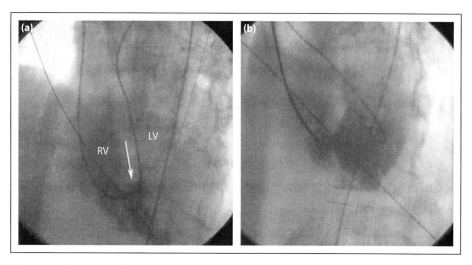

Figure 72.8   Right ventricular approach. The arrow shows the Terumo guide wire passing through the VSD (a). The catheter was introduced from the right internal jugular vein and passed into the right ventricle. The right ventricular approach was used in this particular patient to introduce a 24 mm post-MI VSD device (b) without the need for an AV guide wire loop. LV, left ventricle; RV; right ventricle.

Recent literature

To date, there are no published prospective randomized controlled trials directly comparing morbidity and mortality outcomes of surgical repair with transcatheter closure of PMIVSDs. Furthermore, outcome data for intention-to-treat basis are lacking, that is, mortality rates for those who were turned down for intervention as well as those who underwent intervention.

The largest trial reporting on the incidence and outcomes of PMIVSDs is the GUSTO-1 trial. This trial reported on 84 patients from their original cohort of 41,021 patients (0.2%), who developed VSD following thrombolysis for ACS between 1990 and 1993. These patients had a higher mortality compared with those who did not develop PMIVSDs (73.8% vs. 6.8%). There was also a significantly higher mortality in those with PMIVSDs managed medically as opposed to surgically (30-day mortality 94% vs. 47%).[1]

Despite advances in surgical techniques, the mortality rates in recent publications remain high. One of the largest series of 2876 patients reports an operative mortality of 54.1% if repair was performed within 7 days of myocardial infarction.[18]

The 30-day mortality rates for patients who undergo transcatheter closure for PMIVSDs range between 28% and 65%.[19,20] Both surgical and transcatheter techniques report higher mortality rates for patients undergoing intervention as an emergency procedure or within 24 h of VSD occurrence and for those with cardiogenic shock at the time of intervention.

The study published by Thiele et al. in 2008 probably represents one of the most realistic outcomes of patients with PMIVSDs undergoing transcatheter closure. They included all comers and report on the outcomes of 29 consecutive patients, who underwent closure with Amplatzer devices. Overall, 30-day mortality was reported at 65.5%; however, when this was divided into those with and without cardiogenic shock, the 30-day mortality for those without cardiogenic shock was found to be 38%.[19]

Maltais et al. compared the outcomes of 51 patients, who underwent either transcatheter (12 patients) or surgical closure (39 patients) of PMIVSDs. Eighty-eight percent of their cohort had systemic shock prior to intervention. They reported a 30-day mortality for the surgical repair group of 33%, with those undergoing percutaneous treatment having a 30-day mortality of 42%. It should be noted that those who underwent transcatheter closure had a longer time to diagnosis following MI compared with those who underwent surgical repair (6.1 days ± 3.7 vs. 5.5 days ± 6.2) and a longer time to treatment (6.1 days ± 3.7 vs. 3.7 days ± 4.2; $p = 0.08$). The factors that were found to predict hospital stay or 30-day mortality were residual VSD following treatment, time from MI to PMIVSD diagnosis, and time from diagnosis to treatment. On the basis of their experience, they have proposed a treatment algorithm where those with PMIVSDs ≤15 mm undergo transcatheter treatment while those with defects >15 mm undergo surgical repair. Repair should be followed by a repeat TTE and those with residual VSDs deemed to be severe should undergo a repeat procedure, either transcatheter or surgical as appropriate.[21]

Residual VSDs in surgical series are reported in 28–35% of cases.[6,7] Transcatheter series report successful implantation of devices in 73.6–89% of cases; however, they also record the presence of residual VSDs in up to 85% of cases, although these are classified as "trivial" or "small" in over 60% of cases.[20,22]

Although many other surgical and transcatheter series include patients with cardiogenic shock, they rarely

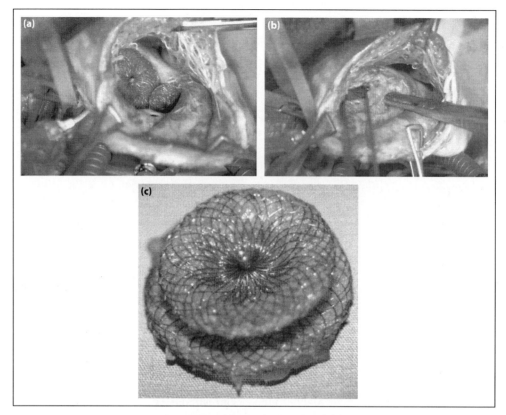

Figure 72.9 Crossover to surgery. An interoperative photograph via the left ventriculotomy shows the previously placed 20 mm atrial septal defect and 14 mm congenital muscular devices (a). Neither device appears to have developed much "endothelialization." After device removal, two well-circumscribed VSDs can be seen with surgical forceps inside each of them (b). The relatively incomplete "endothelialization" can be seen on the right ventricular aspect of the congenital muscular device (c).

comment on the sickest patients, who were deemed unsuitable for any form of intervention and thus have an inherent selection bias.

Long-term follow-up data for transcatheter techniques are for the large part missing, with most series reporting a follow-up of <2 years. Thiele et al.[19] reported that in their cohort, those who survived for the first 30 days, had a 90% survival at a median follow-up of 2 years. For those who survive for the first 30 days, surgical series have reported a 5-year survival of between 46% and 67%.[6,8]

Conclusions

Although surgical repair remains the gold standard for primary PMIVSDs, transcatheter closure is probably the treatment of choice for recurrent postinfarction VSD following patch repair. Primary catheter closure of PMIVSDs following acute myocardial infarction is an evolving technique that may avoid surgery or serve as a bridge to subsequent elective lower risk surgery. The outcomes in patients with acute PMIVSDs should improve with larger diameter, less porous devices (Figure 72.9), simpler delivery techniques, clearer imaging, and increased experience.

However, while this approach is good for the technique, it may not necessarily produce the best results for the entire group of patients presenting with PMIVSD. An earlier aggressive approach may salvage more patients, particularly in centers where a policy of "trial of life" is also adopted by the surgical team. To this end, the availability of less porous larger-diameter devices coupled with improved delivery systems is urgently required.

References

1. Crenshaw BS, Granger CB, Birnbaum Y, Pieper KS, Morris DC, Kleiman NS et al. Risk factors, angiographic patterns, and outcomes in patients with ventricular septal defect complicating acute myocardial infarction. GUSTO-I trial investigators. *Circulation* 2000;101:27–32.
2. Steg G, James SK, Atar D, Badano LP, Blomstrom-Lundqvist C, Borger M et al. ESC guidelines for the management of acute myocardial infarction in patients presenting with ST-segment elevation. *Eur Heart J* 2012;33:2569–619.
3. O'Gara PT, Kushner FG, Ascheim DD, Casey DE, Chung MK, DeLemos JA et al. ACCF/AHA guideline for the management of ST-elevation myocardial infarction: A report from the American College of Cardiology Foundation/American Heart Association Task Force on Practical Guidelines. *Circulation* 2013;127:529–55.

4. Edwards BS, Edwards WD, Edwards JE. Ventricular septal rupture complicating acute myocardial infarction: Identification of simple and complex types in 53 autopsied hearts. *Am J Cardiol* 1984;54:1201–5.

5. Labrousse L, Choukroun E, Chevalier JM, Madonna F, Robertie F, Merlico F et al. Surgery for post infarction ventricular septal defect: Risk factors for hospital death and long term results. *Eur J Cardiothorac Surg* 2002;21:725–32.

6. Jeppsson A, Liden H, Johnsson P, Hartford M, Radegran K. Surgical repair of post infarction ventricular septal defects: A national experience. *Eur J Cardiothorac Surg* 2005;27:216–21.

7. Fukushima S, Tesar PJ, Jalali H, Clarke A, Sharma H, Coudary J et al. Determinants of in-hospital and long-term surgical outcomes after repair of postinfarction ventricular septal rupture. *J Thorac Cardiovasc Surg* 2010;140:59–65.

8. Deja MA, Szostek J, Widenka K, Szafron B, Spyt TJ, Hickey MSJ et al. Post infarction ventricular septal defect—Can we do better? *Eur J Cardiothorac Surg* 2000;18:194–201.

9. Landzberg MJ, Lock JE. Transcatheter management of ventricular septal rupture after myocardial infarction. *Semin Thorac Cardiovasc Surg* 1998;10:128–32.

10. Pienvicht P, Piemonte TC. Percutaneous closure of post-myocardial infarction ventricular septal defect with the Cardioseal septal occluder implant. *Catheter Cardiovasc Interv* 2001;54:490–4.

11. Lee EM, Roberts DH, Walsh KP. Transcatheter closure of a residual post-myocardial infarction ventricular septal defect with the Amplatzer septal occluder. *Heart* 1998;80:522–4.

12. Demkow M, Ruzyllo W, Konka M, Wilczynski J, Dzielinska Z, Kochman J. Staged transcatheter closure of chronic post-infarction ventricular septal defects with the Amplatzer septal occluder. *Int J Cardiovasc Intervent* 2001;4:43–46.

13. Rodes Cabau J, Figueras J, Pena C, Barrabes J, Anivarro I, Soler-Soler J. Communication interventricular postinfarto de miocardio tratada en fase aguda mediante cierre percutaneo con el dispositivo Amplatzer. *Rev Esp Cardiol* 2003;56:623–5.

14. Mullasari AS, Umesan Ch V, Krishan U, Srinvasan S, Ravikumar M, Raghuraman H. Transcatheter closure of post-myocardial infarction ventricular septal defect with Amplatzer septal occluder. *Catheter Cardiovasc Interv* 2001;54:484–7.

15. Szkutnik M, Bialkowski J, Kusa J, Banaszak P, Baranowski J, Gasior M et al. Post-infarction ventricular septal defect closure with Amplatzer occluders. *Eur J Cardiothorac Surg* 2003;23:323–7.

16. Goldstein JA, Casserly IP, Balzer DT, Lee R, Lasala JM. Transcatheter closure of recurrent post-myocardial infarction septal defects utilizing the Amplatzer post-infarction VSD device: A case series. *Catheter Cardiovasc Interv* 2003;59:238–43.

17. Attia R, Blauth C. Which patients might be suitable for a septal occluder device closure of postinfarction ventricular septal rupture rather than immediate surgery? *Int Cardiovasc Thorac Surg* 2010;11:626–9.

18. Arnaoutakis GJ, Zhao Y, George TJ, Sciortino CM, McCarthy PM, Conte JV. Surgical repair of ventricular septal defect after myocardial infarction: Outcomes from the Society of Thoracic Surgeons National Database. *Ann Thorac Surg* 2012;94:436–43.

19. Thiele H, Kaulfersch C, Daehnert I, Schoenauer M, Eitel I, Borger M et al. Immediate primary transcatheter closure of postinfarction ventricular septal defects. *Eur Heart J* 2009;30:81–8.

20. Holzer R, Balzer D, Amin Z, Ruiz CE, Feinstein J, Bass J et al. Transcatheter closure of postinfarction ventricular septal defects using the new Amplatzer muscular VSD occluder: Results of a U.S. Registry. *Catheter Cardiovasc Interv* 2004;61:196–201.

21. Maltais S, Ibrahim R, Basmadjian AJ, Carrier M, Bouchard D, Cartier R et al. Post infarctation ventricular septal defects: Towards a new treatment algorithm? *Ann Thorac Surg* 2009;87:687–93.

22. Bilkowski J, Szkutnik M, Kusa J, Kalarus Z, Gasior M, Prybylski R, et al. Transcatheter closure of postinfarction ventricular septal defects using Amplatzer devices. *Rev Esp Cardiol* 2007;60:548–51.

73

Patent ductus arteriosus (PDA): Background and indications for closure

Jamie Bentham and Neil Wilson

Introduction

Failure of the arterial duct to close in the weeks following birth results in a common form of congenital heart disease affecting around 1 in 2000 term newborn infants and a greater proportion of preterm infants.[1,2] Confusion surrounding this condition stems from a number of causes, starting with the fact that this normal fetal structure only becomes abnormal if it fails to close. Further, failure to close has a varied clinical impact: it may be asymptomatic ("silent"), symptoms may be deferred until later in life, or it may be overtly symptomatic as early as the first days of life in a preterm infant. Understanding the background to the debate surrounding failed ductal closure and when to intervene is important for the interventionist where indications for intervention need to be clearly defined. This is the objective of this chapter.

Background

Ductal patency is maintained during fetal life predominantly by the combination of circulating prostaglandins and a reduced oxygen tension, both contributing to vasodilatation of the smooth muscle within the ductus. In full-term infants, failure of the ductus to close in the hours to weeks following birth is secondary to a relative failure of smooth muscle development and is caused by a combination of factors, both genetic and environmental. In the preterm infant, the situation is more complex in that both the physiological state of the preterm infant and developmental immaturity contribute significantly in maintaining ductal patency. Given the precarious hemodynamic state of the preterm infant, a significant left-to-right shunt can have a potentially devastating effect. In view of these differences, it is useful to consider the indications for ductal closure by age. Transcatheter closure of the patent ductus using an Ivalon plug was first reported by Portsmann some 28 years after reports of surgical ligation of the ductus emerged

(1967[3]). It was not until the introduction of Gianturco coils in 1992, however, that transcatheter closure of the patent ductus became a routine, technically achievable, and successful procedure.[4]

Clinical indications for transcatheter duct closure

Term infants and children

Duct closure is indicated in any child demonstrably symptomatic from significant left-to-right ductal shunting. In the term infant, signs of cardiac failure alongside evidence of significant ductal shunting (left ventricular and left atrial volume overload) make for a straightforward clinical decision with clear benefit to be derived from ductal closure. Concomitant viral respiratory infection may even result in failure to wean from respiratory support. Unfortunately, this is a relatively uncommon situation and in the absence of symptoms both in childhood and adulthood, the indications for duct closure become more difficult to define.[5] Given that the majority of patent ducts will be closed in asymptomatic infants or children, it becomes important to have a good understanding of the natural history of a significant patent ductus and how this is practically defined.

The long-term clinical significance of an untreated patent arterial duct undoubtedly relates to the degree of left-to-right shunt as well as the duration of exposure to the shunt. Multiple factors govern the degree of shunt and many of these are difficult to characterize in a noninvasive manner with a degree of accuracy. Ductal size is easily assessed on transthoracic echocardiography measured at the point of maximal constriction. Flow will also be dependent, however, on the systemic and pulmonary pressure and resistance differences as well as ductal resistance (ductal length and profile will thus also be important). It is no surprise, therefore, that surrogate markers of potentially important ducts have arisen, including left heart volume load, left atrial size, and whether a duct murmur is clinically audible.

The natural history of an untreated significant ductal shunt includes congestive cardiac failure, atrial fibrillation, and pulmonary vascular disease.[6] In the setting of an acquired cardiac disease, a previously well-tolerated ductal shunt may become symptomatic. As a consequence of these clear associations, significant shunts should undoubtedly be closed when identified in childhood, and few would disagree. Debate begins when we attempt to define what is significant, especially given the problems of assessing shunts discussed above. It is for this reason, as well as the association, however small, of patent ducts with endarteritis, that some interventionists advocate closure of all ducts, even those deemed clinically "silent." This is a defensible position though a middle ground is preferred by the majority, namely closing only those ducts that are clinically audible, since objective signs of a duct murmur are likely to represent significant ductal flow.[7] The reason that the authors prefer this position is that the evidence for the association of small ducts with an increased risk of endarteritis is limited and closure of small ducts is not unlikely to generate complications. They can be difficult to cross and may require small coils that are notoriously difficult to retrieve from small vessels should they embolize. However, it is important to acknowledge the possibility of encountering a duct that appears too small to be significant during a case. We would support closure in these circumstances as failure to do so introduces many difficulties with managing parental expectation and a reluctance to discharge the patient "untreated." Occasionally, such a duct may be in spasm and placing a device reveals the true ductal size. This should be apparent if careful clinical and transthoracic assessment took place prior to catheterization. Contraindications to closure in children would be established and irreversible pulmonary vascular disease, management of which is discussed below.

Preterm infants

A persistent patent arterial duct complicates the neonatal course of around 30% of preterm infants. Delayed closure of the duct is associated with an increase in neonatal morbidity. Hemodynamically significant ducts with high left-to-right flow have been associated with an increased incidence of intraventricular hemorrhage, necrotizing enterocolitis, pulmonary hemorrhage, chronic lung disease, and poor weight gain. It is generally agreed that closing arterial ducts in selected infants reduces the length of ventilation and improves their neonatal course. However, there are no universally accepted criteria to identify ducts most likely to be pathogenic. The difficulties with these assessments are discussed above, though in recent years cardiac biomarkers have begun to show promise in preterm infants in aiding identification of potentially significant shunts. In spite

of increasing experience in catheterizing sick newborn infants, there remain substantial difficulties to be overcome when catheterizing small preterm infants and most centers still regard the indication for transcatheter duct closure to be a weight of over 5 kg. Although the indications for duct closure in preterm infants remain controversial, those infants receiving significant ventilatory support and in whom pharmacological measures have failed or are contraindicated frequently undergo surgical ligation by lateral thoracotomy. It seems reasonable to extrapolate from this similar indications for transcatheter closure though the interventionist will need to become comfortable with catheterizing such small infants and generally equipment-related difficulties will increase below 1.5 kg by virtue of the infant's small size. As a consequence, preterm duct closure remains a relatively rare procedure performed by few operators.[8]

Adults

Occasionally, ducts evade detection and present in later life with an asymptomatic cardiac murmur, endarteritis, atrial fibrillation, or rarely with impaired cardiac function or pulmonary hypertension.[5,6,9] Closure of patent arterial ducts in adults is a relatively rare procedure. As a consequence, in the absence of symptoms, in adulthood, the indications for duct closure become more difficult to define.[5] Following an absence of sequelae from the patent duct in the preceding decades of life, a symptomatic presentation as a procedural indication can occur but would be uncommon. As discussed above, indicating closure on the basis of a reduction in endarteritis risk would be considered by some to be inadequate, especially for small ducts.[7] Elevation of pulmonary artery pressure would seem a stronger and justifiable indication for closure of significant ducts in adult patients with an obvious reluctance to leave even mildly elevated pulmonary artery pressure lifelong.[6,10] There may also be arguable logic for closing an asymptomatic duct in an adult in the context of comorbidity of systemic hypertension and or ischemic heart disease or chronic obstructive pulmonary disease. The argument here being that even a relatively small shunt is likely to contribute in the long term to overall morbidity. In practical terms, few adult patients are denied closure once the diagnosis is made.

Irreversible elevation of pulmonary artery pressure remains a clear contraindication to duct closure to avoid hastening right ventricular failure. Not infrequently, especially in children born preterm with concomitant chronic lung disease, significantly elevated pulmonary artery pressure will be encountered. Determining the degree and direction of shunt, a balloon occluding the ductus and assessing pharmacologically for reversibility are all important steps in establishing operability. Even here, some cases of pulmonary vascular disease will continue to progress following ductal closure.

Device-related indications

The very existence of an ever-increasing number of devices available for transcatheter closure of the patent ductus implies that each has its limitations. Given the important anatomic variability that exists, it is essential to be familiar with and have available a range of devices. Detachable coils are still frequently used, particularly in small ducts, though they have predominantly given way to occluding devices. This is primarily because multiple coils are required in larger ducts and even then residual shunt, hemolysis, and coil embolizations occurred

occasionally. The Amplatzer Duct Occluder (ADO) is the most established device and the only one approved by the Food and Drug Administration (FDA) in the United States for transcatheter PDA closure (AGA Medical Corporation, Plymouth, MN, USA). There is considerable clinical experience with this device and its limitations are well known to the interventionist. It is a stiff asymmetric device that may only be delivered from a venous approach. Although it has an excellent safety profile,[11] there are concerns using this device in small infants, particularly those with large ducts, due to the potential for distortion and compression of the left pulmonary artery

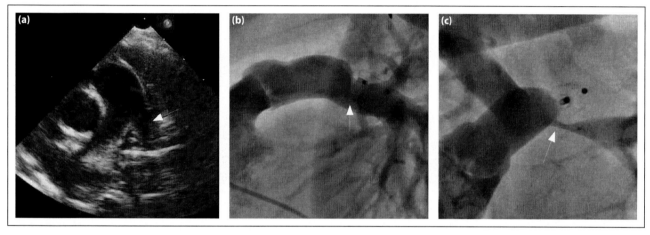

Figure 73.1 Left pulmonary artery compression resulting from the placement of an 8/6 Amplatzer Duct Occluder I (ADO I) device in a 1-year-old 7 kg infant with a large duct (4 mm) and moderate pulmonary artery hypertension (65 mmHg vs. systemic pressure of 120 mmHg). (a) Short-axis transthoracic echocardiogram through the pulmonary artery. The left pulmonary artery is of a respectable size prior to duct closure (arrow). (b and c) Following placement and release of an 8/6 ADO I, severe left artery compression is evident (arrow) in this lateral view (b) and steep cranial left anterior oblique view (c).

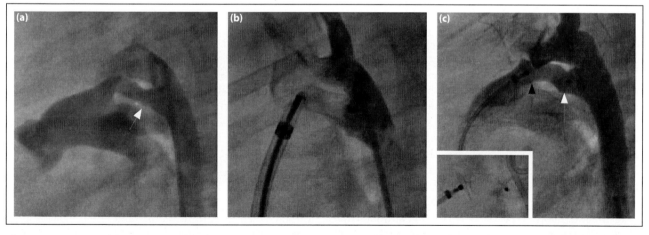

Figure 73.2 Placement of a 6/4 Amplatzer Duct Occluder I device in a moderate-sized tubular duct in a 5 kg infant with moderately elevated pulmonary artery pressure (52 mmHg vs systemic pressure of 74 mmHg). (a) Lateral angiogram demonstrates a long tubular, type C, ductus (arrow). (b) A 6/4 ADO I device has been placed though not released. The device is appropriately positioned though the aorta is small. A pullback pressure gradient from either side of the device was 15 mmHg. The device may have altered its position following release given the tension from the delivery cable but we elected to remove it and placed an ADO IIAS device. (c) The ADO IIAS device (5/6, see inset figure) is better placed with aortic disk (white arrow) and pulmonary disk (black arrow) appropriately placed. There is no pullback gradient and the device is released.

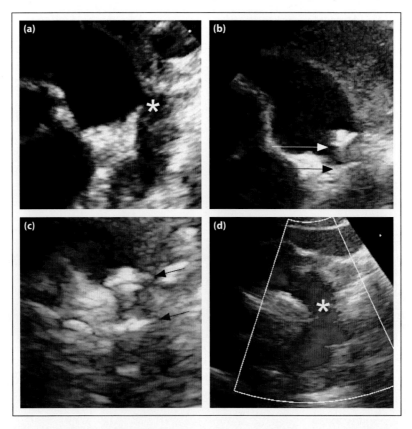

Figure 73.3 **(See color insert.)** Echocardiography-guided placement of an ADO IIAS device in an infant. (a) A moderate-sized duct is assessed at the beginning of the procedure for suitability for device closure, device size, and device type. The constriction of the duct at the pulmonary end measures 3 mm. There is sufficient ductal length to place a device without risking protrusion of the device into the aorta or causing left pulmonary artery obstruction. (b) An ADO IIAS 5/4 device has been uncovered within the duct. The device is not suitably placed, with the pulmonary disk of the device (white arrow) protruding into the main pulmonary artery and the aortic disk (black arrow) deployed within the duct. (c) The device has been repositioned and its position is now appropriate, with both disks clearly seen on echocardiography (black and blue arrows). The device has been correctly sized with constriction from the duct on the central waist of the device (between the two arrows). (d) Before and following device release, careful assessment of the aorta and left pulmonary artery is performed to ensure no obstruction and that the device has been placed correctly. There is no flow turbulence on color-flow Doppler in the aortic isthmus (*).

or aorta (Figures 73.1 and 73.2). Nevertheless, the ADO I has emerged around the world as reliable and easy to use, well suited to larger children and to ducts with large ampullas (type A[12]). A newer-generation Amplatzer Duct Occluder (ADO II) addressed some of the concerns with the ADO I with modifications supporting lower-profile delivery owing to the absence of a central fabric, with symmetrical disks enabling delivery via either a retrograde or antegrade approach.[13] This device seemed to find its place in more variable ductal morphologies, including long tubular ducts (type C[12]).[13] However, although the ADO II has been used effectively in small infants,[8] the disks are 6 mm larger than the central waist and recommended use is in infants ≥6 kg or with a descending aortic diameter of ≥10 mm, again in order to minimize the potential for aortic and left pulmonary artery obstruction in these smaller infants. The relatively recent introduction of the ADO II AS device aims to address this deficit

(Figure 73.2). It is similarly suited to varying duct morphology, but will likely find its place in small infants with long tubular ducts. Closure under echocardiographic guidance alone in the neonatal intensive care unit using this device from an arterial approach has been reported (Figure 73.3).

Conclusions

There are good natural history studies to support transcatheter duct closure in infants and children with a significant shunt. New devices lend themselves to a more streamlined technical approach allowing ever-smaller infant ducts to be closed. Evidence to support duct closure in adults and preterm infants is more confusing and indications are generally extrapolated from other sources calling for consideration on a case-by-case basis by a multidisciplinary team. Although transcatheter duct closure is an effective and low-risk procedure, it can, on occasion, be technically demanding, requiring multiple devices and the armamentarium to deal with difficulties that arise during the procedure.

References

1. Hoffman JI. Incidence of congenital heart disease: I. Postnatal incidence. *Pediatr Cardiol* 1995;16:103–13.
2. Schneider DJ, Moore JW. Patent ductus arteriosus. *Circulation* 2006;114:1873–82.
3. Porstmann W, Wierny L, Warnke H. Closure of persistent ductus arteriosus without thoracotomy. *German Medical Monthly* 1967;12:259–61.
4. Cambier PA, Kirby WC, Wortham DC, Moore JW. Percutaneous closure of the small (less than 2.5 mm) patent ductus arteriosus using coil embolization. *Am J Cardiol* 1992;69:815–6.
5. Fortescue EB, Lock JE, Galvin T, McElhinney DB. To close or not to close: The very small patent ductus arteriosus. *Congenit Heart Dis* 2010;5:354–65.
6. Campbell M. Natural history of persistent ductus arteriosus. *Br Heart J* 1968;30:4–13.
7. Sullivan ID. Patent arterial duct: When should it be closed? *Arch Dis Child* 1998;78:285–7.
8. Bentham J, Meur S, Hudsmith L, Archer N, Wilson N. Echocardiographically guided catheter closure of arterial ducts in small preterm infants on the neonatal intensive care unit. *Catheter Cardiovasc Interv* 2011;77:409–15.
9. Bessinger FB, Jr., Blieden LC, Edwards JE. Hypertensive pulmonary vascular disease associated with patent ductus arteriosus. Primary or secondary? *Circulation* 1975;52:157–61.
10. Fisher RG, Moodie DS, Sterba R, Gill CC. Patent ductus arteriosus in adults—long-term follow-up: Nonsurgical versus surgical treatment. *J Am Coll Cardiol* 1986;8:280–4.
11. Pass RH, Hijazi Z, Hsu DT, Lewis V, Hellenbrand WE. Multicenter USA Amplatzer patent ductus arteriosus occlusion device trial: Initial and one-year results. *J Am Coll Cardiol* 2004;44:513–9.
12. Krichenko A, Benson LN, Burrows P, Moes CA, McLaughlin P, Freedom RM. Angiographic classification of the isolated, persistently patent ductus arteriosus and implications for percutaneous catheter occlusion. *Am J Cardiol* 1989;63:877–80.
13. Morgan G, Tometzki AJ, Martin RP. Transcatheter closure of long tubular patent arterial ducts: The Amplatzer Duct Occluder II—A new and valuable tool. *Catheter Cardiovasc Interv* 2009;73:576–80.

Patent ductus arteriosus (PDA): PDA occlusion with the Amplatzer-type devices

Zaheer Ahmad and Mazeni Alwi

Isolated patent ductus arteriosus (PDA) is one of the more common congenital heart lesions comprising approximately 10% of congenital heart disease.[1] Most patients are asymptomatic, as the PDA tends to be small or moderate in size (<3.5–4.0 mm). Diagnosis is suspected on the presence of a continuous murmur. Large PDAs may present with high-output cardiac failure, frequent chest infections, and failure to thrive. Bounding pulses and a continuous murmur are characteristic, though with the development of pulmonary hypertension, the diastolic component of the murmur may disappear and the second heart sound may become loud. The diagnosis of PDA, and the evaluation of its size and hemodynamic impact is easily made by 2D and Doppler echocardiography.

Those with significant left-to-right shunt manifest features of left heart volume overload, that is, dilatation of the left atrium and ventricle. Doppler is helpful in assessing pulmonary artery pressure, but accurate direct measurement is an integral part of the closure procedure. It is recommended that all PDAs be closed to prevent infective endocarditis, relieve heart failure symptoms, and prevent progression to irreversible pulmonary vascular disease. Opinion is divided with regard to the small, silent PDA, which is defined as a duct identified echocardiographically but without a typical continuous murmur.

Small PDAs (<2.5–3.0 mm) can be easily closed with Gianturco or Cook detachable (Flipper) coils with minimal complications and excellent results.[2,3] Those with a significant shunt from a large PDA, that is, patients who are symptomatic and with obvious evidence of LV volume overload and pulmonary hypertension are generally not good candidates for PDA closure with coils because of the technical difficulty in achieving a stable position of the coils and the attendant complication of embolization. The large number of coils required for effective closure can also deform and obstruct adjacent structures such as the left pulmonary artery and descending aorta. Until fairly recently, surgical ligation used to be the most appropriate treatment for such large ducts.

The Amplatzer Ductal Occluder or ADO (St. Jude Medical, Plymouth, MN, USA), first introduced in 1997, shares the modular design features of Amplatzer Septal Occluder (ASO), that is, retrievability for repositioning or change to more appropriate-sized device before release. It was initially developed in a canine model with encouraging results.[4] The ADO has made transcatheter closure of moderate to large PDA a safe and efficacious procedure.[5–9]

The cylindrical, slightly tapered device has a thin retention disk 4 mm larger in diameter than its body to ensure secure positioning in the ductal ampulla. The polyester fibers sewn into the device induce thrombosis and rapid complete occlusion. Platinum marker bands are applied to the wire ends and are laser-welded. A stainless steel sleeve with a female thread is then welded to the marker band (Figure 74.1). The delivery system consists of a delivery cable with a male thread to which the device is screwed, a loading device, a long Mullins-type delivery sheath, and a pin vise to unscrew and release the device. The designation of device sizes 6/4, 8/6, 10/8 mm, and so on, refers to the body of the device. The first number denotes the larger distal (aortic) end of the device at the retention disk whereas the second number, 2 mm smaller, denotes the size of the proximal (pulmonary) end where the stainless steel sleeve for screwing onto the cable is located in its recess. It is important to remember that the retention disk at the distal (aortic) end of the device is always 4 mm larger in diameter than the larger of the quoted sizes. For example, the aortic retention disk on a 6/4 mm device is 10 mm diameter. The device sizes available are in increments of 2 mm, with a range from 5/4 to 16/14 mm. The smallest two sizes are 7 mm in length and the remainder are 8 mm.[5]

The ADO II and ADO II AS are the newest generation from the ADO family, which have broadened the spectrum to close ducts with different anatomic variations. The ADO II has been in use in Europe since January 2008. It is a lower-profile device, which consists of a lattice of nitinol, two very-low-profile disks, and an articulated connecting

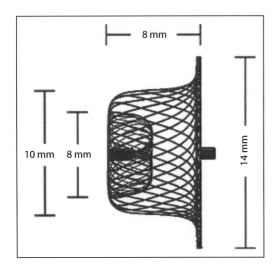

Figure 74.1 The Amplatzer Duct Occluder device. In this example of a 10/8 mm device, the "10" refers to the aortic end of the device and "8" refers to the pulmonary end. The retention disk on the aortic end is 4 mm larger in diameter than the aortic end's diameter. (With permission from St. Jude Medical Inc.)

waist. The absence of fabric inside the device is another major feature that helps lower the device profile. The central waist is designed to fill the ductus and the two retention disks are deployed on the aortic and pulmonary sides. The diameter of each retention disk is 6 mm larger than the connecting waist. The central waist of the device ranges in size from 3 to 6 mm. Each device is available in 4 and 6 mm length.

The ADO II AS (additional sizes) was developed to improve the delivery and profile of the occluder for small to moderate sized ductus in smaller children. It is a self-expanding nitinol lattice device of 144 wires. The central waist of the device fills the ductus and flat retention disks are deployed at pulmonary and aortic end. The ADO II AS has a disk diameter only 1–1.5 mm larger than the central waist, making it attractive for the closure of PDA in small infants. Although the instructions for use designate a weight limit of 6 kg, it has been successfully used to close PDAs in preterm infants less than 2 kg.[10]

Patient selection, hemodynamics, and angiographic evaluation

Patients with small PDA—asymptomatic patients with no clinical, ECG, chest x-ray, and echo evidence of left heart volume overload—may be treated effectively by coil occlusion. For symptomatic infants who weigh less than 5 kg with severe failure to thrive and heart failure due to a large PDA, surgical ligation is the most appropriate treatment. Interventional treatment for these infants is likely to

require a relatively large device and the risk of protrusion of the retention disk into the aortic lumen causing obstruction precludes its use. Additionally, the passage of a large and stiff delivery sheath and dilator through the heart may compromise patient hemodynamics by splinting open the tricuspid valve, inducing tricuspid regurgitation. The tight radius imposed on the curve of the delivery sheath because of the small AP diameter of the thorax may also result in kinking when the device is being advanced.

We would recommend a weight limit of 5 kg for infants with significant symptoms. However, in patients who are only mildly symptomatic, it is preferable, where possible, to perform the procedure when they attain 7–8 kg in weight. Rarely, adult patients are referred late with advanced pulmonary vascular disease and this clinical problem is dealt in the later part of this chapter.

Procedure

Policies vary with regard to the use of general anesthesia in different institutions. It is recommended that the procedure is done under general anesthesia in infants and small children if at all possible. Both femoral artery and vein—usually the right groin—are cannulated using a 4 F sheath in the artery and a 5 or 6 F sheath for the vein. For the initial hemodynamics evaluation, a 5–6 F diagnostic catheter (NIH or multipurpose) is used for pressure and oximetry studies. A 4 F pigtail is used for left heart study and aortography.

Ductal morphology

After the hemodynamic study has been completed, an aortogram using the pigtail catheter is performed aiming to have the loop of the pigtail catheter at the level of or slightly above the PDA ampulla. The lateral projection is the most useful and if a biplane system is available, the other projection can be straight frontal or with some right anterior oblique (30–35°). The great majority of isolated PDAs arise in the distal arch/proximal descending aorta just beyond and opposite the origin of the left subclavian artery. They tend to be a short, conical-shaped structure rather than long and tube-like. The aortic end is a wide ampulla, whereas the narrowest part is where it inserts to the superior aspect of the main pulmonary artery close to the origin of the left pulmonary artery. The PDA runs in a postero-anterior, with a slightly leftward direction, and slightly infero-superiorly from the aorta to the pulmonary artery. For the selection of an appropriate device size, the important measurements are the diameter of the ampulla, the length of the PDA, and most importantly, its narrowest diameter. In a PDA with a large shunt, a large volume of contrast of 2 cc/kg over 1 s may be needed to outline the PDA morphology well. Occasionally, having a large

Mullins sheath across the PDA during aortography may be useful in outlining the ductus, particularly in adult patients. Balloon-sizing techniques have occasionally been employed to accurately outline the PDA in adults.[11] On the lateral projection, the narrowest part of the PDA is usually seen overlapping with the tracheal air column and this serves as a useful landmark at the time of deployment. The short conical ductus is most suited for the ADO. This is designated as type A ductus in the Krichenko angiographic classification.[12] Further subgrouping according to where the narrowest diameter is in relation to the tracheal air column (A1, A2, A3) is perhaps superfluous. A small number of isolated PDAs have a less typical morphology, chiefly the long tubular ductus with or without a constriction at the pulmonary insertion (types C and E, respectively, in the Krichenko classification) and even less common is the window-type short ductus with virtually no ampulla (type B). The long tubular ducti requires some modification of technique or choice of device. ADO II and ADO II AS are the devices of choice in these ductus because of the two retention disks, but the range of sizes available for use is mainly for smaller diameter and shorter length. There are also reports of using Amplatzer vascular plug II and IV in these ducti with good results. In adult patients with large PDA, although the morphology is usually the typical conical type, the actual ductal length may be far in excess of device length, rendering the ADO unsuitable.

Selection of device size and long sheath

For the great majority of PDAs, especially those with conical shape, the device size selected (the pulmonary end) should be at least 2 mm larger than the narrowest PDA diameter. For example, if the narrowest PDA diameter is 3.6 mm, an 8/6 mm device should be selected. In practice, the sizes used are overwhelmingly 8/6 and 10/8 mm, taking into consideration that ducts measuring less than 2.5 mm are generally closed with coils. However, the "2 mm rule" may not be applicable to the larger ducts. For instance, in an adult patient with a 7 mm PDA, the 12/10 mm device may easily slip through into the pulmonary artery as the ratio of the retention disk diameter to the distal device diameter becomes increasingly smaller with increasing device size (the retention disk is always 4 mm larger than the distal device diameter regardless of size). In such large PDAs, 1 or 2 sizes larger may need to be chosen. Another factor for failure of implantation is the relatively longer PDA in adult patients whereas the device length remains 8 mm even in the largest size available (see below). For the 8/6 mm device, we recommend a 7 F long sheath and 8 F for the 10/8 mm device to facilitate easy advancement during device delivery.

Procedure

Once the measurements of the duct from the descending aortogram have been made and a device size selected, a 5 F or 6 F multipurpose catheter is advanced from the venous side through the PDA and into the descending aorta. This catheter is exchanged for the delivery sheath and dilator over a 0.035 inch exchange guide wire. The dilator is then removed, leaving the sheath in the descending aorta.

To load the device, the delivery cable is passed through a short cannulation sheath ("loading pod") with a side port 1 F size smaller than the delivery sheath. The device is screwed onto the tip of the delivery cable and pulled into the loading pod. The side port allows easy flushing of the loaded device within the sheath. The loading pod is introduced into the delivery sheath and the cable is then pushed to advance the device. To prevent inadvertent unscrewing, rotation of the cable should be avoided when the device is being advanced.

Under fluoroscopy, the device is advanced by pushing the delivery cable until it reaches the tip of the delivery sheath in the descending aorta. Gently withdraw the sheath to deploy the retention disk only, following the cable and delivery sheath, which is pulled as one unit, under lateral fluoroscopy until the retention disk is against the ductal ampulla. This can be observed by fluoroscopy using the tracheal air column as a landmark from the diagnostic aortogram previously or felt as a tugging sensation in synchrony with the aortic pulsation. Once the position has been affirmed based on the location of the narrowest diameter in relation to the tracheal air column, the cylindrical portion of the device is deployed by retracting the delivery sheath while applying slight tension on the cable.

An aortogram is then performed to verify correct positioning of the device. This is evident by the retention disk being well opposed to the ampulla and a slight waist seen in the middle portion of the device induced by constriction at the narrowest part of the PDA. If the position is satisfactory, the device is then released by screwing the plastic vise on the delivery cable and rotating it counterclockwise as indicated by the arrow on the vise. It is common to see residual shunt through the device, sometimes described as "foaming" on the immediate postimplantation aortogram. This is acceptable and it is usually unnecessary to repeat the aortogram 5–10 min later to document complete closure. However, if a definite jet is seen, usually above the body of the device, this indicates that the device is not "stenting" the narrowest part of the PDA either due to inappropriate device size or incorrect positioning. In the case of unusual PDA morphology, the ADO may not be the suitable device to use (see below). In this case, the device should be recaptured into the sheath by pulling on the cable while fixing the delivery sheath with the other hand and the steps repeated or a more suitable device selected.

Problems and complications

1. *Small infants with large PDA.* The indication to close a PDA in small infants is the presence of significant "cardiac failure" symptoms and failure to thrive due to a relatively large ductus. In these infants, the forced passage of a stiff delivery sheath and dilator in the right ventricular outflow tract (RVOT) may cause hemodynamic compromise. Tracking the sheath–dilator ensemble over an extra stiff exchange guide wire may streamline the passage by reducing the pressure against the RVOT as the sheath is being advanced. In these infants, the long sheath forms a tight curvature as it conforms to the RVOT, main pulmonary artery, and descending aorta. The sheath may kink as the device is advanced at the RVOT level as the stiffer cable conforms less to the curvature than the device, causing its tip to push against the wall of the sheath. This may be overcome by using a kink-resistant sheath, but a 2 F size or bigger is required, or alternatively the curvature of the delivery sheath can be reduced by placing its tip at the level of the ductal ampulla instead of lower in the descending aorta (Figure 74.2).

As noted above, in these symptomatic infants, a relatively large device is often required, usually 8/6 mm or 10/8 mm. The large retention disk may sit against the aortic wall rather than on the rim of the ductal ampulla, causing a mild gradient. This mild hemodynamic problem is, however, transient and becomes insignificant with somatic growth (Figure 74.2d). In general, problems and complications are more common in children weighing less than 10 kg.[13]

Newer devices such as the ADO II AS have the advantage of being low profile and, hence, they can be deployed via 4 F sheath from the venous or arterial side. The major advantages of this device are the lack of protrusion in the vessel lumen and the capability of closing

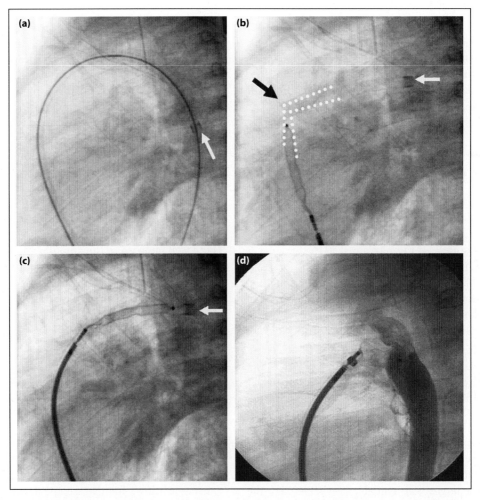

Figure 74.2   A 5.2 kg infant with a 4.5 mm PDA. (a) Tight curvature of delivery sheath with its tip (white arrow) in the descending aorta. (b) Kinking of delivery sheath (black arrow). (c) Curvature of delivery sheath is reduced by placing its tip at the level of the ductal ampulla to prevent kinking. (d) Upper rim of the retention disk (8/6 mm device) protrudes into the aorta causing a 10 mm gradient.

the PDA without major tension on vascular structures. Ductus length should be more than 3 mm and the diameter should be less than 4 mm. The symmetrical design allows delivery from the arterial side and this approach may be preferable in preterm infants, avoiding the hemodynamic impacts of relatively stiff sheaths within a small heart.[10,14] However, in younger children, extra caution should be taken to avoid injury to the femoral artery because of its impact on the growth.

2. *Undersizing and embolization to pulmonary artery.* Embolization of the ADO is rare. In the typical PDA morphology, this may be due to undersizing the device or positioning the device too deep within the ductus before its release. Ideally, in the conical-shaped PDA, the retention disk should be seated within the ampulla rim. When the device is pulled too deep, which may be partly due to undersizing, a "bump" caused by the retention disk is seen on the top part of the PDA. Although complete occlusion is achieved in the laboratory, the device may embolize later probably due to the "milking" action of the ductal wall (Figure 74.3). It is safer to reposition the device and if the same appearance caused by the retention disk is seen, a device 1 size larger is probably more appropriate (Figure 74.4).

An embolized ADO device into the pulmonary artery is difficult to retrieve because the female screw thread is located in a recess. However, if necessary, the device can be removed at the time of surgical ligation.

3. *Long tubular PDAs.* Ducts that are long and tubular may or may not have a constriction at the site of pulmonary insertion. Those with definite constriction do not pose a major problem, as the device may be pulled deep into the ductus before release. The device will be elongated and the retention disk will not configure fully due to the limited space, but embolization to the pulmonary artery is not likely to occur because of the constriction (Figure 74.5).

However, the long, large tubular ductus without a definite constriction may not be suitable for closure with the ADO because the device is relatively short (7 or 8 mm) and only has one retention disk. As illustrated in Figure 74.6, if the retention disk is correctly positioned on the rim of the ductal orifice, the proximal (pulmonary) end of the device is still well within the long PDA. Releasing the device in this position will likely cause embolization to the descending aorta or protrusion of the retention disk into the aorta causing a significant gradient.[15] On the other hand, pulling the device too deep to bring the proximal end into the main pulmonary artery will likely cause embolization to the right side in the absence of a definite constriction.

In this uncommon type of PDA, a device like the AMVO (Amplatzer Muscular VSD Occluder)—though equally short—has two retention disks that confer the advantage of ensuring stable positioning and reduce

the risk of embolization. The ASO, having similar features, may also be used, but the "connecting waist" or body of the device is shorter (4 mm). Apart from the large, long tubular ductus without constriction, the double-disk device is also appropriate for the short, window-type PDA with no ampulla. In this case, the ASO is more suitable as its short waist would conform to the PDA length.[11]

ADO II is an attractive option as it has two equal retention disks. These symmetrical disks have better maneuverability and are able to adapt to different angles and may conform better to the anatomy of the long tubular duct.[16] Because of the relatively larger retention disks, there is a risk of protrusion in the aorta

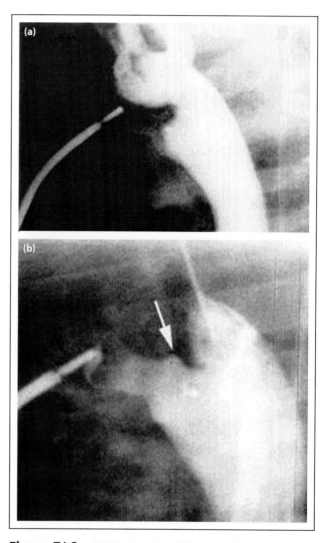

Figure 74.3 (a) The retention disk of the device seated on the rim of the ductal ampulla. The ductus is completely occluded and the device is not likely to embolize. (b) A completely occluded ductus but the device is too small, causing the retention disk to be pulled deep into the ductus, resulting in a "bump" (arrow) on the upper wall. This device embolized to the right pulmonary artery after 24 h.

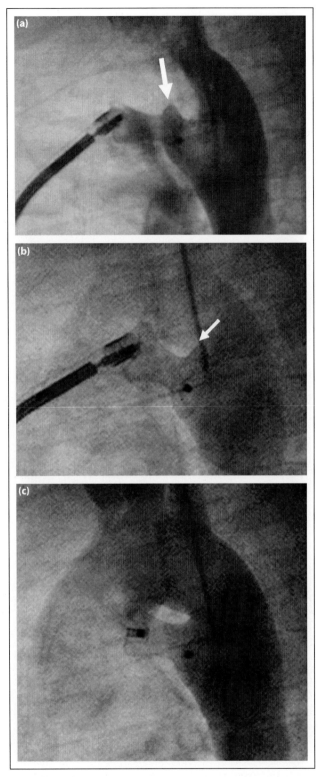

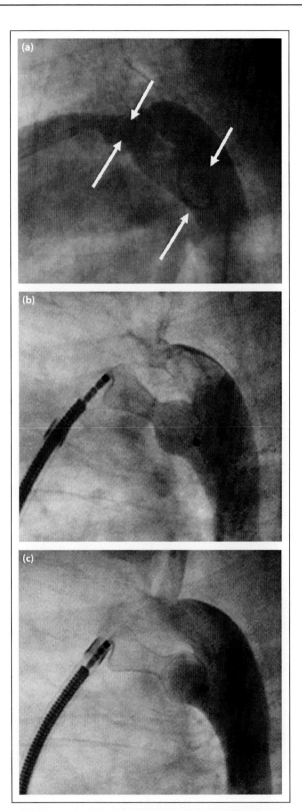

Figure 74.4 (a) The narrowest part of the PDA is well stented by the device, but the "bump" (arrow) indicates that the retention disk has been pulled too deep into the ductus. (b, c) The device was recaptured and repositioned with the retention disk correctly seated in the ampulla.

Figure 74.5 (a) A long tubular ductus with constriction at the pulmonary end. Length 17 mm, aortic end diameter 8 mm, pulmonary end 4.2 mm. (b, c) 8/6 mm device pulled deep into the tubular ductus. The retention disk does not reconfigure fully due to limited space but the ductus is completely occluded and the device does not protrude into the aorta.

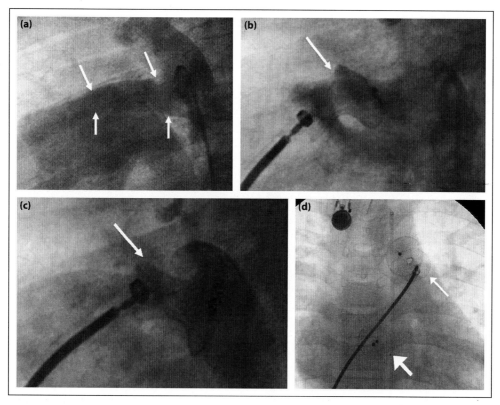

Figure 74.6 (a) A large, long tubular ductus with no constriction at the pulmonary end. Length 18 mm, aortic end diameter 12 mm, pulmonary end 7 mm. (b) 12/10 mm device properly "stents" the pulmonary end of the ductus but as the device is 8 mm in length, the retention disk is inevitably pulled deep into the PDA as indicated by the "bump" (arrow). The device will likely embolize to the pulmonary artery if released. (c) The device is repositioned to have the retention disk seated in the ampulla but the pulmonary end of the ductus is not stented because the device is too short. There is likelihood of embolization to the descending aorta if released. (d) ASO device implanted to close this PDA (small arrow). A membranous VSD was closed prior to the PDA (large arrow).

or pulmonary artery if they are used in shorter ducts, especially in young children.

In smaller infants with tubular ducts, Amplatzer vascular plugs (II and IV) can also be an alternative option as they have two retention disks that are of smaller size and are low-profile devices.[17,18] However, the use of these devices in bigger children with large and longer tubular ducts is limited because of a small range of sizes and length.

If an ADO embolizes to the descending aorta, it is probably unwise to remove it percutaneously through the femoral artery. For reasons mentioned above, it may be extremely difficult to snare the stainless steel sleeve housing the female screw. It is perhaps safer to snare the body of the device and push it back to the level of the ductal ampulla and remove it surgically with the PDA being ligated at the same time. However, aortic embolization and successful retrieval using a snare from the venous side has been described.[8]

4. *Large PDA in adults.* A large PDA in adult patients, although typically conical in shape, tends to be longer than the ADO length. Such large PDAs may be successfully closed with the largest of the ADO devices.[19]

However, to have the proximal (pulmonary) end correctly positioned may result in the device being pulled too deep into the ductus. The retention disk thus "stents" the PDA instead of the body of the device, causing a residual jet above it (Figure 74.7). There is the likelihood of embolization to the pulmonary artery when the device is released in this position. In this situation, a device with two retention disks like the AMVO would be more suitable.

5. *Large PDA with advanced pulmonary vascular disease.* Occasionally, an adult patient may present symptomatically with severe pulmonary hypertension due to a large PDA. The PDA may not be apparent on clinical and echo examination, and only diagnosed at cardiac catheterization in the course of an evaluation of a patient with pulmonary hypertension. The hemodynamic data at this stage would normally reveal advanced pulmonary vascular disease with PA/Ao pressure ratio >0.8 and Qp:Qs <1.5:1. Surgical ligation is usually considered inappropriate. We would treat the patient with the vasodilator sildenafil for 6 months and then, subject to an observed fall in pulmonary vascular resistance, proceed to trial closure with either an

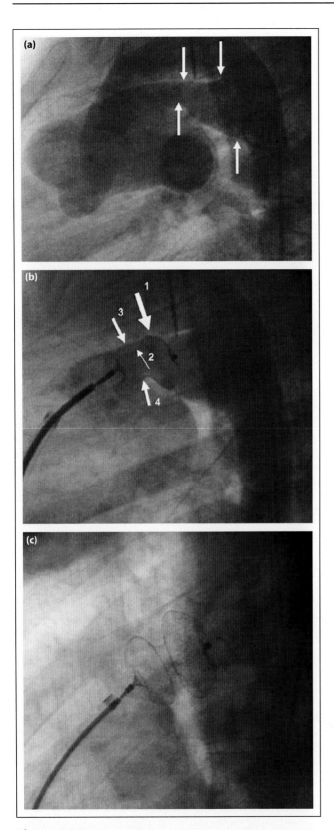

Figure 74.7 (a) An adult with large conical PDA. Ampulla 17 mm, narrowest diameter 7.1 mm, and length 16 mm. (b) Retention disk of 12/10 mm device "stenting" the PDA causing a jet above the body of the device. (c) ASO device implanted.

ASO or an AMVO, where the device is deployed but not released. The patient is then stressed with dobutamine to achieve maximum heart rate while observing the hemodynamics—recording of blood gases and aortic and PA pressures. If the PA pressure does not exceed the systemic, the patient is further observed in the intensive care unit with the cable remaining attached to the device. The patient is kept immobile under full sedation and the hemodynamics closely monitored for 48–72 h. If the hemodynamics and blood gases deteriorate, the device is recaptured into the sheath and removed. Otherwise, it is released permanently and the patient is maintained on sildenafil.

Conclusion

The ADO has made transcatheter closure of moderate and large PDA a reliably safe and effective procedure. It is particularly suited to the conical-shaped duct, which is the most common morphological type of PDA. Its use should be limited to those above 5 kg as in such small severely symptomatic infants, a hemodynamic compromise may be encountered with passage of a stiff sheath and dilator, with the additional hazard of the relatively large device that may partially obstruct the aorta. For the less common ductal morphology where the PDA is long, tubular, and has no definite constriction at the pulmonary end, the relatively short ADO with only one retention disk may not be the most suitable device. Recent results of newer-generation devices like ADO II, ADO II AS, and Amplatzer vascular plugs in these small patients have extended the scope of device closure of PDA and are also valuable addition to the inventory for tubular ducts. The same limitation may apply with a large PDA because of its relative length, though the PDA has a typically conical shape. In both situations, the AMVO is the more suitable device. For the short window-type PDA with no ampulla, the ASO is more suitable.

Recent advances in technology, particularly the emergence of the ADO II AS device, have resulted in some operators closing PDAs in smaller, premature babies.[20] Even more recently, safe, effective closure in preterm babies in the neonatal intensive care unit performed under echo guidance in the incubator has been reported.[21]

The management of adult patients with pulmonary vascular disease due to a large PDA is controversial. Priming with vasodilators and trial closure with ASO or AMVO and observing the hemodynamics response for up to 72 h may have a role in this small number of patients.

References

1. Benson LN. The arterial duct: Its presence and patency. In: Anderson RH, Baker EJ, Penny DJ, Redington AN, Rigby ML, Wernovsky G, Eds. *Paediatric Cardiology*. 3rd ed. London: Churchill Livingstone, 2009. pp. 875–93.

2. Hijazi ZM, Geggel RL. Results of anterograde transcatheter closure of patent ductus arteriosus using single or multiple Gianturco coils. *Am J Cardiol* 1994;74:925–9.

3. Tometzki AJP, Arnold R, Peart I, Sreeram N, Abdulhamed JM, Godman MJ et al. Transcatheter occlusion of the patent ductus arteriosus with Cook detachable coils. *Heart* 1996;76:531–4.

4. Sharafuddin MJ, Gu X, Titus JL, Sakinis AK, Pozza CH, Coleman CC, Cervera-Ceballos JJ, Aideyan OA, Amplatz K. Experimental evaluation of a new self-expanding patent ductus arteriosus occluder in a canine model. *J Vasc Interv Radiol* 1996;7:877–87.

5. Masura J, Walsh KP, Thanopoulous B, Chan C, Bass J, Goussous Y et al. Catheter closure of moderate-large sized patent ductus arteriosus using the new Amplatzer duct occluder: Immediate and short-term results. *J Am Coll Cardiol* 1998;31:878–82.

6. Bilkis AA, Alwi M, Hasri S, Haifa AL, Geetha K, Rehman MA et al. The Amplatzer duct occluder: Experience in 209 patients. *J Am Coll Cardiol* 2001;37:258–61.

7. Thanopoulos BD, Hakim FA, Hiari A, Goussous Y, Basta E, Zarayelyan AA et al. Further experience with transcatheter closure of the patent ductus arteriosus using the Amplatzer duct occluder. *J Am Coll Cardiol* 2000;35:1016–21.

8. Faella HJ, Hijazi ZM. Closure of the patent ductus arteriosus with the Amplatzer PDA device: Immediate results of the international clinical trial. *Catheter Cardiovasc Interv* 2000;51:50–4.

9. Pass RH, Hijazi ZM, Hsu DT, Lewis V, Hellenbrand WE. Multicenter USA Amplatzer patent ductus arteriosus occlusion device trial. *J Am Coll Cardiol* 2004;44:513–19.

10. Kenny D, Morgan GJ, Bentham JR, Wilson N, Martin R, Tometzki A, Oslizlok P, Walsh KP. Early clinical experience with a modified Amplatzer ductal occluder for transcatheter arterial duct occlusion in infants and small children. *Catheter Cardiovasc Interv* 2013 Oct 1;82(4):534–40.

11. Pedra CA, Sanches SA, Fontes VF. Percutaneous occlusion of the patent ductus arteriosus with the Amplatzer device for atrial septal defect. *J Invasive Cardiol* 2003;15(7):413–7.

12. Krichenko A, Benson LN, Burrows P, Möes CA, McLaughlin P, Freedom RM Angiographic classification of the isolated, persistently patent ductus arteriosus and implications for percutaneous catheter occlusion. *Am J Cardiol* 1989;63(12):877–80.

13. Ata JA, Arfi AM, Hussain A, Kouatli AA, Jalal MO. The efficacy and safety of the Amplatzer ductal occluder in young children and infants. *Cardiol Young* 2005;15:279–85.

14. Agnoletti G, Marini D, Villar AM, Bordese R, Gabbarini F. Closure of the patent ductus arteriosus with the new duct occluder II additional sizes device. *Catheter Cardiovasc Interv* 2012;79(7):1169–74.

15. Duke C, Chan KC. Aortic obstruction caused by device occlusion of patent arterial duct. *Heart* 1999; 82(1):109–11.

16. Bhole V, Miller P, Mehta C, Stumper O, Reinhardt Z, DeGiovanni JV. Clinical evaluation of the new Amplatzer duct occluder II for patent arterial duct occlusion. *Catheter Cardiovasc Interv* 2009;74(5):762–9.

17. Gross A, Donnelly JP. Closure of tubular patent ductus arteriosus in infants with the Amplatzer Vascular Plug II. *Catheter Cardiovasc Interv* 2013 Jun 1;81(7):1188–93.

18. Prsa M, Ewert P. Transcatheter closure of a patent ductus arteriosus in a preterm infant with an Amplatzer Vascular Plug IV device. *Catheter Cardiovasc Interv* 2011;77(1):108–11.

19. Kanter JP, Hellenbrand WE, Pass RH. Transcatheter closure of a very large patent ductus arteriosus in a pregnant woman at 22 weeks of gestation. *Catheter Cardiovasc Interv* 2004;61(1):140–3.

20. Roberts P, Adwani S, Archer N, Wilson N. Catheter closure of the arterial duct in preterm infants. *Arch Dis Child Fetal Neonatal Ed* 2007;92(4):F248–50.

21. Bentham J, Meur S, Hudsmith L, Archer N, Wilson N. Echocardiographically guided catheter closure of arterial ducts in small preterm infants on the neonatal intensive care unit. *Catheter Cardiovasc Interv* 2011;77:409–15.

Patent ductus arteriosus (PDA): PDA occlusion with coils

R. Krishna Kumar

Introduction

Gianturco coils were originally developed in the late 1970s and have been used successfully in a variety of situations by interventional radiologists and later by pediatric cardiologists. Since the publication of initial reports in the early 1990s,[1] coil occlusion is now almost universally established as a simple, safe, and effective technique for occlusion of the small (<2 or 3 mm) patent ductus arteriosus (PDA).

Coil occlusion of larger ducts is technically challenging because of a greater tendency for coil embolization. Technical modifications that have been suggested to reduce the risk of embolization include the use of detachable coils, deployment of thicker (0.052") coils, simultaneous deployment of two or more coils, snare-assisted delivery, and bioptome-assisted delivery.[2] Occlusive devices overcome many limitations of the coils for closure of large PDAs and allow for better control. Most institutions now prefer occlusive devices for PDAs that are >3 mm in their narrowest diameter. These devices are, however, considerably more expensive than coils. The bioptome-assisted coil occlusion technique has emerged as a less expensive alternative to the Amplatzer Duct Occluder (ADO).[2] With careful attention to case selection and technique, it is possible to coil occlude a majority of ducts. Furthermore, in specific instances, such as in selected small infants, including preterms, coil occlusion may have an advantage over the ADO.[3] This chapter will describe case selection strategies and the coil occlusion techniques in detail for small as well as large ducts.

Anatomy

The PDA is typically shaped like an asymmetric, truncated cone with considerable variations in its size, shape, and attachment to the aorta (Figure 75.1). The narrowest part of the duct is typically close to the pulmonary arterial (PA) end of the duct, perhaps because of the natural tendency of the duct to close from the PA end. Variations in the size of the ampulla often determine the suitability for coil occlusion. The ampulla in the majority of ducts is large enough to accommodate coils of appropriate size for occluding the PA end. In some instances, however, the ampulla is shallow (Figure 75.1) or absent altogether. The broader aortic end of the ampulla typically originates from the leftward aspect of the aorta. There are variations such as the ductal ampulla being situated entirely to the left of the aorta. Such ducts are typically profiled in the right anterior view (RAO) of the aortogram and may be completely overlapped by the aorta in the left lateral view. Some ducts, particularly the ones seen in early infancy, are tubular (Figure 75.1h) and may be constricted in the middle and, in rare instances, toward the aortic end.

Pathophysiology

Unless the pulmonary vascular resistance is considerably elevated, the PDA shunts continuously from aorta to PA. The duct size and relative resistances of the systemic and pulmonary artery circuits determine the extent of flow reversal that occurs in the proximal descending aorta (Figure 75.2). From the standpoint of coil occlusion, the flow reversal is a useful phenomenon because it can be used for angiographic definition (see section on "Angiography") and for deposition of the coils. The hemodynamic and, therefore, clinical significance of the duct is determined by size, length (longer ducts are likely to offer greater resistance to flows), and age at presentation.

Clinical symptoms and indication for treatment

Moderate or large ducts often require attention in infancy because of symptoms of heart failure, frequent respiratory infections, and failure to thrive. The size of the duct needs to be viewed in the context of the weight and the age of the patient. A 2-mm duct can result in symptoms in a preterm

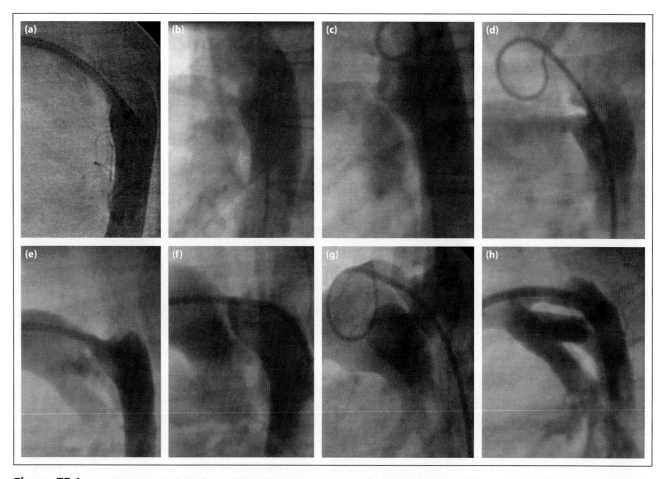

Figure 75.1   Angiograms obtained from eight patients are shown to illustrate the wide variety encountered with the anatomy of the ampulla of the PDA. The angiograms are arranged according to the size of the ampulla from the most shallow (a) to the relatively generous (e, f, g). (h) is an example of a tubular duct. (Also available online at http://www.crcpress.com/product/ISBN/9781482215632, under "Downloads/Updates.")

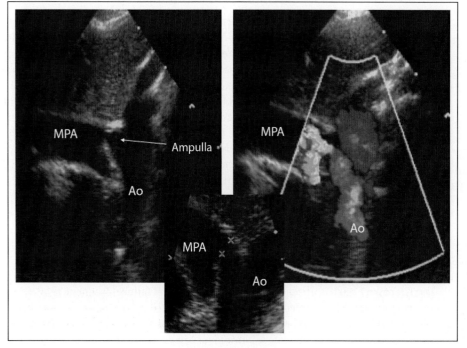

Figure 75.2   (See color insert.) Echo definition of the patent ductus arteriosus. This is a high left parasternal view (ductal view) obtained in an infant. The duct insertion as well as the ampulla is clearly defined. Measurement of the duct insertion site is made in the magnified view (bottom insert). Note the retrograde flow of blood in the color Doppler picture (right). MPA, main pulmonary artery; Ao, aorta. (Also available online at http://www.crcpress.com/product/ISBN/9781482215632, under "Downloads/Updates.")

infant weighing 2 kg or less, whereas a 40 kg adolescent with a 4 mm duct can be symptom-free. Hemodynamically significant ducts (moderate or large) often have symptoms, a wide pulse pressure, active precordial pulsations and, a loud continuous or systolic murmur. These ducts require closure early in infancy.

The hemodynamically insignificant are typically referred because of detection of a continuous or systolic murmur on routine evaluation. Such ducts need not be closed in infancy. The only indication to close these is for the prevention of endarteritis. The timing and indications for closure of small ducts are controversial. Most pediatric cardiologists would hesitate to close clinically silent ducts picked up by color Doppler notwithstanding isolated case reports of ductal endarteritis in patients with a silent PDA. Some pediatric cardiologists recommend closure only if the murmur is continuous.

Precatheter assessment

Clinical evaluation, chest x-ray, and ECG: A good clinical evaluation provides valuable clues on the likely size of the duct and pulmonary blood flow (Table 75.1).

Echocardiography: A detailed echocardiographic evaluation of the duct anatomy and physiology is mandatory for all patients undergoing coil occlusion. Excellent definition of anatomy is feasible in almost all infants and children and in many adults. The duct diameter should be measured in a high parasternal long-axial view at the point of entry into the pulmonary artery (Figure 75.2). The measurement should be made using the zoomed two-dimensional echocardiographic image (Figure 75.2) and not the width of the color Doppler jet. Subtle adjustments in the transducer position and angulations are required for precise definition of the PDA at its pulmonary artery insertion. The maximum diameter at pulmonary artery insertion should be reported. The ductal ampulla is often defined in the high parasternal long-axial or in the suprasternal long-axis view (Figure 75.2). The ductal ampulla is considered adequate if its maximal dimension along the long axis is greater than twice the measured ductal diameter (Figure 75.2). Essentially, one needs to visualize whether a coil that is large enough to occlude the duct can occupy the ampulla without protrusion into the aorta. It is often possible to plan the strategy for coil occlusion based on the echocardiographic anatomy.[2]

Echocardiography provides many clues about the physiologic significance of the duct (Table 75.1). Low velocities in both directions across the PDA together with the absence of flow reversal in the descending aorta suggest elevation in pulmonary vascular resistance. These ducts are typically very large and coil occlusion is often not an acceptable option.

Table 75.1 Precatheter assessment of hemodynamic significance of PDA

Clinical, EKG, x-ray and echo features	Small duct	Large duct with large left-to-right shunt	Large duct with elevated pulmonary vascular resistance
Clinical assessment			
Pulse pressure	Normal	Wide	Normal
Precordium	Normal	Pulsatile, thrill of PDA murmur	Palpable pulmonary artery pulsations and P2
Second heart sound	Normal	Paradoxical	Single, loud P2
Murmur	Continuous (<3/6)	Continuous (>3/6) eddy sounds, apical middiastolic murmur	None or short systolic murmur
ECG	Normal	LV forces, "q" in lateral chest leads	Right ventricular hypertrophy
Chest x-ray			
Heart size, contour	Normal	Enlarged, prominent LV and aorta	Normal heart size, PA prominence
Lung vasculature	Normal	Increased	Prominent hilar vessels, peripheral pruning
Oxygen saturation and blood gas	Normal	Normal	Lower limb desaturation or low PO_2
Echocardiography			
Chamber enlargement	Mild LA, LV enlargement	Significant LA and LV enlargement	LA and LV often normal, RA and RV may be enlarged
Doppler flow across duct	Continuous with diastolic gradients >30 mmHg	Entirely left to right, low diastolic gradients (<300 mmHg)	Bidirectional, right to left during systole, left to right in diastole
Descending aortic flow	Normal or minimal flow reversal in diastole	Prominent flow reversal in diastole	Normal

Additionally, the origins of the branch pulmonary arteries should be carefully inspected for stenosis at their origins. Any internal inconsistencies between duct size estimation and hemodynamic correlates (above) should prompt reassessment of size through repeat measurements.

Case selection

The decision on the closure strategy for PDA is determined by the following considerations:

1. Duct size at its narrowest point (usually at PA insertion)
2. Size of the ampulla
3. Shape of the ampulla
4. Age and weight of the patient

For coil occlusion to be successful, the coil diameters typically have to be greater than or equal to twice the smallest diameter of the duct and the ampulla should be large enough to accommodate the coil(s) (maximum dimension ≥ twice the smallest duct diameter). A conical or funnel-shaped ampulla is best suited for coil occlusion because it allows the coil loops to pack themselves without protrusion into the aorta. Fortunately, the vast majority of ducts have this shape. Tubular ducts have a relatively small diameter at the aortic end. This may prevent some of the coil loops from entering the ampulla as the coil(s) are pulled toward the pulmonary arterial end.

The age and weight of the patient determines the diameter of the descending aorta, which needs to be large enough for the coils to form without straightening up. The maximum size of the delivery system is also determined by the age and weight of the patient. Based on these considerations, the following "rules of thumb" can be used as approximate guides:

1. *Adults and older children (>15 kg):* It is possible to coil occlude most ducts <5 mm in adults and older children and the size of the ampulla is seldom a major consideration. The duct occluder is a better option for ducts >5 mm in diameter, but coil occlusion can be attempted in situations where cost matters.
2. *Infants and young children (5–15 kg):* Ducts that are greater than 5 mm in diameter are often difficult to coil occlude irrespective of the size of the ampulla. Ducts that are 3 mm or smaller can be coil occluded even when the ampulla is small. For ducts that are 3–5 mm in diameter, the size of the ampulla matters (Figure 75.1). The maximum diameter of the ampulla should be greater than or equal to twice the smallest duct diameter. The ADO usually works well as an alternative to coils for this category of patients.
3. *Small infants (<5 kg):* This is a challenging subset of patients. In these patients, coils are often a better alternative to the conventional ADO since they do not protrude into the aorta. An important additional

consideration is the size of the descending aorta. In general, it is difficult to deploy coils larger than 8 mm in diameter. Therefore, ducts larger than 3.5 mm diameter are usually not suited for coil occlusion irrespective of the size of the ampulla. For ducts smaller than 3.5 mm, the same rules (above) apply.

4. *Very small infants and preterm newborns (<2 kg):* Here, the size of the delivery system is an additional concern. Typically, only 4 F delivery systems can be used. Such systems allow a single 0.052 inch coil or two 0.038 inch coils. Coil diameters of 6 mm or more often cannot be used because of the size of the descending aorta. In these babies, ducts >3 mm in diameter should undergo surgery.[3]

Anesthesia

Conscious sedation is usually adequate for most PDA coil occlusion.

Access

For infants and young children with good echocardiographic windows, a venous access with a 5 or 6 F introducer is usually adequate initially and arterial access need not be obtained. After coil occlusion, it is usually possible to evaluate the results through echocardiography in the catheterization laboratory. The advantages of avoiding arterial access include avoiding heparin and thereby potentially accelerating occlusion of the duct, and elimination of inherent risks of arterial puncture such as bleeding and femoral artery thrombosis. If additional coils have to be delivered, it is necessary to obtain arterial access. For this purpose, a 4F introducer sheath is sufficient.

Antibiotic prophylaxis

We prefer to use a single dose of a second-generation cephalosporin (cephazolin) soon after access is obtained.

Hardware

The hardware requirements for PDA coil closure using the techniques described in this chapter are listed in Table 75.2. With an increasing use of magnetic resonance imaging (MRI) in recent years, it is perhaps no longer advisable to use the stainless steel coils. Gianturco coils that are MRI compatible are now available in 0.035 and 0.038 inch diameters in a wide range of sizes.

Hemodynamic evaluations

The pressure in the main pulmonary artery (MPA) often tends to be spuriously high if the catheter tip is close to the duct orifice. The descending aortic pressure should be

Table 75.2 Hardware requirements for coil occlusion of patent ductus arteriosus

Hardware item	Purpose
0.038 inch coils, 4, 5, 6, and 8 mm diameters	Smaller ducts, tubular ducts, additional coils
0.052 inch coils, 6, 8, 10, 12, and 15 mm diameters	Large ducts, they are not generally recommended because they are made of stainless steel and are therefore not MRI compatible
Jackson detachable coils with delivery wire (5–8 mm in diameter)	For operators who prefer controlled release coils for small ducts
Multipurpose catheter 5 F	Crossing the duct initially, free coil delivery
0.038 inch straight-tip, Teflon-coated wire	Crossing the duct initially, free coil delivery
0.038 inch glide wire	Recrossing the duct for additional coil delivery
Right coronary catheter, 4 F, JR 4	Delivering additional coils from the arterial route
Balkan contralateral sheath (Cook) 5.5 F, 6 F, 45-cm-long	Well suited for infants and small children
Mullin sheaths, 7, 8, and 9 F	Older children with large ducts, and F can be used for selected infants and smaller children (>5 kg)
Bioptomes (120 cm long), 3 and 5 F	3 F bioptome can be passed via a 4 F sheath and is well suited for very small infants (<3 kg), for all other situations, the 5 F bioptome is adequate
Amplatz gooseneck snares, 5 and 10 mm	Coil retrieval
Vascular retrieval forceps (3 F)	Coil retrieval

MRI, magnetic resonance imaging.

recorded after the duct is crossed. For calculation of flows and resistances, it is necessary to obtain oxygen saturations from superior vena cava (SVC), branch pulmonary artery, and descending aorta. Again oxygen saturations from the MPA are spuriously high and, thus, shunt quantification in the presence of a duct is often inaccurate.

If the pulmonary vascular resistance is elevated and there are doubts as to whether the PDA closure would reverse the pulmonary artery hypertension, it may be wise to balloon occlude the duct and measure the pulmonary artery pressures. Such ducts are seldom suited for coil occlusion. Few data are currently available on how balloon-occlusion data can be interpreted in hypertensive ducts. From our preliminary experience with 20 patients who had hypertensive ducts, that a decline in PA mean and PA diastolic pressures to less than 25% of the baseline appears to predict a good long-term outcome after duct closure.

Angiography

Aortography for profiling the PDA: If arterial access is obtained, a conventional aortogram in the left lateral view and 45° RAO views with the pigtail catheter in the proximal descending aorta positioned just distal to the ampulla usually allows reasonable definition of the PDA. Large volumes (1–2 mL/kg) at the maximum possible flow rates recommended for the catheter should be used. If the pulmonary arterial end of the duct is not profiled using the conventional aortogram, the pigtail catheter may be passed across the duct and placed in the proximal descending

aorta just beyond the ampulla. Rarely, temporary balloon occlusion of the descending aorta may allow better definition of the PA insertion.

Angiography when arterial access is not obtained: In our institution, we do not routinely obtain arterial access for coil occlusion of PDA in infants and small children.[3] It is still possible to obtain a satisfactory angiographic profile of the PDA without arterial access using techniques outlined below (Videos 75.1 and 75.2).

Angiography before free coil delivery in small ducts: A 5 F multipurpose catheter is used to cross the duct from the MPA with the help of the straight end of a 0.038 inch guide wire. Crossing the duct is usually straightforward. Rarely, difficulty may be encountered if the duct inserts on the superior aspect of the MPA. The duct is profiled in the left lateral view with the tip of the catheter positioned within the ductal ampulla or the proximal descending aorta. The retrograde blood flow into the pulmonary artery (Figure 75.2) and proximal descending thoracic aorta often allows definition of the pulmonary artery insertion of the duct and the ampulla. In patients with very small ducts, where the catheter completely occludes the duct, the injection has to be made in the ductal ampulla close to the pulmonary artery insertion. The relation of the ductal ampulla and its pulmonary artery insertion to the tracheal air shadow should be noted. This injection may be repeated in the 45° RAO view if the ampulla overlaps the aorta.

Angiography before bioptome-assisted coil delivery (Figure 75.3): After obtaining baseline hemodynamic information, a long sheath passed via the femoral vein is positioned across the PDA in the descending aorta over a

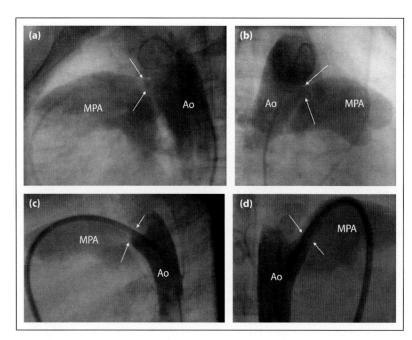

Figure 75.3 Angiograms from selected ducts. Frames (a) and (b) are from an older patient with a relatively shallow duct. Frames (c) and (d) are from an infant. Frame (a) shows a left lateral view of an aortogram. The ampulla is better profiled in this view as compared with frame (b). In the second example, the ampulla appears larger in the right anterior oblique (RAO) view (frame (d)) as compared to the left lateral view (frame (c)). (Also available online at http://www.crcpress.com/product/ISBN/9781482215632, under "Downloads/Updates.")

0.038-inch guide wire (Figure 75.3). Guidelines for selecting the size of the long sheath are shown in Table 75.3. The 45-cm Balkin contralateral introducer sheath (Cook, Bloomington, IN, USA) can be used for the PDA in infants and small children. This sheath has a shape that is well suited for the PDA and comes in sizes from 5.5 F to 7 F. Once the sheath is in the descending aorta, the dilator of the long sheath is removed. With the guide wire in place, the sheath is withdrawn until the aortic end of the ductal ampulla. A hand injection of 5–10 mL of contrast into the sheath in the lateral and 45° RAO views usually allows excellent definition of the ductal ampulla and measurement of duct diameter at pulmonary insertion.

Measurements: The maximum diameter of the PA end of the PDA should be measured. The lateral view is usually better suited for this purpose. The diameter of the pulmonary arterial end of the duct varies with the cardiac cycle and the largest diameter should be identified through careful frame-by-frame evaluation.

Ductal spasm: Ductal spasm is not infrequent in infants and may be provoked by attempts to cross it, although on occasions it may occur spontaneously.

We prefer to use the echocardiographic measurement of the duct size to guide the choice of coil diameter unless the angiographic measurement is larger.

Deployment technique

Free coil delivery: This is essentially applicable for the small duct (<2.5 mm in diameter). An MRI-compatible Gianturco

Table 75.3 Coil combination and sheath sizes for bioptome-assisted occlusion of patent arterial ducts larger than 2.5 mm

Duct size	Suggested coil combination[a]	Minimum size of the long sheath
2.5–3 mm	Two 0.038 inch 6 mm–6 cm coils	4 F[b]
3–3.5 mm	Two 0.038 inch 8 mm–8 cm coils	4 F[b]
3.5–4 mm	Three 0.038 inch 8 mm–8 cm coils	6 F
4–5 mm	Duct occluder preferred, four coils 8–10 mm in diameter may be considered in exceptional circumstances	7 F
>5 mm	Usually not suited for coil occlusion	

Note: F, French.

[a] Coils should all be magnetic resonance imaging compatible. Coil lengths have not been specified; usually, coil lengths (in cm) that are same as the coil diameters (in mm) are adequate. For PDA with a shallow ampulla in infants and small children; however, coil turns have to be cut to ensure that the coil turns fit into the ampulla.

[b] 3 F bioptome will need to be used if a 4 F sheath is to be used. For all other situations, a 5 F bioptome is adequate.

coil with a diameter of at least twice the measured ductal diameter is chosen. Typically, this is a 5-mm-diameter coil. The length of the coil is determined by the size of the ampulla. Shorter coils, such as the 3–4-cm-long coils, are chosen for patients with relatively shallow ampullae to prevent coil loops from protruding into the aortic lumen. We prefer coil deployment from the venous route as it allows better control of coil deployment than the arterial route. The technique for arterial delivery of coils is described below in the section "Delivery of additional coils."

The duct is crossed from the pulmonary artery using a 5 F multipurpose catheter. After the catheter is advanced into the descending aorta, it should be flushed to clear the contrast. The coil is introduced into the catheter and advanced to its tip. Between one and a half to two turns of the coil are released into the descending aorta. The coil/catheter assembly is then pulled together as one unit to the mouth of the ampulla using the tracheal air shadow as the visual landmark for the position of the ampulla and pulmonary arterial insertion. A pulsatile flow in the aorta causes oscillatory movement of the coil turns in the descending aorta. As the coil is pulled toward the pulmonary end of the ductal ampulla, abrupt cessation of oscillations of the coil occurs and this can be used as an indicator that the coil is positioned in the ductal ampulla. At this point, additional turns of the coil should be delivered. The catheter should then be pulled back into the pulmonary artery when less than half a turn remains in the catheter. The coil should be released by gently pulling back the catheter into the MPA. Three minutes after the successful release of the coil, echocardiography should be performed for assessment of residual flow across the duct as well as turbulence at the origin of the left pulmonary artery. If there is a clearly defined color jet of residual flow at 3 min, additional coils (see section on "Delivery of additional coils") may need to be delivered. For patients with small, poorly defined residual color flow, imaging can be repeated on the table every few minutes. If the flow shows a tendency to diminish over the next 10 min, catheters may be removed.

Detachable coils: To decrease the incidence of coil embolization, the controlled-release modified Jackson detachable coils (Cook PDA coils) are a useful but more expensive alternative to free coils for small ducts. The spring coil (similar in shape and size to the Gianturco coils) has a central lumen through which the delivery wire or mandrill is passed. Interlocking screws between the spring coil and the delivery wire help in holding the coil until the correct position is achieved in the duct. The delivery wire is introduced into the sleeve housing the coil and rotated clockwise until the screw locks with the coil. The coil is deployed in a manner identical to that of free coils, but by withdrawal of the mandrill, which allows coil loops to form. The coil is released by unscrewing the wire (counterclockwise rotation) once the position is deemed satisfactory.[4]

Bioptome-assisted coil delivery

Coil selection (Table 75.3): Gianturco coils (Cook) with diameters at least twice the measured duct diameters at the PA end are chosen. We prefer to use the echocardiographic measurement to guide coil selection unless the duct diameter by angiography is larger than the echo measurement. It is preferable to use simultaneously delivered multiple coils for ducts that measure more than 2.5 mm in diameter. This usually results in a higher immediate occlusion rates. Suggested coil diameters and coil combinations for various duct sizes are shown in Table 75.3.

Coil preparation (Figure 75.4): Coils are housed in steel tubing with a black sleeve at one of its ends. A wire introduced from the end with the black sleeve pushes out the coil. The round ball at the tip of the coil that emerges from the tube is stretched out by about 2 mm using a hemostat. If multiple coils are used, the stretched-out ends are secured together using 3-0 prolene suture. A 120-cm-long bioptome (3 F for preterms and 5 F for older infants) passed via a short introducer sheath (one size smaller than the long sheath used for deployment of the coils in the PDA). The secured end of the coils is grasped by the bioptome. It is important to ensure that the coil is firmly held by the jaws of the bioptome. The coils are then pulled into the short sheath by the bioptome. The short sheath essentially serves as an introducer for delivering the coils into the long sheath that is previously positioned across the duct. If it is anticipated that the coil turns would not fit into the ampulla, between 1/2 to 2 coil turns should be cut with a scissor. The cut end of the coil should be inspected for sharp edges and a few more millimeters of the coil can be cut to ensure smoothness. Cutting off the end of the coil is often necessary in infants.

Deployment of coils (Figure 75.5): Videos 75.3–75.7 show the deployment sequence. Videos 75.8–75.13 show deployment sequence in preterm infants. The coils are delivered via the long sheath until one to two loops are extruded out of the tip of the sheath in the descending thoracic aorta. The side arm of the sheath should be connected to the pressure transducer. The entire assembly is pulled back toward the pulmonary artery until the sheath tip is just beyond the ductal ampulla. Coils are almost entirely brought out of the sheath. Typically, the retrograde flow across the duct pushes the entire coil mass into the ampulla. There is an abrupt cessation of oscillatory movements together with compaction of the coils as they enter the ductal ampulla. All coil turns should compact in the ampulla. This is sometimes difficult to ensure when coil diameters are very large. The tracheal air shadow serves as an additional landmark to guide the coil placement. The relationship of the tracheal air shadow to the ductal ampulla and the pulmonary arterial end of the duct is previously identified in the ductal angiogram. Once the coils compact in the ampulla, the sheath is slowly pulled

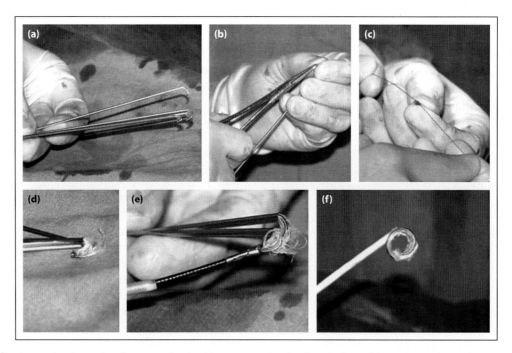

Figure 75.4 **(See color insert.)** Coil preparation for bioptome-assisted coil occlusion. This sequence shows the preparation of four coils for simultaneous deployment in a 6 mm duct. The deployment sequence is shown in Figure 75.5. A small segment of each coil is brought out of the steel tubing (a). The ends of the coil are stretched out using a hemostat (b). The stretched-out ends are secured together using a 3-0-prolene suture (c and d). A 5 F bioptome is passed through a short (8 F) introducer (e), the secured end of the coil is held by the jaws of the bioptome and pulled into the introducer (f). (Also available online at http://www.crcpress.com/product/ISBN/9781482215632, under "Downloads/Updates.")

back until the pressure recorded from the side arm of the sheath declines, indicating that the tip of the sheath is now in the pulmonary artery. At this point, the bioptome is slowly pulled back until a small part of the coil protrudes into the pulmonary artery. Some resistance is felt at this stage. There is further compaction of the coil turns in the ampulla. Efforts should be made, as far as possible, to leave less than half a turn to protrude into the pulmonary artery. Contrast injection through the side arm can be made to ensure that the coils are correctly positioned and there is free flow into the branch pulmonary arteries. The jaw of the bioptome should be released soon after a satisfactory position is obtained. Attempts to hold the coils for longer periods should be avoided because this often results in one or more coil turns being inadvertently pulled into the pulmonary artery. In the event that the coils are too small for the duct, one or more turns or the entire coil mass can be pulled into the pulmonary artery by the bioptome. The coils can be withdrawn into the sheath and redeployed after the addition of another larger coil to the coil mass. An echocardiogram or aortogram (if arterial access was obtained) should be performed after 3 min. Additional 0.038 inch coils are delivered if a well-defined jet of residual flow was demonstrable by either color Doppler or angiography (see section on "Delivery of additional coils"). Small diffuse whiffs of flow often disappear over the next 12–24 hours.

Delivery of additional coils

Delivery of additional coils is contemplated whenever there is an unacceptable amount of residual flow (a clearly defined color jet on Doppler, or filling of the entire MPA on angiography). It is advisable to obtain arterial access if the duct needs to be recrossed. A 4 F introducer sheath can be used for this purpose. Heparin needs to be administered at this stage. The duct is crossed from the aortic aspect using a 0.035 inch glide wire (Terumo or Roadrunner, Cook) and a 4 F right coronary catheter. The regular hydrophilic guide wire should not be used because of the possibility of the Dacron fibers of the previously deployed coils getting entangled with the wire. Once the wire is across the duct, the catheter should be gently advanced over the wire. Some resistance is usually encountered when the catheter crosses the previously deployed coils. The catheter position should be confirmed through pressure measurement or contrast injection. Irrespective of the initial size of the duct, additional coils should be 5 mm in diameter. The length of the coil is determined by the size of the ampulla. In general, 5-cm-long coils work well as additional coils in most situations. The technique of coil delivery from the arterial route is different from the venous route. Half a turn of the coil is brought out of the tip of the 4 F catheter positioned in the MPA across the duct. The catheter is slowly pulled back until the protruding half turn reaches the PA end of

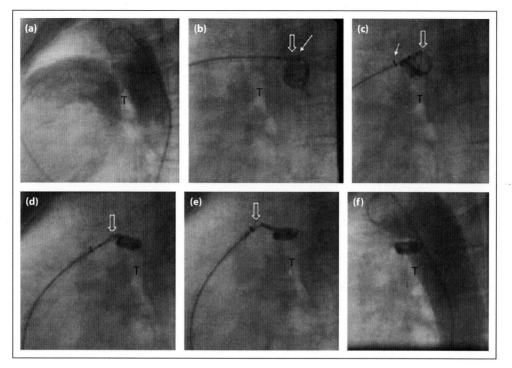

Figure 75.5 Bioptome-assisted simultaneous deployment of multiple coils. Frame (a) shows an aortogram in the left lateral view. The duct measured 6 mm. Four coils (two 12 mm 0.052 inch coils and two 8 mm 0.038 inch coils are simultaneously held by a 5 F bioptome and brought out of a 9 F long sheath placed across the duct in the descending aorta (b). The block arrow points at the jaws of the bioptome and the smaller arrow indicates the tip of the sheath. The assembly is pulled back until the tip of the sheath is in the MPA. This is recognized by a decline in pressure in the side arm of the long sheath. This event coincides with the coils moving into the ampulla. The coils start to compact at this stage (c). The bioptome is then gently pulled into the MPA (d) and the jaws of the bioptome are opened after a small length (< half a turn) of coil protrudes into the MPA (e). Frame (f) shows an angiogram obtained 3 min after release. The tracheal air shadow (T) serves as an additional guide for the coil positioning. (Also available online at http://www.crcpress.com/product/ISBN/9781482215632, under "Downloads/Updates.")

the duct. The coil is then delivered by slowly withdrawing the catheter while keeping the guide wire in the catheter in close contact with the coil. Catheter withdrawal tends to pull the protruding coil out of the MPA and guide wire advancement may result in excessive coil protrusion. Coil delivery has to be accomplished in small steps, ensuring at all times that the coil length protruding out into the MPA is kept constant at half a turn until a substantial length of coil is exposed out of the catheter. Advancing the catheter toward the ampulla usually results in the formation of coil turns that should be positioned in the ampulla. Hand injections of contrast 3 min after coil delivery should be made to assess residual flows.

Troubleshooting

Difficulty in crossing the duct from the pulmonary arterial end: Difficulties may occasionally be encountered in adult patients and in ducts inserted onto the proximal MPA on its superior aspect. These ducts may be crossed from the aortic end using a right coronary or multipurpose catheter. A guide wire can be passed through this catheter and its tip can be held with a snare passed from the venous catheter.

The venous catheter is simply advanced through the PDA while holding the wire tip.

Unsatisfactory coil position in the PDA: This may result from excessive deployment of the coil turns in either the aortic or pulmonary end of the PDA. With excessive deployment at the aortic end, aortic embolization is likely, especially if the coil turns oscillate with pulsatile aortic flows. Rarely, the coil turns may protrude into the aorta sufficiently to result in a gradient in the descending aorta. Excessive coil turns in the pulmonary artery may result in stenosis of the left pulmonary artery at its origin. If the coil position is deemed unsatisfactory, the coils should be retrieved (below) and redeployed.

Embolization to the branch pulmonary arteries: Typically, this happens soon after coil release. The dislodged coils usually embolize to the proximal right or left pulmonary arteries if they are large and if multiple coils are used. Single coils usually embolize distally to smaller branches. There is no need to panic because hemodynamic instability does not usually result from the event. The long sheath should be retained in the MPA. A 4 F multipurpose catheter or the 4 F snare catheter should be passed via the long sheath and positioned near the embolized coil mass with the help of a glide wire. Small contrast injections in multiple views allow precise determination of the vessel into which the coil has embolized. An Amplatz gooseneck snare (5 mm for children and small vessel embolization, 10 mm for other situations) should be used to grasp the coil tip. When multiple coils have been used for PDA closure, it is important to hold the coils at the sutured end. The coils must be captured into the long sheath in the pulmonary artery because it is important to prevent the coil mass from being entangled in the tricuspid valve tensor apparatus.

Embolization to the descending thoracic aorta: When the coil(s) embolize into the aorta, the duct should be immediately recrossed with a 5 F multipurpose catheter or snare catheter. A 10 mm Amplatz gooseneck snare (Microvena, MN, USA) should be used to hold the end of the coil(s) and the same coil(s) can be deployed in the duct once again as the catheter is pulled back toward the MPA.

Loss of grip on the coil mass: The jaws of the bioptome may occasionally lose their grip on the coil mass when coils are being pulled back into the long sheath after an initial unsatisfactory deployment. A variable part of the coil remains in the sheath. Attempts to recapture the coils with the bioptome may push the coils out of the sheath. A 3 F vascular retrieval forceps (Cook) works well in this situation. The tip of the vascular retrieval forceps has a short (3 cm), soft guide wire that can be positioned adjacent to the coil tip in the sheath. The jaws of the forceps open adequately enough to grasp the coil tip and retrieve the coil mass.

Inability to release the coil after bioptome jaws are opened: Occasionally, a coil tip remains in the jaws after they are opened. The coils can be released by slow rotation of the bioptome with the jaws open. Alternatively, advancing the long sheath to the partially open jaws of the bioptome helps in the release of the coil.

Hemolysis from residual flow: Hemolysis is a rare but serious complication of coil occlusion.[5] For hemolysis to occur, there often has to be clearly defined residual flow at the end of the procedure together with an audible murmur. Once hemolysis is established, it is often difficult to eliminate flows and many additional coils may be required. It is therefore important to be aggressive, and early intervention should be considered if residual flows are significant

Postprocedure management

The patient may be sent home 6–8 hours after the procedure once recovery from sedation or anesthesia is complete, especially if arterial access has not been used. We consider it mandatory to obtain an echocardiogram just prior to discharge for residual flows across the PDA, left pulmonary artery (LPA) turbulence, and aortic flows and

ventricular function. A small fraction of patients develop varying degrees of left ventricular dysfunction immediately after duct closure. We suggest antibiotic prophylaxis for endocarditis 6 months after the procedure. We also recommend follow-up echocardiography, 3 months after the procedure and yearly thereafter.

Long-term concerns

Compatibility with MRI: The conventional stainless steel coils are not MR compatible and likely to produce artifacts during imaging. Most manufacturers have started to make coils using materials that are MRI compatible. The 0.052 inch coils are still made of stainless steel. This is an important limitation that needs to be overcome by manufacturers in the future.

Stenosis of the left pulmonary artery origin: It is important, particularly in infants, to avoid excess coil protrusion into the left pulmonary artery; both after initial deployment and during follow-up, the LPA flows should be carefully evaluated by color Doppler.

Residual flows and recanalization: Residual flows at 24 hours may occasionally persist. In addition, a small proportion of completely occluded ducts (0.3% our experience) may recanalize. The indication for repeat coil occlusion is not clear. We recommend coil occlusion if a murmur is audible.

Acknowledgments

The author wishes to acknowledge assistance from Dr. BRJ Kannan, Dr. SR Anil, Dr. K. Sivakumar, and Dr. Balu Vaidyanathan for their inputs, which have helped refine the technique; Arun and the catheter laboratory staff in their assistance with illustrations; and Dr. Prakash Kamath for reviewing the manuscript.

References

1. Lloyd TR, Fedderly R, Mendelsohn AM, Sandhu SK, Beekman RH III. Transcatheter occlusion of patent ductus arteriosus with Gianturco coils. *Circulation* 1993;88:1412–20.
2. Kumar RK, Anil SR, Philip A, Sivakumar K, Bioptome-assisted coil occlusion of moderate-large patent arterial ducts in infants and small children. *Catheter Cardiovasc Interv* 2004;62:266–71.
3. Francis E, Singhi A, Srinivas L, Kumar RK, Transcatheter occlusion of patent ductus arteriosus in preterm infants. *J Am Coll Cardiol Interv* 2010;3:550–5.
4. Tometzki AJP, Arnold R, Peart N et al. Transcatheter closure of patent ductus arteriosus with Cook detachable coils. *Heart* 1996;76:531–5.
5. Anil SR, Sivakumar K, Philip A, Francis E, Kumar RK, Management strategies for hemolysis after transcatheter closure of the patent arterial duct, *Catheter Cardiovasc Interv* 2003;59:538–43.

76

Patent ductus arteriosus (PDA): Aortopulmonary window

Shakeel A. Qureshi

Introduction

Aortopulmonary window is a relatively uncommon congenital cardiac abnormality. It is characterized by an abnormal communication between the ascending aorta and the pulmonary trunk or the right pulmonary artery.[1] Aortopulmonary window has also been termed "aortopulmonary septal defect," but there is usually no septum between the arterial trunks.[1-3] It usually occurs just above the two normally formed aortic and pulmonary valves and always above the aortic sinuses. It may occur as an isolated lesion and may also occur in association with a variety of other congenital cardiac defects.[4-6] The most common associated defect is interruption of the aortic arch or severe preductal aortic coarctation. Other defects include origin of the right pulmonary artery from the ascending aorta, tetralogy of Fallot, pulmonary atresia with ventricular septal defect or ventricular septal defect, aortic atresia and interruption of the aortic arch.[7-11]

The incidence of this defect is about 0.2%.[12,13] Although there is a recognized association between aortic arch abnormalities and 22q11 deletion, this has rarely been reported with aortopulmonary window.[14]

Morphology and classification

The aortopulmonary septum is formed during early embryogenesis by the opposing truncal cushions, which fuse to divide the truncus arteriosus into aortic and pulmonary channels. An aortopulmonary window is the result of malformation in the division of this trunk.[15] Kutsche and Van Mierop defined three types of aortopulmonary window[12]:

1. A defect with a circular border between the arterial valves and the bifurcation of the main pulmonary artery

2. A similarly located fenestration in which the border represents a helix
3. A large defect with no posterior or distal border

Kutsche and Van Mierop proposed a different pathogenesis for these three types, such as nonfusion of the embryonic aortopulmonary and truncal septums in the first, malalignment of the aortopulmonary and truncal septums in the second, and total absence of the embryonic aortopulmonary septum in the third.[12]

Other classifications are based on the pathologic and angiographic anatomy and have undergone modifications.[2,7]

Mori et al. categorized aortopulmonary windows into three types[7]:

Type I: These defects occur in the proximal part of the aortopulmonary septum and are located just above the arterial valves. These occur in 70–96% of cases.
Type II: These defects occur in the distal part of the aortopulmonary septum adjacent to the right pulmonary artery. These occur in 14–25% of cases and may also be associated with interruption of the aortic arch.
Type III: These are large confluent defects with total absence of the aortopulmonary septum and occur in about 5% of cases.

This classification was modified into four types by Ho et al.[2,6,16]:

Type I: These are proximal defects ascending aorta and the main pulmonary artery, with little inferior rim separating the window from the arterial valves.
Type II: Distal defects are located in the upper part of the ascending aorta and involve the origin of the right pulmonary artery or the pulmonary artery bifurcation. These have a well-formed inferior rim, but very little superior rim. This defect may be associated with the origin of the right pulmonary artery from the aorta.

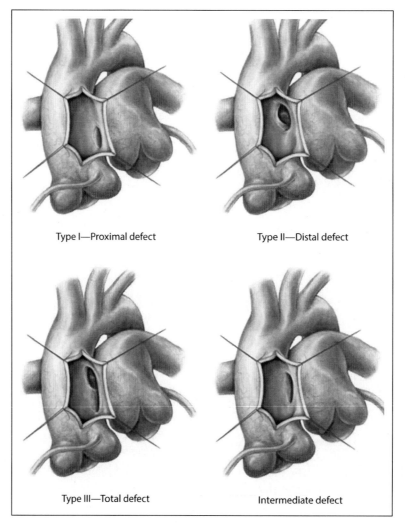

Type I—Proximal defect

Type II—Distal defect

Type III—Total defect

Intermediate defect

Figure 76.1 **(See color insert.)** Classification of aortopulmonary windows. (Reprinted from *Eur J Cardiovasc Surg*, 21, Backer CL, Mavroudis C., Surgical management of aortopulmonary window: A 40 year experience, 773–9, Copyright 2002, with permission from Elsevier.)

Type III: A confluent defect, which is a combination of type I and II defects. These have little superior and inferior rims.

Type IV: Intermediate defects with adequate superior and inferior rims, which tend to be suitable for possible transcatheter device closure (Figure 76.1).

Presentation and management

An aortopulmonary window results in a significant systemic-to-pulmonary artery shunt at the arterial level, which is hemodynamically similar to a large patent arterial duct. The clinical presentation depends on the size of the defect, the timing of the fall of pulmonary vascular resistance after birth, and the presence of other congenital cardiac defects. The symptoms and signs of congestive cardiac failure include failure to thrive, recurrent chest infections, and the development of pulmonary hypertension.[13] Newborn babies may present with these symptoms during the first few weeks of life. The signs of a large window include tachypnea, wide

pulse pressure, a loud second sound, while in a small to moderate window, there may be a continuous murmur at the upper left sternal border with a normal second sound. These patients with small- to medium-sized defects may either be asymptomatic and present with a murmur or have recurrent chest infections. The patients with uncorrected defects may die during the first few years of life from congestive cardiac failure. The signs have to be differentiated from a patent arterial defect.

Treatment is usually needed as soon as the diagnosis is confirmed in order to prevent the development of irreversible pulmonary vascular disease. Occasionally, patients with smaller aortopulmonary windows with good superior and inferior rims may be managed conservatively until they are old enough to undergo transcatheter treatment. However, reports on the treatment and outcome are limited to relatively small group of patients, who have usually undergone surgery.[6,17–22]

In most centers, surgery is performed as soon as the diagnosis is confirmed after birth.[5,6,16,21,23] In patients in whom the diagnosis is made late, pulmonary vascular resistance should be estimated during cardiac catheterization to assess operability.[5,6,17]

Since the first successful repair by Gross in 1952,[8] several surgical techniques have been used, from less invasive simple ligation or division without cardiopulmonary bypass to patch closure of the defect under direct vision, using cardiopulmonary bypass.[5,6,18–21,24,25] Simple ligation or division is associated with a relatively high complication rate, such as recanalization, bleeding, pulmonary artery narrowing, distortion of the arterial valves, and impinging on the left coronary artery. This may be due to inadequate preoperative definition of the defect morphology, combined with dissection around the window. Nowadays, division of the window is reserved for the simple types of relatively small-sized defects located midway between the arterial valves and pulmonary artery bifurcation. However, these defects may be amenable to transcatheter closure with a device. This was first reported in a residual defect by Stamato et al.[26] The larger defects are better treated surgically using a Dacron patch from the aortic end, especially if the presentation is in the newborn period. The prognosis in those patients treated early in infancy is excellent.

The diagnosis can be confirmed by cross-sectional and color Doppler echocardiography.[10,27] Occasionally, magnetic resonance imaging and computerized tomographic scanning may be needed, especially when there are other associated defects. Cardiac catheterization is only needed if there are concerns about the development of pulmonary vascular disease or when operability of the defect needs to be determined. On transthoracic echocardiography, the defect may be visualized with a high parasternal short-axis views with cranial angulation.[26] The size and the location of the defect as well as its relationship to the surrounding structures such as the pulmonary valve, origin of the right pulmonary artery, and left coronary artery also need to be assessed (Figure 76.2). The high pulmonary artery pressure and pulmonary vascular resistance results in a low-velocity flow across the defect, which may be difficult to detect with color Doppler flow. If the patient is given a high concentration of oxygen for several minutes, this may decrease the pulmonary vascular resistance and increase left-to-right shunting on color Doppler echocardiography. Nowadays, cardiac catheterization should be reserved for the determination of pulmonary vascular resistance, or if catheter closure is to be attempted.

Transcatheter closure

Suitability for device closure of aortopulmonary windows should be determined by a combination of echocardiography, magnetic resonance imaging, and computerized tomographic scanning (Figure 76.3a–c). These will help to exclude those patients in whom device closure should not be attempted because of the size of the defect and its proximity to the arterial valves, the left coronary artery in

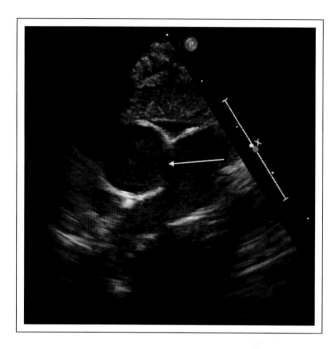

Figure 76.2   Cross-sectional echocardiographic image of an aortopulmonary window (arrow).

particular, and the pulmonary arteries. Various devices have been used to close aortopulmonary windows. In the past, a double-umbrella occluder system or a buttoned device has been used, but nowadays, better and more suitable devices include the Amplatzer Duct Occluder I (ADO I), Amplatzer Septal Occluder (ASO), or ventricular septal defect closure device, or devices of similar shapes.[28–34]

For device closure, the aortopulmonary window should be located in the middle of the two great arteries at least 5 mm from the origin of the left coronary artery and the bifurcation of the pulmonary artery and there should be no anomalous origin of the right or left pulmonary arteries from the aorta.[28]

Technique

Cardiac catheterization is performed either under sedation and regional anesthesia or general anesthesia. General anesthesia may be better, as the technique can be complex. Transesophageal echocardiographic guidance during the procedure is extremely important and if used, the procedure should be performed under general anesthesia. Access is obtained in the right femoral vein and artery and sheaths of 4–6 Fr are inserted, depending on the age and weight of the patient. Heparin 50–100 units/kg should be given intravenously and activated clotting time should be maintained at 200–250 s. Hemodynamic measurements and blood samples for oximetry are obtained from all the right and left heart chambers to determine the Qp:Qs ratio.

Angiography is performed in the aortic root using a pigtail catheter in a 20–30° left anterior oblique projection

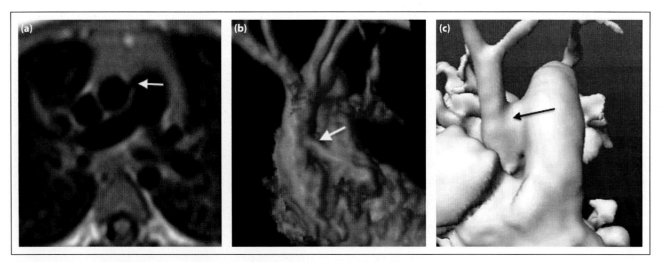

Figure 76.3 **(See color insert.)** (a) A black blood magnetic resonance image of an aortopulmonary window (arrow). (b) A 3D reconstruction magnetic resonance image of the same patient showing the window (arrow). This patient was suitable for transcatheter device closure. (c) 3D magnetic resonance image of another patient with a large window, which needed surgical repair.

with cranial angulation of about 15–20 degrees combined with a 20–30° right anterior oblique projection (Figure 76.4). Although various measurements should be obtained by other forms of imaging before the procedure, measurements are repeated to determine the angiographic size of the defect, its distance from the origin of the left coronary artery, and from both the arterial valves and the bifurcation of the pulmonary trunk. A 4 or 5 Fr Judkins right coronary or Amplatz right coronary catheter is used to cross the defect from the ascending aorta. At the same time, a 5 or 6 Fr snare catheter is positioned in the pulmonary artery, with a snare of 10–20 mm diameter, depending on

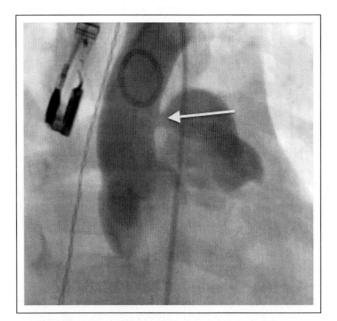

Figure 76.4 An ascending aortogram in a right anterior oblique projection. There is a small aortopulmonary window away from both arterial valves (arrow).

the size of the main pulmonary artery (Microvena, White Bearlake, MN, USA) (Figure 76.5a). A 260-cm-long 0.035 inch Terumo guide wire (Terumo Medical Corporation, Tokyo, Japan) or Bentson wire (Cook, Bloomington, IN, USA) are introduced through the arterial catheter to cross the defect and enter the main pulmonary artery. Usually, the guide wire enters the main pulmonary artery and passes toward the bifurcation, where it can be snared (Figure 76.5b). Occasionally, it may cross the pulmonary valve and enter the right ventricle, in which case attempts could be made to pass across the tricuspid valve through the right atrium into the superior vena cava, where it can also be snared. If the latter option is taken, care should be taken to assess that the catheter does not entangle with the tricuspid valve chordae. Once the right heart end of the guide wire has been snared, it is withdrawn carefully out of the femoral vein to establish an arteriovenous guide wire circuit. Either this guide wire can be used to pass a sheath appropriate for the device or the guide wire may be exchanged for a stiff Amplatz 0.035 inch exchange length J-tipped guide wire. Very occasionally, it may be possible to cross the window from an antegrade venous route, but in either case, obtaining an arteriovenous guide wire circuit helps to perform the procedure more rapidly.

Sizing of the defect

Although sizing of the defect may be performed by balloon occlusion or a static balloon technique, this information should be available from the previous imaging techniques.[29] Occasionally, an end-hole balloon wedge catheter, which can accommodate a 0.035 inch guide wire, such as a 6 or 7 Fr Swan–Ganz catheter, is passed over the guide wire from the femoral vein across the defect into the ascending aorta. The balloon is inflated with diluted contrast to a

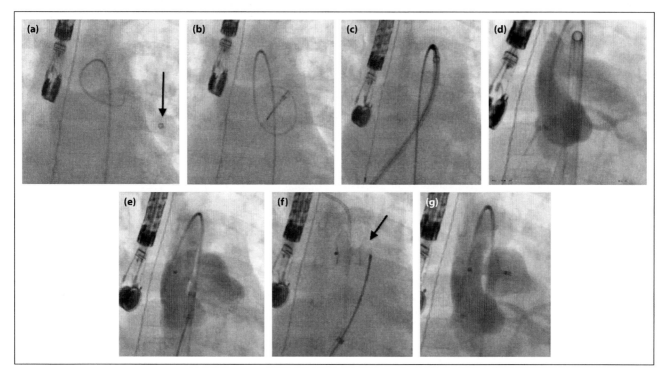

Figure 76.5   (a) A catheter passed from the femoral artery across the aortopulmonary window in the main pulmonary artery. There is a snare catheter already positioned in the left pulmonary artery (arrow). (b) Guide wire snared in the main pulmonary artery. (c) A device-delivery sheath, which has been passed from the femoral vein over the arteriovenous guide wire circuit into the ascending aorta. (d) An ascending aortogram with a delivery sheath having been passed over the guide wire circuit and positioned in the descending aorta. (e) An ascending aortogram after one disk of an Amplatzer Septal Occluder has been opened in the aortic side of the window. (f) Both disks of the Amplatzer Septal Occluder across the aortopulmonary window (arrow). (g) An ascending aortogram after release of the occluder in the aortopulmonary window. Some residual flow is present, which usually disappears within 24 hours.

size bigger than the defect. It is slowly withdrawn into the defect. If transesophageal echocardiography is used, this will help in determining balloon occlusion of the defect. If not, transthoracic echocardiography with color Doppler will also provide important information. Otherwise, a second arterial access may be useful to perform additional angiograms with the balloon inflated or a smaller 4 Fr pigtail catheter is passed through the original femoral arterial sheath alongside the circuit guide wire. By applying gentle traction on the balloon catheter to slow deflation, the catheter is withdrawn slowly until it pops through the defect. The size of the inflated balloon, as it pops through the defect can be measured from fluoroscopy by using catheter calibration or by inflating the exteriorized balloon with the same volume of contrast, on a sizing plate to obtain.

Alternatively, a static balloon method may be helpful.[29] An Amplatzer sizing balloon of 18 mm diameter is passed from the femoral vein over the guide wire circuit and is positioned across the defect. However, this method requires a larger sheath to be placed in the femoral vein. The balloon is inflated to 1–1.5 atmospheres to avoid stretching the defect. A further alternative is to use a low-pressure valvoplasty balloon, such as Tyshak (NuMED, Hopkinton, NY, USA), but care needs to be applied not to overdilate

the defect. The waist on the balloon is then measured. The static balloon method requires speedy inflation and deflation, as the inflated balloon may obstruct both the aorta and the pulmonary artery. It is preferable to avoid balloon sizing, if at all possible.

Selection of device

Nowadays, devices such as the double-umbrella types are not available and the buttoned device is rarely used. A wider choice of improved devices is available but none are specific to the aortopulmonary window. These devices are normally used to close patent arterial defects, ventricular septal defects, or atrial septal defects.[28,29,31–35] The selection may be an operator preference, but is also determined by the space available in the main pulmonary artery. Devices with two disks are likely to be better than a device with a disk only on the aortic side. Nevertheless, Amplatzer Duct Occluder (ADO I) has been used to close aortopulmonary windows, although the device protrudes into the pulmonary artery.[29,34–41] Better alternatives may be the Amplatzer muscular ventricular septal defect occluder or ASO, or similarly shaped devices available from several other manufacturers.[31,39] The device selected should be about 2–3 mm larger than the measured defect.

Delivery of the device

Once the type and the size of the device has been chosen, either an appropriate sized 6–8 Fr Mullins sheath or a kink-resistant sheath that is available with the device is introduced over the guide wire circuit from the femoral vein. It is advanced well into the ascending aorta or the aortic arch and even into the descending aorta, before the guide wire circuit is broken and removed. After breaking the guide wire circuit, a pigtail catheter is passed to the ascending aorta for subsequent angiography (Figure 76.5d). The selected device is then attached to the delivery cable and slowly advanced to the tip of the sheath in the aorta. The retention disk of the ADO I or the distal disk of the ASO or VSD occluder is opened in the aorta and the entire assembly is withdrawn slowly to the opening of the defect under fluoroscopic and echocardiographic guidance. An ascending aortogram is performed to confirm the position of the device in relation to the origin of left coronary artery (Figure 76.5e). Keeping steady traction on the delivery cable, the remaining part of the device is opened in the pulmonary artery by slowly withdrawing the sheath (Figure 76.5f). Correct positioning of the device and occlusion of the defect are confirmed by a combination of echocardiography and angiography and the device is released (Figure 76.5g). After removal of the sheaths, hemostasis is achieved by manual pressure.

As an alternative to ASO device, the ADO I device may be used in a native aortopulmonary window (Figure 76.6a and b) and indeed ADO II has also been used in a postsurgical window.[41]

After the procedure, the patient should be carefully monitored for 24 hours. Very occasionally, because of some residual flow, hemolysis may occur but this should settle very quickly with fluid hydration and conservative management. Prior to discharge, a chest x-ray and echocardiogram are repeated to confirm satisfactory results. The possibility of device embolization, although small, exists.

Antiplatelet agents such as aspirin 75 mg once daily alone or in combination with clopidogrel 75 mg once daily are given for at least 6 months.

Use of antibiotics during and after the procedure depends on the local practice, but generally the procedure should be covered by antibiotics.

Follow-up involves clinical and cross-sectional and color Doppler echocardiography at 1 month and approximately 6–12 months, after which the clinician needs to determine the frequency of follow-up visits. The follow-up is important to assess the presence of a residual shunt, possible stenosis of the pulmonary artery, and thrombus formation.

Discussion

Although patent arterial defects have been closed with devices for over two decades, aortopulmonary windows are rare and so only case reports have been published.[26,29,31–41] Most infants presenting with aortopulmonary windows require early correction at the time of diagnosis.[5,6,16–19,21,23,25] Results of surgical correction of windows over a 40 year period have revealed a steady decline in mortality from 37% to almost 0% with the advances in both diagnostic and the operative techniques.[6] Nowadays, most children are treated in the neonatal period or early infancy, thus preventing late complications such as pulmonary vascular disease. McElhinney et al. reported on 24 patients, who had surgery at a mean age of 34 days and all the patients were under 6 months of age. In the 12 patients with an isolated window, there were no early or late deaths.[5] The risk of morbidity from sternotomy and cardiopulmonary bypass is low. In addition, operative scar, blood transfusion, psychological trauma, acceptability, need for intensive care, and long hospital stay for recovery are the disadvantages of surgery. With the availability of better catheter closure devices and delivery systems, in patients with smaller aortopulmonary windows

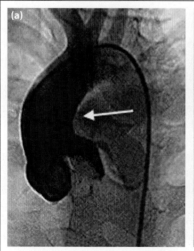 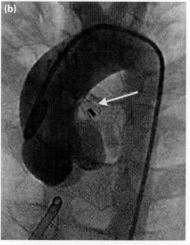

Figure 76.6   (a) Aortogram in a left anterior oblique projection showing a small aortopulmonary window (arrow). (b) Aortogram after release of an ADO I (arrow) showing complete occlusion of the window. (From Atiq M et al. *Pediatr Cardiol* 2003;24:298–9. With Permission.)

with rims suitable for device closure, catheter methods may be an acceptable alternative to surgery.[29,31,34-41] The defect is small in only about 10% of cases with adequate superior and inferior rims as well as a reasonable distance from the other important structures such as the ostium of the left coronary artery, both arterial valves, and the origin of the right pulmonary artery.[34-41] There are no large series of catheter closures of aortopulmonary windows, so only a few case reports have been published.[34-41] Large aortopulmonary windows without adequate rims usually need surgery and small- to medium-sized ones may need surgery if associated with other complex congenital heart defects, which themselves need surgery. Stamato et al. (1995) described the first transcatheter closure of an aortopulmonary window with a modified double-umbrella occluder in a 3-year-old child who had a residual shunt following previous surgery, thus avoiding the need for a second operation.[26] Tulloh and Rigby reported closure of a native 3-mm aortopulmonary window in a 6-month-old child weighing 8 kg using a 12-mm Rashkind double-umbrella device.[32] Jureidini et al. used a buttoned device for the closure of a window in an adult.[33] All these defects were small and complete occlusion was achieved without any complication. With the availability of the Amplatzer Duct Occluder, Richens and Wilson closed a postsurgical residual window.[34] Naik et al. reported closure of isolated native windows in two patients.[29] In one, a 3.7-mm aortopulmonary window was successfully closed with ADO I 6/4 device. In the second case, the stretched diameter of the window was 7 mm and a 10/8 ADO I was attempted but pulled through, so a 14 mm diameter of ASO was successfully used to close the window.

The optimum distance from the important surrounding structures for device closure depends on the size of the defect as well as the type of the occluder and its disk diameters. All the measurements need to be determined accurately by prior imaging such as echocardiography, magnetic resonance imaging, and computerized tomographic scanning to determine the suitability for device closure. Balloon sizing of the defect may be difficult and also because of the angles involved, it may not be very accurate.

There are many embolization devices available, but the Amplatzer Duct Occluder I (ADO I) is easy to use and can be recaptured and repositioned if needed. There is a high complete closure rate in lesions such as the arterial duct.[30] The device needs to be oversized by about 2–3 mm. A small disadvantage of using an ADO I is that it will protrude significantly into the main pulmonary artery and so the presence of any stenosis by echocardiography prior to release should be assessed. As an alternative, a muscular ventricular septal defect occluder or atrial septal defect occluder may be used, especially if there is pulmonary hypertension present. These devices will then have retention disks on both sides of the defect in order

to reduce the possibility of embolization.[31] Immediately following deployment of the device, hemolysis may occur, but the residual shunting through the device usually disappears within a day or so and rarely results in clinically significant hemolysis.[31]

Conclusion

Aortopulmonary windows are easily diagnosed with imaging techniques such as cross-sectional and color Doppler echocardiography combined with magnetic resonance imaging and computerized tomographic scanning. These methods help to select those patients who should have surgery and those who may be suitable for catheter device closure. A small number of case reports have demonstrated that catheter closure of small aortopulmonary windows with devices is feasible and may be considered an alternative to surgery, but larger series are needed.

References

1. Dadds JH, Hoyle C. Congenital aortic septal defect. *Br Heart J* 1949;11:390–7.
2. Ho SY, Gerlis LM, Anderson C, Devine WA, Smith A. The morphology of aorto-pulmonary window with regard to their classification and morphogenesis. *Cardiol Young* 1994;4:146–55.
3. Richardson JV, Doty DB, Rossi NP, Ehrenhaft JL. The spectrum of anomalies of aortopulmonary septation. *J Thorac Cardiovasc Surg* 1979;78:21–7.
4. Blieden LC, Moller JH. Aorticopulmonary septal defect. An experience with 17 patients. *Br Heart J* 1974;36:630–5.
5. McElhinney DB, Reddy MV, Tworetzky W, Silverman NH, Hanley FL. Early and late results after repair of aorto-pulmonary septal defect and associated anomalies in infants <6 months of age. *Am J Cardiol* 1998;81:195–201.
6. Backer CL, Mavroudis C. Surgical management of aorto-pulmonary window: A 40 year experience. *Eur J Cardiovasc Surg* 2002;21:773–9.
7. Mori K, Ando M, Takao A, Ishikawa S, Imai Y. Distal type of aorto-pulmonary window: Report of 4 cases. *Br Heart J* 1978;40:681–9.
8. Redington AN, Rigby ML, Ho SY, Gunthard J, Anderson RH. Aortic atresia with aortopulmonary window and interruption of the aortic arch. *Pediatr Cardiol* 1991;12:49–51.
9. Meisner H, Schmidt-Habelmann P, Sebenning F, Klinner W. Surgical correction of aorto-pulmonary septal defects. A review of the literature and report of eight cases. *Dis Chest* 1968;53:750–8.
10. Rein AJ, Gotsman MS, Simcha A. Echocardiographic diagnosis of interrupted aortic arch with an aortopulmonary communication. *Int J Cardiol* 1989;24:238–41.
11. Deverall PB, Lincoln JCR, Aberdeen E, Bonham-Carter RE, Waterston DJ. Aortopulmonary window. *J Thorac Cardiovasc Surg* 1969;57:479–86.
12. Kutsche LM, Van Mierop LHS. Anatomy and pathogenesis of aorto-pulmonary septal defect. *Am J Cardiol* 1987;59:443–7.
13. Rowe RD. Aorto-pulmonary septal defect. In: Keith JD, Rowe RD, Vlad P. Eds. *Heart Disease in Infancy and Childhood.* 3rd ed. New York: McMillan, 1978.
14. Takahashi K, Kido S, Hoshino K, Ogawa K, Ohashi H, Fukushima Y. Frequency of a 22q11 deletion in patients with conotruncal cardiac malformations: A prospective study. *Eur J Pediatr* 1995;154:878–81.
15. Van Mierop LH, Kutsche LM. Embryology of the heart. In: Hurst JW. Ed. *The Heart.* 6th ed. New York: McGraw-Hill, 1986.

16. Barnes ME, Mitchell ME, Tweddell JS. Aortopulmonary window. *Semin Thorac Cardiovasc Surg Pediatr Card Surg Annu* 2011;14:67–74.

17. Tkebuchava T, Von Segesser LK, Vogt PR et al. Congenital Aorto-Pulmonary Window: Diagnosis, Surgical Technique and Long Term Results. *Eur J Cardiothorac Surg* 1997;11:293–7.

18. Schmid FX, Hake U, Iversen S, Schranz D, Oelert H. Surgical closure of aorto-pulmonary window without cardiopulmonary bypass. *Pediatr Cardiol* 1989;10:166–9.

19. Van Son JAM, Puga FJ, Danielson GK et al. Aortopulmonary window: Factors associated with early and late success after surgical treatment. *Mayo Clin Proc* 1993;68:128–33.

20. Bertolini A, Dalmonte P, Bava GL, Moretti R, Cervo G, Marasini M. Aortopulmonary septal defects. A review of the literature and report of ten cases. *J Cardiovasc Surg* 1994;35:207–13.

21. Castaneda AR, Jonas RA, Mayer JE, Hanley FL. *Cardiac Surgery of the Neonate and Infant*. Philadelphia: WB Saunders Company, 1994;295–300.

22. Tiraboschi R, Salmone G Crupi G et al. Aorto-pulmonary window in the first year of life: Report on 11 surgical cases. *Ann Thorac Surg* 1988;46:438–41.

23. Erez E, Dagan O, Georghiou GP et al. Surgical management of aorto-pulmonary window and associated lesions. *Ann Thorac Surg* 2004;77:484–7.

24. Gross RE. Surgical closure of an aortic septal defect. *Circulation* 1952;5:858–63.

25. DiBella I, Gladstone DJ. Surgical management of aorto-pulmonary window. *Ann Thorac Surg* 1998;65:768–70.

26. Stamato T, Benson LN, Smallhorn JF, Freedom RM. Transcatheter closure of an aorto-pulmonary window with a modified double umbrella occluder system. *Catheter Cardiovasc Diagn* 1995;35:165–7.

27. Balaji S, Burch M, Sullivan ID. Accuracy of cross-sectional echocardiography in diagnosis of aorto-pulmonary window. *Am J Cardiol* 1991;67:650–3.

28. Arora R. Aorto-pulmonary window. In Sievert H, Qureshi SA, Wilson N, Hijazi Z. Eds. *Percutaneous Interventions for Congenital Heart Disease*. London, UK: Informa Healthcare, 2007.

29. Naik GD, Chandra SV, Shenoy A et al. Transcatheter closure of aortopulmonary window using Amplatzer device. *Catheter Cardiovasc Interv* 2003;59:402–5.

30. Faella HJ, Hijazi ZM. Closure of the patent ductus arteriosus with the Amplatzer PDA device: Immediate results of the international clinical trial. *Catheter Cardiovasc Interv* 2000;51:50–4.

31. Demkow M, Ruzyllo W, Siudalska H, Kepka C. Transcatheter closure of a 16 mm hypertensive patent ductus arteriosus with the Amplatzer muscular VSD occluder. *Catheter Cardiovasc Interv* 2001;52:359–62.

32. Tulloh RM, Rigby ML. Transcatheter umbrella closure of aorto-pulmonary window. *Heart* 1997;77:479–80.

33. Jureidini SB, Spadaro JJ, Rao PS. Successful transcatheter closure with buttoned device of aorto-pulmonary window in an adult. *Am J Cardiol* 1998;81:371–2.

34. Richen T, Wilson N. Amplatzer device closure of a residual aorto-pulmonary window. *Catheter Cardiovasc Diagn* 2000;50:431–3.

35. Atiq M, Rashid N, Kazmi KA, Qureshi SA. Closure of aortopulmonary window with Amplatzer duct occluder device. *Pediatr Cardiol* 2003;24:298–9.

36. Trehan V, Nigam A, Tyagi S. Percutaneous closure of nonrestrictive aortopulmonary window in three infants. *Catheter Cardiovasc Interv* 2008;71:405–11.

37. Sivakumar K, Francis E. Transcatheter closure of distal aortopulmonary window using Amplatzer device. *Congenit Heart Dis* 2006;1:321–3.

38. Kosmac B, Eicken A, Kuhn A, Heinrich M, Ewert P. Percutaneous device closure of an aortopulmonary window in a small infant. *Int J Cardiol* 2013;168:e102–3.

39. Srivastava A, Radha AS. Transcatheter closure of a large aortopulmonary window with severe pulmonary arterial hypertension beyond infancy. *J Invasive Cardiol* 2012;24:E24–E26.

40. Viswanathan S, Vaidyanathan B, Krishna Kumar R. Transcatheter closure of the aortopulmonary window in a symptomatic infant using the Amplatzer ductal occluder. *Heart* 2007;93:1519.

41. Noonan PM, Desai T, Degiovanni JV. Closure of an aortopulmonary window using the Amplatzer Duct Occluder II. *Pediatr Cardiol* 2013;34:712–4.

77

Systemic arteriovenous fistulas

Grazyna Brzezinska-Rajszys

Systemic arteriovenous fistulas are a group of vascular anomalies characterized by abnormal communications between systemic arteries and veins without normal capillary development. This situation results in shunting of blood from the high-pressure arterial to the low-pressure venous system. This abnormal circuit steals blood from the normal capillary bed and can result in tissue ischemia. Increased flow in the afferent artery and efferent vein causes dilatation, thickening, and tortuosity of the vessels. Depending on the shunt volume, it may cause right ventricular volume overload and decrease of the peripheral vascular resistance, leading to increased stroke volume and cardiac output. Such hemodynamics can lead to heart failure.

Systemic arteriovenous fistulas may be congenital or acquired resulting from injury or infection. Congenital systemic arteriovenous fistulas are relatively rare lesions, the majority of which do not present with symptoms until adult life. They may become progressively larger throughout childhood, but occasionally spontaneous thrombosis and closure may occur. These fistulas may be found most often in the brain, spinal cord and liver, but occur anywhere in the body.

Clinical manifestation of systemic arteriovenous fistulas depends on their location, pathophysiology, and hemodynamic effects and on the size, number, and nature of the vessels within the lesions. In infants and children, large systemic arteriovenous fistulas involving the brain or liver can present with congestive heart failure.

Embolization is an accepted primary therapeutic approach in the majority of systemic arteriovenous fistulas, sometimes needing to be combined with surgery. The optimal technique of embolization depends on the type of vascular connection to be occluded and the specific defect and preference of the operator for the type of equipment.

Generally, vascular embolization may be undertaken

- To occlude the entire arterial tree in a part or all of an organ—frequently for management of diseased organs prior to their surgical removal. It requires microvascular embolization techniques (mostly liquid embolic agents such as Onyx and *n*-butyl cyanoacrylate).

- To occlude only the large arterial branches—for example, vessels feeding an arteriovenous malformation. It requires different embolization techniques and the use of different coils, devices, and particulate agents such as gelfoam, ivalon, or a combination of these.
- To occlude a vessel at a very localized point—for example, major aorto-pulmonary collaterals and patent ductus arteriosus. Precise, localized interruption of vascular flow using coil embolization or device closure techniques are most commonly used in the practice of the pediatric interventional cardiologist.

The decision concerning embolization of a fistula should be taken by clinicians responsible for the patients who refer their patients for therapy for interventions. Owing to a lack of formal guidelines of the interventional standards, embolization of different arteriovenous malformations are performed in different countries by interventionists from different specialities. The interventional cardiologists perform embolization of systemic arteriovenous fistulas more commonly in pediatric patients, especially in centers where cardiologists share catheterization theaters with radiologists. In such situations, cooperation between pediatric cardiologists and radiologists is mandatory to achieve good results. From a technical point of view, embolization can be performed by specialists familiar with interventional procedures and with the available embolization materials and who have an understanding of the clinical indications for these procedures. It should be stressed that due to the complexity of the intracranial arteriovenous malformations, embolization is most commonly performed by interventional radiologists, interventional neuroradiologists, or neurosurgeons. Some interventional procedures may necessitate joint interventional–surgical approach (e.g., transtorcular approach to close intracranial arteriovenous malformations, umbilical vein approach in the neonate to close patent ductus venosus—personal experience).

Neurological manifestation of the intracranial arteriovenous malformations present at any age, but only when the damage they cause to the brain or spinal cord reaches a critical level. This damage occurs by reducing the amount of oxygen delivered to the neural tissues, by causing bleeding into surrounding tissues, and by compressing parts of the brain or spinal cord. Detailed analysis of the angioarchitecture of malformation is imperative for planning the appropriate treatment. The diagnosis is based on ultrasound, computed tomography, and magnetic resonance imaging studies.

Endovascular therapy is the standard treatment for aneurysms of the vein of Galen, dural arteriovenous malformations in different locations, and other intracranial and spinal arteriovenous malformations.[1-3]

Vein of Galen aneurysm is a type of arteriovenous malformation characterized by the presence of dilated midline deep venous structure, fed by abnormal arteriovenous communications. Vein of Galen malformations have been variably referred to as "aneurysms of the vein of Galen," "arteriovenous aneurysms of the vein of Galen," "vein of Galen aneurysmal malformations," and "vein of Galen malformations." The nomenclature is imprecise, as the dilated venous structure characteristic of these malformations has been demonstrated to represent the embryonic median prosencephalic vein of Markowski, and not the vein of Galen.[4,5]

Several systems of classification have been used to describe malformations of the vein of Galen.[4-7] These malformations should be differentiated from the dilatation of a normally formed vein of Galen, secondary to outflow obstruction. Correct diagnosis is important due to the different treatment that should be used.

Vein of Galen aneurysm is a rare congenital abnormality (1% of all intracranial vascular malformations) that can cause severe morbidity and mortality, particularly in neonates but also in infants and older children.[5] It represents 30% of vascular malformations presenting in the pediatric age group and is the most common cerebrovascular arteriovenous malformation presenting with cardiac symptoms.[8] Vein of Galen malformation associated with capillary malformation–arteriovenous malformation (CM–AVM) is a recognized autosomal dominant disorder caused by mutations in the *RASA1* gene.[9]

The clinical presentation of vein of Galen aneurysm depends on the age of the patient and the severity of the lesion.[4,5,10,11] While *in utero*, these malformations can be detected, but cardiac failure may be absent. Cardiac failure is related to the coexisting low-resistance cerebral and placental circulations. After birth with the exclusion of the low-resistance placental circulation, flow is directed toward the cerebral malformation.[12-14] The cerebral circulation may have 80% or more of the cardiac output, resulting in a large left-to-right shunt and severe congestive heart failure in neonates. The shunt through the malformation increases the pulmonary blood flow and may cause pulmonary hypertension. Increased systemic venous return to the right atrium promotes right-to-left shunt through the foramen ovale. In many patients, right-to-left

shunt also occurs at the level of the ductus arteriosus. These shunts may cause cyanosis in some patients. A large shunt significantly reduces the diastolic pressure within the aorta, causing reduced coronary arterial blood flow. This, combined with increased cardiac output, reduces the subendocardial blood flow and may promote myocardial ischemia.[4,15,16]

Hydrocephalus, seizures, subarachnoid hemorrhage, or venous congestion of the scalp and facial veins are clinical symptoms occurring later in infancy. Older children are more likely to present with mild cardiac failure, hydrocephalus, headache, or focal neurological signs. Neurological deterioration is due to a steal phenomenon resulting in insufficient cerebral perfusion and compression by an aneurysm on the brain tissue.[17]

These malformations can be detected with two-dimensional combined with color Doppler cranial ultrasound techniques. Computed tomography and magnetic resonance demonstrate the nature and location of the intracerebral arteriovenous malformations, morphology of the dural sinuses, and associated pathology such as ventriculomegaly and ischemic infarction[4,5,11,18] (Figure 77.1). Selective arteriography is the "gold standard" required to provide precise information about the anatomy of the malformation, with a detailed assessment of the deep cerebral venous drainage, necessary for planning the most effective therapy[4,7,10,11] (Figure 77.2).

Manifestation of the vein of Galen aneurysm may give a clue in a chest x-ray showing cardiomegaly with right heart dilation, increased pulmonary vascularity, retrosternal fullness, and retropharyngeal soft tissue thickening due to dilatation of the ascending aorta and brachiocephalic vessels. On echocardiography, it is possible to demonstrate normal cardiac anatomy, dilated hyperdynamic cardiac chambers

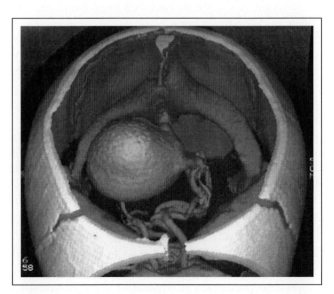

Figure 77.1 Vein of Galen aneurysm. Spiral computed tomography, 3D reconstruction.

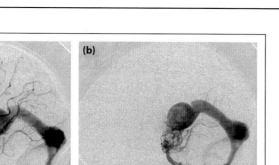

Figure 77.2   Vein of Galen aneurysm. Internal carotid arteriogram, lateral projection (a) and vertebral arteriogram, lateral projection (b).

with increased runoff to the upper half of the body, abnormal dilatation of the superior vena cava, ascending aorta, aortic arch, and brachiocephalic vessels. On Doppler echocardiography, it is possible to show retrograde diastolic flow in the descending aorta with the continuous forward flow in the aortic arch and brachiocephalic vessels. Contrast echocardiography may show recirculation of microbubbles from the left side of the heart to the superior vena cava.

Neurosurgical treatment is associated with a fatal outcome in 80–100% of cases. The results have improved over recent years with endovascular management and may depend on the patient population and the operator experience.[3,5,7,10,11] In the largest reported study, the overall mortality was 10.6%, whereas in the neonatal group, it was 52%, in infants, it was 7.2%, and in children, it was 0%. Importantly, 74% of the surviving patients were neurologically normal, 15.6% were moderately retarded, and 10.4% had severe mental retardation during 4.4 years follow-up.[6]

Morbidity can be reduced by selecting patients with no evidence of cerebral parenchymal damage or severe multisystem failure.

In patients with persistent cardiac failure (mostly neonates), urgent endovascular treatment should be performed and should be directed toward correcting cardiac failure and cerebral ischemia.

The transarterial approach is favored for the endovascular management of the vein of Galen aneurysm. The transvenous or transtorcular approach is reserved for selected patients.[4–7,10,11,19–22] (Figures 77.3 and 77.4). The staging treatment using multiple embolization strategies offers the gradual and more controlled process of devascularization, reducing the risk of adverse events. Although embolization may be effective in controlling the shunt and the symptoms of congestive heart failure in 90% of patients, it may not always completely obliterate the lesion. Leaving the part of malformation untreated in a patient with favorable neurological and developmental outcomes is widely accepted.

The major complications of the interventional procedure include intraventricular bleeding and inadvertent occlusion of an uninvolved vessel. Close follow-up with serial cranial ultrasound and color Doppler techniques, magnetic resonance, or computed tomography is important.

Arteriovenous malformations of the liver are an important group of systemic arteriovenous fistulas. A variety of vascular lesions arise within the liver. Hepatic hemangiomas or hemangio-endotheliomas are benign vascular tumors, that may be part of multinodular hemangiomatosis of the liver. The syndrome consists of hepatomegaly, congestive heart failure, and cutaneous hemangioma, and is associated with consumptive coagulopathy, thrombocytopenia, and liver dysfunction. More than 50% of the total cardiac output may be shunted through the liver, causing congestive heart failure, which is often the dominant clinical and prognostic

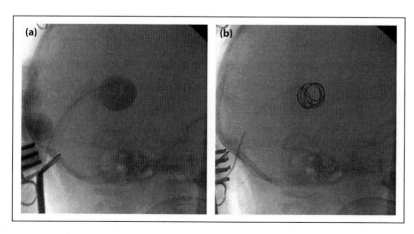

Figure 77.3   Vein of Galen aneurysm. Transtorcular approach. Angiography (a), coil embolization (b).

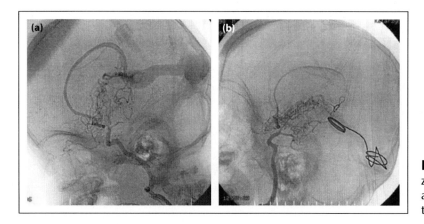

Figure 77.4 Vein of Galen aneurysm. Embolization. Internal carotid arteriogram before (a) and after coil embolization (b). Coils introduced using transfemoral arterial and transtorcular approach.

feature in patients with hepatic hemangio-endotheliomas.[23–26] The hepatic hemangiomas involute in many cases, but those presenting with congestive heart failure have a poor prognosis. Hepatic arteriovenous malformations may be single, multiple, or diffuse over a large spectrum of diameters from a few millimeters to several centimeters. Hepatic arteriovenous malformations presenting with congestive heart failure include the direct arteriovenous fistulas between the hepatic arteries and hepatic veins.

The diagnosis of hepatic arteriovenous malformations is confirmed by hepatic ultrasonography, computed tomography, and magnetic resonance imaging. Aortography and selective arteriography is necessary if arterial embolization or surgical intervention is planned (Figure 77.5).

The treatment depends on the anatomy of the malformation and its hemodynamic effects. Different embolization techniques using different materials (e.g., coils, radiolabeled polyvinyl alcohol particles, or combination of different materials) have been used to embolize hepatic arteriovenous fistulas.[23–29] Prednisone in combination with anticongestive therapy may be an effective treatment of diffuse hemangiomas. Surgical resection is reserved for localized tumors. It should be stressed that a combination of all treatment modalities may need to be used in some patients. In some cases with diffuse arteriovenous malformations and significant symptoms, liver transplantation is the only therapeutic option.

Hepatic arteriovenous malformations are relatively common and often asymptomatic in hereditary hemorrhagic telangiectasia.

Hereditary hemorrhagic telangiectasia (Osler–Weber–Rendu syndrome) is a genetic vascular disorder with autosomal dominant inheritance and an estimated frequency of 1–2:100,000. It is characterized by telangiectasias, arteriovenous fistulas, and aneurysms, and may involve skin, mucosa, and blood vessels of the liver, lungs, and central nervous system.[30] Hepatic arteriovenous malformations occur in approximately 30% of patients, pulmonary in 15–20%, and central nervous system in less than 10%. The treatment depends on the clinical symptoms; percutaneous embolization techniques play an important role in the treatment of these malformations. Arterial embolotherapy of hepatic arteriovenous fistulas can improve the clinical condition of patients with heart failure,[31–33] but transplantation remains the treatment of choice for hepatic arteriovenous malformations with significant symptoms.

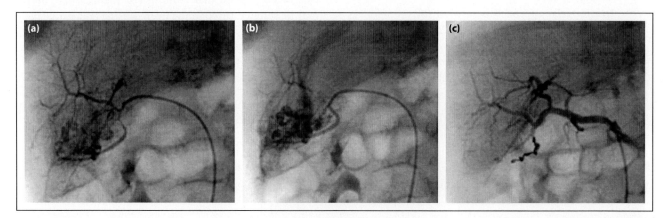

Figure 77.5 Occlusion of hepatic arteriovenous malformations localized in the right lobe of the liver (V and VI segments) presenting with congestive heart failure. Selective arteriography to feeding vessel of malformation, (a) arterial phase, (b) venous phase, (c) arteriovenous fistulas occluded with microcoils (Hilal Embolization Microcoils, Cook Europe).

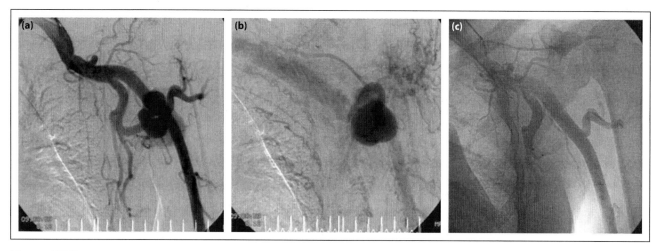

Figure 77.6 Congenital arteriovenous fistula between the axillary artery branch (subscapular artery) and axillary vein occluded with Amplatzer Duct Occluder (AGA Medical Corporation). Subclavian arteriogram, (a) arterial phase, (b) venous phase, (c) arteriogram after occlusion.

Miscellaneous arteriovenous malformations, congenital and acquired, can occur anywhere in the body. In the developing embryo, there are multiple communications between arteries and veins. Persistence of these channels may be the basis for congenital arteriovenous fistulas. Different locations of congenital systemic arteriovenous fistulas are reported mostly as case reports, for example, the common carotid artery and the internal jugular vein, between the descending aorta and the superior vena cava, the azygos vein, and the innominate vein, between the ascending aorta and the superior vena cava—are all very uncommon (Figure 77.6).[34–39] The majority of peripheral fistulas occur as a result of trauma. These acquired fistulas usually occur mostly in the legs or arms, where an artery and vein that are side-by-side are damaged. The healing process results in the two vessels becoming linked. A second group of acquired fistulas are iatrogenic, such as after cannulation of vessels with different catheters and cannulas, after surgery.[40,41] After cardiac catheterization, arteriovenous fistulas may occur as a complication of the arterial puncture in the leg or arm.[42] Clinically significant symptoms from all types of the systemic arteriovenous fistulas are an indication for treatment, which should be based on the detailed analysis of the anatomy of the fistula.

Occlusion of systemic arteriovenous fistulas

All therapeutic decisions should be made on a case-by-case basis. For a particular lesion, the optimal closure technique is best determined by considering its anatomy in the context of the specific goals of the occlusion.

Vessel occlusion may be achieved using a variety of transcatheter methods, including coil embolization (e.g., different types of Gianturco coils, detachable coils,

microcoils), device closure (e.g., Amplatzer Duct Occluder, Amplatzer Vascular Plug; St. Jude Medical, St. Paul, MN, USA), gelfoam embolization, particulate embolization, and liquid agents embolization (absolute ethanol, ivalon, agents consisting of cyanoacrylate monomers). The choice of occlusion material is important for embolization. Systemic arteriovenous fistulas are mostly occluded with coils and devices.

Coils

Coils are available in guide wire diameters from 0.018 inch to 0.052 inch and extruded coil diameter from 2 to 20 mm, of almost any length, different shapes and materials. Also, controlled release coils can be used.

The Gianturco coils (Cook Medical Europe, Limerick, Ireland) are made from stainless steel wire with Dacron fibers attached to increase their thrombogenicity.

A detachable coil-delivery system using the same type of coils is also available (e.g., Flipper detachable embolization coil, from Cook Medical Europe). This can result in more control during the coil placement. The detachable coil is particularly useful when there is a high risk of inappropriate coil positioning or its inadvertent migration during deployment either because of difficult vessel anatomy or because the site of occlusion is particularly critical.

Hilal Embolization Microcoils (Cook Medical Europe) are platinum coils (0.018 inch) with spaced synthetic fibers. They are available in different shapes and lengths. These coils are delivered through 3 F delivery catheters (e.g., Microferret, Cook Medical Europe) passed through a guiding catheter with an inner diameter of 0.038 inch to selectively occlude very tortuous vessels.

Fibered Platinum Coils (Boston Scientific, Natick, MA, USA) are available in a simple helical shape made of 0.035

inch wire and complex cloverleaf shapes made of 0.018 inch wire that are available with a system of coil pushers and delivery tracker microcatheters that fit in the lumen of any catheter with an inner diameter of 0.038 inches..

Guglielmi Detachable Coils (GDC) (Boston Scientific) are coils with different two-dimensional and complex three-dimensional shapes, utilizing an electrolytic detachment for coil deployment.

Devices

The Amplatzer Vascular Plugs (AVP, AVP II, AVP III, AVP 4) (St. Jude Medical) are self-expandable devices made from nitinol wire mesh and are indicated for arterial and venous embolization in the peripheral vasculature. They are available in different shapes and sizes from 3 to 22 mm, delivered through a 4–7 F sheath. Each device is preloaded, attached to a delivery wire with a stainless steel screw. Because of their controlled-release mechanism, plugs can be recaptured and repositioned, if necessary. Amplatzer Vascular Plug 4 (AVP 4) is a low-profile device, available in 4–8 mm diameter, which can be delivered through a 0.038-inch lumen of a diagnostic catheter.

The Amplatzer Duct Occluder (St. Jude Medical) is another type of self-expandable device made from a nitinol wire mesh with polyester fabric sewn into the occluder to induce thrombosis. This device is very effective in the closure of different vessels, including systemic arteriovenous fistulas.

Covered stents are not typical embolization material but some mostly posttraumatic fistulous communications between big arteries and veins can be treated with balloon-expandable or self-expandable covered stents implanted into the artery.

Technique of embolization

The use of anesthesia depends on the age of the patient, the complexity of the procedure, and the local preferences. Intracranial, spinal malformation, and procedures in younger patients should be performed under general anesthesia. Antibiotics are administered intravenously. Embolization can be performed by the retrograde arterial approach, but the transvenous approach has also been used. The choice depends on the lesion. As a rule, the approach should provide the straightest and least complicated course to the systemic arteriovenous fistula. Usually, femoral artery and femoral vein access are used. Venous or arterial access can also be used for the introduction of balloon catheters for temporary occlusion of the flow through the fistula. This can be helpful during embolization of high-flow fistulas with coils or other solid material.

An appropriate-diameter (usually 5–7 F) introducer sheath should provide access to a wide range of catheters, which might be needed for embolization.

Anticoagulation with heparin 100 international units per kilogram is usually given.

From the arterial approach, an angiographic catheter (multipurpose or pigtail) is used for angiography to show the location of the fistula and its relation to the main vessels. With the multipurpose catheter advanced into the branch of the artery feeding the lesion, further selective angiography is performed. Different projections and magnified views are helpful in delineating the exact anatomy of the fistula. Embolization is performed after selective catheterization of the feeding branch with the delivery catheter. The inner diameter of the delivery catheter should be equal to or at most only slightly larger than the coil diameter. If the delivery catheter has a lumen that is too large for the coil, then the guide wire may wedge itself inside the coil and it may be difficult to advance the coil inside the catheter. Easy passage of the wire through the tip of the delivery catheter should be checked before insertion of the coil. The 0.018 inch and 0.025 inch coils can be delivered through 3 F catheters and 0.035 inch and 0.038-inch coils through 4 F catheters.

If the lesion is accessed by the delivery-guiding catheter, then stainless steel coils are deployed through it. The embolization material should be positioned in the vessels feeding the arteriovenous fistula, within the fistula, or a combination of these.

The size of the coil should be 10–30% larger than the vessel diameter. A smaller coil will not cause complete occlusion, while a larger coil straightens out and may extend beyond the site of embolization.

The coils, preloaded in stainless steel or plastic tubes, are passed from the tube into a delivery catheter using an appropriate-size guide wire. When extruded from the catheter, the coil forms to its stated size and shape.

After implantation of the coils, occlusion of the vessel occurs as the result of thrombus formation and its subsequent organization. If the lesion is peripherally located and follows a tortuous course, a coaxial microcatheter system is used to reach the appropriate site. Some microcatheters, such as Tracker (Boston Scientific, Natick, MA, USA) or Microferret (Cook Europe) and compatible guide wires can be introduced through a guiding catheter with an inner diameter of 0.038 inches. Complex helical fibered platinum coils or other microcoils are then deployed depending on the size of the vessel to be occluded.

Intermittent check angiography is needed with hand injections approximately 5 min after deployment of each coil to look for the degree of occlusion, any inadvertent non-target embolization, and additional feeding vessels; also to check the catheter position for subsequent coil deployment. Temporary occlusion of flow by a balloon catheter may help with occlusion too. If satisfactory occlusion is not achieved with coils, this may be combined with the injection of gelatine sponge (Gelfoam, Upjohn, Kalamazoo, MI, USA). Gelfoam particles are mixed with contrast and saline and injected slowly by hand, so that there is no reflux into the adjacent normal vessels.

Systemic arteriovenous fistulas may have multiple feeding vessels and so after the occlusion of the main vessel, additional feeding arteries should be sought and occluded.

The catheter occlusion technique may require many coils to occlude the solitary malformation. Usually, several coils have to be tightly packed in order to achieve complete occlusion, especially if there is a high flow in a vessel. In general, the first coil should be the largest, to prevent distal embolization.

The feeding vessels can be embolized with the new Amplatzer vascular plugs or the Amplatzer duct occluder. The choice between coils or devices is dependent on the anatomy of the fistula as well as on the experience and preference of the operator. Plugs can be delivered through an appropriate diameter-guiding catheter, depending on the plug. The duct occluder may need a long 5–6 F sheath.

Complications

Inadvertent migration of the embolization material is the most common complication. Embolization material may move distally into the arterial tree, in most instances to the distal pulmonary arteries. Materials such as coils or devices are relatively easy to remove with vascular retrieval techniques.

Hemolysis is a serious complication occurring only in cases of significant residual flow. This complication should be treated with additional embolization, if it is impossible to remove previously used material to exchange it for a different one.

After the procedure

Patients may experience postembolization syndrome, with transient fever, pain, and leucocytosis, which is usually self-limiting and treated symptomatically. Ultrasonography with Doppler study, spiral computed tomography, and/or magnetic resonance imaging should document the result of embolization prior to or soon after the patient is discharged from the hospital. The follow-up protocol of patients with intracranial malformation should be discussed with neurosurgeons.

Conclusions

Embolization is an accepted primary therapeutic approach in the majority of systemic arteriovenous fistulas. Vessel occlusion may be achieved using a variety of transcatheter techniques.

The choice of occlusion material is important for the optimal embolization and depends on the anatomy of fistulas.

All therapeutic decisions on treatment of systemic arteriovenous fistulas should be made on a case-by-case basis.

References

1. Berenstein A, Lasjaunias P. Arteriovenous fistulas of the brain. In: *Surgical Neuroangiography 4. Endovascular Treatment of Cerebral Lesions*. Berlin: Springer-Verlag, 1992. pp. 267–317.
2. Humphreys RP, Hoffman HJ, Drake JM et al. Choices in the 1990s for the management of pediatric cerebral arteriovenous malformations. *Pediatr Neurosurg* 1996;25:277–85.
3. Lasjaunias P, Hui F, Zerah M et al. Cerebral arteriovenous malformations in children. Management of 179 consecutive cases and review of the literature. *Childs Nerv Syst* 1995;11:66–79.
4. Gupta AK, Varma DR, Vein of Galen malformations: Review. *Neurol India* 2004;52:43–53.
5. Recinos PF, Rahmathulla G, Pearl M et al. Vein of Galen malformations: Epidemiology, clinical presentations, management. *Neurosurg Clin N Am* 2012;23:165–77.
6. Lasjaunias PL, Chng SM, Sachet M et al. The management of vein of Galen aneurysmal malformations. *Neurosurgery* 2006;59:S184–94.
7. Pearl M, Gomez J, Gregg L et al. Endovascular management of vein of Galen aneurysmal malformations. Influence of the normal venous drainage on the choice of a treatment strategy. *Childs Nerv Syst* 2010;26:1367–79.
8. Pellegrino PA, Milanesi O, Saia OS et al. Congestive heart failure secondary to cerebral arterio-venous fistula. *Childs Nerv Syst* 1987;3:141–4.
9. Revencu N, Boon LM, Mulliken JB et al. Parkes Weber syndrome, vein of Galen aneurysmal malformation, and other fast-flow vascular anomalies are caused by RASA1 mutations. *Hum Mutat* 2008;29:959–65.
10. Li AH, Armstrong D, terBrugge KG. Endovascular treatment of vein of Galen aneurismal malformation: Management strategy and 21-year experience in Toronto. *J Neurosurg Pediatr* 2011;7:3–10.
11. Berenstein A, Fifi JT, Niimi Y et al. Vein of Galen malformations in neonates: New management paradigms for improving outcomes. *Neurosurgery* 2012;70:1207–13.
12. Vintzileos AM, Eisenfeld LI, Campbell WA et al. Prenatal ultrasonic diagnosis of arteriovenous malformation of the vein of Galen. *Am J Perinatol* 1986;3:209–11.
13. Reiter AA, Huhta JC, Carpenter RJ Jr et al. Prenatal diagnosis of arteriovenous malformation of the vein of Galen. *J Clin Ultrasound* 1986;14:623–8.
14. Rodesch G, Hui F, Alvarez H et al. Prognosis of antenatally diagnosed vein of Galen aneurysmal malformations. *Childs Nerv Syst* 1994;10:79–83.
15. Cumming GR. Circulation in neonates with intracranial arteriovenous fistula and cardiac failure. *Am J Cardiol* 1980;45:1019–24.
16. Garcia-Monaco R, de Victor D, Mann C et al. Congestive cardiac manifestations from cerebrocranial arteriovenous shunts: Endovascular management in 30 children. *Childs Nerv Syst* 1991;7:48–52.
17. Zerah M, Garcia-Monaco R, Rodesh G et al. Hydrodynamics in vein of Galen malformations. *Childs Nerv Syst* 1992;8:111–7.
18. Seidenwurm D, Berenstein A, Hyman A. Vein of Galen malformation: Correlation of clinical presentation, arteriography and MR imaging. *Am J Neuroradiol* 1991;12:347–54.
19. Dowd CF, Halbach VV, Barnwell SL et al. Transfemoral venous embolization of vein of Galen malformations. *Am J Neuroradiol* 1990;11:643–8.
20. Mickle JP, The transtorcular embolization of vein of Galen aneurysms and update on the use of this technique in twenty four patients. In: Marlin AE. Ed. *Concepts in Pediatric Neurosurgery*. Karger: Basel, 1991. pp. 69–78.

21. Mitchell PJ, Rosenfield JV, Dargaville P. Endovascular management of vein of Galen aneurysmal malformations presenting in the neonatal period, *Am J Neuroradiol* 2001;22:1403–9.

22. Fourie PA, Potze FP, Hay N et al. Trans-cranial placement of an Amplatzer device to control intractable cardiac failure in an infant with a vein of Galen anomaly A case report. *Intervent Neuroradiol* 2010;16:191–7.

23. Gallego C, Miralles M, Maŕ C et al. Congenital hepatic shunts. *RadioGraphics* 2004; 24:755–72.

24. Boon LM, Burrows PE, Paltiel HJ et al. Hepatic vascular anomalies in infancy: A twenty-seven-year experience. *J Pediatr* 1996;129:346–54.

25. Raghuram L, Korah IP, Jaya V et al. Coil embolization of a solitary congenital intrahepatic hepatoportal fistula. *Abdom Imaging* 2001;26:194–6.

26. Lima M, Lalla M, Aquino A et al. Congenital symptomatic intrahepatic arteriovenous fistulas in newborns: Management of 2 cases with prenatal diagnosis. *J Pediatr Surg* 2005;40:1–5.

27. Norton SP, Jacobson K, Moroz SP et al. The congenital intrahepatic arterioportal fistula syndrome: Elucidation and proposed classification. *J Pediatr Gastroenterol Nutr* 2006;43:248–55.

28. Stanley P, Grinnell VS, Stanton RE et al. Therapeutic embolization of infantile hepatic hemangioma with polyvinyl alcohol. *Am J Roentgenol* 1983;141:1047–51.

29. Subramanyan R, Narayan R, Costa DD et al. Transcatheter coil occlusion of hepatic arteriovenous malformation in a neonate. *Indian Heart J* 2001;53:782–4.

30. Abdalla SA, Geisthoff UW, Bonneau D et al. Visceral manifestations in hereditary haemorrhagic telangiectasia type 2. *J Med Genet* 2003;40:494–502.

31. Derauf BJ, Hunter DW, Sirr SA et al. Peripheral embolization of diffuse hepatic arteriovenous malformations in a patient with hereditary hemorrhagic telangiectasia, *Cardiovasc Intervent Radiol* 1987;10:80–3.

32. Whiting JH Jr, Morton KA, Datz FL et al. Embolization of hepatic arteriovenous malformations using radiolabeled and nonradiolabeled polyvinyl alcohol sponge in a patient with hereditary hemorrhagic telangiectasia: Case report, *J Nucl Med* 1992;33:260–2.

33. Stockx L, Raat H, Caerts B et al. Transcatheter embolization of hepatic arteriovenous fistulas in Rendu-Osler-Weber disease: A case report and review of the literature. *Eur Radiol* 1999;9:1434–7.

34. Soler P, Mehta AV, Garcia OL et al. Congenital systemic arteriovenous fistula between the descending aorta, azygos vein, and superior vena cava. *Chest* 1981;80:647–9.

35. Gutierrez FR, Monaco MP, Hartmann AF et al. Congenital arteriovenous malformations between brachiocephalic arteries and systemic veins. *Chest* 1987;92:897–9.

36. Romero M, Pan M, Suarez de Lezo J et al. Congenital fistula between the left subclavian artery and the innominate vein. A rare cause of intractable insufficiency in the newborn infant. *Rev Esp Cardiol* 1988;41:630–2.

37. Oomman A, Mao R, Krishnan P et al. Congenital aortocaval fistula to the superior vena cava. *Ann Thorac Surg* 2001;72:911–3.

38. Ramsay DW, McAuliffe W. Traumatic pseudoaneurysm and high flow arteriovenous fistula involving internal jugular vein and common carotid artery. Treatment with covered stent and embolization. *Australas Radiol* 2003;47:177–80.

39. Uchida Y, Kawano H, Koide Y et al. Arteriovenous fistula of internal thoracic vessels. *Intern Med* 2003;42:987–90.

40. Droll KP, Lossing AG, Carotid-jugular arteriovenous fistula: Case report of an iatrogenic complication following internal jugular vein catheterization. *J Clin Anesth* 2004;16:127–9.

41. Thiel R, Bircks W, Arteriovenous fistulas after median sternotomy—Report of 2 cases and review of the literature. *Thorac Cardiovasc Surg* 1990;38:195–7.

42. Onal B, Kosar S, Gumus T et al. Postcatheterization femoral arteriovenous fistulas: Endovascular treatment with stent-grafts. *Cardiovasc Intervent Radiol* 2004;27:453–8.

78

Pulmonary arteriovenous fistulas

Miltiadis Krokidis and John Reidy

Pulmonary arteriovenous fistulas

Introduction

Pulmonary arteriovenous fistulas (PAVFs) or pulmonary arteriovenous malformations (PAVMs) are usually classified as simple or complex based on the angiographic findings (Figure 78.1).[1] Simple PAVMs are more common (80%) and have a single feeding artery and draining vein, whereas complex PAVMs have multiple feeding arteries and more than one draining vein and may appear as cirsoid with multiple septations.[1] PAVMs may also be solitary or diffuse; the latter occurs more commonly in the context of hereditary hemorrhagic telangiectasia (HHT).[2] HHT is a congenital disease that has a closed link with PAVMs; more than 80% of patients with HHT have PAVMs.[3,4]

Clinical presentation and diagnosis

PAVMs may occur at any age, but often present in adult life. They may be present at a younger age and cause dyspnea and fatigue, however they may be undiagnosed for many years. Cyanosis and polycythemia may be noted.[3] Some cases may present with a brain abscess or a cerebrovascular accident (CVA); the latter is due to thrombosis secondary to the associated polycythemia or due to paradoxical embolism consequent on venous thrombosis. Even in the absence of any known clinical CVA, an occult CVA may have occurred, so it makes sense to do a baseline head computed tomography (CT) scan prior to any embolization procedure. Occasionally, PAVMs are noted as an incidental finding on a routine chest x-ray (Figure 78.2). In all symptomatic PAVMs, treatment is indicated. Very small PAVMs, especially in older patients, can probably be left safely, but

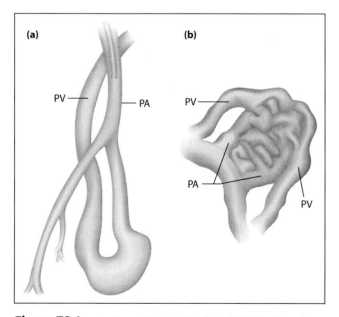

Figure 78.1 Angiographic classification of PAVMs. PA, pulmonary artery; PV, pulmonary vein.

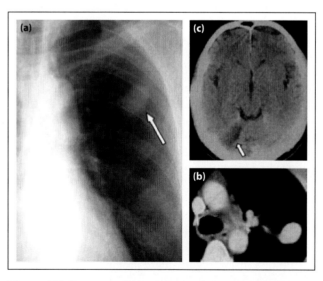

Figure 78.2 Presentation of a large simple single PAVM in an adult. (a) Chest x-ray shows a round opacity in the left upper zone (arrow). (b) CT scan confirms the diagnosis. (c) Brain CT is included in the diagnostic work-up and shows a cerebellar infarct (arrow).

any PAVM with a feeding artery diameter greater than 3 mm on CT should be treated.

Up until 1977, the only treatment available for PAVMs was surgery. This was an effective treatment, but aside from a significant morbidity, it was associated with a mortality of about 4–5%. The first reported case of PAVM embolization was in 1977. Nowadays, embolization is the treatment of choice for PAVMs offering a reliable management for single or multiple lesions with a short hospital stay.

The diagnosis is made in the majority of the cases with contrast echocardiography.[5] PAVMs are detected as bubbles appearing in the left atrium at least four beats after their presence in the right atrium (to exclude patent foramen ovale and other intracardiac causes of right-to-left shunting). CT angiography helps to confirm the diagnosis, delineate the anatomy, and measure the diameter of the feeding vessels, as well as identify multiple malformations. The CT angiography usually follows a positive contrast echocardiogram. Some centers also perform contrast-enhanced magnetic resonance imaging (MRI).

Pulmonary angiography

This is carried out using a femoral vein approach. Infants and children will clearly need a general anesthetic, but this is not necessary for adults. The aim of the pulmonary angiography is to confirm the presence and location of the PAVMs and demonstrate the feeding arteries clearly.[6] Normally, selective right and left pulmonary arteriograms are performed using a pigtail catheter. When the PAVM is identified, usually a 6 or 7 Fr long (90 cm) sheath or a guiding catheter is introduced. More detailed and more selective arteriograms are then needed, focusing on the malformation and its feeding artery, until a selective injection is made directly into the feeding artery in the case of a simple PVAM or one of the arteries in the complex lesions. As the same catheter will then be needed for the embolization procedure, it is important that this has only an end hole with no side holes. More commonly, malformations are situated in the lower lobes and sometimes it may prove quite difficult to identify the feeding artery. Using an angled hydrophilic guide wire can prove particularly useful in this situation. The aim is to position the catheter in the feeding artery in a view where the angulation shows the length of the artery at its best advantage. Magnified views are important and it is not necessary to have subtraction images. It is important to position the embolizing catheter (5 Fr is a good size) in an optimal and stable position. To achieve this, it is advantageous to place a long sheath with its tip in a major, slightly more proximal, branch. One of the concerns about embolizing PAVMs and placing catheters directly into the malformation is that any embolic particles will pass immediately into the systemic circulation, so giving some systemic heparinization may reduce this risk.

Embolization procedure

In the most common form of PAVM (simple type) with a single feeding artery, the aim should be to occlude this artery immediately before it enters the aneurysmal part of the PAVM (Figure 78.3). Embolizing more proximally would occlude branches to the normal lung parenchyma and possibly result in some pulmonary infarction. It is important to assess the diameter of the feeding artery, as this must not be bigger than the diameter of the coil or the device. If the diameter of the extruded coil or device is less than that of the feeding artery, the device could migrate with high flow into the nonseptated aneurysmal part of the AVM and then into the single draining vein, which is usually larger than the feeding artery. This could result in embolism with potentially catastrophic consequences. Thus, it is very important that the tip of the catheter is precisely placed and in a stable position, and that this is checked immediately before delivering any coils. A long floppy-tipped guide wire should be used to push out and deliver the coils. The aim of coil embolization is to produce a localized mass or nest of coils immediately proximal to the malformation that will produce a critical mass and thus effect occlusion of the artery. If a coil diameter is significantly bigger than the diameter of the artery, it could then end up being extended along the length of the vessel and not occlude the artery.[7,8]

To obtain better control on the placement of coils, detachable coils were developed.[9] The advantage of these coils is that they can be fully deployed, but are still attached to the pusher wire and are only detached if the position is satisfactory (Figure 78.4). When aiming to achieve a localized nest of coils, the most critical coil to be placed is the first

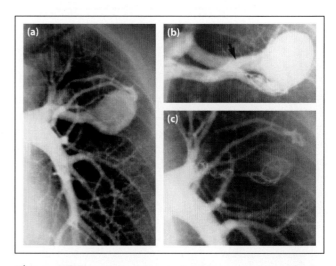

Figure 78.3 Same patient as in Figure 78.2. (a) A selective injection into the LPA (early arterial) shows a single feeding artery. (b) A superselective injection shows the PAVM more clearly with a mass of coils just beyond a small branch to normal lung parenchyma. (c) Despite this, the flow was such that a second procedure was necessary to effect occlusion.

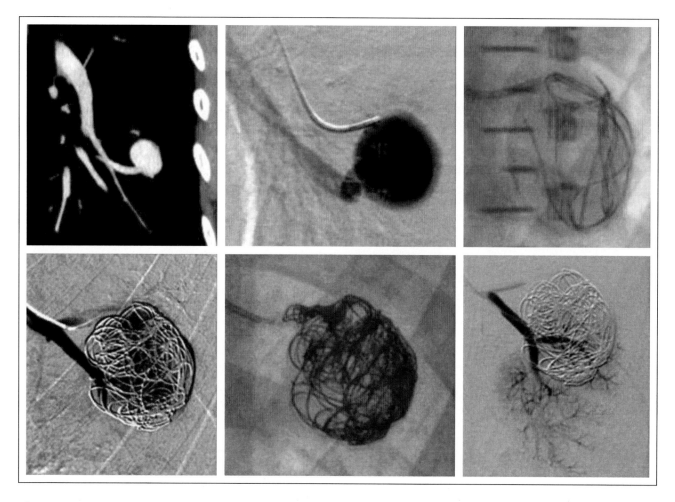

Figure 78.4   PAVM with a single feeding artery. The lesion was treated with multiple detachable coils in order to avoid coil migration in the draining vein.

coil or anchor coil. Once this is satisfactorily placed, it is possible to place further coils usually of a slightly smaller size next to it. If the feeding artery to the PAVM is of a large size and short neck, a further technique to effect occlusion is to pass the catheter into the aneurysmal sac and to deploy large-diameter coils (such as 20 mm) directly into it. These will then prevent any coils in the distal artery migrating through the malformation sac. Very large PAVMs may present a particular problem, as the right-to-left shunt will be very large and there are particular concerns regarding systemic embolism. Good long-term results have been reported, but in such cases, a second embolization procedure is sometimes necessary.[10] New devices such as the vascular plug (AGA Medical Corporation) can be a very effective and safe means of achieving occlusion.[11] The largest device available has a diameter of 22 mm offering a vessel coverage range between 2 and 16 mm. Vascular plugs AVP I and II require an 8 Fr catheter for their delivery; however, the recently developed Amplatzer Vascular Plug (AVP) IV may be delivered through a 4–5 Fr catheter with a 0.038 inch lumen (Figure 78.5). Similar to the

controlled-release coils, these devices also have a release mechanism, so the device is not finally detached from its delivery cable until its position is satisfactory, offering very good embolization results.[12]

After completion of the embolization procedure with coils, it is important to demonstrate on check arteriography that the feeding artery is occluded or severely restricted. Anything less than this is likely to not achieve a permanent occlusion. It is also important to check that there are not other smaller feeding arteries; sometimes there may be a small accessory artery that may need to be occluded.

Complications and how to avoid them

If marked polycythemia is a feature of the PAVM, then venesection to lower the hemoglobin level has been advocated to reduce the risk of spontaneous thrombosis. The most serious complication is systemic or paradoxical embolism. This is more likely to occur in the more common simple PAVMs. With correct sizing of coils and controlled-release devices, this risk may be minimized.

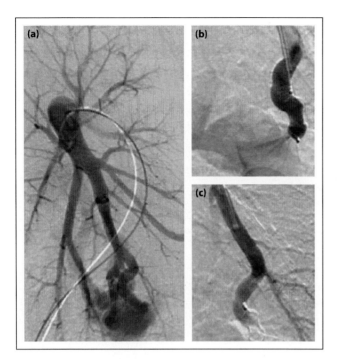

Figure 78.5 Treatment of a PAVM with the use of a type IV vascular plug. (a) Pigtail angiogram shows the PAVM. (b) The feeding artery was selectively catheterized and an 8 mm vascular plug was advanced though a 0.038 inch lumen catheter. Angiogram from the sheath prior to the release of the plug confirmed the appropriate size and position. (c) The plug was then released.

The other concern relates to the use of large end-hole catheters and the possibility of micro air embolism. When the catheter has been carefully positioned using a guide wire and the guide wire is removed, it is sometimes difficult to obtain good backflow from the catheter due to the tip being pushed up against the arterial wall. There is then a risk that small amounts of air can be introduced. An effective means of avoiding this is to have the end of the catheter and guide wire in a bowl of water prior to removal of the guide wire. This will prevent any possible air getting into the system so that if aspiration of blood is not possible, then this will not be a problem.

By identifying and selectively catheterizing the feeding artery to a PAVM and embolizing immediately proximal to the malformation, the PAVM should be occluded with little or no loss of normal parenchyma. Even with such a careful approach, there is the likelihood of a small amount of normal lung being infarcted and this may then result in some pleuritic chest pain. Such pain usually lasts only a few days and is associated with full recovery.

A particular problem occurs when there are multiple and diffuse PAVMs.[13] In such cases, embolizing all the lesions is not possible and the aim should be to embolize the significant localized PAVMs. If a small PAVM is coming off the same branch as normal parenchyma, then this is probably best left alone.

Pleuritic chest pain may be a persistent problem. The best method of following up on these patients is with a CT scan with contrast. This will confirm exclusion of the PAVM.

Postprocedure and follow-up

It should only be necessary for patients to spend one to two nights in the hospital following embolization procedures; nowadays some groups even perform the embolization on an outpatient basis.

Pulmonary artery aneurysms
Anatomy and pathophysiology

Pulmonary artery aneurysms (PAAs) and pulmonary artery pseudoaneurysms (PAPSs) are relatively rare. By definition, they are focal dilatations of the pulmonary artery.[14] If all three wall layers are included, the lesion is characterized as a PAA, otherwise as PAPS. The etiology may be congenital or acquired (Table 78.1). The most common acquired causes are vasculitis (most commonly Behcet's and Hughes–Stovin syndrome), neoplasm (due to erosion into the pulmonary arteries), infection (tuberculosis, pyogenic bacteria, and fungi), and trauma (usually iatrogenic, i.e., postsurgical).

Clinical symptoms and Indications for treatment

Though PAA and PAPS may occasionally be asymptomatic, they are more likely to be symptomatic and may present with dramatic symptoms, such as massive hemoptysis. The most common symptoms are dyspnea, cough, and chest pain.[15] Chest pain may be due to secondary pulmonary hypertension; however, chest pain may also be related to rupture and in such cases massive hemoptysis is also present.[16]

The diagnosis is usually based on clinical examination and CT findings. PAAs and PAPSs may present as a hilar or mediastinal mass on a chest x-ray when located centrally. In such cases, transthoracic echocardiography may be useful to reveal the aneurysmal dilatation. In cases where the lesion is located more peripherally, the diagnosis is made with contrast-enhanced CT.

Table 78.1	Causes of PAA/PAPS from Nguyen et al.[14]
Congenital	• Deficiency of the vessel wall • Valvar and postvalvar stenosis • Increased flow due to left-to-right shunts
Acquired	• Pulmonary arterial hypertension • Vasculitis • Mycotic aneurysms and pseudoaneurysms • Neoplasm • Iatrogenic causes

Owing to the risk of rupture, right heart failure, and pulmonary emboli, PAAs require treatment, which may be mainly surgical or endovascular. Central lesions, such as poststenotic dilatation of the main stem of the PA may be treated surgically on an elective basis with satisfactory results.[17] The surgical options in such cases are mainly Dacron or pericardial patch repair, graft interposition, or plication of the aneurysm.[17,18]

The results of surgery for more peripheral PAAs are less encouraging due to the high risk of bleeding and the development of recurrent pseudoaneurysms at the sites of the anastomoses.[19] In the case of massive hemoptysis (>300 mL in 24 hours), emergency surgery is associated with morbidity and mortality above 40%.[20] In such cases, the treatment of choice is endovascular. The use of cytostatic agents and corticosteroids may also be helpful in the cases of PAAs due to vasculitis when detected in an early stage.[21]

Pulmonary angiography

Access from the femoral vein with a 6 Fr sheath and pigtail angiogram at the bifurcation of the right or left pulmonary artery was performed to demonstrate the PAA in the pre-CT era. The angiogram is usually performed with 30 mL of iodinated contrast at a rate of 15 mL/s. Having the CT information on the location of the PAA, selective catheterization of the segmental and subsegmental branches of the right or left pulmonary artery with a curved multipurpose catheter and angiography at low rate of 3–4 mL/s with 8–10 mL of contrast is performed. The shape and the neck of the aneurysm need to be defined angiographically in order to decide on the treatment options.

Embolization procedure

The main difference in technique compared with a PAVM is that there is no fistula and draining vein and so there is no risk of systemic embolism; the technique usually involves occluding the feeding artery. In case of saccular PAAs in a large branch, a covered stent may be deployed to preserve the supply to the normal lung parenchyma. The reported endovascular treatment options include using coils[22–25] or microcoils,[26] the use of vascular plugs,[27] the use of liquid embolic materials,[28–30] and the deployment of covered stents.[31]

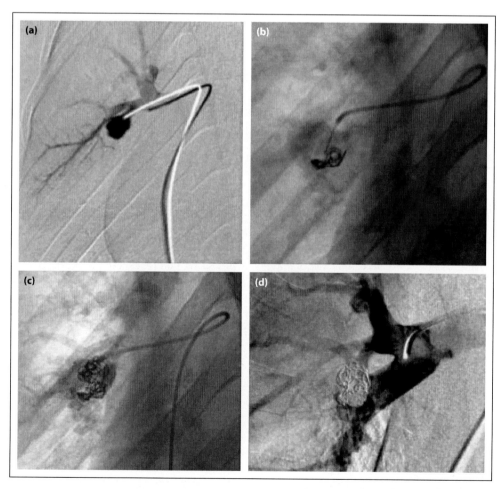

Figure 78.6   (a) Angiogram confirms the presence of a PAA in a patient with Behcet's disease. (b, c) The 4 Fr catheter was advanced in the aneurysmal sac and gradual deployment of coils followed. (d) Angiogram confirmed the complete exclusion of the PAA.

Coils appear to be the most common endovascular option for the treatment of PAA/PAPS because the originating pulmonary artery may be preserved. The cost of conventional coils is relatively low and in the reported series, no complications occurred. The technique requires that the device-carrying catheter is positioned within the aneurysm or at the aneurysm neck and that the coils are deployed inside the aneurysm (Figure 78.6). In case of a wide neck, a bare stent may be deployed across the neck in the pulmonary artery branch in order to prevent coils from migration ("caging technique").

Another solution may be the use of a vascular plug.[27] Liquid embolic agents like glue, ethylene vinyl alcohol copolymer, or thrombin are also used.[28–30] However, the liquid agents carry a risk of systemic artery embolization with potential dramatic complications, they require a longer preparation time, and do not appear to offer any true benefit compared with the traditional embolic materials. Finally, covered stents may offer a solution when the aneurysmal neck is very large.[31] In such cases, the covered stent is deployed to cover the neck.

In the case of PAAs that are not related to infectious processes, such as neoplasm and trauma, embolization of the feeding pulmonary arteries is enough to control the bleeding. In cases of PAAs and PAPSs that are related to infectious lung disease, bronchopulmonary shunts may exist and embolization through both pulmonary and systemic circulation may be required.[22] In such cases, selective catheterization of the bronchial arteries and embolization with particles is performed.

References

1. White R, Mitchell S, Barth K. Angioarchitecture of pulmonary arteriovenous malformations: An important consideration before embolotherapy. *AJR Am J Roentgenol* 1983;140:681–6.
2. Marianeschi SM, McElhinney DB, Reddy VM. Pulmonary arteriovenous malformations in and out of the setting of congenital heart disease. *Ann Thorac Surg* 1998;66(2):688–91.
3. Trerotola S, Pyeritz R. PAVM embolization: An update. *AJR Am J Roentgenol* 2010;195:837–45.
4. Guttmacher A, Marchuck D, Pyeritz R. Hereditary hemorrhagic telangiectasia. In: Rimoin D, Conner J, Pyeritz R, Korf B. Eds. *Principles and Practice of Medical Genetics*. 5th ed. Philadelphia, PA: Churchill Livingstone, 2007. pp. 1200–13.
5. Zukotynski K, Chan RP, Chow CM, Cohen JH, Faughnan ME. Contrast echocardiography grading predicts pulmonary arteriovenous malformations on CT. *Chest* 2007;132:18–23.
6. White RI Jr, Pollak JS, Wirth JA. Pulmonary arteriovenous malformations: Diagnosis and transcatheter embolotherapy. *J Vasc Interv Radiol* 1996;7(6):787–904.
7. Sagara K, Miyazono N, Inoue H. Recanalization after coil embolotherapy of pulmonary arteriovenous malformations: Study of long-term outcome and mechanism for recanalization. *AJR Am J Roentgenol* 1998;170:727–30.
8. Milic A, Chan RP, Cohen JH. Reperfusion of pulmonary arteriovenous malformations after embolotherapy. *J Vasc Intervent Radiol* 2005;16(12):1675–83.
9. Coley SC, Jackson JE. Endovascular occlusion with a new mechanical detachable coil. *AJR Am J Roentgenol* 1998;171:1075–9.
10. Lee DW, White RI, Egglin, TK. Embolotherapy of large pulmonary arteriovenous malformations: Long-term results. *Ann Thorac Surg* 1997;64:930–40.
11. Hill SL, Hijazi ZM, Hellenbrand WE. Evaluation of the AMPLATZER vascular plug for embolization of peripheral vascular malformations associated with congenital heart disease. *Catheter Cardiovasc Interv* 2006;67(1):113–9.
12. Cil B, Canyigit M, Ozkan OS, Pamuk GA, Dogan R. Bilateral multiple pulmonary arteriovenous malformations: Endovascular treatment with the Amplatzer vascular plug. *J Vasc Interv Radiol* 2006;17:141–5.
13. Pollak JS, Saluja S, Thabet A. Clinical and anatomic outcomes after embolotherapy of pulmonary arteriovenous malformations. *J Vasc Interv Radiol* 2006;17(1):34–5.
14. Nguyen E, Silva S, Seely J, Chong S, Lee KS, Muler N. Pulmonary artery aneurysms and pseudoaneurysms in adults: Findings in CT and radiography. *AJR Am J Roentgenol* 2007;188:126–34.
15. Deb SJ, Zehr KJ, Shields RC. Idiopathic pulmonary artery aneurysm. *Ann Thorac Surg* 2005;80:1500–2.
16. Butto F, Lucas RV, Edwards JE. Pulmonary arterial aneurysm. A pathologic study of five cases. *Chest* 1987;91:237–41.
17. Tuncer A, Tuncer E, Gezer S, Erdem H, Polat A. Repair of pulmonary artery aneurysms. *J Card Surg* 2011;26:501–5.
18. Nair KKS, Cobanoglu AM. Idiopathic main pulmonary artery aneurysm. *Ann Thorac Surg* 2001;71:1688–90
19. Hamuryudan V, Yurdakul S, Moral E et al. Pulmonary arterial aneurysms in Behcet's syndrome: Report of 24 cases. *Br J Rheumatol* 1994;33:48–51.
20. Conlan AA, Hurwitz SS, Krige L, Nicolaou N, Pool R. Massive hemoptysis: Review of 123 cases. *J Thorac Cardiovasc Surg* 1983;85(1):120–4.
21. Tunaci M, Ozkorkmaz B, Tunaci A et al. CT findings of pulmonary artery aneurysms during treatment for Behcet's disease. *AJR Am J Roentgenol* 1999;172:729–33.
22. Remy J, Lemaitre L, Lafitte JJ et al. Massive hemoptysis of pulmonary arterial origin: Diagnosis and treatment. *AJR Am J Roentgenol* 1984;143(5):963–9.
23. Sbano H, Mitchell AW, Ind PW et al. Peripheral pulmonary artery pseudoaneurysms and massive hemoptysis. *AJR Am J Roentgenol* 2005;184(4):1253–9.
24. Santelli ED, Katz DS, Goldschmidt AM et al. Embolization of multiple Rasmussen aneurysms as a treatment of hemoptysis. *Radiology* 1994;193:396–8.
25. Mouas H, Lortholary O, Lacombe P. Embolization of multiple pulmonary arterial aneurysms in Behcet's disease. *Scand J Rheumatol* 1996;25:58–60
26. Shin S, Shin TB, Choi H et al. Peripheral pulmonary arterial pseudoaneurysms: Therapeutic implications of endovascular treatment and angiographic classifications *Radiology* 2010;256(2):656–64.
27. Jagia P, Sharma S, Juneja S et al. Transcatheter treatment of pulmonary artery pseudoaneurysm using a PDA closure device. *Diagn Interv Radiol* 2011;17:92–4.
28. Khalil A, Parrot A, Fartoukh M et al. Pulmonary artery occlusion with ethylene vinyl alcohol copolymer in patients with hemoptysis: Initial experience in 12 cases. *AJR Am J Roentgenol* 2012;198(1):207–12.
29. Cantasdemir M, Kantarci F, Mihmanli I et al. Emergency endovascular management of pulmonary artery aneurysms in Behcet's disease: Report of two cases and review of the literature. *Cardiovasc Intervent Radiol* 2002;25:533–7.
30. Lee K, Shin T, Choi J, Kim Y. Percutaneous injection therapy for a peripheral pulmonary artery pseudoaneurysm after failed transcatheter coil embolization. *Cardiovasc Intervent Radiol* 2008;31:1038–41.
31. Park A, Cwikiel W. Endovascular treatment of a pulmonary artery pseudoaneurysm with a stent graft: Report of two cases. *Acta Radiol* 2007;48:45–7.

79

Coronary artery fistulas

Shakeel A. Qureshi

Introduction

Coronary artery fistulas are connections between one or more of the coronary arteries and a cardiac chamber or great vessel. They are rare and usually occur in isolation.[1] Although usually congenital, they may occur after cardiac surgery, such as valve replacement, coronary artery bypass grafting, and after repeated myocardial biopsies in cardiac transplantation.[2,3]

The fistula is usually a dilated, long, and tortuous feeding artery taking a course around the heart before terminating in a cardiac chamber or a vessel. It may drain from a main coronary artery or one or several branches of a coronary artery to a cardiac chamber or into a vessel. Multiple feeding arteries to a single coronary artery fistula may exist.[2] More than 55% of the fistulas originate from the right coronary artery, with the left anterior descending coronary artery being the next most frequently involved.[4] A more recent review has reported a different incidence with about 55% originating from the left coronary artery, about 37% from the right, and 8% from both.[5] Over 90% of the fistulas from either coronary artery drain to the right side of the heart. The remainder drain to either the left atrium or the left ventricle.[6] In the review by Holzer et al., 65% drained to the right heart, 23% to the pulmonary arteries, 11% to the left heart, and rarely to multiple sites.[5] The differences in the sites of origin and drainage is probably due to different eras with different methods of investigation. The sites of drainage in the right heart include the right atrium, the vena cavae, the right ventricle, or the pulmonary trunk. Multiple fistulas between the three major coronary arteries and the left ventricle have also been reported.[7]

Pathophysiology

When the coronary artery fistulas drain to the right side of the heart, the volume load is increased to the right heart as well as the pulmonary vascular bed, the left atrium, and the left ventricle. When the fistula drains into the left atrium or the left ventricle, there is volume overloading of these chambers but no increase in the pulmonary blood flow.

Clinical features

Although the majority of the fistulas are congenital, they do not usually cause symptoms or complications in the first two decades, especially if they are small. After this age, the frequency of both symptoms and complications increases.[8] The complications include "steal" from the adjacent myocardium, thrombosis and embolism, cardiac failure, atrial fibrillation, rupture, endocarditis/endarteritis, and arrhythmias.[1,4,9–11] Thrombosis within the aneurysm of the feeding artery, while rare, may cause acute myocardial infarction, paroxysmal atrial fibrillation, and ventricular arrhythmias.[12] Spontaneous rupture of the aneurysmal fistula causing hemopericardium has also been reported.[13]

Some fistulas may be large during the neonatal period, but others may increase in size over time. Very occasionally, they may be detected prenatally.[14] They vary from short and direct connections of a coronary artery with a chamber or a large vessel to complex aneurysms, in which blood may stagnate, clot, and calcify. The largest shunts tend to occur in those fistulas in which the coronary artery connects to the right side of the heart rather than the left heart chambers.

The majority of the patients are asymptomatic. Symptoms, when present, may include exercise intolerance because of dyspnea, angina, and arrhythmias. Patients with large left-to-right shunts may have symptoms of congestive cardiac failure, especially in infancy and occasionally in the neonatal period.[14] Some patients may have angina and electrocardiographic evidence of myocardial ischemia.[2] Angina may occur because of a "steal phenomenon."[15] The most common presentation is with the detection of an asymptomatic continuous murmur over the praecordium. The murmur is heard over the midchest rather than below the left clavicle and typically peaks in middiastole rather than systole, which occurs when the murmur originates from the arterial duct.

Investigations

The electrocardiogram and chest x-ray are unlikely to help in the diagnosis. The electrocardiogram may be normal in small fistulas or may show the effects of left ventricular volume overload and ischemic changes. However, in the presence of a normal electrocardiogram, if the patient is old enough to exercise on the treadmill with electrocardiographic monitoring, then ischemic ST-segment changes may become apparent.[15] The chest x-ray is usually normal, but occasionally moderate cardiomegaly may be present, when there is a large left-to-right shunt. Magnetic resonance imaging or computerized tomography has been used to diagnose coronary artery fistulas, define the morphology, and plan the treatment.[16]

Selective coronary angiography of both the coronary arteries is essential for confirming the diagnosis, the detailed anatomy of the fistula, and the presence of multiple fistulas. However, this should only be performed when definitive treatment such as an interventional procedure or surgery is planned. During such an intervention, a preliminary aortic root angiogram in a "laid-back view" helps in determining which coronary artery to selectively catheterize.[17] Coronary angiography in several planes assumes great importance and should be performed in the same views as in adults. These views include right anterior oblique, straight anteroposterior, left anterior oblique, left anterior oblique with caudo-cranial angulation, and left lateral projections.

Treatment

The treatment of coronary artery fistulas is determined by the age of the patient, the size of the fistula, and the severity of symptoms. The indications for treatment include the presence of a large or increasing left-to-right shunt, evidence of left ventricular volume overload, myocardial ischemia, left ventricular dysfunction, congestive cardiac failure, and rarely for the prevention of endocarditis/endarteritis. Large coronary artery fistulas may cause cardiac failure, but medical management should be attempted initially, especially in infancy in order to delay the timing of intervention. With medical treatment, some newborns may improve with regard to their symptoms, with possible reduction of the size of the fistula over time.[18]

Surgical closure of coronary artery fistulas is performed by external ligation or intracardiac repair on cardiopulmonary bypass. Surgery is associated with a low morbidity and mortality rate, ranging from 0 to 6%.[19,20] Myocardial infarction has been reported in less than 5% of cases and there is a low but significant risk of persistence or recurrence of the fistula.[21] Over the last two decades, transcatheter closure of coronary artery fistulas has emerged as an effective and safe alternative to surgery and so should be considered as the treatment of choice.[2,22,23] Surgery may be considered if the normal coronary arteries are in close proximity to the site of device closure, posing a risk of occlusion of a main coronary artery.

The aim of catheter closure is to occlude the fistulous artery as distally as possible or as close to its termination point as possible, avoiding any possibility of occluding branches to the normal myocardium. If, however, embolization is achieved too distally, the embolization device could pass inadvertently beyond the fistula into the draining vessel or chamber and into the pulmonary circulation, in particular if there is no constriction present. Thus, it is important that whichever technique is used, the occlusion is achieved at a very precise point. In practice, this involves the use of different types of embolization materials such as detachable balloons, stainless steel coils, or platinum microcoils.[2,23–27] The technique employed is influenced by several factors, including the age of the patient, the morphology of the feeding arteries, their size and degree of tortuosity, and the location of the fistulous connection. Detachable balloons are now rarely used, as a wider variety of better devices has become available.

Equipment

Availability of a wide variety of equipment in the catheterization laboratory is essential for transcatheter closure of the fistula (Figure 79.1). This includes a selection of nontapered catheters, Berman or Swan–Ganz balloon catheters, 3 Fr Tracker or Ferret catheters, a variety of floppy or superfloppy coronary guide wires of 0.014 inch caliber, a range of different types and sizes of coils (conventional Gianturco coils and controlled-release coils), and a variety of closure devices used to close atrial septal defects or patent arterial ducts or vascular plugs.

The choice of the equipment and the technique depends on the tortuosity of the fistula vessels, the presence of a high flow in the fistula, the presence of aneurysmal dilation of the feeding vessel and the point of intended occlusion. Other factors influencing the choice include the age and size of the patient, the catheter size that can be used in the patient, the size of the vessel to be occluded and the tortuosity of the catheter course to reach the intended point of occlusion. For example, if the access artery is small, then a technique needing smaller sheaths and catheters should be chosen. If the target vessel to be occluded is large, then a large device that fits in the smallest guiding catheter or sheath is chosen. If the route to the target vessel is tortuous, then superfloppy guide wires and 3 Fr Tracker, Ferret, or Progreat catheters are preferable. If there is a high flow through the target vessel, then a stop-flow technique is used, in which a balloon inflated proximally stops the blood flow through the fistula. Because of the need for precise occlusion, a potentially reversible technique is preferred.

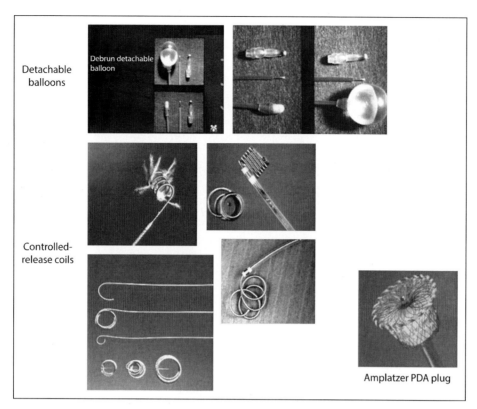

Figure 79.1   A variety of equipment for use in embolization.

Technique

The procedure is usually performed under general anesthesia, especially in infants and children. Conscious sedation may be used in adults. Generally, access is obtained via both the femoral arteries and a femoral vein, in which 5 Fr sheaths are inserted. Heparin (100 units/kg) is given and activated clotting time is maintained between 200 and 250 s during the interventional procedure. Both the femoral arteries are cannulated because coils are deployed through one of the catheters, while check angiograms can be performed through a catheter from the other femoral artery. Alternatively, a balloon catheter can be inflated through the second arterial access to aid in coil deployment in cases of high blood flow. Judkins left and right coronary catheters are used for selective angiography and subsequently a balloon catheter (Berman or Swan–Ganz or balloon wedge catheter) is passed and the balloon inflated with contrast or carbon dioxide to temporarily occlude the vessel. The balloon is kept inflated for 5–10 min to assess whether any ECG changes of ischemia occur.

If there are no ischemic changes, then a guiding coronary catheter appropriate for the coronary artery is positioned in the artery. If the fistula drainage point is fairly proximal and has a straight course, then with the help of a 0.035 inch standard guide wire advanced into the fistula, the catheter can be passed to the point of intended occlusion. Through this catheter, either Gianturco or Cook PDA coils can be

used to achieve occlusion. Stainless steel Gianturco coils of 0.038 inch caliber have been widely used and require standard nontapered catheters of 5 Fr or 6 Fr size for the delivery of the coils (Figure 79.2). The size of the coil should be up to 30% larger than the vessel diameter and in particular the drainage point, so that the coil does not pass through and embolize inadvertently. If this method is used, the first coil is the most important one, as once this is in correct position, different sizes of coils can be deployed subsequently to form a tight nest, which will promote occlusion

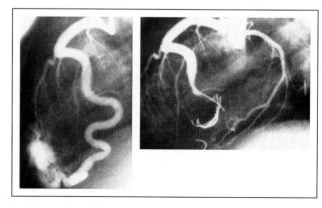

Figure 79.2   A fistula between the diagonal branch of the left anterior descending coronary artery and the right ventricle. The vessel is moderately tortuous and has been closed with Gianturco coils.

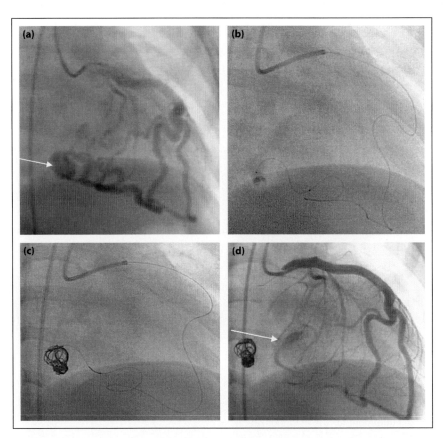

Figure 79.3 (a) A fistula between a branch of the left anterior descending coronary artery and the right ventricle. There are possibly two feeding vessels with a very tortuous course. Arrow points to the presence of an aneurysm at the point of entry into the right ventricle. (b) Tracker catheter having been passed through the guiding catheter around the tortuous course into the aneurysm at the point of occlusion. (c) A nest of controlled-release coils packed into the aneurysm. (d) Complete occlusion of the main fistulous vessels, but now there is a tiny residual fistula from another vessel draining into the left ventricle (arrow).

of the vessel. Positioning such catheters satisfactorily in a distal location in a coronary artery fistula may be both difficult and hazardous. The tortuosity of the fistula may prevent attempts at passing larger catheters distally into the coronary artery. Therefore, this method may be used safely only in those patients in whom the fistulas have a short, relatively less tortuous course and in whom there may be aneurysmal dilation present in the fistulous vessel.

In those patients in whom the fistulous vessel is tortuous with multiple bends that need to be negotiated or when the guiding catheter cannot reach the point of occlusion or when there is a high flow, it may be more appropriate to use controlled-release platinum microcoils of 0.018 inch caliber, which can be deployed using a coaxial 3 Fr Tracker, Ferret, or Progreat catheter passed through the guiding catheter. Such catheters, when used with super-floppy, steerable 0.014 inch coronary guide wires, can be manipulated through tortuous arteries into very distal locations and through them interlocking-detachable coils (IDC) or detachable coil system (DCS) coils can be used (Figure 79.3a–d). These coils have controlled-release mechanisms and so make the procedure reversible and more

controlled. If there is a high flow, then temporary balloon occlusion will be needed during the deployment of the coils (Figure 79.4).[24,25] Multiple coils can be deployed serially through these catheters. When passing these catheters through multiple bends, it is important to use a torque device to manipulate the guide wire around the various curves in the fistula. A short distance of the guide wire is passed, followed by gentle and gradual movement forward

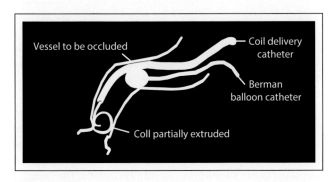

Figure 79.4 Diagrammatic illustration of the stop-flow technique using a balloon catheter.

of the 3 Fr catheter, until this catheter has reached the point of occlusion. By gentle manipulation, it is surprising how relatively easily and how far distally into the fistula the 3 Fr catheter can be passed. It is important to use a Tuohy–Borst adapter or a hemostatic valve connected to the guiding catheter as well as the 3 Fr catheter for prevention of gradual blood loss. The coil will then need to be passed through the hemostatic valve using an introducer provided with the coil.

Very high-flow fistulous arteries present a particular problem because there will be a tendency for the coils to be pushed by the coronary blood flow into the right heart circulation. This difficulty can be overcome by using temporary occlusion of the proximal fistulous artery with a Berman balloon occlusion or a balloon wedge catheter, which stops the blood flow in the vessel. While the balloon is kept inflated, several coils can be deployed to form a nest before deflating the balloon.[28,29] This technique has allowed an occluding mass of these coils to be safely and satisfactorily positioned to achieve complete occlusion (Figure 79.5).

A high-flow artery can be difficult to occlude, so a mass of platinum coils is necessary. Availability of controlled-release coils has made the procedure more practical and safe. These coils can be withdrawn back into the catheter, if the final position is not satisfactory. The coils are not fibered and this results in very little resistance to passage through the microcatheters around the many curves that are normally encountered. However, the disadvantage of these coils is that thrombosis takes a considerably longer time than the fibered coils.

More frequently, devices other than coils are used nowadays to close the fistulas. If the fistula morphology is such that it can be accessed easily from the right side of the heart and when there is a large aneurysmal fistula near the drainage point into the right side of the heart (most often such fistulas drain into the right atrium), then these may be suitable for occlusion with an Amplatzer duct occluder or atrial septal occluder device and some with vascular plugs.[14,30] The fistula vessel needs to be large, have straight access from the right heart, even if an arteriovenous guide

wire circuit is needed, and allow a guiding sheath to be passed into the vessel before deploying a device. In such cases, either femoral venous or internal jugular venous access is needed over an arteriovenous guide wire circuit (Figure 79.6a–c). Creation of a circuit facilitates the passage of an appropriate sheath over the guide wire.

Detachable balloons have been deployed in the past as they can be floated out with the arterial flow and achieve immediate occlusion, which is reversible until the balloon is detached.[24,27] They are, however, complex to use and require large-caliber nontapered introducer catheters (6–8 Fr). This presents a limitation to their use in infants and young children. Early deflation and premature detachment of these balloons are further problems and so they are rarely used.

After occluding the main fistulous vessel, it is imperative to repeat selective coronary angiography in both the coronary arteries, as on occasions a second branch feeding the fistula may be visualized, which may then need to be occluded at the same procedure.

With transcatheter techniques, complete occlusion of the fistula may be achieved in >95% of the patients. The main complications (albeit of low frequency) encountered include premature deflation (in the case of detachable balloons), inadvertent coil embolization (Figure 79.7a and b), transient T-wave changes, transient bundle branch block, and myocardial infarction (Figure 79.8). Some of the inadvertent embolizations may occur as a result of high flow in the large fistulas or with selection of undersized coils.[28]

A particular challenge is encountered when dealing with marked aneurysmal dilation within the feeding artery of the fistula. Although on most occasions, closing the exit point into the right heart is adequate, other strategies may be needed. The expectation is that a device placed at the exit point will result in thrombosis of the aneurysm and its feeding vessel. On some occasions, this may not occur because of multiple exit points and rarely, the aneurysm may continue to enlarge. These will need to be dealt with by repeat procedures. A better alternative strategy is to place a device or a vascular plug in the dilated feeding artery through a

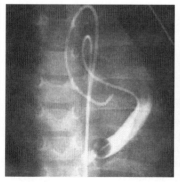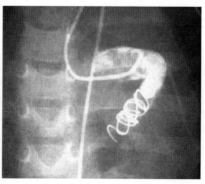

Figure 79.5 A fistula between the left coronary artery and the right atrium. A balloon has been placed for test occlusion and subsequently Gianturco coils have been deployed, resulting in complete occlusion of the fistula.

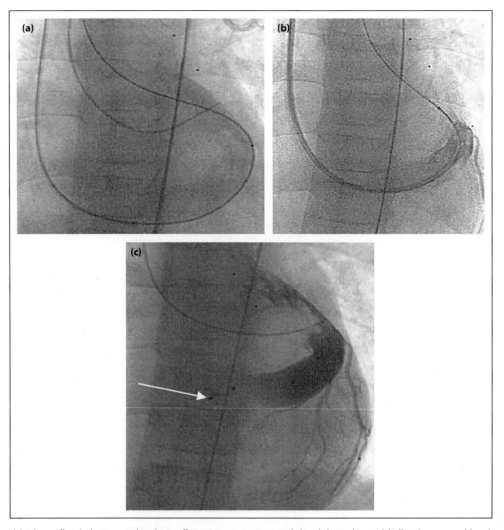

Figure 79.6 (a) A large fistula between the circumflex coronary artery and the right atrium. This fistulous vessel has been approached from the right internal jugular vein and an arteriovenous guide wire circuit has been established. (b) A sheath having been passed from the internal jugular vein into the dilated fistulous vessel, with improved filling of the native coronary artery. (c) An angiogram after implantation of an Amplatzer duct occluder (arrow) resulting in complete occlusion of the fistula and improved filling of the native coronary arteries. (Courtesy of Dr. Masood Sadiq, Lahore, Pakistan.)

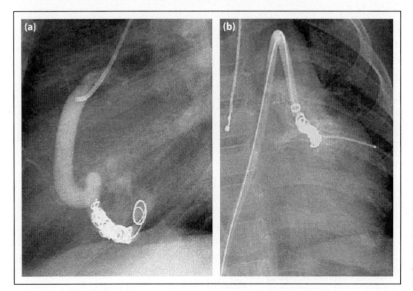

Figure 79.7 (a) A nest of coils released in the right coronary artery to the right ventricle fistula resulting in near complete occlusion. (b) The coils have embolized to the left pulmonary artery. A sheath has been placed close to the coils for retrieval with a snare catheter.

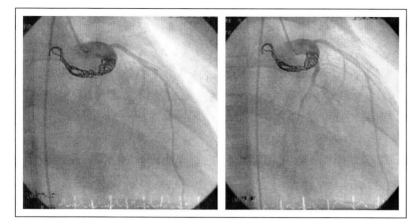

Figure 79.8 Coils implanted into a branch of circumflex coronary artery (fistula between this and the right atrium) have produced complete occlusion of the main circumflex coronary artery. After thrombolysis with r-TPA, there is now a patent circumflex coronary artery. (Courtesy of Dr. Grazyna Brzezinska-Rajszys, Warsaw, Poland.)

sheath positioned over a guide wire circuit and then to withdraw the sheath into the aneurysm. Here, another device can be delivered at the exit point. This approach has the major advantage of completely excluding the aneurysm and occluding the fistula (Figure 79.9a–d).

The patients need to be kept hospitalized for about 3 days, with daily repeat electrocardiograms and cardiac enzymes. There should be a low threshold for repeat angiography, if there is evidence of myocardial infarction, in case thrombolysis is needed. After discharge, the patients are usually maintained on antiplatelet therapy for 3–6 months, in case of small feeding arteries and distal occlusion, or maintained on anticoagulants such as warfarin for about 1 year, if the feeding artery is considerably dilated. If there is an aneurysm as well as a dilated feeding artery, then anticoagulants are maintained for about 1 year, after which coronary angiography should be repeated to decide whether to convert the medication from anticoagulants to antiplatelet agents.[31]

Special considerations

Although a majority of feeding arteries of coronary artery fistulas are side branches, occasionally, the feeding artery is actually the native coronary artery (left anterior descending or circumflex or right coronary artery rather than their branches). In these cases, caution is needed on their closure. Figure 79.10a–e shows an example of a right coronary artery fistula draining into the coronary sinus. The feeding artery is the native coronary artery, which is extremely tortuous. Although this was successfully occluded with a device and full anticoagulation was maintained subsequently, the patient died several months

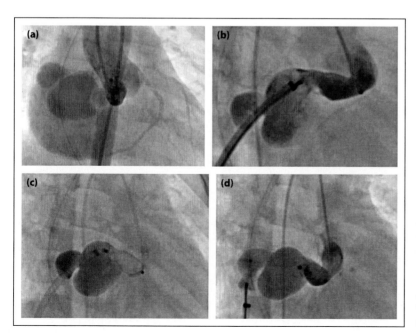

Figure 79.9 (a) An anteroposterior projection of aortogram showing a coronary artery fistula between the right coronary artery and the right atrium. There are multiple aneurysms seen. (b) An angiogram with a delivery sheath in place with an Amplatzer vascular plug (AVP II) being delivered through it proximal to a large aneurysm. (c) An angiogram after release of AVP II but with the delivery sheath still within the aneurysm. (d) A selective coronary angiogram after deploying an Amplatzer duct occluder (ADO I) at the exit point into the right atrium. With such a method, both the vessel feeding the aneurysm and the exit point into the right atrium distal to the aneurysms are occluded with devices. This method excludes the aneurysms. (Courtesy of Dr. K Sivakumar, Chennai, India.)

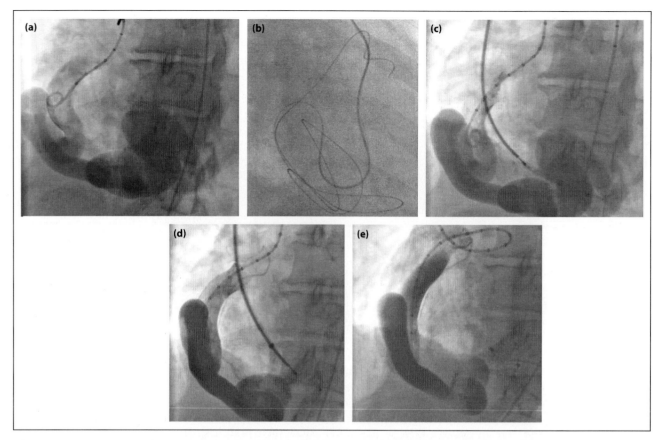

Figure 79.10 (a) Selective right coronary angiogram in left anterior oblique projection with a pigtail catheter showing a complex tortuous coronary artery fistula between the right coronary artery and coronary sinus. (b) A soft exchange length 0.035 inch guide wire has been passed retrogradely from the aorta through the right coronary artery into the right heart. (c, d) A selective right coronary angiogram after a sheath with an Amplatzer muscular ventricular septal defect occluder in position at the exit point into the coronary sinus and fully deployed. Sluggish flow is seen within the coronary artery. (e) A selective right coronary angiogram with muscular ventricular septal defect occluder in place and extremely sluggish flow through the tortuous course of the fistula.

later from an arrhythmia. The arrhythmia was presumed to be secondary to myocardial ischemia from occlusion of a side branch, even though at autopsy the feeding artery remained patent. Other authors have also advised caution in similar situations.[32,33]

Discussion

A majority of coronary artery fistulas are asymptomatic in the early years. When large, they can result in symptoms of congestive cardiac failure or angina; this may be the cause at the extremes of life in infants or middle-aged or older adults. Coronary fistulas have been detected prenatally too, in which case, because of a large left-to-right shunt, they may cause congestive cardiac failure soon after birth.[34] If the congestive cardiac failure cannot be controlled, transcatheter closure may be needed early after birth.[14] If fistulas are detected in infancy and the infants are asymptomatic, conservative management is appropriate, as very rarely, spontaneous closure of a small fistula has been reported.[35]

Even if the fistula does not close, the older the patient, the fewer the technical complications encountered when the catheter procedure is attempted. Some authors recommend closure even in the absence of symptoms on the grounds that with increasing age, the incidence of complications increases.[7]

As these fistulas are infrequently encountered, most operators will only deal with a small number of cases of coronary artery fistulas each year. The aim of the catheter procedure should be to achieve complete occlusion as distally as possible in the fistulous vessel and this can be achieved with meticulous attention to the details of the technique. Specialized techniques and equipment are needed for catheter closure of these fistulas. Occasionally, a combination of techniques is required, but the procedure has become easier with the availability of controlled-release platinum coils and the range of devices or occluders or vascular plugs, and any complexity of the fistulous vessel can be treated. The main complication is inadvertent embolization of the devices. However, even if any of these devices embolize, they can be retrieved by snares.

Conclusions

Excellent results can be achieved by the transcatheter embolization techniques to treat coronary artery fistulas. Furthermore, the technique of catheter closure allows further arterial feeding vessels to be discovered by selective coronary angiography at the end of the procedure and if such a dual supply is noted, this vessel can also be occluded.

It is vital to select an embolization technique suitable for the size and the location of the fistula. A wide range of equipment should be available to cope with the great variety of fistulas as well as possible complications of the techniques. Nowadays, no patient should be referred for surgical ligation unless transcatheter closure has been considered or has been attempted and failed.

References

1. Wilde P, Watt I. Congenital coronary artery fistulae: Six new cases with a collective review. *Clin Radiol* 1980;31:301–11.
2. Reidy JF, Anjos RT, Qureshi SA, Baker EJ, Tynan MJ. Transcatheter embolization in the treatment of coronary artery fistulas. *J Am Coll Cardiol* 1991;18:187–92.
3. Somers JM, Verney GI. Coronary cameral fistulae following heart transplantation. *Clin Radiol* 1991;44:419–21.
4. McNamara JJ, Gross RE. Congenital coronary artery fistula. *Surgery* 1969;65:59–69.
5. Holzer R, Johnson R, Ciotti G, Pozzi M, Kitchiner D. Review of an institutional experience of coronary arterial fistulas in childhood set in context of review of the literature. *Cardiol Young* 2004;14:380–5.
6. Levin DC, Fellows KE, Abrams HL. Hemodynamically significant primary anomalies of the coronary arteries. *Circulation* 1978;58:25–34.
7. Black IW, Loo CK, Allan RM. Multiple coronary artery-left ventricular fistulae: Clinical, angiographic, and pathologic findings. *Eur J Cardiothorac Surg* 1991;23:133–5.
8. Liberthson RR, Sagar K, Berkoben JP, Weintraub RM, Levine FH. Congenital coronary arteriovenous fistula: Report of 13 patients, review of the literature and delineation of management. *Circulation* 1979;59:849–54.
9. Alkhulaifi AM, Horner SM, Pugsley WB, Swanton RH. Coronary artery fistulas presenting with bacterial endocarditis. *Ann Thorac Surg* 1995;60:202–4.
10. Skimming JW, Walls JT. Congenital coronary artery fistula suggesting a "steal phenomenon" in a neonate. *Pediatr Cardiol* 1993;14:174–5.
11. Misumi T, Nishikawa K, Yasudo M, et al. Rupture of an aneurysm of a coronary arteriovenous fistula. *Ann Thorac Surg* 2001;71:2026–7
12. Ramo OJ, Totterman KJ, Harjula AL. Thrombosed coronary artery fistula as a cause of paroxysmal atrial filbrillation and ventricular arrhythmia. *Cardiovasc Surg* 1994;2:720–2.
13. Bauer HH, Allmendinger PD, Flaherty J, Owlia D, Rossi MA, Chen C. Congenital coronary arteriovenous fistula: Spontaneous rupture and cardiac tamponade. *Ann Thorac Surg* 1996;62:1521–3.
14. Khan MD, Qureshi SA, Rosenthal E, Sharland GK. Neonatal transcatheter occlusion of a large coronary artery fistula with Amplatzer duct occluder. *Catheter Cardiovasc Interv* 2003;60:282–6.
15. Oshiro K, Shimabukuro M, Nakada Y et al. Multiple coronary LV fistulas: Demonstration of coronary steal phenomenon by stress thallium scintigraphy and exercise haemodynamics. *Am Heart J* 1990;120:217–9.
16. Zenooz NA, Habibi R, Mammen L et al. Coronary artery fistulas. CT findings. *Radiographics* 2009;29:781–9.
17. Hofbeck M, Wild F, Singer H. Improved visualisation of a coronary artery fistula by the "laid-back" aortogram. *Br Heart J* 1993;70:272–3.
18. Hsieh KS, Huang TC, Lee CL. Coronary artery fistulas in neonates, infants and children: Clinical findings and outcome. *Pediatr Cardiol* 2002;23:415–9.
19. Mavroudis C, Backer CL, Rocchini AP, Muster AJ, Gevitz M. Coronary artery fistulas in infants and children: A surgical review and discussion of coil embolization. *Ann Thorac Surg* 1997;63:1235–42.
20. Rittenhouse EA, Doty DB, Ehrenhaft JL. Congenital coronary artery-cardiac chamber fistula. *Ann Thorac Surg* 1975;20:468–85.
21. Kirklin JW, Barrat-Boyes BG. *Cardiac Surgery*. New York: John Wiley, 1987. pp. 945–55.
22. Reidy JF, Jones ODH, Tynan MJ, Baker EJ, Joseph MC. Embolization procedures in congenital heart disease. *Br Heart J* 1985;54:184–92.
23. Perry SB, Rome J, Keane JF, Baim DS, Lock JE. Transcatheter closure of coronary artery fistulas. *J Am Coll Cardiol* 1992;20:205–9.
24. Reidy JF, Sowton E, Ross DN. Transcatheter occlusion of coronary to bronchial anastomosis by detachable balloon combined with coronary angioplasty at the same procedure. *Br Heart J* 1983;49:284–7.
25. Van den Brand M, Pieterman H, Suryapranata H, Bogers AJ. Closure of a coronary fistula with a transcatheter implantable coil. *Eur J Cardiothorac Surg* 1992;25:223–6.
26. De Wolf D, Terriere M, De Wilde P, Reidy JF. Embolization of a coronary fistula with a controlled delivery platinum coil in a 2-year old. *Pediatr Cardiol* 1994;15:308–10.
27. Skimming JW, Gessner IH, Victorica BE, Mickle JP. Percutaneous transcatheter occlusion of coronary artery fistulas using detachable balloons. *Pediatr Cardiol* 1995;16:38–41.
28. Qureshi SA, Reidy JF, Alwi MB, Lim MK, Wong J, Tay J, Baker EJ, Tynan M. Use of interlocking detachable coils in embolization of coronary arteriovenous fistulas. *Am J Cardiol* 1996;78:110–3.
29. Quek SC, Wong J, Tay JS, Reidy J, Qureshi SA. Transcatheter embolization of coronary artery fistula with controlled release coils. *J Paediatr Child Health* 1996;32:542–4.
30. Sadiq M, Wilkinson JL, Qureshi SA. Successful occlusion of coronary arteriovenous fistula using an Amplatzer duct occluder. *Cardiol Young* 2001;11:84–7.
31. Latson L. Coronary artery fistulas: How to manage them. *Catheter Cardiovasc Interv* 1997;70:110–6.
32. Gowda ST, Latson LA, Kutty S, Prieto LR. Intermediate to long-term outcome following congenital coronary artery fistulae closure with focus on thrombus formation. *Am J Cardiol* 2011;107:302–8.
33. Gowda ST, Latson LA, Kutty S, Prieto LR. Remodeling and thrombosis following closure of coronary artery fistula with review of management: Large distal coronary artery fistula—To close or not to close? *Catheter Cardiovasc Intervent* 2013;82:132–42.
34. Sharland GK, Tynan M, Qureshi SA. Prenatal detection and progression of right coronary artery to right ventricle fistula. *Heart* 1996;76:79–81.
35. Muthusamy R, Gupta G, Ahmed RA, de Giovanni J, Singh SP. Fistula between a branch of left anterior descending coronary artery and pulmonary artery with spontaneous closure. *Eur Heart J* 1990;11:954–6.

80

Obstructions of the inferior and superior vena cava

Marc Gewillig

Anatomy and pathophysiology

Obstruction of caval veins is rare, and usually iatrogenic. Any surgical procedure involving the caval veins, including cannulation for bypass, may be complicated with caval vein obstruction. It was a common complication of the Mustard operation during early and long-term follow-up, with restrictive venous pathways in the majority of the patients.[1,2] It has been reported after a Senning-type procedure, after a Glenn shunt or other cavopulmonary connections, after transplantation with stricture of the anastomosis,[3] or after repair of abnormal pulmonary venous return with subdivision of the superior vena cava (SCV).

Multiple pacing leads or other long-term catheters may lead to progressive narrowing, especially during growth. Thrombosis of a caval vein may occur after endothelial damage during traumatic puncture for central lines, after a long period of low cardiac output with hypertonic IV fluids, or after recurrent and long-term central venous line[4] infections. Any hypercoagulable state may exacerbate this problem (protein C or S, antithrombin 3, Leiden factor, etc.).

Congenital membranous obstruction of the inferior vena cava (ICV) at the junction with the right atrium or a restrictive Eustachian valve has been described.[5] An obstructed ICV may present as Budd–Chiari syndrome.

External compression by a tumor (lung cancer, lymphoma), aneurysmal dilation of the ascending aorta, pseudoaneurysm of a venous coronary graft,[6] goiter, mediastinal fibrosis, constrictive pericarditis, bile bladder distention, polycystic kidneys, hydatid cyst, and hematoma after blunt liver trauma have been reported. Vasculitis such as Behcet's disease may lead to shrinkage and obstruction of the caval veins.[7]

Clinical symptoms, indications for treatment, and alternatives

Clinical symptoms will depend on onset and obstruction rate, the development of collateral flow, and the functionality of the other caval vein.

Obstruction of the SCV may clinically result in superior caval vein syndrome: congestion, swelling, and cyanosis of the head and the upper limbs, headaches or cerebral venous hypertension, (pre)syncope, cough, and airway obstruction. Pemberton's sign involves jugular vein distension in upright position, which progresses to cyanosis and facial edema while keeping both arms elevated. Retrograde congestion of the thoracic duct may lead to leakage of chyl into the gut (protein losing enteropathy), into the pleural space (chylothorax[8] or chylopericardium), or into the bronchial tree (plastic bronchitis).

Obstruction of the ICV may lead to abdominal congestion, chronic hepatic congestion leading to fibrosis, varices, exercise intolerance, fatigue or swelling of the legs, renal insufficiency with proteinuria,[9] or Budd–Chiari syndrome.[10,11]

If inflow to the heart is severely limited from all sides, this will result in decreased cardiac output, which can be very difficult to detect clinically. The heart will typically have no preload reserve; tachycardia or exercise will decrease stroke volume, which may result in hypotension, vertigo, syncope, or sudden death.

Alternative treatment to interventional catheterization depends on the etiology: mass resection or debulking, thrombolysis, anticoagulation, treatment with anti-inflammatory, antibiotic, or oncologic drugs, or radiation treatment may result in fast relief.

History of the procedure

Surgery has for a long time been the therapy of choice for caval vein obstruction; however, it is not well tolerated, with significant morbidity. Stents have changed the treatment strategies enormously; it is currently the technique of choice. The procedure has evolved from bailout for significant stenosis or obstruction, to electively altering flows to the heart, where currently percutaneous Fontan completion with rerouting of the ICV to the SCV or hemi-Fontan is being evaluated.

Precatheter imaging/ assessment and indications

A high clinical suspicion for caval obstruction is mandatory in patients with previous caval vein surgery. Because of sharp angles of Mustard patches when entering the pericardium, a subobstruction can easily be missed. Similarly, Fontan conduits may be difficult to visualize. Even good clinicians may clinically miss obstruction of major caval veins, as this may not result in retrograde congestion, but in low-flow cardiac output.

Prior to the catheterization, the interventionalist should know which vessels are open and can be punctured, and whether a thrombus in either SCV or ICV is present. All information usually can be obtained with echo or preferably computed tomography/magnetic resonance (CT/MR). If a recent thrombus is present, thrombolysis should be given followed by anticoagulation, as any manipulation near or through the thrombus may cause multiple (paradoxical) embolizations.

Anesthesia/supporting imaging

Interventions of the SCV or ICV can best be approached from the femoral and/or jugular vein. After cannulation, a distal angiogram through the sheath should be made to exclude thrombi. If the caval vein is completely obstructed, both the femoral and/or jugular vein should be cannulated, as this will allow the interventionalist to visualize the "target" from both ends; occasionally, this may reveal "hidden" hypoplastic but patent pathways.

Stenting the ICV has been reported as being performed under echographic guidance only from centers with no or limited access to radiographic equipment.[12]

Protocol of hemodynamic assessment

Gradients across obstructions can be obtained, but because of collateral circulation with low flow and low cardiac output, the clinical significance of the obstruction can be severely underestimated.

Angiography catheter selection

Good angiographic visualization in standard perpendicular planes proximal and distal to the stenosis obstruction is important. If the vessel is no longer patent, the lesion should be approached from both ends (cannulation of groin and neck vein). This will allow accurate determination of the length of the obstruction and the desired diameter of the final stent.

Catheter/wire interchange for delivery of balloon/stent/device

After visualization of the (sub)obstruction, a wire must be positioned across the lesion. If the caval vein is still patent, this is usually easy. If a segment has thrombosed or is atretic, a new route must be made.

Frequently, a mini vein may bridge partially the thrombosed distance; this vein should be probed with a thin wire, preferably a microcatheter system (Prograde: 0.018" hydrophilic wire in 2.4 F coaxial catheter system, used through a 4 F end-hole catheter).[13] A final segment can be completely obliterated, making a new route necessary. The most common technique is puncturing with a straightened Brockenbrough needle within a 6 or 8 French dilator transseptal sheath. It must be determined from which cannulation point (groin or neck) the puncture will be easiest. Preference will be given to the side that allows a straight route. When puncturing from one end, it is wise to provide a target at the other side: deployment of a 5 or 10 mm snare perpendicular to the needle direction provides a vessel-centered and radiopaque marker; it also allows it to snare and exteriorize the wire once grabbed, creating a veno-venous loop. Alternatively, a new route can be made with radio-frequency ablation (Figures 80.1 through 80.3).

Once the lesion is crossed, an extra stiff wire should be used to give optimal support and steering of the balloon during deployment.

Balloon dilation alone may occasionally give good relief,[14] however, with frequent early recurrence of obstruction.[15,16] Most interventionalists therefore will prefer stent implantation. Predilation with small balloons may be indicated in order to get the stent or delivery system in place. Predilation or low-pressure balloon interrogation with big balloons may facilitate assessment of the contours of the stenotic site, the stretchability, and the recoil.

A choice must be made from two different types of stents: self-expanding or balloon-expandable.

A self-expanding stent is more flexible; it will continuously push radially to reach its nominal value; it will

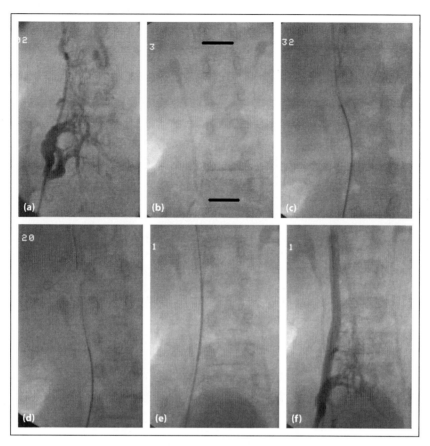

Figure 80.1   (a) A 10-year-old patient with obstruction of inferior caval vein between iliac vein and insertion of renal veins. (b) The distance to cover between catheter in iliac vein and catheter from jugular vein down to the obstruction (solid lines). (c) A 10 mm snare was used as target for the Brockenbrough needle within a 6 F long sheath; (d) A 0.014" wire was inserted through the Brockenbrough needle and grasped by the snare. (e) Partial opening of a 10/80 SMART Cordis self-expandable stent, which was lengthened with a 10/60 SMART Cordis stent. (f) Final result after balloon dilation with an 8 mm balloon; good patency and runoff were documented 8 years after this procedure.

reexpand after external compression (resuscitation, blunt thoracic trauma). A self-expanding stent is limited in maximal diameter, and cannot be dilated beyond nominal value. Such stents are good for long lesions, not ideal for short discrete lesions (obstruction in Mustard repair).[17]

Balloon-expandable stents have high radial strength, and are ideal for short lesions. External force may deform such stents, thereby decreasing or obliterating the lumen; this is rarely a problem in the SCV, but any stent in the ICV may be compressed by the liver.

Both types of stents can come with a cover (graft stents). Covered stents are indicated if rupture to an adjacent cavity vessel is likely or has occurred, such as pulmonary pathway (in Mustard with patch leak, rupture to pleura), or if endothelial reaction or tumor invasion is likely.

Multiple case reports or small series can be found in the world literature.[18–31]

Postdeployment protocol

Angiography post deployment of the stent must be made prior to removal of the wire (injection through sheath, or via multitrack [NuMed]). If extravasation of contrast is observed, a covered stent can still be positioned and deployed. If blood loss is significant, gentle balloon occlusion may temporarily obliterate the tear while preparing the covered stent.

Pitfalls, problems, and complications

Dilation of the caval veins may be complicated by rupture to the pleura with hemothorax, a tear to the pericardium with tamponnade, a tear to the pulmonary pathway allowing right–left or left–right shunting, a tear to the ascending aorta, compression or damage of phrenic or vagal nerve, compression or elongation of the sinus node artery with loss of stable sinus rhythm, compression of the thoracic duct, or compression of the ureter.

Caval veins can significantly stretch and may show some contractility—peristalsis; this may lead to stent migration within minutes or hours after deployment, and embolization to the right ventricle or into the pulmonary artery. Self-expanding stents can be recaptured with a lasso at

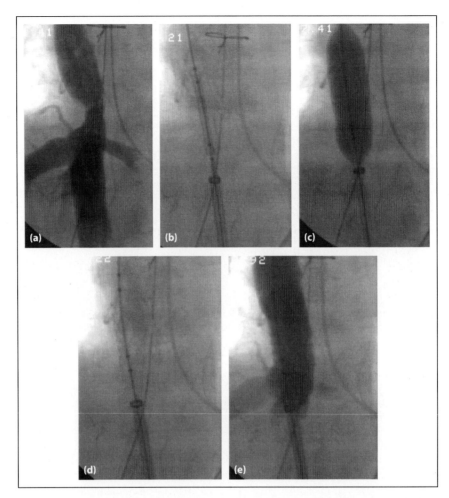

Figure 80.2 (a) A 4-year-old patient 1 hour after TCPC Fontan completion: a significant stenosis at the caudal junction of the inferior caval vein with an 18 mm Goretex conduit is demonstrated. (b) A 25 mm Genesis stent (Johnson and Johnson) mounted on a 14 mm BIB balloon (NuMed) is positioned through an 11 F long Mullins sheath (COOK). (c) Full inflation of outer BIB balloon. (d) Stent well deployed. (e) Cavogram through the sheath demonstrating good relief of the stenosis. This stent was fully expanded up to 18 mm 6 months later.

one end, and refolded into a big sheath;[32] balloon-expandable stents are much more difficult to retrieve, and should be parked/expanded/left in the circulatory system, or retrieved surgically.

Recurrent stenosis or thrombosis may occur; appropriate anticoagulation should be given. However, large stents in large veins in patients with good cardiac output have a low tendency to thrombose. When in doubt, it is safer to give antiaggregation or anticoagulation, at least early after the procedure, allowing the endothelium to cover most of the bare metal.

During long-term follow-up, a stent may fracture, or may be compressed by a blunt external trauma. Radiographic control in two perpendicular dimensions or CT will easily reveal this complication.

When deployed next to pacing wires, the pacing lead may be submitted to concentrated movements in one limited region, resulting in metal fatigue and lead fracture;

damage to the insulation may cause a current leak of the pacemaker leads with dysfunction of the pacing system.

References

1. Moons P, Gewillig M, Sluysmans T, Verhaaren R, Viart P, Massin M et al. Long term outcome up to 30 years after the Mustard or Senning operation: A nationwide multicenter study in Belgium. *Heart* 2004;90:307–13.
2. Michel-Behnke I, Hagel KJ, Bauer J, Schranz D. Superior caval venous syndrome after atrial switch procedure: Relief of complete venous obstruction by gradual angioplasty and placement of stents. *Cardiol Young* 1998;8(4)443–8.
3. Jayakumar A, Hsu DT, Hellenbrand WE, Pass RH. Endovascular stent placement for venous obstruction after cardiac transplantation in children and young adults. *Catheter Cardiovasc Interv* 2002;56:383–6.
4. O'Mahony M, Skehan S, Gallagher C. Percutaneous stenting of the superior vena cava syndrome in a patient with cystic fibrosis. *Ir Med J* 2005;98(3):85–6.

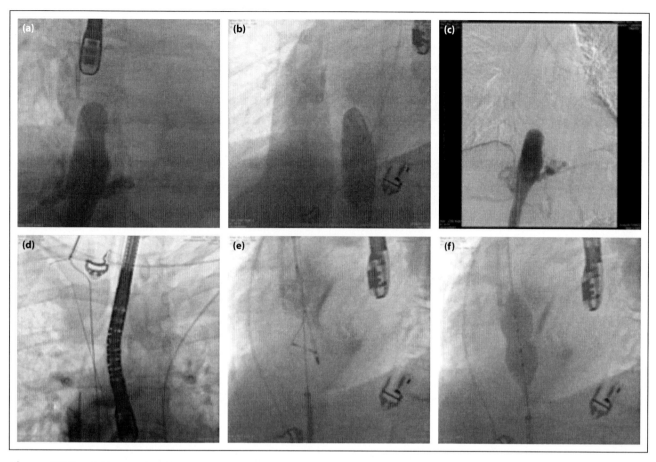

Figure 80.3   (a,b) Frontal and lateral views of cavogram showing complete obstruction of ICV by Eustachian valve. (c) Extensive collateral circulation. (d) Under TEE guidance, the Eustachian valve was punctured with a Brockenbrough needle and a wire was snared in the RA and exteriorized through the jugular vein. (e) Enlargement of opening with blade. (f) Tearing the opening with a 25-mm Mullins balloon to get an unobstructed connection from ICV to the right atrium.

5. Gandhi S, Pigula F. Congenital membanous obstruction of the inferior caval vein. *Ann Thorac Surg* 2004;78:1849.

6. Kavanagh E, Hargaden G, Flanagan F, Murray J. CT of a ruptured vein graft pseudoaneurysm: An unusual cause of superior vena cava obstruction. *Am J Radiol* 2004;183:1239–40.

7. Ousehal A, Abdelouafi A, Thrombati, Kadiri R. Thrombosis of the superior vena cava in Behcet's disease. Apropos of 13 cases. *J Radiol* 1992;73:383–8.

8. Rao PS, Wilson AD. Chylothorax, an unusual complication of baffle obstruction following Mustard operation: succesfull treatment with balloon angioplasty. *Am Heart J* 1992;123(1):244–8.

9. Stecker MS, Casciani T, Kwo PY, Lalka SG. Percutaneous stent placement as treatment of renal vein obstruction due to inferior vena caval thrombosis. *Cardiovasc Intervent Radiol* 2005;8; [Epub].

10. Sanchez-Recalde A, Sobrino N, Galeote G, Calvo Orbe L, Merino JL, Sobrino JA. [Budd-Chiari syndrome with complete occlusion of the inferior vena cava: Percutaneous recanalization by angioplasty and stenting] *Rev Esp Cardiol* 2004;57(11):1121–3.

11. Han SW, Kim GW, Lee J, Kim YJ, Kang YM. Successful treatment with stent angioplasty for Budd-Chiari syndrome in Behcet's disease. *Rheumatol Int* 2005;25(3):234–7.

12. Zhang C, Fu L, Zhang G, Jia T, Liu J, Qin C et al. Long-term effect of stent placement in 115 patients with Budd-Chiari syndrome. *World J Gastroenterol* 2003;9:2587–91.

13. Brown SC, Boshoff DE, Eyskens B, Mertens L, Gewillig M. Use of a microcatheter in a telescopic system to reach difficult targets in complex congenital heart disease. *Catheter Cardiovasc Interv* 2009;73(5):676–81.

14. Berg A, Norgard G, Greve G. Haemoptisis as a late complication of a Mustard operation treated by balloon dilation of a superior caval venous obstruction. *Cardiol Young* 2002;12:298–301.

15. Lock JE, Bass JL, Castaneda W, Fuhrman BP, Rashkind WJ, Lucas RV. Dilation angioplasty of congenital or operative narrowings of venous channels. *Circulation* 1984;70:457–64.

16. Abdulhamed JM, Yousef S, Khan MA, Mullins C. Balloon dilatation of complete obstruction of the superior vena cava after Mustard operation for transposition of great arteries. *Br Heart J* 1994;72(5):482–5.

17. Brown S, Eyskens B, Mertens L, Stockx L, Dumoulin M, Gewillig M. Self expandable stents for relief of venous baffle obstruction after the Mustard operation. *Heart* 1998;79:230–3.

18. Ing FF, Mullins CE, Grifka RG, Nihill MR, Fenrich AL, Collins EL et al. Stent dilation of superior vena cava and innominate vein obstructions permits transvenous pacing lead implantation. *Pacing Clin Electrophysiol* 1998;21(8):1517–30.

19. MacLellan-Tobert SG, Cetta F, Hagler DJ. Use of intravascular stents for superior vena caval obstruction after the Mustard operation. *Mayo Clin Proc* 1996;71(11):1071–6.

20. Castelli P, Caronno R, Piffaretti G, Tozzi M, Lomazzi C, Lagana D et al. Endovascular treatment for superior vena cava obstruction in Behcet disease. *J Vasc Surg* 2005;41:548–51.

21. Bansal N, Deshpande S. Novel use of Brockenbrough needle in relieving membranous obstruction of the inferior vena cava. *Heart* 2005;91:e38.

22. Ward CJ, Mullins CE, Nihill MR. Use of intravascular stents in systemic venous and systemic venous baffle obstructions: Short term follow-up results. *Circulation* 1995;91:2948–54.

23. Trerotola SO, Lund GB, Samphilipo MA, Magee CA, Newman JS, Olson JL et al. Palmaz stent in the treatment of central venous stenosis: Safety and efficacy of rdilation. *Radiology* 1994;190:379–85.

24. Stavropoulos GP, Hamilton I. Severe superior vena caval syndrome after the Mustard repair in a patient with persistent left superior vena cava. *Eur J Cardiothorac Surg* 1994;8(1):48–50.

25. Ro PS, Hill SL, Cheatham JP. Congenital superior vena cava obstruction causing anasarca and respiratory failure in a newborn: Successful transcatheter therapy. *Catheter Cardiovasc Interv* 2005;65(1):60–5.

26. Bolad I, Karanam S, Mathew D, John R, Piemonte T, Martin D. Percutaneous treatment of superior vena cava obstruction following transvenous device implantation. *Catheter Cardiovasc Interv* 2005;65(1):54–9.

27. Kanzaki M, Sakuraba M, Kuwata H, Ikeda T, Oyama K, Mae M et al. [Stenting in obstruction of superior vena cava; clinical experience with the self-expanding endovascular prosthesis]. *Kyobu Geka*. 2004;57(5):347–50; discussion 350–2.

28. Sharaf E, Waight DJ, Hijazi ZM. Simultaneous transcatheter occlusion of two atrial baffle leaks and stent implantation for SCV obstruction in a patient after Mustard repair. *Catheter Cardiovasc Interv* 2001;54(1):72–6.

29. Schneider DJ, Moore JW. Transcatheter treatment of ICV channel obstruction and baffle leak after Mustard procedure for d-transposition of the great arteries using Amplatzer ASD device and multiple stents. *J Invasive Cardiol* 2001;13(4):306–9.

30. Mohsen AE, Rosenthal E, Qureshi SA, Tynan M. Stent implantation for superior vena cava occlusion after the Mustard operation. *Catheter Cardiovasc Interv* 2001;52(3):351–4.

31. El-Said HG, Ing FF, Grifka RG, Nihill MR, Morris C, Getty-Houswright D et al. 18-year experience with transseptal procedures through baffles, conduits, and other intra-atrial patches. *Catheter Cardiovasc Interv* 2000;50(4):434–9; discussion 440.

32. Srinathan S, McCafferty I, Wilson I. Radiological management of superior vena caval stent migration and infection. *Cardiovasc Intervent Radiol* 2005;28(1)127–30.

81

Right ventricular outflow tract obstruction

Jamie Bentham and Neil Wilson

Right ventricular outflow tract obstruction occurs as an isolated congenital lesion, though more typically is associated with other intracardiac pathology. Atretic or obstructed outflow tracts can be opened up by the interventionist in the neonatal period to palliate cyanotic lesions and augment pulmonary blood flow. Pulmonary atresia intact ventricular septum is a relatively rare example that can, at times, be exclusively managed by the interventionist. More commonly, intervention is in the setting of recurrence of obstruction or incomplete surgical relief in the older child and adult. The majority of patients will have tetralogy of Fallot or pulmonary atresia with ventricular septal defect. A significant number, however, will have acquired right ventricular outflow tract disease resulting from surgical placement of a right ventricular outflow tract to pulmonary artery conduit. Such conditions in order of decreasing frequency will include the Ross operation for aortic valve disease, repair of complex double outlet right ventricle or transposition with the Rastelli operation, and repair of common arterial trunk (Figures 81.1 and 81.2).

The first reports of complex intervention to open atretic right ventricular outflow tracts were reported relatively recently by Gibbs[1] and later by Hausdorf.[2] What followed was an acknowledgment that stenting, rather than perforation and angioplasty alone, would frequently be an integral part of a more lasting result, including in the very young.[3] The exception to this general rule is pulmonary atresia intact septum where perforation and angioplasty with or without ductal stenting may be all that is required, at least initially. This is discussed in detail elsewhere. The futility of balloon angioplasty to manage stenosed conduits is not dissimilar to angioplasty on native muscular right ventricular outflow tracts.[4] Although stenotic gradients are modestly reduced by high-pressure balloons acutely, this is a short-lived result and the majority will proceed to surgical conduit replacement unless combined with a stenting procedure.[5,6] Stenting of conduits offers a better and longer-lasting result that can offer extremely useful palliation in delaying or circumventing the need for further conduit exchange. There are however important caveats to this that need to be discussed.

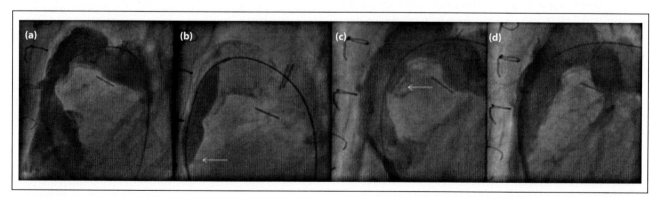

Figure 81.1 Right ventricular outflow tract 90 degree LAO angiograms of a severely obstructed 18-mm right ventricle to pulmonary artery conduit in a 25-year-old patient. The underlying diagnosis is transposition of the great arteries with ventricular septal defect and pulmonary stenosis. The Rastelli operation was performed to restore left ventricle to aortic continuity. In (a), severe obstruction of the heavily calcified conduit is evident so much so that in (b), a 12-mm Atlas balloon ruptures presumably on a calcified spicule (arrow). (c) The conduit is sequentially dilated with high-pressure balloons (12, 14, and 16 mm) and the integrity of the conduit is compromised with contained rupture clearly evident (arrow). (d) Stent placement restores the integrity of the conduit and subsequently a Melody percutaneous pulmonary valve is placed in the stent scaffold (not shown).

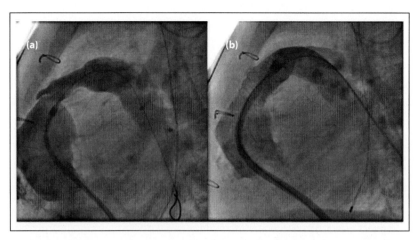

Figure 81.2   Right ventricular outflow tract 90 degree LAO angiograms of a moderately obstructed 12-mm right ventricle to pulmonary artery conduit in a 4-year-old patient. The underlying diagnosis is common arterial trunk. Following reparative surgery, conduit stenosis has progressed over time and the moderate obstruction and calcification is evident in (a). In (b), the conduit was first balloon dilated with a high-pressure balloon and was then stented with an 8-mm Genesis stent with the intention of delaying the need for conduit change to allow time for further somatic growth.

Procedural indications

Like other areas of congenital cardiology, procedural indications for right ventricular outflow tract disease are difficult to define and have a poor evidence base. There is a strong and increasing consensus that right ventricular preservation is a key part of a good, long-term management strategy, especially when this is contrasted against the difficulties encountered when managing a dilated and poorly functioning right ventricle. Right ventricular pressure greater than 0.75 systemic is unlikely to be tolerated well for a prolonged period of time. Exercise testing where possible, with objective cardiopulmonary documentation of anaerobic threshold, oxygen consumption, and ventilator equivalents, can be extremely useful. This is most helpful when applied in a longitudinal comparison as symptoms are notoriously subjective in this group of patients who may well have led a very sedentary lifestyle for many years. QRS dispersion also has some role though it is difficult to define absolute numbers that can be used to justify intervention. Magnetic resonance imaging (MRI) and transthoracic echocardiography are the mainstay assessment tools and changes in right ventricular function, interval increases in right ventricular end diastolic volumes, along with potential treatable stenotic lesions form the indications for cardiac catheterization. Symptoms would be a late sign as would ventricular and atrial dysrhythmia, but are clear-cut indications for intervening. Although hotly debated, for neonatal right ventricular outflow tract procedures, there is some early evidence to suggest that the stented outflow tract may afford more equal flow to both pulmonary arteries than the obvious flow discrepancy introduced by a surgically placed shunt onto either pulmonary artery.[7] This fact, alongside the avoidance of a thoracotomy or occasionally a

sternotomy, is resulting in an increasing number of centers preferring to palliate with a stent (right ventricular outflow tract or ductal stent) in selected cases rather than perform a surgical systemic to pulmonary artery shunt.[8]

Technique

Venous sheath selection should take into consideration the possible use of the diagnostic and subsequent balloon catheters. Oversizing the venous sheath facilitates using a multi-track catheter for hemodynamic and angiographic data. Use of this catheter ensures that once a stable guide wire is in position, repeated catheter and wire replacement is not necessary. Some operators prefer to modify their own monorail-type system by cutting off the end of a pigtail catheter and running it along the wire by means of the cut end hole and one of the side holes. Others use a long sheath from early in the case, including for angiography, which reduces the number of exchanges and allows for frequent angiograms while maintaining wire position. Venous access is usually from the femoral vein, but in chronic patients, thrombosis and collateralization of the iliofemoral veins may have occurred and alternative access via the right or left internal jugular or subclavian veins, or exceptionally transhepatic access, may be necessary. Early change in approach from a femoral to a jugular or subclavian route is recommended when it is proving problematic to cross an anteriorly positioned stenosed conduit. Arterial access for comparison of hemodynamics and beat-to-beat monitoring is essential.

Right ventricular pressure and simultaneous systemic pressure should be measured and both the absolute values and ratio expressed and interpreted in the context of cardiac output. At the end of a long procedure, cardiac output may be compromised and a numerically lower right ventricular pressure may only be so because cardiac output is also reduced. Cardiac output is easily estimated at key points during the case to allow for this. It is important too to have some assessment of pulmonary regurgitation, which often coexists. This too will tend to play a part in maintaining right ventricular pressure despite good relief of obstruction. Branch pulmonary artery anatomy is important; discrete, single, multiple level, proximal, and distal stenotic lesions may maintain right ventricular hypertension when the proximal right ventricular outflow tract obstruction (RVOTO) is relieved. Branch pulmonary artery stenosis is dealt with elsewhere in this book, but it is clear that when there is coexisting significant pathology of this type, it should be dealt with at the time of or before relief of the RVOTO. It is generally our practice to deal with distal lesions first, but this is a point of discussion. Hemodynamic data need to be accurately acquired using an end hole or a wedge catheter or a slow pullback of a long sheath over a wire to determine the true sites of obstruction. The catheter should then be positioned distally in either pulmonary artery branch. It may be necessary to use a hydrophilic wire or some other torque wire to first achieve a distal and lateral position. A hand angiogram can facilitate localizing a larger more distal pulmonary artery segmental branch that might afford a stable wire position.

Wire selection and positioning

A heavy-duty exchange-length 0.035-inch guide wire of 260 cm is then exchanged down the catheter. Our preference is for the Amplatz range of stiff guide wires, such as the superstiff, extrastiff, or ultrastiff (Boston Scientific, Natick, MA, USA). These wires have a floppy end. Stability of the wire can be a potential problem as their own rigidity when under tension around the contours of the right ventricle and pulmonary arteries can induce recoil and wire position can be lost. "Buckling" of the soft tip in the distal pulmonary artery can go some way to prevent this as can manufacturing a bend on the guide wire (estimated from the angiogram) to attempt to reduce the spring effect of the stiff unbent guide wire. Time spent on securing a good distal stable wire position is a worthwhile maneuver in the long run. Smaller patients will require narrower gauge wires, though support strength is still a consideration. Angiography is best performed biplane in a lateral or left anterior oblique (LAO) projection and for normal sites and connections, a right anterior oblique (RAO) projection with some cranial tilt. Angiograms in multiple projections may be necessary to profile the stenotic lesion sufficient to guide the intervention and minimize the impact on surrounding vessels.

Balloon selection

The next decision is selecting the size of the balloon and stent to use. When dealing with conduits of any sort, a high-pressure balloon is recommended. The Z Med balloon series has a good combination of balloon strength and shaft size (NuMed, Hopkinton, NY, USA). The Mullins balloon is exceptionally strong, though it has the drawback that if used with a stent, the balloon profile after inflation can make for considerable traction on removal (NuMed, Hopkinton, NY, USA). For this reason, Atlas balloons are increasingly being used as they are exceptionally strong and lower profile (Bard, Tempe, AZ, USA; Figure 81.1). Balloon size is chosen according to the anticipated required diameter of the outflow tract. If dealing with a conduit, there is clearly no need to be larger than its known diameter. Predilation of lesions in severe chronic obstruction is a debatable point. Unless using a BiB balloon that has a "built-in" predilation, I favor predilating to 50–75% of the anticipated final balloon size (NuMed, Hopkinton, NY, USA). Some operators will serially dilate an obstruction starting with relatively small balloon waists with high-pressure balloons and sequentially dilating a lesion with multiple graded balloons until the lesion is close to the final size on which to place a stent.

Long sheath positioning

The next stage is placement of a long intracardiac sheath to a position well into either pulmonary artery along the guidewire. Sheath caliber is crucial. I choose to oversize 2–3 Fr gauges above the shaft size of the balloon catheter being used. This facilitates passage of the balloon–stent assembly through the heart without friction, minimizing the possibility of stent displacement from the balloon as it is advanced. It also aids removal of the balloon catheter through the long sheath after dilation. Maintaining long sheath position stabilizes wire position, facilitates passage of the multitrack catheter, and is a useful back-up if a larger-diameter balloon catheter is required to complete full deployment. Currently, the most appropriate large bore, long sheaths are the curved Mullins series (Cook, Bloomington, IN, USA) or the Arrowflex (Arrow, Inc., Reading, PA, USA) or Flexor sheaths (Cook, Bloomington, IN, USA). Arrowflex and Flexor sheaths are kink-resistant, though their structure of metallic braided reinforcement can lead to "dragging" of the balloon–stent assembly as it passes through it. On the other hand, the dilator is finely tapered and runs well over the guide wire for positioning. Unfortunately, these sheaths are not currently available in sizes over 12 French. Some operators have confidence in advancing the balloon–stent assembly through the circulation without long sheath protection, merely utilizing the short venous sheath at the groin. This technique can be successful in very small children and in the event of having difficulty positioning a long sheath, but it does carry a serious risk of stent dislodgement as it is advanced within the heart. It also limits the recovery strategy in the event of complication and should not be used as a first choice technique.

Choice of stents

Currently, only balloon-expandable stents are appropriate for the right ventricular outflow tract. These are of three types: stainless steel, chromium cobalt, or platinum. Of the stainless-steel series, a stent with high radial strength is recommended: either the Palmaz series (Cordis J and J Interventional Systems)[9] or the Intrastent Max LD (eV3 Plymouth, MN, USA).[10] The Andrastent (Andramed, Reutlingen, Germany) is a newer high-strength open and closed cell design chromium stent. The platinum/iridium stent (CP Stent, NuMed, Hopkinton, NY, USA) is more radiopaque and capable of large-diameter dilation, and, in some countries outside the United States, available covered with expanded polytetrafluoroethylene and can be supplied premounted.[11] In young children, premounted stents such as the Palmaz Genesis range (Cordis J and J Interventional Systems) continue to be an important resource to have available as their low profile enables them to be positioned to relieve obstruction without the need for large sheaths and stiff guide wires (Figure 81.2). The length of stent is chosen to cover the stenotic area, taking into consideration the effect of shortening on the initial deployment and for subsequent balloon dilation, should that be necessary to keep pace with somatic growth in children. Longer stents may be difficult to pass through the sheath as it turns through the tricuspid valve and curves anteriorly to the outflow tract (a frequent site of sheath kinking). Longer stents also risk jailing either pulmonary artery branch, the stent "milking" off the balloon or the whole assembly "kicking back" during inflation especially if there is significant protrusion into a small distal pulmonary artery. Prior to mounting a stent on a balloon it is useful to denature the balloon material to somewhat enhance the security of the stent crimped down onto the balloon. "Teasing" open the ends of the stent using the tip of a dilator as it is mounted on the balloon avoids the sharp tines of the stent puncturing the balloon. An unrecognized punctured balloon that fails to fully deploy a stent may result in a very difficult-to-manage complication of stent embolization to the right ventricle. The stent is then hand crimped with a guide wire in the balloon catheter lumen to avoid crushing, which might hinder its running on the guide wire. The balloon–stent assembly is then advanced over the wire through the long sheath as far as the main pulmonary artery, perhaps a little distal in position to that judged ideal. The sheath is then withdrawn, uncovering the stent. Angiograms are performed through the side arm of the sheath to facilitate accurate positioning. The balloon is then inflated slowly using an inflation device. One operator should be in control of the balloon catheter shaft, ready to make small adjustments of advancing or withdrawal should the balloon appear to recoil or advance away from the target. Prolonged inflation is usually not necessary, though deployment to nominal balloon pressure is almost always required to ensure proper seating of the stent. After deflating the balloon, I usually wait a few seconds to ensure the balloon material has folded well. If the stent appears well applied to the lesion, there is probably little need to inflate a second time, but many operators choose to do so. After the balloon has deflated fully, it is removed and hemodynamics and angiograms assessed. A second balloon can be then used if further dilation of the stent is deemed necessary. Cardiac output in the absence of an atrial shunt is clearly significantly compromised during stent deployment. Swift deflation of the balloon as well as being prepared to advance the balloon into either pulmonary artery following partial deflation may be necessary. Management of balloon inflation as well as deflation should be discussed as a team prior to deployment.

Right ventricular outflow tract stenting in the neonate and infant

In the small child, the technique, although essentially the same as in an adult, utilizes coronary guide wires and stents to enable the procedure to be performed with the smallest possible gauge of equipment available (Figure 81.3). This equipment helps minimize the potential for significant hemodynamic instability frequently encountered when crossing obstructed pulmonary outflow tracts. Stent positioning can be difficult with the need to depend on hand angiograms. It may be necessary to use two stents delivered serially and telescoped within each other to ensure that the length of the obstructed region is covered. Extreme care is required on removing the deflated balloon to avoid compromising the deployed stent(s).

Potential problems and complications

Difficulty in positioning a long sheath can be experienced on two accounts. First, the large bore sheath may not run over even the stiffest of support guide wires, and second, as the sheath is positioned, cardiac output is compromised and systemic blood pressure falls. In the first instance, consider changing to a more flexible, less stiff guide wire, repositioning the guide wire in the contralateral pulmonary artery or placing a curve on the wire. The logic for this is that sometimes the wire tension presses so forcefully on the margin of the stenotic lesion that the sheath cannot advance between the lesion wall and the wire. Alternatively, consider a different venous approach, say from the right internal jugular vein. In the second instance of loss of cardiac output, this is usually a consequence of the tricuspid valve being splinted open by the sheath. Again, a less stiff wire may help, as might a volume infusion or commencing inotropes. Another tactic

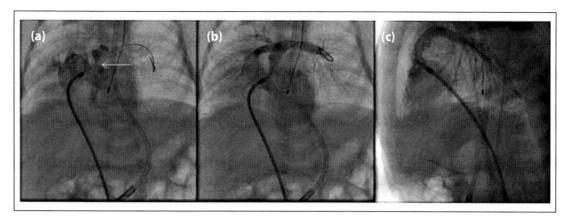

Figure 81.3 Angiograms in a newborn with Pentalogy of Cantrell and with a complex double outlet right ventricle and severe subpulmonary stenosis. (a) A right ventricular angiogram through a 4 French long sheath demonstrates severe subvalve muscular pulmonary outflow obstruction (arrow). (b and c) A 5-mm coronary stent is positioned and deployed over a 0.014-inch stabilizer wire. The PA and lateral angiograms demonstrate the relief of obstruction with flow seen to both distal pulmonary arteries.

to overcome either of these issues is to "front load" the balloon stent assembly through the long sheath, effectively using the tip of the balloon as a dilator. This can be performed starting outside the body or alternatively the sheath can be positioned, say in the high inferior vena cava, the balloon–stent assembly advanced to the tip of the sheath and then the two advanced together into position, taking care not to allow the balloon–stent assembly to protrude too far out of the end of the sheath.

Stent displacement on the balloon during advancement to the field of interest can be minimized by following the methods above to ensure good adherence of the stent by inflating the balloon prior to mounting to slightly denature the balloon fabric. Inflating the balloon a very small amount can also be used to ensure fixation of the stent and improve stability. "Glueing" of the stent with a small amount of viscous contrast is anecdotally favored by some operators. Even so, and especially if the long sheath is already kinked, the stent can migrate off the balloon and the long sheath, balloon, and stent need to be removed with care from the patient while maintaining wire position and the procedure repeated.

Displacement or embolization

Providing the wire position is not lost, it may be possible to secure the stent back on the balloon by advancing the balloon, partially inflating, and advancing or withdrawing to position appropriately. After stent deployment, balloon removal can occasionally dislodge it. To avoid this, it is recommended to keep the long sheath advanced as the balloon is first inflated than deflated as the sheath is advanced over it.[11] Displacement or embolization once inflated is a more difficult prospect and, unless the stent can be recaptured by a slightly larger balloon and manipulated into position, referral for surgical retrieval is probably prudent.

Stent compression/fracture

In the presence of pulmonary artery stenosis, which maintains high right ventricular pressure, it is possible that an RVOT stent may be compressed and subsequently fractured, resulting in recurrence of obstruction. Fracture has been reported with every known type of balloon-expandable stent. In most instances, the fracture per se is not harmful as the stent struts are secured within the wall of the outflow tract. Fracture or compression can be treated by implanting a second or third stent within the existing one.

Homograft fracture

Calcified homografts probably undergo minor fractures quite frequently during balloon angioplasty (Figure 81.1). Major fractures can lead to disruption and dehiscence of the conduit, resulting in severe hemorrhage and death. Though a major fracture can be unpredictable, it is appropriate to consider staged predilation in patients with extensive homograft calcification and significant stenosis, and to have a covered balloon-expandable stent such as the covered CP stent as a possible rescue strategy.[12] Such cases should be discussed with surgical colleagues and rescue strategies discussed and planned in the event of conduit rupture.

Coronary artery compression

Anomalous and aberrant courses of the coronary arteries are not unusual in many of the patients undergoing angioplasty procedures to the right ventricular outflow tract. In such patients, stent angioplasty can rarely lead to temporary or permanent occlusion of the coronary arteries (Figure 81.4). This is a particular hazard in patients who have undergone Rastelli-type operations for complex forms

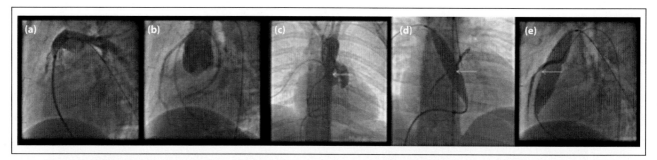

Figure 81.4 Angiograms in an 18-year-old patient with an underlying diagnosis of transposition of the great arteries with ventricular septal defect and pulmonary stenosis who has undergone the Rastelli operation. (a) Right ventricular outflow tract 90 degree LAO angiogram. Right ventricle to pulmonary artery conduit is moderately obstructed and moderately calcified. (b and c) Aortic angiogram (PA and lateral) is suspicious for coronary compression. A wedge catheter was positioned astride the right ventricle to pulmonary artery conduit to profile its course. The right coronary artery is seen to run across the course that the wedge catheter takes. (d and e) Simultaneous inflation of a 16-mm Atlas balloon and an aortic angiogram clearly demonstrates coronary compression (arrow). This conduit cannot therefore be stented.

of transposition of the great arteries. It is prudent therefore in such patients to delineate coronary artery anatomy relative to the RVOT, by either magnetic resonance imaging or angiography. If there is ongoing concern, then a predilation strategy with particular attention to signs of ischemia on the ECG is recommended. Simultaneous selective coronary angiography and balloon dilatation of the lesion is prudent.

Conclusions

Stenting offers good relief of right ventricular outflow tract obstruction in the native or conduit setting. Potential risks and complications can be kept to a minimum by meticulous technique and experience. Although essentially a palliative procedure, when combined with pulmonary valve implantation,[13,14] surgery can often be delayed or avoided altogether, making this a satisfying procedure and a significant advance to the management of right ventricular disease.

References

1. Parsons JM, Rees MR, Gibbs JL. Percutaneous laser valvotomy with balloon dilatation of the pulmonary valve as primary treatment for pulmonary atresia. *Br Heart J* 1991;66(1):36–8.
2. Hausdorf G, Schneider M, Schulze-Neick I, Lange PE. Pulmonary valve atresia with ventricular septum defect: Interventional recanalization of the right ventricular outflow tract. *Zeitschrift für Kardiologie* 1992;81(9):496–9.
3. Gibbs JL, Uzun O, Blackburn ME, Parsons JM, Dickinson DF. Right ventricular outflow stent implantation: An alternative to palliative surgical relief of infundibular pulmonary stenosis. *Heart* 1997;77(2):176–9.
4. Sanatani S, Potts JE, Human DG, Sandor GG, Patterson MW, Gordon Culham JA. Balloon angioplasty of right ventricular outflow tract conduits. *Pediatr Cardiol* 2001;22(3):228–32.
5. Sreeram N, Hutter P, Silove E. Sustained high pressure double balloon angioplasty of calcified conduits. *Heart* 1999;81(2):162–5.
6. Ovaert C, Caldarone CA, McCrindle BW, Nykanen D, Freedom RM, Coles JG et al. Endovascular stent implantation for the management of postoperative right ventricular outflow tract obstruction: Clinical efficacy. *J Thorac Cardiovasc Surg* 1999;118(5):886–93.
7. Barron DJ, Ramchandani B, Murala J, Stumper O, De Giovanni JV, Jones TJ et al. Surgery following primary right ventricular outflow tract stenting for Fallot's tetralogy and variants: Rehabilitation of small pulmonary arteries. *Eur J Cardiothorac Surg* 2013;44(4):656–62.
8. Stumper O, Ramchandani B, Noonan P, Mehta C, Bhole V, Reinhardt Z et al. Stenting of the right ventricular outflow tract. *Heart* 2013;99(21):1603–8.
9. O'Laughlin MP, Slack MC, Grifka RG, Perry SB, Lock JE, Mullins CE. Implantation and intermediate-term follow-up of stents in congenital heart disease. *Circulation* 1993;88(2):605–14.
10. Rutledge JM, Mullins CE, Nihill MR, Grifka RG, Vincent JA. Initial experience with intratherapeutics Intrastent Doublestrut LD stents in patients with congenital heart defects. *Catheter Cardiovasc Interv* 2002;56(4):541–8.
11. Recto MR, Ing FF, Grifka RG, Nihill MR, Mullins CE. A technique to prevent newly implanted stent displacement during subsequent catheter and sheath manipulation. *Catheter Cardiovasc Interv* 2000;49(3):297–300.
12. Ewert P, Schubert S, Peters B, Abdul-Khaliq H, Nagdyman N, Lange PE. The CP stent—short, long, covered—for the treatment of aortic coarctation, stenosis of pulmonary arteries and caval veins, and Fontan anastomosis in children and adults: An evaluation of 60 stents in 53 patients. *Heart* 2005;91(7):948–53.
13. Sugiyama H, Williams W, Benson LN. Implantation of endovascular stents for the obstructive right ventricular outflow tract. *Heart* 2005;91(8):1058–63.
14. Khambadkone S, Coats L, Taylor A, Boudjemline Y, Derrick G, Tsang V et al. Percutaneous pulmonary valve implantation in humans: Results in 59 consecutive patients. *Circulation* 2005;112(8):1189–97.

82

Pulmonary artery stenosis

Larry Latson

Anatomy and pathophysiology

Stenotic lesions of the pulmonary arterial tree occur in at least 2–3% of patients with congenital heart disease (CHD).[1] They are most common in conotruncal abnormalities, such as tetralogy of Fallot/pulmonary atresia with ventricular septal defect, but have been seen in almost all forms of CHD. Stenoses may be discrete or associated with long-segment hypoplasia, and may be congenital or secondary to a surgical procedure. Postsurgical stenosis is most commonly due to scarring, especially at the site of a shunt, at the ends of a patch arterioplasty, or at the anastomotic sites of unifocalized vessels. Torsion, stretching, or compression of a pulmonary artery may also occur after procedures such as the arterial switch or Norwood operations. Rarely, stenosis can be caused by mediastinal inflammatory disorders (radiation or fibrosing mediastinitis) or extrinsic compression from neoplasm.

The pulmonary artery system allows for parallel flow to both lungs and to all lung segments. Thus, isolated stenosis of one pulmonary artery branch reduces flow to the affected downstream area, but may have little effect on right ventricular pressure. In most cases, however, there are multiple affected pulmonary arteries and right ventricular pressure becomes elevated. The pathophysiologic effects of pulmonary artery stenosis can be secondary to reduced segmental pulmonary flow (dyspnea, poor lung growth), or to right ventricular hypertension (right heart failure, arrhythmia, sudden death), or both.

Clinical symptoms, indications for treatment, and alternatives

Indications for treatment and symptoms of pulmonary artery branch stenosis may vary with age and associated cardiovascular defects. Congenitally stenotic lesions may improve with age, and even severe diffuse pulmonary artery stenosis unassociated with other congenital cardiovascular abnormalities rarely causes symptoms in young children.[2]

We generally do not recommend treatment at less than five years of age in such asymptomatic patients. Patients with associated CHD, however, especially if they require repair with a Fontan-type circulation, may not tolerate even relatively mild degrees of pulmonary artery stenosis. These patients may need early aggressive therapy. Older patients with otherwise normal circulation and severe pulmonary artery stenosis affecting only one lung may have symptoms due to the ventilation/perfusion mismatch (primarily dyspnea on exertion), and the potential growth of the affected lung may be reduced. In the absence of right ventricular hypertension, a large perfusion abnormality may warrant a low-risk intervention, but the degree of acceptable risk must be tempered with the generally good outlook without treatment.

Older patients with otherwise normal circulation and severe bilateral proximal stenoses or multiple areas of distal stenosis may have normally distributed perfusion, but severely elevated main pulmonary artery and right ventricular pressures. The right ventricular hypertension may cause symptoms similar to those in patients with primary pulmonary hypertension, including limited ability to increase cardiac output with exercise, and a significant risk for sudden death.[3] Treatment is generally indicated in such patients if right ventricular pressure is more than 65–75% systemic, and in some patients with lower pressures if they have significant symptoms.[4]

History of the procedure

Balloon angioplasty of stenotic pulmonary arteries is one of the earliest transcatheter interventions performed for pediatric and CHD. Lock reported on the results of balloon dilation in an experimental lamb model in 1981.[5] The first "large" (seven patients) human experience with balloon angioplasty was reported from Boston Children's Hospital in 1983.[6] Since then, there have been numerous articles on transcatheter treatment of various forms of pulmonary artery stenosis. Significant advances in technique included the use of high/ultra-high pressure balloons, stents, and cutting balloons.

Precatheter imaging/assessment

The primary effects of pulmonary artery stenosis are maldistribution of blood flow to the lung parenchyma and/or elevation of right ventricular systolic pressure. The pressure gradients across stenotic vascular lesions are the easiest parameters to measure in the cath lab, but the goal of this therapy is to increase flow to underperfused regions of the lung. The determination of relative flow to the lung segments is strongly recommended prior to catheterization in all patients with planned pulmonary artery dilation in order to target regions of the pulmonary vasculature that are most severely affected as the primary targets. In patients with normal circulation, the regional pulmonary blood flow is best assessed with a radionuclide quantitative perfusion scan.[7] MRI is preferable in patients with Fontan circulations because of differential streaming of flow from the upper- and lower-body circulations in these patients. The flow determinations can be readily repeated after the catheterization procedure to assess the immediate and long-term results.

Right ventricular pressure and function can often be conveniently evaluated by echocardiography. Right ventricular pressure can be estimated by the velocity of a tricuspid insufficiency jet if present. Proximal stenotic lesions in the pulmonary arteries may be detectable by echocardiography but distal lesions will not be visible. CT or MRI scan can give excellent visualization of pulmonary artery anatomy, and MRI can quantitate regional flow in some patients.[8] Nonstandard imaging planes and careful analysis is necessary to make accurate assessment of multiple stenotic vessels.

Anesthesia

The choice of sedation versus general anesthesia is usually not critical. The younger the patient and the larger the number of lesions likely to need treatment, the more likely we are to recommend general anesthesia. Procedures requiring treatment of multiple lesions can take several hours. Patients with systemic or near-systemic pressure may be in danger of acute events, such as pulmonary artery rupture or abrupt decrease in cardiac output if a tricuspid or pulmonary valve is held open by the catheter. General anesthesia in these situations is an advantage. Assessments of acute success during the catheterization procedure are generally made by angiographic measurements, pre- and postdilation pressure gradients, and changes in right ventricular to systemic pressure ratios. These values are not dramatically affected by the use of relatively light general anesthesia.

Catheterization procedure

For most cases with complex pulmonary artery stenosis requiring treatment, we recommend placement of two venous sheaths and an arterial monitoring line. Arterial monitoring is optional for simple low-risk procedures, but is important for high-risk patients requiring prolonged procedures.

One venous catheter is used for dilation and/or stent placement in the stenotic region. The second venous catheter is used as a convenient way to perform angiograms immediately after an intervention or as a good reference during balloon dilation and stent placement. In situations where "kissing balloons" are needed, the second sheath is utilized for placement of the second balloon. The presence of a second venous catheter is also extremely helpful in patients who suffer catastrophic complications such as vessel disruption. The second catheter provides a way to deliver drugs or blood and perform angiograms without the danger of losing the wire position of the original dilating catheter. The primary sheath is chosen to accommodate the largest anticipated balloon catheter. The secondary sheath size is chosen to be large enough for the desired angiographic catheter, or for the second balloon if simultaneous balloon inflations are anticipated.

As a routine, we perform a complete right heart catheterization to obtain accurate baseline pressure measurements in the right atrium and right ventricle. Angiographic assessment is best done with the most selective catheter position possible. We do not perform an angiogram in the main pulmonary artery with conventional imaging systems if the site of stenosis has been determined to be more peripheral by previous angiography or noninvasive evaluation. We prefer to use biplane angiography. Selective angiograms that result in filling of vessels in only the left or right lungs make it possible to more precisely determine vascular distribution using the lateral view. For more peripheral and smaller vessels, it is often advantageous to perform the angiographic injections with a catheter that has both endholes and a side-hole such as a Goodale–Lubin or other multipurpose-type catheter.

The best view of the central pulmonary arteries from a main pulmonary artery angiogram is usually with the frontal imaging system in steep cranial angulation (30+ degrees) (Figure 82.1). The right pulmonary artery courses relatively horizontally across the right thorax and straight AP or slight right anterior oblique angulation of the frontal radiographic imaging system, combined with a lateral projection of the lateral imaging system, provides excellent visualization (Figure 82.2). The left pulmonary artery courses leftward in a relatively steep angle from anterior to posterior. Left anterior oblique (LAO) and possibly slight caudal angulation of the frontal imaging system is usually best to evaluate the length of the major portions of the left pulmonary artery. A steep caudal view with some LAO angulation may show the pulmonary artery bifurcation better in some patients, but we find catheter manipulation in this view more difficult due to foreshortening of the image of the main pulmonary artery (Figure 82.3, Videos

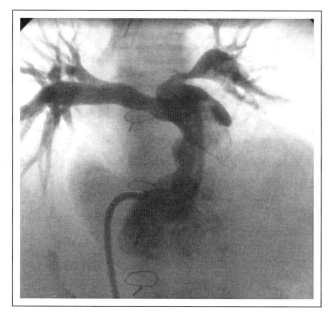

Figure 82.1 Main pulmonary arteriogram in a patient with bilateral proximal pulmonary artery stenosis. The frontal imaging system is angulated 35° cranially and slightly leftward. The length of the right pulmonary artery is well visualized. The origin of the left pulmonary artery is well seen, but this angulation results in foreshortening of the midportion of the vessel.

82.1 and 82.2). Different angulations of the image intensifiers may be needed for specific portions of either the right or left pulmonary artery. At least one of the views should be varied to attempt to image the longest length of the affected vessel. A Tuohy–Borst valve allows angiography to be performed with the guide wire in place and the catheter tip immediately proximal to the stenotic lesion. Newer generations of radiographic systems with rotational angiography and 3D reconstructions of the entire vascular tree (with or without live overlay) from a single angiogram may alter the initial approach.[9,10]

Selected cannulation of the desired stenotic vessels may be challenging because of the sometimes tortuous course through the right ventricle, right ventricular outflow tract, and into sharply angulated branch vessels. Flow-directed balloon catheters may tend to pass to areas of high flow rather than through stenotic lesions. Catheters with excellent torque control and a relatively tight angle at the tip (such as a right coronary artery shape) may be helpful in directing the guide wire in the appropriate direction. We have also found a co-axial combination of multipurpose guide catheter through which a hydrophilic sharply angled catheter (such as a 4 French JR or Terumoangled Glide catheter) may be advanced to be especially helpful. The guide catheter can be shortened by cutting the proximal end. A side-arm sheath (one French size smaller than the guide catheter) can be cut near its hub and carefully advanced onto the cut end of the guide catheter to provide a hemostasis valve and a port for pressure monitoring or dye injection. The guide catheter provides support for the initial direction in the major branch. The sharply angled hydrophilic inner catheter can then be advanced and rotated in any direction to point to the desired branch. A hydrophilic guide wire such as a Terumo Glidewire can then be advanced through the stenotic vessel and the hydrophilic catheter will often follow this type of wire through even tight stenoses.

It is essential to have excellent wire support for placement of dilating balloons or stents. If a flexible hydrophilic wire is used to guide a small catheter across the stenotic area, the wire should generally be replaced with a stiffer wire once the initial catheter is adequately positioned. The time and effort to place a stiff wire in an excellent position provides a significant advantage in many cases.

Stenoses may be treated by simple balloon angioplasty, cutting balloon angioplasty, or placement of a stent. Simple balloon angioplasty or cutting balloon angioplasty is preferable in young patients in whom there is an expectation of continued growth.[11] Placement of a stent in such patients

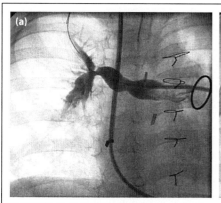 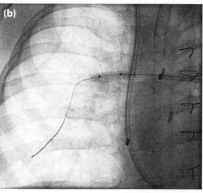 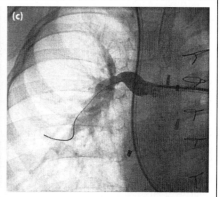

Figure 82.2 (a) Severe stenosis at the anastomosis of a central pericardial roll anastomosed to the right pulmonary artery hilum in a patient with originally discontinuous pulmonary arteries. (b) Cutting Balloon inflated in the area of stenosis. Note that the three blades arranged along the length of the balloon are not readily visible. (c) Final result after dilation with a cutting balloon and then a slightly larger high pressure angioplasty balloon. The patient improved clinically after the procedure.

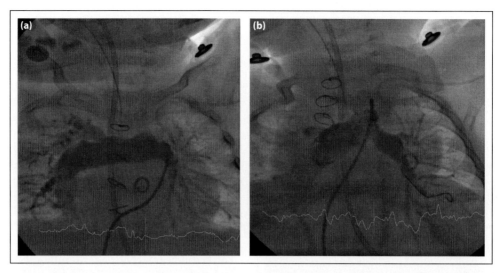

Figure 82.3   **(See color insert.)** (a) Cranial angulation fails to demonstrate the proximal left pulmonary artery stenosis because of opacification of the dilated main pulmonary artery on this pulmonary arteriogram. (b) Caudal and slightly LAO angulation demonstrates the proximal left pulmonary artery stenosis much better.

will mandate the need for later dilation of the stent, but successful balloon angioplasty often results in continued growth of the affected area. Restenosis may occur in as few as 12% of vessels when a good initial result is obtained in a small child. Balloon dilation of pulmonary artery stenoses generally requires a relatively high-pressure balloon for best results.[12] For tight distal lesions less than 3 mm in diameter, we often use large, high-pressure noncompliant coronary angioplasty catheters. The initial balloon diameter generally needs to be 3–3.5 times the diameter of the stenoses to be effective.[13] We feel that care must be taken, however, that the balloon is not larger than 1.5 times the normal vessel diameter immediately adjacent to the stenosis. Use of larger balloons extending into the distal "normal" portions of the vessel increases the risk of rupture or aneurysms. For larger vessels, we prefer to use high-pressure balloons that are relatively flexible and that have a relatively short "shoulder." Examples include the Zmed (NuMed), OptaPro or Savvy (Cordis), and Admiral (Medtronic) balloon dilation catheters.

The dilating balloon is advanced over the guide wire and positioned. A road map image from a prior angiogram is helpful in accurate positioning. A separate angiographic catheter can also be used to confirm that the balloon and guide wire have not shifted the original position of the stenosis. It is vital to ensure that the tip of the balloon is not protruding into a small side branch. Ruptures have been caused by the balloon tip being lodged in a very small adjacent distal vessel. The balloon can be inflated relatively slowly. Blocking one pulmonary artery branch seldom results in severe hemodynamic instability. If there appears to be a resistant waist in the balloon that is less than half of the expected diameter, we recommend against full inflation under high pressure initially. Such a tight

waist, which is subsequently eliminated under high pressure, is more often associated with vascular complications. The next size smaller balloon can be used initially to assess the results, or a smaller Cutting Balloon may be utilized. If the waist in the balloon is not too tight, we generally inflate the balloon to the rated burst pressure. Pressures are monitored with an inflation device, and the rated burst pressure is not exceeded by more than 10%. Rupture of a balloon in a tight vascular stenosis is more likely to lead to vascular complications, and the balloon may be difficult to retrieve if it bursts in a transverse direction. The maximal pressure is maintained for 5–30 s if the patient is hemodynamically stable. A postdilation angiogram is performed to assess the results and possible complications. We do not recommend recrossing dilated segments except with a catheter over the original guide wire because of the possibility of advancing the catheter into an intimal tear. Proximal and distal pressures can be measured with a catheter over the guide wire using a Tuohy–Borst type of side-arm adaptor or Multi-Track (NuMed) catheter. For small vessels, the catheter may be nearly as large as the vascular opening and pressure gradients may not be accurate. The primary assessment of the result in small vessels (<5 mm) is therefore the angiographic appearance. An increase of 50% in diameter is generally considered a reasonable marker of success.

If simple high-pressure balloon angioplasty is unsuccessful or has been unsuccessful in the past, we would proceed to the use of the Cutting Balloon (Boston Scientific). This balloon has 3 or 4 microtome blades fastened along the length of the balloon. The balloon is specially designed to fold over the blades during deflation. With inflation, the blades protrude approximately 10 thousandths of an inch above the surface of the balloon. These blades will create equally spaced micro-incisions that ideally extend through the thickened intima and into the media of the vessel. These equally spaced weakened areas should then be the areas of expansion during angioplasty. Without these incisions, vessels may expand in only the single weakest area around the circumference. We and others have found the Cutting Balloons to be efficacious for lesions that have not responded to simple balloon angioplasty.[14,15] The recommended Cutting Balloon diameter is generally slightly less than the diameter recommended for a simple angioplasty balloon and should not exceed 10% larger than the diameter of the adjacent normal vessel. The diameter and lengths of the Cutting Balloon are limited and they are applicable primarily to smaller vessels. The blades along the balloons make them more difficult to maneuver along tortuous courses. We recommend delivering the Cutting Balloons through a long transseptal sheath or a guide catheter in order to minimize the possibility of damage from the blades as the balloon traverses the tricuspid and pulmonary valves. Cutting Balloons should be inflated and deflated slowly to allow for proper conformational changes in the specially configured balloon. Extreme care must be taken with withdrawal of Cutting Balloons into the sheath or guide catheter to ensure that the microtome blades are not inappropriately caught on the edge of the sheath or catheter and avulsed from the balloon. These blades are extremely difficult or impossible to visualize fluoroscopically (Figure 82.2) and have the potential for significant damage if they embolize distally.

In postpubertal patients in whom surgical intervention in the region of the stenosis is not anticipated in the near future, we will use stenting as the primary treatment for larger vessels that are not immediately adjacent to important branches. If the desired effect cannot be achieved by angioplasty alone in a growing child, then placement of a stent in the stenotic vessel is the next option. For any given balloon diameter, stenting is definitely more effective than angioplasty alone because it prevents all, or nearly all, vessel elastic recoil. Stents generally result in better stenosis relief with less risk than the alternative of using a significantly oversized balloon.[16] The primary consideration against the use of stents in all stenotic lesions is that stents will not grow. If stents are placed in younger children, there must be a plan for dealing with the stenosis that will develop due to somatic growth. In many cases we specifically use a stent that can, in the future, be expanded to the full expected diameter of an adult-sized vessel. Proximal main branch pulmonary arteries in adults generally grow to 16–20 mm and may be significantly larger in some patients. Primary lobar branch pulmonary arteries typically reach 5–10 mm in diameter but may be larger in some patients. Placement of a stent that is incapable of expansion to more than 10–12 mm in a proximal branch pulmonary artery will result in eventual stenosis. Use of such a stent is reasonable if future surgery is anticipated

for other reasons, and the stent can be dealt with at that time. Later disruption of a small stent with an ultra-high-pressure balloon may be feasible, but experience is limited at present.[17]

In general, we prefer to use high-radial-strength balloon-expandable stents with the shortest possible length that can be dilated to the largest anticipated eventual diameter of the normal vessel. We do not recommend the use of self-expanding stents. Such stents cannot be expanded beyond their nominal diameter, and use of oversized self-expanding stents results in continual expansion pressure on the vessel wall that seems to encourage neointimal hyperplasia. Premounted stents (such as the Genesis or Valeo stents) are easy to use and advantageous in some situations because a long delivery sheath is not required. However, maintaining an inventory of premounted stent systems of every possible balloon diameter and stent length is very costly. Premounted stents may also have a more limited range for later expansion. We most frequently therefore use stents that are hand crimped onto an appropriate balloon and delivered through a long sheath. The sheath extends through the tricuspid and pulmonary valves in order to be certain that the stents do not become entangled or embedded in the valves or right ventricular outflow tract as the balloon traverses these regions.

The balloon size for stent implantation is chosen to be equal to or to very slightly exceed the diameter of the normal vessel adjacent to the stenosis. Accurate placement of the balloon and stent is absolutely essential and far more important than positioning a balloon for simple angioplasty. Image intensifiers should be angled to provide the best view of the length of the vessel in which the stent will be implanted. Viewing the stent at an angle (end on) greatly reduces the accuracy of positioning. A long delivery sheath or second catheter may be extremely useful to perform small injections of contrast medium to confirm accurate placement. Stents should be deployed with the catheter over a stiff guide wire to minimize the movement of the system during inflation. When deploying stents in a large high-flow central vessel, delivering the stent on a BIB balloon (NuMed) may allow for more precise placement (Figure 82.4). In some instances, placement of the stent will result in the end of the stent encroaching on, or covering, the orifice of an adjacent important branch vessel. In this situation, it may be best to deploy stents in the two vessels simultaneously. This "kissing balloon" technique results in a "double-barrel" opening into the adjacent pulmonary artery branches.[18] In order to perform this type of intervention, it is necessary to have adequate personnel to hold both catheters in position while two other operators inflate the balloons simultaneously.

Once stents have been deployed, extreme care must be used in removing the balloon catheter. It is often helpful to advance the long sheath over the balloon if the deflated balloon seems to be catching on the stent. Inadvertent

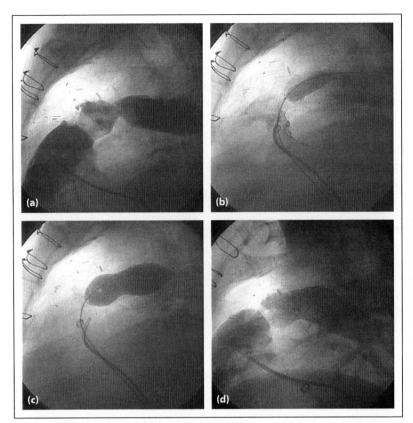

Figure 82.4   (a) Lateral view of severe supra-valve main pulmonary stenosis after arterial switch procedure. (b) First stage of stent deployment using the BIB balloon. The inner balloon has been inflated to its maximal diameter and the stent has a uniform diameter that is small enough to allow slight repositioning before full deployment. (c) The outer balloon of the BIB catheter has been inflated to its maximal pressure. This step must be accomplished expeditiously since the main pulmonary artery is completely occluded by the balloon at this point. (d) The final stent location is excellent with significant improvement in right ventricular pressure and no compromise of the pulmonary valve.

embolization of a stent caused by careless withdrawal of the balloon is a most unfortunate event.

Pitfalls and complications

The major immediate complication of balloon angioplasty is vascular damage or even disruption. Luminal irregularities are seen in nearly all successful angioplasties, especially if evaluated by intravascular ultrasound.[19] The experimental studies have suggested that angioplasty is unlikely to be successful unless there is disruption of the intima that extends into the media.[5] Disruption of the inner layers of the vessel, however, may result in the formation of vascular flaps that can cause severe stenosis or occlusions. These flaps are indicated by a curtain within the vessel lumen angiographically after dilation. As long as the guide wire has not been removed, the dilating balloon can be re-advanced past the flap, then partially inflated under low pressure and withdrawn to attempt to "tack" the disrupted inner layer back into position. The balloon can be maintained with low-pressure inflation for at least 3–5 min and a repeat angiogram can be performed to see if the curtain reforms. If the intimal flap persists, placement of a stent may be necessary. Extension of the vascular disruption past the media may result in extreme thinning of the remaining circumference of the vessel with only the

adventitial layer containing the disruption. An aneurysm is frequently seen in this circumstance. Any aneurysm seen immediately after angioplasty should be reevaluated after 5–30 min to be certain that the aneurysm is not enlarging (Figure 82.5). If an aneurysm is enlarging rapidly or if there is disruption of a pulmonary artery seen with pulmonary imaging, the balloon catheter should be immediately reinflated at or slightly proximal to the region of previous stenosis. Tamponading the affected vessel will reduce the chance of an urgent catastrophe. If the pressure proximal to the disruption is relatively low, coagulation parameters can be quickly normalized and the balloon can be deflated after 15–30 min with angiographic reassessment. If there is continued expansion of the aneurysmal area or continued bleeding, the vessel may need to be permanently occluded with a device such as a Gianturco coil or an Amplatzer vascular plug. If a covered stent is available, this may be another alternative treatment, but placement may be difficult under emergency circumstances.

Aneurysms that remain stable during the procedure still require follow-up evaluation by repeat catheterization or CT/MRI.[20] Some aneurysms have significantly expanded over days to months. These aneurysms may rupture catastrophically.[21] Significantly enlarging aneurysms require close follow-up.

A further serious complication of stent placement is stent migration. Aneurysms or vascular disruptions are

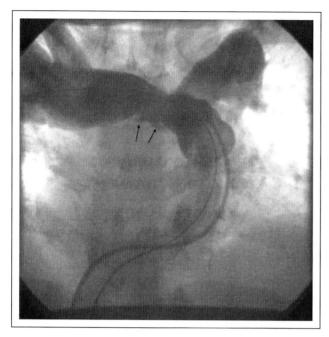

Figure 82.5 Small irregular aneurysm (arrows) at the origin of the right pulmonary artery after balloon angioplasty. In this patient, the area was unchanged 10 min later and also, by CT scan, 1 month later.

also possible, but should be less likely than with angioplasty alone if appropriate (smaller) balloons are utilized. The possibility of stent migration can be minimized by ensuring that the stent delivery balloon is adequate in size to result in apposition of the stent to the vessel wall over as much of its length as possible. The stent should be at least 30–50% larger than the stenotic area in most cases. Accurate measurements are absolutely essential. If a stent migrates, it is essential that the guide wire position be maintained. As long as the stent does not slip off of the guide wire, it may be possible to reposition it by partially inflating a balloon in the stent and then either retracting or advancing the stent to a favorable location. In most instances, a reasonable alternative position for the stent can be found, and the stent can be further dilated to maintain the new position. More sophisticated stent-retrieval techniques are beyond the scope of this chapter.

Postprocedure protocol

Following pulmonary artery dilation or stent deployment, most patients will be observed overnight. If stenosis relief has been successful, there will be increased flow into the affected lung segments. A reperfusion type of injury, with flash edema in portions of the lung, may occur if the pulmonary artery pressure is elevated and

the stenosis has been very effectively relieved.[22] In rare instances, the degree of edema may be sufficient to lead to hemoptysis or even the need for transient mechanical ventilation. The effects of dilation of proximal areas of stenosis can often be seen echocardiographically. A decrease in Doppler peak systolic velocity and normalization of the waveform on spectral Doppler indicates a good outcome. The effects of right ventricular pressure and size can be estimated. The best method to assess the effect on flow to the affected region is a quantitative radionuclide pulmonary perfusion scan. We generally prefer to wait for approximately 1 month to perform this scan after the procedure. This time frame allows for remodeling of the vasculature and resolution of any areas of mild edema that may affect the regional flow. Long-term echocardiography and an occasional radionuclide perfusion scan may be sufficient for the follow-up of simple, proximal stenotic lesions. CT or MRI or repeat angiography may be necessary for evaluation of more distal lesions. In most cases with more than one stenotic area, and certainly if a stent is implanted, a follow-up cardiac catheterization is often needed months to years after the procedure. Timing depends upon factors such as the residual right ventricular pressure, symptoms, and the results of noninvasive studies.

Catheter techniques to improve areas of stenosis in the pulmonary artery system have greatly improved outcomes over surgical management alone. Incorporation of the catheter techniques into the management plan of difficult patients has expanded surgical options for treatment of many forms of complex congenital cardiovascular malformations.

References

1. Trivedi KR, Benson LN. Interventional strategies in the management of peripheral pulmonary artery stenosis. *J Interv Cardiol* 2003;16(2):171–88.
2. Kim YM, Yoo SJ, Choi JY, Kim SH, Bae EJ, Lee YT. Natural course of supravalvar aortic stenosis and peripheral pulmonary arterial stenosis in Williams' syndrome. *Cardiol Young* 1999;9(1):37–41.
3. Kreutzer J, Landzberg MJ, Preminger TJ et al. Isolated peripheral pulmonary artery stenoses in the adult. *Circulation* 1996;93(7):1417–23.
4. Feltes TF, Bacha E, Beekman RH et al. Indications for cardiac catheterization and intervention in pediatric cardiac disease: A scientific statement from the American Heart Association *Circulation* 2011;123:2607–52.
5. Lock JE, Niemi T, Einzig S, Amplatz K, Burke B, Bass JL. Transvenous angioplasty of experimental branch pulmonary artery stenosis in newborn lambs. *Circulation* 1981;64(5):886–93.
6. Lock JE, Castaneda-Zuniga WR, Fuhrman BP, Bass JL. Balloon dilation angioplasty of hypoplastic and stenotic pulmonary arteries. *Circulation* 1983;67(5):962–7.
7. Sabiniewicz R, Romanowicz G, Bandurski T. Lung perfusion scintigraphy in the diagnosis of peripheral pulmonary stenosis in patients after repair of Fallot tetralogy. *Nucl Med Rev Cent East Eur* 2002;5(1):11–3.

8. Roman KS, Kellenberger CJ, Farooq S, MacGowan CK, Gilday DL, Yoo SJ. Comparative imaging of differential pulmonary blood flow in patients with congenital heart disease: Magnetic resonance imaging versus lung perfusion scintigraphy. *Pediatr Radiol* 2005;35(3):295–301.

9. Fagan T, Kay J, Carroll J, Neubauer A. 3-D guidance of complex pulmonary artery stent placement using reconstructed rotational angiography with live overlay. *Catheter Cardiovasc Interv* 2012;79:414–21.

10. Berman DP, Khan DM, Gutierrez Y, Zahn EM. The use of three-dimensional rotational angiography to assess the pulmonary circulation following cavo-pulmonary connection in patients with single ventricle. *Catheter Cardiovasc Interv* 2012;80:922–30.

11. Mori Y, Nakanishi T, Niki T et al. Growth of stenotic lesions after balloon angioplasty for pulmonary artery stenosis after arterial switch operation. *J Cardiol* 2003;91(6):693–8.

12. Gentles TL, Lock JE, Perry SB. High pressure balloon angioplasty for branch pulmonary artery stenosis: Early experience. *J Am Coll Cardiol* 1993;22(3):867–72.

13. Kan JS, Marvin WJ Jr, Bass JL, Muster AJ, Murphy J. Balloon angioplasty—branch pulmonary artery stenosis: Results from the valvuloplasty and angioplasty of congenital anomalies registry. *Am J Cardiol* 1990;65(11):798–801.

14. Rhodes JF, Lane GK, Mesia CI, Moore JD, Nasman CM, Latson LA. Cutting balloon angioplasty for children with small-vessel pulmonary artery stenoses. *Catheter Cardiovasc Interv* 2002;55(1):73–7.

15. Bergersen L, Gauvreau K, Justino H et al. Randomized trial of cutting balloon compared with high-pressure angioplasty for the treatment of resistant pulmonary artery stenosis. *Circulation* 2011;124:2388–96.

16. Bacha EA, Kreutzer J. Comprehensive management of branch pulmonary artery stenosis. *J Interv Cardiol* 2001;14(3):367–75.

17. Maglione J, Bergersen L, Lock JE, McElhinney DB. Ultra-high-pressure balloon angioplasty for treatment of resistant stenoses within or adjacent to previously implanted pulmonary arterial stents. *Circ Cardiovasc Intervent* 2009;2:52–8.

18. Stapleton GE, Hamzeh R, Mullins CE et al. Simultaneous stent implantation to treat bifurcation stenoses in the pulmonary arteries: Initial results and long-term follow up. *Catheter Cardiovasc Interv* 2009;73:557–63.

19. Nakanishi T, Tobita K, Sasaki M et al. Intravascular ultrasound imaging before and after balloon angioplasty for pulmonary artery stenosis. *Catheter Cardiovasc Interv* 1999;46(1):68–78.

20. Simmons PL, Scavetta KL, McLeary MS, Kuhn MA. Pulmonary artery pseudoaneurysm after percutaneous transluminal angioplasty in a pediatric patient. *Pediatr Radiol* 1997;27(9):760–2.

21. Zeevi B, Berant M, Blieden LC. Late death from aneurysm rupture following balloon angioplasty for branch pulmonary artery stenosis. *Catheter Cardiovasc Diagn* 1996;39(3):284–6.

22. Rothman A, Perry SB, Keane JF, Lock JE. Early results and follow-up of balloon angioplasty for branch pulmonary artery stenoses. *J Am Coll Cardiol* 1990;15(5):1109–17.

83

Pulmonary vein stenosis

Lee Benson

Introduction

Individual pulmonary vein stenosis, hypoplasia, or atresia is a rare congenital cardiac lesion that may cause pulmonary hypertension. Both stenosis and atresia can occur in the same patient, and one or more veins can be involved. The obstruction may be localized to the venoatrial junction, or may extend into the lung parenchyma for some distance. It may occur in isolation or in combination with other cardiac lesions (e.g., scimitar syndrome [Figure 83.1] or due to compression from the left atrium and descending aorta, or from an extracardiac Fontan conduit [right vein compression]).[1,2] It may evolve with time and affect additional pulmonary veins. For the interventionalist, the commonest indication will be after surgery for total anomalous pulmonary venous connection.[3-5] Thereafter, follow the ablation techniques to address atrial fibrillation, in which pulmonary vein stenosis occurs in 1.3% of procedures.[6-9]

In infants, despite improved surgical repair, there continues to be a significant incidence of relentless pulmonary vein stenosis,[3-5,10] particularly common in the setting of infracardiac and mixed drainage. There have been a number of reports, primarily with short-term follow-up of the impact of balloon dilation alone or in combination with endovascular stent implantation with mixed results. Although the majority of reports document acute reduction in flow obstruction, long-term follow-up has generally found restenosis, in-stent stenosis, or progression of the disease process.[11-19] These observations are in contrast to the effect of stent implantation in a swine model with essentially normal pulmonary vein histology.[20] This may be due to the intrinsically abnormal histopathology noted in the congenital lesion,[21] where there is significantly increased thickness of the media of the arteries and upstream veins, the worst examples being in those infants presenting with obstruction.[22] Recent studies from our laboratory have documented the role of increased TGF-β expression, resulting in the loss of endothelial and gain of mesenchymal marker expression upstream from obstructed pulmonary veins. This implies that the endothelial to mesenchymal cell transition contributes to the propagation of the disease into the upstream pulmonary veins.

This poor longer-term outcome applies to acquired pulmonary vein stenosis after attempted radio-frequency ablation as well,[6,8] despite initial early enthusiasm in short-term follow-up.[7,9] It appears that final stent diameter is critical, with smaller (<5 mm) implants developing in-stent restenosis sooner. Whether adjunctive therapies (brachytherapy, sonotherapy) have a place in the growing child is a matter for future study. The concept of recurrent interventions to manage restenosis is not appealing.[3,4,6] The application of drug eluting-biodegradable stents, however, may result in a renewed interest in the form of percutaneous therapy, but presently, studies are lacking to support human application.

One short-term application of stent management of pulmonary vein stenosis is in the preoperative patient with an obstructed vein, particularly if the child is not a good surgical candidate for whom short-term palliation can be achieved[23,24] (Figure 83.2).

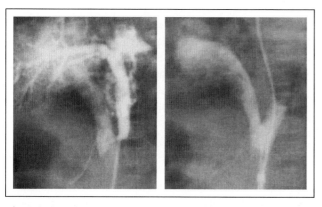

Figure 83.1 Left panel, from an angiogram of a child with scimitar syndrome taken in the left lateral projection showing the obstructed connection to the inferior caval vein. A 3.5 mm bare-metal coronary stent was implanted (right panel) for short-term palliation, to avoid surgery in this 2.5 kg infant with respiratory distress syndrome and an obstructed anomalous right pulmonary vein to the inferior caval vein.

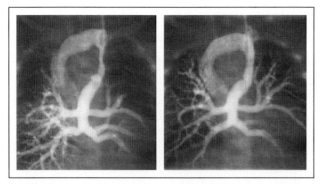

Figure 83.2   This 3 kg infant had obstructed supracardiac total anomalous venous return, complicating an unbalanced atrioventricular septal defect and right isomerism. The anatomical vertical vein obstruction was due to the left pulmonary artery anteriorly, duct or ductal ligamentum medially, and the left bronchus posteriorly. A 3 mm coronary stent was placed from the left internal jugular vein, as a bridge to a bidirectional cavopulmonary anastomosis. The angiograms shown were obtained in the frontal projection, although the left lateral was valuable for device positioning as well.

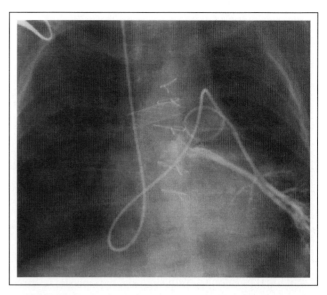

Figure 83.3   A frontal projection of a left pulmonary artery wedge injection demonstrating long segment left lower pulmonary vein stenosis, in a previously stent vein (in-stent stenosis).

Indications

The limited success in effective long-term relief of pulmonary vein stenting restricts the application of this technique to specific situations. If there is only one affected vein, and right ventricular pressure is not elevated, then intervention may not be indicated versus the potential complications of the interventional and known outcomes.

Congenital lesions:
- The infant with obstructed total or partial anomalous pulmonary venous return before surgical repair as short-term palliation (Figures 83.1 and 83.2).

Acquired lesions:
- The child after attempted repair of obstructed postoperative pulmonary vein stenosis, in the setting of anomalous venous return.[3-5] In this situation, a suture-line discrete stenosis may be present that might respond to angioplasty. If the lesion is not discrete, but extends into the hilar pulmonary veins, then endovascular stents can be considered, but outcomes are generally poor (Figure 83.3). The decision to place a stent must weigh against the eventual need for treatment of in-stent stenosis, and factor in the absolute diameter that the implant can be dilated, as the child grows.
- Mediastinal fibrosis
- After attempted ablation of atrial fibrillation. In this setting the results are mixed; early studies reflect acute improvement, but most studies demonstrate the need for repeat catheter intervention to maintain stent patency.

Imaging

- A variety of imaging modalities can be used to perform surveillance for the development of pulmonary vein stenosis or confirm its presence if the clinical situation demands. Transthoracic echocardiography with Doppler flow examination of pulmonary vein flow should be performed as the initial imaging modality. The practice in our unit for infants after total anomalous pulmonary vein repair is to perform an early postoperative echocardiogram between 2 and 3 months after discharge. Early studies are performed if the suspicion is raised in the immediate post-repair period of clinical symptoms that suggest obstruction.
- Other noninvasive imaging studies of value include cardiac magnetic resonance (cMR) volume-rendering imaging; cMR angiography, and spiral computed tomographic (CT) studies. As radiation exposure is an issue, MR imaging is preferred despite the need of general anesthesia to perform the study in infants (Figure 83.4). Although a previous report[25] has suggested that cMR is superior to transesophageal echocardiography, there are few data comparing MRI to spiral CT scans.
- Pulmonary artery angiography with a balloon wedge injection is the definitive diagnostic modality and will define the extent of the lesion, and catheterization is recommended even if the vessel is thought occluded by other techniques. Initial scout views can be

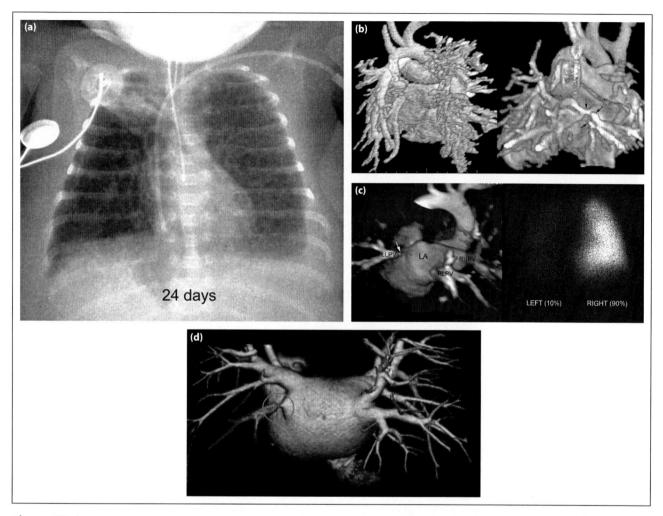

Figure 83.4   (**See color insert.**) In (a), a typical appearance to the chest x-ray (frontal projection) shortly after surgical repair in an infant with anomalous pulmonary venous return and persistent pulmonary vein obstruction. Note the hyperinflation and reticulated pattern of venous hypertension in the right lung. (b) A volume-rendered reconstruction of the venous confluence showing right pulmonary vein stenosis in the left panel, and stenosis of the confluence (all veins-arrows) in the right panel. In (c), left panel, a computed tomographic angiogram shows the reconstructed pulmonary confluence and left lower pulmonary vein (LLPV) stenosis. (d) This is a volume-rendered image of an isolated LLPV stenosis (red circle) after attempted radio-frequency ablation for atrial fibrillation. LA = left atrium, RUPV, RLPV = right upper and lower pulmonary vein. In the right panel, a perfusion scan after surgery in an infant with acquired pulmonary vein stenosis, defining little flow into the right lung.

obtained with pulmonary artery wedge injections (see "Catheterization Procedure" below). Generally, this is performed in the frontal and left lateral projections, but if the target lesion is known, then appropriate angulations can be performed. For right pulmonary veins, generally the frontal view is adequate, while for left veins, either the hepatoclavicular or long-axis oblique view will suffice, with a left lateral (Figure 83.5). Although noninvasive imaging such as spiral CT scans are accurate in defining mild to severe degrees of stenosis, vessels deemed occluded by these methods have been found to be patent by the use of the balloon wedge angiogram technique. This perhaps is related to the dye being forced

through the collapsed and stenotic vessel, with otherwise undetectable flow under normal conditions.[8]

Catheterization procedure

The goals of the procedure should be well defined beforehand. A right heart study should be performed, with selective pulmonary artery wedge injections to define the overall anatomy. Entry to the left atrium will be required, and selective pulmonary vein cannulation is required. Whether no intervention, balloon angioplasty alone, or stent implantation is performed, will depend on the anatomy so imaged, and management goals.

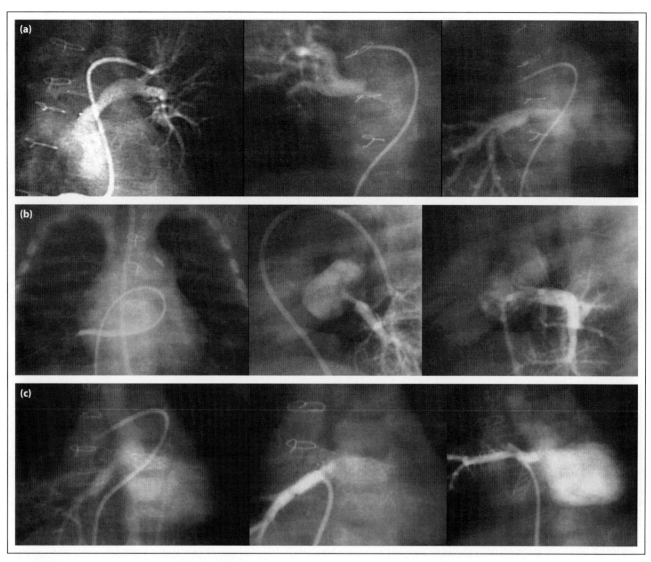

Figure 83.5 In (a), left panel, a right pulmonary artery wedge injection in a long-axis oblique view defines mild narrowing of the left upper vein as it enters the left atrium. In the middle panel, the frontal projection shows the right upper vein, and in the left panel, the right lower pulmonary vein, which are stenotic as they enter the atrium, is shown in those infants after anomalous vein surgery. In (b), left panel, the course of a catheter to cannulate the right lower pulmonary vein is shown, while in the middle and right panels, the left lateral view of a left lower pulmonary vein lesion before (middle) and after stent angioplasty is shown. In (c), left panel, multiple stents are seen in this infant after anomalous vein surgery, in the left lower, and right lower and upper veins, from a right pulmonary artery wedge injection. The frontal detector was adjusted to be in profile with the right lower lobe vein stent, to avoid foreshortening. In the middle panel, a selective injection shows evidence of restenosis within and distal to the implanted stent. In the right panel, a selective injection into the right upper vein, in-stent restenosis is evident.

Preparation and access

Procedures should be performed under general endotracheal anesthesia. Access must be from the femoral vein(s); if there is an intact atrial septum, a transseptal puncture must be performed. The puncture should be performed such that the ultimate catheter or sheath course avoids tight curves. This can be assisted using intracardiac echocardiography imaging and a steerable transseptal sheath (Agilis™, St. Jude Medical, Saint Paul, MN, USA). The internal jugular vein can be used if no other access is available, and if there is an atrial defect. Cannulation of the right veins may be difficult from the neck. Systemic and left heart pressures should be monitored with a retrograde femoral artery catheter. Patients should be given intravenous heparin sulfate (our dose: 100 IU/kg, no maximum). The activated clotting times (ACT) should be monitored throughout the procedure with the goal to maintain an ACT of >250 s.

Hemodynamics and angiography

Right heart hemodynamic data can be obtained with a balloon wedge catheter (6 or 7 Fr). This catheter can be used to perform both pulmonary artery wedge pressures and a wedge angiogram for mapping the individual pulmonary vein flow and to determine if any segments were completely occluded (Figure 83.5). Axially angulated angiography will be required, depending on the vein under evaluation. Generally, the right veins are best imaged in the frontal and left lateral views, while the right veins are profiled in the four-chamber and left lateral views. The wedge injections can be used to improve the angulations for subsequent selective injections. The technique for obtaining a wedge angiogram is as follows:

1. Cannulate the segmental branch feeding the venous segment of interest.
2. Connect the catheter to a 20 cc syringe with 10 cc of contrast, and prior to wedging the catheter tip withdraw 10 cc of the patient's blood, and hold the syringe upright; the contrast and blood layer will form, with the contrast lower than the blood.
3. Wedge the catheter, and by hand inject the 20 cc of fluid. The contrast will fill the capillary-venous circulation, and the injected blood will force the contrast into the pulmonary vein, avoiding overlap of arterial and venous phases.

Pulmonary vein cannulation

The left atrium is then entered by a transseptal technique with a 6 or 7 Fr long sheath, depending upon the diameter of the subsequent balloon or stent anticipated for the intervention. Entry to the left veins follows a gentle curve from the inferior caval vein, through the atrial puncture. Lesions in the right veins are more difficult to address, particularly in the smallest of patients if the right middle or lower vein requires cannulation. To cannulate this vessel, a cobra or right coronary-shaped catheter or one that is shaped as a hockey stick can be deflected off the lateral atrial wall to allow a direct position into the right lower pulmonary vein (Figure 83.5b). For left veins, a right coronary artery catheter with a 2 or 2.5 curve, or a cobra-shaped catheter (4 or 5 Fr), can be used to probe the individual vessels, with or without the assistance of a floppy-tipped wire (e.g., 0.035 inch Glidewire wire Terumo, or V-18™ Boston Scientific). This catheter or a 5 Fr angled glide catheter (Medi-tech, Boston Scientific) can be used to measure the mean pressure gradient across the target lesion, angiographically study the individual pulmonary venous anatomy, and position an exchange wire into the distal pulmonary vein. A different protocol is used to engage the right lower pulmonary vein. To cannulate this vessel, a modified hockey stick-shaped coronary guide catheter (Medtronic/AVE)

can be used within the left atrium and deflected off the lateral wall to allow a direct position toward the right lower pulmonary vein. This catheter is then used to place a guide wire as described above. For a rare instance, for example, the ostium of the vein is atretic, techniques to cross the lesion can be attempted using a variety of guide wires such as a Whisper™ (Abbott Vascular, Santa Clara, CA, USA), Fielder XT™, or Miracle 3™ (Asahi-Intecc, Aichi, Japan), which is usually reserved for coronary total occlusions. Often a small dimple is noted in the left atrium on non-invasive imaging, and fusion-imaging using previously obtained images should be overlaid, if possible, on live fluoroscopy to assure the correct location of entry.

Preparation for the intervention

The diameter and length of the obstructive lesion and the distal pulmonary vein should be measured digitally, using the catheter diameter for magnification correction. Other techniques such as marker catheters can also be employed.

Angioplasty intervention

An angioplasty balloon, chosen not to exceed the diameter of the stenotic lesion by 3–4 mm or the distal vessel by a factor of 2 can be initially chosen, with standard angioplasty performed in each lesion. Stent implantation can be considered if there is elastic recoil of the lesion; in the absence of a fixed lesion, a flap occurs or when there is in-stent restenosis noted in the follow-up. A variety of stents are available. In small infants, coronary stents, which can be placed through a 4 Fr guide, and dilated to 5 or 6 mm, are generally used. These stents, while giving early relief for the obstruction, tend to restenose, and their effectiveness is limited by the child's growth. In the older patient and adult, a larger stent (e.g., Genesis, Cordis), can be used, which can be dilated to 10 mm in diameter. If a fixed lesion is present (i.e., persistence of a waist at high inflation pressures [>8 atm]), Cutting Balloon angioplasty can be considered (Boston Scientific).[25] In general, the lesions should be dilated or stented to the same diameter of the distal, noninvolved vessel.

Postintervention assessment

After balloon angioplasty or stenting, a mean pressure gradient across the lesion should be measured. Angiography should also be performed to measure the residual lesion diameter and assess the degree of vessel injury.

Follow-up studies are recommended due to the high restenosis rate. Echocardiography appears the best initial modality to follow patient course, with flow determination in the affected vein, and measurement of right ventricular pressures. CT and cMR imaging may not be useful if the vein is stented due to the metal artefact. Repeat catheterization at 8 months to 1 year as a routine may be considered.

Intraoperative placement

In the very small infant, and in those children who have difficult vein access, intraoperative placement has been performed.[14-16] However, these procedures were performed at a time when the balloons and stents available were stiff and difficult to maneuver through tight turns; these are probably not needed with today's technology. Surgical techniques such as sutureless vein repairs have been adopted with reasonably good short-term results.[33]

Summary and outcomes

In both acquired and congenital forms of pulmonary vein stenosis, the lesion has been uniformly frustrating to treat for cardiac surgeons and interventional cardiologists, with restenosis being a common occurrence.[3-5,11,12] Various surgical approaches have been attempted, with variable results, depending on the technique used, anatomy, and timing of surgery, although recent experience with a sutureless technique is promising.[27,28] In children, balloon angioplasty has been uniformly unsuccessful[11,12] and endovascular stenting has met with little clinical success.[14-16,29-31] On the other hand, stent placement in the pulmonary veins after extrinsic compression in adults has yielded some clinical success.[18] In the setting of acquired stenosis after attempted radio-frequency ablation for atrial fibrillation, the situation may be different. The application of energy near the orifice of the pulmonary veins results in the formation of thrombus, necrotic myocardium, and proliferation of elastic lamina and intimal proliferation.[32] This may provide a substrate for angioplasty or stent placement different from other acquired or congenital vein lesions and, hence, transcatheter therapy could potentially be successful. However, recent long-term follow-up studies have demonstrated restenosis and the need for frequent reintervention.[6] Children and adults with this lesion require lifetime follow-up and potentially multiple procedures to prevent the loss of lung segments.

References

1. O'Donnell CP, Lock JE, Powell AJ, Perry SB. Compression of pulmonary veins between the left atrium and the descending aorta. *Am J Cardiol* 2003;91:248–51.
2. Freedom RM, Yoo SJ, Mikailian H, Williams W. Eds. *The Natural and Modified History of Congenital Heart Disease*. New York: Blackwell Publishing, 2004. p. 466.
3. Caldarone CA, Najm HK, Kadletz M, Smallhorn JF, Freedom RM, Williams WG, Coles JG. Relentless pulmonary vein stenosis after repair of total anomalous pulmonary venous drainage. *Ann Thorac Surg* 1998;66:1514–20.
4. Hyde JA, Stumper O, Barth MJ, Wright JG, Silove ED, deGiovanni JV, Brawn WJ, Sethia B. Total anomalous pulmonary venous connection: outcome of surgical correction and management of recurrent venous obstruction. *Eur J Cardiothorac Surg* 1999;15:735–40.
5. Michielon G, DiDonato RM, Pasquini L, Giannico S, Brancaccio G, Mazzera E, Squitieri C, Catena G. Total anomalous pulmonary venous connection: Long-term appraisal with evolving technical solutions. *Eur J Cardiothorac Surg* 2002;22:184–91.
6. Packer DL, Keelan P, Munger TM et al. Clinical presentation, investigation, and management of pulmonary vein stenosis complicating ablation for atrial fibrillation. *Circulation* 2005;111:546–54.
7. Purerfellner H, Aichinger J, Martinek M, Nesser HJ, Cihal R, Gschwendtner M, Dierneder J. Incidence, management, and outcome in significant pulmonary vein stenosis complicating ablation for atrial fibrillation. *Am J Cardiol* 2004;93:1428–31.
8. Qureshi AM, Prieto LR, Latson LA et al. Transcatheter angioplasty for acquired pulmonary vein stenosis after radiofrequency ablation. *Circulation* 2003;108:1336–42.
9. Vance MS, Bernstein R, Ross BA. Successful stent treatment of pulmonary vein stenosis following atrial fibrillation radiofrequency ablation. *J Invasive Cardiol* 2002;14:414–6.
10. Ricci M, Elliott M, Cohen GA, Catalan G, Stark J, de Leval MR, Tsang VT. Management of pulmonary venous obstruction after correction of TAPVC: Risk factors for adverse outcome. *Eur J Cardiothorac Surg* 2003;24:28–36.
11. Driscoll DJ, Hesslein PS, Mullins CE. Congenital stenosis of individual pulmonary veins: clinical spectrum and unsuccessful treatment by transvenous balloon dilation. *Am J Cardiol* 1982;49:1767–72.
12. Lock JE, Bass JL, Castaneda-Zuniga W, Fuhrman BP, Rashkind WJ, Lucas RV Jr Dilation angioplasty of congenital or operative narrowings of venous channels. *Circulation* 1984;70:457–64.
13. Tomita H, Watanabe K, Yazaki S, Kimura K, Ono Y, Yagihara T, Echigo S. Stent implantation and subsequent dilatation for pulmonary vein stenosis in pediatric patients: Maximizing effectiveness. *Circ J* 2003;67:187–90.
14. Coles JG, Yemets I, Najm HK et al. Experience with repair of congenital heart defects using adjunctive endovascular devices. *J Thorac Cardiovasc Surg* 1995;110:1513–9; discussion 1519–20.
15. Ungerleider RM, Johnston TA, O'Laughlin MP, Jaggers JJ, Gaskin PR. Intraoperative stents to rehabilitate severely stenotic pulmonary vessels. *Ann Thorac Surg* 2001;71:476–81.
16. Mendelsohn AM, Bove EL, Lupinetti FM et al. Intraoperative and percutaneous stenting of congenital pulmonary artery and vein stenosis *Circulation* 1993;88(5 Pt 2):II210–7.
17. McMahon CJ, Mullins CE, ElSaid HG. Intrastent sonotherapy in pulmonary vein restenosis: A new treatment for a recalcitrant problem. *Heart* 2003;89:E6.
18. Doyle TP, Loyd JE, Robbins IM. Percutaneous pulmonary artery and vein stenting: A novel treatment for mediastinal fibrosis. *Am J Respir Crit Care Med* 2001;164:657–60.
19. Dieter RS, Nelson B, Wolff MR, Thornton F, Grist TM, Cohen DM. Transseptal stent treatment of anastomotic stricture after repair of partial anomalous pulmonary venous return. *J Endovasc Ther* 2003;10:838–42.
20. Hosking M, Redmond M, Allen L, Broecker L, Keaney M, Lebeau J, Walley V. Responses of systemic and pulmonary veins to the presence of an intravascular stent in a swine model. *Cathet Cardiovasc Diagn* 1995;36:90–6.
21. Haworth SA, Reid L. Structural study of pulmonary circulation and of heart in total anomalous pulmonary venous return in early infancy. *Br Heart J* 1977;39:80–92.
22. Yamaki S, Tsunemoto M, Shimada M, Ishizawa R, Endo M, Nakayama S, Hata M, Mohri H. Quantitative analysis of pulmonary vascular disease in total anomalous pulmonary venous connection in sixty infants. *J Thorac Cardiovasc Surg* 1992;104(3):728–35.

23. Michel-Behnke I, Luedemann M, Hagel KJ, Schranz D. Serial stent implantation to relieve in-stent stenosis in obstructed total anomalous pulmonary venous return. *Pediatr Cardiol* 2002;23(2):221–3.

24. Coulson JD, Bullaboy CA. Concentric placement of stents to relieve an obstructed anomalous pulmonary venous connection. *Cathet Cardiovasc Diagn* 1997;42(2):201–4.

25. Yang M, Akbari H, Reddy GP et al. Identification of pulmonary vein stenosis after radiofrequency ablation for atrial fibrillation using MRI. *J Comput Assist Tomogr* 2001;25:34–35.

26. Sugiyama H, Veldtman GR, Norgard G, Lee KJ, Chaturvedi R, Benson LN Bladed balloon angioplasty for peripheral pulmonary artery stenosis. *Catheter Cardiovasc Interv* 2004;62:71–7.

27. Najm HK, Caldarone CA, Smallhorn J, Coles JG. A sutureless technique for the relief of pulmonary vein stenosis with the use of *in situ* pericardium. *J Thorac Cardiovasc Surg* 1998;115:468–70.

28. Lacour-Gayet F, Rey C, Planche C Pulmonary vein stenosis. Description of a sutureless surgical procedure using the pericardium in situ. *Arch Mal Coeur Vaiss* 1996;89:633–6.

29. Wax DF, Rocchini AP. Transcatheter management of venous stenosis. *Pediatr Cardiol* 1998;19:59–65.

30. O'Laughlin MP, Perry SB, Lock JE, Mullins CE. Use of endovascular stents in congenital heart disease. *Circulation* 1991;83:1923–39.

31. Cullen S, Ho SY, Shore D et al. Congenital stenosis of pulmonary veins failure to modify natural history by intraoperative placement of stents. *Cardiol Young* 1994;4:395–8.

32. Taylor GW, Kay GN, Zheng X et al. Pathological effects of extensive radiofrequency energy applications in the pulmonary veins in dogs. *Circulation* 2000;101:1736–1742.

33. Azakie A, Lavrsen MJ, Johnson NC, Sapru A. Early outcomes of primary sutureless repair of the pulmonary veins. *Thorac Surg* 2011;92:666–71.

84

Balloon dilation of aortic coarctation and recoarctation

Rui Anjos and Inês Carmo Mendes

Introduction

Aortic coarctation may occur as a discrete lesion or be associated with a variable degree of aortic arch hypoplasia, and should be considered as part of a diffuse arteriopathy. Surgical repair of coarctation was established over 60 years ago, and balloon dilation was introduced 30 years later. The best approach in the treatment of coarctation has been the subject of intense debate for the past few decades.

Indication for treatment

In infants and children, the indication for treatment of aortic coarctation includes a pressure gradient >20 mmHg between the upper and lower limbs and the presence of upper body hypertension. Left ventricular hypertrophy secondary to hypertension is another indication, but is rarely seen in infants and small children. In adolescents and adults, the European Society of Cardiology (ESC) guidelines for coarctation treatment are summarized in Table 84.1. In practice, the indications for treatment almost always include criteria which are class I recommendations,[1,2] and only very rarely a decision is based on class II recommendations. The criteria defined by the ESC have a C level of evidence, reflecting the ethical and logistical difficulty of performing randomized trials in this area.

Mechanism of balloon dilation of aortic coarctation

Balloon dilation of resected coarctation segments[3,4] demonstrated that the mechanism of effective relief of the stenosis was the tearing of the intimal and medial layers of the aortic wall. Similar findings were observed after dilation of surgically created coarctation lesions in lambs, with complete healing of the intimal lesions without aneurysm formation within 2 months.[5] Intravascular ultrasound studies

confirmed the occurrence of intimal tears after aortic balloon angioplasty, revealing a higher diagnostic sensitivity over angiography.[6,7] At follow-up, intravascular ultrasound evaluation revealed disappearance or reduction of most arterial wall lesions with evidence of healing, remodeling, and resolution of the intimal tears.[6] Long-term complications, such as the late development of aneurysms, may occur years after the procedure.[8]

Technique

Careful assessment of the patient before the procedure is extremely important. Echocardiography provides confirmation of the diagnosis, including location and extent of

Table 84.1 Indications for treatment of coarctation in adolescents and adults

Criteria	Class of recommendation	Level of evidence
Gradient >20 mmHg between upper and lower limbs	I	C
Upper limb hypertension		
Pathological BP response to exercise		
Significant LV hypertrophy		
Hypertension and aortic coarctation diameter <50% of the diameter of aorta at diaphragm level	IIa	C
Aortic coarctation diameter <50% of the diameter of aorta at diaphragm level	IIb	C

Source: Adapted from Baumgartner H et al. ESC. *Eur Heart J* 2010;31: 2915–57.

BP: blood pressure; LV: left ventricular.

coarctation, and assessment of other left-sided lesions. The ascending aorta, pattern, and dimensions of the aortic arch and branches can be assessed echocardiographically,[9] especially in younger patients. Echocardiographic measurements of the aortic arch are useful noninvasive predictors of outcome of coarctation balloon dilation.[9] In adolescents and adults, because of the acoustic windows, echocardiographic imaging and quantification of the distal aortic arch and isthmus may be challenging and sometimes impossible. Doppler gradients may be unreliable in the presence of extensive collaterals, but a diastolic runoff is a consistent sign of significant coarctation.

Magnetic resonance imaging (MRI) provides exceptional anatomic and functional evaluation of the aortic arch, and 3D reconstruction is useful to plan the procedure, particularly if there is a tortuous aortic arch.[10] MRI is also extremely useful to diagnose irregularities of the aortic wall, including aneurysms, which may be present in native lesions[11,12] but also after any type of previous surgical or interventional treatment. Patient selection for percutaneous or surgical approach of coarctation and procedure planning is therefore a noninvasive process.

Informed consent should include information on the expected results and the immediate and long-term risks associated with balloon dilation or surgery, including the risks and benefits of both options.

The procedure is usually performed under general anesthesia, although deep sedation can be used in adolescents and adults.[13] It is prudent to have a unit of blood cross-matched. The femoral artery is the usual approach, although in infants, the axillary or carotid arteries are possible alternatives. A 4 to 6 Fr introducer is selected, depending on the patient's weight.

Heparin is administered (100–150 IU/kg intravenously, with a maximum dose of 5000 IU), with activated clotted times monitored regularly and maintained at >200 s. A catheter is advanced retrogradely to the ascending aorta and a pullback gradient is obtained. A multipurpose catheter with two side holes provides an accurate evaluation of the gradient location, which is particularly important when there are multiple stenoses or there is a marked tortuosity of the aortic arch. The initial gradient can also be evaluated through a separate arterial line placed in the radial or contralateral femoral artery, which has the advantage of providing continuous monitoring during the procedure. Pressure monitoring can also be obtained through the side arm of the introducer.

An alternative to the retrograde approach is transseptal entry to the left atrium from the right atrium, with a balloon-tipped or angiographic catheter, which is then advanced to the left ventricle, ascending aorta, and transverse arch. Through this catheter, positioned proximal to the coarctation, gradients can be recorded initially without a catheter crossing the coarctation and hemodynamic and angiographic evaluation can be obtained before and after balloon dilation without removing the balloon from the area and without having to reposition catheters.

The anatomy of the transverse arch and the coarctation is defined by aortograms performed in the transverse aortic arch, to show the narrowest part of the lesion in two different views (Figure 84.1). Angiographic projections usually include lateral and a left anterior oblique (15° to 20°) or straight anteroposterior view. A caudal tilt of 10° to 20° on the left anterior oblique view may improve delineation of the lesion, if the isthmus overlaps the descending aorta. A pigtail catheter with multiple markers or an angiographic catheter with calibration marks is used for accurate measurement of the diameter and length of the coarctation, the diameters of the transverse arch, isthmus, aorta proximal and distal to the coarctation and the aorta at diaphragm level. The origins of the brachiocephalic, carotid, and subclavian arteries are noted and irregularities or aneurysms of the aortic wall are carefully excluded.

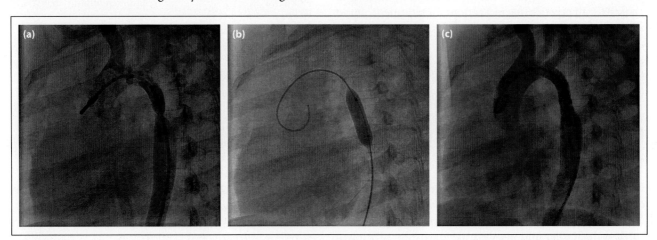

Figure 84.1 The left anterior oblique view of aortic coarctation (a), in a 3-year old patient with discrete coarctation, with no hypoplasia of the aortic arch, treated with balloon angioplasty (b). Angiography after dilation shows a good result with no residual stenosis and no aortic wall abnormalities (c).

A stiff 0.035 inch exchange guide wire is placed through the retrograde catheter, with the tip in a secure position. If the left subclavian artery arises some distance away from the coarctation or has a large diameter, it is the best option for anchoring the guide wire. If not, other alternatives are the ascending aorta or the right subclavian artery, the latter allowing for a straight and secure position of the guide wire. The tip of the guide wire should always be kept away from the coronary, carotid, or vertebral arteries.

There is no consensus regarding optimal selection of the balloon diameter. In native aortic coarctation, the usual initial option is a balloon diameter equal to or 1 mm smaller than the diameter of the aorta immediately distal to the origin of the subclavian artery, and not larger than the diameter of the aorta at the diaphragm level.[14,15] In aortic recoarctation, the same rules are applied by some authors, or a balloon two to three times the minimum diameter of the coarctation, not exceeding 150% of the transverse arch,[16] and not exceeding the diameter of the aorta at the diaphragm.[16,17] No "safe" upper limit of balloon size has been defined. The shortest possible balloons for the specific anatomy should be selected, covering the entire length of the coarctation and ideally with small shoulders.

The arterial introducer sheath is replaced by a larger size, if necessary, to accept the balloon selected. It is preferable to use a slightly larger vascular sheath than a balloon catheter inserted directly over a wire, which may increase the risk of arterial damage.[18] The balloon is advanced to just distal to the coarctation, and purged. It is then centered at the coarctation level and inflated using a pressure-monitored inflation device, until the waist disappears or the maximum recommended pressure is achieved. The inflation/deflation times are variable but usually short, under 10 s. Balloon inflation is then repeated two to four times. The balloon should be kept away from the carotid and vertebral arteries, to minimize the risk of trauma. Balloon rupture should be avoided, as this causes a sudden increase in shear forces with the possibility of additional aortic trauma[19] and also increases the risk of femoral damage.

Once the coarctation has been dilated, the balloon is removed and a multipurpose catheter attached to a valve or hemostatic adaptor, or a Multi-Track™ catheter, is used. Gradients are recorded while crossing the coarctation area, maintaining the guide wire in position or assessed by simultaneous pressure recording through a catheter positioned above the coarctation, antegradely or retrogradely, and a femoral arterial line or the side arm of the introducer.

Repeat final angiograms in two different image views are obtained. The guide wire should not be withdrawn across the dilation site until the procedure is complete. A pigtail catheter should only be removed over a guide wire, avoiding potential contact of the free tip with an intimal tear, which could cause additional trauma to the arterial wall.

If there is still angiographic narrowing at the coarctation site or a significant residual gradient is seen, and the aortic wall shows no damage, a balloon 1 to 2 mm larger may be used, not exceeding 10–15% of the normal size of the adjacent aorta.[14] The use of oversized balloons (more than three times the coarctation diameter) should be avoided to prevent excessive stretching of the coarctation segment and adjacent aorta, which has been associated with arterial wall damage.[5]

Balloon dilation of aortic coarctation in neonates and small infants

Aortic coarctation present in the neonatal group is frequently associated with hypoplasia of the aortic arch and very commonly to a patent arterial duct. Neonates may present in a life-threatening condition, with ventricular dysfunction and multiorgan failure. Early reports of balloon dilation of coarctation in stable neonates revealed low morbidity and mortality rates,[20–22] but persistence or recurrence of coarctation was reported in 41–83% of cases.[20–24] In most studies, more than half of the patients required reintervention. The mechanism for recurrence of coarctation in neonates is elastic recoil of ductal tissue surrounding the coarctation, isthmus hypoplasia, intimal proliferation, and arterial remodeling.[25] Femoral arterial occlusion or stenosis after balloon dilation in this age group is frequent.[21,22,26] In one report, 38% of patients had aortic aneurysms after neonatal balloon dilation.[24]

As a result of the high recurrence rates, the risk of arterial damage, and aneurysm formation, balloon dilation of coarctation is not performed routinely as a primary treatment in neonates or small infants. Surgical repair in this age group has produced good results in most recent series,[27–29] but surgical risk is increased in neonates with severe heart failure.[30,31] In case of no response to medical treatment, balloon angioplasty may be a good option promoting clinical stability and if necessary, acting as a bridge to surgery.[32,33]

Children, adolescents, and adults with coarctation

In many centers, balloon dilation is the primary approach for native or recurrent coarctation after infancy.

Early results after balloon dilation for coarctation

Only two prospective randomized studies have compared the results of balloon dilation and surgery for *native aortic coarctation* in children: one with 36 and the other with 58 patients.[34,35] Balloon angioplasty and surgery provided similar acute gradient reduction and decrease in systolic blood pressure in both studies.[34,35] Other reports of transcatheter treatment for native coarctation in children are retrospective. There are usually excellent immediate angiographic results in most patients (Figure 84.1) and an effective gradient reduction obtained with intervention, with increase in coarctation diameters, and immediate reduction of gradient to <20 mmHg in 80–90% of the patients.[15,36–42] The risk factors for a poor immediate response include a higher initial gradient, a small transverse arch, a lower immediate gradient reduction,[15,36,42] and older age at the time of balloon dilation.[42] Procedure-related complications are lower and the hospital stay is shorter with angioplasty compared to surgery.[34–36]

In patients with *recoarctation*, the acute results of balloon dilation are similar to those of native coarctation.[42] An immediate gradient reduction to <20 mmHg has been described in 65–93% of patients after balloon dilation for recoarctation,[16,17,42–46] with suboptimal risk factors, including earlier procedure date, low volume institution, older age, and higher initial gradient.[17,42] Frequently, a residual obstruction is caused by unsuspected transverse arch hypoplasia,[16,44] which reinforces the importance of a detailed morphological assessment.

Late results after balloon dilation for coarctation

Intermediate and late follow-up prospective studies are limited after balloon angioplasty in *native coarctation*. Hernandez-Gonzales[35] documented a higher rate of recoarctation after angioplasty than after surgery (50% vs. 21% at 1 year follow-up). In Cowley's prospective 10 year follow-up study, blood pressure, gradient, and the need for repeat interventions were similar for the two approaches but more aneurysms were noted in the balloon dilation group, requiring surgery.[8] Reintervention rates after balloon dilation for native coarctation in two retrospective studies comparing both approaches were 26–44%, with no reintervention after surgery.[36,37] Recurrent stenosis after balloon angioplasty of native coarctation in other retrospective studies varies from 3 to 42%,[8,13,38,41,47–51] with very good results in adolescents and young adults with discrete lesions.[13,49] The rates of reintervention after surgery in children with native coarctation have been reported to be 0–13%.[36,37]

Late reintervention after balloon dilation for *recurrent coarctation* has been described in 6–33% of patients at 5–12 years.[16,17,45,46] Surgical approach to recoarctation is associated with a higher mortality of up to 7%[52] than for native coarctation, with a need for reintervention between 4 and 30% of patients.[53–55]

Left ventricular hypertrophy[56] regresses after balloon dilation and there is normalization of blood pressure in 63–79% of the patients.[57–59] In most patients who remain hypertensive, there is a reduction in the number of antihypertensive medications required to control the blood pressure.[57,58]

Determinants of hemodynamic results

A significant gradient at follow-up due to a suboptimal initial result or late restenosis has been associated with young age,[38,48,50,60,61] aortic arch hypoplasia,[9,21,48,50,61] very narrow coarctation,[48,61] high initial gradient,[15,38,60] and low immediate gradient reduction.[15] Based on these results, the selection of candidates for coarctation angioplasty can be improved with a meticulous aortic arch analysis by echocardiography or MRI.[9,10] A poor result with angioplasty is more likely in the presence of an aortic isthmus diameter <70% of the descending aorta,[50] <2/3 the ascending aorta,[48,61] or with a z-score lower than −2.[9] The best candidates for balloon dilation of native aortic coarctation are those with a discrete and moderately severe lesion.[9,50,54,61] In *recoarctation*, the type of previous surgery did not influence the outcome[17,46] but angioplasty[17] and transverse arch hypoplasia[16] at an older age were associated with a higher incidence of reinterventions.

Markers of biophysical response of the arterial wall subjected to dilation, such as stretch, gain, and recoil were studied to evaluate a possible relation with outcome.[15,62,63] A higher rate of restenosis was found in patients with larger stretch and gain.[15,62] Stretch causes an exponential increase in the area and circumference gain, especially in severe coarctations, and possibly more extensive wall damage by reduction of elastic properties of the aorta.[15,62] Ovaert et al.[15] suggested aiming at a circumferential stretch of 60–70%, which is achieved with a balloon diameter two to three times the coarctation, and in line with early experimental studies.[5] Rao et al., in a young population, showed a greater immediate recoil in patients without recoarctation,[63] which might imply preservation of the elastic properties of the aorta or a less severe cystic medial necrosis.[11]

Complications

Mortality

The valvuloplasty and angioplasty congenital anomalies (VACA) registry reported mortality rates of 0.7% for dilation of native coarctation[40] and 2.5% for recoarctation.[43] More recent publications report no or very low mortality rates for balloon dilation of coarctation and recoarctation in children, in most cases less than 1%.[15,17,36–39,42]

Aortic wall damage

Concerns about balloon angioplasty for coarctation are particularly focused on arterial damage. Aortic rupture is the most serious complication, with an incidence of 0–2% in large reports of dilation of native[36,40,42] and recurrent coarctation.[19,43,64]

As the mechanism of dilation of the stenosed segment involves tearing of the intimal and medial layers, some degree of damage to the arterial wall is expected and is in fact inherent to balloon dilation. Spontaneous healing of intimal and medial tears or dissections present after angioplasty of coarctation occurs at late follow-up in most patients.[7] In an animal model,[5] normal aortas were stretched by at least 30% without any visible vascular injury. Balloon diameters greater than three times the coarctation diameter produced vascular tears and mediastinal haemorrhage.[5]

Cystic medial necrosis is present in the aortic wall of patients with coarctation.[11,65] It is more frequent in older patients, in whom there is a higher incidence of wall thinning, marked tortuous segments, and calcification,[66] increasing the probability of wall injury after angioplasty.

The reported rates of aneurysms after balloon dilation for native coarctation have been highly variable, from 1.5%[15] to 43%,[41] possibly as a result of different interventional techniques, a lack of agreement on the definition of aneurysm,[37,41,67,68] and the type of follow-up. The highest rates were reported from the earlier series, and recent publications describe an incidence under 7% for native,[15,36,37,47,49,51] and 0–4% for recurrent coarctation.[17,45,46] Stenting may result in less vascular injury than balloon angioplasty, by tacking intimal flaps to the aortic wall, reducing intimal dissection, and reinforcing weakened areas. Nevertheless, aneurysms have been reported in 9% of patients after bare stent implantation, with prestent angioplasty being an additional risk factor.[69] Aneurysms may also occur after surgery, especially after Dacron patch repair, with an incidence of 5–50%.[70–73]

Imaging of the aorta by MR or CT scans should be performed regularly after balloon dilation of coarctation and recoarctation (Figure 84.2). The optimal timing for a first imaging scan and how often it should be repeated is not clearly defined. Late development of aneurysms, sometimes more than 5 years after intervention[8,74] supports the recommendation of long-term regular imaging of the aortic arch.

The clinical significance of small-to-moderate aneurysms (Figure 84.3) and their best management remain unclear.[39,41,47,67] Most patients are managed conservatively, but larger aneurysms are usually referred for surgery[75] or covered stent implantation.[76]

Other complications

Femoral artery injury after balloon dilation for coarctation, including thrombosis or other lesions requiring treatment, was reported in 2–10% of children.[15,32,34–36] Serial MRI assessment revealed progression of some lesions.[18] The incidence of significant injury was higher in earlier reports, when balloon catheters were introduced directly into the vessel over a wire. The use of low-profile balloons and arterial access through small introducers has significantly reduced this complication.

Paradoxical hypertension occurring after balloon dilation of coarctation is rare and usually not severe, with an occurrence of less than 1.5%,[15,36,39] in contrast with surgical patients with a reported incidence of 25–36%.[36,77]

Persistent systemic hypertension was found at late follow-up in 15–50% of patients without residual stenosis after dilation of aortic coarctation.[15,49] Systemic hypertension was also documented in 10–33% of patients after effective stent implantation[78,79] and in 25–72% after surgery.[80,81] Ambulatory blood pressure monitoring and exercise testing shows hypertensive responses in the majority of patients on late follow-up, irrespective of the type of treatment.[81–83]

Cerebrovascular accidents have been reported in less than 2% of patients[42,84] and are usually secondary to thromboembolic events. Careful anticoagulation and control of guide wire and balloon position, avoiding trauma or occlusion of the neck vessels, minimizes this problem.

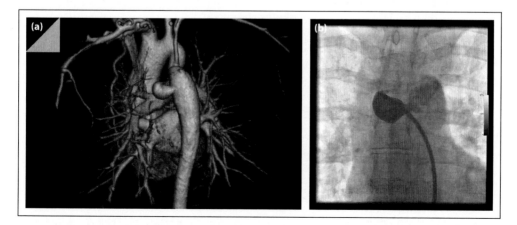

Figure 84.2 A saccular aortic aneurysm detected 5 years after balloon dilation of aortic coarctation, on a routine MRI in an asymptomatic adult (a). The aneurysm is far from the tortuous and hypoplastic arch, and gives rise to an intercostal artery, best seen with selective angiography (b), so this may have started as a lesion at the origin of the intercostal artery.

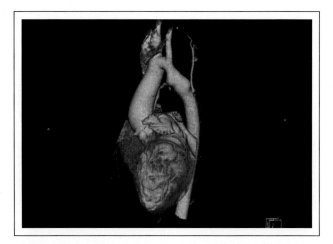

Figure 84.3 **(See color insert.)** Two aneurysms detected by routine imaging of the aortic arch 1 year after balloon dilation of coarctation. These are mild lesions, being managed conservatively.

Conclusion

Balloon angioplasty of native and recurrent aortic coarctation provides similar acute results. There is a small but definite risk of acute complications, and a sustained relief of the obstruction in the majority of patients treated with percutaneous angioplasty. The ideal candidates are patients after the first months of life, with discrete and moderately severe coarctation, with a normal or near-normal-sized transverse arch. An adequate selection of the ideal patients for balloon dilation is therefore of paramount importance. In some centers, stent implantation has become a preferred approach to aortic coarctation in older children and adults, as its results are less unpredictable than balloon dilation and stents can provide sustained dilation while supporting the aortic wall.

Comparison of outcome and complications between percutaneous intervention and surgery for native and recurrent coarctation is difficult, as there are no large prospective randomized studies, and the evaluation of an unselected series of patients, who frequently are not comparable, is biased. Long-term follow-up data on a large series of patients is required for all therapeutic approaches to native and recurrent coarctation.

References

1. Baumgartner H, Bonhoeffer P, De Groot NM et al. ESC guidelines for the management of grown-up congenital heart disease. *Eur Heart J* 2010;31:2915–57.
2. Warnes CA, Williams RG, Bashore TM et al. ACC/AHA 2008 guidelines for the management of adults with congenital heart disease: Executive summary. *Circulation* 2008;118:2395–451.
3. Lock JE, Castaneda-Zuniga WR, Bass JL et al. Balloon dilation of excised aortic coarctations. *Radiology* 1982;143:689–91.
4. Ho SY, Somerville J, Yip WC et al. Transluminal balloon dilation of resected coarcted segments of thoracic aorta: Histological study and clinical implications. *Int J Cardiol* 1988;19(1):99–105.
5. Lock JE, Niemi T, Burke BA et al. Transcutaneous angioplasty of experimental aortic coarctation. *Circulation* 1982;66:1280–6.
6. Sohn S, Rotham A, Shiota T et al. Acute and follow-up intravascular ultrasound findings after balloon dilation of coarctation of aorta. *Circulation* 1994;90:340–7.
7. Erbel R, Görge G, Gerber T et al. Dissection following balloon angioplasty of aortic coarctation: Review of the literature. *J Interv Cardiol* 1992;5(2):99–109.
8. Cowley CG, Orsmond GS, Feola P et al. Long-term, randomized comparison of balloon angioplasty and surgery for native coarctation of the aorta in childhood. *Circulation* 2005:28;111(25):3453–6.
9. Kaine SF, O'Brian Smith E et al. Quantitative echocardiographic analysis of the aortic arch predicts outcome of balloon angioplasty of native coarctation of the aorta. *Circulation* 1996;94:1056–62.
10. Bank ER, Aisen AM, Rocchini AP et al. Coarctation of the aorta in children undergoing angioplasty: Pretreatment and post treatment MR imaging. *Radiology* 1987;162:235–40.
11. Isner JM, Donaldson RF, Fulton D et al. Cystic medial necrosis in coarctation of the aorta: A potential factor contributing to adverse consequences observed after percutaneous balloon angioplasty of coarctation sites. *Circulation* 1987;75(4):689–95.
12. Oliver JM, Gallego P, Gonzalez A et al. Risk factors for aortic complications in adults with coarctation of the aorta. *J Am Coll Cardiol* 2004;44(8):1641–7.
13. Walhout RJ, Suttorp MJ, Mackaij GJ, Ernst JM, Plokker HW. Long-term outcome after balloon angioplasty of coarctation of the aorta in adolescents and adults: Is aneurysm formation an issue? *Catheter Cardiovasc Interv* 2009;73(4):549–56.
14. Mullins, CE. *Cardiac Catheterization in Congenital Heart Disease: Pediatric and Adult.* Malden, Massachusetts: Blackwell Publishing, 2006. pp. 454–71.
15. Ovaert C, McCrindle BW, Nykanen D et al. Balloon angioplasty of native coarctation: Clinical outcomes and predictors of success. *J Am Coll Cardiol* 2000;35(4):988–96.
16. Yetman AT, Nykanen D, McCrindle BW et al. Balloon angioplasty of recurrent coarctation: A 12-year review. *J Am Coll Cardiol* 1997;30:811–6.
17. Reich O, Tax P, Bartáková H, Tomek V et al. Long-term (up to 20 years) results of percutaneous balloon angioplasty of recurrent aortic coarctation without use of stents. *Eur Heart J* 2008;29(16):2042–8.
18. Burrows PE, Benson LN, Babyn P et al. Magnetic resonance imaging of the iliofemoral arteries after balloon dilation angioplasty of aortic arch obstructions in children. *Circulation* 1994;90:915–20.
19. Balaji S, Oommen R, Rees PG. Fatal aortic rupture during balloon dilation of recoarctation. *Br Heart J* 1991;65:100–1.
20. Redington AN, Booth P, Shore DF et al. Primary balloon dilation of coarctation of the aorta in neonates. *Br Heart J* 1990;64:277–81.
21. Rao PS, Chopra PS, Koscik R et al. Surgical versus balloon therapy for aortic coarctation in infants < or = 3 months old. *J Am Coll Cardiol* 1994;23:1479–83.
22. Park Y, Lucas VW, Sklansky MS et al. Balloon angioplasty of native aortic coarctation in infants 3 months of age and younger. *Am Heart J* 1997;134:917–23.
23. Patel HT, Madani A, Paris YM et al. Balloon angioplasty of native coarctation of the aorta in infants and neonates: Is it worth the hassle? *Pediatr Cardiol* 2001;22:53–7.
24. Fiore AC, Fischer LK, Schwartz T et al. Comparison of angioplasty and surgery for neonatal aortic coarctation. *Ann Thorac Surg* 2005;80:1659–64.
25. Ino, T., Ohkubo, M. Dilation mechanism, causes of restenosis and stenting in balloon coarctation angioplasty. *Acta Paediatrica* 1997;86:367–71.

26. Lee CL, Lin JF, Hsieh KS et al. Balloon angioplasty of native coarctation and comparison of patients younger and older than 3 months. *Circ J* 2007;71(11):1781–4.

27. Burch PT, Cowley CG, Holubkov R et al. Coarctation repair in neonates and young infants: Is small size or low weight still a risk factor? *J Thorac Cardiovasc Surg* 2009;138(3):547–52.

28. Wright GE, Nowak CA, Goldberg CS et al. Extended resection and end-to-end anastomosis for aortic coarctation in infants: Results of a tailored surgical approach. *Ann Thorac Surg* 2005;80(4):1453–9.

29. Barreiro CJ, Ellison TA, Williams JA et al. Subclavian flap aortoplasty: Still a safe, reproducible, and effective treatment for infant coarctation. *Eur J Cardiothorac Surg* 2007;31(4):649–53.

30. Quaegebeur JM, Jonas RA, Weinberg AD et al. Outcomes in seriously ill neonates with coarctation of the aorta. A multi-institutional study. *J Thorac Cardiovasc Surg* 1994;108:841–51.

31. McGuinness JG, Elhassan Y, Lee SY et al. Do high-risk infants have a poorer outcome from primary repair of coarctation? Analysis of 192 infants over 20 years. *Ann Thorac Surg* 2010;90(6):2023–7.

32. Suárez de Lezo J, Pan M, Romero M et al. Percutaneous interventions on severe coarctation of the aorta: A 21-year experience. *Pediatr Cardiol* 2005;26(2):176–89.

33. Bouzguenda I, Marini D, Ou P et al. Percutaneous treatment of neonatal aortic coarctation presenting with severe left ventricular dysfunction as a bridge to surgery. *Cardiol Young* 2009;19(3):244–51.

34. Shaddy RE, Boucek MM, Sturtevant JE et al. Comparison of angioplasty and surgery for unoperated coarctation of the aorta. *Circulation* 1993;87:793–9.

35. Hernandez-Gonzalez M, Solorio S, Conde-Carmona I et al. Intraluminal aortoplasty vs. surgical aortic resection in congenital aortic coarctation. A clinical random study in pediatric patients. *Arch Med Res* 2003;34(4):305–10.

36. Rodés-Cabau J, Miró J, Dancea A et al. Comparison of surgical and transcatheter treatment for native coarctation of the aorta in patients > or = 1 year old. The Quebec Native Coarctation of the Aorta study. *Am Heart J* 2007;154(1):186–92.

37. Fruh S, Knirsch W, Dodge-Khatami A et al. Comparison of surgical and interventional therapy of native and recurrent aortic coarctation regarding different age groups during childhood. *Eur J Cardiothorac Surg* 2011;39(6):898–904.

38. del Cerro MJ, Fernández-Ruiz A, Benito F et al. Balloon angioplasty for native coarctation in children: Immediate and medium-term results. *Rev Esp Cardiol* 2005;58(9):1054–61.

39. Morrow WR, Vick III GW, Nihill MR et al. Balloon dilation of unoperated coarctation of the aorta: Short-term and intermediate-term results. *J Am Coll Cardiol* 1988;11:133–8.

40. Tynan M, Finley JP, Fontes V, Hess J, Kan J. Balloon angioplasty for the treatment of native coarctation: Results of valvuloplasty and angioplasty of congenital anomalies registry. *Am J Cardiol* 1990;65(11):790–2.

41. Cooper RS, Ritter SB, Rothe WB et al. Angioplasty for coarctation of the aorta: Long-term results. *Circulation* 1987;75:600–4.

42. McCrindle BW, Jones TK, Morrow WR et al. Acute results of balloon angioplasty of native coarctation versus recurrent aortic obstruction are equivalent. Valvuloplasty and angioplasty of congenital anomalies (VACA) registry investigators. *J Am Coll Cardiol* 1996;28:1810–7.

43. Hellenbrand WE, Allen HD, Golinko RJ et al. Balloon angioplasty for aortic recoarctation: Results of valvuloplasty and angioplasty of congenital anomalies registry. *Am J Cardiol* 1990;65(11):793–7.

44. Anjos R, Qureshi SA, Rosenthal E et al. Determinants of hemodynamic results of balloon dilation of aortic recoarctation. *Am J Cardiol* 1992;69:665–71.

45. Hijazi ZM, Fahey JT, Kleinman CS et al. Balloon angioplasty for recurrent coarctation of aorta. Immediate and long-term results. *Circulation* 1991;84:1150–6.

46. Siblini G, Rao PS, Nouri S et al. Long-term follow-up results of balloon angioplasty of postoperative aortic recoarctation. *Am J Cardiol* 1998;81:61–7.

47. Rao PS, Galal O, Smith PA, Wilson AD. Five to nine-year follow-up results of balloon angioplasty of native coarctation in infants and children. *J Am Coll Cardiol* 1996;27:462–70.

48. Rao PS, Thapar MK, Kutayli F et al. Causes of recoarctation after balloon angioplasty of unoperated aortic coarctation. *J Am Coll Cardiol* 1989;13(1):109–15.

49. Fawzy ME, Fathala A, Osman A, Badr A et al. Twenty-two years of follow-up results of balloon angioplasty for discreet native coarctation of the aorta in adolescents and adults. *Am Heart J* 2008;156(5):910–7.

50. Fletcher SE, Nihill MR, Grifka RG et al. Balloon angioplasty of native coarctation of the aorta: Midterm follow-up and prognostic factors. *J Am Coll Cardiol* 1995;25:730–4.

51. Walhout RJ, Suttorp MJ, Mackaij GJ, Ernst JM, Plokker HW. Long-term outcome after balloon angioplasty of coarctation of the aorta in adolescents and adults: Is aneurysm formation an issue? *Catheter Cardiovasc Interv* 2009;73(4):549–56.

52. Ralph-Edwards AC, Williams WG, Coles JC et al. Reoperation for recurrent aortic coarctation. *Ann Thorac Surg* 1995;60:1303–7.

53. Sweeney MS, Walker WE, Duncan JM. Reoperation for aortic coarctation: Techniques, results and indications for various approaches. *Ann Thorac Surg* 1985;40:46–9.

54. Beekman RH, Rocchini AP, Behrendt DM et al. Reoperation for coarctation of the aorta. *Am J Cardiol* 1981;48:1108–14.

55. Brown JW, Ruzmetov M, Hoyer MH et al. Recurrent coarctation: Is surgical repair of recurrent coarctation of the aorta safe and effective? *Ann Thorac Surg* 2009;88(6):1923–30.

56. Hassan W, Awad M, Fawzy ME et al. Long-term effects of balloon angioplasty on left ventricular hypertrophy in adolescent and adult patients with native coarctation of the aorta. Up to 18 years follow-up results. *Catheter Cardiovasc Interv* 2007;70:881–6.

57. Schräder R, Bussmann WD, Jacobi V, Kadel C. Long-term effects of balloon coarctation angioplasty on arterial blood pressure in adolescent and adult patients. *Cathet Cardiovasc Diagn* 1995;36:220–5.

58. Hassan W, Malik S, Akhras N et al. Long-term results (up to 18 years) of balloon angioplasty on systemic hypertension in adolescent and adult patients with coarctation of the aorta. *Clin Cardiol* 2007;30(2):75–80.

59. Fawzy ME, Awad M, Hassan W et al. Long-term outcome (up to 15 years) of balloon angioplasty of discrete native coarctation of the aorta in adolescents and adults. *J Am Coll Cardiol* 2004;43(6):1062–7.

60. Beekman RH, Rocchini AP, Dick M 2nd et al. Percutaneous balloon angioplasty for native coarctation of the aorta. *J Am Coll Cardiol* 1987;10(5):1078–84.

61. Rao PS, Koscik R. Validation of risk factors in predicting recoarctation after initially successful balloon angioplasty for native aortic coarctation. *Am Heart J* 1995;130:116–21.

62. Ino T, Ohkubo M, Akimoto K et al. Angiographic assessment of the stretch-recoil-gain relation after balloon coarctation angioplasty and its relation to late restenosis. *Jpn Circ J* 1996;60(2):102–7.

63. Rao PS, Waterman B. Relation of biophysical response of coarcted aortic segment to balloon dilation with development of recoarctation following balloon angioplasty of native coarctation. *Heart* 1998;79(4):407–11.

64. Roberts DH, Bellamy CM, Ramsdale DR. Fatal aortic rupture during balloon dilation of recoarctation. *Am Heart J* 1993;125:1181–2.

65. Niwa K, Perloff JK, Bhuta SM et al. Structural abnormalities of great arterial walls in congenital heart disease: Light and electron microscopic analyses. *Circulation* 2001;103:393–400.

66. Oliver JM, Gallego P, Gonzalez A et al. Risk factors for aortic complications in adults with coarctation of the aorta. *J Am Coll Cardiol* 2004;44(8):1641–7.

67. Marshall AC, Lock JE. Leaving never land: A randomized trial for coarctation shows pediatric interventional cardiology is growing up. *Circulation* 2005;111(25):3347–8.

68. Pedra CA, Fontes VF, Esteves CA et al. Stenting versus balloon angioplasty for discrete unoperated coarctation of the aorta in adolescents and adults. *Catheter Cardiovasc Interv* 2005;64(4):495–506.

69. Forbes TJ, Moore P, Pedra CA et al. Intermediate follow-up following intravascular stenting for treatment of coarctation of the aorta. *Catheter Cardiovasc Interv* 2007;70(4):569–77.

70. delNido PJ, Williams WG, Wilson GJ et al. Synthetic patch angioplasty for repair of coarctation of the aorta: Experience with aneurysm formation. *Circulation* 1986;74(3 Pt 2):I32–6.

71. Parks WJ, Ngo TD, Plauth WH Jr et al. Incidence of aneurysm formation after Dacron patch aortoplasty repair for coarctation of the aorta: Long-term results and assessment utilizing magnetic resonance angiography with three-dimensional surface rendering. *J Am Coll Cardiol* 1995;26(1):266–71.

72. von Kodolitsch Y, Aydin MA, Koschyk DH et al. Predictors of aneurysmal formation after surgical correction of aortic coarctation. *J Am Coll Cardiol* 2002;39(4):617–24.

73. Bromberg BI, Beekman RH, Rocchini AP et al. Aortic aneurysm after patch aortoplasty repair of coarctation: A prospective analysis of prevalence, screening tests and risks. *J Am Coll Cardiol* 1989;14(3):734–41.

74. Aydogan U, Dindar A, Gurgan L et al. Late development of dissecting aneurysm following balloon angioplasty of native aortic coarctation. *Cathet Cardiovasc Diagn* 1995;36(3):226–9.

75. Brandt B III, Marvin WJ Jr, Rose EF et al. Surgical treatment of coarctation of the aorta after balloon angioplasty. *J Thorac Cardiovasc Surg* 1987;94:715–19.

76. Butera G, Heles M, Mc Donald S et al. Aortic coarctation complicated by wall aneurysm: The role of covered stents. *Catheter Cardiovasc Interv* 2011;78(6):926–32.

77. Sealy WC. Paradoxical hypertension after repair of coarctation of the aorta: A review of its causes. *Ann Thorac Surg* 1990;50(2):323–9.

78. Eicken A, Pensl U, Sebening W et al. The fate of systemic blood pressure in patients after effectively stented coarctation. *Eur Heart J* 2006;27(9):1100–5.

79. Morgan GJ, Lee KJ, Chaturvedi R et al. Systemic blood pressure after stent management for arch coarctation implications for clinical care. *J Am Coll Cardiol Cardiovasc Interv* 2013;6(2):192–201.

80. Kaemmerer H, Oelert F, Bahlmann J et al. Arterial hypertension in adults after surgical treatment of aortic coarctation. *Thorac Cardiovasc Surg* 1998;46(3):121–5.

81. Hager A, Kanz S, Kaemmerer H, Schreiber C et al. Coarctation long-term assessment (COALA): Significance of arterial hypertension in a cohort of 404 patients up to 27 years after surgical repair of isolated coarctation of the aorta, even in the absence of restenosis and prosthetic material. *J Thorac Cardiovasc Surg* 2007;134:738–45.

82. Lee MG, Kowalski R, Galati JC et al. Twenty-four-hour ambulatory blood pressure monitoring detects high prevalence of hypertension late after coarctation repair in patients with hypoplastic arches. *J Thorac Cardiovasc Surg* 2012;144(5):1110–6.

83. Galvão P, Matos Silva M, Amador P et al. Freedom from antihypertensive medication after balloon dilation with stent implantation in patients with coarctation of the aorta. *Cardiol Young* 2012;22(Suppl 1):S6.

84. Benson LN, Freedom RM, Wilson GJ et al. Cerebral complications following balloon angioplasty of coarctation of the aorta. *Cardiovasc Intervent Radiol* 1986;9:184–6.

85

Stenting in aortic coarctation and transverse arch/isthmus hypoplasia

Shakeel A. Qureshi

Introduction

Aortic coarctation is a fairly common congenital heart defect. There are many morphological variations. These vary from hypoplasia of the transverse aortic arch and isthmus to a very localized stenosis just beyond the left subclavian artery. The former variants are frequent in neonates, whereas the latter is noted in older children and adults. Very occasionally aortic arch interruption is seen in adults, although it is more frequently seen in neonates in association with other defects, such as ventricular septal defect. In older patients with untreated coarctation, the natural history may be adversely affected by consequences of hypertension.[1,2] Treatment of coarctation, whether surgical or interventional, improves the control of the blood pressure and may impact on the long-term survival.[3]

Stent implantation in aortic coarctation has been increasingly used to treat patients, who were previously treated by balloon angioplasty or surgery. Balloon dilation in native aortic coarctation and recoarctation has been controversial since its introduction in 1982.[4] Histological and intravascular ultrasound[5–10] studies have demonstrated that the mechanism of angioplasty involves tearing of the intima and media. Deficient elastic and muscular lamellae have been noted in ballooned sections of aorta at the time of surgery.[11] Although some of the intimal and medial tears may heal, there is concern that some may progress to aneurysms. Cystic medial necrosis may exist in the coarctation segment, suggesting that the aortic wall may be weak at the point of the stenosis.[12] A relatively high incidence of aneurysm formation of 2–20% has been reported.[13–17]

Stenting of aortic coarctation was first performed in 1991.[17] Stents tack intimal flaps to the aortic wall after tearing of the intima and media, allowing healing to occur without dissection.[18,19] They further reinforce the weakened areas within the aortic wall, which may later predispose to formation of a pseudoaneurysm. Where intimal tears occur, the stent provides a surface for formation of neointima over the tear, allowing healing to occur without intimal dissection. Furthermore, intimal and medial damage may not occur to the same extent following stenting compared with balloon dilation, as overdilation of the aorta is avoided during stent implantation.

Initially, stent implantation was used only for cases where surgery and balloon angioplasty had failed.[20] However, as experience increased, stenting has gradually become the treatment of choice in aortic coarctation. This is especially the case when coarctation coexists with hypoplasia of the aortic isthmus or transverse arch, when balloon dilation tends to have a high failure rate. This and other morphological variations such as a tortuous coarctation, long segment coarctation, or mild discrete coarctation may all be considered suitable for stenting. In other cases, in whom the anatomy is more straightforward, stenting may reduce the gradient at the coarctation site more effectively than balloon dilation. In adult patients, stenting is now considered as the treatment of choice in any variant of aortic coarctation, because growth is not an issue and so there is no need to keep up with somatic growth. At the other end of the scale, in children less than 10 years of age, it is preferable to avoid stenting, as several redilations may be required, until the child is fully grown and there remain questions about the feasibility of redilation.

Equipment

Palmaz (Cordis, Johnson and Johnson), Intratherapeutics Doublestrut, or LD Max and LD Mega (EV3), or Cheatham-Platinum (C-P) (NuMED) stents have been used the most in clinical practice (Figure 85.1a–f). Other stents such as Andrastents (Andramed) or Valeo (Bard) are recent introductions and are being used with increasing frequency. These are all balloon expandable and so need to be mounted on the appropriate balloon diameter. They are available in different lengths and so can be selected as

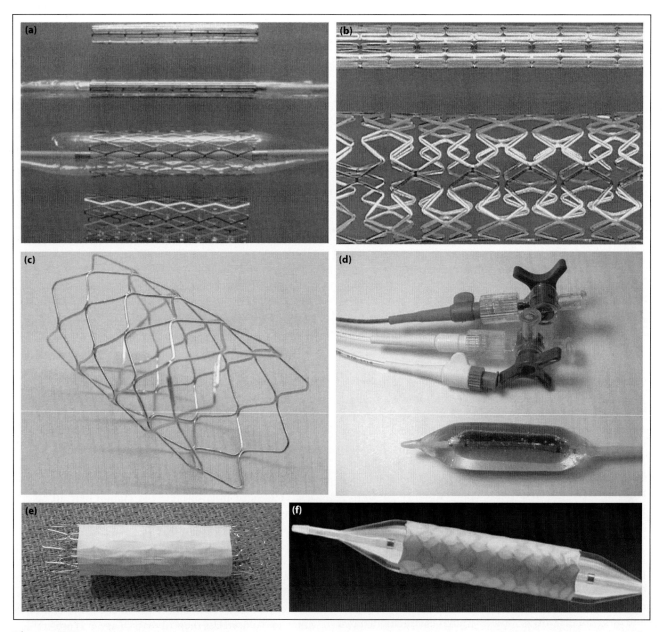

Figure 85.1 (a) Palmaz stent unexpanded, then mounted on a balloon, inflated, and then finally fully expanded. (b) Intrastent double-strut stent unexpanded and fully expanded. (c) Expanded Cheatham-Platinum (C-P) stent. (d) A BIB (balloon-in-balloon) system, which requires two inflation devices to inflate the balloons separately. (e) A covered C-P stent (with expanded polytetrafluoroethylene covering). (f) A covered Advanta V12 stent.

appropriate for a particular patient. Selection of balloons such as the Opta, Powerflex (Cordis, Johnson and Johnson), BIB (NuMED), Cristal balloons (Merck), or Z-Med balloons (NuMED) need to be kept in stock in catheter laboratories. On occasions, higher-pressure balloons such as the Mullins (NuMED) or Atlas balloons (Bard) may be needed. A range of sizes of covered stents such as C-P or Advanta V12 (Atrium) stents also need to be stocked for emergency cases, as there may be the rare complication of dissection and even aortic rupture. However, covered stents are almost routinely used now for the treatment of aortic coarctation in adolescents and adults.[21] Occasionally,

self-expanding stents may have some role to play, but these have a limited use in pediatric cardiology practice. They have the disadvantage of lower radial strength. The choice of a stent depends on the experience and the preferences of the operator and the local cost considerations.

Technique

The procedure is performed under general anesthesia, as it is painful for the patient when the balloon is inflated to deploy the stent in the aorta. Access is obtained in the femoral artery as well as in the femoral vein. The venous access is required for the insertion and the use of a temporary pacemaker during stent implantation, if needed. This is of importance in adults with a high stroke volume, such as when aortic regurgitation is present. Rapid right ventricular pacing reduces the cardiac output in a controlled manner, during the deployment of the stent, facilitating its precise positioning. In the presence of a very tight or nearly atretic or even atretic aortic segment, access may be needed in the right radial or brachial artery, so that a catheter can be passed from above into the descending aorta. If there is a pinhole opening present, the coarctation segment can be crossed from above, as it may be difficult to cross from below. Rarely, carotid arterial access by a surgical arteriotomy may be required for access to the descending aorta. A Perclose/Proglide (Abbott Vascular) suture may be inserted after local angiography of the femoral arteries. This helps to produce hemostasis at the end of the procedure and may prevent complications, such as hemorrhage from the arterial puncture site. This is a major advance in the method of hemostasis. Either a single suture or occasionally two sutures are used to repair the femoral arteries, in which up to 14 Fr sheaths have been inserted for the stent deployment. These sutures have to be inserted prior to the introduction of the larger sheath.

Heparin at a dose of 50–100 IU/kg is given after access is obtained to maintain the activated clotting time >200–250 s during the procedure.

A 5 or 6 Fr end-hole catheter is negotiated with a Terumo guide wire through the aortic coarctation and positioned in the ascending aorta. With a tight or tortuous coarctation, it is preferable to use a straight tip guide wire to cross the coarctation from below and this is followed by the catheter being passed over the guide wire. An Amplatz stiff exchange guide wire of 0.035 inch caliber is exchanged for the previous guide wire and over this, a Multi-Track catheter (NuMED) is passed. This catheter has a monorail system and is used to measure withdrawal gradients across the coarctation, without losing the guide wire position. In addition, angiography can be performed with this catheter, which has a 1 cm marker, allowing accurate calibration and the exact measurements of the aorta. Alternatively, a pigtail catheter with 1 cm radiopaque markers is used for angiography. Angiography is performed in the left lateral and either shallow left anterior oblique or right anterior oblique views (if biplane facilities are available). A better way of profiling the aortic coarctation is to pass the catheter into the ascending aorta and move the antero-posterior camera to the right anterior oblique projection until the catheter course in ascending and descending aorta is superimposed. The lateral camera should then be positioned at right angles to the antero-posterior camera. Accurate measurements are essential. The diameters of the distal transverse arch (just proximal to the origin of the left subclavian artery), the aortic isthmus (just distal

to the origin of the left subclavian artery), the site of coarctation, and the descending aorta above the diaphragm are measured, using catheter magnification or the calibration markers on the catheters. The diameter of the aorta at maximum systolic expansion is measured and is used to select the appropriate diameter balloon.

The length of the chosen stent is based on the distance from the left subclavian artery (or the left common carotid artery, if the subclavian artery has been used at previous surgery or if the subclavian artery is intimately related to the site of coarctation) to about 15 mm beyond the site of the coarctation. The maximum balloon diameter on which the stent is mounted is based on either the transverse or the distal arch diameter, whichever is the greater, and on occasions 1–2 mm greater.

The types of stents in use for this procedure include the Palmaz 2910 (29 mm long, nominal diameter 3.4 mm, dilates to 8–12 mm), 4014 (4 cm long, nominal diameter 4.6 mm, dilates to 14–25 mm), and 5014 (5 cm long, nominal diameter 4.6 mm, dilates to 14–25 mm), the various sizes of the Intratherapeutics doublestrut (LD Max or LD Mega) stents, Andrastents, Advanta V12, and the C-P stents available in 22 mm, 28 mm, 34 mm, 39 mm and 45 mm. All are available as bare-metal stents and the latter two are available as covered stents. The C-P stents have a slighter higher profile and are more rigid with higher radial strength than other stents and so are preferable in adult patients and those with aortic recoarctation after previous surgery, although any of the above stents may be used.

A long Mullins sheath (75 cm long) is passed over a 0.035 inch stiff exchange length guide wire positioned in the ascending aorta for stent delivery. As an alternative, the guide wire may be positioned in either the innominate artery or the left subclavian artery. However, if the distance between the origin of the left subclavian artery and the coarctation is less than 10 mm, then placing the guide wire in this location should be avoided. This is because on full inflation, the balloon may be pushed downward, resulting in possible stent malposition and even migration. The sheath size ranges between 10 and 14 Fr for bare stents or covered stents, and is generally 2–3 Fr larger than that required for the introduction of the balloon catheter alone. The stent is manually crimped onto the selected balloon tightly enough to ensure that it does not slip off the balloon during insertion through the tight diaphragm of the sheath. To avoid the stent from slipping off the balloon, a small piece of sufficient length of a similar size short sheath is cut to cover the stent and this covering is used to pass the stent/balloon assembly through the diaphragm of the sheath. This is even more important when introducing a covered stent through the diaphragm of the sheath. The various steps of the technique are shown in Figure 85.2a–f. In the past, adenosine was used to produce transient asystole during balloon inflation, but rapid right ventricular pacing has been used with good effect. The rate of pacing

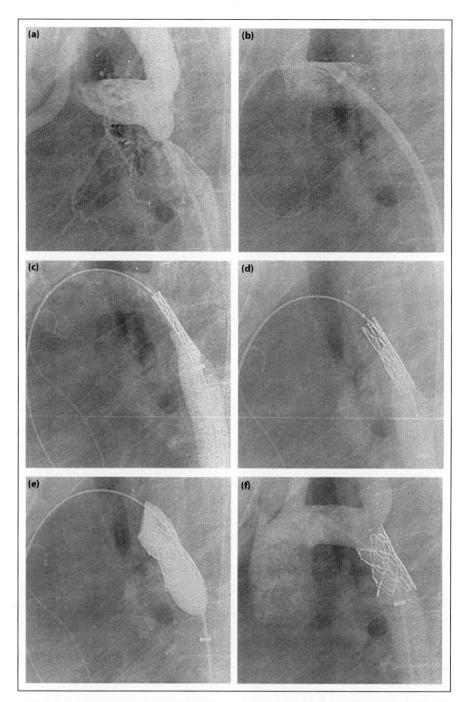

Figure 85.2   (a) A discrete aortic coarctation just beyond the left subclavian artery with mild distal isthmic hypoplasia. (b) The guide wire is positioned in the ascending aorta and the Mullins sheath is placed in the transverse aortic arch. (c) The stent/balloon assembly is positioned at the site of coarctation and the Mullins sheath is withdrawn to expose the stent. (d) The inner BIB balloon is inflated and an angiogram performed to check for the satisfactory position of the stent. (e) The outer BIB balloon is inflated to deploy the stent fully. A mild residual waist is kept on the balloon on occasion, especially if a tight coarctation is present to reduce the possibility of a dissection. (f) An angiogram after stent implantation showing good position of the stent and excellent relief of coarctation.

varies between 180 and 240 beats per minute. The exact rate can be determined at the outset, by monitoring the pressure in the ascending aorta, while pacing the heart at different rates. The rate for pacing, which reduces the blood pressure in the ascending aorta to less than 50 mmHg, is used.

The stent/balloon assembly is advanced through the long sheath and positioned across the site of the coarctation. Optimal positioning is confirmed by small hand injections of contrast through the side arm of the Mullins sheath or alternatively by hand injections through a second catheter placed in the descending aorta. While maintaining the balloon catheter and wire in position, the Mullins sheath is withdrawn to expose the stent/balloon assembly in position at the site of the coarctation. Rapid right ventricular pacing is initiated and the balloon is inflated with an inflation device, so that pressures up to the balloon burst pressure can be delivered. The final part of stent expansion may sometimes occur slowly with sustained pressure. Once the stent is deployed, the balloon is deflated and then pacing is stopped. Further dilation with a larger balloon may be performed in some cases, until satisfactory relief of the stenotic waist is attained. If a BIB balloon is used, then two inflation devices are needed. As soon as rapid pacing is started, one operator inflates the inner balloon first and after check angiography, the other operator inflates the outer balloon. For deflation, the same sequence is followed.

Although a bare stent can be expanded to the diameter of the normal vessel on either side of the coarctation, in a tight coarctation, either an undersized balloon is chosen or the balloon is not fully expanded to the normal vessel diameter, to reduce the likelihood of aortic wall damage and dissection. The stent is expanded to approximately 70–80% of the diameter of the descending aorta at the diaphragm at implantation. Flaring of the ends of the stent to achieve contact with the aortic wall at all points is not usually performed, although in some cases, flaring may be beneficial in securing the stent in a good position (Figure 85.3a–c).

After deflation, the balloon is withdrawn carefully so as not to dislodge the stent. The gradient across the stent is re-measured, by recording simultaneous pressures from the angiographic catheter passed over the guide wire to above the stent and the long sheath placed below the stent. An aortogram is repeated to exclude dissection or aneurysm formation. The guide wire and catheter are removed under fluoroscopy to ensure that these have not been trapped in the stent struts. After removal of the sheath, hemostasis is achieved with the Perclose/Proglide suture.

After the procedure, subcutaneous low-molecular-weight heparin is administered for 24 h. However, there is no consensus about this, as the diameters of the stents are large enough to preclude the use of anticoagulation. Antibiotics (flucloxacillin and gentamycin or cefuroxime) are given at the beginning of the procedure and may be continued for 24 h, according to local protocols. Aspirin is administered to all the patients the evening prior to the procedure at a dose of 3–5 mg/kg and continued for up to 6 months. Once again, there is a lack of evidence of the efficacy of aspirin. If a Perclose/Proglide suture has not been used to achieve hemostasis, manual pressure is needed, but reversal of heparin with protamine may be needed.

Follow-up is arranged 4 weeks, 6 months, and 1 year after the procedure, and spiral CT scanning is performed 4–6 weeks after the procedure to exclude aneurysm formation, dissection, and stent thrombosis. Recatheterization is performed only if there is clinical recoarctation, continuing hypertension, or CT evidence of aneurysm formation. Elective recatheterization is only performed after 6–12 months to carry out stent redilation, when there is a residual stenosis as a result of the stent having been intentionally underinflated initially.

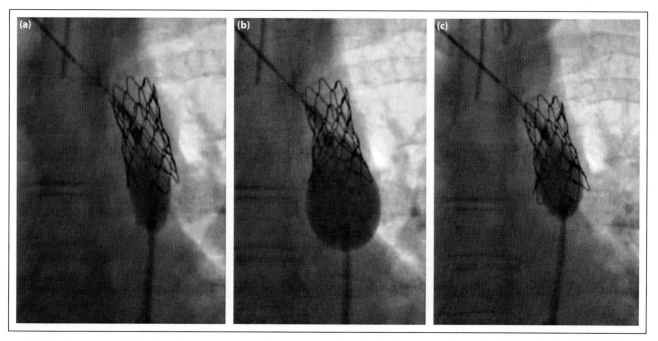

Figure 85.3   (a) A stent has been implanted at the site of aortic coarctation. (b) Coda balloon is inflated in the distal part of the stent. (c) The distal part of the stent has been flared.

Disadvantages of stenting

Relatively large 10–14 Fr Mullins delivery sheaths are used to deliver the stent/balloon assembly across the coarctation. While there may be a higher risk of femoral artery occlusion with stenting than with balloon angioplasty, this has not been a problem in adult patients.[22,23] If it was crucial to avoid a larger sheath and the coarctation was tight enough, then the stent could initially be deployed using an 8 or 10 mm diameter balloon (introduced through an 8 or 9 Fr sheath) and then expanded to the final size with a larger balloon, thereby minimizing the sheath size and trauma to the femoral artery.[24] Stenting should, if possible, be deferred in children until above 10 years of age, unless surgery is contraindicated.[25] However, children weighing less than 30 kg have received stents to treat aortic coarctation with excellent results.[26] A possible disadvantage with unknown consequences may be the introduction of a noncompliant and nonpulsatile section in the aorta at the stent site and its possible effects on the systolic blood pressure on exercise in the future.[27–30]

Complications of stenting

Complications of the stenting procedure include femoral artery disruption or thrombosis, stent migration at implantation, delayed stent migration, acute aortic rupture, paradoxical hypertension, thrombotic occlusion of the stent (described in stenting of the abdominal aorta), and endocarditis.[26–37] Deaths from stenting of aortic coarctation are rare, but have been reported in 0–1.4% of cases. Other complications such as embolic strokes may occur in 0–3.7% of patients[38] and aneurysm formation in 0–17%, when bare stents have been implanted.[38–44] The commonest complication related to femoral arterial access is occlusion, although avulsion and development of a false aneurysm of the femoral artery may occasionally occur. Use of closure devices may help, although complications can occur after these also.[45]

Most of the complications can be dealt with by medical treatment or catheter techniques. Stent thrombosis can be treated with local thrombolysis. Stent migration, which may occur in about 5% of procedures, may be dealt with by implanting and dilating the stent in an alternative safe location. If a dissection occurs, this can be managed conservatively, if small or by implanting a bare or a covered stent, if large. The occurrence of an aneurysm can also be treated similarly (Figure 85.4a–c). Rarely, if aortic rupture occurs, then availability of covered stents, which can be rapidly inserted percutaneously, can save the day and avoid the need for emergency surgery. Paradoxical hypertension can be treated by aggressive medical treatment. With covered stents, the experience is limited but even then, aneurysm formation is rare.[21,46,47]

Measures of success

In the adult population, the initial gradient across the coarctation may not reflect its severity as there may be extensive collateral vessels decompressing the aorta proximal to the stenosis. Resolution of hypertension cannot necessarily be used as a measure of efficacy because the incidence of hypertension may be masked by antihypertensive treatment. Some adult patients without residual stenosis at the coarctation site will continue to be hypertensive.[48–51] However, their blood pressure control may become easier

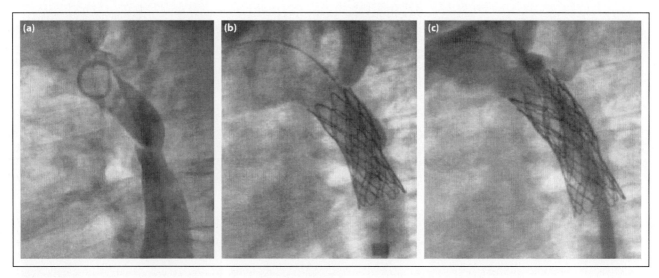

Figure 85.4 (a) An unusual native aortic coarctation with a small duct ampulla and moderate distal arch/isthmic hypoplasia. (b) After implantation of a Cheatham-Platinum (C-P) stent, there is evidence of a small aneurysm posteriorly related to upper edge of the stent. (c) Angiogram after implantation of an overlapping covered C-P stent showing exclusion of the small aneurysm.

after stenting. Stenting appears to be effective in reducing resting blood pressure to normal levels in the majority of children and adults.[32,48–52] There is no information on how stenting affects exercise tolerance or how well the stented coarctation segment responds to the increased cardiac output in pregnancy. However, some studies have shown that up to one-third of patients continue to have an abnormal blood pressure response to exercise and so will continue to need antihypertensive treatment.[28–30]

Staged dilation

Aortic rupture, although rare, is well documented after balloon angioplasty.[53,54] The risk of pseudoaneurysm formation after balloon angioplasty may be associated with overdilation.[55] Although stenting avoids overdilation, there may still be insufficient vascular tissue to stretch to a normal aortic diameter when the coarctation is tight. There is, therefore, a risk of rupture and aneurysm formation when a severely stenotic coarctation is stretched to the diameter of the adjacent vessel. Staged dilation, where expanding stents to a diameter less than the adjacent aorta and redilating a few months later may overcome the possible risks of disruption. A controlled injury is allowed time to heal and the arterial wall to remodel before full expansion is attempted. However, even with this approach, aneurysm formation may not be avoidable.

Aneurysm formation after stenting

The incidence of aneurysms following bare-metal stenting is low.[32,33,37,38,40–42] It is possible that medial injury from compression by the stent struts or intimal and medial tears at the time of stent implantation create a substrate for late aneurysm formation. Several reports describe cases of aneurysm formation.[33,34,37,38,43,44] Predilation may be a risk factor for subsequent aneurysm formation.[40,41] If aneurysm occurs after redilation of a previously implanted stent, this can now easily be treated with a covered stent, as can any aneurysms (Figure 85.5a,b). More and more operators now implant covered stents as the primary procedure for coarctation of the aorta, rather than saving these for complications for bare-metal stenting.

Allowance for growth/redilation

If stents are implanted in smaller patients, somatic growth of the patient will require redilation and so it is best to avoid stenting in infants and smaller children, unless it is unavoidable.[25,26] In this age group, stenting should be reserved for exceptional clinical indications rather

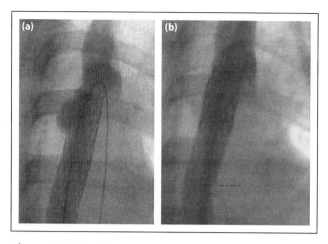

Figure 85.5   (a) An angiogram showing an aneurysm after redilation of a previously implanted Palmaz stent. (b) This was treated by implantation of an overlapping covered C-P stent.

than routine use because excellent surgical results can be obtained with extended arch repair.

Covered stents

Covered stents have almost replaced bare-metal stents in the treatment of aortic coarctation in adults. Although covered stents should prevent formation of aneurysms, there is some concern that they may occlude aortic side branches to the spinal cord and therefore carry a risk of paraplegia. However, arterial supply to the spinal cord usually originates below the aortic isthmus in the region of T9–T12 vertebrae and so in the usual location of aortic coarctation, there should not be any incidence of paraplegia. Indeed, this was the case in two recent small series after stent-graft insertion.[56,57] However, a larger series reported a 3.6% paraplegia rate after stent grafting,[58] suggesting that there is a small but significant risk. This is supported by data from surgical series in which the risk of paraplegia from surgery has been reported to be under 1% for procedures at the upper end of the aorta, but over 10% for procedures in the midportion of the aorta just above the diaphragm.[59] Nevertheless, stent grafts have now established an important role in the treatment of thoracic aortic aneurysms.[60]

Covered stents to treat aortic coarctation are being used predominantly in adults, but they have been rarely used in children.[61,62] The recent introduction of the C-P stent is an example of an ePTFE covered stent in the early phase of clinical trials and is now becoming an important part of the stock of catheter laboratories (Figure 85.1e).[42–44] Another covered stent that has also been used for similar indications is Advanta V12 stent (Atrium) (Figure 85.1f).[63] These may be indicated in adults with very tight aortic coarctation, in atretic or subatretic coarctation, in complex tortuous coarctation, with hypoplasia of the isthmus, or when there is an aneurysm, either native or after previous

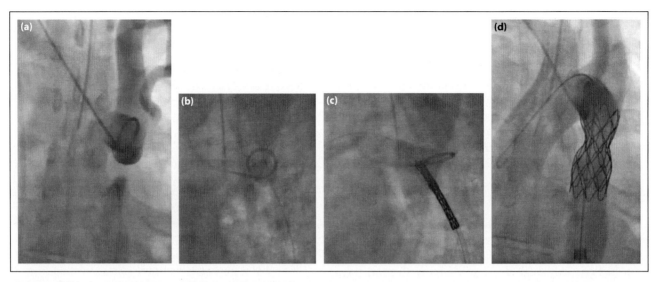

Figure 85.6 (a) Simultaneous aortogram in the distal arch and descending aorta in antero-posterior projection in an adult showing complete interruption at the site of coarctation. (b) Left anterior oblique projection showing a radio-frequency guide wire passed from descending aorta into the transverse aortic arch. (c) Positioning of a covered Cheatham-Platinum stent at the site of the interruption. (d) Arch aortogram in the antero-posterior projection showing an excellent result of covered stent implantation.

balloon dilation or surgery or after redilation of a previously implanted stent. It may rarely be indicated when there is a native coarctation associated with a patent arterial duct in an adolescent or an adult, (Figures 85.4 and 85.5).[64-67]

Covered stents can be implanted using the same technique as described above for the bare stents. A Mullins sheath of 1–2 Fr larger than that needed for implantation of a bare stent is used. A short covering sheath is important to allow introduction of the covered stent through the diaphragm of the Mullins sheath, otherwise the covering may be stripped off from the stent if it is introduced without a protective covering. Experience with stent grafts for thoracic aortic aneurysms suggests that the origin of the left subclavian artery can be covered with a covered stent to treat coarctation without any ill effects, although it is best avoided.[60,64] However, it is important to avoid covering the origins of the left common carotid artery. If needed, blood flow can be restored by perforation of the stent covering, if it has covered the origin.[68]

Occasionally complete interruption of the aorta may be encountered in adult patients. These present particular challenges in the interventional treatment. Covered stents are then essential. On some occasions, a fine 0.014 inch coronary guide wire may be negotiated slowly through the interruption via radial artery access, following which an arterioarterial guide wire circuit can be established. A covered stent is implanted in a similar method to that described earlier. However, if there is a long segment interruption, either a stiff end of a coronary guide wire or 0.018 inch radio-frequency may be used to perforate from below into the distal aortic arch from above into the descending aorta. Once perforated, angiogram checks are performed to ensure that the guide wire is in the aorta, after which

a circuit is established and a covered stent is implanted (Figure 85.6a–d).

Stenting for transverse aortic arch/isthmic hypoplasia

While the most common indication for stenting is discrete aortic coarctation, there are some patients in whom there is a residual gradient because of associated transverse arch or isthmic hypoplasia. Indeed, it has been shown that the aortic arch anatomy (in particular transverse and distal arch hypoplasia) plays an important role in a less than optimal result such as risk of recoarctation or residual coarctation.[35,69,70-72] There may also be occasional patients in whom the coarctation is diffuse and located in the transverse arch (Figure 85.7a–c). Treatment for these patients is difficult. The surgical treatment option for transverse arch hypoplasia is to perform an extended arch repair, which frequently requires cardiopulmonary bypass and is not without risk. It is easier in the neonate rather than adults. Thus, if such lesions can be treated in the adult patients with nonsurgical means, such as by using a stent, then clearly there are benefits for the patient. A small series of patients, in whom transverse arch stenting has been performed with good results, has been reported in the literature.[71,72] A considerable amount of information can be obtained about the anatomy and the diameters of the aortic arch by magnetic resonance imaging prior to the interventional procedure.

The technique of stent implantation is similar to that described above for conventional implantation of a stent in aortic coarctation. An ascending angiogram is performed in the left lateral and either left anterior oblique or a right

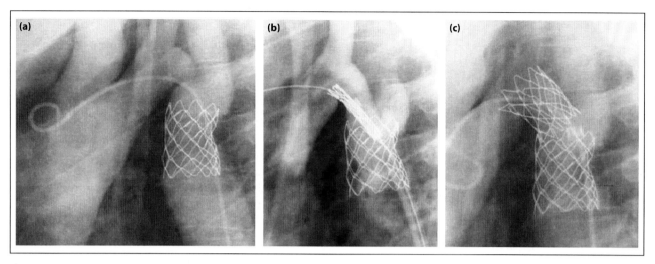

Figure 85.7   (a) An angiogram of an unusual native aortic coarctation. The usual typical coarctation site has been treated with a bare C-P stent just distal to the origin of the left subclavian artery. There is additional severe transverse arch hypoplasia between the origins of the left common carotid and left subclavian arteries with a tortuous aorta. (b) A further bare C-P stent is positioned in the transverse aortic arch. (c) Angiogram after full inflation of the bare C-P stent showing a good result. The residual gradient was abolished.

anterior oblique projection, with the aim of defining the arch anatomy as well as the origins of the innominate, the left common carotid, and the left subclavian arteries. Accurate measurements of the aortic arch at different locations are crucial in the decision making. The largest diameter of the aortic arch (usually just beyond the left carotid artery or between the innominate artery and the left common carotid artery) is used as a guide for the selection of the stent and the balloon. The distance between the origins of these vessels is also measured and this helps in the selection of an appropriate-length stent. The balloon needs to be 1–2 mm larger than the largest diameter of the aortic arch and the stent needs to be about 3–5 mm longer than the distance between the origins of the vessels where the aorta is to be stented. The size of the Mullins sheath is determined by the diameter and the type of the balloon on which the stent is to be mounted. The sheath should be at least 2 Fr larger than that needed to introduce the balloon alone in order to allow the stent to pass through it when mounted on the same balloon. It is preferable to use open-cell, bare-metal stents in the transverse arch, as the main risk is covering the origin of the head and neck vessels, in particular the left common carotid artery. If this were to happen, then a catheter and guide wire can be passed through the open cell of the stent and balloon dilation performed to make the cell round so that there is no metal across the origin of the vessel.[68] Stents such as LD Mega or LD Max or Andrastents are preferred because of their open-cell design. Rapid right ventricular pacing is essential during the placement of the stent, as it is possible to displace the stent/balloon assembly distally during inflation of the balloon, because of a relatively large stroke volume in an adult patient and because of the relatively mild narrowing.

The stiff Amplatz exchange length guide wire is positioned in the ascending aorta. Once the Mullins sheath is in place across the hypoplastic arch, the stent/balloon assembly is passed through this (using a short covering sheath during passage through the diaphragm of the Mullins sheath) until it is at the tip of the sheath. Frequent angiograms are performed through the side arm of the Mullins sheath to check for accurate positioning of the stent. In case of hypoplasia of the arch between the left common carotid artery and the left subclavian artery (the most frequently encountered lesion), the stent is positioned such that only about 2–3 mm of the stent is protruding across the origin of the left carotid artery. On balloon inflation, the stent will tend to shorten and so will be clear of the origin of the carotid artery. Stent struts covering the origin of the left subclavian artery are not of concern (Figure 85.8a–d). Even if the origin of the left carotid artery is covered, the open cell can be opened with a further balloon (Figure 85.9a–d). The Mullins sheath is withdrawn while keeping the stent/balloon assembly in position so as to expose the stent. After accurate positioning has been checked, rapid right ventricular pacing is initiated and the balloon is inflated rapidly to a pressure recommended by the manufacturer so as to deploy the stent. After full inflation is achieved, pacing is terminated and gradually the balloon is deflated and gently withdrawn back into the Mullins sheath. As a further precaution, a BIB balloon is used for gradual and accurate placement of the stent. An angiogram is repeated either through the Mullins sheath or through a pigtail catheter advanced over the guide wire into the ascending aorta. The pigtail catheter is withdrawn over the guide wire and an end-hole multipurpose catheter is advanced over the wire in order to remove the guide wire from the ascending

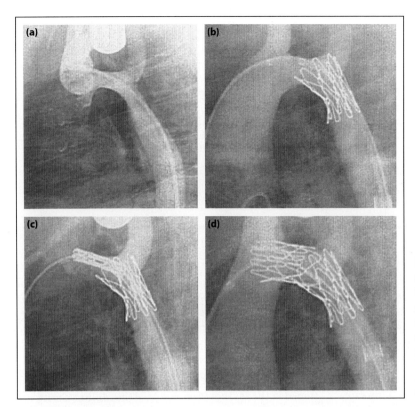

Figure 85.8 (a) An angiogram of a post-surgical aortic recoarctation combined with transverse arch hypoplasia (between the left common carotid artery and the innominate artery). (b) A bare C-P stent has been implanted across the recoarctation site. (c) A further C-P stent positioned in the transverse aortic arch. (d) After inflation of the stent, angiogram showing a good result. A few millimeters of the stent protrude into the origin of the left common carotid artery.

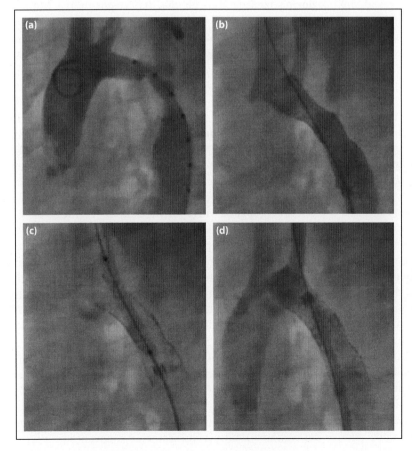

Figure 85.9 (a) An ascending aortogram in left anterior oblique projection, showing a complex recoarctation combined with distal arch hypoplasia. (b) Two overlapping open-cell stents (LD Max) have been implanted to treat the complex coarctation. The origin of the left common carotid artery is covered by the proximal stent. (c) A guide wire is passed through an open cell of the stent into the left common carotid artery and a balloon is passed over the guide wire to open the cell such that it is round. (d) Finally, an aortogram showed a good result with patent left common carotid artery. (Courtesy of Dr. Alan Magee, London, UK.)

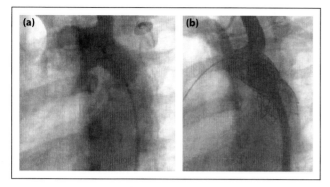

Figure 85.10   (a) An angiogram showing arch hypoplasia distal to the left common carotid artery—treated with a covered C-P stent. (b) The diameter of the stent matches the aorta proximal to the left common carotid artery.

aorta and then to measure the pressure gradient across the stented vessel. If a covered stent is used, then it can be inflated to its full size without too much concern about dissection (Figure 85.10a,b).

Conclusions

Stents are an important advancement in the treatment of aortic coarctation. Their use should be limited to older children, preferably more than 10 years old, and adults. While stents can be used to treat localized aortic coarctation, they are also indicated in adolescents and adults with long segment coarctation, or when there is associated hypoplasia of the isthmus or transverse arch, or in a tortuous aortic coarctation, in recoarctation after previous balloon or surgery, or when an aneurysm has developed after previous treatment. With any form of treatment for aortic coarctation, there is a small incidence of aneurysm formation that is inevitable in all forms of treatment. However, most of these complications can be treated with covered stents, which are gradually becoming the treatment of choice in adolescents and adults.

References

1. Campbell M. Natural history of coarctation of the aorta. *Br Heart J* 1970;32:633–40.
2. Hoimyr H, Christensen TD, Emmertsen K. Surgical repair of coarctation of the aorta: Up to 40 years of follow-up. *Eur J Cardiothorac Surg* 2006;30:910–6.
3. English KM. Stenting the mildly obstructive aortic arch: Useful treatment or oculo-inflatory reflex? *Heart* 2006;92:1541–3.
4. Singer MI, Rowen M, Dorsey TJ. Transluminal aortic balloon angioplasty for coarctation of the aorta in the newborn. *Am Heart J* 1982;103:131–2.
5. Ho SY, Somerville J, Yip WC et al. Transluminal balloon dilation of resected coarcted segments of thoracic aorta: Histological study and clinical implications. *Int J Cardiol* 1988;19:99–105.
6. Lock JE, Castaneda-Zuniga WR, Bass JL et al. Balloon dilatation of excised aortic coarctations. *Radiology* 1982;143:689–91.
7. Ino T, Kishiro M, Okubo M et al. Dilatation mechanism of balloon angioplasty in children: Assessment by angiography and intravascular ultrasound. *Cardiovasc Intervent Radiol* 1998;21:102–8.
8. Rothman A, Ricou F, Weintraub RG et al. Intraluminal ultrasound imaging through a balloon dilation catheter in an animal model of coarctation of the aorta. *Circulation* 1992;85:2291–5.
9. Sohn S, Rothman A, Shiota T et al. Acute and follow-up intravascular ultrasound findings after balloon dilation of coarctation of the aorta. *Circulation* 1994;90:340–7.
10. Ino T, Ohkubo M. Dilation mechanism, causes of restenosis and stenting in balloon coarctation angioplasty. *Acta Paediatr* 1997; 86:367–71.
11. Brandt Bd, Marvin WJ, Jr., Rose EF et al. Surgical treatment of coarctation of the aorta after balloon angioplasty. *J Thorac Cardiovasc Surg* 1987;94:715–9.
12. Isner JM, Donaldson RF, Fulton D et al. Cystic medial necrosis in coarctation of the aorta: A potential factor contributing to adverse consequences observed after percutaneous balloon angioplasty of coarctation sites. *Circulation* 1987;75:689–95.
13. De Lezo JS, Sancho M, Pan M et al. Angiographic follow-up after balloon angioplasty for coarctation of the aorta. *J Am Coll Cardiol* 1989;13:689–95.
14. Shaddy RE, Boucek MM, Sturtevant JE et al. Comparison of angioplasty and surgery for unoperated coarctation of the aorta [see comments]. *Circulation* 1993;87:793–9.
15. Rao PS, Galal O, Smith PA et al. Five- to nine-year follow-up results of balloon angioplasty of native aortic coarctation in infants and children. *J Am Coll Cardiol* 1996;27:462–70.
16. Fletcher SE, Nihill MR, Grifka RG et al. Balloon angioplasty of native coarctation of the aorta: Midterm follow-up and prognostic factors. *J Am Coll Cardiol* 1995;25:730–4.
17. O'Laughlin MP, Perry SB, Lock JE et al. Use of endovascular stents in congenital heart disease. *Circulation* 1991;83:1923–39.
18. Trent MS, Parsonnet V, Shoenfeld R et al. A balloon-expandable intravascular stent for obliterating experimental aortic dissection. *J Vasc Surg* 1990;11:707–17.
19. Ohkubo M, Takahashi K, Kishiro M et al. Histological findings after angioplasty using conventional balloon, radiofrequency thermal balloon and stent for experimental aortic coarctation. *Pediatr Int* 2004;46:39–47.
20. Rosenthal E, Qureshi SA, Tynan M. Stent implantation for aortic recoarctation. *Am Heart J* 1995;129:1220–1.
21. Qureshi SA. Use of covered stents to treat coarctation of the aorta. *Korean Circ J* 2009; 39:261–3.
22. Lee HY, Reddy SC, Rao PS. Evaluation of superficial femoral artery compromise and limb growth retardation after transfemoral artery balloon dilatations. *Circulation* 1997;95:974–80.
23. Burrows PE, Benson LN, Babyn P et al. Magnetic resonance imaging of the iliofemoral arteries after balloon dilation angioplasty of aortic arch obstructions in children. *Circulation* 1994;90:915–20.
24. Bjarnason H, Hunter DW, Ferral H et al. Placement of the Palmaz stent with use of an 8-F introducer sheath and Olbert balloons. *J Vasc Interv Radiol* 1993;4:435–9.
25. Bouzguenda I, Marini D, Ou P, Boudjemline Y, Bonnet D, Agnoletti G. Percutaneous treatment of neonatal aortic coarctation presenting with severe left ventricular dysfunction as a bridge to surgery. *Cardiol Young* 2009;19:244–51.
26. Mohan UR, Danon S, Levi D et al. Stent implantation for coarctation of the aorta in children <30 kg. *J Am Coll Cardiol Cardiovasc Interv* 2009;2:877–83.
27. Xu J, Shiota T, Omoto R et al. Intravascular ultrasound assessment of regional aortic wall stiffness, distensibility, and compliance in patients with coarctation of the aorta. *Am Heart J* 1997;134:93–8.

28. Eicken A, Pensl U, Sebening W et al. The fate of systemic blood pressure in patients after effectively stented coarctation. *Eur Heart J* 2006;27:1100–5.

29. Chen S, Donald A, Storry C et al. Impact of aortic stenting on peripheral vascular function and daytime systolic blood pressure in adult coarctation. *Heart.* 2008;94:919–24.

30. Oechslin E. Does a stent cure hypertension? *Heart.* 2008;94:828–9.

31. Suarez de Lezo J, Pan M, Romero M et al. Balloon-expandable stent repair of severe coarctation of aorta. *Am Heart J* 1995;129:1002–8.

32. Magee AG, Brzezinska-Rajszys G, Qureshi SA et al. Stent implantation for aortic coarctation and recoarctation. *Heart* 1999;82:600–6.

33. Thanopoulos BD, Hadjinikolaou L, Konstadopoulou GN et al. Stent treatment for coarctation of the aorta: Intermediate term follow up and technical considerations. *Heart* 2000;84:65–70.

34. Marshall AC, Perry SB, Keane JF et al. Early results and medium-term follow-up of stent implantation for mild residual or recurrent aortic coarctation. *Am Heart J* 2000;139:1054–60.

35. Pihkala J, Pedra CA, Nykanen D et al. Implantation of endovascular stents for hypoplasia of the transverse aortic arch. *Cardiol Young* 2000;10:3–7.

36. Brzezinska-Rajszys G, Qureshi SA, Ksiazyk J et al. Middle aortic syndrome treated by stent implantation. *Heart* 1999;81:166–70.

37. Suarez de Lezo J, Pan M, Romero M et al. Percutaneous interventions on severe coarctation of the aorta: A 21-year experience. *Pediatr Cardiol* 2005;26:176–89.

38. Harrison DA, McLaughlin PR, Lazzam C et al. Endovascular stents in the management of coarctation of the aorta in the adolescent and adult: one year follow up. *Heart* 2001;85:561–6.

39. Godart F. Intravascular stenting for the treatment of coarctation of the aorta in adolescent and adult patients. *Arch Cardiovasc Dis* 2011;104:627–35.

40. Forbes TJ, Garekar S, Amin Z et al. Procedural results and acute complications in stenting native and recurrent coarctation of the aorta in patients over 4 years of age: A multi-institutional study. *Catheter Cardiovasc Interv* 2007;70:276–85.

41. Forbes TJ, Moore P, Pedra CA et al. Intermediate follow-up following intravascular stenting for treatment of coarctation of the aorta. *Catheter Cardiovasc Interv* 2007;70:569–77.

42. Qureshi AM, McElhinney DB, Lock JE et al. Acute and intermediate outcomes, and evaluation of injury to the aortic wall, as based on 15 years' experience of implanting stents to treat aortic coarctation *Cardiol Young* 2007;17:307–18

43. Mahadevan VS, Vondermuhll IF, Mullen MJ. Endovascular aortic coarctation stenting in adolescents and adults: Angiographic and haemodynamic outcomes. *Catheter Cardiovasc Interv* 2006;67:268–75.

44. Holzer R, Qureshi S, Ghasemi A et al. Stenting of aortic coarctation: Acute, intermediate, and long-term results of a prospective multi-institutional registry—Congenital cardiovascular interventional study consortium (CCISC). *Catheter Cardiovasc Interv* 2010;76:553–63.

45. Derham C, Davies JF, Shahbazi R et al. Iatrogenic limb ischemia caused by angiography closure devices. *Vasc Endovascular Surg* 2006;40:492–4.

46. Tzifa A, Ewert P, Brzezinska-Rajszys G et al. Covered Cheatham-platinum stents for aortic coarctation: Early and intermediate-term results. *J Am Coll Cardiol* 2006;47:1457–63.

47. Butera G, Piazza L, Chessa M et al. Covered stents in patients with complex aortic coarctations. *Am Heart J* 2007;154:795–800.

48. Kaemmerer H, Oelert F, Bahlmann J et al. Arterial hypertension in adults after surgical treatment of aortic coarctation. *Thorac Cardiovasc Surg* 1998;46:121–5.

49. Gunthard J, Buser PT, Miettunen R et al. Effects of morphologic restenosis, defined by MRI after coarctation repair, on blood pressure and arm-leg and Doppler gradients. *Angiology* 1996;47:1073–80.

50. Guenthard J, Zumsteg U, Wyler F. Arm-leg pressure gradients on late follow-up after coarctation repair. Possible causes and implications. *Eur Heart J* 1996;17:1572–5.

51. Gardiner HM, Celermajer DS, Sorensen KE et al. Arterial reactivity is significantly impaired in normotensive young adults after successful repair of aortic coarctation in childhood. *Circulation* 1994;89:1745–50.

52. Bulbul ZR, Bruckheimer E, Love JC et al. Implantation of balloon-expandable stents for coarctation of the aorta: Implantation data and short-term results. *Cathet Cardiovasc Diagn* 1996;39:36–42.

53. Balaji S, Oommen R, Rees PG. Fatal aortic rupture during balloon dilatation of recoarctation. *Br Heart J* 1991;65:100–1.

54. Rao PS. Aortic rupture after balloon angioplasty of aortic coarctation. *Am Heart J* 1993;125:1205–6.

55. Fletcher SE, Cheatham JP, Froeming S. Aortic aneurysm following primary balloon angioplasty and secondary endovascular stent placement in the treatment of native coarctation of the aorta. *Cathet Cardiovasc Diagn* 1998;44:40–4.

56. Kato N, Dake MD, Miller DC et al. Traumatic thoracic aortic aneurysm: Treatment with endovascular stent-grafts. *Radiology* 1997;205:657–62.

57. Rousseau H, Soula P, Perreault P et al. Delayed treatment of traumatic rupture of the thoracic aorta with endoluminal covered stent. *Circulation* 1999;99:498–504.

58. Mitchell RS, Miller DC, Dake MD. Stent-graft repair of thoracic aortic aneurysms. *Semin Vasc Surg* 1997;10:257–71.

59. Connolly JE. Hume Memorial lecture. Prevention of spinal cord complications in aortic surgery. *Am J Surg* 1998;176:92–101.

60. Taylor PR, Gaines PA, McGuinness CL, Beard JD, Cooper G, Reidy JF. Thoracic aortic stent grafts—early experience from two centers using commercially available devices. *Eur J Vasc Endovasc Surg* 2001;22:70–6.

61. Gunn J, Cleveland T, Gaines P. Covered stent to treat co-existent coarctation and aneurysm of the aorta in a young man. *Heart* 1999;82:351.

62. Khan MS, Moore JW. Treatment of abdominal aortic pseudoaneurysm with covered stents in a paediatric patient. *Cathet Cardiovasc Intervent* 2000;50:445–48.

63. Bruckheimer E, Birk E, Santiago R, Dagan T, Esteves C, Pedra CAC. Coarctation of the aorta treated with the Advanta V12 large diameter stent: Acute results. *Catheter Cardiovasc Interv* 2010;75:402–6.

64. Qureshi SA, Zubrzycka M, Brzezinska-Rajszys G, Kosciesza A, Ksiazyk J. Use of covered Cheatham-Platinum stents in aortic coarctation and recoarctation. *Cardiol Young* 2004;14:50–54.

65. Ewert P, Abdul-Khalid H, Peters B, Nagdyman N, Schubert S, Lange PE. Transcatheter therapy of long extreme subatretic aortic coarctations with covered stents. *Catheter Cardiovasc Interv* 2004;63:236–9.

66. Forbes T, Matisoff D, Dysart J et al. Treatment of coexisting coarctation and aneurysm of the aorta with covered stent in a pediatric patient. *Pediatr Cardiol* 2003;24:289–91.

67. Sadiq M, Malick NH, Qureshi SA. Simultaneous treatment of native coarctation of the aorta combined with patent ductus arteriosus using a covered stent. *Catheter Cardiovasc Interv* 2003;59:387–90.

68. Tsai S, Hill S and Cheatham J. Treatment of aortic arch aneurysm with a NuMed-covered stent and restoration of flow to excluded left subclavian artery: Perforation and dilation of e-PTFE can be done! *Catheter Cardiovasc Interv* 2009;73:385–9.

69. Kaine SF, Smith EO, Mott AR et al. Quantitative echocardiographic analysis of the aortic arch predicts outcome of balloon angioplasty of native coarctation of the aorta. *Circulation* 1996;94:1056–62.

70. Walhout RJ, Lekkerkerker JC, Ernst SM, Hutter PA, Plokker TH, Meijboom EJ. Angioplasty for coarctation in different aged patients. *Am Heart J* 2002;144:180–6.

71. Boshoff D, Budts W, Mertens L et al. Stenting of hypoplastic aortic segments with mild pressure gradients and arterial hypertension. *Heart* 2006;92:1661–6.

72. Pushparajah K, Sadiq M, Brzezińska-Rajszys G, Thomson J, Rosenthal E, Qureshi SA. Endovascular stenting in transverse aortic arch hypoplasia. *Catheter Cardiovasc Interv* 2013;82:E491–E499.

86

Middle aortic syndrome

Grazyna Brzezinska-Rajszys and Shakeel A. Qureshi

Middle aortic syndrome (MAS), also known as abdominal coarctation, or midaortic dysplastic syndrome, and first described in 1963,[1] is an uncommon cause of arterial hypertension in children and young adults. It is characterized by segmental narrowing of the distal thoracic and/or abdominal aorta (Figure 86.1).[2-7] It accounts for 0.5–2% of cases of coarctation of the aorta. Stenosis of the aorta may be associated with stenoses of aortic side branches, mostly renal and visceral arteries (Figure 86.2).

The exact etiology of MAS remains unknown, but most often it is acquired, caused by nonspecific inflammatory arteritis, or Takayasu's disease, fibromuscular dysplasia, retroperitoneal fibrosis, radiation-induced arterial fibrosis, or a congenital disease (developmental anomaly in the fusion and maturation of the paired embryonic dorsal aortas). MAS may occur in association with neurofibromatosis, Alagille syndrome, and Williams syndrome.[2,3,5,7-13]

Stenosis of the aorta causes upper limb hypertension. Additionally, reduction of perfusion to one or both kidneys causes severe renovascular hypertension. MAS is considered to be life-threatening as a result of the complications associated with severe hypertension. The prognosis in untreated patients is poor, with death usually occurring in the fourth decade.

Whatever the etiology of MAS, assuming that active aortic inflammation has been medically treated and is in a burnt-out state, patients with aortic narrowing, who have clinical symptoms such as severe arterial hypertension, lower extremity claudication, or mesenteric ischemia, will need revascularization treatment.[2-4,13,14]

Depending on the experience of the center and the anatomical forms of MAS, several management strategies are used. Surgery is widely accepted, especially in older patients and in complex MAS associated with renal and visceral arterial stenosis.[2,3,6-8,15-18] The type of surgery may involve thoracoabdominal to infrarenal aortic bypass, with renal artery reimplantation, splenorenal bypass, aortorenal bypass, and autotransplantation. In children, surgical bypass using conduits is difficult and complex and the tube graft may need to be replaced at a later date.[5,7,8,13,17]

Experience over the last decade has shown that MAS can be treated with percutaneous techniques, such as either balloon angioplasty or stent implantation, depending on the anatomy and the age of the patient.[12,19-30]

The mechanism of relief of narrowing after balloon dilation is similar to that of dilation of aortic coarctation and so intimal tears may be seen on intravascular ultrasound.[19] Percutaneous transluminal balloon angioplasty is reported to be effective in relieving short-segment stenosis (<3 cm) of the aorta due to aortic arteritis in children,[14,20,21] but the results may be unpredictable and unsatisfactory in other forms of MAS. Stent implantation for long segment lesions or after unsuccessful angioplasty of the aorta, in which there may be incomplete relief of stenosis or dissection, is associated with good early and immediate results (Figure 86.3). Indeed in some centers, it may be the primary therapy of MAS.[20,23-26] As the risk of dissection, aneurysm, and

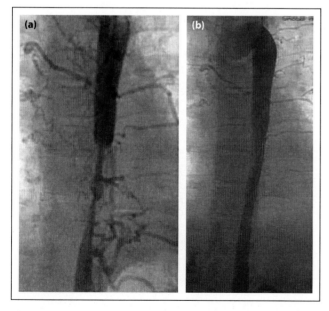

Figure 86.1 A patient with middle aortic syndrome demonstrating narrowing of the distal thoracic aorta before (a) and after (b) stent implantation.

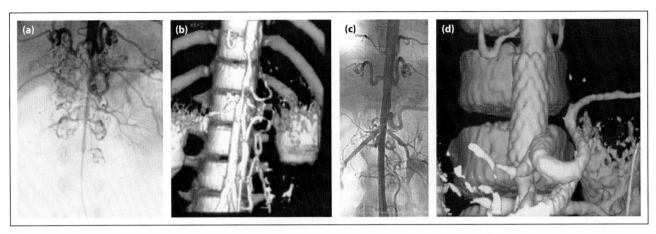

Figure 86.2 A patient with middle aortic syndrome demonstrating narrowing of the abdominal aorta associated with stenoses of renal and visceral arteries. Angiography (a) and computed tomography angiography (3D reconstruction) (b) before treatment. Angiography (c) and computed tomography angiography (3D reconstruction) (d) after stent implantation into aorta.

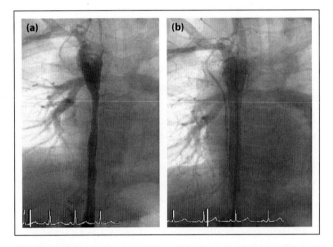

Figure 86.3 A patient with ventricular septal defect with pulmonary atresia after two Blalock-Taussig shunts with severe long segment stenosis of thoracic aorta. Aortography 1 year after two balloon angioplasties (a). Aortography after implantation of two stents into aorta (b).

rupture of aorta exists with this type of treatment, covered stents for bailout purposes should be available. In some patients covered stents may be used as primary therapy. In carefully selected cases of severe aortic narrowing in very small children, cutting balloons have been used.[31]

In complex forms of MAS, for example those associated with additional renal artery stenosis, dilation of the aorta should be combined with the treatment of renal artery stenosis. In patients with discrete renal artery stenosis, balloon angioplasty of the stenotic renal arteries is highly effective, but in diffuse stenosis, renal autotransplantation may be associated with better results (Figure 86.4).[14,27,30] Besides the good immediate results of treatment, progression of the arterial occlusive process may occur afterward, so careful follow-up of patients with MAS is mandatory.[11,12,28]

The report of using a tissue expander to induce longitudinal growth of the normal distal abdominal aorta and iliac arteries in child with the midaortic syndrome is a new concept, which may allow autologous arterial replacement.[32]

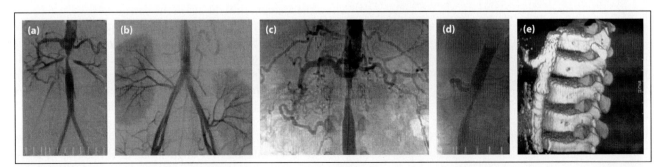

Figure 86.4 A patient with middle aortic syndrome showing narrowing of the abdominal aorta and diffuse stenosis of both renal arteries, angiography before treatment (a). Angiography after renal autotransplantation. Both renal arteries transplanted to iliac arteries (b). Severe stenosis of abdominal aorta (c) and celiac artery (d). Computed tomography angiography 3 years after stent implantation into aorta and celiac artery (e).

Pre-intervention imaging

The site and type of obstruction of the aorta and additional arterial stenosis can be shown in detail by magnetic resonance imaging (MRI), computed tomography (CT), or aortography.

MRI and CT accurately illustrate the site and extent of the obstruction of the aorta, and also the involvement of its branches and collaterals. Analysis of MRI or CT angiography may reduce the need for angiography in the planning of the required treatment. Angiography should be reserved for interventional treatment rather than for diagnostic purposes.

Breath-hold gadolinium-enhanced MRA and contrast-enhanced CT angiography demonstrate thickening of the arterial wall with crescents and indistinct outlines typical for acute phase of arteritis, which can be demonstrated as the vessel wall hypermetabolism on positron emission tomography. It may be important for the timing of interventions.[33–36]

Modern spiral and multidetector CT, which can be used for rapid imaging of large scan volumes using thin-section collimation, is useful for the evaluation of the arterial system, without anesthesia even in small children (Figure 86.5).

Ultrasonography usually demonstrates vascular stenoses in the accessible areas, and their location may help in diagnosing MAS, but ultrasonography is mostly important for the follow-up assessment of the results of interventions.

The technique of interventional therapy (balloon angioplasty and stent implantation in aorta)

Dilation of the aorta should be performed under sedation or general anesthesia, depending on the experience of the center and the age of the patient. The standard access is by femoral arterial percutaneous puncture. In small children, surgical cutdown onto the iliac artery or carotid artery may be needed. In complex MAS, femoral artery access is used also for dilation of the renal and celiac arteries. The brachial artery approach may be helpful in some cases. The vascular access depends on the anatomy of the stenosed vessels and should facilitate the intervention.

Heparin is administered intravenously, a dose of 100 IU/kg, with a maximum of 5000 units given and repeated as needed to maintain the activated clotted times (ACT) above 200 s during the procedure.

Immediately prior to the intervention, the diagnostic procedure consists of obtaining hemodynamic and angiographic data. From the femoral arterial approach, a multipurpose catheter is used to cross the stenosis in the aorta with the help of a guide wire, which is positioned in a stable position across the stenosis and located in the ascending or descending thoracic aorta, depending on the location of the narrowing. A J-curve guide wire may be helpful to avoid entering the collateral arteries. An angiographic catheter, such as a pigtail or multipurpose or Multi-Track catheter (NuMED, Hopkinton, NY, USA), is introduced over the guide wire into the aorta above the stenosis. The advantage of using the Multi-Track catheter is that the guide wire position can be maintained while repeated pullback measurements and angiography are performed. Hemodynamic measurements are recorded with the aortic pressures in the ascending and descending aorta and the gradient is obtained. Aortography in antero-posterior and lateral projections, and in complex cases in left anterior oblique or right anterior oblique projections, are performed using any of the previously mentioned angiographic catheters. The projection is variable and depends on the anatomy. It should be planned after considering CT, MRI, or rotational angiography pictures.

Measurements of the anatomical details are performed. The measurements, which are needed to determine the size of the balloon, should be accurate, as errors in the measurements may lead to complications.

These include the minimum diameter of the stenotic aorta and the diameter above and below the stenosis. In patients in whom there are coexisting additional stenoses of the aortic branches (e.g., renal or celiac arteries),

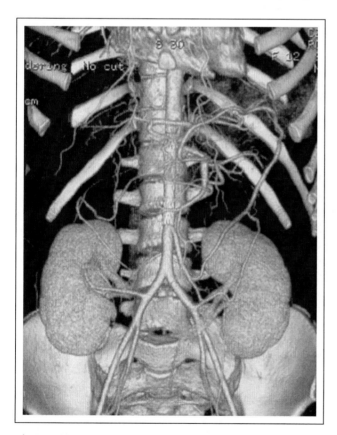

Figure 86.5 Computed tomography (3D reconstruction). Middle aortic syndrome after renal autotransplantation and stent implantation into aorta.

measurements of these vessels, with minimum diameter of the stenosis and the diameter of the normal vessel, should be performed. A stiff exchange length guide wire (such as an Amplatz wire) is positioned across the stenosis with the soft J-curve in the ascending or in the thoracic aorta, depending on the anatomy.

Balloon angioplasty of MAS

Balloon angioplasty of MAS is based on the same rules as balloon angioplasty of coarctation of the aorta. Low-pressure balloon catheters such as Tyshak balloons (NuMED) may be effective in discrete stenoses and in younger children, but high-pressure balloons are usually more effective. The balloon diameter should not exceed the diameter of the aorta above the stenosis and also should not exceed three times the diameter of the stenosis. The guide wire lumen of the balloon catheter is flushed and air is also removed from the balloon with a syringe by creating a vacuum. Over the wire, the angiography catheter is exchanged for the balloon catheter. A correct-sized sheath, according to the recommendation of balloon catheter manufacturer, should be introduced into the artery. The side port of the sheath should be connected to the pressure-monitoring system for the immediate assessment of hemodynamic result. The balloon catheter is placed at the level of the stenosis. The balloon is inflated with diluted contrast material (25% contrast + 75% saline). An inflation device is useful to control and monitor the balloon pressure, but manual inflation may be performed in low-pressure balloons. This choice depends on the experience of the individual operator. Appearance of a waist on the balloon indicates the site of stenosis. The balloon is inflated until the waist caused by the stenosis disappears. The balloon is kept inflated for approximately 10–30 s, after which it is deflated as quickly as possible. Additional inflations may be required if the balloon slips during inflation or the waist has not been completely abolished. Occasionally, rapid right ventricular pacing may be useful for stabilization of the balloon position during inflation, in particular in older patients. After dilation, the contrast material is removed from the balloon, which is then withdrawn through the sheath. Continuous negative pressure applied on the balloon lumen should diminish its profile and allow for easy withdrawal. The wire position should be maintained and a Multi-Track catheter inserted over the wire into the aorta above the area of dilation. It is important to avoid manipulation of the tip of the catheter or guide wire in the dilated area and avoid losing guide wire position and avoid trying to recross the recently dilated lesion.

Final aortography is performed in the same projections as before balloon dilation to check the anatomical result of dilation and the diameter of the stenosis as well as the hemodynamic measurements with pressures in the aorta. A reduction of the pressure gradient below 10 mmHg secondary to an increase in the diameter of aorta at the level of the stenosis constitutes a good result of the angioplasty.

Stent implantation in MAS

In patients with suboptimal reduction of the gradient, or those with long segment stenosis of the aorta, or those accepted for primary stent implantation into the aorta, the technique of implantation is very similar to that used in the typical coarctation of the aorta. After the diagnostic part of the procedure, consisting of hemodynamic and angiographic data acquisition, an appropriate sized balloon catheter and stent are selected. The selected balloon diameter should be similar to the diameter of the aorta above the stenosis. A long segment narrowing of the aorta may mimic serial vessel obstructions. Low-pressure balloon inflation may show a beady appearance with multiple waists due to the multiple stenoses. These waists can be a marker for precise placement of a stent. The length of the balloon should be similar to the length of the stent and certainly not shorter than the stent. The BIB ("balloon in balloon") catheter (NuMED) is preferable for stent implantation in the aorta, but other types of high-pressure balloons may also be used. Premounted or manually crimped stents can be used. Nowadays, stents used in this situation include the Palmaz, Palmaz Genesis (Johnson and Johnson Interventional Systems, Warren, NJ, USA), LD Max (EV3, Plymouth, MN, USA), Andrastent (Andramed, Reutlingen, Germany), or the Cheatham-Platinum stents (NuMED). In some situations, self-expanding stents have also been used (Figure 86.6). The choice of the stent depends on the technical properties of the stent and, in particular, the need for the stent to be dilatable to the diameter of the adult aorta. The guide wire lumen of the balloon catheter is flushed, and the air is removed from the balloon with a syringe by creating a vacuum. The BIB catheter preparation is similar, but the air should be removed from both the inner and outer balloons with syringes by creating a vacuum, after which both hubs are connected to the inflation devices. The appropriate stent is mounted on the balloon between the markers on the balloon catheters. If there is any uncertainty, the position of the stent on the balloon should be checked under fluoroscopy prior to the final crimping. The stent is crimped manually onto the balloon. An appropriate diameter and length sheath with a radiopaque marker at its tip (such as the Mullins sheath) is placed in the aorta. The sheath should be at least 1–2 French sizes larger than that recommended for the introduction of the balloon catheter. This usually depends on the type of the stent being used. The sheath and its dilator are flushed with saline and introduced over the guide wire and the sheath is placed across the stenosis with the marker above the stenosis. For insertion of the stent/balloon assembly

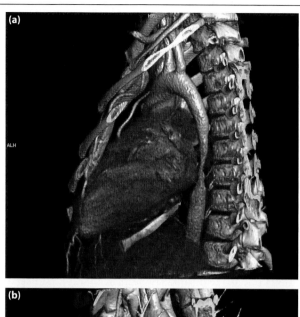

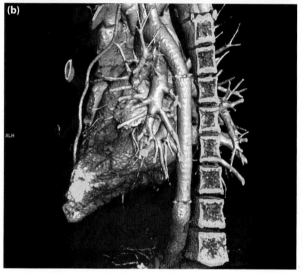

Figure 86.6 A patient with middle aortic syndrome showing narrowing of the thoracic aorta, computed tomography angiography before (a) and after self expandable stent implantation (b).

using the BIB balloon, initial inflation of the inner balloon is performed with the inflation device to reach the pressure recommended by the manufacturer. After inflation, the stopcock connected to the inner balloon should be closed and aortography performed through the long sheath or through a second catheter, if inserted, to check the position of the stent. If needed, the position of the stent may be adjusted at this stage. The outer balloon is then inflated with the inflation device also to reach the pressure recommended by the manufacturer. Full inflation of balloons should be maintained for approximately 10–30 s. The stent position should be checked under fluoroscopy during the balloon inflation. The inner balloon is deflated first, followed by the outer balloon. With continuous negative pressure applied on both balloons, the balloon catheter is carefully withdrawn under fluoroscopy. Occasionally, it is helpful to advance the sheath over the balloon while taking care not to push the stent upward. A Multi-Track catheter is inserted over the exchange wire into the aorta above the dilated area and aortography is repeated in the same projection as prior to stent implantation to assess the anatomical result of dilation and measure the diameter of the stent. Finally, the postprocedure pressures in the aorta with a pullback method are recorded. A reduction of pressure gradient below 10 mmHg and an increased diameter of the stented aorta at the level of stenosis is considered a good result of the procedure. After balloon angioplasty or stent implantation, aspirin at a dose of 3–5 mg/kg is given daily for 3–6 months and antihypertensive treatment is maintained or started.

Spiral CT or MRI assessment should be performed preferably before discharge, if there are any complications during the procedure or 1 year later if the procedure was uncomplicated. In complex forms of MAS with stenosis of the aorta coexisting with the stenosis of the renal and other branches of the abdominal aorta, interventional dilation of these should be considered. In discrete forms of renal artery stenosis, balloon angioplasty usually produces good results. In long segment renal artery stenosis, balloon angioplasty may be ineffective and the risks of damage of the arterial wall, spasm, dissection, and rupture are higher. In such cases, surgery should be considered. Celiac trunk stenosis or mesenteric artery stenosis can be treated with balloon angioplasty, but in some cases, stent implantation should be considered. In some variants, immediate implantation of stents into the aorta and its branches may be needed. In cases of aortic narrowing in the region of the renal orifices, balloon angioplasty of renal arteries should be the first step in the procedure followed by stent implantation in the aorta. It should be stressed that balloon angioplasty of renal arteries, especially their orifices, may be the origin of a dissection of aorta. Balloon angioplasty of the aorta with guide wires positioned in the renal arteries to protect their flow after tear of the aortic intima has been reported.

into the long sheath, a small piece of tubing of appropriate similar French size is prepared to cover the stent/balloon assembly. This will protect the stent against slipping off the balloon during its introduction through the diaphragm of the long sheath. The tubing may be the cut piece of a short sheath or the plastic or metal tube included in the stent package. The stent/balloon assembly is advanced through the sheath under fluoroscopic guidance and placed across the stenosis. Special care should be taken to maintain the guide wire position throughout the procedure. Once in position, the long sheath is withdrawn to completely uncover the stent/balloon assembly. Accurate positioning of the stent is checked with hand injections of contrast through the side port of the sheath. The balloon is inflated with diluted contrast (25% contrast + 75% saline). When

Complications

The main complications of balloon angioplasty of MAS relate to aortic wall damage. A small aortic dissection should be treated with additional prolonged balloon inflation maintained for approximately 1–2 min or even longer. If the repeat spiral CT or MRI scans show progress of the dissection, implantation of a bare or a covered stent should be performed. A large dissection should be treated with a bare or a covered stent implanted during the same procedure.[20]

Follow-up of a small aneurysm should be with repeat spiral CT or MRI scans. If necessary, when the diameter of the aneurysm increases or when there is an aneurysm, implantation of a bare or covered stent should be performed. A large or increasing aneurysm should be treated immediately with the implantation of a covered stent.

Aortic rupture is an indication for emergency surgery or implantation of a single or multiple covered stents.[37] Another complication is damage to the femoral artery, which should be treated with thrombolysis or surgical repair.

The main complications of stent implantation into the aorta in MAS are mostly related to stent migration and malposition, even though these are rare. Implantation of the migrated stent below or above the stenosis, depending on the anatomy, allows for the completion of the procedure. Migration of the stent to the ascending aorta has been reported and may be more difficult to treat. An expanded stent can be retrieved percutaneously, but this may be very difficult and requires a combination of snares, tip-deflectors, forceps, and large sheaths for retrieval. In some situations, surgery is recommended. Aortic wall complications are less frequent during stent implantation in MAS. In such situations, treatment is the same as discussed earlier.

During the follow-up period, restenosis of the stent may occur due to neointimal hyperplasia or growth of the patient. This can generally be treated successfully with balloon redilation.

Stent fracture may occur rarely in patients in whom the stent is only partially expanded. If this results in stent restenosis, a further stent or a covered stent is implanted.

Our experience

In the Children's Memorial Health Institute, Warsaw, 24 children (aged 3–17 years, mean 11.6) with severe arterial hypertension and a diagnosis of MAS, and resistant to multidrug therapy underwent interventional treatment. There were no inflammatory signs or symptoms suggesting Takayasu disease in the group.

Twenty-five had narrowing of the thoracic and/or abdominal aorta (length of the stenosis varied between 2 and 12 cm, minimum diameter 1.5–6 mm), and one

had aortic atresia below the origin of a stenosed left renal artery. Aortic narrowing was isolated in 12 patients and coexisted with renal, celiac, mesenteric artery stenosis in 13 patients. The aortic narrowing was treated in 25 with stent implantation (20 as primary treatment and 5 after previous balloon angioplasty). Additional interventional or surgical procedures were performed (renal arterial balloon angioplasty in 7 patients, renal artery autotransplantation in 4 patients, celiac artery balloon angioplasty in 5 patients, mesenteric artery balloon angioplasty in 3 patients, stent implantation in the celiac trunk in 1 patient, and heminephrectomy in 1 patient). Good hemodynamic and anatomical results of stent implantation with reduced gradient from mean 43 mmHg to mean 11 mmHg and increased diameter of the aorta from mean 3 mm to mean 9.8 mm was achieved. During mean 8.5 years follow-up, 8 patients had elective stent redilation, 6 successful redilations due to neointimal hyperplasia, and 2 had second stent implantation because of aneurysm formation, and progressive aortic narrowing in 1 patient. Balloon angioplasty of the aorta was performed in a complex form of MAS or in very young patients as a primary treatment, which improved the blood pressure control temporarily. The antihypertensive medication was continued in all the patients, but the dosage was reduced with improved control of the blood pressure during follow-up. Progression of vascular changes was observed in 4 patients, 3 of whom had neurofibromatosis.

Conclusion

MAS is an uncommon cause of arterial hypertension. Based on our experience, the interventional treatment of children with MAS is effective in early and midterm follow-up. Due to the complexity of the disease, combined interventional and surgical treatment may be necessary.

References

1. Sen PK, Kinare SG, Engineer SD et al. The middle aortic syndrome. *Br Heart J* 1963;25:610–8.
2. Graham LM, Zelenock GB, Erlandson EE et al. Abdominal aortic coarctation and segmental hypoplasia. *Surgery* 1979;86:519–29.
3. Lewis VDIII, Meranze SG, McLean GK et al. The midaortic syndrome: Diagnosis and treatment. *Radiology* 1988;167:111–3.
4. Poulias GE, Skoutas B, Doundoulakis E. The middle aortic dysplastic syndrome: Surgical considerations with a 2 to 18 year follow-up and selective histopathology study. *Eur J Vasc Surg* 1990;4:75–82.
5. Sumboonnanonda A, Robinson BL, Gedroyc WM et al. Middle aortic syndrome: Clinical and radiological findings. *ADIC* 1992;67:501–5.
6. Panayiotopoulos YP, Tyrrell MR, Koffman G et al. Mid-aortic syndrome presenting in childhood. *Br J Surg* 1996;83:235–40.
7. Connolly JE, Wilson SE, Lawrence PL et al. Middle aortic syndrome: Distal thoracic and abdominal coarctation, a disorder with multiple etiologies. *J Am Coll Surg* 2002;194:774–81.

8. Stanley JC, Criado E, Eliason JL et al. Abdominal aortic coarctation: Surgical treatment of 53 patients with a thoracoabdominal bypass, patch aortoplasty, or interposition aortoaortic graft. *J Vasc Surg* 2008;48:1073–82.

9. Pagni S, Denatale RW, Boltax RS. Takayasu's arteritis: The middle aortic syndrome. *Am Surg* 1996;62:409–12.

10. Shefler AG, Chan MK, Ostman-Smith I. Middle aortic syndrome in a boy with arteriohepatic dysplasia (Alagille syndrome). *Pediatr Cardiol* 1997;18:232–4.

11. Radford DJ, Pohlner PG The middle aortic syndrome: An important feature of Williams' syndrome. *Cardiol Young* 2000;10:597–602.

12. Criado E, Izquierdo L, Lujan S et al. Abdominal aortic coarctation, renovascular, hypertension, and neurofibromatosis. *Ann Vasc Surg* 2002;16:363–7.

13. Delis KT, Gloviczki P. Middle aortic syndrome: From presentation to contemporary open surgical and endovascular treatment. *Perspect Vasc Surg Endovasc Ther* 2005;17:187–203.

14. D'Souza SJ, Tsai WS, Silver MM et al. Diagnosis and management of stenotic aorto-arteriopathy in childhood. *J Pediatr* 1998;132:1016–22.

15. Stanley JC, Graham LM, Whitehouse WM et al. Developmental occlusive disease of the abdominal aorta and the splanchnic and renal arteries. *Am J Surg* 1981;142:190–6.

16. Reiher L, Sandmann W. Coarctation of the thoracoabdominal aorta. *Chirurg* 1998;69:753–8.

17. Upchurch GR. Jr, Henke PK, Eagleton MJ et al. Pediatric splanchnic arterial occlusive disease: Clinical relevance and operative treatment. *J Vasc Surg* 2002;35:860–7.

18. Terramani TT, Salim A, Hood DB et al. Hypoplasia of the descending thoracic and abdominal aorta: A report of two cases and review of the literature. *J Vasc Surg* 2002;36:844–8.

19. Kashani IA, Sklansky MS, Movahed H et al. Successful balloon dilation of an abdominal coarctation of the aorta in patient with presumed Takayasu's aortitis. *Catheter Cardiovasc Diagn* 1996;38:406–9.

20. Tyagi S, Kaul UA, Arora R: Endovascular stenting for unsuccessful angioplasty of the aorta in aortoarteritis. *Cardiovasc Intervent Radiol* 1999;22:452–6.

21. Tyagi S, Khan AA, Kaul UA et al. Percutaneous transluminal angioplasty for stenosis of the aorta due to aortic arteritis in children. *Pediatr Cardiol* 1999;20:404–10.

22. Minson S, McLaren CA, Roebuck DJ et al. Infantile midaortic syndrome with aortic occlusion. *Pediatr Nephrol* 2012;27:321–4.

23. Brzezinska-Rajszys G, Qureshi SA, Ksiazyk J et al. Middle aortic syndrome treated by stent implantation. *Heart* 1999;81:166–170.

24. Bali HK, Bhargava M, Jain AK. De novo stenting of descending thoracic aorta in Takayasu arteritis: Intermediate-term follow-up results. *J Invasive Cardiol* 2000;12:612–7.

25. Keith D.S., Markey B., Schiedler M. Successful long-term stenting of an atypical descending aortic coarctation. *J Vasc Surg* 2002;35:166–7.

26. Sharma BK, Jain S, Bali HK. A follow-up study of balloon angioplasty and de-novo stenting in Takayasu arteritis. *Int J Cardiol* 2000;75 Suppl 1:S147–52.

27. Tyagi S, Singh B, Kaul UA. Balloon angioplasty for renovascular hypertension in Takayasu's arteritis. *Am Heart J* 1993;125:1386–93.

28. Liang P, Tan-Ong M, Hoffman GS. Takayasu's arteritis: Vascular interventions and outcomes. *J Rheumatol* 2004;31:102–6.

29. Tummolo A, Marks SD, Stadermann M et al. Mid-aortic syndrome: Long-term outcome of 36 children. *Pediatr Nephrol* 2009;24:2225–32.

30. Brzezinska-Rajszys G, Zubrzycka M, Rewers B et al. Mid-term follow-up of treatment of middle aortic syndrome in children. *Cardiol Young* 2010;20,Supl.2:S23–4.

31. Ozawa A, Predescu D, Chaturvedi R et al. Cutting balloon angioplasty for aortic coarctation. *Invasive Cardiol* 2009;6:295–9.

32. Kim HB. A novel treatment for the midaortic syndrome. *N Engl J Med* 2012;367:2361–2.

33. Choe YH, Han BK, Koh EM. Takayasu's arteritis: Assessment of disease activity with contrast-enhanced MR imaging. *Am J Roentgenol* 2000;175:505–11.

34. Yamada I, Nakagawa T, Himeno Y et al. Takayasu arteritis: Diagnosis with breath-hold contrast-enhanced three-dimensional MR angiography. *J Magn Reson Imaging* 2000;11:481–7.

35. Akin E, Coen A, Momeni M. PET-CT findings in large vessel vasculitis presenting as FUO, a case report. *Clin Rheumatol* 2009;28:737–8.

36. Pacheco Castellanos MD, Mínguez Vega M, Martínez Caballero A et al. Early diagnosis of large vessel vasculitis. Usefulness of positron emission tomography with computed tomography. *Rheumatol Clin* 2013;9:65–8.

37. Deshmukh HL, Rathod KR, Sheth RJ et al. Fatal aortic rupture complicating stent plasty in a case of aortoarteritis. *Cardiovasc Intervent Radiol* 2003;26:496–8.

87

Catheter intervention for hypertrophic obstructive cardiomyopathy

Stéphane Noble, Haran Burri, and Ulrich Sigwart

Introduction

About 30% of patients with hypertrophic cardiomyopathy have left ventricular outflow tract (LVOT) obstruction under resting conditions.[1-3] Medical therapy with negative inotropic drugs effectively alleviates symptoms in many patients but 5–10% remain refractory to drug therapy.[4] Since the 1960s, surgical septal myectomy (SSM) has been shown to reduce outflow obstruction and relieve symptoms. However, some patients are unfavorable candidates for surgery because of advanced age, concomitant medical conditions, or previous cardiac surgery. In 1994, Sigwart introduced a catheter treatment that uses ethanol to create a localized and controlled septal infarction, thus mimicking the anatomic and hemodynamic effects of SSM. Since the first series of three patients reported in 1995,[5] the number of cases performed worldwide has been growing rapidly and, currently, the estimated number of alcohol septal ablations (ASA) is several-fold higher than the reported number of surgical myectomies.[6]

Patient selection

ASA represents an alternative to SSM in selected patients who are considered poor surgical candidates due to comorbidities and/or advanced age (class IIa), or prefer SSM after a balanced and objective discussion of both therapies (class IIb).[7] ASA may be considered when all of the following are present: drug refractory symptoms, significant LVOT obstruction (peak gradient ≥50 mmHg), and an appropriate cardiac morphology (Table 87.1). The septal wall thickness should be at least ≥15 mm in order to reduce the risk of an iatrogenic ventricular septal defect, and the septal perforator branches should be adequately sized and accessible. Studies have shown that the clinical success of ASA in patients with provocable obstruction (exercise is considered the standard provocation method) is comparable to that in patients with obstruction at rest.[8]

So far, little experience with ASA has been reported in patients with midventricular obstruction, although this is technically feasible.

SSM is preferable to ASA in patients with severe septal hypertrophy (e.g., ≥30 mm), septal anatomy unfavorable for alcohol delivery, or concomitant cardiac conditions requiring surgery such as extensive coronary artery disease or valvular heart disease. Finally, apical hypertrophy—hypertrophy limited to the free left ventricular (LV) wall—and absence of obstruction are contraindications for ASA.

Mechanisms of treatment efficacy

ASA induces a well-demarcated subaortic infarct—corresponding to approximately 10% of the left ventricular muscle mass by MRI[9,10]—with a histopathological myocardial appearance typical of necrosis and healed infarction similar to that caused by coronary occlusions in addition to direct injury (coagulative necrosis) to the septal vasculature.[11]

The LVOT gradient usually falls immediately after ASA as a result of a loss of septal contractility caused by ischemia, necrosis, and stunning of the septal myocardium. One-third of patients have a triphasic evolution of the gradient.[12] After the initial reduction, an early reappearance of the gradient (≥50% of the pre-ASA value) can be observed reflecting edema as well as the recovery of the septal myocardium from stunning. At 3 months a subsequent gradient reduction (≤50% of the pre-ASA value) is caused by the thinning of the ablated area and scar formation.[12]

The long-term relief in outflow obstruction is mainly the result of LVOT remodeling due to myocardial scar formation.[13,14] In addition to the relief in LVOT obstruction, a reduction in the severity of mitral regurgitation and more favorable diastolic properties contribute to reported improvements in long-term hemodynamic results and clinical status.[15–18] Furthermore, LV hypertrophy of areas remote from the basal septum—the consequence of increased afterload—can be reduced by an effective reduction of the LV gradient after ASA. Lastly, outflow obstruction relief may increase coronary blood flow, thereby decreasing the likelihood of ischemia and anginal symptoms.[15]

The technique

Measurement of outflow gradient

Most operators continuously monitor the outflow gradient invasively during the procedure, however, some centers only measure the gradient noninvasively using echocardiography. A 5-F pigtail or multipurpose catheter with distal side holes can be used to measure the prestenotic pressure. Some centers prefer the transseptal approach for hemodynamic monitoring.[5] It is important to place the catheter close to the apex, particularly in cases with midventricular hypertrophy. Attention should be paid to avoid entrapment in the myocardium, as this may exaggerate the true LVOT gradient. Injection of small volumes of contrast via the catheter while checking for brisk dye clearance can verify the absence of entrapment.

The poststenotic pressure is measured through a 7-F guiding catheter (e.g., Judkins type or another appropriate

curve) placed in the ascending aorta. A 6-F catheter is suboptimal, as it causes excessive pressure damping with concomitant use of an over-the-wire (OTW) balloon catheter required for alcohol injection later during the procedure. After the exclusion of a valvular gradient, the peak gradient should be measured at rest, during isoproterenol infusion, and after extrasystoles. Isoproterenol with a bolus of 4–12 mcg (1–3 cc of 200 mcg diluted in 50 cc of saline) may be administered and supplemental boluses carefully added until a heart rate of 100 bpm is reached or if the patient reports symptoms.

Routine placement of a temporary pacing lead is mandatory to ensure backup pacing in the event of an AV block.[19,20] The pacing lead may also serve to measure the postextrasystolic gradient by programmed stimulation, if extrasystoles are not observed spontaneously.

Identification of the appropriate septal perforator artery

A left coronary angiogram is performed (Figure 87.1a). High-quality images (30 frames per second) may be required to improve visualization of septal perforator arteries (SPAs). The 30° right anterior oblique projection (±30° cranial) and 45° left anterior oblique projection with cranial angulation generally provide adequate visualization of most SPA and their anatomic variations. Milking of the SPA supplying the hypertrophied target segment can frequently be seen and typically identifies the corresponding target vessel. Usually, the wire will first be inserted in the most proximal accessible SPA of the left anterior descending (LAD) artery.

Positioning of the guide wire in the SPA may sometimes be difficult due to a perpendicular takeoff. Preshaping the guide wire with the help of the introducer needle with two angles (Figure 87.2), rather than a single curve may help. A floppy guide wire should be tried first, and advanced distally into the SPA to provide stability and support. Stiffer guide wires may be necessary to allow OTW balloon delivery. In exceptional cases, a 4-F guiding catheter with a sharp angle (e.g., internal mammary catheter) may be used as an inner catheter to selectively engage a SPA with extremely steep takeoff, facilitating placement of a 0.014 inch guide wire. However, extreme caution must be used during catheter manipulation to avoid parent vessel (typically LAD) dissection. As a last resort, a balloon may be briefly inflated at low pressure just distal to the SPA, thus directing the 0.014 inch guide wire into the target vessel.

The target SPA should be at least 1.5 mm in diameter. The shortest available balloon (2.0 × 10 mm OTW balloon is suitable for most cases) is then placed as close as possible in a stable position after intravenous administration of weight-adjusted heparin. The balloon should be slightly oversized (usually a 2 up to 3 mm OTW balloon). In case

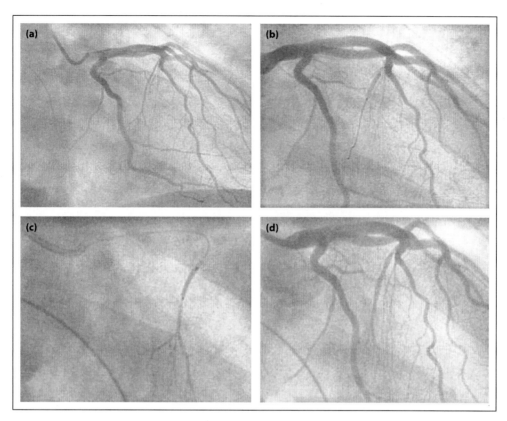

Figure 87.1   (a) An LAO angiogram of the left coronary artery. (b) Balloon catheter inflated and positioned in the first septal branch over a 0.014 inch guide wire. (c) Contrast dye is injected via the balloon catheter to confirm the absence of retrograde leakage. (d) Angiogram after alcohol injection. Note that the first septal branch is patent.

of proximal branching of the SPA, a shorter OTW balloon may be used. The guiding catheter may then have to be positioned more deeply, in order to provide more support for the balloon and avoid recoil during injection. The balloon should be inflated with a pressure of 4–6 bars and correct positioning is verified by contrast injection into the left coronary artery (Figure 87.2b), and subsequently (via the OTW balloon lumen) into the SPA using approximately 1 cc of contrast (Figure 87.2c). Absence of retrograde leakage and stability of balloon position should be verified attentively.

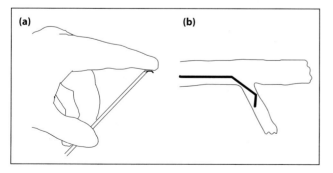

Figure 87.2   (a) Preshaping the 0.014 inch guide wire with two angles through a blunt introducer needle. (b) Positioning of the guide wire in a septal branch.

It is very important to inject the contrast *forcefully* via the inflated balloon catheter to assure balloon stability and a complete seal within the SPA. Furthermore, the extent of myocardium supplied by the SPA and shunting through collateral circulation between SPA branches can also be analyzed, ideally using two different projections.[21] Contrast injection may also promote ischemia to the territory of the SPA. The outflow gradient should be monitored continuously to check for a drop in the resting or postextrasystolic gradient within 5 min of balloon occlusion. If there is no drop in peak gradient (in about 20% of patients[22]), the balloon catheter may be positioned in another SPA. In up to 10% of patients, the appropriate SPA does not originate from the LAD, but from an intermediate or diagonal branch,[23,24] or from the posterior descending artery.

Myocardial contrast echocardiography (MCE) has been proven to be extremely useful in targeting the desired SPA, increasing the success rates while limiting the infarct size and associated complications.[23,25–28] Before injecting alcohol, 1–2 mL of echo contrast (e.g., Definity®, Sonovue®, Optison®) is injected via the inflated OTW balloon during trans-thoracic echocardiography (TTE) imaging in the apical four- and five-chamber views (Figure 87.3a). This serves to determine whether the opacified myocardium is adjacent to the region of anterior mitral leaflet septal contact

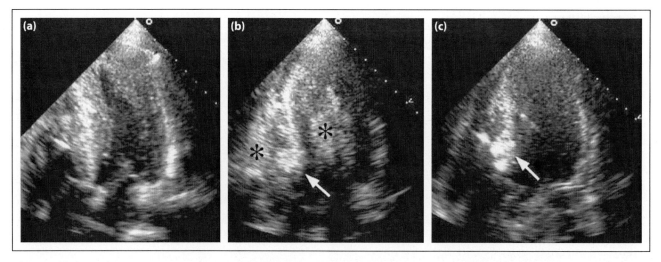

Figure 87.3 (a) An Apical four-chamber echocardiogram showing the hypertrophied septum. (b) Injection of echo-contrast (Levovist®) via the occluded balloon catheter positioned in the first septal perforator, with opacification of the basal septum (arrow). Note the presence of echo-contrast (asterisks) within both ventricles due to transcapillary passage. (c) After alcohol injection, the area of necrosis becomes echodense (arrow).

and maximal flow acceleration, and to withhold alcohol injection in case of a suboptimal irrigation pattern (e.g., predominant opacification of the right side of the interventricular septum).[24] This technique also helps to delineate the infarct zone and rule out retrograde leakage or involvement of myocardium distant from the expected target region[29] (i.e., involvement of the ventricular free wall[26,27] or papillary muscles).[27,30] In ~5% of cases, no target SPA can be identified and the procedure is aborted.

With echo-contrast volumes >1 mL, transcapillary passage of the contrast medium into the ventricles, more often the right than the left, is usually observed during the injection (Figure 87.3b). If echo contrast is not available, regular angiographic contrast dye injection into the SPA via the inflated OTW balloon may also provide sufficient echocardiographic myocardial opacification. Finally, if resistance is encountered while injecting through the OTW balloon, it might be related to a kink of the balloon catheter at the SPA origin. An option is to insert a 0.009 inch rotawire in the OTW balloon to correct the kinking.

Alcohol injection

Once the SPA is considered suitable and the inflated balloon is in a stable position without retrograde spilling, 0.7–3 mL of 96% ethanol may be slowly injected through the inflated balloon catheter under fluoroscopic guidance. The indeflator pressure should be visible throughout the procedure in order to prevent unintended pressure loss. Analgesics may be given before alcohol administration for chest pain control. The volume injected depends on the size of the vessel and volume of the targeted myocardium (approximately 1 mL for every 10 mm of septum thickness[28]). The electrocardiogram should be monitored closely,

and the injection is aborted if an atrio-ventricular block occurs. Over the last few years, there has been a tendency to limit the amount of alcohol injected to a maximum of 2 mL,[22,31,32] which may reduce complications. The balloon should be kept inflated for at least 10 min to enhance contact of alcohol with the tissue, and to avoid reflux into the LAD. A left coronary angiography should be repeated after balloon deflation to confirm LAD patency (Figure 87.1d). The target SPA may not necessarily be occluded, although flow is usually sluggish. It is not known whether this has an impact on treatment efficacy. Echocardiographically, the injection of alcohol results in a significant myocardial opacification, much stronger than that observed with currently available echo-contrast agents (Figure 87.3c).

The hemodynamic objective is a gradient reduction by >50% (80% in certain centers[34]) to ≤10 mmHg at rest in cases with provocable gradient. If the residual gradient after alcohol injection remains >30 mmHg at rest after 5–10 min following the last injection of alcohol, the balloon may be positioned more proximally inside the same SPA, or a shorter balloon is used if branches of the SPA were occluded by the balloon inflation during the first injection. Alternatively, a second SPA may be targeted. Most patients will require one target SPA only, especially since the advent of MCE. Some operators prefer a priori a "one vessel per session" approach, and it is still unclear whether more than a single SPA should be targeted initially.

Postprocedural management

Heparin at the therapeutic level should be discontinued at the end of the procedure. All patients should receive aspirin before the procedure and subsequently for 1 month. Creatinine kinase levels should be checked every 4 h. Peak

Table 87.2 Score system to predict the risk of pacemaker dependency after percutaneous septal ablation

Parameter ($n = 11$)	Cutoff value	Score points
Baseline PQ interval (ms)	>160	+2
Baseline minimal heart rate (Holter, bpm)	<50	+2
Baseline LVOT gradient (echo, mmHg)	>70	+2
AV block III during ASA (any time)	Yes	+2
AV block III at CCU admission	Yes	+2
Recovery of AV conduction at 12 h	Yes	−2
No recovery after 12 h	Yes	+1
No recovery after 24 h	Yes	+2
No recovery after 48 h	Yes	+3
Maximum QRS width during the first 48 h (ms)	>155	+3
Timing of GOT peak (h)	>16 >20	+1 +3
Risk group	**Score points**	**Procedure**
Low	<8	Discharge from monitoring
Intermediate	8–12	Prolonged monitoring
High	>12	Prepare for early PM implantation

Source: Reproduced from Faber L et al. *Int J Cardiol* 2007;119(2):163–7. ASA: Alcohol septal ablation, AV: Atrio-ventricular, Bpm: Beat per minute, LVOT: Left ventricular outflow tract.

rises are usually observed in the range of 750–1500 U/L (~500 U/L per 1 mL ethanol injected). Patients should be observed in the coronary care unit for 24–48 h, with removal of the temporary pacing lead at the end of this period in the absence of predictive factors for definite pacemaker need[19] (Table 87.2).

Treatment efficacy

Evidence from nonrandomized trials and meta-analysis indicates that ASA is comparable to SSM with respect to hemodynamic and functional improvements.[17,31–40] A gradient reduction can be achieved in about 80% of the patients.[18,23,34,41] However, the above-cited studies show a slightly higher residual gradient (perhaps related to the triphasic gradient evolution[12]) and a higher incidence of pacemaker implantation after ASA.[42] Unfortunately, an adequately powered randomized trial comparing long-term results of ASA and SSM is unlikely to be undertaken considering the large number of patients required.[43]

Table 87.3 Clinical variables that predicted acute hemodynamic success

Age ≥65 years
Resting LVOT gradient <100 mmHg
Septal hypertrophy at site of SAM ≤18 mm
LAD diameter <4.0 mm

Soure: According to Sorajja P et al. *Catheter Cardiovasc Interv* 2013;81(1):E58–67.
LAD: left descending coronary artery; LVOT: left ventricular outflow tract. Patients with ≥3 characteristics had superior 4-year survival free of death and severe symptoms.

The Mayo Clinic group recently reported predictors of success[33] (Table 87.3) and the longest follow-up (median 5.7 years) of an ASA series.[34] This latter series shows that long-term survival after ASA is similar to the expected survival for a similar age-matched general US population, and comparable to age- and sex-matched patients who underwent SSM. Furthermore, it shows that ASA in selected patients can result in durable symptom relief and that the severity of the residual gradient after ASA is an important determinant of long-term outcome.[34]

Procedures may need to be repeated in some patients (up to 25%[6]), mainly due to the fact that the basal part of the septum is supplied by more than one SPA,[44] while a minority is ultimately referred to surgery for gradient reduction.

Procedural risks

The mortality associated with the procedure is low, ranging from 0–4%, comparable to that reported with SSM. In the registry of the German Cardiac Society (264 patients),[45] the in-hospital mortality was 1.2% and in the Mayo Clinic experience (177 patients) it was 1.1%.[34] There are also reports of death due to stroke,[41,46] complete heart block,[41,46] dissection of the LAD,[18] and right coronary artery thrombosis.[18] A dreaded complication is retrograde leakage of alcohol into the LAD (Table 87.4), which may result in a massive

Table 87.4 Alcohol leakage: The cause and how to avoid it

Cause of alcohol leakage
Incomplete sealing of the septal branch by the inflated balloon
Slippage of the balloon
Too early deflation and retraction of the balloon
Anterograde flow due to collateralization between septal branches that has been overloaded

How to avoid it
Slightly oversized balloon
Sufficient support by the guiding catheter
Timely deflation of the balloon (no earlier than 10 min after alcohol injection)

Table 87.5   Most frequent complications of alcohol septal ablation

Complete atrio-ventricular block
Bradyarrhythmias in patients without permanent pacemaker
Sustained ventricular tachycardia
Puncture site complications
    Pseudoaneurysm
    Arterio-venous fistula
Death related to
    Spontaneous ventricular fibrillation
    Cardiac tamponade
    Cardiogenic shock
Remote acute infarction
    LAD or left main dissection
    Alcohol leakage and/or misplacement
Pulmonary embolism

infarct.[47,48] This complication is, however, extremely rare and avoidable. The importance of checking for leakage before alcohol injection cannot be overemphasized.

The most frequent complications of ASA are summarized in Table 87.5. Spontaneous ventricular fibrillation and tachycardia have been reported to occur within 48 h of the procedure.[34,41,47] The most frequent complication of ASA, however, is transient (up to 70%) or permanent (now approximately 10%) complete atrio-ventricular block.[23] The block is usually observed shortly after alcohol injection (but may appear up to 72 h[49]) and is most often transient. Complete heart block may resolve within the first 12 h of ASA, and then recur within the following week, requiring pacemaker implantation.[22] We and others[8,50] implant a pacemaker if the block persists for >48–72 h, although with longer observation, atrio-ventricular conduction may recover in some patients. The German registry[45] reported implantation of a pacemaker in 9.6% of patients due to complete heart block.

Baseline conduction abnormalities (especially preexisting left bundle branch block) may increase the risk for complete heart block after ablation.[19,50,51] The other factors found to be independently predictive of pacemaker implantation are female gender, bolus injection of ethanol, high volume of ethanol used, and injection into more than one septal artery.[50–52] The use of MCE helps limit infarct size, and in one series reduced the need for permanent pacemaker implantation from 17% to 7%,[23] which is still higher than the reported 2% incidence with SSM.[53]

Right bundle branch block (RBBB) following the procedure may be observed in over half of the patients.[22,51,54] This is not surprising, as the right bundle is supplied by septal branches from the LAD in 90% of patients, whereas the left bundle receives a dual blood supply via perforator branches from both the LAD and posterior descending arteries. Since ASA often causes RBBB and SSM often

causes left bundle branch block, patients undergoing the two procedures will be exposed to a very high risk of complete atrio-ventricular requiring a permanent pacemaker.

ASA may result in loss of capture in patients in whom the ventricular lead is placed near the septum.[55] It may be prudent to deliver a maximal output during the first days following the procedure in these patients.

There was no evidence for the creation of an arrhythmogenic substrate by ASA as assessed by serial electrophysiological studies before and after the procedure in a total of 78 patients in two different series,[22,41] and none of the published reports indicate an increase in incidence of ventricular arrhythmias or sudden death at follow-up.[34]

Conclusion

Data indicate that procedural success rates with ASA are high and comparable to those reported for SSM. The advantage of ASA is that it may be performed in high-risk surgical candidates. MCE has contributed to our ability to cause smaller and more targeted infarctions with lower doses of alcohol, leading in turn to fewer complications while maintaining therapeutic efficacy. The need for permanent pacemaker implantation has decreased to ~10% and periprocedural mortality is very low in experienced centers. However, ASA has an important learning curve with potentially serious complications and should be performed in carefully selected patients by experienced operators in appropriate centers.

References

1. Maron BJ, Olivotto I, Spirito P et al. Epidemiology of hypertrophic cardiomyopathy-related death: Revisited in a large non-referral-based patient population. *Circulation* 2000;102:858–64.
2. Maron MS, Olivotto I, Betocchi S et al. Effect of left ventricular outflow tract obstruction on clinical outcome in hypertrophic cardiomyopathy. *N Engl J Med* 2003;348:295–303.
3. Maron MS, Olivotto I, Zenovich AG et al. Hypertrophic cardiomyopathy is predominantly a disease of left ventricular outflow tract obstruction. *Circulation* 2006;114(21):2232–9.
4. Maron BJ, Bonow RO, Cannon RO, 3rd et al. Hypertrophic cardiomyopathy. Interrelations of clinical manifestations, pathophysiology, and therapy (1). *N Engl J Med* 1987;316:780–9.
5. Sigwart U. Non-surgical myocardial reduction for hypertrophic obstructive cardiomyopathy. *Lancet* 1995;346:211–4.
6. Maron BJ. Surgical myectomy remains the primary treatment option for severely symptomatic patients with obstructive hypertrophic cardiomyopathy. *Circulation* 2007;116:196–206.
7. Gersh BJ, Maron BJ, Bonow RO et al. 2011 ACCF/AHA Guideline for the Diagnosis and Treatment of Hypertrophic Cardiomyopathy: Executive Summary: A Report of the American College of Cardiology Foundation/American Heart Association Task Force on Practice Guidelines. *Circulation* 2011;124:2761–96.
8. Gietzen FH, Leuner CJ, Obergassel L et al. Role of transcoronary ablation of septal hypertrophy in patients with hypertrophic cardiomyopathy, New York Heart Association functional class III or IV, and outflow obstruction only under provocable conditions. *Circulation* 2002;106:454–9.

9. Talreja DR, Nishimura RA, Edwards WD, et al Alcohol septal ablation versus surgical septal myectomy: Comparison of effects on atrioventricular conduction tissue. *J Am Coll Cardiol* 2004;44:2329–32.

10. Pedone C, Vijayakumar M, Ligthart JM et al. Intracardiac echocardiography guidance during percutaneous transluminal septal myocardial ablation in patients with obstructive hypertrophic cardiomyopathy. *Int J Cardiovasc Interv* 2005;7:134–7.

11. Baggish AL, Smith RN, Palacios I, Vlahakes GJ, Yoerger DM, Picard MH et al. Pathological effects of alcohol septal ablation for hypertrophic obstructive cardiomyopathy. *Heart* 2006;92(12):1773–8.

12. Yoerger DM, Picard MH, Palacios IF et al. Time course of pressure gradient response after first alcohol septal ablation for obstructive hypertrophic cardiomyopathy. *Am J Cardiol* 2006;97(10):1511–4.

13. Flores-Ramirez R, Lakkis NM, Middleton KJ et al. Echocardiographic insights into the mechanisms of relief of left ventricular outflow tract obstruction after nonsurgical septal reduction therapy in patients with hypertrophic obstructive cardiomyopathy. *J Am Coll Cardiol* 2001;37:208–14.

14. Henein MY, O'Sullivan CA, Ramzy IS et al. Electromechanical left ventricular behavior after nonsurgical septal reduction in patients with hypertrophic obstructive cardiomyopathy. *J Am Coll Cardiol* 1999;34:1117–22.

15. Nagueh SF, Lakkis NM, Middleton KJ et al. Changes in left ventricular diastolic function 6 months after nonsurgical septal reduction therapy for hypertrophic obstructive cardiomyopathy. *Circulation* 1999;99:344–7.

16. Nagueh SF, Lakkis NM, Middleton KJ et al. Changes in left ventricular filling and left atrial function six months after nonsurgical septal reduction therapy for hypertrophic obstructive cardiomyopathy. *J Am Coll Cardiol* 1999;34:1123–8.

17. Sitges M, Shiota T, Lever HM et al. Comparison of left ventricular diastolic function in obstructive hypertrophic cardiomyopathy in patients undergoing percutaneous septal alcohol ablation versus surgical myotomy/myectomy. *Am J Cardiol* 2003;91:817–21.

18. Lakkis NM, Nagueh SF, Dunn JK et al. Nonsurgical septal reduction therapy for hypertrophic obstructive cardiomyopathy: One-year follow-up. *J Am Coll Cardiol* 2000;36:852–5.

19. Faber L, Welge D, Fassbender D, Schmidt HK, Horstkotte D, Seggewiss H. Percutaneous septal ablation for symptomatic hypertrophic obstructive cardiomyopathy: Managing the risk of procedure-related AV conduction disturbances. *Int J Cardiol* 2007;119(2):163–7.

20. Noble S, Roffi M, Burri H. Use of an explanted pacemaker connected to a regular screw-in lead for temporary pacing. *Rev Esp Cardiol* 2011;64(12):1229–30.

21. Rigopoulos A, Sepp R, Palinkas A et al. Alcohol septal ablation for hypertrophic obstructive cardiomyopathy: Collateral vessel communication between septal branches. *Int J Cardiol* 2006; 113(2):e67–9.

22. Boeksteegers P, Steinbigler P, Molnar A et al. Pressure-guided nonsurgical myocardial reduction induced by small septal infarctions in hypertrophic obstructive cardiomyopathy. *J Am Coll Cardiol* 2001;38:846–53.

23. Faber L, Seggewiss H, Gleichmann U. Percutaneous transluminal septal myocardial ablation in hypertrophic obstructive cardiomyopathy: Results with respect to intraprocedural myocardial contrast echocardiography. *Circulation* 1998;98:2415–21.

24. Noble S, Frangos C, L'Allier PL. Alcohol septal ablation for obstructive hypertrophic cardiomyopathy: The perfect septal branch may originate from an atypical location. *Can J Cardiol.* 2012;28(2):245 e1–3.

25. Lakkis NM, Nagueh SF, Kleiman NS et al. Echocardiography-guided ethanol septal reduction for hypertrophic obstructive cardiomyopathy. *Circulation* 1998;98:1750–5.

26. Nagueh SF, Lakkis NM, He ZX et al. Role of myocardial contrast echocardiography during nonsurgical septal reduction therapy for hypertrophic obstructive cardiomyopathy. *J Am Coll Cardiol* 1998;32:225–9.

27. Faber L, Seggewiss H, Ziemssen P et al. Intraprocedural myocardial contrast echocardiography as a routine procedure in percutaneous transluminal septal myocardial ablation: Detection of threatening myocardial necrosis distant from the septal target area. *Catheter Cardiovasc Interv* 1999;47:462–6.

28. Faber L, Seggewiss H, Welge D et al. Echo-guided percutaneous septal ablation for symptomatic hypertrophic obstructive cardiomyopathy: 7 years of experience. *Eur J Echocardiogr* 2004;5(5):347–55.

29. Faber L, Ziemssen P, Seggewiss H. Targeting percutaneous transluminal septal ablation for hypertrophic obstructive cardiomyopathy by intraprocedural echocardiographic monitoring. *J Am Soc Echocardiogr* 2000;13:1074–9.

30. Harada T, Ohtaki E, Sumiyoshi T. Papillary muscles identified by myocardial contrast echocardiography in preparation for percutaneous transluminal septal myocardial ablation. *Acta Cardiol* 2002;57:25–7.

31. Kuhn H, Lawrenz T, Lieder F et al. Survival after transcoronary ablation of septal hypertrophy in hypertrophic obstructive cardiomyopathy (TASH): A 10 year experience. *Clin Res Cardiol* 2008;97:234–243.

32. Veselka J, Prochazkova S, Duchonova R et al. Alcohol septal ablation for hypertrophic obstructive cardiomyopathy: lower alcohol dose reduces size of infarction and has comparable hemodynamic and clinical outcome. *Catheter Cardiovasc Interv* 2004;63:231–235.

33. Sorajja P, Binder J, Nishimura RA et al. Predictors of an optimal clinical outcome with alcohol septal ablation for obstructive hypertrophic cardiomyopathy. *Catheter Cardiovasc Interv* 2013;81(1):E58–67.

34. Sorajja P, Ommen SR, Holmes DR et al. Survival after alcohol septal ablation for obstructive hypertrophic cardiomyopathy. *Circulation* 2012;126(20):2374–80.

35. Faber L, Meissner A, Ziemssen P et al. Percutaneous transluminal septal myocardial ablation for hypertrophic obstructive cardiomyopathy: long term follow up of the first series of 25 patients. *Heart* 2000;83:326–31.

36. Seggewiss H, Faber L, Meissner A et al. Improvement of acute results after percutaneous transluminal septal myocardial ablation in hypertrophic obstructive cardiomyopathy during mid-term follow-up. *J Am Coll Cardiol* 2000;35:188A. [Abstract].

37. Firoozi S, Elliott PM, Sharma S et al. Septal myotomy-myectomy and transcoronary septal alcohol ablation in hypertrophic obstructive cardiomyopathy. A comparison of clinical, haemodynamic and exercise outcomes. *Eur Heart J* 2002;23:1617–24.

38. Nagueh SF, Ommen SR, Lakkis NM et al. Comparison of ethanol septal reduction therapy with surgical myectomy for the treatment of hypertrophic obstructive cardiomyopathy. *J Am Coll Cardiol* 2001;38:1701–6.

39. Qin JX, Shiota T, Lever HM et al. Outcome of patients with hypertrophic obstructive cardiomyopathy after percutaneous transluminal septal myocardial ablation and septal myectomy surgery. *J Am Coll Cardiol* 2001;38:1994–2000.

40. Agarwal S, Tuzcu EM, Desai MY et al. Updated meta-analysis of septal alcohol ablation versus myectomy for hypertrophic cardiomyopathy. *J Am Coll Cardiol* 2010;55(8):823–34.

41. Gietzen FH, Leuner CJ, Raute-Kreinsen U et al. Acute and long-term results after transcoronary ablation of septal hypertrophy (TASH). Catheter interventional treatment for hypertrophic obstructive cardiomyopathy. *Eur Heart J* 1999;20:1342–54.

42. Fifer MA, Sigwart U. Controversies in cardiovascular medicine. Hypertrophic obstructive cardiomyopathy: alcohol septal ablation. *Eur Heart J.* 2011;32(9):1059–64.

43. Olivotto I, Ommen SR, Maron MS, Cecchi F, Maron BJ. Surgical myectomy versus alcohol septal ablation for obstructive hypertrophic cardiomyopathy. Will there ever be a randomized trial? *J Am Coll Cardiol* 2007;50(9):831–4.

44. Lee JM, Moon JC, Pennell DJ, Sigwart U, Clague JR. Late recurrence of outflow tract obstruction seven years after septal ablation in hypertrophic cardiomyopathy. *Int J Cardiol* 2005;100(2):341–2.

45. Kuhn H, Seggewiss H, Gietzen FH et al. Catheter-based therapy for hypertrophic obstructive cardiomyopathy. First in-hospital outcome analysis of the German TASH Registry. *Z Kardiol* 2004;93:23–31.

46. Oomman A, Ramachandran P, Subramanyan K et al. Percutaneous transluminal septal myocardial ablation in drug-resistant hypertrophic obstructive cardiomyopathy: 18-month follow-up results. *J Invasive Cardiol* 2001;13:526–30.

47. Knight C, Kurbaan AS, Seggewiss H et al. Nonsurgical septal reduction for hypertrophic obstructive cardiomyopathy : outcome in the first series of patients. *Circulation* 1997;95:2075–81.

48. Dimitrow PP, Dudek D, Dubeil JS. The risk of alcohol leakage into the left anterior descending coronary artery during non-surgical myocardial reduction in patients with obstructive hypertrophic cardiomyopathy. *Eur Heart J* 2001;22:437–8.

49. Kern MJ, Holmes DG, Simpson C et al. Delayed occurrence of complete heart block without warning after alcohol septal ablation for hypertrophic obstructive cardiomyopathy. *Catheter Cardiovasc Interv* 2002;56:503–7.

50. Chang SM, Nagueh SF, Spencer I, William H et al. Complete heart block: determinants and clinical impact in patients with hypertrophic obstructive cardiomyopathy undergoing nonsurgical septal reduction therapy. *J Am Coll Cardiol* 2003;42:296–300.

51. Runquist LH, Nielsen CD, Killip D et al. Electrocardiographic findings after alcohol septal ablation therapy for obstructive hypertrophic cardiomyopathy. *Am J Cardiol* 2002;90:1020–2.

52. Qin JX, Shiota T, Lever HM et al. Conduction system abnormalities in patients with obstructive hypertrophic cardiomyopathy following septal reduction interventions. *Am J Cardiol* 2004;93:171–5.

53. ten Berg JM, Suttorp MJ, Knaepen PJ et al. Hypertrophic obstructive cardiomyopathy. Initial results and long-term follow-up after Morrow septal myectomy. *Circulation* 1994;90:1781–5.

54. Kazmierczak J, Kornacewicz-Jach Z, Kisly M et al. Electrocardiographic changes after alcohol septal ablation in hypertrophic obstructive cardiomyopathy. *Heart* 1998;80:257–62.

55. Valettas N, Rho R, Beshai J et al. Alcohol septal ablation complicated by complete heart block and permanent pacemaker failure. *Catheter Cardiovasc Interv* 2003;58:189–93.

88

Hypertrophic obstructive cardiomyopathy: Radio-frequency septal reduction

Joseph DeGiovanni

Pathophysiology

Hypertrophic cardiomyopathy (HCM) consists of severe myocardial hypertrophy as a primary disease of the heart muscle. The pattern is variable in that it usually involves the ventricular septum more than the rest of the myocardium, but it can be primarily apical. With the former, around 25% will have a septal bulge that will create a dynamic obstruction giving rise to a very high left ventricular (LV) pressure, limited flow to the circulation and, sometimes, mitral regurgitation. The condition is caused by one of many potential gene mutations that are transmitted in an autosomal dominant way and it can manifest itself by inappropriate hypertrophy of the myocardium due to myocyte hypertrophy and disarray.

There is good systolic function but impaired diastolic function due to poor myocardial relaxation. The outflow obstruction usually involves the LV, but occasionally can involve the right ventricle or both outlets. Additionally, coronary artery compression can occur due to myocardial bridging. A major cause of mortality and morbidity, however, is the propensity to arrhythmias. These arrhythmias include atrial fibrillation but, of more concern, ventricular tachycardia or fibrillation. The link between the severity of obstruction and fatal arrhythmias is not clear-cut but, in general, severe obstruction is considered responsible for symptoms, including syncope and arrhythmias and, when associated with other risk factors, contributes to sudden death and heart failure symptoms.[1,2] Relief of important obstruction, therefore, carries good logic in selected cases. The technique of radio-frequency septal reduction is only one of several treatment modalities and is more applicable and of interest in the pediatric population. Whereas most patients with HCM are diagnosed well into adulthood, some present in childhood and these often have a more severe form of the condition.

Symptoms

Many patients with HCM remain asymptomatic until this condition has progressed to an advanced degree but, eventually, they can develop reduced exercise tolerance, chest pain, exercise-induced syncope, arrhythmias (some potentially fatal), or sudden death. LV outflow tract obstruction contributes to the symptoms.

Treatment options

The condition is incurable and any treatment is directed at management of arrhythmias (anti-arrhythmic drugs, ±pacing, ±implantable cardiovertor defibrillator) or improvement in mechanical function to relieve symptoms. This may happen through pharmacologic (e.g., drugs such as β-blockers, calcium channel blockers, or disopyramide) and surgical (relief of right ventricular [RV] or LV outflow tract by myotomy or myectomy, mitral valve replacement, or relief of myocardial bridging) means (see Box 88.1). Interventional procedures have been used to replace these surgical options. For instance, myocardial bridging can be overcome by placement of a coronary stent, and future

---

BOX 88.1: METHODS FOR RELIEF OF LEFT VENTRICULAR OUTFLOW TRACT OBSTRUCTION

1. Surgery: Myotomy, myectomy, and diathermy.
2. Interventional septal reduction:
   a. Alcohol injection in septal branches of left anterior descending coronary artery (TASH)
   b. Coil embolization of septal branches
   c. Covered stent to exclude septal branches
   d. Radio-frequency directly to ventricular septum (discussed in this chapter)
3. Electrical: Pacing with short AV delay

transcatheter techniques for mitral regurgitation may prove useful in this setting. The main advance in interventional procedures for HCM has been to tackle the outflow tract obstruction, but the use of implantable defibrillators has been responsible for the improved longevity.

Diagnosis and indications for treatment

Initial assessment of HOCM is carried out by echocardiographic and Doppler studies. Apart from making a diagnosis largely based on asymmetric septal hypertrophy, quantitative or semi-quantitative assessment of the LV outflow gradient and mitral regurgitation may also be used. Obstruction within the left ventricle can be multilevel and is usually dynamic. Indications for detailed invasive evaluation and possible intervention include the presence of symptoms (e.g., shortness of breath, chest pain, dizziness, or syncope on exercise) or increasing hemodynamic deterioration (often due to worsening outflow gradient), and mitral regurgitation. In addition, intervention is also indicated in those considered at high risk, for example, those with septal thickness of more than 2 cm, strong family history of sudden death, or documented arrhythmias. It is unusual for symptoms to arise until the LV outflow velocity is more than 4 m/s and, therefore, intervention is usually indicated when the velocity exceeds this and, more often, when it exceeds 4.5 m/s. The radio-frequency technique can be used when there is a contraindication to surgery or alcohol ablation, particularly in children, where TASH is not feasible and surgery carries significant risks; the condition is progressive. The radio-frequency approach does not preclude the use of any other treatment modality and may be repeated if required.

History

The first and most extensively used and evaluated catheter interventional method was pioneered by Sigwart[3] and involved the selective injection of absolute alcohol into the appropriate septal branch/branches of the left anterior descending coronary artery. The territory covered by specific septal branches can be identified by selective injection of ultrasound contrast material into a septal branch and observing its distribution into the myocardium on transesophageal echocardiography (TOE) prior to injecting alcohol; depending on the distribution of the septal branches, the territory supplied by a septal branch may not cover the culprit muscle bulge causing the obstruction, in which case TASH should not be carried out. An alternative to this, however, is the use of radio-frequency to create lesions in the septum; these lead initially to tissue desiccation followed by muscle atrophy and, hence, a reduction

in outflow obstruction as atrophied muscle creates a crater. This latter technique, first used at Birmingham Children's Hospital in the UK in 1998, is of particular benefit to children, whereas alcohol septal ablation is not a practical option in young patients, but very applicable in adults.

The use of electrical energy to treat HOCM was first described by Armistead and Williams[4] when they recommended using diathermy to remove septal muscle that was causing obstruction during open surgery; this was suggested as an alternative to myotomy or myectomy using a traditional scalpel. In 1994, Dalvi[5] proposed using radio-frequency ablation to create left bundle branch block, which was designed to produce paradoxical septal motion (an effect similar to one that results from RV pacing, which gives a left bundle branch block pattern), with the expectation of gradient reduction on the left side. Our recommendation has been to apply radio-frequency energy directly to the septal bulge in the LV outflow tract;[6,7] others have suggested applying radio-frequency to the right side of the ventricular septum and have claimed improvement in the gradient.[8] Conceptually, it is difficult to see how a right-sided approach could improve the left-sided obstruction as the lesions created are unlikely to be more than 6 mm and the septal thickness is usually over 2 cm. Moreover, there are no technical advantages to this over the left-sided approach. Right-sided ablation is, however, applicable if there is a dynamic obstruction involving the infundibulum.

The rest of this chapter concentrates on the technique of radio-frequency septal reduction.

Technique

Invasive assessment and radio-frequency septal reduction can be technically carried out under sedation with local anesthesia, but in children this is usually carried out under general anesthesia as the procedure can take a long time, making it difficult for patient cooperation. It is important for an anesthetist to avoid using potent systemic vasodilators or drugs with positive sympathomimetic action. The procedure can be carried out even in small children and the limitation is the size of the ablation catheter in relation to the size of the femoral vessels. Ideally, therefore, patients should be over 10 kg in weight.

Cardiac catheterization is carried out ideally with biplane fluoroscopy and facilities for intracardiac electrograms as well as disposables and a generator for delivering radio-frequency energy. These are standard equipment in institutions where ablation therapy for arrhythmias is conducted. The procedure requires several steps:

1. TOE obtains detailed assessment of the ventricular outflow obstruction and correlates this with angiography. TOE also helps to target delivery of radio-frequency energy to the site of obstruction, avoiding the mitral valve. When using an irrigation tip catheter, the

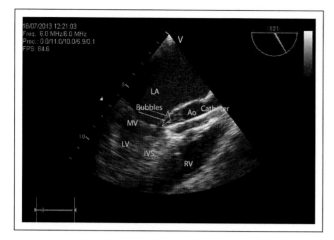

Figure 88.1 TOE during procedure showing catheter through aortic valve reaching the septal bulge with a gentle curve and showing bubbles from the irrigation with saline; these help to identify the catheter tip.

micro-bubbles created help to identify the tip of the ablation catheter (Figure 88.1). The area where ablation has been applied shows a higher echogenicity on TOE, but in the acute stage there is no regression of the septal bulge.

2. Hemodynamic assessment of the right and LV side of the heart, with specific quantitation of the RV outflow and the LV outflow tract gradients usually without pharmacological enhancement, is carried out. This is accompanied by detailed biplane angiography usually in right anterior oblique (RAO) 30° and left anterior oblique (LAO) 60° projections. Angiography will show the level, length, and the number of obstructions within the ventricle and whether this also involves the right side although the usual and more important obstruction is often on the left side (Figure 88.2). In addition, mitral regurgitation can be assessed and selective coronary angiography is carried out to look for coronary artery compression from myocardial bridging, as this may determine whether to proceed with intervention or surgery. Although stent implantation is an option for coronary compression from myocardial bridging,

this is not a recommended option in young patients in whom surgery is preferable.

Having determined the resting gradient, two temporary bipolar pacing wires are introduced through femoral venous sheaths that are usually 5 or 6 French (Fr) in size. One of the temporary wires is placed in the right atrial appendage and one in the apex of the right ventricle in order to assess the effect of pacing on the gradient.[9] In some cases, anatomical mapping using the LocaLisa has been used, in which case a surface reference electrode is placed and the temporary RV lead is screwed in to avoid movement during the procedure; this mapping system is no longer commercially available and if electro-anatomic mapping is desired the CARTO® system is used (Biosense Webster, Diamond Bar, CA, USA). A back plate is used as an indifferent electrode for the radio-frequency generator, and radiolucent defibrillator pads are placed on the chest for remote defibrillation in the event of ventricular fibrillation; the latter can occur with catheter manipulation, but also during the application of radio-frequency. A baseline PR interval is measured in sinus rhythm and ventricular pacing with atrial tracking is carried out while measuring the gradient across the LV outflow tract. The atrioventricular (AV) delay is reduced from baseline by 20 ms increments, while monitoring the change this produces to the LV outflow gradient. The lowest AV delay is usually 60 ms. If the gradient is substantially reduced by altering the AV delay (arbitrarily more than 50% reduction in the gradient), then this can determine how aggressive septal reduction is carried out, particularly if the muscular obstruction is in the vicinity of the HIS bundle. In other words, if the obstruction is close to the HIS bundle and there is improvement in the gradient with a short AV delay pacing, a balanced judgment would be to attempt septal reduction even if this may result in heart block that requires pacing. The temporary wire acts as a backup should heart block occur during ablation.

If the obstruction is significant on the basis of the gradient and angiographic observations, a radio-frequency ablation catheter is introduced into the left ventricle through a femoral artery sheath, which is usually 7 Fr. Standard

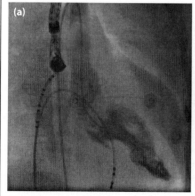
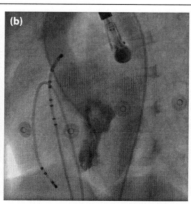

Figure 88.2 Left ventriculogram in RAO and LAO projections showing multiple and long segment muscular obstruction in HOCM. Two temporary pacing wires one in RA and one in RV. Reference electrode for CARTO seen behind the spine in (a).

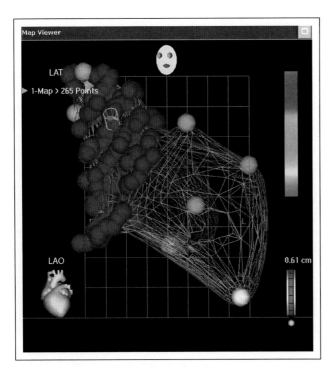

Figure 88.3 **(See color insert.)** A CARTO electro-anatomical map of the left ventricle in LAO projection showing His signal position in yellow, site of radio-frequency energy application on the septal bulge in red, and the mitral valve demarcated by blue.

intracardiac electrograms can be recorded; the alternative is to use an electro-anatomical mapping system, such as the LocaLisa navigation system (no longer available) or CARTO (Biosense Webster) (Figure 88.3). If this is used, the HIS bundle and the left bundle with its anterior and posterior fascicles are identified, mapped, and plotted with the radio-frequency catheter prior to administration of energy. A note is made of the anatomical relationship between the muscular obstruction and the conducting system prior to ablation. A standard or preferably a cool tip irrigation ablation catheter can be used. If a standard radio-frequency ablation catheter is used, a longer tip electrode, such as 8 mm (e.g., Celsius, Biosense Webster, Waterloo, Belgium) is preferable. An irrigation or cool tip catheter

(e.g., Thermocool® from Biosense Webster or Sprinkler® from Medtronic) can theoretically produce a deeper lesion of up to 6 mm compared with a 3 mm lesion when using the standard ablation catheter. With irrigation tip catheters, fluid administration must be kept under control, especially in small children. During mapping and catheter placement, a normal saline infusion is run through an irrigation catheter at 30 cc per hour whereas during ablation this is increased to between 300 and 600 cc per hour. It is important to reduce the flow once ablation has stopped to avoid fluid overload. Intravenous furosemide may be required. Occasionally, the approach to the LV has been through the femoral vein using a transeptal puncture and this may apply to small children or ones where good contact cannot be achieved from an arterial access.

During energy application, the AV conduction is observed closely and the radio-frequency application is stopped if there is evidence of heart block. The energy delivered is between 40 and 60 watts and each application is for 1 minute unless there are conduction problems or arrhythmias.

Radio-frequency delivery is carried out sequentially using the angiographic images of the obstruction, TOE, and electro-anatomical mapping, if this is available, making sure that all the bulges are covered and not leaving any gaps that may cause an arrhythmia substrate. More recently, the procedures have been carried out using intracardiac ultrasound (ICE) in conjunction with CARTO using the CARTO Sound® facility. The radio-frequency application is commenced distally away from the HIS bundle working proximally toward the aortic valve. Prior to each application of energy, the intracardiac ECG is checked for evidence of a HIS bundle signal avoiding energy delivery if at all possible in this region. It is important to appreciate the difference between HIS bundle signals and one produced by a fascicle of the left bundle. A linear application of radio-frequency energy is carried out along different planes of the ventricular septum until the whole area of obstruction is covered, as assessed by biplane fluoroscopy, electro-anatomical mapping, or TOE. The ablation catheter is steerable and can be curved from the handle control and adjusted to obtain maximal contact and stability (Figure 88.4). The ablation

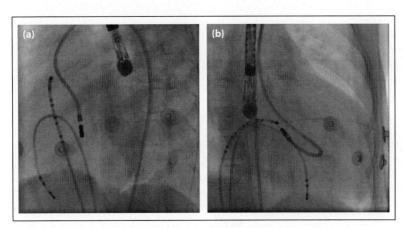

Figure 88.4   A radio-frequency ablation catheter in the LV via femoral artery in LAO with the catheter approaching the septal bulge with a gentle curve adjusted from the steerable handle (a) and in RAO with a larger curve bending the catheter on itself to achieve adequate reach and contact with the septum (b).

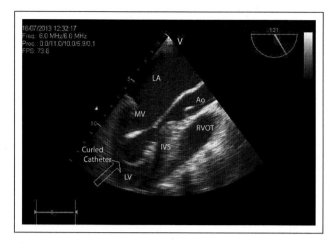

Figure 88.5 TOE image of catheter curved on itself to reach the lower end of the septal bulge to achieve optimal contact. (Courtesy of Dr. V Bhole.)

catheters come in different sizes of curves and a "medium" or D-curve is commonly used, although small children may benefit from a smaller curve. The catheter is negotiated directly within the aorta and LV although, on occasion, the use of a large sheath has been used to stabilize and orientate the catheter tip to the target. For the lower end of the septal bulge, the ablation catheter may have to be curved on itself and then gently released until it is in good contact and in a good position for delivery of radio-frequency (Figure 88.5). With the CARTO Sound mapping, a shell of the LV outflow

tract can be created using ICE and superimposed on this, the conducting system can be marked and the target area for ablation can be identified; the latter is uniformly ablated by several applications of radio-frequency without leaving any gaps, as these can potentially become arrhythmia substrates (Figure 88.6). During the application of energy, it is important to observe the impedance and temperature, bearing in mind that the temperature rise with irrigation catheters is lower than with standard ones; this usually hovers around the mid-40s, but does not rise above 50°C. Using the electro-anatomical mapping system helps to ensure that the treatment area covers the site of obstruction and avoids damage to the HIS bundle; moreover, it reduces the amount of fluoroscopy used. The area of muscle treated by radio-frequency immediately becomes more echogenic compared with the rest of the myocardium. This is not only a helpful observation in directing the ablation catheter toward the obstructing muscle band but also to make sure that coverage has been comprehensive.

During the procedure, the patient is given heparin 100 IU/kg and an ACT is checked 1 to 1.5 hours later. We aim to keep the ACT between 250 and 300 s. The number of radio-frequency applications required depends on the size of the patient, the severity and nature of the obstruction (multiple or long segment), and the appearance of echogenic changes on TOE. Usually, between 20 and 50 radio-frequency applications are required. As the radio-frequency lesions may initially lead to edema before atrophy produces regression, the gradient at the end of

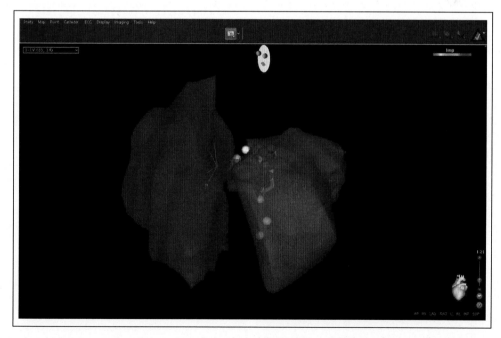

Figure 88.6 (**See color insert.**) A CARTO Sound® image in LAO projection showing the right ventricle shell in green and the left ventricle in gray. The area of septal bulge causing obstruction is highlighted by a pink area and the red dots indicate the sites where radio-frequency was applied. The blue dots indicate the sites where a His signal was identified during mapping. (Courtesy of Drs. Simon Modi and Rob Cooper.)

the procedure is meaningless; indeed, this may be higher, especially for right-sided lesions, because of the anatomy of the infundibulum. An echocardiographic assessment at the end of the procedure consists of the evaluation of the septal lesions, ensuring that there is no aortic regurgitation or worsening of mitral regurgitation and excluding thrombus or pericardial effusion.

The appearance of left bundle branch block is not of concern and may indeed prove an additional benefit by encouraging paradoxical septal motion and, hence, an improvement in the LV outflow tract obstruction.

Postoperative observations

The sites of entry are checked in the usual way for bleeding and for the integrity of the pulses. Cardiac monitoring is advised to make sure that there is no heart block or ventricular arrhythmias. Blood is taken for cardiac enzymes at the end of the procedure and repeated 12 h later; these include troponin and creatine kinase; the higher the figures the more muscle desiccation would have been achieved.

An ECG and an echocardiogram/Doppler are carried out, the former mainly for conduction or ischemic changes; the echocardiogram often shows the area where radio-frequency application has taken place and is shown by a highly echogenic area (however, in early stages the muscle may not have atrophied and the bulge and a gradient may still be present). In addition, it is important to exclude a pericardial effusion and to make sure that any mitral regurgitation is not worse after treatment. It is not uncommon for mitral regurgitation to improve, probably because the LV pressure drops, but there may also be less systolic anterior motion. Aspirin as an anti-platelet dose (5 mg/kg/day for children) is prescribed for 6 months. If heart block results, a short course of steroids is recommended prior to considering permanent pacing.

Patients are usually kept overnight after the procedure prior to discharge. If the radio-frequency application has been successfully delivered to the culprit area, a reduction in gradient is often seen within 2–3 days, but it may take up to 3 months for the maximum effect to be seen until muscle atrophy occurs and is complete; this is best assessed by echo/Doppler (Figures 88.7 and 88.8). Once atrophy sets in, a crater-like lesion occurs giving rise to a recessed area and at the base of this there is an echogenic area caused by the original burn (Figure 88.9).

The benefits of this procedure compared with others include:

1. The technique uses a single radio-frequency catheter and standard equipment usually available in most units that carry out ablation for arrhythmias. Personnel are also already trained.
2. It is a more controlled tissue reduction procedure than alcohol ablation and, therefore, of particular benefit to children. In other words, it can be specifically targeted and one can do as much or as little as deemed necessary.
3. The procedure may be repeated if required.
4. There are minimal complications.
5. It does not preclude any other forms of treatment if required.
6. Minimally traumatic to patients.
7. Constant intracardiac ECG helps to reduce risk of heart block.

Potential complications

Complications are uncommon but are similar to those encountered in most interventional procedures and include thrombo-embolic, vessel thrombosis or damage, cardiac perforation tamponade, aortic/mitral valve damage,

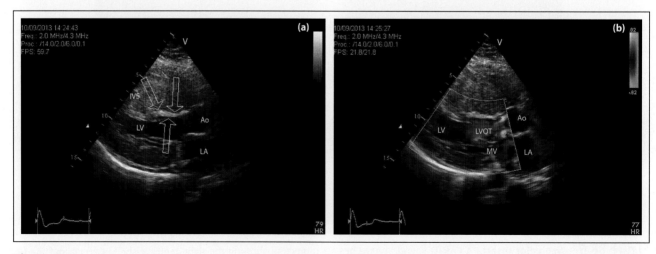

Figure 88.7   **(See color insert.)** A long-axis parasternal TTE during systole 3 years after radio-frequency showing the grossly thickened ventricular septum with recession of the outlet bulge and an area of echogenicity where the ablation took place shown by arrows (a). The LVOT color Doppler shows laminar flow during systole and this was accompanied by a low velocity without a dynamic component (b).

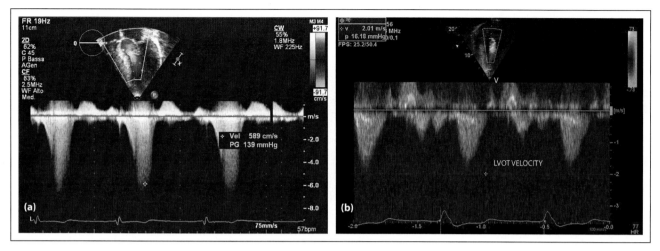

Figure 88.8   **(See color insert.)** A continuous-wave Doppler of the LVOT from the apex showing a velocity of over 6 m/s with a dynamic component (a) and on follow-up with a velocity of 2 m/s without a dynamic trace (b).

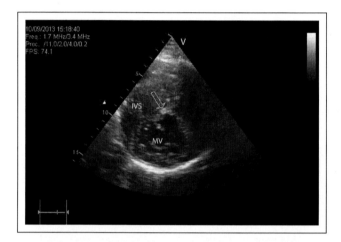

Figure 88.9   The short axis of the LV on TTE shows the excavation created by the radio-frequency as well as the echogenic area at the site of treatment. The usual doughnut appearance is replaced by a pear-shaped LV. The crater and the echogenic area are indicated by an arrow.

inadvertent entry ± radio-frequency application within a coronary artery, heart block (which may require pacing), and ventricular fibrillation.

Results

Since 1998, this procedure has been offered to families with children who have symptoms considered to be secondary to significant LV outflow tract obstruction associated with HOCM. The Birmingham Group, ranging from 4 to 15 years of age, all had left-sided septal reduction (one also had radio-frequency application to the right side of the septum because of bilateral obstruction). Two patients required a second procedure, one after 5 years and another 6.5 years after the original ablation due to gradual recurrence of the

LV outflow tract gradient; these were from the original group when the number of energy applications were far fewer and the irrigation technique had not been used. One patient developed transient heart block and this lasted more than 48 h. As this patient had shown benefit with short AV pacing, it was decided to implant a permanent dual-chamber pacemaker, but the heart block resolved. One patient developed two episodes of ventricular fibrillation during the procedure, one during catheter manipulation and one during application of radio-frequency energy responding to a DC shock each time. Two patients developed left bundle branch block, with no consequence other than potential enhancement of gradient relief. One patient developed a large groin hematoma needing two extra days in hospital, but there was no need for active intervention.

The largest series was published in 2011 from Cologne and Birmingham[5] where 32 children received radio-frequency ablation in the age range of 2.9–17.5 years (median 11.1 years). In this group, the number of energy applications ranged from 10 to 63, with a median of 27. The Doppler gradient prior to the procedure was a mean of 96.9 ± 27 mmHg and once the full effect of the ablation had occurred this dropped to a mean of 32.7 ± 27.1 mmHg ($p < 0.01$). In this group, there was one death, probably due to worsening of an already severe gradient due to the edema cause by the ablations, and one patient with subsequent AV block requiring permanent pacing. The follow-up ranged from 3 to 144 months (median 48). There was an 87.5% freedom from intervention at 10 year follow-up.

Role of radio-frequency

This technique is being increasingly used, particularly in children and young adults, but it has also been used in adults who have failed or have a contraindication to

TASH.[10] While surgery is still an option, this is invasive and not without risk; moreover, remodeling and perhaps limited surgical opportunity for optimal resection in children contributes to the recurrence rate.[11] Recurrence can occur as the condition is progressive and this is more likely to take place in growing children although remarkably 87.5% were free from further intervention at 10 years. The procedure can, however, be repeated if necessary. The experience in adults is limited, mainly as TASH is the treatment of choice and this is feasible in the majority of patients. The difficulties to overcome in adults include good catheter contact and stability, being able to reach all areas of the septal bulge and being able to administer enough energy to cover a larger area than in children. Experience and better mapping has evolved the technique into a more aggressive approach with improved results. If the technique continues to show promise, less symptomatic patients may be considered for treatment on the basis of risk stratification.[12]

The introduction of CARTO Sound not only helps in creating an anatomical replica of the outflow obstruction and its relationship to surrounding structures, for example, the aortic and mitral valves, but it can also be used to identify the position of the His-Purkinje system and create a target area for radio-frequency ablation. Moreover, this modality allows for the procedure to be carried out under conscious sedation if the patient is large enough to have ICE instead of TOE. An additional modality of some radio-frequency catheters is to monitor the pressure being applied to the tissue on contact; this is due to pressure sensors present at the tip, for example, in the CARTO Smart Touch® catheters.

An extension of this technique is envisaged for muscular infundibular stenosis, such as that associated with Fallot's tetralogy, and this could form part of an interventional repair for the condition in selected patients or in patients who develop a recurrence of the muscular obstruction after repair. This is work in progress.

References

1. Maron MS, Olivotto I, Betocchi S et al. Effect of left ventricular outflow tract obstruction on clinical outcome in hypertrophic cardiomyopathy. *N Engl J Med* 2003;348(4):295–303.
2. Elliott PM, Gimeno JR, Tome' MT et al. Left ventricular outflow tract obstruction and sudden death risk in patients with hypertrophic cardiomyopathy. *Eur Heart J* 2006; 27(16):1933–41.
3. Sigwart U. Non-surgical myocardial reduction for hypertrophic obstructive cardiomyopathy. *Lancet* 1995;346(8969):211–4.
4. Armistead SH, Williams BT. Hypertrophic cardiomyopathy. The use of a diathermy loop for septal resection. *J Cardiovasc Surg* 1984;25(2):185–6.
5. Dalvi B. Percutaneous radiofrequency ablation of the left bundle branch: An alternative modality of treatment for patients with hypertrophic cardiomyopathy. *Med Hypotheses* 1994;43(3):141–4.
6. Emmel M, Sreeram N, De Giovanni JV, Brockmeier K. Radiofrequency catheter septal ablation for hypertrophic obstructive cardiomyopathy in childhood. *Z Kardiol* 2005;94(10):699–703.
7. Sreeram N, Emmel M, DeGiovanni JV. Percutaneous radiofrequency septal reduction for hypertrophic obstructive cardiomyopathy in children. *J Am Coll Cardiol* 2011; 58(24):2501–10.
8. Lawrenz T, Kuhn H. Endocardial radiofrequency ablation of septal hypertrophy. A new catheter-based modality of gradient reduction in hypertrophic obstructive cardiomyopathy. *Z Kardiol* 2004;93(6):493–9.
9. Rishi F, Hulse JE, Auld DO et al. Effect of dual chamber pacing for pediatric patients with hypertrophic obstructive cardiomyopathy. *J Am Coll Cardiol* 1997 Mar15;29(4):734–740.
10. Riedlbauchova L, Janousek J, Veselka J Ablation of hypertrophic septum using radiofrequency energy—An alternative for gradient reduction in patient with hypertrophic obstructive cardiomyopathy? *J Invasive Cardiol* 2013;25(6):E128–132.
11. Minakata K, Dearani JA, O'Leary PW et al Septal myectomy for obstructive hypertrophic cardiomyopathy in pediatric patients: Early and late results. *Ann Thorac Surg* 2005;80(4):1424–9.
12. McKenna WJ, Behr ER. Hypertrophic cardiomyopathy; management, risk stratification and prevention of sudden death. *Heart* 2002;87(2):169–176.

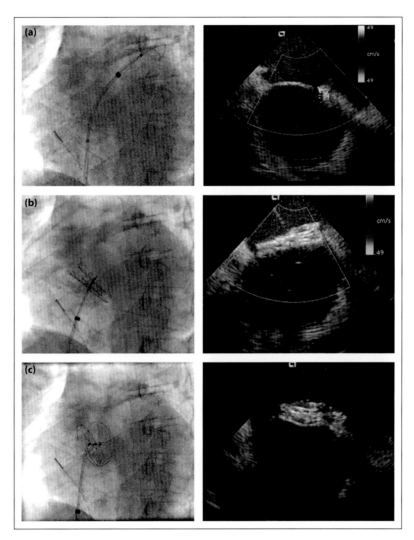

Figure 60.9 Fluoroscopic and intracardiac echo images of the key steps in deployment of the Gore Septal Occluder in a secundum ASD. (a) With the delivery catheter in the left atrium, the device is advanced configuring the left disk first. (b) The device is then drawn back to the septum, and the right disk deployed. (c) The device is then locked and released using the delivery handle. It is normal to see the device realign as it is liberated from the delivery catheter.

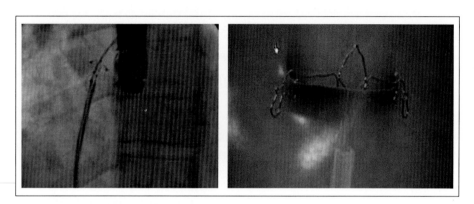

Figure 63.5   Distal anchors open into the left atrium.

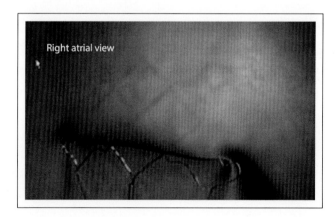

Figure 63.6   Proximal anchors open into the right atrium.

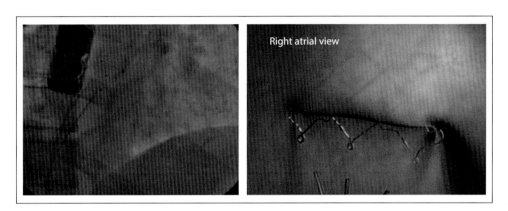

Figure 63.7 CoherexFlatStent EF detached.

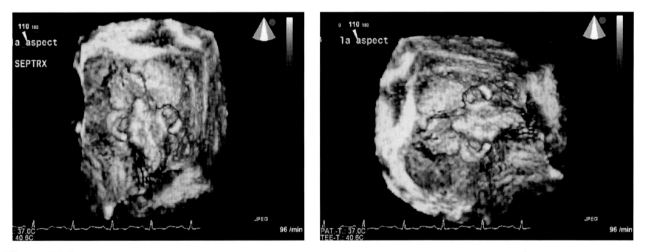

Figure 64.8 3D TEE image: Long-axis view, view from the left atrium to the interatrial septum 3 months after implantation.

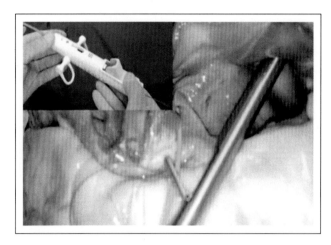

Figure 65.2 The NobleStitch secundum suture-carrying arm being opened in the right atrium with distal tip in the SVC.

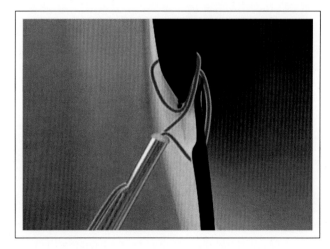

Figure 65.6 The NobleStitch KwiKnot over the 3-0 polypropylene suture forming the "S"-shaped suture that will pull the primum septum into the tunnel forming a "valve-like" effect, closing the tunnel, and eliminating right-to-left shunting.

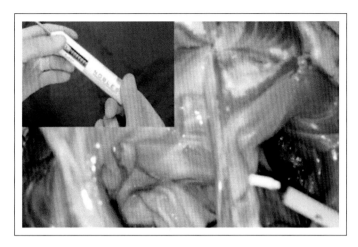

Figure 65.8 The KwiKnot deploying the polypropylene suture knot in the right atrium.

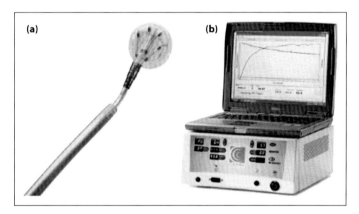

Figure 66.1 PFx Closure System. (a) Radio-frequency electrode, (b) radio-frequency generator. (Courtesy of Cierra, Redwood City, CA, USA.)

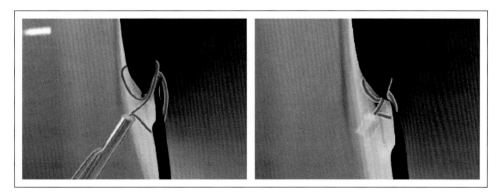

Figure 66.4 NobleStitch suture-mediated PFO closure.

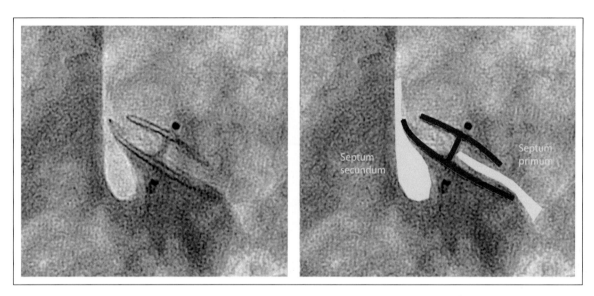

Figure 67.1 Misplaced Amplatzer PFO occluder. The device is anchored in the PFO tunnel, but does not grasp the septum secundum due to a malpositioned right atrial disk at the antero-superior aspect. Potential consequences include device embolization and an increased risk for a significant residual shunt.

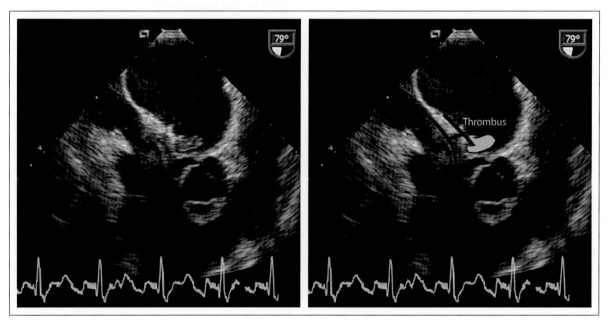

Figure 67.2 Thrombus on the left atrial disk 3 weeks after implantation of an Amplatzer PFO occluder, successfully treated with temporary anticoagulation for 6 months.

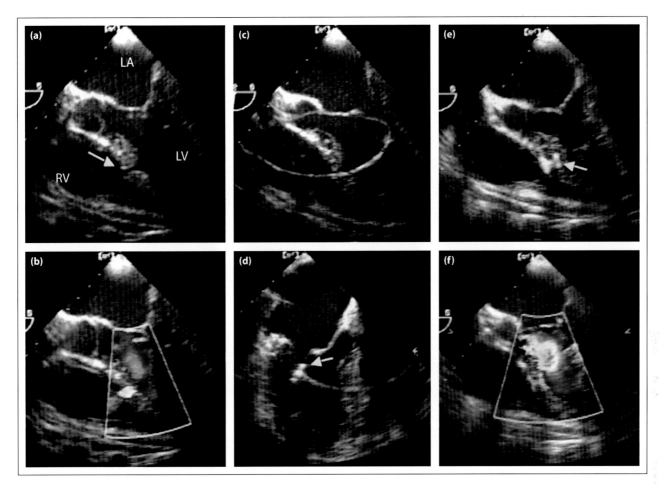

Figure 69.2 Transesophageal echocardiographic images in modified four-chamber views in a 31-year-old male patient with a 5 mm anterior muscular VSD and left-to-right shunt. (a) View demonstrating the VSD (arrow). LV: left ventricle; RV: right ventricle; LA: left atrium. (b) Similar view to (a) with color Doppler demonstrating the shunt. (c) View demonstrating the arteriovenous wire loop (from the aorta, left ventricle, VSD, right ventricle, and out the jugular vein). (d) Deployment of the LV disk of a 6 mm Amplatzer muscular VSD device in mid-LV cavity (arrow). (e) The device has been released (arrow) in the ventricular septum. Note for an adult, the connecting waist is not long enough, but it achieves closure. (f) Final image with color Doppler demonstrating good device position and no residual shunt.

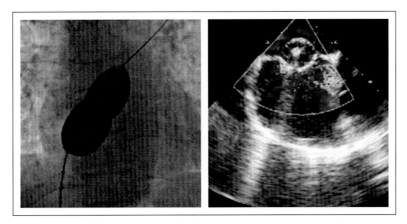

Figure 70.2 Balloon sizing of the defect by fluoroscopy/transesophageal echocardiography (TEE) for measuring the stretched diameter of the atrial septal defect.

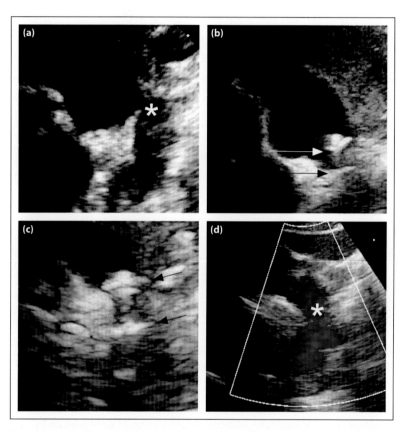

Figure 73.3 Echocardiography-guided placement of an ADO IIAS device in an infant. (a) A moderate-sized duct is assessed at the beginning of the procedure for suitability for device closure, device size, and device type. The constriction of the duct at the pulmonary end measures 3 mm. There is sufficient ductal length to place a device without risking protrusion of the device into the aorta or causing left pulmonary artery obstruction. (b) An ADO IIAS 5/4 device has been uncovered within the duct. The device is not suitably placed, with the pulmonary disk of the device (white arrow) protruding into the main pulmonary artery and the aortic disk (black arrow) deployed within the duct. (c) The device has been repositioned and its position is now appropriate, with both disks clearly seen on echocardiography (black and blue arrows). The device has been correctly sized with constriction from the duct on the central waist of the device (between the two arrows). (d) Before and following device release, careful assessment of the aorta and left pulmonary artery is performed to ensure no obstruction and that the device has been placed correctly. There is no flow turbulence on color-flow Doppler in the aortic isthmus (*).

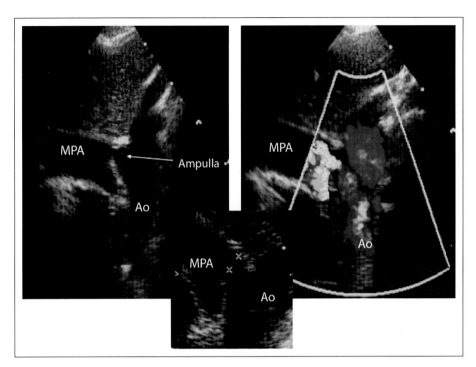

Figure 75.2   Echo definition of the patent ductus arteriosus. This is a high left parasternal view (ductal view) obtained in an infant. The duct insertion as well as the ampulla is clearly defined. Measurement of the duct insertion site is made in the magnified view (bottom insert). Note the retrograde flow of blood in the color Doppler picture (right). MPA, main pulmonary artery; Ao, aorta. (Also available online at http://www.crcpress.com/product/ISBN/9781482215632, under "Downloads/Updates.")

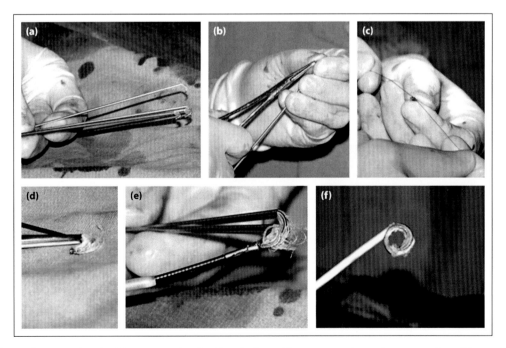

Figure 75.4   Coil preparation for bioptome-assisted coil occlusion. This sequence shows the preparation of four coils for simultaneous deployment in a 6 mm duct. The deployment sequence is shown in Figure 75.5. A small segment of each coil is brought out of the steel tubing (a). The ends of the coil are stretched out using a hemostat (b). The stretched-out ends are secured together using a 3-0-prolene suture (c and d). A 5 F bioptome is passed through a short (8 F) introducer (e), the secured end of the coil is held by the jaws of the bioptome and pulled into the introducer (f). (Also available online at http://www.crcpress.com/product/ISBN/9781482215632, under "Downloads/Updates.")

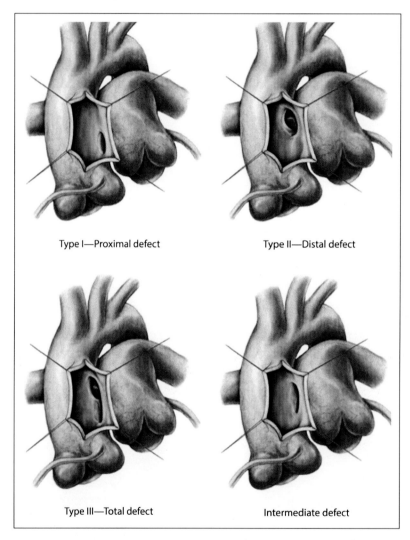

Type I—Proximal defect Type II—Distal defect

Type III—Total defect Intermediate defect

Figure 76.1 Classification of aortopulmonary windows. (Reprinted from *Eur J Cardiovasc Surg*, 21, Backer CL, Mavroudis C., Surgical management of aortopulmonary window: A 40 year experience, 773–9, Copyright 2002, with permission from Elsevier.)

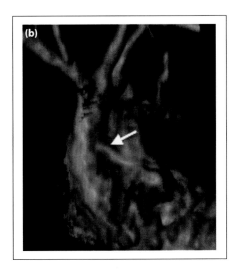

Figure 76.3 (b) A 3D reconstruction magnetic resonance image of the same patient showing the window (arrow). This patient was suitable for transcatheter device closure.

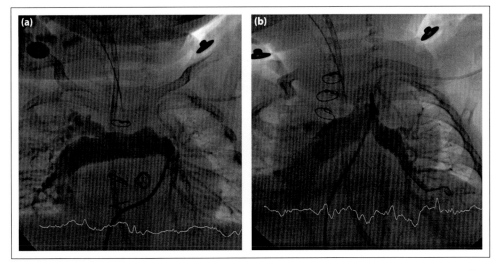

Figure 82.3 (a) Cranial angulation fails to demonstrate the proximal left pulmonary artery stenosis because of opacification of the dilated main pulmonary artery on this pulmonary arteriogram. (b) Caudal and slightly LAO angulation demonstrates the proximal left pulmonary artery stenosis much better.

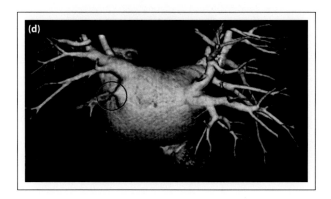

Figure 83.4 (d) This is a volume-rendered image of an isolated LLPV stenosis (red circle) after attempted radio-frequency ablation for atrial fibrillation.

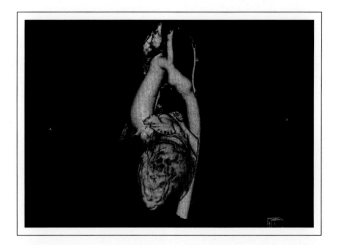

Figure 84.3 Two aneurysms detected by routine imaging of the aortic arch one year after balloon dilation of coarctation. These are mild lesions, being managed conservatively.

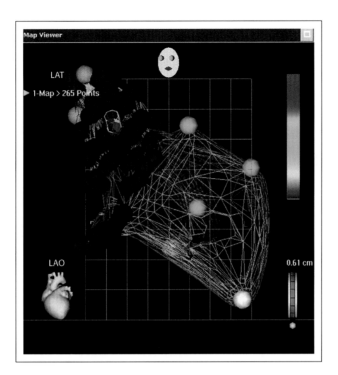

Figure 88.3 A CARTO electro-anatomical map of the left ventricle in LAO projection showing His signal position in yellow, site of radio-frequency energy application on the septal bulge in red, and the mitral valve demarcated by blue.

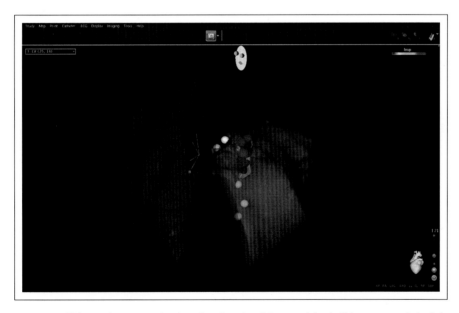

Figure 88.6 A CARTO Sound® image in LAO projection showing the right ventricle shell in green and the left ventricle in gray. The area of septal bulge causing obstruction is highlighted by a pink area and the red dots indicate the sites where radio-frequency was applied. The blue dots indicate the sites where a His signal was identified during mapping. (Courtesy of Drs. Simon Modi and Rob Cooper.)

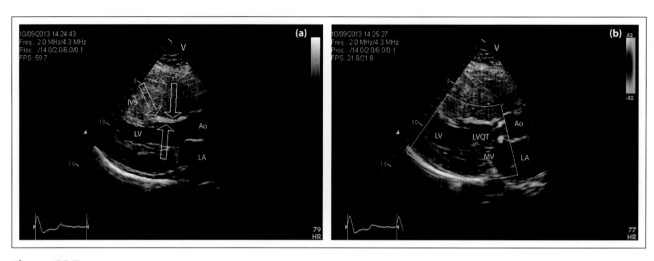

Figure 88.7 The LVOT color Doppler shows laminar flow during systole and this was accompanied by a low velocity without a dynamic component (b).

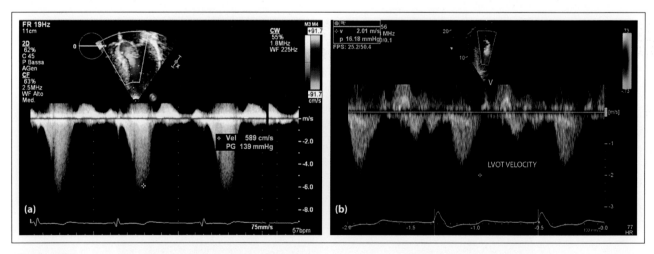

Figure 88.8 A continuous-wave Doppler of the LVOT from the apex showing a velocity of over 6 m/s with a dynamic component (a) and on follow-up with a velocity of 2 m/s without a dynamic trace (b).

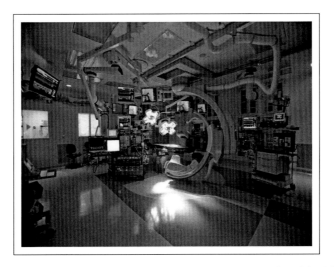

Figure 90.3 A photograph of the specially designed hybrid OR at the Heart Center, Nationwide Children's Hospital.

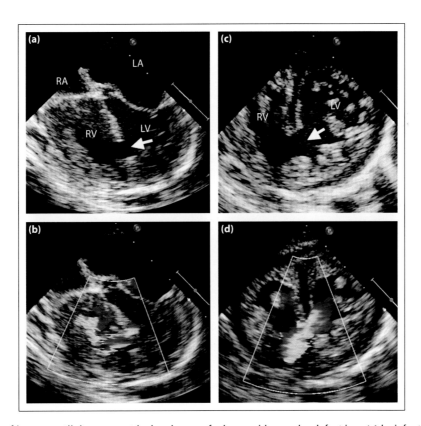

Figure 92.1 Series of images outlining perventricular closure of a large midmuscular defect in a 4.1 kg infant. TEE assessment of the midmuscular defect in two different planes (a and c) with and without color Doppler (b and d).

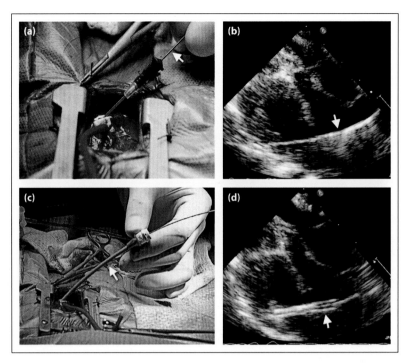

Figure 92.2 Advancement of the wire (a, b) and the sheath (c, d) across the defect.

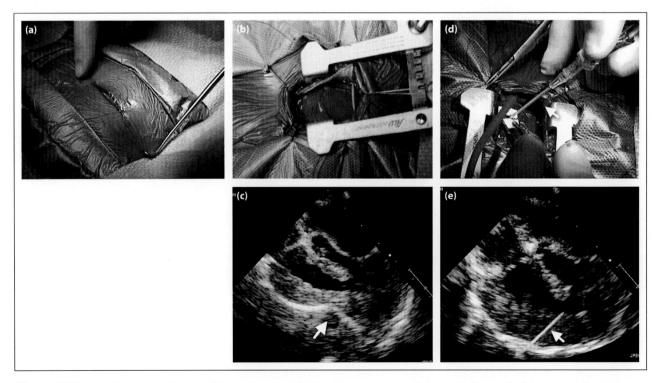

Figure 92.3 (a, b) Sternal and pericardial opening. (c) Digital pressure seen transmitted to the free wall of the RV to define puncture site. (d, e) Needle puncture of the RV with corresponding TEE image.

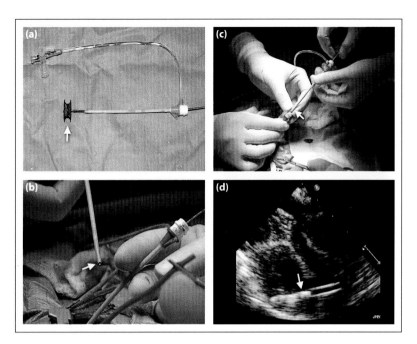

Figure 92.4 Loading the device through a short delivery sheath (a, b) and advancement of the device through the preexisting per-ventricular sheath to the LV.

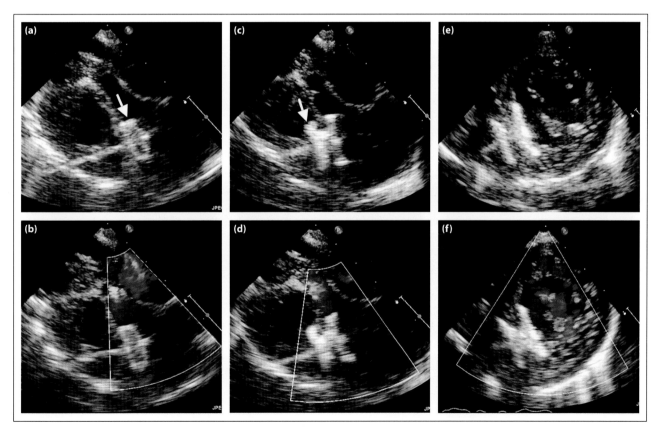

Figure 92.5 Deployment of the left ventricular disk with color assessment on TEE (a, b), following full device deployment (c, d) and following release (e, f).

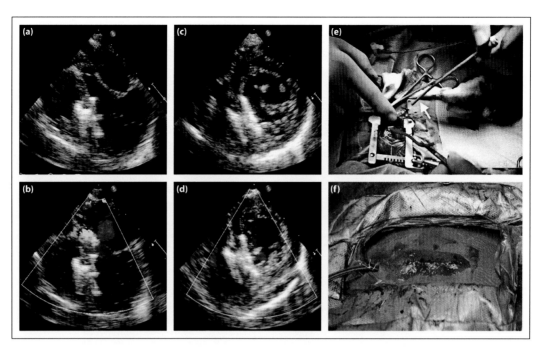

Figure 92.6 Final assessment of the device in two separate planes with no residual leak seen on color Doppler (a–d). Chest closure with sutured wound and chest drain (e, f).

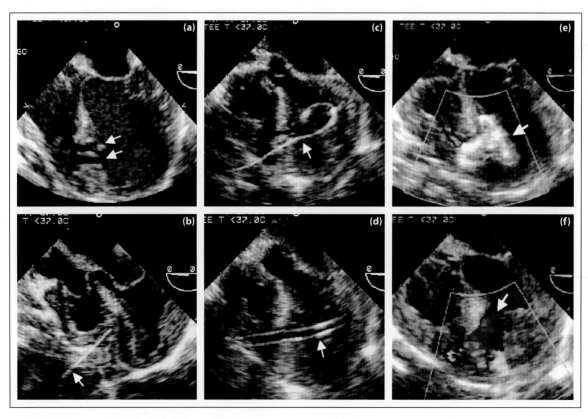

Figure 92.7 Series of TEE and fluoroscopic images demonstrating perventricular closure of two midmuscular VSDs. (a) Initial imaging defines the two defects with needle puncture (b) and crossing of the more inferior defect (c). Advancement of the delivery sheath (d) with device delivery (e) however persisting flow through the separate defect.

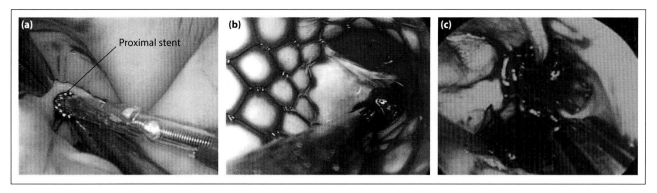

Figure 93.3 (a) Prior to inflation of the balloon, the proximal stent is positioned using videoscopic guidance to cover the most proximal portion of the stenosis. The suction tip (*) is used to stabilize the pulmonary artery during positioning. (b) After stent expansion, apposition to vessel wall as well as position in relation to side branch takeoff (*) are examined. (c) Final result of "adult-sized kissing stents" placed in the 6-month-old seen in Figure 93.1.

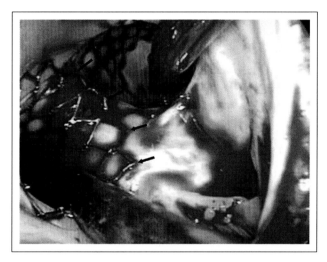

Figure 93.4 Following implantation of left (LPA) and right (RPA) proximal branch pulmonary artery stents, the proximal struts (arrows) of the RPA stent have been flared by the surgeon to facilitate future catheter passage in the RPA as well as limit the cutting effect these struts could have on future angioplasty balloons in the proximal LPA.

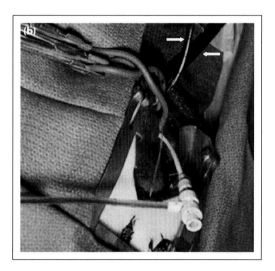

Figure 93.5 Diagrammatic representation (a) and digital photo (b) of sheath placement via an incision into a right ventricle–pulmonary artery homograft conduit of a patient with severe early pulmonary artery stenosis after complete repair of pulmonary atresia and ventricular septal defect. Note the arterial and venous cannulas (white arrows) required to perform this intervention on cardiopulmonary support.

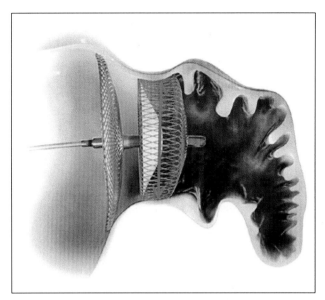

Figure 95.6 The landing zone of the ACP has to ensure that the entire lobe is within the LAA and well anchored. Ideally, albeit not always possible as depicted on the figure, the landing zone for the entire lobe is within the neck of the LAA (green arrow). However, depending on the anatomy, sometimes the lobe will not be perpendicular to the neck axis and reside partially within one of the lobes of the LAA. (Courtesy of St. Jude Medical.)

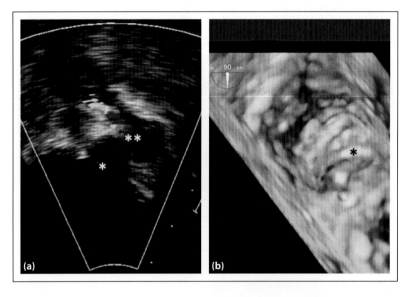

Figure 95.10 Thrombus on the ACP. (a) 2-D TEE image showing a small thrombus on the screw of the disk (*). The ACP does not cover one of the small lobes of the LAA, resulting in a considerable residual shunt (**). If such a large residual shunt persists, implantation of a second ACP or a different device (e.g., Amplatzer Vascular Plug) can be considered. (b) Thrombus on the ACP screw depicted on 3-D TEE (*).

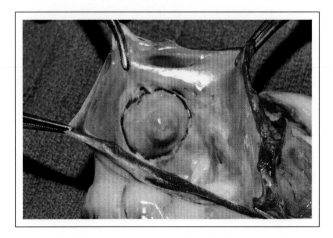

Figure 97.2 180 day animal model with well-endothelialized Coherex LAA occluder.

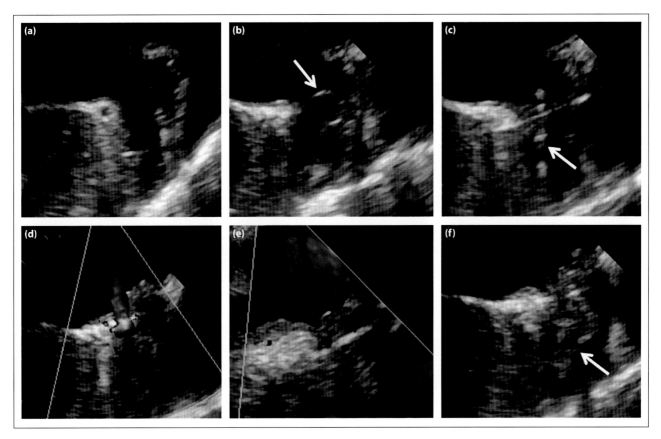

Figure 98.3 Transesophageal echocardiography (TEE) assessment of LAA closure. TEE imaging LAA at baseline (a) and during the placement of the balloon (arrow) at the orifice of the LAA (b). Closure of the LARIAT snare closes the orifice of the LAA around the EndoCATH (arrow) (c). Color Doppler is used to verify the acute closure of the LAA following ligation of the LAA. There is a leak following hand tightening of the suture (d), which disappears following suture tightening with the TenSure device (e). At the end, the LAA is closed and collapsed (arrow), which creates a space within the pericardial cavity (f).

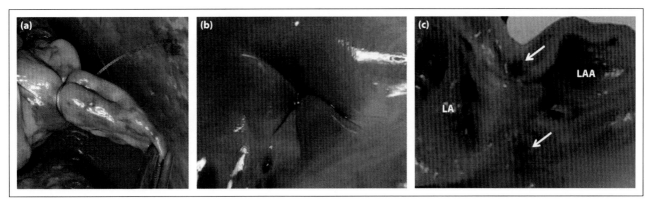

Figure 98.4 Gross anatomy of an LAA following LAA ligation. Examination of the previously ligated LAA during mitral valve replacement taken from the explanted heart of a patient undergoing heart transplantation. Gross examination of the LAA reveals an atretic LAA (a) with a smooth endocardial surface (b). The glutaraldehyde fixed tissue was then sectioned through the suture ligation (c). The blue sutures (arrow) are still present delineating a completely closed closure line, thus resulting in complete exclusion of the LAA. LA, left atrium; LAA, left atrial appendage.

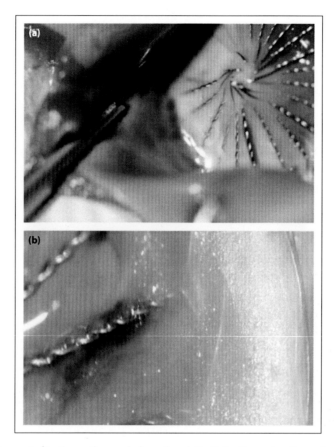

Figures 99.2   (a,b) Cardiac harvest after 1 month revealed good endothelialization using the endocardial device for LAA closure.

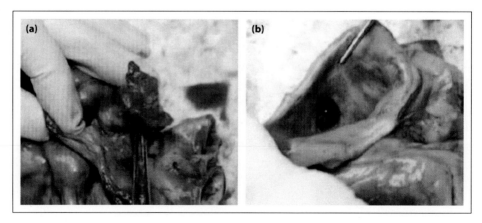

Figure 99.5   (a,b) The first in vitro examination of the Occlutech™ device demonstrates a good fixation and adaption to the tissue.

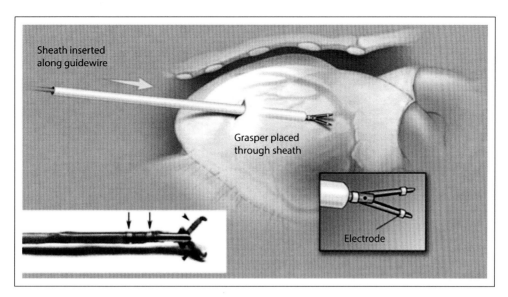

Figure 99.7   The AEGIS system.

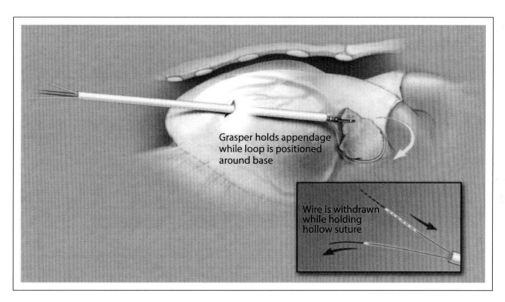

Figure 99.8   The second part of the AEGIS system, the ligator or hollow suture.

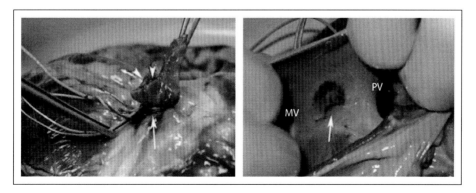

Figure 99.9   Thoracotomy findings after LAA closure with the hollow suture.

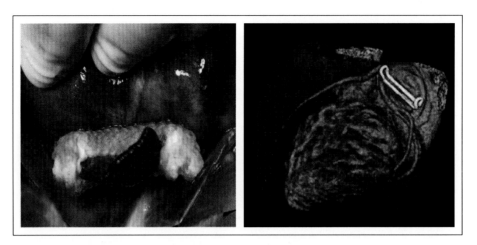

Figure 99.10 The AtriClip system right after placement and on a CT scan.

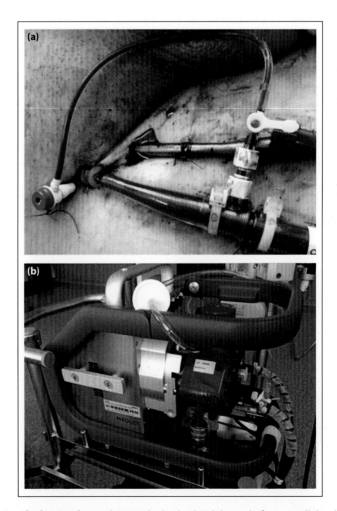

Figure 100.1 (a) Puncture site of a femoro-femoral ECMO device in the right groin from medial to lateral: venous inflow cannula in the common femoral vein, arterial outflow cannula in the common femoral artery, antegrade access sheath in the superficial femoral artery for distal perfusion oft the right leg supplied by a little bypass from the arterial ECMO outflow cannula. (b) CardioHelp core unit with the centrifugal pump and the red-colored gas exchange membrane. (Courtesy of Maquet GmbH und Co. KG, Rastatt, Germany.)

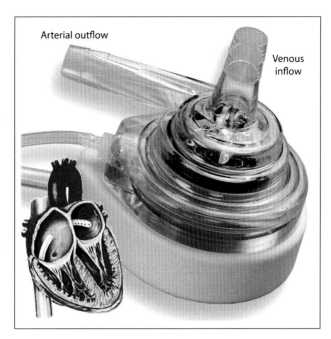

Figure 100.3 The centrifugal pump of the TandemHeart system. The venous inflow tract of the pump is connected to the venous inflow cannula, which is introduced into the left atrium after transseptal puncture. (Figure modified after CardiacAssist Inc., Pittsburgh, Pennsylvania, USA.)

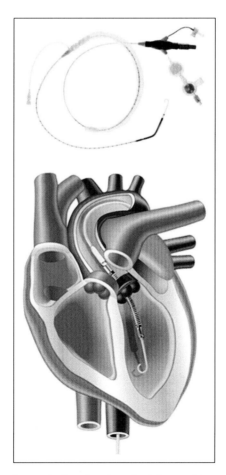

Figure 100.4 The catheter-mounted Impella 2.5 device placed in the left ventricle across the aortic valve. (Figure modified after Abiomed Inc., Danvers, Massachusetts, USA.)

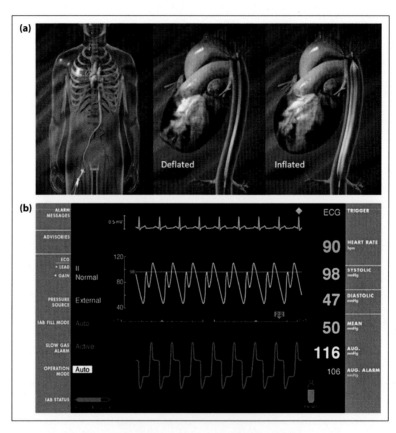

Figure 100.5 (a) Position of the IABP device within the descending aorta. (b) Early-diastolic augmentation (116 mmHg) on balloon inflation immediately following the systolic peak (98 mmHg) before rapid balloon deflation facilitates a decrease of end-diastolic aortic pressure (47 mmHg). (Figure modified after Maquet GmbH und Co. KG, Rastatt, Germany.)

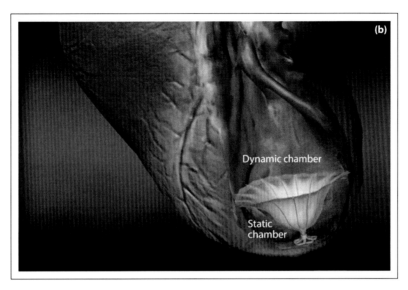

Figure 101.1 (b) The VPD positioned in the aneurysmal apex of the LV. The device has 16 nitinol struts that insert into the endocardium and is covered by an ePTFE membrane. The VPD partitions the ventricle into dynamic and static chambers.

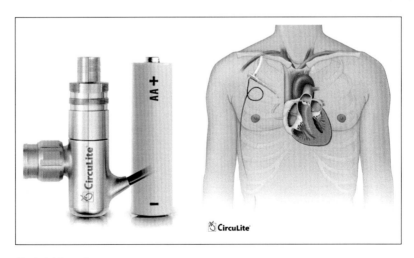

Figure 102.1 Synergy Pocket Micro-Pump.

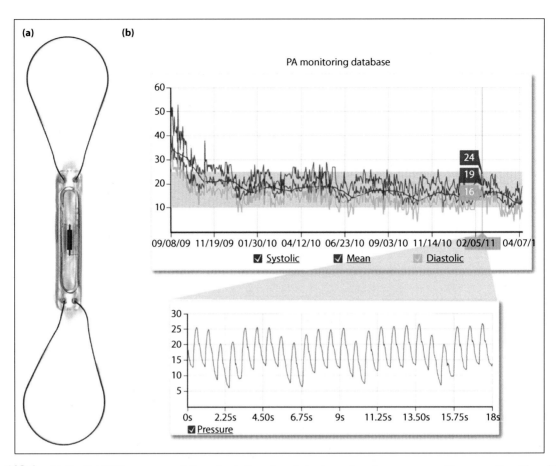

Figure 103.1 (a) CardioMEMS sensor consisting of a battery-free inductor coil and pressure-sensitive capacitor. The nitinol wire loops maintain the device position in a ~10 mm vessel, ensuring unobstructed flow around sensor. (b) High-fidelity pulmonary artery pressure trend with specific waveform. This information is displayed on a secure website accessed by clinicians. (Reproduced with permission from CardioMEMS Inc, Atlanta, Georgia.)

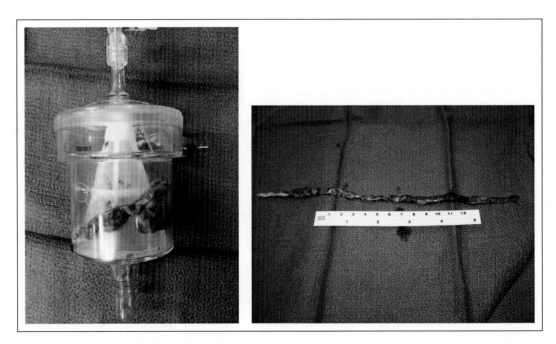

Figure 105.1 A large, chronic thrombus removed from the right atrium via vacuum-assisted catheter retrieval concomitantly with PICC line removal.

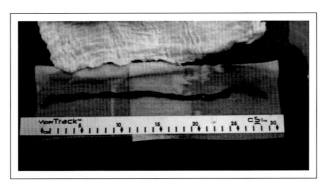

Figure 105.2 A large pulmonary embolism in transit removed using AngioVac catheter retrieval techniques.

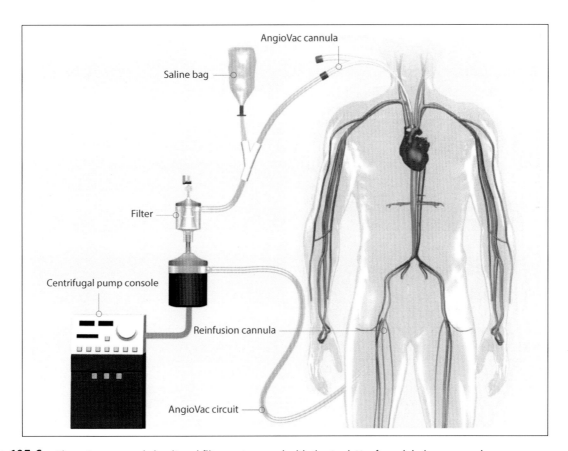

Figure 105.6 The extracorporeal circuit and filter system used with the AngioVac funnel drainage cannula.

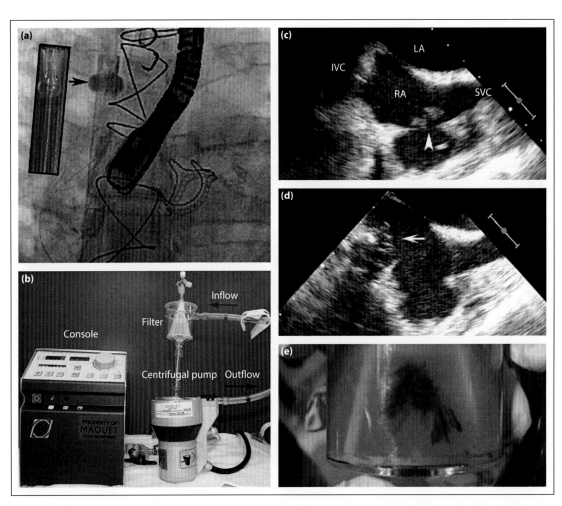

Figure 105.7 Use of the AngioVac platform to remove an infected right atrial vegetation. (a) Insertion of AngioVac cannula under fluoroscopic guidance with the balloon tip inflated (arrow). (b) The circuit consists of a console, filter, centrifugal pump, and standard bypass tubing. The aspirated blood from the AngioVac cannula (inflow) is filtered and then returned to the patient (outflow). (c) TEE demonstrates right atrial mass (arrowhead) before extraction. RA, right atrium; LA, left atrium; SVC, superior vena cava; IVC, inferior vena cava. (d) TEE of the right atrium after mass extraction with the cannula (arrow) in the inferior vena cava. (e) Filter is shown containing the extracted vegetation. (Adapted from Todoran TM, Sobieszczyk P. *Progr Cardiovasc Dis* 2010;52:429–37.)

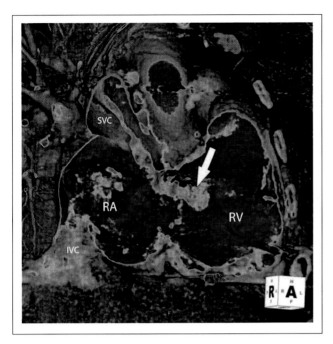

Figure 105.8 A large, mobile mass in the right atrium that tracked up to the superior vena cava and prolapsed into the right ventricle seen on three-dimensional computerized tomography. (Adapted from Todoran TM et al. *J Vasc Interv Radiol* 2011;22(9).)

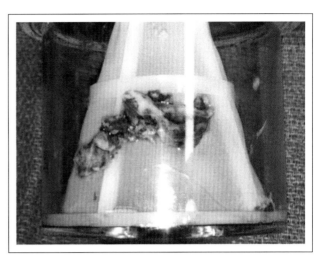

Figure 105.11 Tricuspid valve vegetation after percutaneous catheter retrieval.

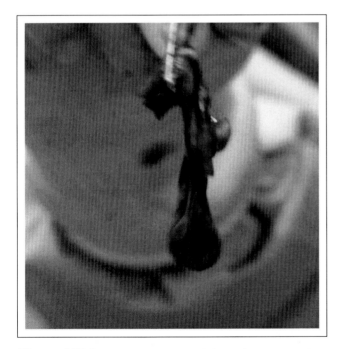

Figure 105.9 Thrombus removed from the same patient using the AngioVac device. (Adapted from Todoran TM et al. *J Vasc Interv Radiol* 2011;22(9).)

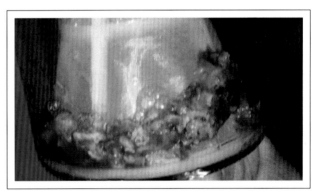

Figure 105.16 Infected vegetation within the filter trap. (Adapted from Pillai JB et al. *Innovations* 2012;7(1):59−61.)

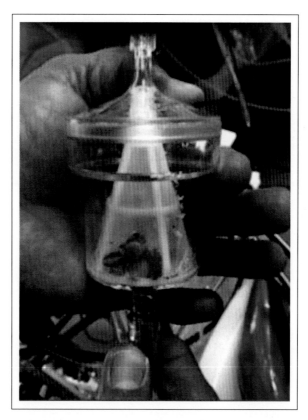

Figure 105.17   A right atrial thrombus retrieved from a PFO closure device. (Adapted from Patel N et al. *J Card Surg* 2013;20:1–4.)

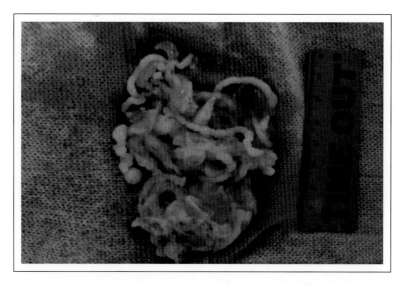

Figure 105.18   An intracardiac tumor removed percutaneously using flow-directed catheter retrieval (AngioVac).

Thoracic aortic aneurysms

Jose Pablo Morales and John Reidy

Introduction

The natural history of untreated descending thoracic aneurysms (DTA) includes progressive expansion, increasing risk of rupture, and ultimately death, usually from rupture of the aneurysm. The 1-year and 5-year actuarial survival rates for patients not operated on had been estimated to be 60% and 20%, respectively.[1] The yearly risk of any occurrence of rupture, dissection, or death in a patient with a thoracic aneurysm >6 cm in diameter is over 14%.[2] As is the case with abdominal aortic aneurysms, the risk of rupture for thoracic aneurysms increases with size, and the 5-year rupture rate is fivefold higher for aneurysms >6 cm in diameter.[3] Because of the risk of lethal rupture, all patients with DTA should be evaluated for potential operative repair. Surgical indications include an urgent operation in symptomatic patients who present with signs of rupture, chest or back pain, hemoptysis, hematemesis, or cardiovascular collapse. In asymptomatic patients, risk/benefit analysis in a large population study supports that for thoracic aneurysms >6.5 cm be repaired electively, with the threshold for Marfan's disease or familial DTAs being >6 cm[2]; therefore, most aneurysms get repaired when they reach 5.5 and 5.0 cm[2], respectively. The latter is done in order to mitigate any risk of aneurysm rupture.

Traditionally, open surgical repair of DTAs involves aortic graft replacement via a left thoracotomy and has been found to improve survival when compared with medical therapy.[4] Despite dramatic advances in the technical expertise for performing these complex thoracic aortic operations using distal perfusion methods and spinal cord protection, open surgery remains a high-risk endeavor, especially given the frequent comorbid cardiovascular and pulmonary disease.[5] The operative mortality rates from centers of excellence are reported between 8% and 20% for elective cases and up to 60% for emergency operations.[6,7] Survivors of open repair of thoracic aneurysms further suffer from morbidity rates of up to 50% related to renal, intestinal, and spinal cord ischemia that substantially limit functional recovery and long-term

survival, with recent 5-year survival rates reported to be about 60–70%.[8,9]

The use of endovascular stent grafts has revolutionized the management of thoracic aortic pathologies since first reported in 1988 by Volodos et al.[10] Thoracic endovascular aneurysm repair (TEVAR) is considered safe and effective in preventing aneurysm rupture through short and intermediate-term follow-up studies; and long-term studies have started to become published. The ascribed benefits of such treatment options center on the lack of the need for a thoracotomy, extensive tissue dissection, and aortic cross-clamping. The acute physiologic insult is much less compared with open surgery, allowing patients considered too ill for traditional surgery to be treated and lessening the risk of morbidity and mortality for those who are candidates for either type of repair.[11]

To date, four second-generation thoracic endograft devices such as Valiant (Medtronics), TX-2 (Cook), TAG (Gore), and Relay (Bolton) have been mainly used, although these manufacturers have continued to modify and improve their devices with more sizes becoming available and in smaller delivery systems.

Symptoms

Most patients with aortic aneurysms have no symptoms attributable to the aneurysm when first diagnosed,[12] explaining why the diagnosis of aneurysms, particularly thoracic, are rarely made on physical examination. It is estimated that before an acute event, 95% of DTAs are asymptomatic. As a result, most aneurysms are detected incidentally through imaging for an unrelated problem (e.g., a computed tomography [CT] scan for a lung nodule). The only common presenting symptom is vague chest pain. The pain may increase steadily as the aneurysm enlarges, or the patient may experience a sudden, sharp pain due to rapid expansion and impending rupture. Occasionally, the aneurysm might compress or erode into adjacent structures, yielding diagnostic clues such as hoarseness, tracheal deviation, hemoptysis, dysphagia, hematemesis, or neurologic and musculoskeletal complaints. Superior vena cava syndrome can also occur secondary to expanding thoracic aneurysm.

Preprocedure imaging

Endovascular aneurysm repair requires a far more detailed assessment than is necessary for open surgery. This is necessary to plan the procedure and to assess the length and diameter of the devices needed. Until recently, CT and angiography were required for the full assessment of aneurysms. CT allows the physician to measure the maximum diameter of the aneurysm, wall thickness, and also to measure the diameters of the aneurysm necks and other landmarks. CT allows the measurement of the diameter of the normal aorta on either side of the aneurysm, which is necessary to plan the endovascular procedure and to select an adequate device size. More sophisticated multislice (MS) CT scans with 3D reconstructions are extremely helpful to assess the aneurysm morphology and can accurately measure aneurysm length and dimensions. Although MS CT scans produce excellent quality pictures, there is a concern, particularly in children, regarding the high x-ray dose and in patients with renal pathology where contrast media is contraindicated. In these cases, magnetic resonance imaging (MRI) and magnetic resonance angiography are used, because they do not utilize ionizing radiation and provide detailed vascular imaging without the use of iodinated contrast media.

Assessment

There are three areas of particular importance in endovascular stent-grafting:

1. *Access:* The currently available 24–46 mm devices can be introduced via 21–28 Fr sheaths. Diseased and tortuous iliac arteries may prevent passage of the delivery system. Endovascular stent-grafting is contraindicated in patients with iliac artery diameter less than 8 mm, tortuosity with more than one >90° angulation, and with heavy calcification. In these cases, an iliac conduit can be performed prior to the endovascular procedure.
2. *Anchorage sites:* Suitable lengths for the proximal and distal stents are normally ≥2 cm in order to enable adequate seal. It is contraindicated when the proximal neck length is less than 1.5 cm, proximal neck angulation ≥60°, and when a tapering neck is present.
3. *Adequate cerebral blood supply:* The graft material of the stent-graft must not cover vital arteries such as the left common carotid artery or innominate artery.

Anesthesia

The anesthesia of choice for endovascular repair of aortic aneurysms in adults is the epidural, as it is easy to

identify any neurological and visceral complications. If the patient develops paraplegia, insertion of cerebrospinal fluid (CSF) drain must urgently be considered. However, general anesthesia is the method of choice in children.

Procedure technique

Arterial access for the devices is usually via a right common femoral arteriotomy (CFA). Unfractionated heparin (adult dose 5000 units) and prophylactic antibiotics are given intravenously before insertion of the delivery sheath. A contralateral percutaneous femoral puncture is used for an angiographic catheter (5 Fr) as well as for the initial angiography to give an overview of the aneurysm. The device is inserted over an extra stiff 0.035 inch guide wire (Lunderquist®; Cook Inc., Bloomington, IN, USA) and advanced through the aortic lumen. The device is oversized by a minimum of 10% relative to the normal aorta at the fixation sites, and deployed in the optimal position with a minimum of 2 cm of normal aorta proximal and distal to achieve a good seal. The positioning of the graft is achieved under digital subtraction angiography and the planning CT or MRI scans enable the optimum angulation to be chosen to demonstrate the aorta. The origin of the left subclavian artery may be covered when necessary to achieve a good seal of the stent-graft. However, the Society for Vascular Surgery (SVS)[13] recommends surgical reconstruction of the left subclavian artery in the following scenarios: (1) In patients who need elective TEVAR where achievement of a proximal seal necessitates coverage of the LSA, (2) in selected patients who have an anatomy that compromises perfusion to critical organs, and (3) in patients who need very urgent TEVAR for life-threatening acute aortic syndromes where achievement of a proximal seal necessitates coverage of the LSA. The SVS suggests that revascularization should be individualized and addressed based on the anatomy, urgency, and availability of surgical expertise. If it is necessary to cover the origin of the left common carotid artery to achieve a good seal, it is then necessary to perform a right-to-left carotid–carotid bypass prior to the stenting. An angiogram is performed on completion of the procedure to confirm adequate placement of the stent-graft and to confirm exclusion of the aneurysm sac.

Basic steps for endovascular procedure

1. Surgical cutdown to access CFA to allow introducer device placement.
2. A 4 Fr or 5 Fr pigtail catheter is placed just proximal to the aneurysm from the contralateral groin.

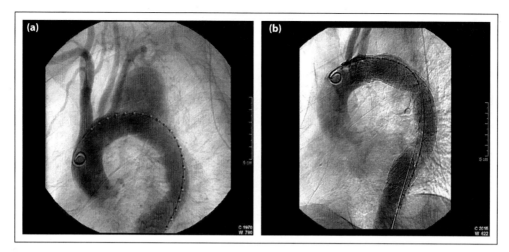

Figure 89.1 (a) Aortography demonstrates a descending thoracic aneurysm proximal to the left subclavian artery. (b) Postprocedure aortography demonstrates successful exclusion of the aneurysm covering the left subclavian artery.

3. Initial angiography performed to give an overview of the aneurysm (Figure 89.1a).
4. Insertion of the delivery system just above the proximal portion of the aneurysm.
5. Magnified angiogram to demonstrate the position of the left common carotid and left subclavian arteries. The table is locked in position.
6. Deploy stent-graft using continuous fluoroscopy.
7. Balloon top and bottom sides of stent, and overlapping joints where there are two or more stents. Ballooning outside the stent-graft should be avoided.
8. Repeat angiogram to confirm satisfactory position of the stent-graft with aneurysm exclusion and to check for endoleaks (Figure 89.1b).

Follow-up

CT or MRI scans should be performed at 6 months (Figure 89.2a) and then yearly thereafter in order to assess aneurysm sac shrinkage (Figure 89.2b and c) as well as detection

of possible device-related complications, such as endoleaks, migration, or stent-fracture.

Conclusion

Proper patient selection and improvements in stent-graft design have allowed an increased number of patients with DTA to be treated endovascularly. The continuous development of these minimally invasive technologies will ultimately allow for the treatment of more complex thoracic aneurysms involving the aortic arch and the ascending aorta.

Disclaimers

The views presented in this chapter do not necessarily reflect those of the Food and Drug Administration. No official support or endorsement of this chapter by the Food and Drug Administration is intended or should be inferred.

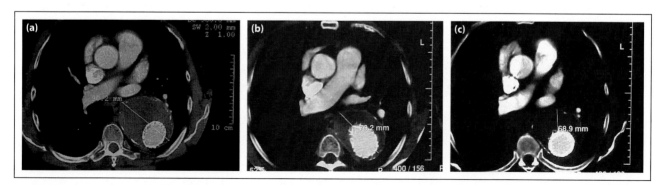

Figure 89.2 (a) Six-month CT scan demonstrates a stent-graft *in situ* with an aneurysm sac measuring 9.02 cm (maximum diameter). (b) One-year CT scan demonstrates a stent-graft *in situ* with an aneurysm sac shrinking and now measuring 7.92 cm (maximum diameter). (c) Two-year CT scan demonstrates a stent-graft *in situ* with an aneurysm sac shrinking and now measuring 6.89 cm (maximum diameter).

References

1. Kouchoukos NT, Dougenis D. Surgery of the thoracic aorta. *N Engl J Med* 1997;336(26):1876–88.
2. Elefteriades JA. Natural history of thoracic aortic aneurysms: Indications for surgery, and surgical versus nonsurgical risks. *Ann Thorac Surg* 2002;74(5):S1877–80.
3. Perko MJ, Norgaard M, Herzog TM, Olsen PS, Schroeder TV, Pettersson G. Unoperated aortic aneurysm: A survey of 170 patients. *Ann Thorac Surg* 1995;59(5):1204–9.
4. Crawford ES, DeNatale RW. Thoracoabdominal aortic aneurysm: Observations regarding the natural course of the disease. *J Vasc Surg* 1986;3(4):578–82.
5. Cambria RP, Davison JK, Carter C et al. Epidural cooling for spinal cord protection during thoracoabdominal aneurysm repair: A five-year experience. *J Vasc Surg* 2000;31(6):1093–102.
6. Svensson LG, Crawford ES, Hess KR, Coselli JS, Safi HJ. Experience with 1509 patients undergoing thoracoabdominal aortic operations. *J Vasc Surg* 1993;17(2):357–68.
7. Coselli JS, Conklin LD, Lemaire SA. Thoracoabdominal aortic aneurysm repair: Review and update of current strategies. *Ann Thorac Surg* 2002;74(5):S1881–4.
8. Clouse WD, Hallett JW, Jr., Schaff HV, Gayari MM, Ilstrup DM, Melton LJ, III. Improved prognosis of thoracic aortic aneurysms: A population-based study. *JAMA* 1998;280(22):1926–9.
9. Rectenwald JE, Huber TS, Martin TD et al. Functional outcome after thoracoabdominal aortic aneurysm repair. *J Vasc Surg* 2002;35(4):640–47.
10. Volodos' NL, Karpovich IP, Shekhanin VE, Troian VI, Iakovenko LF. [A case of distant transfemoral endoprosthesis of the thoracic artery using a self-fixing synthetic prosthesis in traumatic aneurysm]. *Grudn Khir* 1988;(6):84–6.
11. Makaroun MS, Dillavou ED, Kee ST et al. Endovascular treatment of thoracic aortic aneurysms: Results of the phase II multicenter trial of the GORE TAG thoracic endoprosthesis. *J Vasc Surg* 2005;41(1):1–9.
12. Fann JI. Descending thoracic and thoracoabdominal aortic aneurysms. *Coron Artery Dis* 2002;13(2):93–102.
13. Matsumura JS, Lee WA, Mitchell RS et al. The society for vascular surgery practice guidelines: Management of the left subclavian artery with thoracic endovascular aortic repair. *J Vasc Surg* 2009;50(5):1155–8.

90

A hybrid strategy for the initial management of hypoplastic left heart syndrome: Technical considerations

Mark Galantowicz and John P. Cheatham

Introduction

A collaborative interaction between pediatric cardiothoracic surgeons and interventional cardiologists, coupled with new technology, has enabled the development of new hybrid treatment strategies for patients with congenital heart disease. The goal of hybrid therapies is to reduce the accumulated insults of necessary interventions over the lifetime of a child with complex congenital heart disease, thereby improving his or her quantity and quality of life. The short- and long-term outcomes for children with hypoplastic left heart syndrome (HLHS) using traditional staged open heart procedures remain suboptimal.

Despite significant early improvements in outcomes with the traditional surgical staged palliations, the past decade or more has seen very little improvement. A report from the Congenital Heart Surgeon's Society, from 1994 to 2000 involving 29 institutions, demonstrated only a 54% survival after 5 years using conventional palliative techniques for HLHS.[1] In addition, only 28% of patients underwent Fontan completion with another 20% as potential candidates. This report identified the period around the stage 1 Norwood operation as the greatest risk for mortality and morbidity. Then, in 2010, the Pediatric Heart Network reported on a landmark prospective randomized comparison of the two shunt types utilized in a Norwood procedure versus the Sano modification in 555 patients randomized at the 15-member institutions from 2005 to 2008.[2] One year transplant-free survival was 64% versus 74% for the Norwood and Sano cohorts, respectively. Moreover, the rate of serious adverse events, excluding death, was 46% and 37%, respectively, for the two groups representing significant morbidity and resource utilization. These results are revealing for their lack of significant improvement over time despite improvements in our understanding of the anatomy and physiology of HLHS, the overall training, techniques, multidisciplinary teams focused on complex congenital heart disease, and the fact that these studies were carried out at potentially the best prepared institutions for handling these complex procedures. What are the results with these procedures across all institutions? Perhaps, we need to acknowledge that further improvement using these traditional strategies may not be possible given the nature of the disease, the physiology established, and the accumulated insults.

Our hybrid strategy for the initial management of HLHS involves an innovative combination of surgical and transcatheter techniques creating a stable physiology to palliate the neonate until a comprehensive procedure can be performed at around 6 months of age. This new hybrid palliation controls pulmonary blood flow, provides reliable systemic cardiac output through the patent ductus arteriosus (PDA), and creates unobstructed flow from the left atrium all performed without cardiopulmonary bypass. We review the technical aspects of this hybrid procedure from a surgeon's and an interventional cardiologist's perspective. Emphasis is placed on highlighting the lessons learned from our experience,[3,4] so that the significant learning curve may be shortened or avoided by other teams embarking on this hybrid approach.

Preoperative management

The goal of the preoperative management of newborns with HLHS is to balance the systemic, pulmonary, and coronary circulations. There are many strategies to accomplish this goal. Our typical patient is supported with prostaglandin to maintain a PDA, is extubated on room air, receives oral digoxin and lasix, and is beginning enteral feeding. If the patient manifests pulmonary overcirculation, a nitrogen hood is placed over the head to create a subambient inspired oxygen content. During this period of time an echocardiogram is performed to establish the anatomy, to assure an unrestrictive atrial septum, and to rule out retrograde, transverse aortic arch stenosis. A general neonatal survey is performed including a head and abdominal ultrasound. Parental counseling of the nature of HLHS and treatment options is ongoing.

Contraindications to a hybrid

Stage 1 procedure

All forms of HLHS, including aortic atresia/mitral atresia, have been successfully palliated with a hybrid approach. However, there was one death secondary to an unusual anatomic variant that we now consider a contraindication to the hybrid stage 1 procedure. This child had an undetected, congenital stenosis of the retrograde orifice of the transverse arch which was established at autopsy (Figure 90.1). When the PDA stent was deployed it created critical occlusion of retrograde flow into the transverse arch, thereby creating fatal coronary and cerebral ischemia leading to death within hours. Typically, children with HLHS, even aortic atresia/mitral atresia with a diminutive ascending aorta, have an adequate size transverse aortic arch that opens even further at the ductal connection.

This area of connection can be imaged effectively with echocardiography. If there is a small retrograde orifice, or signs of flow acceleration consistent with stenosis, the child is at risk of the stent distorting this orifice, further creating critical or fatal limitation to retrograde perfusion of the heart or brain. We have detected this type of stenosis in approximately 3% of neonates with HLHS. These patients

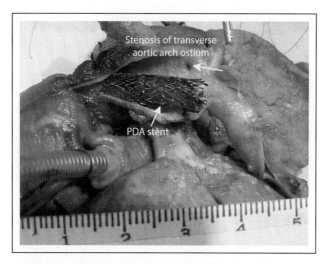

Figure 90.1 This autopsy photograph illustrates the congenital, critical stenosis of the transverse aortic arch. (Reproduced from Galantowicz M, Cheatham JP. *Pediatr Cardiol* 2005;26(3):190–9.)

undergo a traditional Norwood stage 1 procedure in our center. Currently, we have no other contraindications to a hybrid approach including patient size or degree of prematurity.

Hybrid stage 1: Evolution of a novel technique

The evolution of the new initial palliation for HLHS has occurred over the past decade with modifications based on clinical experiences and outcomes. The goals of the initial palliation include (1) unobstructed systemic output through the PDA, (2) balanced pulmonary and systemic blood flows, and (3) an unobstructed atrial septal defect (Figure 90.2). This is currently accomplished by placing bilateral pulmonary artery bands and a PDA stent via a median sternotomy as one hybrid procedure in a specially designed hybrid suite (Figure 90.3), followed by a balloon atrial septostomy several days later prior to discharge. However, this procedure was and can be performed in a traditional operating room or cath lab as sequential procedures or combined in either venue. If a combined hybrid approach is desired in the operating room a portable, a digital C-arm in the lateral position can give adequate angiographic guidance for the PDA stent deployment or in the cath lab the surgeon needs to adapt to the limitations of a cath lab bed for patient positioning and visualization.

Several lessons learned during this experience have led to our current approach. First, placing the bands before the stent is important. The PDA stent does not change the patient's hemodynamics or add any stability over an open PDA secondary to prostaglandin. However, adequately placed branch pulmonary artery bands will improve the hemodynamics by balancing the circulation, improving systemic perfusion, which helps stabilize the patient for any subsequent procedures. Moreover, with the PDA stent in place, the left pulmonary artery is harder to isolate for banding and the stent is at greater risk for distortion or perforation while trying to get around the left pulmonary artery.

Second, any transcatheter wire course through the HLHS heart can lead to hemodynamic compromise secondary to acute tricuspid and pulmonary valve insufficiency from wire distortion. This can lead to end-organ damage or, rarely, valve damage. Therefore, we now avoid any wire course through the heart by placing a sheath directly into the main pulmonary artery above the pulmonary valve, through which the PDA stent can be deployed without crossing any valves.

Finally, creating an unrestrictive, durable atrial septal communication in the HLHS heart is more difficult than a standard balloon septostomy for other anomalies. This has to do with the size and location of the defect, the size of the left atrium, and the stability of the patient. We have varied the timing of the procedure, utilized other techniques

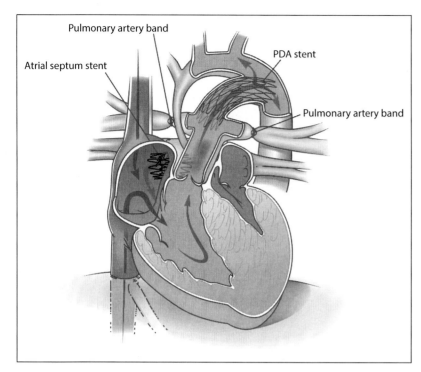

Figure 90.2 The hybrid stage I palliation. Note pulmonary artery (PA) bands on the left and right PAs, proximal to the upper-lobe branches. Stents span the length of the PDA and atrial septum (if necessary). (Reproduced from Galantowicz M, Cheatham JP. *Pediatr Cardiol* 2005;26(3):190–9.)

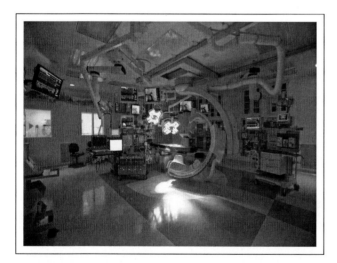

Figure 90.3 (**See color insert.**) A photograph of the specially designed hybrid OR at the Heart Center, Nationwide Children's Hospital.

including static balloon dilatation with and without cutting balloons, and have even placed atrial septal stents. No technique yielded a reliable, reproducible result until our current approach.

Hybrid stage 1: Current technique

The typical neonate comes to the hybrid suite extubated, on prostaglandin as the only intravenous medication. The

goal of the anesthetic management is to extubate the child at the end of the procedure. Appropriate venous and arterial access is established. The surgical team starts with a median sternotomy and creation of a pericardial well to expose the heart. From a standard 3.5 mm Gore-Tex (WL Gore & Associates, Flagstaff, AZ, USA) tube graft an approximately 1-mm-wide ring is cut to serve as the pulmonary artery band material (Figure 90.4). The ring is opened and passed around the right and left pulmonary artery (RPA and LPA). On the right, exposure is straightforward and the band is positioned on the RPA between the ascending aorta and superior vena cava proximal to the right upper pulmonary artery takeoff. Exposure on the left is much more difficult. It is easier to visualize and maneuver a clamp around the LPA with the surgeon standing on the patient's left side. Stay stitches pull the main PA–PDA junction rightward, exposing the takeoff of the left pulmonary artery. A small gauze can help push the left atrial appendage out of its usual position on top of the LPA. Using sharp dissection, the veil of tissue between the LPA and PDA is cleared, allowing a right angle clamp to be passed around the origin of the LPA to position the band. The bands are then tightened by reclosing the band with a 5-0 horizontal mattress suture. An additional stitch is placed through the band and tacked to the local adventitia to resist band migration (Figure 90.5). The tightness of the band is an intraoperative decision based on the child's size, pulmonary artery size, systemic blood pressure, and saturation response to tightening. However, experience has shown that bands closed to approximately 3.1 mm (slightly smaller than the original diameter of the shunt)

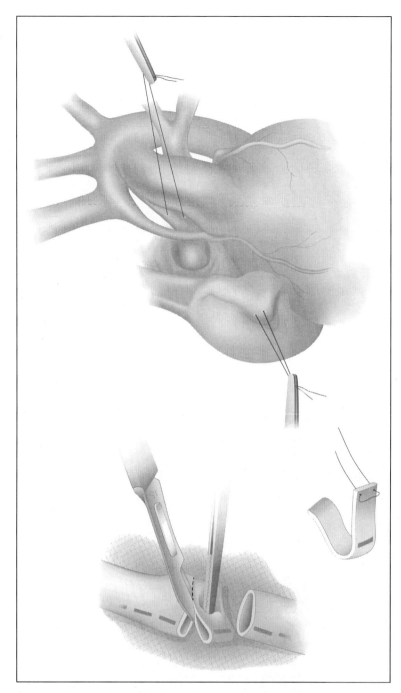

Figure 90.4 (Top) The typical anatomy of HLHS with exposure of the right pulmonary artery. (Bottom) Fashioning a band from a Gore-Tex tube graft.

will adequately balance the circulations and protect the pulmonary bed, while not becoming too tight with resultant cyanosis as the child grows to around 5.5 kg at 4–6 months of age when the comprehensive stage 2 procedure is performed.

After the bands are placed, a 6 Fr sheath with a side arm is prepared. A silk suture is placed around the distal sheath approximately 2 mm from the tip to serve as an external marker for the surgeon as to how far to insert the sheath.

This is important in order to avoid the sheath being inserted too far into the pulmonary artery, hindering deployment of the stent to cover the entire length of the PDA. A purse-string is placed in the main pulmonary artery just above the sinotubular junction and the sheath and dilator advanced through a small incision. After the sheath is advanced to the external suture, the dilator is removed and the snare tightened (Figure 90.6). The side arm of the sheath is then flushed to clear any remaining air or blood.

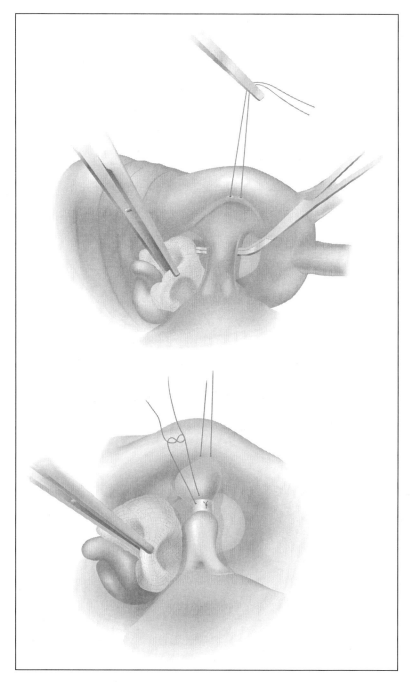

Figure 90.5   (Top) Exposure of the left pulmonary artery. (Bottom) Left band in position tightened and secured with a tacking stitch.

Next, a V-18 Control Wire (Boston Scientific Corporation, Miami, FL) is preshaped and passed through the sheath, into the PDA, and down the descending aorta. A small hand injection of contrast through the side arm of the sheath nicely defines the PDA, left pulmonary artery, descending aorta, and retrograde aortic flow. We prefer to perform the angiogram after the guide wire is in position, simulating any distortion that will be present during stent delivery. In addition, we ask the anesthesiologist to place an NG feeding tube down the esophagus to be used as a

landmark during PDA stent deployment. The PDA diameter is measured at the distal, middle, and proximal ends, and the length is measured to allow the expanded stent to cover the entire length of the PDA in order to avoid stenosis after PGE1 is discontinued. The stent chosen should be approximately 1 mm larger in diameter than the PDA at the PA entrance and the length of the expanded stent must cover the entire length of the PDA.

In our early experience, there were very few appropriate size premounted, balloon-expandable stents (BES)

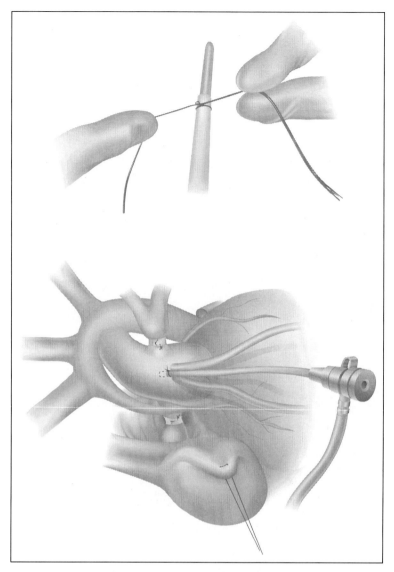

Figure 90.6 (Top) 6 Fr sheath preparation with a silk marker 1–2 mm from the tip. (Bottom) Sheath secured through purse-strings in the main pulmonary artery at the sino-tubular junction.

available in the United States. Therefore, we used self-expandable biliary stents (SES), which were available in diameters from 6 to 10 mm, but in lengths of only 20 mm, 30 mm, and so on. We chose 20-mm-long stents from 7 to 9 mm in diameter, attempting to cover the entire length of the PDA from the junction with the LPA to the aorta distal to the left subclavian artery, where the typical coarctation shelf was located. This necessitated extending the bare stent across the orifice of the transverse aortic arch in most patients, which allows retrograde flow. The self-expandable nitinol stents used were the Smart® or Precise® (Johnson & Johnson, Cordis Division, Miami, FL), Protégé™ GPS™ (eV3, St. Paul, MN), or the Zilver®518 (Cook, Bloomington, IN). All have slightly different delivery systems and characteristics, but the deployment required a slow, controlled

pulling of the outer catheter to allow the nitinol stent to self-expand (Figure 90.7).

Some of the stents above tended to "jump" out of the delivery catheter due to relatively short length. In addition, there was little ability to control or reposition the stent during deployment. Over the years it became apparent that the design of the Protégé SES delivery system had a "tongue-in-groove" technology that eliminated the stent from "jumping" forward in a suboptimal position. The operator could position the stent in the desired location distally and then slowly withdraw the sheath with traction on the partially deployed stent to allow a smooth and controlled placement. Rarely, it is necessary to use two coaxially delivered SES to cover the entire length of a long PDA. It is important that the second stent's distal struts do not also cross the orifice

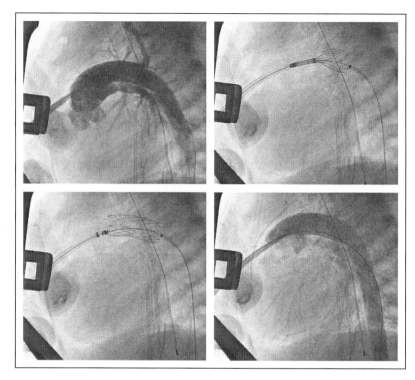

Figure 90.7 In this series of angiograms performed through the side arm of the sheath using the lateral camera, the PDA is nicely demonstrated, along with the banded LPA, as well as the retrograde aortic flow. The Protégé self-expandable stent is deployed by slowly pulling the outer catheter back, allowing the nitinol stent to expand. A follow-up angiogram demonstrates the stent to be completely covering the entire PDA.

of the retrograde aortic arch, avoiding an excessive number of cells that could contribute to reduced flow. The advantage of the SES is its ability to conform to the anatomy of the PDA. However, if there is native PDA stenosis, then a BES is necessary.

After the premounted Palmaz® Genesis stents (Johnson & Johnson) and Cook Formula 418 stents (Cook) became available in the United States, we began to use these balloon-expandable stainless steel stents with variable lengths from 12 to 24 mm and diameters from 4 to 8 mm. We found these stents easier and more familiar to deploy, with more precise placement and a greater choice of stent lengths (Figure 90.8). However, either the self-expandable or balloon-expandable stents may be used successfully and should be left to the

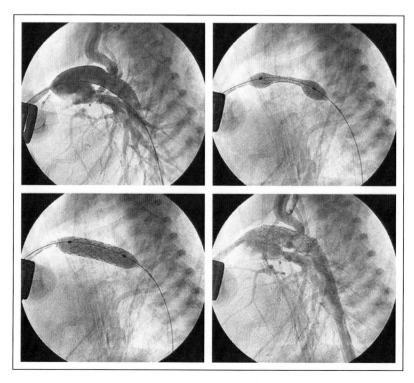

Figure 90.8 The balloon-expandable, pre-mounted Genesis stent is shown here being deployed to cover the entire PDA. Note the stent crossing the origin of the aortic arch with retrograde flow filling the atretic ascending aorta and coronary arteries.

hybrid team's discretion. In our experience, the SES Protégé stents are used in about 75% of patients, while BES stents are used in all patients with native PDA stenosis or that need a shorter length than the 20-mm-long SES. In the premature patient less than 2 kg, a BES is usually necessary because of the short length of the PDA. With the hybrid approach, the size of the patient is not an issue with PDA stent delivery. We have successfully performed this several times in 1 kg newborns. Regardless of which stent is chosen, a 6 Fr sheath placed through the purse-string suture in the MPA will allow deployment.

Finally, after the stent is deployed, the delivery catheter or balloon is removed and a final angiogram is performed. Although we typically remove the guide wire before the angiogram is performed, it can be left in place until enough experience is gained by the hybrid team. Once the stent position is confirmed to completely cover the ductus the sheath is removed and the purse-string suture tied. After hemostasis is assured, the pericardium, sternum, and skin are closed. Typically there is no need for inotropic support, the prostaglandin is stopped, and the child is extubated prior to transport to the cardiac intensive care unit.

A baseline echocardiogram is performed on the first postoperative day. Observation for 2–4 days in the cardiac ICU is typical, during which time oral feeding is started as well as digoxin, lasix, and aspirin therapy. Once reliable caloric intake is established and the child is a day or two away from being discharged home he or she returns to the cath lab for a balloon atrial septostomy.

While it is tempting to perform transcatheter creation of a larger atrial septal defect (ASD) at the time of the hybrid procedure, there are several caveats. Some surgeons will choose to perform PA banding in the conventional operating room, followed by PDA stent placement in the cath lab. Performing balloon atrial septostomy at the same time seems like a natural choice. However, creation of an adequate ASD that will last long enough until the comprehensive stage 2 repair is performed can be problematic. The left atrium in the newborn with HLHS is extremely small. The latex Miller–Edwards balloon atrial septostomy catheter and the 2 mL (13.5 mm) NuMED balloon atrial septostomy catheter (NuMED, Hopkinton, NY) will not "fit" in the small left atrium. Therefore, as a compromise, the 1 mL (9.5 mm) NuMED catheter was used. However, the ASD typically becomes too restrictive within 2–3 months and creates a scenario of either repeat balloon atrial septostomy or early comprehensive stage 2 repair. We also attempted static balloon atrial septoplasty with and without Cutting Balloon™ (Boston Scientific Corporation, Murrieta, CA) septoplasty as an alternative in these newborns. However, an ASD large enough to last until 6 months was rare. Therefore, we changed to our current protocol and elected to defer balloon atrial septostomy until the day before the patient was to be discharged or after discharge when the mean Doppler gradient was >5–8 mmHg. At this time, the 2 mL NuMED balloon atrial septostomy can be used (Figure 90.9). The left atrium is large enough to accommodate the 2 mL (13.5 mm) balloon at this time. In our experience, this creates an unrestrictive ASD that lasts until the comprehensive stage 2 repair can be performed at 6 months in over 90% of patients. Usually the atrial tissue around the defect is thin enough to allow safe and successful creation

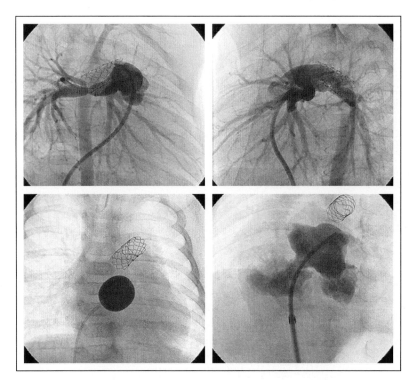

Figure 90.9 The day prior to discharge, the neonate returns to the hybrid suite for a short hemodynamic study, angiography, and balloon atrial septostomy. The right pulmonary artery band is best shown in the RAO projection, while the left pulmonary artery band and PDA stent are seen in the LAO view. A 2 mL (13.5 mm) NuMED balloon atrial septostomy catheter is used to create an ASD that will remain unrestrictive until the comprehensive stage 2 repair at 6 months.

of an adequate ASD. This anatomic characteristic should be remembered when considering stent therapy.

While it is tempting to stent all patients with HLHS to ensure unrestricted atrial flow for a length of time until comprehensive stage 2 repair is performed, there are reasons to be cautious. Typically, and as mentioned earlier, the atrial septum is thin adjacent to the fossa ovalis defect, while the septum inferiorly near the atrioventricular valves is quite thick. The secure placement of a stent relies on the adjacent thickness of the septum, as well as the length of stent able to be used. Stent embolization is more likely in this scenario with the thin septum primum being pushed downward during balloon expansion of the stent, only to recoil with deflation and guide wire removal, thus "pushing" the stent from the LA to the RA. Therefore, our prejudice is to only implant stents in the atrial septum when there is a severely restrictive ASD or intact atrial septum as a newborn. This is an urgent or emergent situation that must be addressed shortly after birth and before the PA bands or PDA stent is placed. We prefer to perform this procedure in the hybrid suite using transvenous access from the right femoral vein and echo guidance during radio-frequency perforation of the septumusing the Nykanen catheter (Baylis Medical Company, Montreal, Canada). This is much easier and safer than attempting transseptal puncture in these critically ill newborns with a small "flat" left atrium. A premounted Genesis Palmaz Stent is then delivered over the 0.018 inch guide wire and expanded. Typically a 12-mm-long stent premounted on an 8 mm balloon is used (Figure 90.10). We have also used a Cutting Balloon after successful RF perforation followed by static balloon septoplasty, but now feel

stent therapy is the best choice (Figure 90.11). Regardless, be cautious of stenting the atrial septum as a "routine" procedure and reserve it for specific indications. After the child is discharged home, close interstage monitoring is critical.

Interstage monitoring

Close interstage monitoring has been important in minimizing interstage mortality, as well as perioperative complications at the comprehensive stage 2 procedure. After discharge home, the infants are followed closely with a minimum of every-other-week cardiology assessment. Echocardiography is used liberally to monitor for obstruction through the PDA stent, retrograde into the transverse aortic arch, at the atrial septum or decreased right ventricular function or increased tricuspid regurgitation as another indicator of obstruction. Any evidence of obstruction or decreased ventricular function leads to a catheterization to diagnose and treat the level of obstruction.

Given the volume load on the heart after the initial palliation, any increased afterload leads to the rapid development of right ventricular dysfunction with or without tricuspid regurgitation. Early detection and treatment of obstruction of flow through the PDA stent related to coarctation to antegrade or retrograde aortic flow is mandatory. Restriction of the atrial septum may manifest as tachypnea and/or cyanosis. Maintaining ventricular function has been the key to survival through the comprehensive stage 2 procedure. The patientsare scheduled for their comprehensive stage 2 surgery at 4–6 months of age.

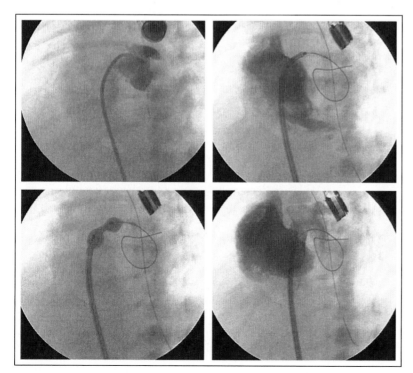

Figure 90.10 A 12-mm-long premounted Genesis stent on an 8-mm-diameter Slalom balloon is delivered through a 6 Fr long sheath over a 0.018 inch guide wire. TEE is used to help guide placement of the interatrial stent. Follow-up angiography demonstrates a widely patent ASD and small decompressed LA.

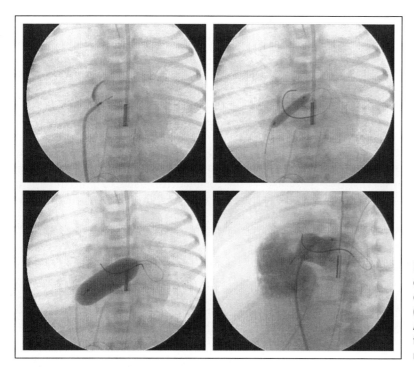

Figure 90.11 Radio-frequency perforation of the intact atrial septum using the Nykanen RF catheter with an intracardiac echocardiography (ICE) probe placed transesophageal is shown here. A 4-mm-diameter Cutting Balloon is expanded, followed by a 10 mm static balloon septoplasty, resulting in a moderate ASD.

Comprehensive stage 2

This is a formidable operation. Despite the magnitude, the resultant circulation in series rather than in parallel, outside of the neonatal period has been well tolerated. Unexpected benefits of the new initial hybrid palliation have been the growth of the native pulmonary arteries and the transverse aortic arch. Because the transverse arch/innominate artery junction has grown, the aortic cannula can be positioned into the innominate artery during arch reconstruction, thereby removing the need for circulatory arrest with its associated risks. Moreover, much of the procedure can be done with the heart beating on bypass without aortic cross-clamping, thereby minimizing the period of cardiac ischemia. And in many patients an additional small aortic cannula can be placed in the aortic root, even with aortic atresia, allowing continuous coronary perfusion throughout the entire procedure.

The open–heart surgery consists of removal of the PDA stent and PA bands, repair of the aortic arch and pulmonary arteries (if necessary), division of the diminutive ascending aorta with reimplantation into the pulmonary root, main PA to reconstructed aorta anastomosis, atrial septectomy with removal of the atrial stent (if present), and a modified cavopulmonary anastomosis (Figure 90.11). All of these steps are familiar to a pediatric cardiothoracic surgeon with single-ventricle experience, except for the removal of the PDA stent. This is the most intimidating aspect of the procedure because of the delicate nature of removing the distal part of the stent that continues into the descending thoracic aorta. Moreover, injury of the aorta at this level has very few reasonable bailout options. Therefore, widespread acceptance of the hybrid stage 1 procedure will be dependent on surgeons' comfort with the comprehensive stage 2 procedure. Hopefully, with future stent development specifically designed for this procedure, stent removal or better yet absorbable stents will make this significant technical hurdle obsolete for surgeons.

Conclusion

Given the seemingly limited improvement in outcomes for the initial management of babies with HLHS over the past decade there are many reasons to continue to evolve an alternative strategy such as the hybrid approach.[5] The goal of the hybrid stage 1 for the initial management of HLHS is to effectively palliate patients through the neonatal period with minimal morbidity and mortality, preserving ventricular function, while allowing normal growth and development, especially of the pulmonary vascular bed. Thus, the patient is prepared for a comprehensive open heart procedure that yields a circulation in series rather than parallel, with expected improved hemodynamic stability resulting in reduced morbidity and mortality. This hybrid approach combining surgical and transcatheter techniques can achieve acceptable short- and intermediate-term outcomes in patients with

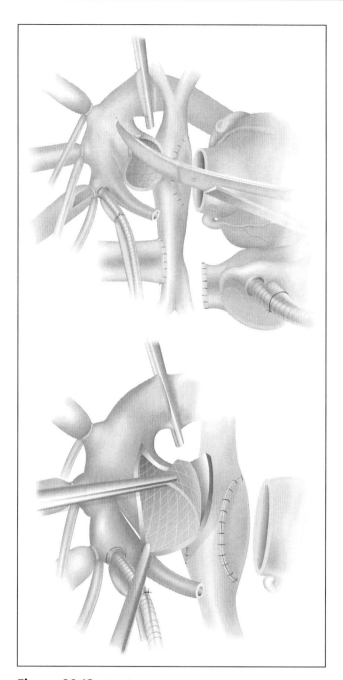

Figure 90.12   (Top) Comprehensive stage 2 using regional cerebral perfusion during aortic arch reconstruction after pulmonary artery band removal and cavopulmonary anastomosis as well as proximal ascending aortic implantation into the pulmonary root. (Bottom) Establishing a plane between the PDA stent vessel wall for complete stent removal.

HLHS. Long-term studies will be necessary. Continued collaboration between cardiothoracic surgeons, interventional cardiologists, and industry is necessary to further develop innovative hybrid management strategies for HLHS as well as other congenital heart anomalies (Figure 90.12).

References

1. Ashburn DA, McCrindle BW et al. Outcomes after the Norwood operation in neonates with critical aortic stenosis or aortic valve atresia. *J Thorac Cardiovasc Surg* 2003;125(5):1070–82.
2. Ohye RG, Sleeper LA, Mahony L et al. Comparison of shunt types in the Norwood procedure for single-ventricle lesions. *N Engl J Med* 2010;362(21):1980–92.
3. Galantowicz M, Cheatham JP. Lessons learned from the development of a new hybrid strategy for the management of hypoplastic left heart syndrome. *Pediatr Cardiol* 2005;26(3):190–9.
4. Galantowicz M, Cheatham JP et al. Hybrid approach for hypoplastic left heart syndrome: Intermediate results after the learning curve. *Ann Thorac Surg* 2008;85(6):2063–70.
5. Galantowicz M. In favor of the Hybrid Stage 1 as the initial palliation for hypoplastic left heart syndrome. *Semin Thorac Cardiovasc Surg* 2013;16:62–4.

Further reading and additional sources

Akintuerk H, Michael-Behnke I, Valeske K et al. Stenting of the arterial duct and banding of the pulmonary arteries. Basis for combined Norwood stage 1 and 2 repair in hypoplastic left heart. *Circulation* 2002;105:1099–103.

Gibbs JL, Wren C, Watterson KG et al. Stenting of the arterial duct combined with banding of the pulmonary arteries and atrial septectomy or septostomy: A new approach to palliation for the hypoplastic left heart syndrome. *Br Heart J* 1993;69:551–5.

Hill SL, Galantowicz M, Cheatham JP. Emerging strategies in the treatment of HLHS: Combined transcatheter and surgical techniques. *Pediatr Cardiol Today* 2003;1(3):1–5.

91

Alternative procedures for hypoplastic left heart syndrome as a bridge to transplantation

Ryan R. Davies and Jonathan M. Chen

Introduction

Hypoplastic left heart syndrome (HLHS) is a lethal congenital malformation of the left ventricle, aorta, and associated valves that occurs at a rate of approximately 0.23 per 1000 live births or 1500 cases per year in the United States.[1,2] Prior to 1980, HLHS was uniformly fatal, with most infants dying within 1 month of birth. Following the pioneering efforts of Norwood and Bailey, two treatment options are now available: staged reconstruction and cardiac transplantation.[3]

Although Norwood's procedure represented an important advance in the management of infants with HLHS, initial survival was poor, ranging only from 9% to 47% in early series.[4–6] Such results led Bailey and colleagues to advocate cardiac allotransplantation as primary therapy for infants with HLHS. However, neonatal transplantation for HLHS requires lifelong immunosuppression and is associated with a waiting list mortality of 20–25% owing to a distinct shortage of donors of appropriate size. Improvements in pretransplant survival are thus necessary before cardiac transplantation can be an epidemiologically viable therapeutic alternative for all newborns with HLHS.

Staged reconstruction: The Norwood principle

The concept of the Norwood procedure is predicated upon many of the same principles that underlie catheter-based procedures for the palliation of HLHS. The essential components of the Norwood procedure are: (1) unobstructed pulmonary venous return, (2) unobstructed systemic blood flow from the single ventricle to the systemic circulation, (3) adequate pulmonary blood flow without volume overload, and (4) unobstructed mixing at the atrial level.[7] Most commonly, this is accomplished through construction of a neo-aorta consisting of pulmonary artery and aortic tissue,

closure of the patent ductus arteriosus (PDA), atrial septectomy, and creation of a modified Blalock–Taussig shunt (or Sano RV-PA connection) to provide regulated pulmonary blood flow.

Stage 2 is performed between 4 and 6 months of age; it consists of a hemifontan or bidirectional Glenn procedure, and involves removal of the systemic (or RV)-pulmonary shunt and creation of a cavopulmonary shunt.[8] The Fontan procedure, which completely separates the pulmonary and systemic circulations, is typically performed between 18 months to 3 years of age.[9] Transplantation may be performed at (or between) any of these stages, often with outcomes comparable to patients transplanted for primary cardiomyopathy. However, those transplanted after a failed "high-risk" Glenn or Fontan procedure have impaired outcomes when compared with those undergoing interval transplantation in lieu of staged succession.

Outcomes

Over the 25 years since the introduction of the Norwood procedure, significant changes in both surgical technique and perioperative management have resulted in improved survival to Fontan completion. However, operative mortality remains high, and is primarily related to the stage 1 repair.[10] Data from the early 1990s described a 1 year survival of only 36–42% in patients undergoing staged repair of HLHS. Continued improvement in techniques and experience has resulted in significant improvements over time, but overall 1 year survival remains only 70–85% in even the best series.[11–15]

Because HLHS includes a range of anatomic defects, from mitral or aortic stenosis through complete atresia of one or both valves with variable atrial septal anatomy, attempts at improving outcomes with staged reconstruction have focused on improved patient selection and perioperative management based on preoperative anatomic and physiologic factors predictive of poor outcomes following

Table 91.1 Predictors of poor outcome following stage 1 Norwood reconstruction

Low operative weight[15,18,19] or low birth weight[10]

Atresia of one or both of the left ventricular valves[10,11]

Preoperative ventricular dysfunction[24]

Moderate or severe tricuspid regurgitation[17,21]

High preoperative creatinine[10]

Preoperative acidosis[11,18]

Highly restrictive atrial septal defect[22] or need for preoperative septostomy[10]

Severe pulmonary venous obstruction[23]

Significant noncardiac congenital conditions[23]

repair. Such research has identified several factors that increase the risk to children undergoing the Norwood procedure. Patients with larger ascending aortic arch diameter have improved survival.[11,14,16–18] Older patients tend to have significantly higher mortality rates, especially those with age >1 month at the time of operative repair.[15,19] Patients with increased PVR are particularly prone to lethal pulmonary vascular crises.[20]

A variety of other risk factors have been identified for poor outcomes following stage 1 reconstruction (Table 91.1).[10,11,15,17–19,21–24] However, despite this extensive list of risk factors, an analysis of the causes of death following stage 1 found that most (77%) were related to largely correctable surgical technical problems associated with perfusion of the lungs, myocardium, and systemic organs,[21] thus explaining the improved survival in the most recent series. Long-term survival should improve dramatically as the higher short-term survival following stage 1 in contemporary series is translated into intermediate and long-term improvements after subsequent stages.[15,25]

Cardiac transplantation for HLHS

Following the first report of cardiac transplantation in HLHS by Bailey and colleagues in 1986, transplantation has become the preferred method of surgical treatment at some institutions.[26] It offers several obvious advantages over staged reconstruction, most notably a single, definitive operative repair with return to normal circulatory physiology. The transplant procedure is performed in a fashion similar to transplants into patients with normal physiology, although donor aorta is used to reconstruct the ascending aorta and aortic arch under deep hypothermic circulatory arrest.[27,28]

Both short- and long-term outcomes following transplantation have been excellent. Early postoperative survival approaches 90% in some series,[11,29] and long-term survival in those surviving the first 2 years of life is excellent.[29] The main limitation, therefore, to the use of transplantation in all infants with HLHS has been the relative

shortage of donor organs, and the resultant waiting list mortality for those unpalliated infants awaiting transplantation approaches 30%.[30] In addition to an increased risk of death on the wait list, longer waiting times result in a higher risk of removal from the list for organ failure and may result in impaired long-term survival following transplantation.[10,31–33] Furthermore, if an infant waits on the transplant list without receiving an organ and ultimately requires surgical palliation, survival following the Norwood procedure is likely to be compromised.[16,19,31]

Mechanical devices as a bridge to transplantation have been used extensively in adult patients and have lately been extended to select groups of pediatric patients with heart failure. Until recently, the device size limited the use of ventricular assist devices to adolescents, precluding their use in the neonatal and infant population. In addition, congenital physiology may limit the application of either ventricular support or extracorporeal membrane oxygenation (ECMO). In general, patients with single-ventricle physiology have poor outcomes with ECMO support, where delivering an adequate mechanically supported systemic cardiac output without causing pulmonary volume overload makes the use of ECMO or ventricular assist devices particularly challenging.[34] Thus, although only limited data are available, prospects for an effective mechanical bridge-to-transplant technique in this population are poor.

Catheter-based interventions in HLHS

The high mortality associated with waiting for donor organ availability, as well as the surgical mortality that continues to be associated with stage 1 reconstruction, demonstrates that there is significant room for improvement in the early management of infants with HLHS. Several catheter-based techniques have been proposed both as measures to increase survival prior to transplantation and—more recently—as alternatives to stage 1 palliation (to be covered elsewhere in Chapter 90). Advances in interventional techniques and in prenatal diagnostic methods have also enabled the treatment of some of the anatomic defects associated with HLHS *in utero*.

Fetal interventions

Balloon atrial septostomy

Surgical reconstruction with the Norwood procedure (and ultimately the hemi-Fontan and Fontan procedures) requires low pulmonary vascular resistance in order to enable adequate pulmonary blood flow and normal systemic pressures.[3,14,35–36] Similarly, the risk of cardiac transplantation has been directly associated with reversibility and/or a lower baseline pulmonary vascular resistance. The presence of a restrictive atrial communication in infants with HLHS results in higher left atrial pressures, which when transmitted to the pulmonary vascular bed, may lead to pulmonary venous hypertension *in utero*.[22,37] While some infants may benefit from early postnatal atrial septostomy[38] or open atrial septectomy, the resultant pulmonary vascular changes may be only partially reversible.[22,37] In addition, balloon atrial septostomy can be technically difficult in these patients, owing to the posterior deviation of the interatrial septum and its thick integrity. Moreover, staged open septectomy with subsequent Norwood procedure (or transplantation) naturally also carries an increased risk of morbidity and mortality.

Accordingly, some investigators have proposed enlargement of the foramen ovale *in utero* in patients with HLHS who have an apparent restrictive atrial communication.[39] Marshall and colleagues recently published a report of seven fetuses with prenatally diagnosed HLHS demonstrating the feasibility of *in utero* atrial septostomy.[39] Their technique draws both on experience with neonatal atrial septostomy as well as fetal valvuloplasty and cardiocentesis. In this procedure, an introducer is advanced through the maternal abdominal wall and the uterus, then through the fetal chest wall and ultimately into the right atrium. A needle is then passed through the atrial septum and an angioplasty balloon advanced and used to perform the septostomy.

In Marshall's series, the procedure was technically successful in six of seven fetuses, however, one of the six died within 4 h due to procedural complications (right hemothorax, small hemopericardium), potentially related to the use of a larger introducer in this patient to enable creation of a larger atrial septal defect (ASD). The size of the ASD remains one of the primary drawbacks of the technique, as an ASD of >2 mm could only be created in four of the fetuses. Only two patients remained alive and well following Norwood stage 1. Obviously, significant work remains both in surpassing the technological hurdles and in demonstrating survival advantages to this technique; however, the poor outcome in patients with restrictive ASDs with either cardiac transplantation or surgical reconstruction,[38,40] argue in favor of continued attempts to mitigate the pulmonary vascular damage occurring prior to birth.[37]

Aortic valvuloplasty. HLHS consists of a wide range of anatomic defects from complete mitral and aortic atresia without an appreciable left ventricular (LV) cavity, to those with severe aortic stenosis and a diminutive LV. Those in the latter category may in fact have had a morphologically normal LV outflow tract early in gestation, but with reduced flow consequently evolved either poor LV development or a hypoplastic outflow tract and aortic arch.[41–42] Some have suggested that the ability to identify patients with critical prenatal aortic stenosis and perform valvuloplasty *in utero* might allow for more normal left ventricular growth with the potential to allow a postnatal two-ventricle repair with its attendant improved survival.[17,37,42] Naturally, an incomplete result with this technique still allows for subsequent procedures. However, the creation of significant valvar insufficiency could render the staged procedure unlikely to succeed and thus render transplantation the only remaining option postnatally.

To date, several case reports have been published describing the use of prenatal aortic valvuloplasty.[43–45] The results of these studies, comprising a total of 12 human fetal patients were analyzed in 2000 by Kohl and colleagues.[46] As with atrial septostomy described above, fetal cardiac access is obtained via insertion of a needle through the maternal abdominal wall and uterus and then into the fetal chest and the hypoplastic ventricle. Coronary artery balloons are used to perform the valvuloplasty. Of the 12 patients, 3 required emergency C-sections for either sustained bradycardia or chorioamnionitis. Four fetuses (25%) died within 24 h of the procedure either from bleeding, sustained bradycardia, or in one case at open operative valvotomy following emergency delivery. Only one patient with a technically successful valvuloplasty survived long term.[46] Despite the need for multiple subsequent valvuloplasties in the postnatal period, by 4 years of age, this patient had near-normal cardiac contractility and ejection fraction.[43] Further advances in the equipment, techniques, and, most importantly, in patient selection are necessary before the wider adoption of prenatal intervention to treat critical aortic stenosis. Furthermore, fetoscopic or open procedures may have higher success rates than ultrasound-guided direct cardiac punctures.[46] However, the anecdotal results in this patient population combined with the growing understanding of flow-dependent cardiac chamber growth *in utero* suggests that prenatal intervention could potentially have a role in the treatment of patients along the spectrum of HLHS.

Neonatal interventions

Preoperative preparation of patients with HLHS for either surgical palliation or for transplantation requires optimization of the balance between systemic and pulmonary circulations, maintenance of ductal patency, adequate restriction of pulmonary blood flow, and creation of unobstructed atrial mixing. Several noninterventional therapies have been used to achieve this goal: maintenance of ductal patency via prostaglandin–E1 infusion as well as adjustment of the ratio of systemic to pulmonary vascular resistances using inspired hypoxic air, nitrogen, carbon dioxide, or the use of inotropes and vasodilators.[47–49] Although these treatments may be successful, in some patients, pharmacologic and inhalational techniques may not provide adequate resuscitation. Accordingly, several investigators have developed mechanical techniques for improving systemic blood flow and limiting pulmonary flow, including balloon atrial septostomy (described previously), mechanical stenting of the ductus arteriosus and pulmonary artery banding.

Stenting of the ductus arteriosus

Successful stenting as a palliative procedure in anticipation of transplantation was first reported by Ruiz and colleagues at Loma Linda in 1993.[50] Four of the five infants reported in the series were successfully bridged to transplantation. Access was first obtained with a 6 French sheath through which a 5 French Berman catheter was introduced and advanced through the main pulmonary artery into the ductus. A 7 French sheath was then introduced and a 2.5 mm × 2 cm premounted Palmaz–Schatz balloon-expandable stent was placed. The sheath was retracted, the balloon (5 French Medi-tech PE-MT balloon) was inflated, and the stent was deployed. In this technique, the authors note that particular care must be made to prevent protrusion of the device into either the pulmonary artery, or isthmus of the descending aorta, and while stent migration is unlikely, it did occur in one patient who died. Additionally, balloon inflation naturally compromises cardiac output during stent expansion. Later studies by Gibbs and colleagues in the United Kingdom were less favorable, owing partially to progressive endothelialization of the stent and procedural morbidities.[51]

Subsequent technological advances have allowed for the use of self-expanding nitinol stents, which may be delivered through smaller sheaths (5 or 6 French) and whose delivery does not impair cardiac output (Figure 91.1). A more recent review of the 4 year experience at Denver Children's Hospital demonstrated 40 patients to have been successfully stented.[52] The mean age of the patients was 1.6 ± 1.2 months, with a mean weight of 3.8 ± 0.9 kg (the smallest weighing 2.1 kg). Stent deployment was performed with sedation and under fluoroscopic guidance. A 4 French Berman catheter was placed and the ductal size and diameter measured using biplane angiography. The lateral projection was the most useful during positioning of the stent

delivery sheath. Biplane imaging was helpful in infants with a distal, inferior insertion of the aortic end of the ductus arteriosus. A stent was then chosen at least 2 mm larger than the minimal ductal diameter and 1 mm larger than the maximum ductal diameter, and deployed through a 6 or 7 French sheath; ideally, the stent was opened in the aortic ampulla of the ductus and the distal aspect of the stent was allowed to flare into both the aortic isthmus and descending aorta. In the lateral projection the distal end of the stent was at the anterior border of the spinal bodies.

Angiography was also useful to demonstrate ductal anatomy. Approximately 70% of infants with HLHS were found to have favorable ductal anatomy that would allow the distal end of the stent to be placed in the aortic ampulla and avoid placement into the descending aorta. About 25% of infants with HLHS had transitional ductal anatomy that could require stent placement beyond the aortic ampulla into the descending aorta. In 5% of infants the ductal anatomy was felt to be unsuitable for stenting.

Of interest, heparinization to an ACT >200 s was employed, as were six doses of 1 mg/kg of dipyridamole therapy and two doses of 0.5 mg/kg enoxaparin postprocedurally, as well as 5–10 mg/kg of acetylsalicylic acid daily until stent removal.

There were no deaths in this series related to the ductal procedure, with a mean follow-up of 65 ± 65 days; however, there was one late death possibly related to stenting at 3 months (during readmission for coarctation angioplasty). Only one patient was deemed unstentable, owing to a short ductus measuring less than 10 mm, and a posterior ductal ridge. In six patients, two stents were required for complete coverage of ductal tissue (the mean length of the ductus in these patients was 22.4 mm, the mean length for the entire population was 16.3 ± 4.4 mm). One patient required a second stent due to stent migration. The mean ductal diameter of the entire population was 6.6 ± 1.2 mm. Procedural complications included bradycardia (3), hypotension (4), respiratory arrest (1), and transient heart block (1). Of note, morbidity was significantly higher among patients with

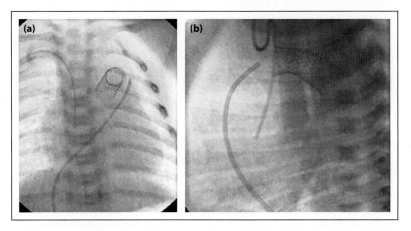

Figure 91.1 Ductal stent deployed in postero-anterior and lateral projections.

either type 2 or 3 ductal anatomy (ductal orientation ≤10° leftward from the vertical plane),[52] suggesting that certain anatomic variants may be better managed with earlier surgical palliation or transplantation. Two patients developed coarctation adjacent to the distal stent, one of whom underwent successful balloon angioplasty, the other of whom died preprocedurally.

Longer-term follow-up has been reported in 20 patients undergoing combined ductal stenting and pulmonary artery banding by Michel-Behnke and colleagues.[53] In their series, two patients died during the stent insertion or PA banding. Two patients received heart transplantation (57 and 331 days following stenting), although two also died awaiting transplantation at similar time periods (58 and 193 days).[53] Ten patients had undergone a combined stage 1 and 2 Norwood surgical repair with only 10% mortality in these patients. Perhaps most encouragingly, two patients with multiple left heart obstructive lesions (one with HLHS, the other with interrupted aortic arch and hypoplastic aortic valve annulus) were successfully palliated with DA stenting and PA banding enabling eventual biventricular repair with its attendant improved long-term prognosis.[17,54]

Pulmonary artery banding

Several investigators have recently promoted the concept of a hybrid first-stage procedure (ductal stenting, open pulmonary artery banding) as an alternative to the Norwood procedure for HLHS (to be discussed in Chapter 90).[53] These same strategies to allow for ductal patency but limited pulmonary blood flow may also be adopted as a means to

"bridge" such patients to transplantation. In fact, the banding of the pulmonary arteries has been a strategy employed in older infants with HLHS who have experienced prolonged severe pulmonary overcirculation, but who may not have yet developed fixed pulmonary hypertension.[55]

Mitchell and colleagues performed open bilateral pulmonary artery banding with 2 mm PTFE bands. These were placed on the branch pulmonary arteries and secured to reduce pulmonary arterial pressure to 50% of systemic. The distal pulmonary arterial pressures were measured with 3 French catheters advanced into the distal pulmonary arteries, the right directly, and the left via a purse-string suture on the pulmonary trunk. Subsequently, intravascular branch pulmonary artery flow-limiting devices delivered via femoral venous techniques were employed. The flow-limiting devices are constructed of nitinol mesh and sized to fit securely in the proximal right and left pulmonary arteries. The device has a fixed internal lumen that reduces the effective orifice: reducing distal pressure and flow in a predictable fashion (Figure 91.2). Figure 91.3 shows a fluoroscopic image of a patient who received the percutaneous pulmonary artery bands.

The order in which the ductal stent and pulmonary banding procedures are done varies. Some have suggested performing a one-time procedure in the neonatal period.[53] Others have supported a staged procedure, unless the child is to undergo balloon atrial septostomy. These authors have suggested that waiting for pulmonary banding until 3–4 months of age can allow for good distal pulmonary artery growth prior to band procedures, and does not appear to impact upon pulmonary vasoreactivity.[55] Children in their

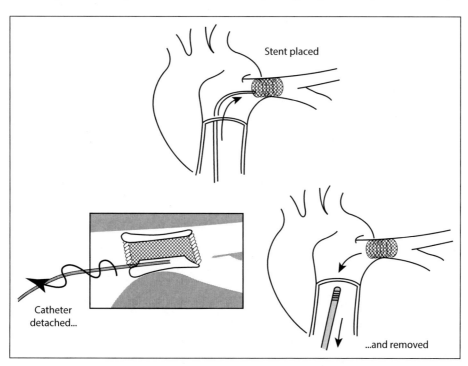

Figure 91.2 Schematic of percutaneous pulmonary band placement and deployment.

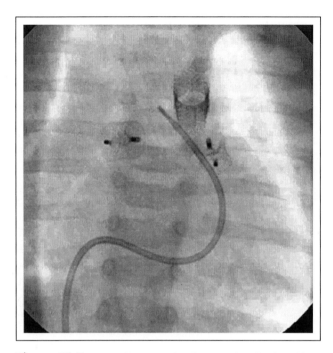

Figure 91.3 Ductal stent and pulmonary bands placed in a patient with HLHS.

study demonstrated a mean interval from PDA stent to band placement of 76 ± 52 days. With the use of internal bands the mean age of banding decreased and procedures were performed in the first several weeks of life. One caveat noted by several groups in palliating those with HLHS and other high-risk single ventricle variants is that application of the bands may confer a significant afterload to the single ventricle, and require substantial inotropic support or rapid ductal stent deployment.[56]

As experience develops with internal bands one would anticipate routine use during interventional catheterization by two weeks of age. Internal bands may also provide an option for patients who were diagnosed late or were unsuitable for early palliative surgery before 1 month of age. A follow-up study by the Denver group evaluating their long-term experience with internal bands as a bridging strategy toward heart transplantation demonstrated no evidence of pulmonary artery reconstruction necessary at the time of transplant, and moreover the very attractive possibility of rapid home discharge for the duration of the waiting time.[57] Most notably, for those with internal bands, the route of surgical access for the transplant is a primary sternotomy (not reoperative).

Transplantation

Orthotopic heart transplantation for HLHS following any of the prior interventional palliative procedures must be performed under deep hypothermic circulatory arrest (usually limited to the aortic arch reconstruction). In PA band patients, often the bands are removed and the branch

pulmonary arteries snared to prevent runoff. Alternatively, the ductus can be clamped or snared if a self-expanding stent had been placed in the ductus. These stents do not crush and will reexpand if the clamp needs to be removed. The internal bands are then removed from the branch pulmonary arteries by separating the devices from the intimal surface of the artery. After circulatory arrest, the ductal stent is removed by dividing the ductus (and stent) at its midpoint. The remaining stent in the aorta is carefully removed during the arch reconstruction; all residual ductal tissue within the descending aorta must be excised (often requiring removal of the isthmus and anastomosis of the posterior wall of the aorta from the distal descending aorta to the underside of the left subclavian artery). The branch pulmonary arteries should be dilated (5–7 mm Hegar dilators) prior to pulmonary arterial anastomosis. Any residual stenosis should be addressed by patch arterioplasty at the time of transplantation.

For those with internal pulmonary arterial flow limiters, the stent and ductus are clamped in their midpoint after bypass is initiated. The stent in the ductus must be removed first, the internal flow limiting devices extracted through the divided pulmonary trunk and again dilators passed to confirm the patency and integrity of the branch pulmonary arteries.

In all cases, it is essential to assure that the donor procurement team retrieve all of the donor aortic arch and branch pulmonary arterial vessels so that arch reconstruction can be completed with donor aorta and that, in the event that pulmonary artery reconstruction must occur, donor pulmonary artery tissue may be used for onlay patch angioplasty.[58] Of note, in the cases reported by Mitchell using internal bands, none required pulmonary artery reconstruction or repair after band removal. Furthermore, none of these patients developed late branch pulmonary artery stenosis, and 1 year after transplant, follow-up catheterizations documented appropriate pulmonary arterial growth.[55] Moreover, concerns about the possible long-term aortic consequences of patients transplanted after a prior Norwood reconstruction extend to those who underwent prior hybrid procedures, and argues in favor of lifelong monitoring with ongoing vigilance.[59]

Norwood or cardiac transplant, which for whom?

Several recent studies have attempted to establish whether the Norwood procedure or primary transplantation affords the greatest survival to infants with HLHS. The rapidity with which (1) percutaneous strategies for interval palliation as well as (2) technical advances in the management of Norwood patients have evolved has rendered the results of these earlier decision analyses somewhat difficult to interpret in the current era. Importantly, however, while a recent transplant multicenter analysis demonstrated a 25% waiting list mortality for infants with HLHS, the posttransplant survival of this subgroup did not differ from those patients with other pretransplant diagnoses.[56] Five-year survival from listing through transplantation in this series was 54% for infants with HLHS, a finding comparable to the long-term survival after the Norwood procedure in recent reports.[60]

Recent evolving data would suggest that there may be certain anatomic variants of HLHS who have significantly impaired results after a Norwood procedure, in particular those born with aortic atresia-mitral stenosis (AA-MS) and coronary artery fistula. The AA-MS subgroup has been demonstrated to have a mortality as high as 29% compared with other anatomic variants.[61] As some have suggested, the presence of this diagnosis alone may favor the exploration of other therapeutic alternatives (hybrid bridge to transplant) in lieu of standard Norwood palliation. Indeed, the poor survival statistics for "rescue" cardiac transplantation in those who have failed Norwood palliation would endorse this strategy as well.[62] Moreover, those born with HLHS and restrictive atrial septa, if bridged toward transplantation, should undergo some interventional procedure to encourage atrial mixing so as not to adversely affect results posttransplant.[63]

Jenkins reported the results of a comparison study between infants undergoing staged palliation or transplantation for HLHS.[29] Here, with 118 patients intended for staged surgery, and 124 intended for transplantation, transplantation resulted in greater survival rates at 1 and 5 years (61% and 55%) when compared with staged surgery (42% and 38%). A later comparison study evaluated a decision analysis involving six strategies: staged surgery, transplantation, stage 1 surgery as an interim to transplantation, listing for transplant for 1, 2, or 3 months before performing surgery if a donor was unavailable.[10] In this study, it was suggested that the optimal strategy for individual centers should be guided by their center's historical donor organ availability and stage 1 surgical mortality, since optimal outcome necessarily involves a balance of these risks. In centers where <10% of patients receive an organ within 3 months of birth, and where stage 1 operative mortality is <20%, staged surgery appears to offer the higher survival.[10] In contrast, where organ donation rates exceed 30% in 3 months, optimal treatment would include waiting 1 month on the transplant list followed by stage 1 surgery if an organ fails to become available.[10] Their analysis suggested that performing stage 1 surgery before listing, or performing it after a 2 or 3 month wait on the transplant list were rarely optimal choices.

In order to more accurately delineate optimal treatment in individual patients (versus treatment preferences in programs overall), the group from Loma Linda has developed a scoring system to predict those patients with higher mortality risk after stage 1 repair. Their scoring system used several factors known to increase the risk of surgical palliation (Table 91.2); patients with scores greater than 7 were

selected for early surgical palliation, while transplant was used in those with lower scores. Following the implementation of this system (as well as modifications in the perioperative care of all patients with HLHS), they reported significant increases in postoperative survival with the Norwood procedure (48 hour survival 88% vs. 40% and 1 year survival 50% vs. 10%), while transplant outcomes remained unchanged.[13] These reports suggest that the survival of patients following staged reconstruction can be significantly improved through an appropriate treatment algorithm tailored both to the program performing the repairs and to the individual patient.

Importantly, the best timing of hybrid intervention for those awaiting transplantation remains to be delineated clearly. As the group from Toronto Hospital for Sick Children has highlighted, earlier referral presages a better result, and clearly waiting for progression toward hemodynamic instability only compounds the potential risk factors for later transplantation.[64] In most "large" series endorsing this strategy, patients who had elective hybrid palliation were allowed to be discharged home to await transplantation.

Table 91.2 Loma Linda preoperative scoring system

Variable	Points
Ventricular Function	
Poor	0
Marginal	1
Good	2
Tricuspid Regurgitation	
Severe	0
Moderate	1
Mild or less	2
Ascending arch size (mm)	
<3	0
≥3	2
ASD Characteristics	
Restrictive	0
Nonrestrictive	1
Blood type	
A, B, AB	0
O	1
Age at Surgery (days)	
>21	0
14–21	1
<14	2

Source: Based on the recommendations from Checchia PA et al. *Ann Thorac Surg* 2004;77(2):477–83; discussion 483. With permission.
Note: Total score <7 points is a recommendation to proceed to surgical palliation, stage 1 (Norwood procedure); ≤7 points is a recommendation to list for transplantation.
ASD = atrial septal defect.

Summary

The optimal treatment of neonates with HLHS is a process in evolution. The rapid growth and development of hybrid procedures as an alternative to the Norwood procedure as first-stage palliation has also promoted several strategies for catheter-based palliation of neonates as a "bridge" to heart transplantation. A medical program involving maintenance of ductal patency with either PGE1 or ductal stenting, and a limiting of pulmonary blood flow with nitrogen or allowance of a mildly restrictive atrial septum, has even allowed for home discharge in some series, with a reduction in waiting list mortality to 15%.[48] In parallel with these advances are those of the recent Sano modification of the Norwood procedure, which has reportedly improved first-stage survival to as high as 90%. Only with continued reevaluation in light of further evolution of these processes will the optimal treatment strategy for neonates with HLHS become evident.

References

1. Fixler DE, Pastor P, Sigman E, Eifler CW. Ethnicity and socioeconomic status: Impact on the diagnosis of congenital heart disease. *J Am Coll Cardiol* 1993;21(7):1722–6.
2. Fyler DC. Report of the New England Regional Infant Cardiac Program. *Pediatrics* 1980;65(2 Pt 2):375–461.
3. Norwood WI, Lang P, Hansen DD. Physiologic repair of aortic atresia-hypoplastic left heart syndrome. *N Engl J Med* 1983;308(1):23–6.
4. Lang P, Norwood WI. Hemodynamic assessment after palliative surgery for hypoplastic left heart syndrome. *Circulation* 1983;68(1):104–8.
5. Meliones JN, Snider AR, Bove EL et al. Longitudinal results after first-stage palliation for hypoplastic left heart syndrome. *Circulation* 1990; 82(5 Suppl):IV151–6
6. Sade RM, Crawford FA, Jr., Fyfe DA. Symposium on hypoplastic left heart syndrome. *J Thorac Cardiovasc Surg* 1986;91(6):937–9.
7. Norwood WI, Kirklin JK, Sanders SP. Hypoplastic left heart syndrome: Experience with palliative surgery. *Am J Cardiol* 1980;45(1):87–91.
8. Pridjian AK, Mendelsohn AM, Lupinetti FM et al. Usefulness of the bidirectional Glenn procedure as staged reconstruction for the functional single ventricle. *Am J Cardiol* 1993; 71(11):959–62.
9. Bove EL, Ohye RG, Devaney EJ. Hypoplastic left heart syndrome: Conventional surgical management. *Semin Thorac Cardiovasc Surg Pediatr Card Surg Annu* 2004;7:3–10.
10. Jenkins PC, Flanagan MF, Sargent JD et al. A comparison of treatment strategies for hypoplastic left heart syndrome using decision analysis. *J Am Coll Cardiol* 2001;38(4):1181–7.
11. Bando K, Turrentine MW, Sun K et al. Surgical management of hypoplastic left heart syndrome. *Ann Thorac Surg* 1996;62(1):70–6; discussion 76–7.
12. Bu'Lock FA, Stumper O, Jagtap R et al. Surgery for infants with a hypoplastic systemic ventricle and severe outflow obstruction: Early results with a modified Norwood procedure. *Br Heart J* 1995;73(5):456–61.
13. Checchia PA, Larsen R, Sehra R et al. Effect of a selection and postoperative care protocol on survival of infants with hypoplastic left heart syndrome. *Ann Thorac Surg* 2004;77(2):477–83; discussion 483.
14. Bove EL. Current status of staged reconstruction for hypoplastic left heart syndrome. *Pediatr Cardiol* 1998;19(4):308–15.
15. Mahle WT, Spray TL, Wernovsky G et al. Survival after reconstructive surgery for hypoplastic left heart syndrome: A 15-year experience from a single institution. *Circulation* 2000;102(19 Suppl 3):III136–41.
16. Jonas RA, Hansen DD, Cook N, Wessel D. Anatomic subtype and survival after reconstructive operation for hypoplastic left heart syndrome. *J Thorac Cardiovasc Surg* 1994; 107(4):1121–7; discussion 1127–8.
17. Lofland GK, McCrindle BW, Williams WG et al. Critical aortic stenosis in the neonate: A multi-institutional study of management, outcomes, and risk factors. Congenital Heart Surgeons Society. *J Thorac Cardiovasc Surg* 2001;121(1):10–27.
18. Forbess JM, Cook N, Roth SJ et al. Ten-year institutional experience with palliative surgery for hypoplastic left heart syndrome. Risk factors related to stage I mortality. *Circulation* 1995;92(9 Suppl):II262–6.
19. Iannettoni MD, Bove EL, Mosca RS et al. Improving results with first-stage palliation for hypoplastic left heart syndrome. *J Thorac Cardiovasc Surg* 1994;107(3):934–40.
20. Duncan BW, Rosenthal GL, Jones TK, Lupinetti FM. First-stage palliation of complex univentricular cardiac anomalies in older infants. *Ann Thorac Surg* 2001;72(6):2077–80.
21. Bartram U, Grunenfelder J, Van Praagh R. Causes of death after the modified Norwood procedure: A study of 122 postmortem cases. *Ann Thorac Surg* 1997;64(6):1795–802.
22. Graziano JN, Heidelberger KP, Ensing GJ et al. The influence of a restrictive atrial septal defect on pulmonary vascular morphology in patients with hypoplastic left heart syndrome. *Pediatr Cardiol* 2002;23(2):146–51.
23. Bove EL, Lloyd TR. Staged reconstruction for hypoplastic left heart syndrome. Contemporary results. *Ann Surg* 1996;224(3):387–94; discussion 394–5.
24. Andrews R, Tulloh R, Sharland G et al. Outcome of staged reconstructive surgery for hypoplastic left heart syndrome following antenatal diagnosis. *Arch Dis Child* 2001;85(6):474–7.
25. Chang RK, Chen AY, Klitzner TS. Clinical management of infants with hypoplastic left heart syndrome in the United States, 1988–1997. *Pediatrics* 2002;110(2 Pt 1):292–8.
26. Bailey LL, Nehlsen-Cannarella SL, Doroshow RW et al. Cardiac allotransplantation in newborns as therapy for hypoplastic left heart syndrome. *N Engl J Med* 1986; 315(15):949–51.
27. Vricella LA, Razzouk AJ, del Rio M et al. Heart transplantation for hypoplastic left heart syndrome: Modified technique for reducing circulatory arrest time. *J Heart Lung Transplant* 1998;17(12):1167–71.
28. Bailey L, Concepcion W, Shattuck H, Huang L. Method of heart transplantation for treatment of hypoplastic left heart syndrome. *J Thorac Cardiovasc Surg* 1986;92(1):1–5.
29. Jenkins PC, Flanagan MF, Jenkins KJ et al. Survival analysis and risk factors for mortality in transplantation and staged surgery for hypoplastic left heart syndrome. *J Am Coll Cardiol* 2000;36(4):1178–85.
30. Guleserian KJ, SChechtman KB, Zheng J. Outcomes after listing for primary transplantation for infants with unoperated-on non-hypoplastic left heart syndrome congenital heart disease: A multi-institutional study. *J Heart Lung Transplant* 2011;30:1023–32.
31. Razzouk AJ, Chinnock RE, Gundry SR et al. Transplantation as a primary treatment for hypoplastic left heart syndrome: Intermediate-term results. *Ann Thorac Surg* 1996;62(1):1–7; discussion 8.
32. Chiavarelli M, Gundry SR, Razzouk AJ, Bailey LL. Cardiac transplantation for infants with hypoplastic left-heart syndrome. *JAMA* 1993;270(24):2944–7.
33. Tweddell JS, Canter CE, Bridges ND et al. Predictors of operative mortality and morbidity after infant heart transplantation. *Ann Thorac Surg* 1994;58(4):972–7.
34. Morris MC, Ittenbach RF, Godinez RI et al. Risk factors for mortality in 137 pediatric cardiac intensive care unit patients managed with extracorporeal membrane oxygenation. *Crit Care Med* 2004;32(4):1061–9.

35. Jonas RA, Lang P, Hansen D et al. First-stage palliation of hypoplastic left heart syndrome. The importance of coarctation and shunt size. *J Thorac Cardiovasc Surg* 1986;92(1):6–13.
36. Norwood WI, Jacobs ML. Fontan's procedure in two stages. *Am J Surg* 1993;166(5):548–51.
37. Goldberg CS, Gomez CA. Hypoplastic left heart syndrome: New developments and current controversies. *Semin Neonatol* 2003;8(6):461–8.
38. Rychik J, Rome JJ, Collins MH et al. The hypoplastic left heart syndrome with intact atrial septum: Atrial morphology, pulmonary vascular histopathology and outcome. *J Am Coll Cardiol* 1999;34(2):554–60.
39. Marshall AC, van der Velde ME, Tworetzky W et al. Creation of an atrial septal defect in utero for fetuses with hypoplastic left heart syndrome and intact or highly restrictive atrial septum. *Circulation* 2004;110(3):253–8.
40. Canter C, Naftel D, Caldwell R et al. Survival and risk factors for death after cardiac transplantation in infants. A multi-institutional study. The Pediatric Heart Transplant Study. *Circulation* 1997;96(1):227–31.
41. Allan LD, Sharland G, Tynan MJ. The natural history of the hypoplastic left heart syndrome. *Int J Cardiol* 1989;25(3):341–3.
42. Hornberger LK, Sanders SP, Rein AJ et al. Left heart obstructive lesions and left ventricular growth in the midtrimester fetus. A longitudinal study. *Circulation* 1995;92(6):1531–8.
43. Maxwell D, Allan L, Tynan MJ. Balloon dilatation of the aortic valve in the fetus: A report of two cases. *Br Heart J* 1991;65(5):256–8.
44. Allan LD, Maxwell DJ, Carminati M, Tynan MJ. Survival after fetal aortic balloon valvoplasty. *Ultrasound Obstet Gynecol* 1995;5(2):90–1.
45. Lopes LM, Cha SC, Kajita LJ et al. Balloon dilatation of the aortic valve in the fetus. A case report. *Fetal Diagn Ther* 1996;11(4):296–300.
46. Kohl T, Sharland G, Allan LD et al. World experience of percutaneous ultrasound-guided balloon valvuloplasty in human fetuses with severe aortic valve obstruction. *Am J Cardiol* 2000;85(10):1230–3.
47. Mora GA, Pizarro C, Jacobs ML, Norwood WI. Experimental model of single ventricle. Influence of carbon dioxide on pulmonary vascular dynamics. *Circulation* 1994;90(5 Pt 2):II43–6.
48. Tweddell JS, Hoffman GM, Fedderly RT et al. Phenoxybenzamine improves systemic oxygen delivery after the Norwood procedure. *Ann Thorac Surg* 1999;67(1):161–7; discussion 167–8.
49. Bourke KD, Sondheimer HM, Ivy DD et al. Improved pretransplant management of infants with hypoplastic left heart syndrome enables discharge to home while waiting for transplantation. *Pediatr Cardiol* 2003;24(6):538–43.
50. Ruiz CE, Gamra H, Zhang HP et al. Brief report: Stenting of the ductus arteriosus as a bridge to cardiac transplantation in infants with the hypoplastic left-heart syndrome. *N Engl J Med* 1993;328(22):1605–8.
51. Gibbs JL, Uzun O, Blackburn ME et al. Fate of the stented arterial duct. *Circulation* 1999;99(20):2621–5.
52. Boucek MM, Mashburn C, Kunz E, Chan KC. Ductal anatomy: A determinant of successful stenting in hypoplastic left heart syndrome. *Pediatr Cardiol* 2005;26:200–5.
53. Michel-Behnke I, Akintuerk H, Marquardt I et al. Stenting of the ductus arteriosus and banding of the pulmonary arteries: Basis for various surgical strategies in newborns with multiple left heart obstructive lesions. *Heart* 2003;89(6):645–50.
54. de Leval MR. Surgical management of the neonate with congenital heart disease. *Br Heart J* 1986;55(1):1–3.
55. Mitchell MB, Campbell DN, Boucek MM et al. Mechanical limitation of pulmonary blood flow facilitates heart transplantation in older infants with hypoplastic left heart syndrome. *Eur J Cardio-Thoracic Surg* 2003;23(5):735–42.
56. Guleserian KHm Barker GM, Sharma MS. Bilateral pulmonary artery banding for resuscitation in high-risk, single-ventricle neonates and infants: A single-center experience. *J Thorac Cardiovasc Surg* 2013;145:206–14
57 Miyamoto SD, Pietra BA, Chan KC, Ivy DD, Mashburn C, Campbell DN et al. Long-term outcome of palliation with internal pulmonary artery bands after primary transplantation for hypoplastic left heart syndrome. *Pediatr Cardiol* 2009;30(4):419–25.
58. Sebastian VA, Guleserian KJ, Leonard SR, Forbess JM. Heart transplantation techniques after hybrid single-ventricle palliation. *J Cardiac Surg* 2010;25:596–600.
59. Kanter KR, Mahle, WT, Vincent RN, Berg AM. Aortic complications after pediatric cardiac transplantation in patients with a previous Norwood reconstruction. *Semin Thorac Cardiovasc Surg Pediatr Card Surg Ann* 2011;14:24–28.
60. Chrisant MR, Naftel DC, Drummond-Webb J et al. Fate of infants with hypoplastic left heart syndrome listed for cardiac transplantation: A multicenter study. *J Heart Lung Transplant* 2005;24(5):576–82.
61. Vida, VL, Bacha EA, Larrazabal A. Surgical outcome for patients with the mitral-stenosis-aortic atresia variant of hypoplastic left heart syndrome. *J Thorac Cardiovasc Surg* 2008;135:139–46.
62. Jacbos JP, Quintessensa JA, Chai PJ et al. Rescue cardiac transplantation for failed staged palliation in patients with hypoplastic left heart syndrome. *Cardiol Young* 2006;16:556–62.
63. Canter CE, Moorhead S, Huddleston CB, Spray TL. Restrictive atrial septal communication as a determinant of outcome of cardiac transplantation for hypoplastic left heart syndrome. *Circulation* 1993;88(pt II):456–60.
64. Caldarone CA, Benson L, Holtby H et al. Initial experience with hybrid palliation for neonates with single-ventricle physiology. *Ann Thorac Surg* 2007;84:1294–300.

92

Intraoperative VSD device closure

Damien Kenny, Qi-Ling Cao, and Ziyad M. Hijazi

Introduction

Almost all perimembranous and most muscular ventricular septal defects (VSDs) can be closed surgically, regardless of the patient's size or weight. Some muscular VSDs, however, have been a challenge because of their location, the presence of right ventricular trabeculations, and inability to effectively close the defect through the right atrium, necessitating right or left ventriculotomy, which is fraught with its own complications.[1] Among the muscular VSDs, the apical and anterior muscular VSDs are difficult to visualize intraoperatively and, hence, closure maybe incomplete or not possible.[1,2] Surgical closure may be prolonged and this in turn increases the cardiopulmonary bypass (CPB) time, and its associated complications.[3]

On the other hand, transcatheter techniques are being employed with increasing frequency to close muscular and perimembranous VSDs.[4] These techniques, with several advantages when compared with surgery, have limitations primarily because of patient's weight and size. In our practice, we may be able to close muscular VSDs percutaneously in small infants (around 3 kg); however, the procedure is difficult and may carry an added risk, including hemodynamic compromise.

Intraoperative device closure of VSDs was first introduced in 1991.[5-7] After the patient was placed on CPB, a Clamshell device was used to close complicated muscular VSDs under direct visualization. This procedure was, however, inadequate, because visualization of the VSD was difficult, as the heart was flaccid and hence results were suboptimal.[6]

After the introduction of the Amplatzer septal occluder device, attention was redirected to design a muscular VSD device designed specifically for closure of muscular VSDs.[8] During initial experiments in a dog model, a muscular VSD (with 10 mm sharp-punch device) was created on a beating heart through a right ventriculotomy, under epicardial echocardiographic guidance. This experimental process was designed to assess the efficacy of the muscular occluder delivered percutaneously.[8] A further report from the same group followed describing closure through the ventricular wall in a similar fashion to how the defect was created.[9] Utilizing epicardial echocardiography, closure was performed by introducing the delivery sheath through the free wall of the right ventricle. Subsequent successful reports in humans soon followed.[10-12] and the term "perventricular" closure was coined by Amin and colleagues and the application of the technique was extended to perimembranous defects.[13] The evolution of patient selection, procedural technique, and outcome data are presented in this chapter.

Patient selection

Indications from published reports for perventricular closure of muscular defects are low weight, issues with vascular access, inability or failed attempt to close the defect in the catheterization laboratory, concomitant lesions that require a visit to the operating room, and patients who have had pulmonary artery banding in the past for VSD and require de-banding of the pulmonary artery in addition to closure of the defect.[11,12,14-16] More recently, published guidelines for intervention in pediatric cardiac diseases[17] have suggested (as a class IIb recommendation) limitation of this approach for neonates or infants weighing less than 5 kg with a hemodynamically significant muscular VSD undergoing surgery for concomitant defects requiring CPB (level of evidence B). It may be argued that this is overly restrictive and working practice is likely to continue to include small infants with single large muscular defects irrespective of the need for concomitant surgery. In this setting patient selection will continue to be based on transthoracic echocardiography with particular attention paid to the relationship of the defect to the surrounding ventricular and valvar structures including the moderator band, and the ventricular apex.

More recently, attention has been redirected to intraoperative closure of perimembranous defects[18,19] since the original report in an animal model in 2004.[13] Concern for closure in this setting has mirrored concern following percutaneous closure with an unacceptable incidence of complete heart block and potential encroachment on the aortic valve. However, it is unclear whether newer device designs now undergoing clinical trials for percutaneous closure of perimembranous defects will revive further interest in the perventricular approach.

Devices

The majority of reported cases have been attempted using the Amplatzer muscular VSD device (St. Jude Medical, Plymouth, MN). The device is made of 0.005" Nitinol wire that is woven to form two symmetrical disks connected by a waist. The disks are 8 mm larger than the waist with the waist 7 mm in length to accommodate the thickness of the muscular ventricular septum. The available sizes range from 4 to 18 mm in 2 mm increments. For defects that are larger than 18 mm, a postinfarction muscular VSD device can be used with a waist 10 mm in length and disks 10 mm larger than the waist. However, this device is not readily available in the United States due to lack of FDA approval. Experience has also been reported with the CardioSEAL occluder[16] and a number of Amplatzer-like devices developed in China. Further details on the membranous VSD occluder 2 are beyond the scope of this chapter, particularly considering limited percutaneous clinical experience to date[20] and will be discussed in a separate chapter. The CardioSEAL and StarFLEX devices (NMT Medical, Boston, MA) do not exist anymore (the manufacturer went out of business).

The procedure

The key to a successful procedure is collaboration between the surgeon and the interventionalist. For single muscular VSDs, the procedure may be performed in an operating room setting (no need for fluoroscopy) or in a hybrid catheterization suite. However, for multiple muscular defects, fluoroscopy is useful, so a hybrid setting is preferred. Ideally, transesophageal echocardiography (TEE) is used to guide the interventional procedure. Epicardial echocardiography may also be used, however, this further limits availability of space in a potentially cramped environment. Recently, a micro-TTE probe has become available that may be used in infants as small as 1.7 kg.[21] The septum is carefully scanned from apex to the base of the heart and from anterior to posterior dimensions. Particular vigilance should be given to troubled spots such as the apical and the anterior septum. The defect is measured in two views during ventricular diastole, to choose the appropriately sized device (Figure 92.1). Usually a device that is 2 mm larger than the defect is chosen for muscular VSDs (with a device equal to or 1 mm larger than the defect reported for perimembranous VSDs).

After the patient is draped and prepped in sterile fashion, a median sternotomy is performed. The extent and degree of sternal opening is dependent on surgical experience, however, with initial experience greater degrees of exposure are recommended. After the sternum is divided, the pericardium is opened longitudinally and a pericardial cradle made (Figure 92.2). Depending upon the location of the muscular VSD, a purse-string suture is placed (opposite to the defect) on the free wall of the right ventricle. If the defect is apical, it is of paramount importance not to place the purse-string suture close to the apex. In order to be as close to the defect as possible, a gentle tapping on the right ventricular free wall and echocardiographic assistance is helpful in locating an optimal spot for placement of the purse-string suture (Figure 92.3).

Once the purse-string suture is placed on the free wall of the right ventricle, the distance from the right ventricular free wall to the middle of the defect, and the maximum distance from the free wall to the left ventricular free wall (with a straight line passing through the middle of the VSD) is measured. This distance is important because it helps in determining how deep the delivery sheath can be advanced without injuring the left ventricular free wall. "Hybrid" sheaths are available with shorter dilators, which are ideal for use in this setting and may prevent damage to the ventricular free wall.

Once an appropriate puncture site is identified by echocardiography, an 18G angio-catheter is advanced through the purse string over the right ventricle, and once it is in the lumen of the right ventricle, the needle is removed. Under TEE guidance, a short soft-tipped J-wire (Rosen wires are more echogenic than Terumo GlideWires) is advanced through the angio-catheter and directed toward the VSD. The angio-catheter is ideally held by the surgeon as his or her knowledge of the location of the VSD in the operating room is helpful in directing the catheter toward the VSD. Once the wire crosses the defect, it is maneuvered and advanced through the aortic valve or toward the left ventricle. The angio-catheter is removed and an appropriate sized sheath (1 Fr larger than that recommended for delivery of that specific device size) is placed across the defect (Figure 92.2). The dilator is removed after ensuring that the sheath is in the left ventricle or ascending aorta. (Predilation may be carried out with a dilator 1 Fr larger than the delivery sheath chosen to place the device.) The sheath is allowed to back bleed and flushed. Gently pull the sheath back if spontaneous back bleeding does not occur when the dilator is removed. The flushing of the sheath will clear blood from the sheath and also help accurately locate the sheath tip (saline contrast echocardiography). The device is then loaded to an appropriately sized short sheath and advanced to the tip of the sheath. This sheath is then placed into the hemostatic seal of the sheath in the right ventricular free wall and advanced through the sheath to its tip within the LV (Figure 92.4). The whole system is pulled back (for perimembranous VSDs

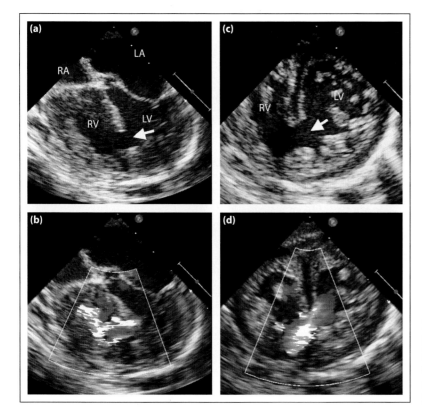

Figure 92.1 (**See color insert.**) Series of images outlining perventricular closure of a large midmuscular defect in a 4.1 kg infant. TEE assessment of the midmuscular defect in two different planes (a and c) with and without color Doppler (b and d).

the tip should be in the ascending aorta), and the left disk is deployed by both pulling on the delivery sheath and advancing the cable to ensure the stiff device again does not damage the left ventricular free wall. Once the left disk is completely deployed, the whole system is pulled toward the ventricular septum and, while keeping the delivery cable stable in one location, the delivery sheath is pulled to deploy the waist and the right disk. If the device appears stable, after gentle pull–push maneuvers, it is released, by anticlockwise rotation of the delivery cable (Figure 92.5). The procedure can be repeated if there are multiple defects. Full TEE reassessment is carried out to ensure the defect is closed and that there is

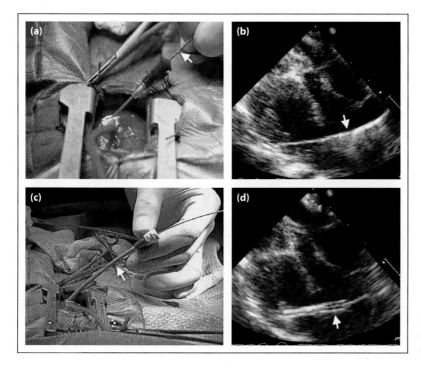

Figure 92.2 (**See color insert.**) Advancement of the wire (a, b) and the sheath (c, d) across the defect.

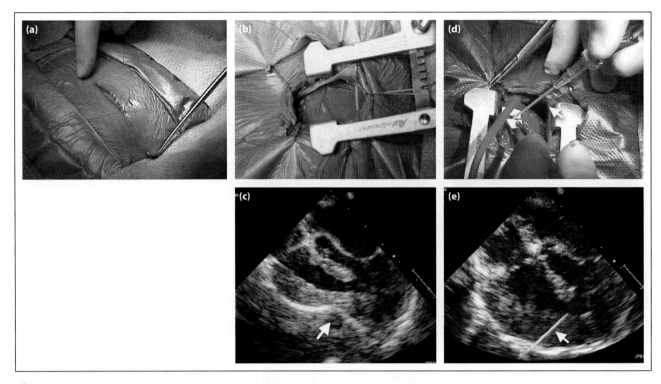

Figure 92.3 (**See color insert.**) (a, b) Sternal and pericardial opening. (c) Digital pressure seen transmitted to the free wall of the RV to define puncture site. (d, e) Needle puncture of the RV with corresponding TEE image.

no impingement on the surrounding structures. The sheath and the cable are removed and the purse-string suture tightened to achieve hemostasis. The chest is closed in the routine fashion (Figure 92.6). If there are multiple defects, as mentioned above, we recommend performing the procedure in a true hybrid lab with fluoroscopy. The first defect is crossed in the usual fashion. Then an attempt is made to cross the

second defect using the perventricular approach. On occasions and due to the proximity of these defects to each other, it may not be possible to cross the second defect from the RV side. In such situations, we perform percutaneous crossing of the second defect from the LV side. We maneuver a wire to the main pulmonary artery. Then we snare the wire from the pulmonary artery using the sheath that is placed in the right

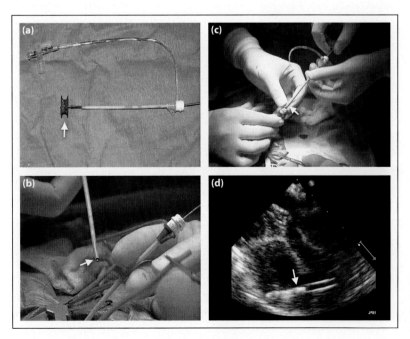

Figure 92.4 (**See color insert.**) Loading the device through a short delivery sheath (a, b) and advancement of the device through the preexisting perventricular sheath to the LV.

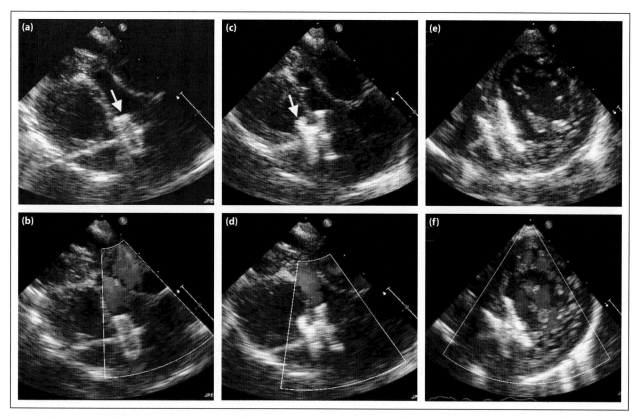

Figure 92.5 (**See color insert.**) Deployment of the left ventricular disk with color assessment on TEE (a, b), following full device deployment (c, d) and following release (e, f).

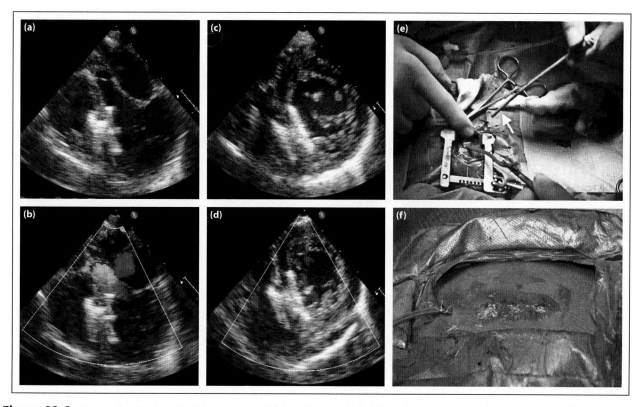

Figure 92.6 (**See color insert.**) Final assessment of the device in two separate planes with no residual leak seen on color Doppler (a–d). Chest closure with sutured wound and chest drain (e, f).

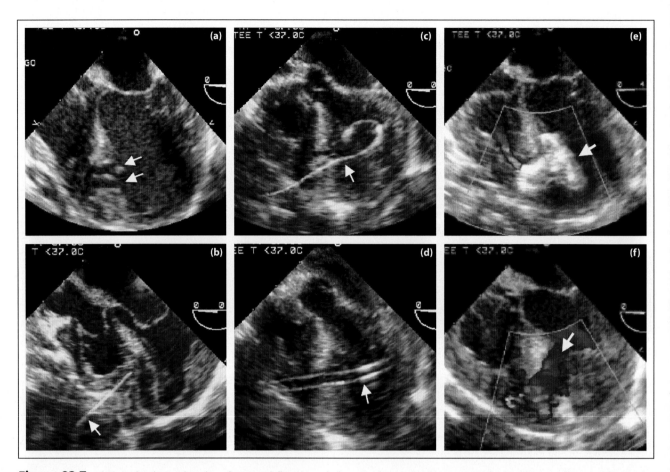

Figure 92.7 (**See color insert.**) Series of TEE and fluoroscopic images demonstrating perventricular closure of two midmuscular VSDs. (a) Initial imaging defines the two defects with needle puncture (b) and crossing of the more inferior defect (c). Advancement of the delivery sheath (d) with device delivery (e) however persisting flow through the separate defect.

ventricle free wall. The wire is exteriorized and the sheath is advanced over the wire to the LV side. Then the device can be deployed similar to the first device deployment (Figures 92.7 and 9.8).

If the defect is apical, it is recommended not to place the purse-string suture adjacent to the defect. The deployment of the right ventricular disk is difficult because as the sheath is withdrawn, the disk may protrude out of the right ventricle free wall. The purse-string suture is placed away from the RV apex, and a loop is made for the delivery sheath as if the device was being deployed from the internal jugular vein. The waist and part of the RV disk is deployed into the left ventricle, and the sheath and the cable is pulled to approximate the left disk to the LV side of the ventricular septum and the right disk is deployed very slowly while advancing the cable and retracting the sheath. If the device protrudes out of the RV free wall, the delivery sheath is advanced over the device and the right disk is repositioned. In some patients, the microscrew of the device has protruded through the RV free wall. In such cases, the surgeon has sutured the microscrew in the free wall and augmented this with some pledgets. In patients

with larger perimembranous or inlet VSDs and associated more apical muscular VSDs, initial perventricular closure of the apical defect may be followed by surgical closure of the more basal defect (Figure 92.9).

Results

The use of the perventricular technique for closure of muscular VSDs has been widespread and currently a multicenter retrospective analysis of the US experience is underway. Initial animal experience demonstrated low complication rates with complete closure of all muscular defects. Residual flow was seen following membranous occlusion in three of five animals and one went on to develop aortic regurgitation. Subsequent studies followed confirming these outcomes in either isolated VSDs or when occurring in conjunction with other congenital cardiac lesions.[15,22–25] Over 60 collective attempted procedures describing perventricular approach to muscular VSDs have been reported with success rates of 85–100% and variable residual shunting rates.[14,15,22–25] Approximately

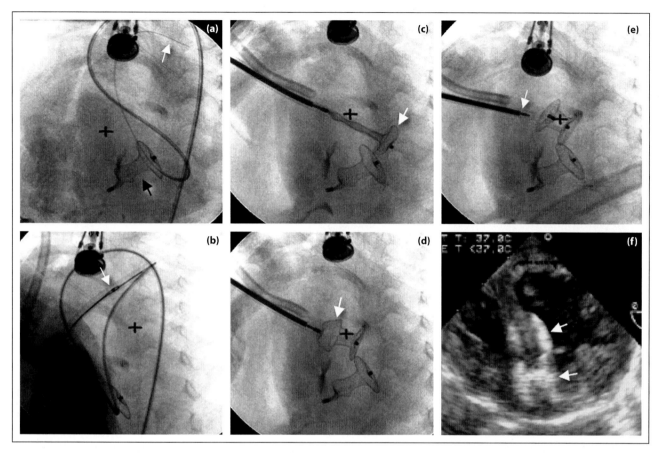

Figure 92.8   As the defect was challenging to cross again from the RV side, retrograde femoral arterial approach facilitated crossing from the less crowded LV (a) and creation of an arteriovenous loop through the wall of the right ventricle (b). The device was then delivered and deployed through the perventricular sheath (c and d). Once in position the device was released (e) with the final result demonstrating satisfactory position of both devices across the ventricular septum (f).

50% of these patients weighed 6 kg or less at the time of the procedure. In one of these studies evaluating exclusive muscular VSD closure in small infants, residual shunting requiring pulmonary artery banding was seen in two of eight patients.[15] Experience with alternative occlusion

devices, namely the CardioSEAL Occluder, have also been published, with successful deployment of the device in four of five attempted cases.[16] There was one device failure with the arms of the device protruding through the right ventricular free wall in a 4 kg neonate requiring surgical

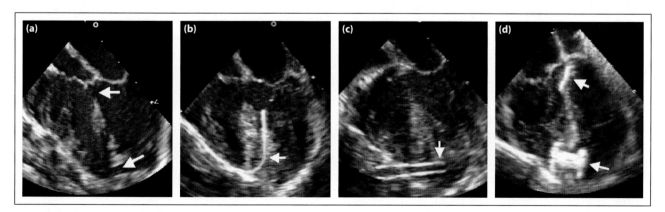

Figure 92.9   Series of images demonstrating perventricular closure of an apical VSD followed by patch closure of a large inlet VSD. (a) Initial TEE imaging demonstrates the two defects as outlined by the white arrows. (b) Crossing the apical defect with a wire and (c) sheath. (d) Final TEE image demonstrating patch closure of the inlet defect with device closure of the apical defect.

removal of the device. A novel approach describing apical VSD closure with the Amplatzer ductal occluder sutured surgically at the RV aspect of the device in small patients undergoing open repair of other cardiac lesions has also been described.[26]

The largest clinical experience with intraoperative perimembranous VSD closure evaluated attempted closure and median follow-up of 22 months in 61 patients using an asymmetric device designed in China (Shanghai Shape Memory Alloy Co, Ltd [SHSMA], Shanghai, China).[27] Patients had a mean weight of 12.6 kg. The defect was closed with a device in 97% of patients with 6% eventually converted into surgical closure. Residual shunt was seen in 6% of patients and two patients developed intraoperative complete heart block, one recovering with removal of the device and another following treatment with steroids.

Experience has also been reported with attempted perventricular closure of doubly committed subarterial VSDs with a specially designed device (Lifetech Scientific, Shenzhen, China).[28] The device is partly designed like a saddle without the protruding superior rim to escape from the aortic and pulmonary valve, with a positioning marker in the opposite side. The device is available in sizes ranging from 5 to 10 mm in 1 mm increments. The connecting waist is 5 mm long, and the inferior rim of the left ventricle and right ventricle disks is only 3 mm larger than the waist. Five of six patients (11–23 kg) underwent successful closure through a left anterior thoracotomy with one patient requiring conversion to full surgical closure. Follow-up of up to 21 months did not demonstrate any residual leak, or conduction or valvar abnormalities.

There has also been limited reported experience with perventricular closure of postinfarct VSDs.[29] This group described plicating the apical RV free wall to the VSD margin by deploying the proximal disk on the exterior surface of the RV serving to minimize the degree of residual shunting in large defects.

Most published data with muscular defects have reported shorter-term outcomes, however, one study evaluating medium term (40 month) follow-up in six infants suggested small residual shunts in two patients and one who had developed a left ventricular pseudoaneurysm thought to be related to trauma of the LV free wall at the time of the intraoperative closure.[25]

Robotic-assisted perventricular closure of perimembranous VSD in an animal model has also been reported, however, this has not evolved into clinical practice as yet.[30]

Conclusions

At the current time, most centers are practicing intraoperative VSD closure for infants with large muscular defects, however, recent reports suggest a broadening application of this approach to other types of VSDs with variations in surgical incision sites. There is no risk of radiation, contrast dye, or cumbersome catheter courses, which may cause arrhythmias, decrease cardiac output, and lead to hemodynamic compromise.

The technique can be done purely in the OR under TEE guidance only or for multiple defects it can be done in a hybrid suite using both TEE and fluoroscopy to guide the closure. The use of the technique can be extended to patients with concomitant lesions to shorten total CPB time. It remains to be seen whether newer device designs will allow widespread extension of the approach to perimembranous defects.

References

1. Serraf A, Lacour-Gayet F, Bruniaux J et al. Surgical management of isolated multiple ventricular septal defects. *J Thorac Cardiovasc Surg* 1992;103:437–43.
2. Singh AK, de Leval MR, Stark J. Left ventriculotomy for closure of muscular ventricular septal defects. *Ann Surg* 1997;186:577–80.
3. Kern FH, Hickey PR. The effects of cardiopulmonary bypass on the brain. In: Jonas RA. Ed. *Cardiopulmonary Bypass in the Neonates, Infants and Young Children.* 1st ed. Boston: Blackwell Science; 1994. pp. 263–78.
4. Chessa M, Carminati M, Cao Q et al. Transcatheter closure of congenital and acquired muscular ventricular septal defects using the Amplatzer device. *J Invas Cardiol* 2002;14:322–7.
5. Bridges ND, Perry SB, Goldstein SA et al. Preoperative transcatheter closure of congenital muscular ventricular septal defects. *N Engl J Med* 1991;324:1312–7.
6. Fishberger SB, Bridges ND, Keane JF et al. Intraoperative device closure of ventricular septal defects. *Circulation* 1993;88(part 2):205–9.
7. Okubo M, Benson LN, Nykanen D et al. Outcomes of intraoperative device closure of muscular ventricular septal defects. *Ann Thorac Surg* 2001;72:416–23.
8. Amin Z, Gu X, Berry JM et al. A new device for closure of muscular ventricular septal defects in a canine model. *Circulation* 1999;100:320–8.
9. Amin Z, Gu X, Berry JM et al. Perventricular closure of ventricular septal defects without cardiopulmonary bypass. *Ann Thorac Surg* 1999;68:149–54.
10. Amin Z, Berry JM, Foker J et al. Intraoperative closure of muscular ventricular septal defect in a canine model and application of the technique in a baby. *J Thorac Cardiovasc Surg* 1998;115:1374–6.
11. Amin Z, Berry JM, Danford D et al. Intraoperative closure of muscular ventricular septal defects without cardiopulmonary bypass: Preliminary results of the perventricular approach. *Circulation* 2001;104(suppl 17):II-710.
12. Maheshwari S, Suresh PV, Bansal M et al. Perventricular device closure of muscular ventricular septal defects on the beating heart. *Indian Heart J* 2004;56:333–5.
13. Amin Z, Danford D, Lof J et al. Intraoperative device closure of perimembranous ventricular septal defects without cardiopulmonary bypass: Preliminary results with the perventricular technique. *J Thorac Cardiovasc Surg* 2004;127:234–41.
14. Bacha E, Cao Q, Starr JP et al. Perventricular device closure of muscular ventricular septal defects on the beating heart: Technique and results. *J Thorac Cardiovasc Surg* 2003;126:1718–23.
15. Crossland DS, Wilkinson JL, Cochrane AD et al. Initial results of primary device closure of large muscular ventricular septal defects in early infancy using perventricular access. *Catheter Cardiovasc Interv* 2008;72:386–9.

16. Lim DS, Forbes TJ, Rothman A et al. Transcatheter closure of high-risk muscular ventricular septal defects with the CardioSEAL occluder: Initial report from the CardioSEAL VSD registry. *Catheter Cardiovasc Interv* 2007;70:740–4.

17. Feltes TF, Bacha E, Beekman RH 3rd et al. Indications for cardiac catheterization and intervention in pediatric cardiac disease: A scientific statement from the American Heart Association. *Circulation* 2011;123:2607–52.

18. Zhang GC, Chen Q, Chen LW et al. Transthoracic echo cardiographic guidance of minimally invasive perventricular device closure of perimembranous ventricular septal defect without cardio pulmonary bypass: Initial experience. *Eur Heart J Cardiovasc Imaging* 2012;13:739–44.

19. Schreiber C, Vogt M, Kühn A et al. Periventricular closure of a perimembranous VSD: Treatment option in selected patients. *Thorac Cardiovasc Surg* 2012;60:78–80.

20. Velasco-Sanchez D, Tzikas A, Ibrahim R, Miró J. Transcatheter closure of perimembranous ventricular septal defects: Initial human experience with the amplatzer membranous VSD occluder 2. *Catheter Cardiovasc Interv* 2013;82:474–9.

21. Zyblewski SC, Shirali GS, Forbus GA et al. Initial experience with a miniaturized multiplane transesophageal probe in small infants undergoing cardiac operations. *Ann Thorac Surg* 2010;89:1990–4.

22. Bacha EA, Cao QL, Galantowicz ME et al. Multicenter experience with perventricular device closure of muscular ventricular septal defects. *Pediatr Cardiol* 2005; 26:169–75.

23. Gan C, Lin K, An Q, Tang H, Song H, Lui RC, Tao K, Zhuang Z, Shi Y. Perventricular device closure of muscular ventricular septal defects on beating hearts: Initial experience in eight children. *J Thorac Cardiovasc Surg* 2009;137:929–33.

24. Michel-Behnke I, Ewert P, Koch A et al. For the investigators of the Working Group Interventional Cardiology of the German Association of Pediatric Cardiology. Device closure of ventricular septal defects by hybrid procedures: A multicenter retrospective study. *Catheter Cardiovasc Interv* 2011;77:242–51.

25. Bendaly EA, Hoyer MH, Breinholt JP. Mid-term follow up of perventricular device closure of muscular ventricular septal defects. *Catheter Cardiovasc Interv* 2011;78:577–82.

26. Neukamm C, Bjørnstad PG, Fischer G, Smevik B, Lindberg HL. A novel method of hybrid intraoperative catheter-based closure of ventricular septal defects using the Amplatzer PDA occluder. *Catheter Cardiovasc Interv* 2011;77:557–63.

27. Tao K, Lin K, Shi Y, Song H, Lui RC, Gan C, An Q. Perventricular device closure of perimembranous ventricular septal defects in 61 young children: Early and midterm follow-up results. *J Thorac Cardiovasc Surg* 2010;140:864–70.

28. Pan S, Xing Q, Cao Q et al. Perventricular device closure of doubly committed subarterial ventral septal defect through left anterior minithoracotomy on beating hearts. *Ann Thorac Surg* 2012;94:2070–5.

29. Love BA, Whang B, Filsoufi F. Perventricular device closure of post-myocardial infarction ventricular septal defect on the beating heart. *J Thorac Cardiovasc Surg* 2011;142:230–2.

30. Amin Z, Woo R, Danford DA et al. Robotically assisted perventricular closure of perimembranous ventricular septal defects: Preliminary results in Yucatan pigs. *J Thorac Cardiovasc Surg* 2006;131:427–32.

93

Intraoperative stent implantation

Sameer Gafoor and Evan M. Zahn

Intraoperative stent implantation

Since 1990, transcatheter implantation of intravascular stents has been extensively described as an effective form of therapy for a variety of acquired and congenital vascular stenoses.[1–7] Congenital lesions treated by stent placement include central and branch pulmonary artery stenosis, native and recurrent coarctation of the aorta, a variety of venous stenoses, intra- or extracardiac baffle obstructions, and conduit narrowing. More recently, stents and covered stents have been utilized as means of creating or maintaining new vascular channels such as transcatheter Fontan baffle placement or long-term maintenance of ductal arteriosus patency.[8–12] Although the effectiveness of stent therapy is well accepted, the technical demands of implantation have at times limited the applicability of these devices, particularly in small critically ill children. While improvements in delivery technique, balloon, stent, and sheath technology have made percutaneous stent implantation a more accomplishable procedure,[13–15] there are numerous clinical scenarios where intraoperative stent implantation may be preferable. In this chapter, we will discuss the techniques utilized for intraoperative implantation of stents in the pulmonary arteries and aorta.

History

Intraoperative stent implantation was first reported in 1992.[16] This description and all other subsequent reports describe stent implantation under direct visualization in the operating room with essentially no immediate postprocedural assessment. Despite the obvious pitfalls of such techniques, the results reported for intraoperative pulmonary artery stent implantation have been good with improvements in vascular diameter (as measured in follow-up) comparable to those reported using standard percutaneous implantation.[17–19] A smaller experience with intraoperative placement of pulmonary vein stents indicate

good initial results with high early restenosis rates, similar to what has been described with the percutaneous treatment of this lesion. Proponents of intraoperative stent implantation tout the speed and ease of implantation as important advantages of this technique.

Indications of intraoperative stent implantation

Previously described[19] indications for intraoperative stent implantation include (1) a need for a concomitant surgical procedure, (2) limited vascular access, (3) small patient size, and (4) as rescue therapy after failed percutaneous stent placement. At one author's institution (EMZ), this approach is advocated in selected patients requiring stent placement in the early postoperative period as an alternative to surgical arterioplasty.[20] One important advantage of intraoperative or hybrid stent implantation is that regardless of patient size, a stent ultimately capable of achieving an adult diameter can nearly always be implanted. The majority of children requiring stent implantation at any age would ideally receive stents capable of being expanded to "adult size" (e.g., 16–20 mm in diameter) as a child grows. Despite dramatic improvements in stent technology, relatively large stiff delivery systems are still required for deployment of "adult-size" stents (e.g., a large XD Genesis typically requires at least an 8 F delivery system). In small infants or children, particularly those with tenuous hemodynamics, the placement of these delivery systems often produces such profound hemodynamic compromise as to preclude safe completion of the procedure. Even stable infants and toddlers (<15 kg) can present significant challenges for percutaneous implantation of adult-size stents across certain lesions (e.g., tortuous left pulmonary artery stenosis in the setting of a redundant outflow tract after repair of tetralogy of Fallot). Additional technical issues that may negatively impact percutaneous stent placement include (1) an excessively tortuous catheter course with numerous acute angles to navigate, (2) pronounced

Table 93.1 Potential indications for intraoperative stenting

Patient	Small patient size
Clinical	Concomitant cardiac surgery (e.g., homograft or Fontan)
	Rescue procedure after percutaneous attempt
Hemodynamic	Marginal hemodynamics that cannot tolerate passage of delivery system across right heart (tricuspid or pulmonary regurgitation with wire in place)
Anatomical	Tortuous vasculature
	Movement due to pulmonary insufficiency
	Proximity of important cardiac structures to lesion
	Stenosis in proximal segment with length too short for shortest stent
	Mechanical pulmonary valve

delivery system movement during implantation (e.g., as a result of pulmonary insufficiency), and (3) close proximity of important vascular structures to the target lesion (e.g., origin of the right pulmonary artery when attempting to stent an ostial stenosis of the left pulmonary artery). Utilizing a hybrid technique in these instances may mean the difference between a successful result versus a "nightmare case." Potential indications for intraoperative stenting are listed in Table 93.1.

Advantages and disadvantages of intraoperative stent implantation

The advantages and disadvantages of intraoperative stent implantation are listed in Table 93.2. The abilities to access the lesion directly, shape the stent, and handle complications are the often-listed advantages behind intraoperative stent implantation. Access is usually through the main pulmonary artery directly to the lesion without need for stiff

Table 93.2 Advantages and disadvantages of intraoperative stent implantation

Advantages	Ease of implant—direct wire and stent course
	Complications can be addressed intraoperatively
	Ability to shape stents to fit anatomy
	Ability to alter stent length
Disadvantages	Imprecise distal positioning
	Results of stent dilatation not known unless concomitant C-arm

wires or delivery systems. The stent can be shaped (e.g., the proximal stent edge can be folded back to appose the back wall of the main pulmonary artery [MPA]) or have a customized length (e.g., tailored to fit the stenotic regions).[20]

The disadvantages of intraoperative stent implantation include imprecise distal positioning. It is difficult to know where the wire location is at times during the implantation of the stent. It may be in a very small distal branch or even in a side branch, with risk of perforation. An x-ray can be required to see the effect of stent dilatation. These disadvantages can be mitigated by fluoroscopy in the operative suite.

Techniques

Over the past decade, two methods have been developed for hybrid stent delivery. The first technique, *videoscopic guided stent implantation*, has been used solely for the treatment of branch pulmonary artery stenosis, and typically is a planned procedure that takes place in the operating room. The second technique, *stent implantation via surgically provided vascular access*, has been used to treat a wide variety of lesions, including branch pulmonary artery stenoses, recurrent aortic arch obstruction (after hypoplastic left heart syndrome (HLHS) palliative surgery), and shunt occlusion/stenosis. This approach can be performed in the catheterization laboratory, a surgical suite, or a hybrid suite.

Videoscopic guided stent implantation

Often, videoscopic guided stent implantation procedures have been performed in conjunction with other surgical procedures, most commonly, right ventricular outflow reconstruction (including conduit replacement) and/or delayed ventricular septal defect closure in the setting of pulmonary atresia and ventricular septal defect. A critical component to the success of this technique is an exhaustive evaluation of the pertinent anatomy *prior* to the operative procedure. To date, this has been done with preoperative angiography although it is likely that preoperative MRI and/or CT angiography will replace the need for this in the near future.[21] During the preoperative catheterization, selective pulmonary angiography using multiple axial angulated views aimed at obtaining optimal images of the target lesion and surrounding vascular structures is performed.

If angiography is not used during videoscopic stent placement, decisions regarding stent type/length, implantation diameter, and precise implant location are decided *prior* to surgery based upon these preprocedural angiograms (Figure 93.1). A stent with the largest future potential diameter (i.e., "an adult-sized stent") is chosen in most cases. An important exception occurs in neonates or small

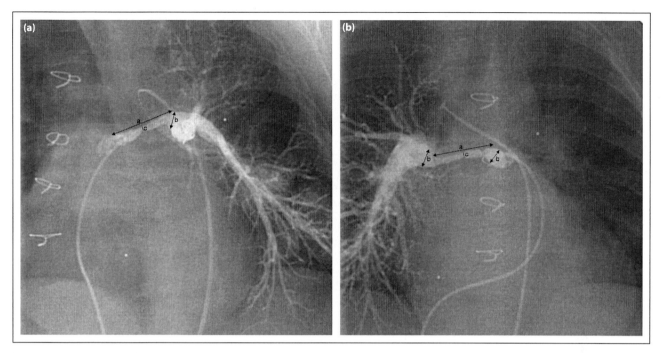

Figure 93.1   Preoperative selective pulmonary angiography is performed in a 6-month-old with bilateral severe branch pulmonary artery hypoplasia associated with pulmonary atresia/VSD, status postneonatal right ventricular outflow reconstruction (VSD left open). Measurements used for stent/balloon selection are vessel length to be stented (a), diameter of adjacent "normal vessel" (b), and narrowest stenosis diameter (c).

infants where implantation diameter is limited by adjacent small native vessel size *and* further future surgery will be required (e.g., conduit replacement). In these cases, smaller stents, with potential diameters less than adult size, may be implanted and either removed or altered surgically at subsequent operations. Sometimes, coronary stents have been used for extreme hypoplasia of the pulmonary arteries or very distal stenosis.[18] The balloon diameter used for implantation is chosen to match the diameter of the nearest adjacent normal vessel (typically distal to the target lesion) regardless of the stenosis diameter. It is recommended to not oversize stent diameter at implantation secondary to concerns regarding accelerated stenosis at transition zones when implant diameters greatly exceed adjacent vessel diameters.[22,23]

Stent length is determined by obtaining the optimal length desired as measured on the preoperative angiogram and using known foreshortened length–diameter relationships provided by the manufacturers. A stent length is selected with a predicted foreshortened length that best approximates the desired ideal length paying careful attention to the location of side branch takeoffs. Crossing side branches should be avoided whenever possible.

Implantation procedures are performed with general anesthesia with the patient maintained on cardiopulmonary bypass. Timing of stent placement in relation to other portions of the operation is decided upon by the cardiac surgeon and varies depending upon the specific anatomy

of the patient, location of the lesion(s) being treated, and the operation being performed. The interventional cardiologist and an experienced catheter laboratory technician scrub into the case and temporarily replace the surgical first assistant at the left side of the table while the cardiac surgeon remains at the right side of the table. A separate sterile "interventional table," easily accessible to the interventional team, is set up on the left side of the table with all of the devices and equipment needed for a particular case. Since in most institutions, the catheterization laboratory and operating room are in separate physical locations, duplicates of catheter-related inventory that could be needed are brought into the operating room as well as a wide range of balloons and stents on either end of the predicted stent and balloon, which were calculated from the preoperative angiograms. This saves precious minutes when an unanticipated finding occurs or equipment fails. Additionally, a second catheter laboratory technician is always present to be used as a "runner" should more supplies be needed from the catheterization laboratory. These issues can be minimized or eliminated when these procedures are performed in a true hybrid suite. The interventional table typically holds a heparinized bowl of saline, a small curved surgical clamp, a 0.035 inch Wholey Hi-torque floppy guide wire (Mallinckrodt, St. Louis, MO, USA), a digitized pressure manometer, and the predetermined stent and balloon.

Prior to implantation, the target vessel is examined externally and internally with a digital videoscope (Image

1 digital camera, Karl Storz Endoscopy, Culver City, CA, USA) operated by the cardiac surgeon. Use of this imaging technique limits the amount of dissection required around the target vessel, thereby minimizing trauma to surrounding structures (e.g., phrenic nerve), shortening operative time, and preserving supporting tissue as the target vessel is forced to expand under the tension of the stent and balloon. The videoscopic images are compared with the preprocedural angiograms, which are available for viewing in the operating room through a digital network (Siemens ACOM NET, Erlangen, Germany) and the location of side branch takeoffs and target vessel length are confirmed or altered accordingly. Based on these observations, the surgeon and interventional cardiologist make a final decision regarding implantation diameter and the length of vessel to be covered by the stent.

The interventional cardiologist and technician then prepare the stent for delivery on the intervention table. The delivery balloon lumen is flushed with saline and the balloon inflated and deflated using a manometer syringe filled with saline (there is no need for contrast media with this method). Refolding the balloon often improves stent adherence to the lower-profile delivery balloons, which may be preferable for this application. Balloons with moderate burst pressures (8–12 atm) and low deflation profiles minimize the possibility of stent dislodgement during balloon removal following implantation. Some examples include Cordis Opta Pro and Power-flex balloons (Cordis Endovascular, Miami Lakes, FL, USA) for this application. Balloons with larger deflation profiles (e.g., Z-Med, Numed, Hopkinton, NY, USA) have been more difficult to remove after stent deployment and on occasion have resulted in intraoperative stent dislodgement requiring stent removal and replacement. It is not recommended to use high-pressure balloons and inflation pressures (>14 atm) with this technique secondary to concerns about

transmural vessel tear or rupture in this setting. The stent is hand crimped onto the delivery balloon in a similar fashion to percutaneous deployment. One author's preferred stent for this application is the Palmaz Genesis XD series (Cordis Endovascular, Miami Lakes, FL, USA) with the length determined by the above-described method. As discussed above, if the implantation diameter is restricted to <6 mm (such as in a small baby or severely hypoplastic vessel and the child will require further surgery), it is recommended to use stents with smaller ultimate diameter potential (Palmaz Genesis medium transhepatic biliary stent, Cordis Endovascular) secondary to concerns regarding early thrombosis and/or rapid neointimal buildup if a large stent is used in that situation.

After crimping the stent onto the balloon, firm but gentle traction is placed on the stent to test for the possibility of stent slippage. This is particularly important since fluoroscopy is not used during stent deployment. Prior to deployment, if the stent slips easily upon the balloon surface, the balloon is inflated slightly to form a "dumbbell" shape thereby further improving stent adherence (Figure 93.2). Since there is no requirement to fit the stent–balloon complex within a delivery sheath, the diameter of this partially inflated balloon is irrelevant. A slight "hockey stick" curve is placed on the soft tip of a Wholey guide wire, which is then advanced through the balloon lumen until a few centimeters extend from the balloon tip. The entire apparatus is then moved over to the operating table with the interventional cardiologist positioned at the head of the patient, handling the front end of the balloon–stent complex and the technician handling the manometer and back end of the balloon and wire toward the patient's feet.

Access to the branch pulmonary arteries is provided by the surgeon either directly at the bifurcation (more distal lesions) or through a proximal anastomosis of a conduit whose distal anastomosis has already been completed. The

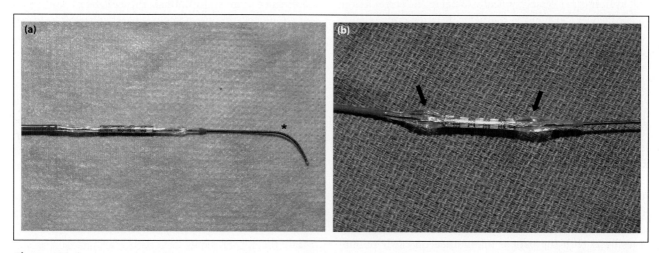

Figure 93.2   Genesis 1910B XD stent mounted on low-profile balloon (Cordis Opta Pro) before (a) and after (b) slight inflation to create a "dumbbell" (black arrows) shape on either side of the stent to secure position on the balloon. Note the soft-tipped curved Wholey wire (*), which has been placed through the catheter lumen to assist with guiding the stent–balloon complex across the stenosis.

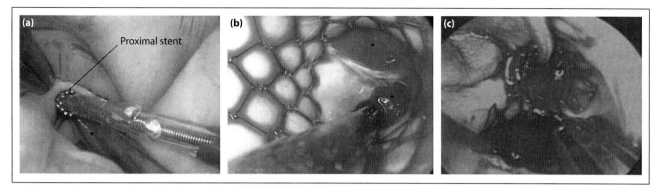

Figure 93.3 **(See color insert.)** (a) Prior to inflation of the balloon, the proximal stent is positioned using videoscopic guidance to cover the most proximal portion of the stenosis. The suction tip (*) is used to stabilize the pulmonary artery during positioning. (b) After stent expansion, apposition to vessel wall as well as position in relation to side branch takeoff (*) are examined. (c) Final result of "adult-sized kissing stents" placed in the 6-month-old seen in Figure 93.1.

balloon tip is positioned by the interventional cardiologist near the vessel orifice using a pair of forceps and the tip of the Wholey wire torqued (by the technician) to align with the course of the vessel to be stented. The wire tip is then gently advanced using the delivery forceps down the vessel lumen. If early resistance is encountered, a different wire angle is tried until several centimeters of wire have been passed down into the distal vessel. With the back of the wire held in place by the technician, the balloon-mounted stent is advanced to the target lesion by the interventional cardiologist being careful not to damage either the stent or balloon with the forceps. Prior to deployment, positioning is checked with the videoscope (Figure 93.3).

The balloon is then inflated to the manufacturer's rated burst pressure. Because it is not possible using this technique to visualize the entire length of the balloon–stent complex during the inflation, a pressure manometer is suggested for this to make sure that the nominal pressure is reached to indicate balloon expansion. The balloon is deflated in the usual fashion and removed over the wire, which is left in place, should further expansion of the stent be needed. The surgeon places gentle pressure on the proximal struts of the stent with forceps during balloon removal to prevent accidental stent dislodgement. With the guide wire still in place, the videoscope is carefully passed down through the stented vessel to examine the result. Particular attention is paid to the appearance of any transmural tears, the degree of apposition of the stent to the vessel wall, the location and patency of any side branches in close proximity to the stent and the integrity of any suture lines, which were crossed by the stent. If further stent expansion is required due to residual stenosis or failure of complete stent apposition to the vessel wall, a second balloon with a higher inflation pressure or larger diameter can be advanced over the guide wire and inflated. For ostial lesions where a small amount of stent must protrude into the main pulmonary artery, the surgeon often will carefully flare the proximal struts by gently bending each cell with forceps to better appose

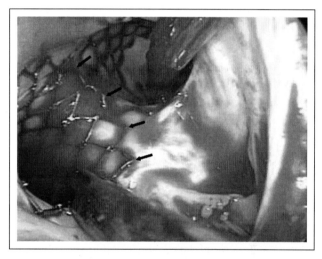

Figure 93.4 **(See color insert.)** Following implantation of left (LPA) and right (RPA) proximal branch pulmonary artery stents, the proximal struts (arrows) of the RPA stent have been flared by the surgeon to facilitate future catheter passage in the RPA as well as limit the cutting effect these struts could have on future angioplasty balloons in the proximal LPA.

the device to the ostium of the vessel (Figure 93.4). Other methods used for proximal flaring include the Hegar dilator or larger angioplasty balloon.[21] This facilitates future catheter entry into the vessel as well as protection against stent migration. It is thought that cutting the stent should be avoided as the sharp edges that result can make further balloon expansion in the catheter laboratory difficult, secondary to balloon rupture. After final assessment with the videoscope, the guide wire is removed and the intervention completed.

Potential pitfalls

While this is a simple technique that offers several potential advantages over the more commonly performed percutaneous technique, this procedure places the interventional cardiology team in what is initially an unfamiliar environment using new types of equipment and eliminating fundamental tools such as angiography and fluoroscopy. Therefore, meticulous attention to detail, careful preprocedural planning, and good cooperation with the surgical team are all essential to a successful outcome. Because intraprocedural angiography is not used, one must be sure that the measurements made prior to the hybrid procedure are accurate. The most common causes for inaccurate vessel measurement are erroneous calibration for magnification and lack of proper profiling of a given vessel. These pitfalls must be avoided to have consistent success with hybrid stent implantation. As an example, a case seen by one of the authors involved underestimation of preprocedural measurement of distal vessel diameter, which resulted in late distal migration of an intraoperatively implanted stent. Use of a soft-tipped guide wire and avoidance of high inflation pressures are important safety measures to prevent vessel perforation, particularly from the distal tip of the balloon, which is not visualized during inflation with this technique. Stents that fail to expand completely secondary to resistant stenoses can be left in place with the intent of proceeding with high-pressure balloon inflation at a later date using percutaneous techniques.

Institutional experience

Between October 1998 and September 2005, physicians at one author's (EMZ) center utilized this approach to implant 33 stents into the pulmonary arteries of 27 patients. The median weight in this group was 16 kg (2.9–67 kg). There was one procedural failure in a child with previously implanted stents that were incompletely removed at another institution. The metal fragments from the partially removed stents repeatedly resulted in rupture of the implantation balloon and prevented hybrid stent placement. All other hybrid stent implant procedures were technically successful (96% success of implantation). There were no instances of excessive postoperative bleeding, suture disruption, or early stent migration. Later follow-up indicates maintenance of improved vessel diameters, minimal tissue buildup within stented vessels, and the consistent ability to further expand hybrid stents in a manner similar to stents placed percutaneously. The one instance of late stent migration was noted above and resulted in no clinical sequelae.

Stent implantation via surgically provided vascular access

A second hybrid approach to stent implantation involves the use of surgical techniques to provide a variety of access ports to place stents into otherwise difficult to reach areas within the vascular system. These procedures can be performed in either the catheterization laboratory or operating room, with or without the use of cardiopulmonary bypass. In our experience, these techniques are typically utilized in two distinct groups of patients: (1) infants and neonates who are critically ill in the early postoperative period or (2) comparatively healthy outpatients presenting with unusual lesions or limited vascular access, which makes conventional stent implantation impossible. The indications and advantages of this approach are similar to those noted above for videoscopic guided stent implantation. These approaches, however, utilize fluoroscopy and angiography and allow access to a wider range of target vessels than the videoscopic hybrid technique.

Using these approaches, stents have been successfully used to treat branch pulmonary artery stenoses, recurrent aortic arch obstruction, modified Blalock–Taussig, and central shunt stenosis/occlusion, and create extracardiac Fontan fenestrations. Cases are performed using general anesthesia with endotracheal intubation. Most cases begin with a diagnostic catheterization performed from a conventional access route (most often femoral artery or vein) if one is available. Based upon the particular lesion being treated and the patient's individual anatomy, the best access route for stent placement is chosen. The cardiac surgical team then enters the case and the appropriately sized introducer sheath (based upon the predicted balloon and stent, which will be utilized) is placed under direct vision through an incision into the chosen access location. Vessels utilized for this purpose have included carotid artery, innominate vein, ascending aorta, and right ventricular outflow tract. Utilization of various vascular access routes are discussed elsewhere in this book and therefore the discussion will be confined to techniques used for stent implantation via surgically provided access through the open chest in a beating heart.

Pulmonary artery stent implantation via the right ventricular outflow tract

Significant residual branch pulmonary artery stenosis may result in unfavorable hemodynamics in the early postoperative period and negatively influence outcome.[5,22] It is our institutional bias that aggressive treatment of these types of stenoses is warranted and may significantly improve outcome in terms of hospital morbidity, mortality, and the long-term fate of the right ventricle. Reoperation in this setting incurs more trauma, is technically difficult, and has limited success. Balloon angioplasty may be effective in the early postoperative period; however, its inherent unreliability coupled with the requirement to oversize balloons in order to achieve an effective result make it an unattractive option in critically ill postoperative patients. Stent implantation with its more predictable result can be hampered by the technical issues of implantation discussed previously. These issues may be compounded when the goal is to put in a stent capable of achieving adult diameter. It has been found that implantation directly via the right ventricular outflow tract greatly facilitates stent placement in this group of patients.

Implantation technique

Often, experience with this procedure is in patients in the early postoperative period who arrive in the catheterization laboratory with their sternum open. At one author's (EMZ) center, a diagnostic catheterization using femoral venous access is performed to delineate the hemodynamics and the postoperative anatomy. The surgical team then scrubs into the case and places a purse-string suture in the proximal right ventricular outflow tract. An arteriotomy is made with an 11 blade and a standard sheath and dilator are directly inserted through the arteriotomy (Figure 93.5). The dilator can be used to approximate the location of the stenosis and length of the stent. The dilator is removed and after confirming proper position with fluoroscopy, the purse-string suture is tightened around the sheath to secure position. Care must be taken to ensure that enough distance exists between the tip of the sheath and the area to be stented so that the delivery balloon can be fully expanded without constraint from the sheath. Repeat angiography is performed through the side arm of the sheath using non-diluted contrast media injected by hand (Figure 93.6). This injection is then used as a road map for performing stent implantation. A soft-tipped guide wire (typically a 0.035 inch Wholey or GlideWire, Terumo Medical Corporation, Somerset, NJ, USA) is then advanced across the stenosis with or without the assistance of a catheter as needed. The wire tip is positioned as far distally into a lower-lobe

branch as possible. This wire can then be exchanged for a slightly stiffer wire (0.035 inch Rosen guide wire, Boston Scientific Corporation, Natick, MA, USA) to be used for stent positioning if needed. An appropriately sized stent is then chosen and hand crimped upon a delivery balloon in the usual fashion. It is best to implant stents with "adult-size potential" whenever possible. Using this technique, sheath size is never a limiting factor.

A delivery balloon diameter equal to the adjacent normal vessel diameter is chosen and overexpansion of the stent is avoided. The stent–balloon complex is then advanced through the sheath, over the guide wire, and across the stenosis. It is often not necessary to "protect" the stent–balloon complex with the sheath since the distance traveled is typically short and the catheter course straight. Serial angiography through the side arm of the delivery sheath aids with precision of stent placement prior to deployment. The balloon is then inflated using a pressure manometer and the stent deployed. Angiography through the side arm of the sheath is used to assess the adequacy of the result and if deemed satisfactory, the delivery balloon is removed over the guide wire. A final angiogram is performed, the guide wire is removed and the surgical team then reenters the case, removes the sheath, and repairs the arteriotomy. Minimal hemodynamics, including pressure measurements, are performed in these cases.

Advantages

Typically, these children are young, small, and hemodynamically unstable with open chests. They may require mechanical cardiopulmonary support. In these instances, it is found that using the right ventricular outflow tract for

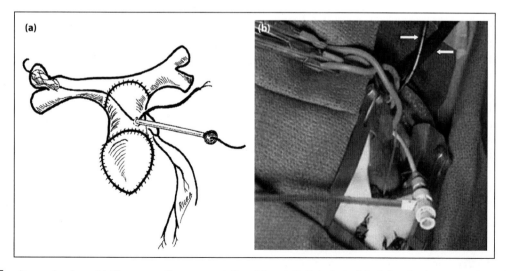

Figure 93.5 (**See color insert.**) Diagrammatic representation (a) and digital photo (b) of sheath placement via an incision into a right ventricle–pulmonary artery homograft conduit of a patient with severe early pulmonary artery stenosis after complete repair of pulmonary atresia and ventricular septal defect. Note the arterial and venous cannulas (white arrows) required to perform this intervention on cardiopulmonary support.

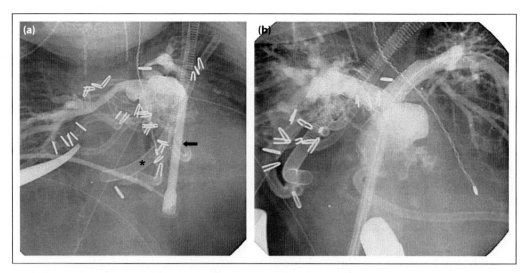

Figure 93.6 (a) Pulmonary angiogram performed through the side arm of a sheath (*) in the right ventricular outflow tract in a 6.2 kg, 9-month-old following complete repair of pulmonary atresia using a homograft conduit. Note the severe hypoplasia of the branch pulmonary arteries as well as the presence of bypass cannulas (arrows) as this child required mechanical cardiopulmonary support for this procedure. (b) Repeat angiogram following placement of adult-sized Genesis stents into both branch pulmonary arteries.

stent placement offers numerous important advantages, including freedom from sheath size constraints; simplification of the catheter course, making passage of the rigid stents much simpler; and avoidance of tension upon the tricuspid valve and right ventricle. This results in the ability to implant larger stents more precisely in a shorter time with more stable patient hemodynamics during the case. It also ensures in-room surgical backup should an untoward event occur.

Results

Between 1999 and 2004, nine patients at the author's (EMZ) center underwent placement of 10 pulmonary artery stents using this technique. The patients were generally small (median weight = 6.2 kg) and all were critically ill, requiring mechanical ventilation, inotropic support, and ON mechanical cardiopulmonary support in several cases. There were no procedural complications or deaths. All stent placements were considered successful as judged by standard criteria as well as clinical improvement. In the follow-up, all stents placed in this fashion have been amenable to further balloon expansion via conventional access routes and there have been no instances of late complications.

Aortic stent implantation via the right ascending aorta

Survival after stage 1 palliative surgery for HLHS has improved remarkably over the past decade; however,

recurrent or residual aortic arch obstruction continues to be a common and serious problem.[23–25] Typically, aortic obstruction occurs in the area of the distal anastomosis of the aortic gusset with the thoracic aorta. In addition to upper-body hypertension, aortic obstruction in this setting may result in a number of other undesirable physiologic effects, including pulmonary overcirculation resulting in ventricular volume overload, systemic atrioventricular valve insufficiency, and diminished cardiac output. This constellation of hemodynamic abnormalities may be poorly tolerated by an already overburdened systemic right ventricle. Surgical revision of the distal aortic arch reconstruction is difficult and may not completely relieve the obstruction. Balloon angioplasty does not always provide long-term relief and may carry an increased risk compared with simple recurrent coarctation angioplasty. In infants who have persistent aortic obstruction despite aortic angioplasty, we have utilized a hybrid approach to place adult-sized stents into the aorta at the time of their cavo-pulmonary anastomosis.

Technique

These procedures are typically performed in the operating room using a portable digital C-arm for imaging, although cases may also be performed in the catheterization laboratory. After dissecting out the neoaortic root, the surgeon places a purse-string suture in the ascending neoaorta. Via a small incision, a standard vascular sheath large enough to accommodate the stent–balloon

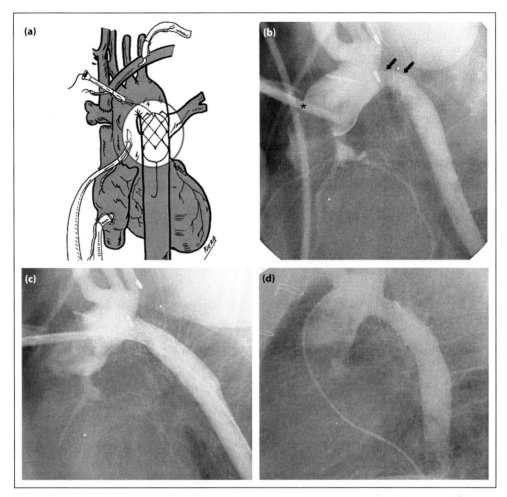

Figure 93.7   Hybrid stent implantation for treatment of resistant aortic reobstruction after hypoplastic left heart palliation. Diagrammatic representation (a) demonstrating the location used for sheath placement in the distal ascending aorta. Aortogram (b) performed through the side arm of the sheath (*) placed in the neoascending aorta demonstrating recurrent/residual distal aortic arch/isthmus hypoplasia (black arrows). Follow-up aortogram (c) after hybrid stent implantation with a large Genesis stent showing improvement in hypoplastic aortic segment. Follow-up aortogram (d) performed following balloon expansion of the hybrid stent 3 years after implantation.

complex is placed a short distance into the aorta (Figure 93.7). It is important that the access site leaves enough room for the sheath to be pulled back proximally enough as to not interfere with balloon inflation. After removing the dilator and de-airing the sheath, an angiogram is performed by hand injection through the side arm of the sheath using 20–30° of left anterior oblique (LAO) angulation. This image is stored to be used as a road map. Stent length and implantation diameter are chosen prior to the intervention based upon the preoperative angiograms. Implant diameter is chosen to match the aortic diameter at the level of the diaphragm. Only stents with the potential to achieve adult diameter are used for this application. Currently, large Genesis XD stents in as short a length as possible due to the small size of these children (typically

between 3–6 months of age) are preferred. The stent is mounted and hand crimped on a delivery balloon in the usual fashion employed for transcutaneous deployments.

Using the initial angiogram as a road map, a 0.035 inch Wholey wire with a curved tip is advanced directly through the sheath, across the stenosis, and down into the descending aorta. Once again, owing to the simplicity of the "catheter course," a catheter is not needed. The balloon-mounted stent is advanced through the sheath over the guide wire until it straddles the stenosis. Because of the short, straight wire path, it is often not necessary to advance the sheath across the stenosis prior to or during passage of the stent. Once the stent is in position, serial angiography is used to confirm precise positioning and then the stent is deployed by manometer guided balloon inflation. After removal of the balloon, one final angiogram is performed and then the sheath and guide wire are removed by the surgeon and the small aortic incision closed. The remainder of the operation is then completed.

Advantages

This is a very simple technique that allows an adult-sized stent to be placed into the aorta of a young infant when balloon angioplasty has not adequately alleviated recurrent aortic obstruction. It is far less traumatic than attempted repeat surgical repair and offers the possibility of a lifetime "cure" with repeated stent expansion as a patient grows.

Results

To date, this procedure has been performed at the author's center (EMZ) in eight children with successful stent implantation in all. There were no procedural complications. In follow-up, all stents have been successfully redilated when needed although the maximum follow-up to date is short. In the single case where a Double Strut LD stent (ev3, Plymouth, MN, USA) was implanted, significant stent distortion was observed when redilation was performed prompting surgical removal of the stent at the time of the Fontan operation. Therefore, this device is no longer used for this application. While there has been no other evidence of stent failure in follow-up, unfortunately, several of the patients who have undergone this procedure have had persistent poor ventricular function. This may represent the cumulative negative effects of early continued arch obstruction after stage I palliation for hypoplastic left heart syndrome.

Review of the literature

There have been a few papers discussing hospital experience with intraoperative stenting, but no known large interhospital data registries. A few selected papers are shown in Table 93.3. The papers span from 1993 to 2011. The number of patients ranges from 4 to 27, with an age range between 1 week and 60 years. The cardiac diagnoses vary, as do the distribution of single pulmonary artery or bilateral pulmonary artery stenting. Some indications include emergency procedures or bailout procedures after an errant percutaneous attempt.

The complications vary between the different papers, both in quantity and type. Some papers report no significant complications or issues during the stenting procedure. However, listed complications include laceration of the pulmonary artery, malposition of the stent, stent dislodgement, and stent migration. There may be a learning curve associated with these procedures, as described by Mitropoulos et al.[26] in referencing two papers from the same institution.[27,28] Follow-up data may show no need for reintervention, but these patients should be closely followed with a combination of mean gradient, luminal diameter, and evaluation for right ventricular systolic function compromise.

The paper with largest group of patients and follow-up period is by Angtuaco et al.,[21] who reported on 67 patients with a total of 96 stents placed intraoperatively and followed for 7.6 ± 4.5 years. Complications at the time of procedure included pulmonary artery rupture in five patients and embolized stent in one patient. The pulmonary artery ruptures happened early in their experience and were addressed surgically and happened in cases with extensive surgical dissection of the pulmonary artery prior to stent implantation. No mortality was noted.

The same paper described follow-up for this group of 7.6 ± 4.5 years. Forty-seven of 96 stents (49%) required reintervention. One patient had reintervention on postop day 0, which was an undiagnosed pulmonary artery (PA) rupture and attempts to repair the PA were unsuccessful so the patient underwent excision of the stented segment with interposition of a tube graft. All cases requiring reintervention were due to recurrent branch pulmonary artery stenosis. Of these, 18 stents (19%) required a second reintervention. The actuarial freedom from reintervention at 2, 5, and 10 years was 68%, 49%, and 40%, respectively. Factors that were significantly associated with reintervention included age <2 years, weight <10 kg, and initial postinflation stent diameter <10 mm; on multivariate Cox regression analysis, the significant factors were age <2 years, diagnosis of tetralogy of Fallot, or truncus arteriosus.

It is important to note that some papers describe the use of intraoperative stent implantation for pulmonary vein stenting.[19,29] These patients often had unfavorable outcomes. The optimal role for pulmonary vein stenting using an intraoperative approach has not yet been elucidated.

Conclusion

Most patients with structural heart disease can undergo successful stent implantation into a wide variety of vascular and intracardiac locations using standard percutaneous techniques. A select group that includes small children and neonates, hemodynamically unstable children, and those with poor vascular access may greatly benefit from the hybrid techniques described in this chapter. With experience, these procedures are relatively simple to perform, require a minimal amount of inventory, and appear to provide excellent results. Careful consideration of the long-term medical and surgical management of these patients as well as excellent communication between the interventional cardiologist and cardiac surgeon are mandatory for ultimate success.

Table 93.3   Literature relating to intraoperative stenting

	Patients	Age range	Cardiac diagnosis	Stented if pulmonary artery (% right, left, bilateral)	Concomitant surgery	Procedural event	Follow-up
Mendelsohn et al. (1993)[17]	15	Mean 3.0 years	n/a	n/a	n/a	No mortality	Mean follow-up 8.7 months in three patients no restenosis thrombosis or aneurysm formation
Fogelman et al. (1995)[28]	4	Mean 6.1 years	Not specifically listed	Not specifically listed	Not specifically listed	Not specifically listed Listed issues for whole data set: 1. Stent straddled side branch with reduced flow 2. Distal left pulmonary art thrombosis 3. Stent in proximal LPA protruded into MPA and removed 4. Stent migration distally treated with dilation	Not specifically listed but noted nonsignificant change in RVEDP, nonsignificant increase in mean systolic pressure gradient, and a small decrease in lumen diameter
Ungerleider et al. (2001)[19]	27	7 days– 14 years	Truncus arteriosus (4) Pulmonary atresia + VSD (7) Tetralogy of Fallot (8) Pulmonary atresia/intact ventricular septum (1) Transposition of the great arteries (1) Complex single ventricle (6)	Pulmonary artery (19%, 37%, 26%)	Conduit change (5) Rastelli (3) VSD or A closure (3) Glenn shunt (1) Pulmonary valve replacement (3) Removal errant stent (4) Aortic arch reconstruction (2)	5 in-hospital deaths 8 stent-related complications— laceration of PA in 2, inadequate balloon dilatation in 1, malposition of stent in 1, stent dislodgment in 2, reperfusion pulmonary edema (1)	Mean follow-up 2.3 years Mean gradient fell from 66 to 28 mmHg

(continued)

Table 93.3   (continued) Literature relating to intraoperative stenting

	Patients	Age range	Cardiac diagnosis	Stented if pulmonary artery (% right, left, bilateral)	Concomitant surgery	Procedural event	Follow-up
Hjortdal et al. (2002)[30]	4	3–18 years	Double-inlet/double-outlet right ventricle (1) Fallot repair with RPA/LPA stenosis and dislodged PA stent (1) Absent right atrioventricular connection, ventriculo-arterial discordance, restrictive VSD, s/p coarctation aorta + PA banding + damus	Pulmonary artery (0%, 75%, 25%)	Reconnection of SVC to RA with Gore-tex (1) Removal of displaced stent in RVOT and homograft from RV-PA (1) Gore-tex repair of SVC-IVC tunnel (1) Surgical enlargement of LPA (1)	No complications noted	Redilation in 1 patient after 2 years
Bockencamp et al. (2005)[18]	11	1 week–6 years	Pulmonary atresia with VSD +/– MAPCA (5) Truncus arteriosus (2) Aortic arch interruption with VSD (1) AVSD/tetralogy of Fallot (1) TGA + VSD + hypoplastic R PA (1) Hypoplastic L heart syndrome (1)	Pulmonary artery (27%, 46%, 27%)	Pulmonary atresia repair (2) RVOT + PA reconstruction (3) Unifocalization of PA (1) Truncus repair revision (1) AVSD/Fallot repair revision (1) Retrieval dislodged stent PA (1) Bidirectional cavopulmonary anastomosis after Norwood I operation for HLHS (1)	No complication Urgent procedure (4)	1 in-hospital death unrelated to stent 4 patients with redilation (one patient having redilation within 2 months) 1 patient having reoperation
Galantowicz et al. (2005)[31]	17	n/a	Hypoplastic left heart syndrome	PDA	n/a	n/a	n/a
Menon et al. (2008)[32]	24	3–67 years	Pulmonary atresia with VSD (9) Tetralogy of Fallot (7) Tricuspid atresia (2) Double-outlet left ventricle (2) Trucus arteriosus (2) D-transposition with pulmonary atresia (1) Accidental ligation of L PA (1)	Pulmonary artery (33%, 54%, 13%)	RVOT reconstruction (2) Conduit replacement (6) PV replacement (7) Dislodged stent removal (1) Fontan revision (2) RVOT reconstruction (1) Conduit replacement (5)	Incomplete inflation (2) Stent migration (2) Emergency procedure (2)	1 patient in 6 months with redilation

Study	n	Age	Diagnosis	Location	Procedure	Results/Complications	Follow-up
Schmitz et al. (2008)[33]	7	3–13 months	Hypoplastic left heart syndrome, s/p Norwood, re-coarctation of aorta (4) Ventricular septal defect, hypoplastic arch, recoarctation of aorta (1) Tetralogy of Fallot, RPA stenosis (1) Tetralogy of Fallot, LAD crossing RVOT (1)	ReCOA (5) RPA (1) RVOT (1)	Glenn operation (4) VSD closure (1) Tetralogy of Fallot repair (2)	n/a	3 patients stents redilated, unknown which ones
Mitropoulos et al. (2007)[26]	22	9 months–24 years	Pulmonary atresia, VSD (5) Pulmonary atresia intact septum (2) Tetralogy of Fallot (3) Truncus arteriosus (4) Double-outlet right ventricle (1) Hypoplastic left heart syndrome (1) Transposition great arteries (3) Aortic valve insufficiency (1) Complex congenital heart disease (1)	Pulmonary artery (59%, 36%, 5%)	Augmentation patch angioplasty (11) Pulmonary valve replacement (13) Conduit repair or augmentation (11)	Mean PA diameter increased from 7.6 to 10.9 mm, decrease gradient from 45.4 to 4.3 mmHg	No reinterventions at mean 22.8 month follow-up
Holzer et al. (2008)	4	n/a	Not specified for these patients	Pulmonary artery (25%, 50%, 25%)	Not specified for these patients	Not specified for these patients	Not specified for these patients
Angtuaco et al. (2011)[21]	67	7 days–23.4 years	Tetralogy of Fallot (22) Truncus arteriosus (7) D-transposition of great arteries (9) Single ventricle anomalies (13) Atrioventricular septal defects (3) Double-outlet right ventricle (4) Supravalvular aortic stenosis with branch pulmonary stenosis (3) Isolated branch pulmonary artery stenosis (6)	n/a	n/a	PA rupture (5) Stent embolization (1)	7.6 ± 4.5 years 49% of stents required reintervention Median time to first reintervention 4.7 years

(continued)

Table 93.3 (continued) Literature relating to intraoperative stenting

Patients	Age range	Cardiac diagnosis	Stented if pulmonary artery (% right, left, bilateral)	Concomitant surgery	Procedural event	Follow-up
22	9 months–24 years	Pulmonary atresia, VSD (5) Pulmonary atresia intact septum (2) Tetralogy of Fallot (3) Truncus arteriosus (4) Double-outlet right ventricle (1) Hypoplastic left heart syndrome (1) Transposition great arteries (3) Aortic valve insufficiency (1) Complex congenital heart disease (1)	59%, 36%, 5%	Augmentation patch angioplasty (11) Pulmonary valve replacement (13) Conduit repair or augmentation (11)	Mean PA diameter increased from 7.6 to 10.9 mm, decrease gradient from 45.4 to 4.3 mmHg	No reinterventions at mean 22.8 month follow-up

References

1. Palmaz JC, Garcia OJ, Schatz RA et al. Placement of balloon-expandable intraluminal stents in iliac arteries: First 171 procedures. *Radiology* 1990;174:969–75.
2. O'Laughlin MP, Perry SB, Lock JE, Mullins CE. Use of endovascular stents in congenital heart disease. *Circulation* 1991;83:1923–39.
3. Moore JW, Kirby WC, Lovett EJ, O'Neill JT. Use of an intravascular endoprosthesis (stent) to establish and maintain short-term patency of the ductus arteriosus in newborn lambs. *Cardiovasc Intervent Radiol* 1991;14:299–301.
4. Beekman RH, Muller DW, Reynolds PI, Moorehead C, Heidelberger K, Lupinetti FM. Balloon-expandable stent treatment of experimental coarctation of the aorta: Early hemodynamic and pathological evaluation. *J Interv Cardiol* 1993;6:113–23.
5. Hosking MC, Benson LN, Nakanishi T, Burrows PE, Williams WG, Freedom RM. Intravascular stent prosthesis for right ventricular outflow obstruction. *J Am Coll Cardiol* 1992;20:373–80.
6. O'Laughlin MP, Slack MC, Grifka RG, Perry SB, Lock JE, Mullins CE. Implantation and intermediate-term follow-up of stents in congenital heart disease. *Circulation* 1993;88:605–14.
7. Benson LN, Nykanen D, Freedom RM. Endovascular stents in pediatric cardiovascular medicine. *J Interv Cardiol* 1995;8:767–75.
8. Akintuerk H, Michel-Behnke I, Valeske K et al. Stenting of the arterial duct and banding of the pulmonary arteries: Basis for combined Norwood stage I and II repair in hypoplastic left heart. *Circulation* 2002;105:1099–103.v
9. Boucek MM, Mashburn C, Chan KC. Catheter-based interventional palliation for hypoplastic left heart syndrome. *Semin Thorac Cardiovasc Surg Pediatr Card Surg Annu* 2005;8(1):72–7.
10. Galantowicz M, Cheatham JP. Fontan completion without surgery. *Semin Thorac Cardiovasc Surg Pediatr Card Surg Annu* 2004;7:48–55.
11. Michel-Behnke I, Akintuerk H, Thul J, Bauer J, Hagel KJ, Schranz D. Stent implantation in the ductus arteriosus for pulmonary blood supply in congenital heart disease. *Catheter Cardiovasc Interv* 2004;61:242–52.
12. Alwi M, Choo KK, Latiff HA, Kandavello G, Samion H, Mulyadi MD. Initial results and medium-term follow-up of stent implantation of patent ductus arteriosus in duct-dependent pulmonary circulation. *J Am Coll Cardiol* 2004;44:438–45.
13. McMahon CJ, El Said HG, Vincent JA et al. Refinements in the implantation of pulmonary arterial stents: Impact on morbidity and mortality of the procedure over the last two decades. *Cardiol Young* 2002;12:445–52.
14. Pass RH, Hsu DT, Garabedian CP, Schiller MS, Jayakumar KA, Hellenbrand WE. Endovascular stent implantation in the pulmonary arteries of infants and children without the use of a long vascular sheath. *Catheter Cardiovasc Interv* 2002;55:505–9.
15. Qureshi SA, Sivasankaran S. Role of stents in congenital heart disease. *Expert Rev Cardiovasc Ther* 2005;3:261–9.
16. Houde C, Zahn EM, Benson LN, Coles J, Williams WG, Trusler GA. Intraoperative placement of endovascular stents. *J Thorac Cardiovasc Surg* 1992;104:530–2.
17. Mendelsohn AM, Bove EL, Lupinetti FM et al. Intraoperative and percutaneous stenting of congenital pulmonary artery and vein stenosis. *Circulation* 1993;88:II210–7.
18. Bockencamp R, Blom NA, De Wolf D, Francois K, Ottenkamp J, Hazekamp MG. Intraoperative stenting of pulmonary arteries. *Eur J Cardiothorac Surg* 2005;27:544–7.
19. Ungerleider RM, Johnston TA, O'Laughlin MP, Jaggers JJ, Gaskin PR. Intraoperative stents to rehabilitate severely stenotic pulmonary vessels. *Ann Thorac Surg* 2001;71:476–81.
20. Ing FF. Delivery of stents to target lesions: Techniques of intraoperative stent implantation and intraoperative angiograms. *Pediatr Cardiol* 2005;26:260–6.
21. Angtuaco MJ, Sachdeva R, Jaquiss RD et al. Long-term outcomes of intraoperative pulmonary artery stent placement for congenital heart disease. *Catheter Cardiovasc Interv* 2011;77:395–9.
22. Chau AK, Leung MP. Management of branch pulmonary artery stenosis: Balloon angioplasty or endovascular stenting. *Clin Exp Pharmacol Physiol* 1997;24:960–2.
23. Soongswang J, McCrindle BW, Jones TK et al. Outcomes of transcatheter balloon angioplasty of obstruction in the neo-aortic arch after the Norwood operation. *Cardiol Young* 2001;11:54–61.
24. Tworetzky W, McElhinney DB, Burch GH, Teitel DF, Moore P. Balloon arterioplasty of recurrent coarctation after the modified Norwood procedure in infants. *Catheter Cardiovasc Interv* 2000;50:54–8.
25. Zeltser I, Menteer J, Gaynor JW et al. Impact of re-coarctation following the Norwood operation on survival in the balloon angioplasty era. *J Am Coll Cardiol* 2005;45:1844–8.
26. Mitropoulos FA, Laks H, Kapadia N et al. Intraoperative pulmonary artery stenting: An alternative technique for the management of pulmonary artery stenosis. *Ann Thorac Surg* 2007;84:1338–41; discussion 42.
27. Coles JG, Yemets I, Najm HK et al. Experience with repair of congenital heart defects using adjunctive endovascular devices. *J Thorac Cardiovasc Surg* 1995;110:1513–9; discussion 9–20.
28. Fogelman R, Nykanen D, Smallhorn JF, McCrindle BW, Freedom RM, Benson LN. Endovascular stents in the pulmonary circulation. Clinical impact on management and medium-term follow-up. *Circulation* 1995;92:881–5.
29. Okubo M, Benson LN. Intravascular and intracardiac stents used in congenital heart disease. *Curr Opin Cardiol* 2001;16:84–91.
30. Hjortdal VE, Redington AN, de Leval MR, Tsang VT. Hybrid approaches to complex congenital cardiac surgery. *Eur J Cardiothorac Surg* 2002;22(6):885–90.
31. Galantowicz M, Cheatham JP. Lessons learned from the development of a new hybrid strategy for the management of hypoplastic left heart syndrome. *Pediatr Cardiol* 2005;26(3):190–9.
32. Menon SC, Cetta F, Dearani JA, Burkhart HA, Cabalka AK, Hagler DJ. Hybrid intraoperative pulmonary artery stent placement for congenital heart disease. *Am J Cardiol* 2008;102(12):1737–41.
33. Schmitz C, Esmailzadeh B, Herberg U, Lang N, Sodian R, Kozlik-Feldmann R, Welz A, BreuerJ. Hybrid procedures can reduce the risk of congenital cardiovascular surgery. *Eur J Cardiothorac Surg* 2008;34(4):718–25.
34. Holzer RJ, Chisholm JL, Hill SL, Olshove V, Phillips A, Cheatham JP, Galantowicz M. *J Invasive Cardiol* 2008;20(11):592–8.

94

Background, indication for LAA closure, and clinical trial results

Stefan Bertog, Laura Vaskelyte, Ilona Hofmann, Jennifer Franke, Simon Lam, Sameer Gafoor, and Horst Sievert

Why do we consider left atrial appendage closure useful?

Strokes are common yet devastating events, both to the individual and the society. They are the third leading cause of death in Western countries and the leading cause of disability.[1] More than 80% of all strokes are ischemic and approximately one-third are considered the consequence of cardiogenic emboli, most commonly caused by atrial fibrillation. In fact, among patients 80–89 years of age, 20% of all ischemic strokes are thought to be the consequence of atrial fibrillation.[2,3] Strokes caused by atrial fibrillation tend to be larger in size with more severe neurological deficit and higher recurrence rate than strokes of other etiologies.[4] The average annual risk of stroke in patients with atrial fibrillation is 5% and increases with age, gender, and presence of clinical risk factors, including diabetes mellitus, congestive heart failure, hypertension, previous thromboembolic events, and vascular disease.[5] This has prompted exploration of anticoagulation for the prevention of thromboembolic events in atrial fibrillation. Anticoagulation with warfarin has been shown to cause a significant and pronounced reduction in stroke risk by up to 84% in patients with nonvalvular atrial fibrillation.[5] It is more effective than aspirin, which is accompanied by a more modest risk reduction of approximately 36%.[5] Therefore, it is undisputed that anticoagulation should be recommended to individuals with atrial fibrillation and at least one additional risk factor and aspirin to patients with atrial fibrillation and no additional risk factors. Traditionally, the agent of choice was warfarin. However, warfarin is associated with a bleeding risk and logistical challenges related to periodic international normalized ratio (INR) assessment with necessary instructions regarding dose adjustments. In addition, drug–drug and drug–diet interactions need to be taken into account while patients are taking warfarin.

Importantly, too low of an INR increases the stroke risk and too high of an INR increases the bleeding risk, including that of intracranial hemorrhage.[6] These downsides, in addition to the narrow therapeutic window may explain why nearly 70% of patients who are at high risk of stroke and would warrant anticoagulation, are not anticoagulated.[7] These disadvantages have fueled the search for new agents. In this context, direct thrombin inhibitors and antifactor Xa agents have been explored. Three agents stand out with good results when compared with warfarin in a randomized fashion: rivaroxaban, apixaban, and dabigatran. Dabigatran, a direct thrombin inhibitor, has been compared to warfarin in patients with atrial fibrillation in the RE-LY (dabigatran vs. warfarin in patients with atrial fibrillation) trial.[8] The stroke risk in patients who received dabigatran 150 mg twice daily was significantly lower than in the control group treated with warfarin (relative risk reduction: 34%, absolute risk reduction: 0.58%, number needed to treat: 178). The risk of major hemorrhage did not differ between the groups at this dose. There was no significant difference in the stroke risk between patients treated with 100 mg of dabigatran twice daily and warfarin, but the risk of major bleeding was significantly lower (relative risk reduction: 19%, absolute risk reduction: 0.65%, number needed to treat: 153).[8] Concerns have been raised regarding a trend toward a higher incidence of myocardial infarction in patients treated with dabigatran ($p = 0.07$). Similarly, in ROCKET-AF (rivaroxaban vs. warfarin in patients with nonvalvular atrial fibrillation), rivaroxaban 20 mg daily was noninferior when compared with warfarin regarding the prevention of embolic events, it is associated with a lower risk of fatal and intracranial hemorrhage while the overall rate of major bleeding did not differ.[9] In the ARISTOTLE (apixaban vs. warfarin in patients with atrial fibrillation) trial, apixaban 5 mg twice daily was associated with a lower stroke or systemic embolism rate and overall mortality compared with warfarin (relative risk reduction: 21%, absolute risk reduction: 0.33%, number needed to treat: 303) and there was a significant reduction in major bleeding (relative risk reduction: 27%).[10] Importantly, though major bleeding rate reductions in the three pivotal trials described are statistically significant, these reductions are small and the remaining annual rates of major bleeding are high regardless of which anticoagulant is used as illustrated in Table 94.1. Moreover, effective and proven reversal agents do not exist. Hence, these agents do not provide a solution for patients who are considered to have a high bleeding risk with or absolute contraindications to warfarin. The inherent bleeding risk of any anticoagulant fostered interest in eliminating the structure thought to be responsible for thromboembolic events in the majority of patients with atrial fibrillation—the left atrial appendage (LAA). Nearly 90% of LAA thrombi in the setting of nonvalvular atrial fibrillation are located in the LAA.[11] The notion is that removal or occlusion of this structure leads to a substantial stroke risk reduction. This has prompted surgical LAA removal in those patients with atrial fibrillation undergoing open-chest surgery for other indications, particularly mitral valve surgery. A number of techniques have been used, including stapling, excision, and suture closure. However, none have ever been compared in a randomized fashion to oral anticoagulants, and residual leaks are very common and potentially associated with a higher risk of thrombus formation.[12,13] Hence, the efficacy of this approach has not yet been proven. Moreover, the risk of open surgical closure (including that of a stroke) in the absence of indications for open-chest surgery for reasons other than atrial fibrillation would offset any potential benefits. Percutaneous closure has the obvious advantage of avoiding open-chest surgery and extracorporeal circulation.

The first closure device used for this purpose was the PLAATO (percutaneous transcatheter left atrial appendage occlusion) device. It was first implanted in 2001[14] followed by a nonrandomized safety and feasibility trial.[15] Taking 359 patients from three observational studies into account (mean follow-up: 9.6, 9.8, and 24 months), the annualized

stroke risk after device implantation was 2.3%, 2.2%, and 0.7%, respectively and, thereby, lower than the stroke rate calculated according to the CHADS-2 score (6.6%, 6.3%, and 4.9%).[15–17] At long-term (5 year) follow-up, the annual stroke rate in one study ($n = 61$) was 3.8% and compared favorably to that calculated based on the CHADS-2 score (6.6%).[17] Of interest, in the described studies, patients were routinely treated with antiplatelet agents only after implantation. Taking data from three studies including 364 patients into account, device embolization, pericardial effusion, and periprocedural stroke occurred in 1%, 2.5%, and 0.5%, respectively.[15–17] The device is no longer manufactured. However, the aforementioned data demonstrated for the first time the safety and feasibility of percutaneous closure. In addition, though none of the data was randomized and controlled, it suggested a stroke reduction compared with historical controls not treated with anticoagulation. Shortly after the first PLAATO implantation, based on the proven low thrombogenicity of Amplatzer devices used for other purposes (mainly interatrial septal closure), the utility of the Amplatzer septal occluder (St. Jude Medical, St. Paul, MN, USA) for LAA occlusion was explored. It was demonstrated that this device could also be used for the purpose of LAA occlusion,[18] but was associated with a relatively high risk of device embolization. The results of the PLAATO trial and studies using nondedicated Amplatzer devices furthered an interest in the development of novel devices including the WATCHMAN device (Boston Scientific, Natick, MA, USA) and the Amplatzer cardiac plug (ACP, St. Jude Medical) both of which currently have a CE mark.

The WATCHMAN LAA occluder design will be discussed in the following chapters. Briefly, it is a nitinol cage covered by an ePTFE membrane facing the LAA and has circumferential anchors that help fixation in the LAA. It is the first device that has been studied in a randomized fashion compared to conventional anticoagulation using warfarin. In the pivotal trial, PROTECT-AF (percutaneous closure of the LAA vs. warfarin therapy for the prevention of stroke in patients with atrial fibrillation: a randomized noninferiority trial),[19] patients with nonvalvular atrial fibrillation and a CHADS-2 score of at least 1 (average 2.2) were randomized to warfarin versus WATCHMAN implantation (in a 1:2 fashion) followed by 45 days of warfarin and, provided there was no or only a small (<5 mm) residual leak, with aspirin and clopidogrel from day 45 to 6 months, and aspirin only thereafter. A total of 707 patients were randomized. At a mean follow-up of 45 months, WATCHMAN implantation was noninferior to warfarin with respect to the overall stroke risk.[20] In addition, there was no difference in adverse event rates. Though the rate of perioperative events was higher for patients who underwent LAA occlusion at 18 months,[19] this was balanced by the cumulative rate of major bleeding in patients treated with warfarin at 45 months.[20] Importantly,

Table 94.1 Bleeding rates in pivotal trials with novel anticoagulants

Study	Treatment	Major bleeding (%)	Hemorrhagic stroke (%)
RE-LY	Dabigatran 110 mg	2.71	0.12
	Dabigatran 150 mg	3.11	0.10
	Warfarin	3.36	0.38
ROCKET-AF	Rivaroxaban	3.60	0.50
	Warfarin	3.40	0.70
ARISTOTLE	Apixaban	2.13	0.24
	Warfarin	3.09	0.47

there was a significant reduction in overall mortality favoring the LAA occlusion arm.[20] In the overwhelming majority of patients, oral anticoagulation could be discontinued at 45 days (86%) and 6 months (92%).[19] However, in some patients, warfarin was continued, most commonly due to the presence of a residual peridevice leak of >5 mm. At 6 months, the peridevice leak rate was 32%. Of patients with residual leaks, it was large (>3 mm) in only 37%. The risks of pericardial hemorrhage and thrombus formation were 4.8%[19] and 4.2%,[21] respectively. Of those with pericardial hemorrhage, the majority (68%) underwent percutaneous drainage and 32% surgical drainage. The risk of device embolization and periprocedural stroke was 0.6% and 1.1%, respectively. Importantly, it became clear that, at later stages of the trial, the complication rate (particularly that of pericardial effusions) was lower than at the beginning of the trial, an attest to a substantial learning curve in this procedure. This finding was further corroborated by the results of the CAP registry, a subsequent nonrandomized registry of 460 patients undergoing WATCHMAN implantation by PROTECT-AF operators who had already gained experience with the device.[21] In order to confirm the results of PROTECT-AF in other operators, the PREVAIL (prospective randomized evaluation of the WATCHMAN LAA closure device in patients with atrial fibrillation vs. long-term warfarin therapy) trial was conducted, the results of which were recently presented at the 2013 American College of Cardiology Annual Scientific Meeting. The trial design was almost identical to PROTECT-AF. Four hundred and seven patients (mean CHADS-2 score: 2.6) were randomized, once again, to warfarin versus LAA occlusion with the WATCHMAN device with identical postprocedural follow-ups. Primary endpoints were procedural complications and a composite of stroke, systemic embolism, or unexplained cardiovascular death. Importantly, the implantation success rate was significantly higher than in PROTECT-AF (95% vs. 91%) and the rate of major procedural complications (composite of cardiac perforation, pericardial effusion with tamponade, stroke, device embolization, and access-related complications) were significantly lower than in PROTECT-AF. Pericardial effusion requiring surgical repair occurred in 0.6% in PREVAIL versus 1.6% in PROTECT-AF. There was no difference in the composite of stroke, systemic embolism, and cardiovascular/unexplained death at 18 months when compared with conventional anticoagulation with warfarin; however, final analysis of the data was incomplete at the time of presentation, given that only 88 patients had completed the 18 month follow-up. The safety of WATCHMAN implantation in the absence of temporary anticoagulation (followed by antiplatelet therapy only) has been examined in the ASAP trial. One hundred and fifty patients (mean CHADS-2 score of 2.8) underwent WATCHMAN implantation followed by 6 months of daily clopidogrel and lifelong daily aspirin. Device-associated thrombi occurred in

six patients (4%) and, therefore, no more frequent than in PROTECT-AF. One of these thrombi caused a stroke; the remainder were discovered incidentally on surveillance transesophageal echocardiographic examinations and resolved with temporary (4–8 weeks) of low-molecular-weight heparin. The annual stroke rate was 1.7%, significantly lower than that calculated based on the CHADS-2 score (7.3%) for patients treated with aspirin only. This suggests that antiplatelet therapy only may be sufficient in patients after WATCHMAN implantation, but it also stresses the importance of surveillance echocardiographic examinations to detect clinically silent thrombi.[22]

The ACP device that will be described in more detail in Chapter 95 consists of a nitinol plug connected by a waist to a nitinol disk (the plug anchors the device in the LAA and the disk covers the ostium). It is delivered into the LAA in a similar fashion as the WATCHMAN device. To date, nonrandomized registry data including well over 600 patients are available. In one of the larger series ($n = 137$), Park et al. reported successful implantation in 96% with a periprocedural complication rate of 7% (stroke in 2.1%, pericardial tamponade requiring drainage in 3.5%, and device embolization with successful percutaneous retrieval in 1.4%). Long-term follow-up has not been reported in this study. Guerios et al.[23] performed successful ACP implantation in 85 of 86 patients (99%). Periprocedural cerebral events occurred in 2.3%, and device embolization (retrieved percutaneously) and pericardial tamponade (drained percutaneously) in 1%, respectively. After 26 patient-years of follow-up, there were no embolic events. At follow-up, the LAA was completely occluded in 97%. In 6 of 69 (9%) patients who underwent transesophageal echocardiographic follow-up, a device-associated thrombus was seen with resolution after anticoagulation. Similarly, Lopez-Minguez et al.[24] described thrombus formation in 5 of 35 patients, 14% with resolution in all after temporary heparin therapy and minor peridevice leaks (not further characterized) in 9%, and Plicht et al.[25] reported thrombus formation in 18% of 34 patients (risk factors for thrombus formation were: high CHADS-2 and CHAD2DS2-VASc score and low ejection fraction). In contrast, Urena et al. did not detect any thrombi at follow-up in 52 patients.[26] In this study, the residual leak rate was 16%. Of note, in all of the latter four studies, temporary dual antiplatelet therapy was only used routinely after LAA closure in the majority of patients. Hence, all periprocedural complications described with the WATCHMAN device can also be encountered with the ACP. There appears to be a slightly lower residual leak rate and a slightly higher device-associated thrombus rate; however, a direct comparison to the WATCHMAN device has not been performed. Several improvements have recently been made in the second-generation ACP (ACP-II or Amulet), the end-screw thought to be responsible for thrombus formation has a lower profile, the anchor plug is longer with fixation barbs proportionate to the lobe perhaps reducing the embolization risk, the disk size is larger with respect to the anchor plug to minimize residual leaks, and the waist is longer, adapting better to nonlinear appendages. First-in-man experience with this device has been described. Further data are pending. Once again, randomized data comparing the first- or second-generation ACP are not yet available. The ongoing ACP trial (www.clinicaltrials.gov, identifier: NCT01118299) with a planned enrollment of 3000 patients and estimated completion in 2017 will compare the device to anticoagulation in a randomized fashion.

Several potential problems that accompany device closure are residual leaks, thrombus formation, and device embolization. In this context, minimally invasive suture closure with the LARIAT device (Sentre Heart, Redwood City, CA, USA) has potential merit as the closure is accomplished by a lasso-like suture delivered via the epicardium with procedural guidance using a rail composed of a wire delivered into the LAA apex that attaches, via a magnet, to a wire delivered to the LAA apex within the pericardial space. Under fluoroscopic and transesophageal echocardiographic guidance, the LAA can be cinched closed and a suture applied. The technique will be discussed in Chapter 98 in detail. The theoretical advantage is closure irrespective of the LAA ostium shape, thereby perhaps allowing more consistent complete closure. Secondly, no foreign body is left behind, perhaps minimizing device-associated thrombus formation and embolization. Four studies have been published.

Bartus et al., who will elaborate on closure techniques with the LARIAT device, first demonstrated the feasibility of LAA closure in a pilot study of patients undergoing open-chest surgery for other reasons.[27] Subsequently, in the largest study published to date,[28] LAA ligation was attempted in 92 patients (CHADS-2 score of 1.9) and completed successfully in 85 (92%). The procedure was aborted in four patients in whom pericardial adhesions were encountered during epicardial access. It was aborted in one patient due to superficial epigastric artery puncture requiring hemostasis and in one patient in whom the right ventricle was punctured requiring pericardial drainage. In one patient, it was aborted because of an inability to perform transseptal puncture. Of those (85) who underwent LAA ligation, a transesophageal echocardiogram was performed in 81 at 1 and 30 days after the procedure, demonstrating complete closure defined as a residual leak <1 mm in 95%. At 1 year, transesophageal echocardiography showed a complete closure rate of 98% (n = 77). Of note, in the remainder of the patients, the residual leak was <3 mm.

One patient mentioned above developed pericardial hemorrhage, requiring drainage and, in one patient, likewise described above, the procedure was aborted due to bleeding from a superficial epigastric artery successfully cauterized. In addition, in one patient a pericardial effusion was noted 2 weeks after the procedure and was drained successfully percutaneously. Three months after the procedure, one patient died of events unrelated to the procedure, and at 6 months, one patient developed an intracranial hemorrhage believed to be the result of cerebral aneurysm. This patient had not been on anticoagulation during the event. One patient died 12 months after the procedure, presumably due to bradycardia with refusal of pacemaker implantation and one patient developed a lacunar stroke. A minor, but more frequent event is the development of postprocedural pleuritic chest pain. This occurred in 23% of patients in the overwhelming majority of whom (90%) were resolved after removal of the pericardial drain the day following the procedure. In two patients, symptoms of pericarditis required treatment with nonsteroidal anti-inflammatory therapy with resolution 2–3 days after the procedure. Of note, 55% of patients remained on anticoagulation at 12 month follow-up. No definitive thromboembolic events occurred.

Two smaller studies recently published describe additional experience with the LARIAT device. Massumi et al.[29] report successful closure (defined as a residual leak of <5 mm), in all patients in whom it was attempted (n = 20, mean CHADS-2 score: 3.2). In those who underwent transesophageal echocardiographic follow-up (n = 17) at a mean of approximately 3 months, the appendage remained completely closed in 16 with minimal residual flow in 1. No thromboembolic events occurred (mean follow-up of 352 days) and oral anticoagulation was used in only 20% of patients after the procedure. In the remainder, either no antiplatelet therapy (20%), aspirin (65%), clopidogrel (20%), and aspirin and dipyridamole (5%) were used. In one patient, emergent surgical pericardial drainage was necessary due to perforation of the right ventricle, and in one more patient, repeat pericardial drainage related to tamponade physiology was required. Three patients developed pericarditis requiring hospitalization, one of whom also had a moderate pericardial effusion requiring drainage. One death occurred at 50 days unrelated to the procedure. Stone et al.[30] reported successful LAA closure in 93% of attempted cases (n = 27, CHADS-2 score: 3.5). In one patient, LAA perforation required pericardial drainage and the appendage was closed nonemergently surgically (in conjunction with a MAZE procedure) and in one patient, placement of the LARIAT loop over the LAA was not possible. There were no residual leaks (defined as color flow <5 mm) in any patient with the exception of the above-mentioned patients who sustained the LAA perforation. A periprocedural stroke due to thrombus adherent to the left atrial sheath occurred in one patient, postprocedural pericarditis in three patients, and a transudative pleural effusion in one patient. At a mean follow-up of 4 months, no deaths or pericardial complications were reported. One patient, at 33 days after the procedure had a stroke that most likely related to aortic arch atheromata based on the absence of a residual leak or thrombus formation in the LAA and presence of significant aortic arch atheromata during transesophageal echocardiography.

Conclusion

Several statements can be made: First, LAA occlusion is feasible and has recently been demonstrated to be superior to long-term anticoagulation with warfarin. Second, currently, prospective randomized data are limited to the WATCHMAN device. A randomized trial using the ACP is underway, the results of which will clarify the utility of this device for LAA occlusion. Nonrandomized data with this device suggest at least equivalent efficacy (measured by residual leak rates) and similar complication rates. Third, both devices are foreign bodies and, therefore, accompanied by the risk of thrombus formation, device embolization, and residual leak. In this context, minimally invasive suture closure has the theoretical advantage of leaving no foreign body behind. The feasibility of LAA closure with the LARIAT device has recently been demonstrated and, based on the limited available data, closure rates appear to be superior to both, the WATCHMAN device and ACP. However, in addition to transseptal access, epicardial access is necessary and poses the risk for right ventricular perforation and pericardial hemorrhage/effusion. The merit of this concept will be determined pending more data. Fourth, though in most centers LAA closure is considered in patients who are not candidates for, or failures of, conventional anticoagulation, it is noteworthy that available data supporting LAA closure is the result of trials that included predominantly patients who are candidates for anticoagulation. This should, therefore, be considered as an alternative rather than a default in patients with nonvalvular atrial fibrillation and appropriate CHADS-2 score. Fifth, with the advent of new and effective anticoagulant agents, it remains to be determined whether LAA closure or a novel anticoagulant is more effective for stroke prevention in patients who are candidates for anticoagulation. Finally, limited data support the safety of LAA occlusion in patients who cannot tolerate even temporary anticoagulation regardless of which of the above-described concepts are chosen.

References

1. Sacco RL, Benjamin EJ, Broderick JP et al. American Heart Association Prevention Conference. IV. Prevention and rehabilitation of stroke. Risk factors. *Stroke* 1997;28:1507–17.
2. Go AS, Mozaffarian D, Roger VL et al. Executive summary: Heart disease and stroke statistics—2013 update: A report from the American Heart Association. *Circulation* 2013;127:143–52.
3. Roger VL, Go AS, Lloyd-Jones DM et al. Heart disease and stroke statistics—2012 update: A report from the American Heart Association. *Circulation* 2012;125:e2–e220.
4. Lin HJ, Wolf PA, Kelly-Hayes M et al. Stroke severity in atrial fibrillation. The Framingham study. *Stroke* 1996;27:1760–4.
5. Atrial fibrillation investigators. Risk factors for stroke and efficacy of antithrombotic therapy in atrial fibrillation. Analysis of pooled data from five randomized controlled trials. *Arch Intern Med* 1994;154:1449–57.
6. Hylek EM, Skates SJ, Sheehan MA, Singer DE. An analysis of the lowest effective intensity of prophylactic anticoagulation for patients with nonrheumatic atrial fibrillation. *N Engl J Med* 1996;335:540–6.
7. Stafford RS, Singer DE. National patterns of warfarin use in atrial fibrillation. *Arch Intern Med* 1996;156:2537–41.
8. Connolly SJ, Ezekowitz MD, Yusuf S et al. Dabigatran versus warfarin in patients with atrial fibrillation. *N Engl J Med* 2009;361:1139–51.
9. Patel MR, Mahaffey KW, Garg J et al. Rivaroxaban versus warfarin in nonvalvular atrial fibrillation. *N Engl J Med* 2011;365:883–91.
10. Granger CB, Alexander JH, McMurray JJ et al. Apixaban versus warfarin in patients with atrial fibrillation. *N Engl J Med* 2011;365:981–92.
11. Blackshear JL, Odell JA. Appendage obliteration to reduce stroke in cardiac surgical patients with atrial fibrillation. *Ann Thorac Surg* 1996;61:755–9.
12. Katz ES, Tsiamtsiouris T, Applebaum RM, Schwartzbard A, Tunick PA, Kronzon I. Surgical left atrial appendage ligation is frequently incomplete: A transesophageal echocardiograhic study. *J Am Coll Cardiol* 2000;36:468–71.
13. Kanderian AS, Gillinov AM, Pettersson GB, Blackstone E, Klein AL. Success of surgical left atrial appendage closure: Assessment by transesophageal echocardiography. *J Am Coll Cardiol* 2008;52:924–9.
14. Sievert H, Lesh MD, Trepels T et al. Percutaneous left atrial appendage transcatheter occlusion to prevent stroke in high-risk patients with atrial fibrillation: Early clinical experience. *Circulation* 2002;105:1887–9.
15. Ostermayer SH, Reisman M, Kramer PH et al. Percutaneous left atrial appendage transcatheter occlusion (PLAATO system) to prevent stroke in high-risk patients with non-rheumatic atrial fibrillation: Results from the international multi-center feasibility trials. *J Am Coll Cardiol* 2005;46:9–14.
16. Park JW, Leithauser B, Gerk U, Vrsansky M, Jung F. Percutaneous left atrial appendage transcatheter occlusion (PLAATO) for stroke prevention in atrial fibrillation: 2-year outcomes. *J Invasive Cardiol* 2009;21:446–50.
17. Bayard YL, Omran H, Neuzil P et al. PLAATO (percutaneous left atrial appendage transcatheter occlusion) for prevention of cardioembolic stroke in non-anticoagulation eligible atrial fibrillation patients: Results from the European PLAATO study. *EuroIntervention* 2010;6:220–6.
18. Meier B, Palacios I, Windecker S et al. Transcatheter left atrial appendage occlusion with Amplatzer devices to obviate anticoagulation in patients with atrial fibrillation. *Catheter Cardiovasc Interv* 2003;60:417–22.
19. Holmes DR, Reddy VY, Turi ZG et al. Percutaneous closure of the left atrial appendage versus warfarin therapy for prevention of stroke in patients with atrial fibrillation: A randomised non-inferiority trial. *Lancet* 2009;374:534–42.
20. In: Annual Scientific Meeting of the Heart Rhythm Society. Denver, CO, USA; 2013.
21. Reddy VY, Holmes D, Doshi SK, Neuzil P, Kar S. Safety of percutaneous left atrial appendage closure: Results from the Watchman Left Atrial Appendage System for Embolic Protection in Patients with AF (PROTECT AF) clinical trial and the Continued Access Registry. *Circulation* 2011;123:417–24.
22. Reddy VY, Mobius-Winkler S, Miller MA et al. Left atrial appendage closure with the Watchman device in patients with a contraindication for oral anticoagulation: The ASAP study (ASA Plavix Feasibility Study With Watchman Left Atrial Appendage Closure Technology). *J Am Coll Cardiol* 2013;61:2551–6.

23. Guerios EE, Schmid M, Gloekler S et al. Left atrial appendage closure with the Amplatzer cardiac plug in patients with atrial fibrillation. *Arq Bras Cardiol* 2012;98:528–36.

24. Lopez-Minguez JR, Eldoayen-Gragera J, Gonzalez-Fernandez R et al. Immediate and one-year results in 35 consecutive patients after closure of left atrial appendage with the amplatzer cardiac plug. *Rev Esp Cardiol* 2013;66:90–7.

25. Plicht B, Konorza TF, Kahlert P et al. Risk factors for thrombus formation on the Amplatzer Cardiac Plug after left atrial appendage occlusion. *J Am Coll Cardiol Cardiovasc Interv* 2013;6:606–13.

26. Urena M, Rodes-Cabau J, Freixa X et al. Percutaneous left atrial appendage closure with the AMPLATZER cardiac plug device in patients with nonvalvular atrial fibrillation and contraindications to anticoagulation therapy. *J Am Coll Cardiol* 2013;62:96–102.

27. Bartus K, Bednarek J, Myc J et al. Feasibility of closed-chest ligation of the left atrial appendage in humans. *Heart Rhythm* 2011;8:188–93.

28. Bartus K, Han FT, Bednarek J et al. Percutaneous left atrial appendage suture ligation using the LARIAT device in patients with atrial fibrillation: Initial clinical experience. *J Am Coll Cardiol* 2013;62:108–18.

29. Massumi A, Chelu MG, Nazeri A et al. Initial experience with a novel percutaneous left atrial appendage exclusion device in patients with atrial fibrillation, increased stroke risk, and contraindications to anticoagulation. *Am J Cardiol* 2013;111:869–73.

30. Stone D, Byrne T, Pershad A. Early results with the LARIAT device for left atrial appendage exclusion in patients with atrial fibrillation at high risk for stroke and anticoagulation. *Catheter Cardiovasc Interv* ePub ahead of print June 13, 2013.

95

Amplatzer cardiac plug

Fabian Nietlispach and Bernhard Meier

Introduction

In 2008, the Amplatzer cardiac plug (ACP) designed for left atrial appendage (LAA) occlusion replaced nondedicated Amplatzer devices, such as atrial and ventricular septal defect occluders and patent foramen ovale occluders, that had been used since 2002 for this purpose (Figure 95.1).[1] While nondedicated devices provided good occlusion of the LAA, the high embolization rate was a concern that was overcome with the new dedicated ACP.[2]

Amplatzer cardiac plug device and delivery system

The nitinol-based ACP device consists of a disk and a lobe connected by a stretchable waist. The lobe has hooks on the outer circumference (Figure 95.2) that serve as anchors to prevent device embolization. The polyester filling of the device enhances endothelialization and prevents blood flow through the device.

The nominal device size is determined by the outer diameter of the lobe. Available sizes currently range from 16 to 30 mm (2 mm steps). The height of the lobe measures 6.5 mm and the disk extends the lobe by 4–6 mm (Figure 95.3).

The delivery system consists of (1) a *loader*, (2) a *pusher cable* that is screwed onto the thread on the inner side of the disk and allows advancing the device through the sheath, and (3) the Amplatzer TorqVue 45° × 45° *delivery sheath* with an obturator. The preformed shape of the sheath features two 45° bends facing anterior (Figure 95.4). A Y-connector enables flushing and contrast medium injections. The sheath is available in three sizes: 9 French (F) for 16 mm ACPs, 10 F for the 16–22 mm ACPs, and 13 F for all ACPs.

Owing to the hooks on the lobe, the device should not be retracted into the loader in a retrograde fashion, as is standard with other Amplatzer devices. Retrograde loading would potentially damage the hooks. Moreover, advancing the device with the hooks looking forward is not recommended. Therefore, the device has two threads at either end that, once attached to the pusher cable and a temporary loading cable, allow for antegrade advancement into the loader (pull on the loading cable) and the sheath (push on the pusher cable; Figure 95.5, Video 95.1).

Amulet

A second-generation ACP II (Amulet) was designed to minimize the risk of device embolization and to further improve LAA sealing. The new features are a lobe that measures 2–3 mm more in height and larger sizes come with 10 rather than 6 pairs of (stiffer) hooks. The lobe diameter range was extended to 34 mm and the disk now outsizes the lobe by

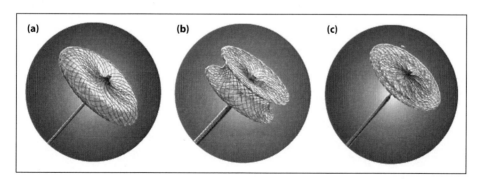

Figure 95.1 Nondedicated Amplatzer devices used for LAA occlusion. Depending on the LAA anatomy, an (a) ASD, (b) VSD, or (c) PFO occluder was used. (Courtesy of St. Jude Medical.)

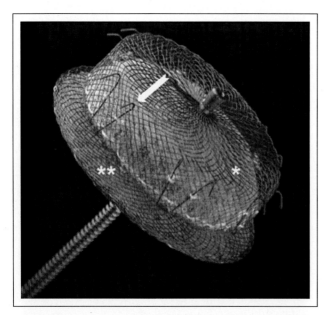

Figure 95.2 The dedicated ACP with a lobe (*) and the disk (**), which are connected by a flexible thin waist. Arrow: hooks on the outer side of the lobe ensure fixation in the LAA. (Courtesy of St. Jude Medical.)

6–7 mm for improved sealing. The device comes preloaded in the delivery system. In order to minimize the risk of thrombus formation, the thread on the disk is retracted not to protrude into the LAA.

Sizing and deployment of the ACP

In many centers, the procedure is performed using guidance with transesophageal echocardiography (TEE) under deep sedation or general anesthesia.[3] The more frugal and time-saving approach using local anesthesia and fluoroscopic guidance is a safe alternative.[4]

Antibiotic prophylaxis and heparin are given before or during the procedure. Femoral venous access is obtained

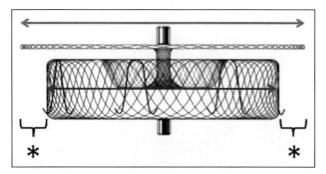

Figure 95.3 The dedicated ACP with the disk (top double arrow) extending the lobe (center double arrow) by 4–6 mm (*). (Courtesy of St. Jude Medical.)

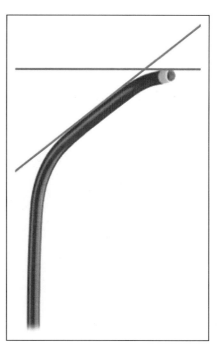

Figure 95.4 The TorqVue 45° × 45° delivery sheath. The particular configuration of the sheath with two 45° bends that face anterior considerably facilitates engagement of the LAA, even in an atypical location or with a high transseptal puncture. (Courtesy of St. Jude Medical.)

and, unless a patent foramen ovale or an atrial septal defect is present and used for passage, a transseptal puncture is performed as explained in Chapter 15. A stiff guide wire (e.g., Backup wire [Boston Scientific, Natick, MA, USA] or Amplatz extra stiff guide wire [Cook Medical Inc., Bloomington, IN, USA]) replaces the transseptal catheter. A stiff guide wire is necessary, since resistance during sheath introduction is often encountered in the groin area and in the atrial septum.

Device sizing orients on the diameter of the landing zone and aims for at least 20% oversizing (e.g., 28 mm device for a landing zone of 23 mm; Figure 95.6). However, given the large intraindividual variability in the shape of the LAA, device sizing needs to take into account different lengths of the neck and oblique lobe positions. Therefore, the LAA is depicted in different views by fluoroscopy (Figure 95.7) and/or by TEE. Ideally, the lobe sits like a pacifier in a baby mouth in the neck of the LAA, with the disk circumferentially adjacent to the left atrial wall like the pacifier plate in front of the mouth according to the so-called pacifier principle (Figure 95.8).

At our center, since the year 2006, a pusher cable with a movable core was used per availability. It allows pulling back the sleeve around the core wire to which the screw is attached. This reveals the stability of the device practically uninfluenced by the attached safety tether. A good device position is confirmed by tugging on the delivery cable and by fluoroscopic imaging in a parallel plane to the LAA occluder.

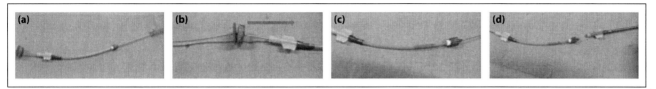

Figure 95.5   Antegrade loading of the ACP using a temporary loading cable (distal) and the pusher cable (proximal) attached at each side. (a) The ACP adjacent to the loader and attached to the temporary loading cable (right). (b) Once the pusher cable is attached to the thread on the disk (left), the lobe of the ACP is pulled into the loader. (c) By pulling on the temporary loading cable, the ACP is pulled to the connector of the loader in antegrade fashion. The hooks are compressed "arms down" rather than "arms up." (d) The temporary loading cable is unscrewed and the connector of the loader is attached to the delivery sheath. When unscrewing the temporary loading cable, it is recommended to grasp the tip of the lobe in order not to unscrew the pusher cable at the same time.

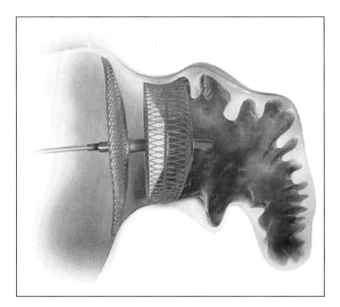

Figure 95.6   **(See color insert.)** The landing zone of the ACP has to ensure that the entire lobe is within the LAA and well anchored. Ideally, albeit not always possible as depicted on the figure, the landing zone for the entire lobe is within the neck of the LAA (green arrow). However, depending on the anatomy, sometimes the lobe will not be perpendicular to the neck axis and reside partially within one of the lobes of the LAA. (Courtesy of St. Jude Medical.)

In case of malpositioning, the device can be (preferentially only partially) reloaded into the delivery sheath and then repositioned (Figure 95.9).

Only once a good position is confirmed, the device is unscrewed from the delivery cable.

Postprocedural care

Postinterventional care involves a transthoracic echocardiogram before discharge (possible the same day) to confirm device position. A follow-up TEE after a few months (typically 4–6 months) confirms exclusion of the LAA and excludes thrombus on the device.

At our center, oral anticoagulation (OAC) is terminated the day of the procedure and antiplatelet therapy is initiated. Acetylsalicylic acid is prescribed until 1 month before the follow-up TEE or is pursued in case of concomitant atherosclerosis. One month of clopidogrel is added.

Complications and possible solutions

If thrombus on the device is found on follow-up TEE (Figure 95.10), short-term OAC is prescribed. A small residual shunt into the LAA does not warrant further

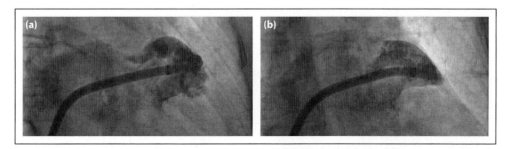

Figure 95.7   Fluoroscopic image of the LAA in a right anterior oblique projection with caudal (a) and cranial (b) angulation. One can appreciate the neck and the lobes of the LAA structures better in the caudal projection (a) with a large interindividual variability.

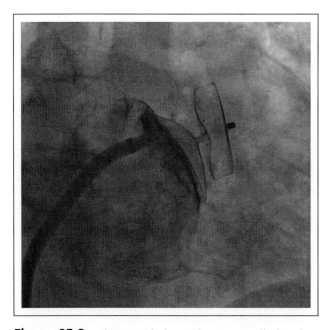

Figure 95.8 Fluoroscopic image in a perpendicular view, showing the lobe in the LAA and the disk adjacent to the left atrial wall (pacifier principle).

measures.[5] If it is large (Figure 95.10), it may warrant OAC or closure with a second device.

Device embolization occurs exclusively within minutes to hours after the procedure and can either be treated percutaneously by snaring and externalization of the device through the femoral artery (Figure 95.11), or by surgical removal of the device. In case this requires thoracotomy, the LAA should be surgically closed on the occasion.

Besides cerebral or coronary air embolism, which typically resolves spontaneously, the most dreaded procedural complication is cardiac tamponade. It can occur during transseptal puncture, or by perforation of the LAA or the left atrial wall. It warrants pericardiocentesis (harvested blood can be reinfused into a vein or artery) or in severe cases surgical evacuation and hemostasis.

Conclusion

LAA closure is a valuable alternative to OAC. It is a rather demanding procedure with a flat learning curve. However, there is a benefit for the patient and it keeps increasing with longer follow-up due to the reduced bleeding risk compared to OAC.

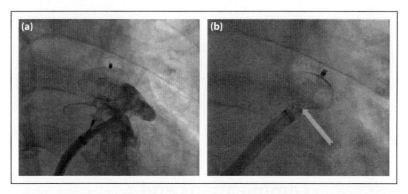

Figure 95.9 LAA occluder inadvertently deployed in the pulmonary vein (a). The device is then partially resheathed, such that the hooks, slightly distal to the markers (arrow, b), remain outside the sheath in order not to get reverted or even damaged.

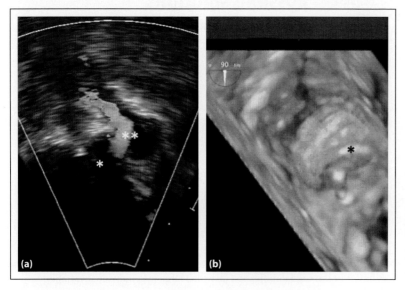

Figure 95.10 (**See color insert.**) Thrombus on the ACP. (a) 2-D TEE image showing a small thrombus on the screw of the disk (*). The ACP does not cover one of the small lobes of the LAA, resulting in a considerable residual shunt (**). If such a large residual shunt persists, implantation of a second ACP or a different device (e.g., Amplatzer Vascular Plug) can be considered. (b) Thrombus on the ACP screw depicted on 3-D TEE (*).

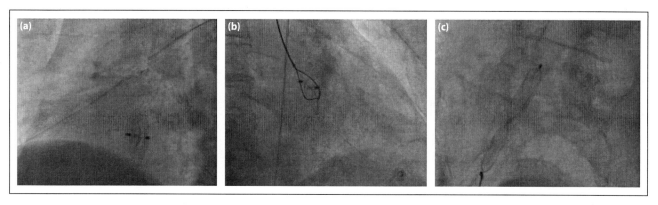

Figure 95.11   Embolization of the device into the left ventricle (a). Snaring the device in the left ventricle (b). Externalization of the device from the femoral artery (c).

References

1. Meier B, Palacios I, Windecker S et al. Transcatheter left atrial appendage occlusion with Amplatzer devices to obviate anticoagulation in patients with atrial fibrillation. *Catheter Cardiovasc Interv* 2003;60:417–22.
2. Park JW, Bethencourt A, Sievert H et al. Left atrial appendage closure with Amplatzer cardiac plug in atrial fibrillation: Initial European experience. *Catheter Cardiovasc Interv* 2011;77:700–6.
3. Rodes-Cabau J, Champagne J, Bernier M. Transcatheter closure of the left atrial appendage: Initial experience with the Amplatzer cardiac plug device. *Catheter Cardiovasc Interv* 2010;76:186–92.
4. Nietlispach F, Gloekler S, Krause R et al. Amplatzer left atrial appendage closure: Single center 10-year experience. *Catheter Cardiovasc Interv* 2013;82:283–9.
5. Viles-Gonzalez JF, Kar S, Douglas P et al. The clinical impact of incomplete left atrial appendage closure with the Watchman Device in patients with atrial fibrillation: A PROTECT AF (Percutaneous Closure of the Left Atrial Appendage Versus Warfarin Therapy for Prevention of Stroke in Patients With Atrial Fibrillation) substudy. *J Am Coll Cardiol* 2012;59:923–9.

96

Watchman device

Peter Sick

Introduction

The Watchman® device (Boston Scientific, formerly Atritech) is one of the best-studied left atrial appendage (LAA) closure devices in the literature and has been used most often worldwide. It is composed primarily of a nitinol frame structure with fixation barbs along the waist and a thin permeable polyterephthalate membrane covering the atrial-facing surface of the device (see Figure 96.1). It can be used in patients with chronic or paroxysmal atrial fibrillation with or without contraindication for oral anticoagulation therapy.

The first procedure was performed in August 2002. Since then, more than 2000 devices have been implanted.

The technique for left atrial appendage occlusion using the Watchman device

The principal procedure is shown in Figure 96.2a–c with measurement of the LAA, implantation of the device, and late results with complete endothelialization on the surface of the device.

Performance of a transesophageal echocardiogram (TOE) within 48 hours before the procedure is strongly recommended to exclude thrombi in the LAA, to measure the LAA ostium, proximal part, and length of the body, as well as to characterize the shape of the LAA, which may have multiple lobes. Other important preprocedural information is the anatomical orientation of the axis of the LAA body, as this has important implications for the transseptal puncture site during implantation. Transesopageal echo (TEE) guidance is also recommended during the implantation procedure to assure correct placement of the device. The procedure is usually performed under conscious sedation with midazolam and propofol or general anesthesia.

The Watchman device is implanted using a three-part system consisting of a transseptal access sheath (Figure 96.3), a delivery catheter, and the device. The principal method and location of the device is shown in Figure 96.3.

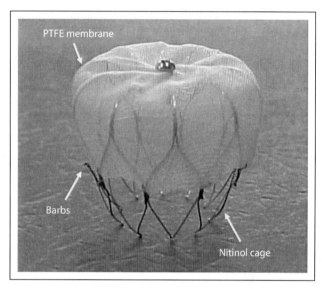

Figure 96.1 The Watchman device with the nitinol cage and the polyterephthalate membrane spanned over the surface in contact with the left atrium. The barbs prevent the device from embolization by fixing in the left atrial appendage wall.

The (14 F) access system and (12 F) delivery catheter are designed to facilitate device placement via femoral venous access and transseptal crossing to the left atrium. The delivery catheter allows retrieval of a deployed Watchman device, prior to release, if the placement is not optimal.

Transseptal puncture may be performed with a Brockenbrough needle and any of the currently available transseptal sheaths as a standard procedure. It is most commonly performed under TOE control; however, some operators prefer intracardiac echocardiography (ICE). The puncture height is dependent on the orientation of the LAA. If the axis is oriented cranially, the puncture site should be low in the interatrial septum, best seen in TOE in the bicaval view (90°). In all cases with anterior or caudal orientation of the LAA axis, the puncture site should be in the upper part of the interatrial septum. In general, puncture should be performed as posterior as possible,

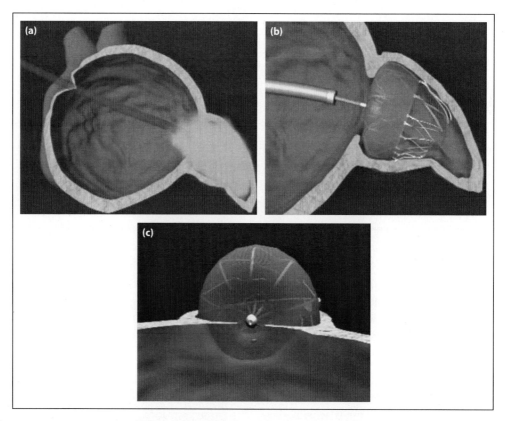

Figure 96.2 A schematic implantation of the Watchman device in the LAA: (a) Injection of contrast dye in the left atrial appendage to measure the size of the body to select the correct size of the device. (b) The implanted device still connected to the delivery system. (c) Schematic endothelialization of the device with complete coverage of the surface to the LA; thus leading to complete occlusion of the LAA usually within 6 months.

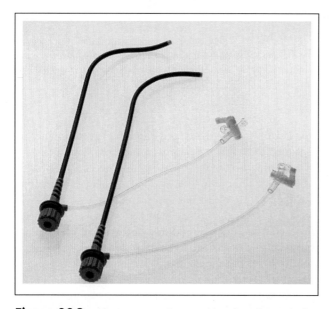

Figure 96.3 The transseptal access sheath, advanced after transseptal puncture over a pigtail catheter to the LAA. There are two different shapes available, one with a single curve and one with a double curve (the latter is used in over 95% of cases). The side arm is used for continuous saline infusion to avoid air suction during pullback of the device.

best confirmed via TOE in the 45° view. After successful transseptal puncture, the Brockenbrough needle and sheath dilator are exchanged for a 0.035 inch wire (e.g., Amplatzer extra-stiff wire) placed into the left upper pulmonary vein, or a transseptal pigtail guide wire GMS (former mitral valvuloplasty guide wire), spirally placed in the left atrium. Over either of the wires, the transseptal sheath is exchanged for the 14 F Watchman access sheath (Figure 96.2). There are two shapes available, a single curve and a double curve. The latter is used in more than 95% of cases. It is very important to have a continuous saline infusion through the side arm of the sheath and to remove the dilator of the sheath very slowly to avoid negative pressure in the sheath, potentially leading to air embolism via air suction through the valve of the sheath during removal of the dilator. Side holes at the tip of the catheter provide backward flow of blood to avoid this problem at least in part, if the tip of the catheter is in direct contact with the atrial wall. Once the access sheath is well located in the left atrium, a 4 F or 5 F pigtail catheter is advanced into the LAA. LAA angiography (either via the access sheath or pigtail catheter) is performed and TOE and angiographic measurements are made.

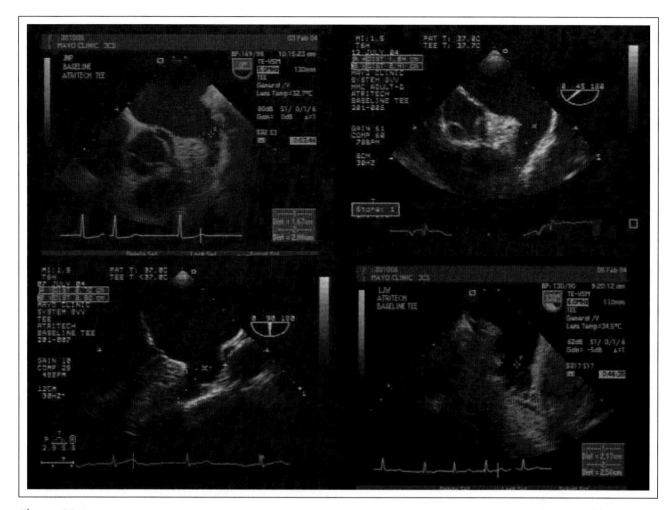

Figure 96.4   Echocardiographic measurement for evaluation of LAA anatomy in four different views (0°, 45°, 90°, 135°).

By TOE, an LAA measurement is performed (see Figure 96.4) in four different views (0°, 45°, 90°, and 135°), always looking for the left circumflex artery as a landmark. Measurements are taken from the edge of the left circumflex artery (LCX) to the opposite wall perpendicular to the axis of the LAA in all four views. Angiographic measurements can be made in two planes by contrast (see Figure 96.5a and b). The best projections are typically RAO/caudal 30/20° or RAO/cranial 30/20° (corresponding to the 45° and 135° TOE views, respectively) (Figure 96.5a). Sometimes, the lateral view is also helpful (Figure 96.5b). The largest size measured determines the size of the device, which should be compressed to about 80% of its nominal size. The 20% compression of the device after implantation is necessary to engage the fixation barbs of the device into the LAA wall, thereby avoiding embolization.

To allow positioning of the access sheath deep in the left atrium in the least traumatic manner, it is advanced over the pigtail catheter. After removal of the pigtail catheter, the Watchman device is delivered in a compressed state (and attached to a delivery cable) via the delivery catheter. It is important to note that the access sheath has one distal

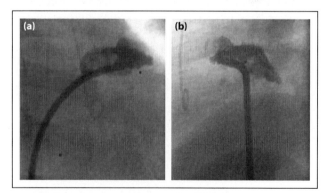

Figure 96.5   (a,b) Angiographic measurement of the LAA in two planes for correct selection of the size of the device.

marker and three more proximal markers. The proximal markers align with the most proximal aspect of the device that will be facing the left atrium once deployed. The most proximal of the three proximal markers aligns with the largest device size (33 mm), the middle marker with the 27 mm device, and the most distal marker with the smallest (21 mm) device. The 30 and 24 mm devices align between

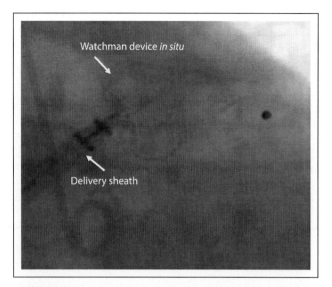

Figure 96.6 An implanted device still connected to the delivery system.

the proximal and midmarker and between the distal and midmarker, respectively. For example, if one is planning to implant a 33 mm device, it is important that the access sheath position is such that the most proximal of the three proximal marker aligns with the imaginary line that connects from the circumflex coronary artery to the opposite appendage wall in a fashion described above (perpendicular to the LAA axis). The delivery catheter that harbors the device is continuously flushed with heparinized saline via a syringe to avoid air bubbles while introducing the delivery system into the access sheath. The delivery catheter also has a distal marker. The delivery sheath and device are advanced under fluoroscopic guidance until the distal marker of the delivery catheter aligns with the distal marker of the access sheath. At this position, the access

sheath is gently pulled back until it locks (a click is felt). This interlocks the access sheath with the delivery catheter. Under fluoroscopic control with contrast injections through the delivery system to assure correct placement, the interlocked access and delivery sheath are pulled back as one unit while holding the delivery cable of the device in a stable position. This allows the device to unfold while still fixed to the delivery system (Figure 96.6). Angiography via the delivery system (Figure 96.7a) and TOE (Figure 96.7b) are performed to assure an optimal device position has been made. Another proof of stability is to perform a tug test by gently pulling the delivery cable simultaneously with contrast injection (to see the movement of the LAA together with the system) and TOE imaging to assure that the LAA moves together with the device and the delivery system.

Now the device can be released from the delivery system by turning it counterclockwise five times (Figure 96.8). Again, TOE control in all four views and final contrast injections are performed, and then the delivery system can be removed from the LAA (Figure 96.9). Under optimal circumstances, there should be no or minimal (<5 mm) residual leak by color flow in all TOE planes. In addition, if there is shoulder overhang, it should not exceed 20% of the device diameter and, as previously mentioned, the compression grade should be 10–20%.

Postinterventional medical treatment

In the PROTECT AF-Trial,[1] warfarin was continued for 45 days with a goal INR (international normalization ratio) between 2 and 3 in parallel with aspirin 100 mg for the presumed duration of device endothelialization. If at 45 days, there was no or <5 mm diameter device leak (measured by

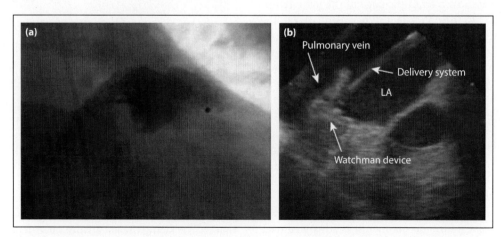

Figure 96.7 (a) Angiographic control of the device implanted in the LAA. Contrast dye is injected through the delivery system and shows the barrier between left atrium and LAA due to the membrane of the device. The tug test is performed during dye injection to visualize the movement of the device and LAA in unison. (b) Echocardiographic control shows complete coverage of the LAA by the device. The tug test can also be assessed echocardiographically.

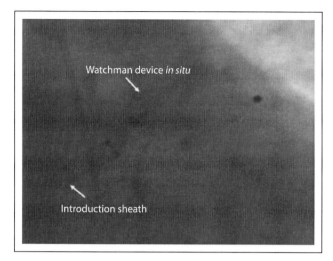

Figure 96.8 After control of stability of the device, the delivery system is removed by counterclockwise rotation. The released device is in stable position in the LAA.

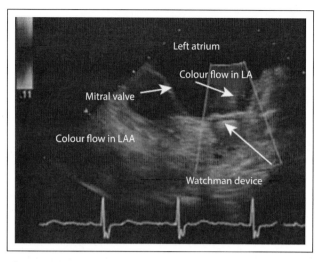

Figure 96.10 Echocardiographic control 45 days after implantation of the device. Color Doppler demonstrates very little flow behind the device in the LAA thus allowing discontinuation of warfarin therapy.

color Doppler) (Figure 96.10), warfarin was discontinued and replaced by clopidogrel therapy 75 mg daily until the 6 month follow-up. This strategy was based on the finding that, in the feasibility study,[2] four patients were found to have device-associated thrombus formation at 6 month follow-up; one such example is demonstrated in Figure 96.10. In this context, there is evidence for complete endothelialization in a patient who died 9 months after implantation due to a rupture of an aortic aneurysm. Figure 96.11 shows the state of the Watchman device at the time of autopsy. If, at 6-month TOE, there was no residual leak or leak <5 mm and no device-associated thrombus formation, clopidogrel therapy was discontinued and aspirin therapy 100 mg

per day continued lifelong. In case of thrombus formation (Figure 96.12), clopidogrel was stopped and anticoagulation with warfarin restarted again, at least for a limited time until thrombus resolution.

It is worth mentioning that more recent registry data in patients with absolute contraindications to even temporary anticoagulation who underwent Watchman implantation followed by temporary (6 months) double antiplatelet (aspirin and clopidogrel) therapy and aspirin only thereafter, demonstrated a low incidence of embolic events or thrombus formation, suggesting that this strategy may be safe in patients who cannot tolerate even temporary anticoagulation.

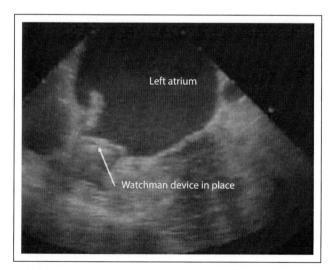

Figure 96.9 Echocardiographic control also shows a well-positioned device with complete coverage of the entrance of the LAA.

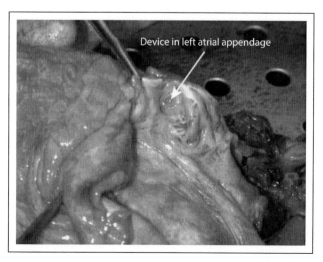

Figure 96.11 A pathological specimen in a patient who died 9 months after implantation of a Watchman device due to an aortic aneurysm. There is complete coverage of the device with new endothelium.

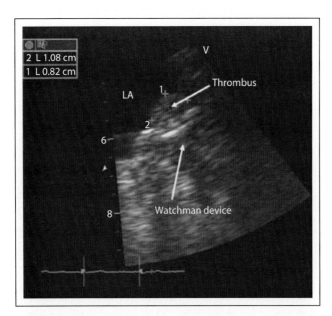

Figure 96.12 Smooth thrombus formation on the surface of a Watchman device in a patient with noncompliance to warfarin therapy.

Possible device-specific complications

Possible complications of heart catheterization and transseptal puncture will not be discussed here, only device-specific complications will be mentioned.

Air embolism, especially in cases of device retrieval, might be a problem, if the catheter tip is in tight contact to the atrial wall, as negative pressure can develop in the introduction sheath during pullback of the device. When removing the delivery system from the access sheath, air might be sucked into the sheath, which could inadvertently be injected into the left atrium with the next contrast dye injection. A continuous infusion of saline solution through the side arm of the sheath helps to avoid this problem as well as a slow pullback of the device and waiting for spontaneous blood return into the guiding catheter.

The risk of perforation of the LAA wall, with the catheter as well as with the device itself leading to pericardial tamponade, can be minimized by advancing the access sheath over the pigtail catheter. Additionally, the correct site of the transseptal puncture helps to avoid perforation with the device during deployment. The tugging test has to be performed very carefully using contrast dye injection for angiographic control and visualizing by TOE.

If all echocardiographic release criteria are fulfilled, embolization of the device is rare. Embolized devices can be retrieved percutaneously by snaring, usually in the descending aorta and being pulled out through a femoral sheath.

References

1. Holmes DR, Reddy VR, Turi ZG et al. Percutaneous closure of the LAA vs warfarin therapy for prevention of stroke in pts with AF: A randomised non-inferiority trial. *Lancet* 2009;374:534–42.
2. Sick PB, Schuler G, Hauptmann KE et al. Initial worldwide experience with the Watchman left atrial appendage system for stroke prevention in atrial fibrillation. *J Am Coll Cardiol* 2007;49:1490–5.

97

Coherex WaveCrest

Brian Whisenant and Saibal Kar

Introduction

The Coherex WaveCrest™ left atrial appendage (LAA) occluder is a catheter-delivered implantable device designed to permanently occlude the LAA and thereby reduce the incidence of atrial fibrillation-mediated stroke. LAA closure has been associated with anatomic challenges, procedural complications, and late thrombus formation on the left atrial surface of occluder devices. The WaveCrest LAA occlusion system is a next-generation device, which separates occlusion and anchoring. It is uniquely designed to address these challenges with an implant that can be safely and confidently deployed in a variety of anatomies to deliver long-term stroke reduction. The WAVECREST I Trial conducted in Europe, Australia, and New Zealand resulted in CE mark approval in August 2013. The WaveCrest LAA occlusion system is available in select countries through a distribution agreement with Biosense Webster.

Device description

WaveCrest occluder

The WaveCrest occluder is designed to be positioned in the ostium of the LAA. It is constructed with expanded polytetrafluoroethylene (ePTFE) facing the left atrium to minimize thrombus formation. A rim of polyurethane on the inner surface and along the occluder margin facilitates early endothelialization and tissue in-growth (Figures 97.1 and 97.2). This combination of minimal thrombogenicity and rapid endothelialization is designed to eliminate the need for postprocedure anticoagulation while reducing the risk of device-associated thrombus and stroke. As the occluder is unsheathed, the leading edge of the device is formed by the polyurethane foam, making it soft and atraumatic (Figure 97.3). After fully unsheathing the occluder within the LAA, its position may be manipulated for an optimal deployment within the LAA ostium prior to engaging the anchors. The device may be fully or partially recaptured and repositioned if necessary. The WaveCrest occluder is available in three sizes with unconstrained diameters of 22, 27, and 32 mm.

WaveCrest anchors

The WaveCrest occluder and the retractable anchors are distinctly separate. The 10 anchor struts are interconnected to provide both conformability and sufficient radial expansion force. After the occluder is ideally positioned within the LAA ostium, the WaveCrest anchors are advanced to engage the LAA walls, becoming the most distal portion of the implant. Each of the 10 interconnected WaveCrest anchors has a bidirectional double microtine and a single microtine (Figure 97.4), creating 30 points of tissue engagement for increased stability. The distal anchor system extends 3 mm or less beyond the microtines. The separation of occlusion from anchoring, along with the distal position of the anchors, allows the physician to precisely position the Coherex occluder in the ostium of even the most challenging LAA anatomies, including short and wide appendages or appendages with a proximal bifurcation of lobes (Figure 97.5). After deployment and tissue engagement, the anchors may be retracted and disengaged from the LAA wall, allowing the occluder to be recaptured within the delivery sheath for removal or repositioning. Anchor deployment and retraction are designed to engage and disengage tissue without tearing or otherwise traumatizing the appendage wall. Radiopaque tantalum markers on 5 of the 10 anchors indicate the distal aspect of the anchors and the microtines (Figure 97.4).

WaveCrest delivery catheter

The distal portion of the delivery catheter is designed with a flexible segment, which allows the occluder to assume a less constrained orientation and enhances tactile feel during push and pull stability testing.

The delivery catheter flush port (Figure 97.6) serves as a conduit for radiographic contrast injection directly into the appendage beyond the occluder. Opacification of the LAA

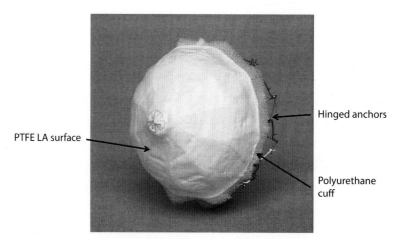

PTFE LA surface

Hinged anchors

Polyurethane cuff

Figure 97.1   The Coherex LAA occluder.

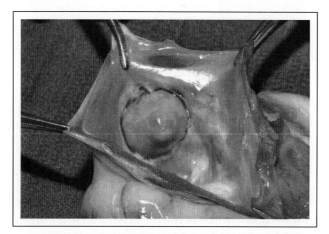

Figure 97.2   (**See color insert.**) 180 day animal model with well-endothelialized Coherex LAA occluder.

with the occluder in place illuminates the relationship of the occluder to surrounding tissue, allowing the physician to assess position and occlusion while minimizing contrast use. Distal LAA contrast opacification also confirms tissue engagement and stability of the WaveCrest anchors during push and pull provocative testing.

The anchor actuator knob of the delivery system handle deploys and retracts the anchors. While the actuator cable is attached to the anchors with a threaded insert, the delivery system is separately connected to the occluder hub. Attachment to the occluder hub allows the physician to push and pull the occluder and test stability without altering anchor engagement. The WaveCrest delivery catheter allows for simple simultaneous detachment from both the anchors and the occluder. Counterclockwise rotation of the anchor actuator unscrews the delivery system from anchors. Withdrawal of the anchor actuator

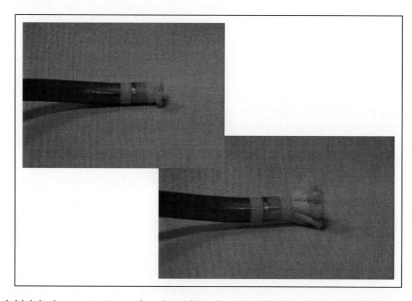

Figure 97.3   During initial deployment, atraumatic polyurethane is unsheathed in advance of nitinol components.

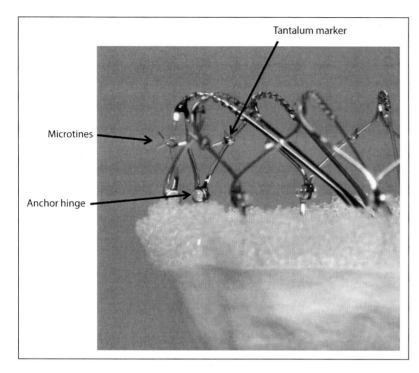

Figure 97.4   Coherex LAA anchors and microtines. Each of the 10 anchors includes a bidirectional double tine and a single retrograde tine.

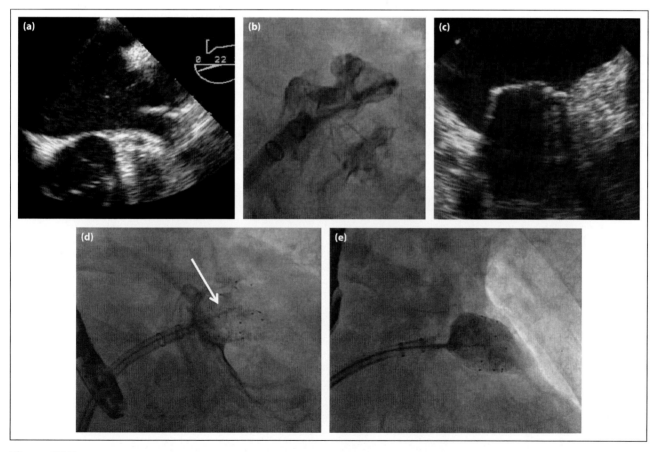

Figure 97.5   The LAA with a proximal bifurcation and an appropriately positioned Coherex occluder: (a) TEE image. (b) Angiographic image. (c) Coherex LAA occluder TEE image and (d) Coherex LAA occluder angiographic image; radiopaque anchor core indicates extended anchors. (e) Distal injection.

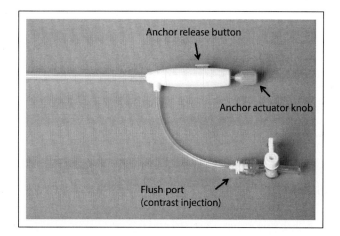

Figure 97.6 The WaveCrest LAA delivery system handle.

proximal to the occluder hub completes the detachment of the device.

WaveCrest delivery sheaths

The 15 Fr WaveCrest delivery sheath is designed to deliver the occluder in a coaxial position in the ostium. The delivery sheaths are labeled 60°, 75°, 90°, and 90°s (distal superior angle), which correspond to the angles between the shaft and the distal tip of the delivery sheath (Figure 97.7). The 75° will be appropriate for most LAA anatomies. The 90° delivery sheath is designed for LAAs with a horizontal or inferior trajectory while the 60° and 90°s shapes are designed for LAAs with a more superior trajectory. The Coherex delivery sheaths have an atraumatic distal tip and side holes in the distal segment to facilitate aspiration and injection. A clear chamber immediately distal to the hemostasis valve allows the operator to inspect for air after the WaveCrest device is introduced into the delivery sheath. The flush port adjacent to the clear chamber allows for the removal of air prior to advancing the occluder, as well as injection of contrast once the occluder is deployed. The two distal marker bands are 5 and 15 mm from the distal tip.

WaveCrest device summary

In summary, unique attributes of the Coherex WaveCrest occluder include the following:

- Designed for proximal placement to avoid difficult distal anatomy and reduce pericardial effusions caused by catheter manipulation deep in the LAA
- Separation of occlusion and anchoring facilitates precise positioning, conformability, and radial expansion
- Minimal length beyond the anchors facilitates deployment in short appendages or appendages with proximal bifurcations
- Ten anchors with 30 bidirectional tines for tissue engagement provide conformability and secure retention
- ePTFE surface eliminates the need for early anticoagulation while helping to prevent late device thrombosis
- Polyurethane material on the underside and along the occluder cuff enhances early endothelialization
- Ability to inject contrast distal to occluder to assess stability, position, and closure while minimizing contrast use and reducing reliance on transesophageal echocardiography (TEE) imaging
- Multiple full recaptures and redeployments with a single device
- Three sizes, 22, 27, and 32 mm, cover 14–30 mm ostial diameters
- Leading edge during device deployment is atraumatic polyurethane

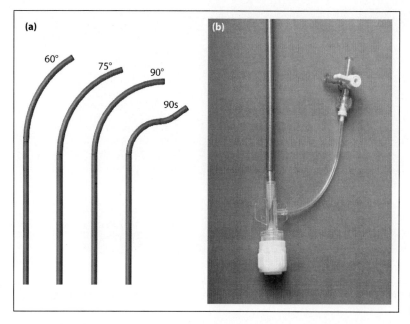

Figure 97.7 (a) The Coherex delivery sheath's distal shapes. (b) The Coherex delivery sheath's proximal visualization chamber.

- Flexible distal delivery shaft allows device to assume less constrained position and enhances tactile feel during push and pull stability testing
- Delivery sheath with an air inspection chamber and atraumatic distal tip helps to improve procedural safety and success

Procedural instructions

LAA size and device selection

While the Coherex occluder accommodates a large range of LAA sizes, selecting the appropriate-size device enhances closure and stability. Mild anchor compression is essential for secure tissue engagement. Excessive oversizing can diminish the stability if the anchors are forced to overlap with inadequate space for expansion. Similarly, occluder folds or pleats may be formed by marked oversizing with inadequate space for expansion. The Coherex sizing recommendations according to TEE-measured anchor landing zone diameters are outlined in Figure 97.8. The average of the largest and smallest anchor landing zone measurements should be 3 mm or less than the labeled device size. No measurement should exceed the labeled device size.

A transesophageal echo should include measurements of the anticipated anchor landing zone at approximately 0°, 45°, 90°, and 135°. Computed tomographic angiography (CTA) may also be useful to determine LAA size and anatomy. The anticipated anchor landing zone generally extends from a point adjacent to the left circumflex on the inferior side to a point distal to the apex of the warfarin ridge, which divides the pulmonary veins from the LAA

(Figure 97.9). The WaveCrest occluder is deployed proximally near the ostium, often occluding the smooth-walled superior pouch. The LAA ostium is not planar, but rather spirals from the posterior wall (border with left pulmonary veins) around to the posterior/inferior wall below the MV annulus (Figure 97.9). When the superior pouch is covered with the occluder, care should be taken to make sure the anchors fully engage the LAA posterior wall. Posterior engagement is best visualized in the 120–135° TEE images and AP/cranial or AP/caudal cine views.

Transseptal puncture and sheath delivery

Transseptal puncture under ultrasound guidance (TEE or intracardiac echocardiography; ICE) is recommended. The fossa ovalis is generally punctured in the mid- to posterior segment along the anterior/posterior axis and mid to low along the superior/inferior axis (Figure 97.10). This facilitates an anterior superior trajectory that optimizes device delivery for most LAAs. Rarely, as with all LAA devices, a second transseptal puncture in an alternate segment of the fossa ovalis may enhance coaxial device delivery when difficult or unusual anatomy is encountered. When present, a patent foramen ovale (PFO) should not be used to access the left atrium as the PFO does not allow the delivery sheath to engage the LAA with a coaxial trajectory.

Anticoagulation with a target ACT of 250–300 s is recommended during the implant procedure. An initial contrast injection with the transseptal catheter may assist with selection of a preferable delivery sheath shape. A support wire is advanced through the transseptal catheter into the left superior pulmonary vein for catheter exchanges. The

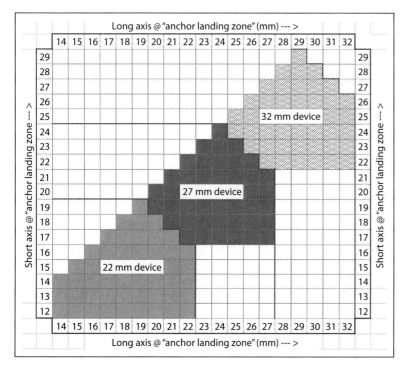

Figure 97.8 Device size selection according to TEE defined LAA ostial measurements.

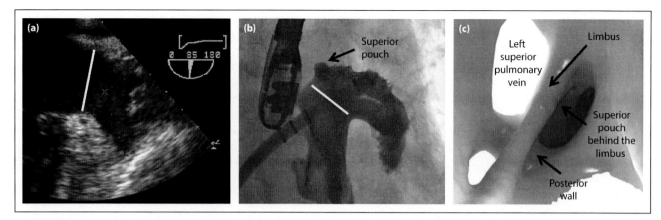

Figure 97.9 Common landing zone for WaveCrest anchors (white lines) extends from the left circumflex artery inferiorly to distal to the limbus superiorly. (a) TEE image. (b) Angiographic image. (c) 3D CT reconstruction demonstrates spiral nature of LAA ostium.

Coherex delivery sheath and dilator are advanced across the interatrial septum. The dilator is fixed and the delivery sheath further advanced over the dilator. The dilator and guide wire are removed and the sheath is flushed before being advanced into the LAA. Deep engagement of the delivery catheter in the LAA is not necessary or recommended. A pigtail catheter may be advanced through the lumen to facilitate positioning of the delivery sheath in the LAA. Initial cine images acquired with contrast injection through the pigtail catheter may limit contrast usage.

Device preparation

After removing the WaveCrest delivery system from the sterile package, the anchors must be retracted before the implant is collapsed into the loader to avoid damaging the anchors. Heparinized saline is flushed through the flush port of the delivery system handle until saline drips from the distal tip. The implant, loader, and the white loader funnel are submerged under heparinized saline while the implant is withdrawn into the loader. While still submerged, the delivery system is again flushed after the implant is collapsed into the loader. With the white funnel removed, the loader is advanced into the hemostatic valve of the delivery sheath. Maintaining a slow heparinized saline drip through the side port of the delivery sheath may help prevent air entrapment as the implant is inserted into the hemostatic valve and advanced through the delivery sheath to the LAA. The delivery catheter is slowly advanced into the clear proximal portion of the sheath. If air is observed, it can be aspirated at this time. The delivery catheter is slowly advanced and the loader removed after the flexible portion is inside the sheath.

Device deployment

With the delivery sheath in the proximal portion of the LAA, the WaveCrest implant is advanced to the sheath tip

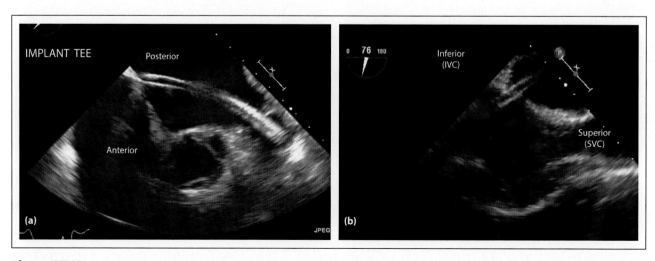

Figure 97.10 TEE guided transseptal puncture. (a) Short-axis TEE image defines septum in the anterior/posterior axis. (b) Bicaval TEE image defines septum in the superior/inferior axis.

and the occluder is unsheathed. If the implant is initially deployed too deep, the unsheathed occluder may be withdrawn to an ideal position under fluoroscopic and echo guidance. Contrast may be injected through the delivery sheath to facilitate device positioning. The anchors may then be extended and the position of the implant fixed within the LAA. The position of the anchors may be best appreciated by the presence of the radiopaque anchor core (Figure 97.5). The core will be visible within the occluder when the anchors are extended, but is hidden within the occluder hub when the anchors are retracted. If position and occlusion are satisfactory, the device is then tested for stability. The delivery sheath should be withdrawn approximately 2 cm from the occluder during stability testing. Contrast can be injected through the flush port of the delivery system and will appear beyond the occluder during push and pull manipulation to assess position, stability, and occlusion. If the implant is not stable or adequately positioned, the anchors may be retracted, and the device recaptured and redeployed. With a typical deployment position, the tantalum anchor markers should be 5–10 mm distal to the LAA ostium with the occluder face extending proximal to the LAA ostium. Prior to detaching the implant, ensure that the anchors are engaged into tissue without anchor entanglement. TEE interrogation should reveal no large gaps adjacent to the occluder.

An appropriately positioned WaveCrest device is shown in Figure 97.5. The angiography demonstrates the tantalum anchor markers ~10 mm distal to the ostium. The occluder face protrudes modestly into the left atrium via both angiographic and TEE imaging.

Device detachment

While holding the implant in a fixed position by immobilizing the position of the handle on the patient, the anchor actuator knob is unscrewed (counterclockwise rotation) with a minimum of five complete rotations. The anchor release button is depressed and the anchor actuator is pulled proximally to a hard stop resulting in implant detachment. Both of these steps should be visualized on fluoroscopy to confirm release before the delivery system is withdrawn into the delivery sheath. Final angiography may be performed, the delivery sheath removed, and hemostasis achieved according to physician preference.

Postprocedure

Dual antiplatelet therapy with aspirin 100–325 mg and clopidogrel 75 mg is recommended for 6 weeks following device deployment. After 6 weeks, clopidogrel may be discontinued while aspirin alone is continued indefinitely. Antibiotic prophylaxis is recommended at implant and following American Medical Association (AMA) guidelines for 6 months. Surveillance TEE 5–6 weeks following device deployment may be considered.

Coherex LAA deployment highlights

Significant oversizing may result in anchor entanglement and is not recommended with the WaveCrest occluder. The average of the largest and smallest anchor landing zone measurements should be 3 mm or less than the labeled device size. No measurement should exceed the labeled device size.

- Echo guided posterior and inferior transseptal puncture usually facilitates coaxial catheter engagement of the LAA.
- Deployment of the WaveCrest occluder does not require deep engagement of the delivery sheath in the LAA. Deep or aggressive delivery sheath manipulation should be avoided.
- Ideally, 5 mm of "headroom" distal to the occluder allows for unimpeded anchor extension. When deployed in a shallow appendage or with a trajectory that pushes the occluder into an LAA side wall, adequate headroom for anchor expansion must be allowed.
- With a typical deployment position, the tantalum anchor markers should be 5–10 mm distal to the LAA ostium with the occluder face extending proximally to the LAA ostium.

Clinical experience

The WAVECREST I Trial has completed enrollment at the time of this submission. The WAVECREST I Trial included 73 patients with a CHADS$_2$ score ≥1 who were either anticoagulant indicated or contraindicated. All patients were followed with TEEs 45 days post-device implantation. If not closed at 45 days, the TEE was repeated at 180 days. All patients were followed clinically for stroke and adverse events until 1 year postprocedure. The primary efficacy endpoint of the trial was LAA occlusion at 45 and/or 180 days postprocedure. The primary safety endpoint was the incidence of major adverse events within 45 days of the index procedure. An independent core lab reviewed all TEE studies and an independent clinical events committee reviewed all serious adverse events. Initial procedural results presented in 2013 suggest excellent procedural safety and closure efficacy. Publication is pending completion of follow-up and core lab adjudication.

Conclusion

The next-generation Coherex WaveCrest LAA occlusion system has been optimized for simple and safe procedures and long-term stroke reduction in even the most challenging anatomies. Unique features include the ability to optimize position in the LAA ostium, the separation of the occluder from the anchors, the ability to completely recapture and reposition the implant at any time prior to release, and the ability to inject contrast distal to the occluder. The ePTFE material facing the left atrium minimizes thrombus formation, while polyurethane along the underside and occluder margin promotes rapid endothelialization. Based on outstanding initial results from the WAVECREST I Trial, a CE Mark was received in August 2013, and commercialization outside of the United States was initiated shortly afterwards. Coherex Medical is planning an OUS (Outside the United States) commercial registry as well as a US pivotal trial, designed to both advance the science of LAA closure as well to vigorously test this device.

Acknowledgments

The authors acknowledge the editorial assistance of John Lundquist, Michael Simmons, and Cliff Montagnoli from Coherex Medical.

98

Sentre heart

Krzysztof Bartus and Randall J Lee

Introduction

Atrial fibrillation (AF) is the most common cardiac arrhythmia. The prevalence of AF increases with age, from 0.1% among adults younger than 55 years to 9.0% in persons aged 80 years or older.[1] After the age of 40, an individual in the United States has a lifetime risk of 1 in 4 of developing AF.[2] Approximately 2.3 million individuals in the United States and 4.5 million in the European Union have AF.[1,3] In developed countries, the number of persons with AF is likely to increase during the next 50 years, owing to the growing proportion of elderly individuals. The incidence in the United States is projected to be in the range of 5.6 to 12.1 million by 2050.[1,4]

As early as the 1940s, the left atrial appendage (LAA) was thought to be a primary source of thrombus formation leading to cardioembolic events. Exclusion of the LAA was utilized as an adjunct to mitral operations in order to prevent cardioembolic events.[5–8] In a review of operative, autopsy, and transesophageal echocardiographic studies, examination of the left atrium (LA) and LAA confirmed that the great majority of thrombi that develop in the LAA (Table 98.1) were attributed to stasis of blood flow within that particular structure.[9] At least two-thirds of the ischemic cerebrovascular events and half of all vascular events in AF are related to the atrial thrombi.

Additionally, the original surgical approaches to "curative" procedures for AF also included LAA exclusion. A study of 178 AF patients who had their oral anticoagulants (OAC) discontinued after a Cox Maze III procedure found that 99% of the patients had no strokes over 10 years.[10] The cumulative body of evidence for the LAA as a primary source of thrombus formation leading to cardioembolic events is highlighted in the 2006 AHA/ACC/ESC Guidelines for Treatment of AF and the AHA/ACC/ESC Guidelines for Treatment of Mitral Disease, which recommend exclusion of the LAA during concomitant procedures as a prophylactic measure to eliminate a primary source of thrombus.[3,11]

Surgical methods of LAA exclusion have included the use of sutures, staples, and clips. Suture ligation from the endocardial surface of the left atrium is often performed during valve replacement surgery, but not all surgeons find a need for LAA exclusion in AF patients. This invasive procedure may require the use of cardiopulmonary bypass and may also be associated with bleeding or injury to the circumflex coronary artery due to its proximity to the LAA. In addition, endocardial suture ligation is incomplete in 10–30% of patients, which itself may predispose the patient to thromboembolic events.[12–14] This high rate of incomplete closure is attributed to several factors: the procedure is performed when the heart is in a flaccid state, the access is generally awkward for traditional suturing, and often transesophageal echocardiography (TEE) is not used to confirm complete intraoperative closure. Only after the heart is reperfused can the closure result be completely assessed. Unfortunately, the opportunity to rectify incomplete closure has passed.

Epicardial ligation or excision can be performed without cardiopulmonary bypass. Epicardial exclusion of the LAA can be accomplished using suture ligation and excising the LAA or with the use of noncutting surgical staples.[15,16] TEE studies of LAA closure using staples suggest that complete closure occurs in 0–80% of cases.[17,18] Grasping of the LAA and pulling traction while applying the staple can lead from bleeding and tissue damage to tearing of the LAA (reported in 7–25% of the cases).[15,19,20] Additionally, staples generally result in a linear closure pattern that may not comply with the line required to close the LAA at its origin. Surgical studies often define successful closure to include a residual diverticulum of 2 cm. A diverticulum of >1 cm is not unusual after surgical stapling and may serve as a nidus for subsequent thrombus formation.[16,18]

Epicardial suture closure of the LAA is performed by placing a tie around the base of the appendage by either directly sewing the appendage closed or by tightening pre-tied suture loops around the LAA base. Success rate of epicardial suture closure ranges from 23% to 100% and is both technique and operator dependent.[15,17,18,20] Incomplete suture ligation is present immediately after the procedure rather than via a degenerative process.[13] Complications rarely arise

820 Interventions in structural, valvular, and congenital heart disease

Table 98.1 Prevalence of cardiac thrombus located in the LA and LAA for patient population with nonvalvular AF[a] in published studies

Detection methods	Patients screened	Patients with heart thrombus	Thrombus in LA cavity		Thrombus in LAA	
TEE[b]	317	67	1	(2%)	66	(98%)
TEE	233	35	1	(3%)	34	(97%)
Autopsy	506	47	12	(26%)	35	(74%)
TEE	52	4	2	(50%)	2	(50%)
TEE	48	13	1	(8%)	12	(92%)
TEE and operation	171	11	3	(27%)	8	(73%)
ACUTE	549	76	9	(12%)	67	(88%)
TEE	272	19	0	(0%)	19	(100%)
TEE	60	6	0	(0%)	6	(100%)
Total	2208	278	29	(10%)	249	(90%)

[a] Modified from Blackshear JL, Odell JA. *Ann Thorac Surg* 1996;61(2):755–9.
[b] 5% of patients in this trial had mitral stenosis or prosthetic valve.
ACUTE, Assessment of Cardioversion Using Transesophageal Echocardiography multicenter trial.

at the suture closure of the LAA, but are generally limited to LAA tearing that occurs either during the suture needle placement or while grasping the LAA as is required in conventional open approaches.[13,20] Table 98.2 summarizes the literature regarding the efficacy and complications of conventional epicardial suture closure of the LAA.

Percutaneous approaches for exclusion of the LAA were developed to decrease the invasive nature and morbidity associated with surgical LAA exclusion. The results of the Protect AF trial provided evidence that LAA exclusion of the LAA provided a similar benefit in preventing neurological events in AF patients as did warfarin.[22] The LARIAT® suture delivery device was adapted from surgical LAA ligation procedures as an alternative to LAA implants for LAA exclusion. Initial preclinical studies starting in 2006 demonstrated the feasibility, safety, and efficacy of a closed-chested LAA ligation procedure.[23] Histological evaluation of the LAA revealed endothelialization of the closure site, resulting in a smooth endocardial surface.[23] In a collaboration between clinicians from the University of California, San Francisco, and Department of Cardiovascular Surgery and Transplantology, Jagiellonian University, John Paul II

Hospital, Krakow, Poland, first-in-man studies were initiated in 2009 with a subsequent single-center observation study that demonstrated efficacy with low access-related complications.[24,25]

LAA ligation with the LARIAT suture delivery device

The LARIAT suture delivery device and associated accessories used to perform the close-chested LAA ligation are shown in Figure 98.1. The procedure utilizes an anterior pericardial access and transseptal approach to allow placement of an endocardial magnet-tipped guide wire into the most anterior lobe of the LAA; this is then connected with an epicardial magnet-tipped guide wire (Figure 98.2b). This connection of the magnet-tipped guide wires allows for stabilization of the LAA and advancement of the LARIAT suture delivery device over the epicardial guide wire in an "over-the-wire" approach to direct the LARIAT snare over the LAA (Figure 98.2c). Proper positioning of the LARIAT snare over the LAA is guided by

Table 98.2 Epicardial suture closure assessed by transesophageal echography summary

Author	n	Closure method	Complete exclusion	Tearing of LAA	Bleeding
Roscoe[18]	11	Epicardial suture	4 (30%)	0 (0%)	0 (0%)
Johnson[20]	391	Epicardial or endocardial suture	–	0 (0%)	0 (0%)
Healy[19]	11	Epicardial encircling or running suture line	5 (45%)	1 (9%)	0 (0%)
Kanderian[17]	73	Epicardial or endocardial suture	17 (23%)	0 (0%)	0 (0%)
Blackshear[21]	8	Epicardial thorascopic pre-tied loop	8 (100%)	1 (12%)	0 (0%)

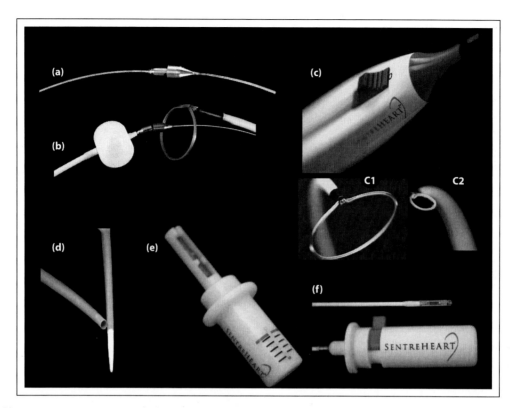

Figure 98.1 LARIAT suture delivery device and accessories. The LARIAT suture delivery device and accessories (SentreHEART, Redwood City, CA) for exclusion of the LAA is based on 0.025″ and 0.035″ magnet-tipped guide wires (FindrWRZ™) (a). The system consists of three components: (1) 0.025″ and 0.035″ magnet-tipped guide wires (FindrWRZ), (2) a 15 mm compliant occlusion balloon catheter (EndoCATH™), and (3) a 12 F suture delivery device (LARIAT), which are put together as a system (b). The LARIAT suture delivery device has an adjustable slide lever to open and close the snare (c). The higher-power insets demonstrate the pre-tied size 0 Teflon-coated, braided polyester suture mounted in the open (C1) and closed (C2) radiopaque adjustable snare. (d) The epicardial SofTIP™ guide cannula with and without the 13.5 French dilator inserted in the guide cannula. (e) The TenSure suture-tightening device. (f) The SureCUT™ suture cutter.

TEE placement of the inflated balloon catheter at the OS of the LAA (Figure 98.3b). Prior to release of the suture, conformation of complete capture of the LAA is confirmed with TEE and contrast LA angiography. If the closure of the snare does not completely capture the entire LAA, the snare can be opened and repositioned to ensure complete LAA capture.

The success of LAA ligation with the LARIAT suture delivery device can be enhanced by following a prescriptive approach. This begins with proper patient selection.[25] The procedure requires enough access to the pericardial space to freely move the LARIAT device over the LAA. Therefore, patients with prior open-heart surgery, pectus excavatum, history of pericarditis, and conditions that may lead to pericarditis or pericardial adhesions should be excluded. Appropriate preprocedural imaging is essential to rule out anatomical limitations, LAA thrombus, and placement of the endocardial magnet-tipped guide wire. LAA anatomical exclusion criteria includes (1) LAA width >40 mm, (2) superiorly oriented LAA with the LAA apex directed behind the pulmonary trunk, (3) bilobed LAA or multilobed LAA

in which lobes were oriented in different planes exceeding 40 mm, and (4) a posteriorly rotated heart.[25]

Proper access to the pericardial space and left atrium is a critical procedural step. An anterior epicardial puncture is required to advance the LARIAT device over the right ventricular surface and approach the tip of the LAA in its most anterior aspect. The anterior–posterior fluoroscopic view is used to align the needle toward the lateral aspect of the cardiac silhouette, while the 90° left lateral fluoroscopic view assures that the epicardial puncture is on the anterior surface of the right ventricle. An epicardial puncture that is too medial will not easily allow the LARIAT device to be directed in an anterior to posterior direction of the surface of the heart and advance over the LAA. The transseptal puncture should occur at the mid to lower aspect of the atrial septum and slightly posterior. A transseptal catheterization entering high on the septum tends to direct the transseptal sheath toward the left pulmonary veins.

A left atrial angiogram is performed either by contrast injection through the transseptal sheath or a pigtail catheter

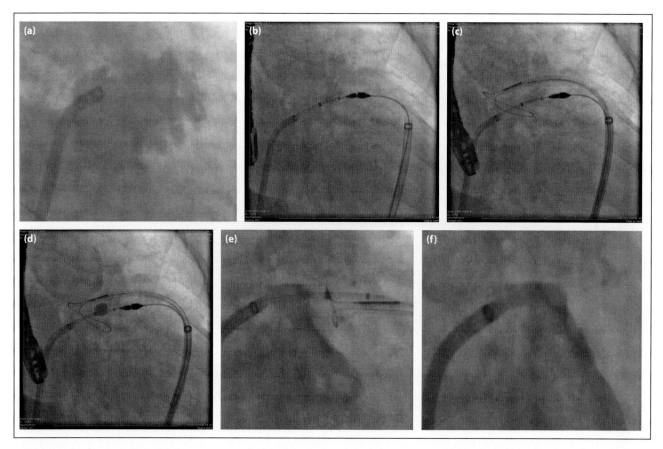

Figure 98.2 Steps of LAA ligation with the LARIAT suture delivery device. All images are in the right anterior oblique fluoroscopic projection. After pericardial and transseptal access has been achieved, a left atrial (LA) angiography identifies the ostium and body of the LAA (a). The attachment of the magnet-tipped endocardial and epicardial guide wires stabilizes the LAA (b) and allows for the LARIAT suture delivery device to be guided over the LAA using an over-the-wire approach (c). Inflation of the occlusion balloon allows for identification of the LAA ostium and proper positioning of the LARIAT snare (d). An LA angiogram is performed prior to release of the pre-tied suture to ensure complete exclusion of the LAA (e). A final LA angiogram verifies LAA exclusion (f).

positioned within the LAA. This helps delineate the LAA ostium and morphology. The placement of the endocardial magnet wire in the most anterior aspect of the LAA allows the epicardial magnet-tipped guide wire to be connected to the endocardial magnet-tipped guide wire for the most direct path of the LARIAT device snare over the LAA. Proper closure of the LARIAT device snare over the LAA is assisted by positioning the catheter balloon at the LAA ostium. Under certain circumstances, the LARIAT device snare can be closed over the balloon to help maintain positioning of the snare at the LAA ostium. The LARIAT snare can be opened and closed multiple times to assure proper closure of the LAA. The position of the LARIAT snare is not committed until release of the suture from the snare is performed. Once the desired position of the LARIAT snare is achieved, the endocardial magnet and balloon catheter are removed from the LAA and the suture is released from the snare to ligate the LAA. The TenSure™ device is used to tighten the knot. Following removal of the LARIAT device from the pericardial space, the suture is cut with only an epicardial suture left in place.

Initial clinical results

PLACE I (Permanent Ligation Approximation Closure of the Left Atrial Appendage in Patients with Atrial Fibrillation) study

First-in-man studies using the LARIAT suture delivery device were initiated in 2009 at John Paul II Hospital, Krakow, Poland (Table 98.3).[24] LAA exclusion using the LARIAT device in the first two patients was performed during mitral valve replacement surgery to test whether the suture could be released from the LARIAT device snare after closure on the LAA. After this was found feasible, a hybrid approach using a pericardial window to allow for epicardial access and a transseptal catheterization for LA access was developed to allow connection of the endocardial and epicardial magnet-tipped guide wires. In these two patients, the LARIAT device snare was advanced over the epicardial magnet-tipped guide wire, allowing successful

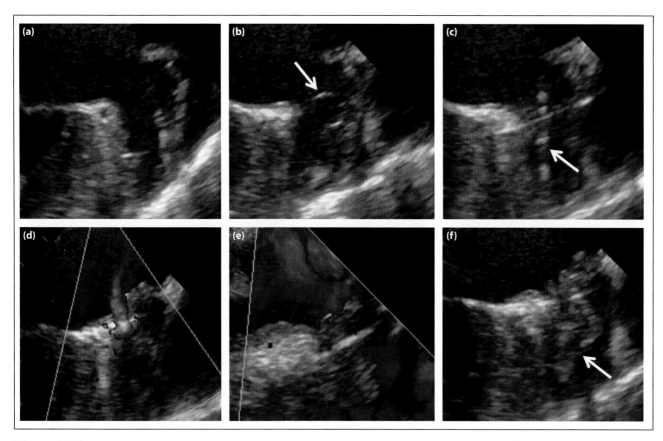

Figure 98.3 **(See color insert.)** Transesophageal echocardiography (TEE) assessment of LAA closure. TEE imaging LAA at baseline (a) and during the placement of the balloon (arrow) at the orifice of the LAA (b). Closure of the LARIAT snare closes the orifice of the LAA around the EndoCATH (arrow) (c). Color Doppler is used to verify the acute closure of the LAA following ligation of the LAA. There is a leak following hand tightening of the suture (d), which disappears following suture tightening with the TenSure device (e). At the end, the LAA is closed and collapsed (arrow), which creates a space within the pericardial cavity (f).

Table 98.3 PLACE I Summary	
Total number of study patients	13
AF type	Persistent: 12 (92%) Paroxysmal: 0 (0%) Atrial flutter: 1 (8%)
Age	Mean 57 years (range of 43–64 years)
Gender	Male: 8 (62%) Female: 5 (38%)
Procedures performed	LAA exclusion with MVR: 2 (15%) LAA exclusion with ablation: 11 (85%)
Exclusion completed	12 (92%)
Major device complications	1 (8%)
Acute closure	12 (100%)
Procedural time	Mean of 85.7 min (range of 22–335 min)
Device-related adverse events	Acute: 0/13 (0%) 1 day–17 months: 0/13 (0%)

Source: Bartus K et al. *Heart Rhythm* 2011;8(2):188–93.

closure of the LAA. To complete the feasibility study, 10 additional patients underwent a completely percutaneous approach with successful closure of the LAA.

One complication occurred in a patient with severe pectus excavatum. The LARIAT was placed in the correct position during LAA capture, resulting in complete LAA closure. However, the LARIAT device could not be removed from the LAA after suture deployment despite reopening the snare. A second 5 cm incision was made to open the pericardium, through which the device was freed with no other sequelae. After the procedure, the LARIAT device was analyzed and found to exhibit normal function. The procedure was considered a successful LAA exclusion with a device complication.

PLACE II study

The encouraging results from the PLACE I study led to the PLACE II study. The PLACE II study was a single-center, observational study designed to test LAA closure efficacy and safety.[25] The patient population consisted of patients with AF, CHADs2 score >1 with contraindications or intolerance

Table 98.4 PLACE II clinical summary

Number of patients screened	119
Number of patients excluded	30
Total number of treated patients	89
Age	Mean of 62 years (range of 35–81 years)
Gender	Male: 51 (57%); female: 38 (43%)
AF type	Paroxysmal: 30 (34%); persistent: 59 (66%)
CHADS$_2$ score	Average of 1.9 ± 0.95 (range of 1–5)
Treatment failure	4/89 (7%)
	• Two preprocedure access complications, nonserious, n = 2
	• Anatomic limitation (dilated RA), n = 1
	• Unable to capture LAA due to localized adhesions on LAA sulcus, n = 1
Acute closure (postprocedure)	Complete <1 mm: 82/85 (96%); ≤1–2 mm: 2/85 (2%); ≤2–3 mm: 1/85 (2%)
90 day chronic closure	Complete <1 mm: 77/81 (95%); ≤1–2 mm: 3/81 (3.7%); ≤2–3 mm: 1/81 (1.2%)
1 year chronic closure	Complete <1 mm: 64/65 (98%); ≤1–2 mm: 1/65 (2%); ≤ 2–3 mm: 0/65 (0%)
Procedural time	Mean of 53.7 ± 28.8 min
Acute complications	Total: 3/85 (3.5%)
	Access related: 3/85 (3.5%); nonserious
	Device related: 0/85 (0%)
Adverse events	Acute: 0/85 (0%)
	Follow-up: chest pain 20/85 (23.5%); postoperative pericarditis 2/20 (10%) did not resolve after 2 days
Serious adverse events	Acute: 0/85 (0%)
	Follow-up: pericardial effusion: 1/85 (1.2%)
	Death: 2/85 (1.2%)
	Stroke: 2/85 (1.2%)

Source: Bartus K et al. *J Am Coll Cardiol* 2013;62(2):108–18.

to warfarin therapy. Serial TEE was performed during 1 day, 30 days, 90 days, and 1 month after LAA ligation with the LARIAT device. Complete closure defined as TEE color flow Doppler of ≤1 mm was achieved in 96% of patients. A clinical summary demonstrates the efficacy of LAA closure with the LARIAT device with acceptably low procedural and periprocedural adverse events (see Table 98.4).

Long-term consequences of LAA ligation

Preclinical studies have demonstrated that LAA ligation with the LARIAT suture delivery device results in atrophy of the LAA with endothelization of the site of closure resulting in a smooth endocardial surface.[23] A similar phenomenon most

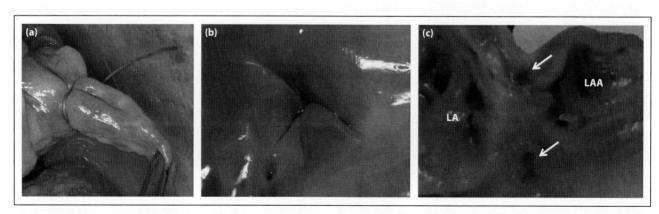

Figure 98.4 (**See color insert.**) Gross anatomy of an LAA following LAA ligation. Examination of the previously ligated LAA during mitral valve replacement taken from the explanted heart of a patient undergoing heart transplantation. Gross examination of the LAA reveals an atretic LAA (a) with a smooth endocardial surface (b). The glutaraldehyde fixed tissue was then sectioned through the suture ligation (c). The blue sutures (arrow) are still present delineating a completely closed closure line, thus resulting in complete exclusion of the LAA. LA, left atrium; LAA, left atrial appendage.

likely occurs in patients following suture ligation of the LAA. Recently, a patient with prior LARIAT device LAA ligation underwent heart transplantation. Gross examination of the LAA revealed an atretic structure with a completely closed orifice at the site of suture ligation (Figure 98.4c).

Summary

The LARIAT suture delivery device provides a novel, stand-alone catheter-based approach for permanent closure of the LAA. The initial clinical results demonstrate a highly effective procedure for LAA exclusion with low procedural complications.

References

1. Go AS et al. Prevalence of diagnosed atrial fibrillation in adults: National implications for rhythm management and stroke prevention: The AnTicoagulation and Risk Factors in Atrial Fibrillation (ATRIA) Study. *JAMA* 2001;285(18):2370–5.
2. Lloyd-Jones DM et al. Lifetime risk for development of atrial fibrillation: The Framingham heart study. *Circulation* 2004;110(9):1042–6.
3. European Heart Rhythm Association et al. ACC/AHA/ESC 2006 guidelines for the management of patients with atrial fibrillation—Executive summary: A report of the American College of Cardiology/American Heart Association Task Force on Practice Guidelines and the European Society of Cardiology Committee for Practice Guidelines (Writing Committee to Revise the 2001 Guidelines for the Management of Patients with Atrial Fibrillation). *J Am Coll Cardiol* 2006;48(4):854–906.
4. Miyasaka Y et al. Secular trends in incidence of atrial fibrillation in olmsted county, Minnesota, 1980–2000, and implications on the projections for future prevalence. *Circulation* 2006;114(2):119–25.
5. Bailey CP et al. Commissurotomy for mitral stenosis; technique for prevention of cerebral complications. *JAMA* 1952;149(12):1085–91.
6. Belcher JR, Somerville W. Systemic embolism and left auricular thrombosis in relation to mitral valvotomy. *Br Med J* 1955;2(4946):1000–3.
7. Longmire WP, Jr., Beal JM, Leake WH. Resection of the auricular appendages. *Dis Chest* 1951;19(3):307–18.
8. Madden JL. Resection of the left auricular appendix; a prophylaxis for recurrent arterial emboli. *JAMA* 1949;140(9):769–72.
9. Blackshear JL, Odell JA. Appendage obliteration to reduce stroke in cardiac surgical patients with atrial fibrillation. *Ann Thorac Surg* 1996;61(2):755–9.
10. Damiano RJ, Jr. et al. The long-term outcome of patients with coronary disease and atrial fibrillation undergoing the Cox maze procedure. *J Thorac Cardiovasc Surg* 2003;126(6):2016–21.
11. American College of Cardiology et al. ACC/AHA 2006 guidelines for the management of patients with valvular heart disease: A report of the American College of Cardiology/American Heart Association Task Force on Practice Guidelines (writing Committee to Revise the 1998 guidelines for the management of patients with valvular heart disease) developed in collaboration with the Society of Cardiovascular Anesthesiologists endorsed by the Society for Cardiovascular Angiography and Interventions and the Society of Thoracic Surgeons. *J Am Coll Cardiol* 2006;48(3):e1–148.
12. Fisher DC, Tunick PA, Kronzon I. Large gradient across a partially ligated left atrial appendage. *J Am Soc Echocardiogr* 1998;11(12):1163–5.
13. Katz ES et al. Surgical left atrial appendage ligation is frequently incomplete: A transesophageal echocardiograhic study. *J Am Coll Cardiol* 2000;36(2):468–71.
14. Rosenzweig BP et al. Thromboembolus from a ligated left atrial appendage. *J Am Soc Echocardiogr* 2001;14(5):396–8.
15. DiSesa VJ, Tam S, Cohn LH. Ligation of the left atrial appendage using an automatic surgical stapler. *Ann Thorac Surg* 1988;46(6):652–3.
16. Odell JA et al. Thoracoscopic obliteration of the left atrial appendage: Potential for stroke reduction? *Ann Thorac Surg* 1996;61(2):565–9.
17. Kanderian AS et al. Success of surgical left atrial appendage closure: Assessment by transesophageal echocardiography. *J Am Coll Cardiol* 2008;52(11):924–9.
18. Roscoe A. Left atrial appendage closure for the prevention of stroke. Abstract 2005.
19. Healey JS et al. Left atrial appendage occlusion study (LAAOS): Results of a randomized controlled pilot study of left atrial appendage occlusion during coronary bypass surgery in patients at risk for stroke. *Am Heart J* 2005;150(2):288–93.
20. Johnson WD et al. The left atrial appendage: Our most lethal human attachment! Surgical implications. *Eur J Cardiothorac Surg* 2000;17(6):718–22.
21. Blackshear JL et al. Thoracoscopic extracardiac obliteration of the left atrial appendage for stroke risk reduction in atrial fibrillation. *J Am Coll Cardiol* 2003;42(7):1249–52.
22. Holmes DR et al. Percutaneous closure of the left atrial appendage versus warfarin therapy for prevention of stroke in patients with atrial fibrillation: A randomised non-inferiority trial. *Lancet* 2009;374(9689): 534–42.
23. Lee RJ, Bartus, K, Yakubov SJ. Catheter-based left atrial appendage (LAA) ligation for the prevention of embolic events arising from the LAA: Initial experience in a canine model. *Circul Cardiovasc Interv* 2010;3(3):224–9.
24. Bartus K et al. Feasibility of closed-chest ligation of the left atrial appendage in humans. *Heart Rhythm* 2011;8(2):188–93.
25. Bartus K, Han FT, Bednarek J, Myc J, Kapelak B, Sadowski J, Lelakowski J, Bartus S, Yakubov SJ, Lee RJ. Percutaneous left atrial appendage suture ligation using the LARIAT device in patients with atrial fibrillation: Initial clinical experience. *J Am Coll Cardiol* 2013;62(2):108–18.

99

Other new endocardial and epicardial techniques

Annkathrin Braut, Jennifer Franke, Stefan Bertog, and Horst Sievert

Introduction

Atrial fibrillation is one of the leading causes of stroke in elderly patients. Over 90% of left atrial thrombi are located in the left atrial appendage (LAA). So far, oral anticoagulation has been the standard therapy, but over the past few years LAA occlusion has proven to be a viable alternative to long-term oral anticoagulation for stroke prevention in patients with atrial fibrillation. Closure of the LAA can be performed either endocardially, requiring transseptal puncture, or epicardially via pericardial access. The range of available devices is under continuous development. While some have already made it into clinical practice, a number of devices are still in the preclinical phase.

New endocardial techniques

The majority of devices for LAA closure are delivered via the endocardial approach.

pfm™

The endocardial device for LAA closure by pfm medical is made of a nitinol wire mesh and consists of three main parts: an anchor to grab the LAA tissue, a flexible middle part of variable length to adjust to the LAA anatomy, and an occluder disk to ensure sealing of the LAA orifice, as seen in Figure 99.1. The device is delivered through a 8 or 9 French sheath.

Feasibility and efficacy have been tested in a canine model. The implant was performed under general anesthesia and fluoroscopy as well as ICE or TEE guidance. A Baylis RF perforation of the atrial septum was performed. Heparin was administered during the procedure. After device implantation, ASA was given to all subjects.

One, three, or six months after the procedure, ICE and subsequent cardiac harvest were performed to assess closure rate and the endothelialization process. Thirty-nine dogs were treated and a total number of 48 devices were used as two or three devices were required in seven

animals. For the last 13 cases, an improved self-centering design of the device was used. The results for the last 13 specimens are shown in Table 99.1.

In two cases, the device embolized but could be successfully retrieved via an 8 French sheath. Femoral hematoma occurred in four cases; one of the dogs died 24 h after the procedure due to continuous bleeding. After the sixth case, the long 8 Fr delivery sheath was advanced through a short 10 Fr sheath and no more access site bleeding

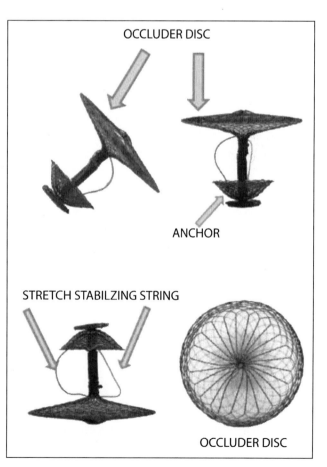

Figure 99.1 A construction sketch of the pfm medical LAA closure device.

Table 99.1   Results for the last 13 specimen of the pfm canine model

Complete closure	7
Small residual leak	4
Large residual leak	2

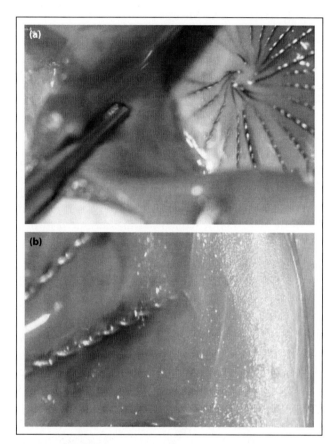

Figures 99.2 **(See color insert.)** (a,b) Cardiac harvest after 1 month revealed good endothelialization using the endocardial device for LAA closure.

complications occurred thereafter. There was one case of an aortic perforation due to the transseptal puncture without sequelae. Transient atrial flutter during the procedure occurred in one case.

There were no device-related deaths and no pericardial effusions during the procedure. In follow-up, there were no cases of late death, arrhythmia, effusion and embolization, or device-associated thrombus formation. The device proved to be adjustable to the LAA length and the occlusion disk adjusted well to the LAA wall in most cases. The embolization rate was low and device retrieval could be performed without difficulty. No stretching or distending of the LAA due to the device was noted and there was no case of LAA perforation or compression of the circumflex artery. Cardiac harvest after 1 month revealed good endothelialization (see Figure 99.2a and b).

Occlutech™

Another new endocardial LAA closure device currently under development is designed by Occlutech. The main body of the device consists of a self-expanding, flexible nitinol wire mesh with loops instead of barbs for fixation in the LAA to reduce the risk of perforation. The included PET patch is covered in a special coating to ensure quick endothelialization and lower the risk of thrombus formation on the device (for device design, see Figure 99.3). The connector between the device and the delivery cable is designed to be extra flexible—its ball-like shape (see Figure 99.4) allows a maximum angle of 45° between device and delivery cable without applying stress or tension on the device.

The device will be available in seven sizes (for details, see Table 99.2) and can be delivered through a 12 French delivery sheath in single- or double-curve design.

The first *in vitro* examination of the device demonstrates a good fixation and adaption to the tissue as seen in Figure 99.5a and b as well as no LAA perforation. Animal studies are planned to further evaluate its safety.

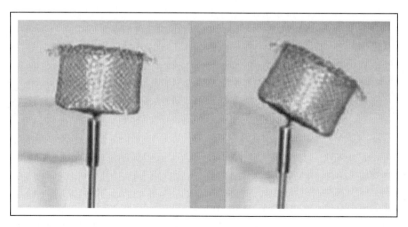

Figure 99.3   Design of the Occlutech device.

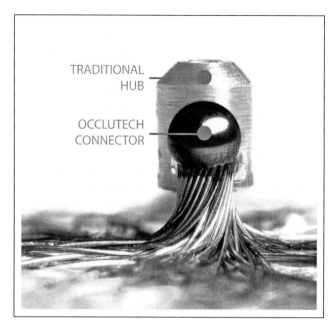

Figure 99.4   Ball-like shape of the Occlutech™ connector between device and delivery cable.

Table 99.2   Available device sizes for the Occlutech™ device
15 mm
18 mm
21 mm
24 mm
27 mm
30 mm
33 mm

Lifetech™

The endocardial closure device by Lifetech also consists of a coated nitinol wire mesh with a PET membrane inside the occlusion disk. The distal anchors have small barbs to hook into the LAA tissue for fixation and the tips of the anchors are rounded to lower the risk of perforation. For details, see Figure 99.6. The barbs are able to fold inward and, therefore, allow multiple device retrievals and repositioning if necessary to ensure complete coverage of the LAA ostium. The device is delivered through 7–10 French delivery sheaths.

The device was evaluated in a canine model from June 2011 to August 2012 and 24 dogs underwent LAA closure. All procedures were successful. Evaluation with echo was performed immediately after closure, after 3 days, and prior to cardiac harvest. Cardiac harvest was performed 1–3 days, post procedure and after 1, 3, or 6 months. Complete LAA closure was achieved in 16 dogs.

The first human implantations were performed in October and November 2012.

New epicardial techniques

AEGIS™

One of the novel epicardial techniques is the AEGIS system. It consists of two parts. One is the appendage grasper—a small forceps with special electrodes for ECG recordings. An ECG recording helps monitor the forceps location and facilitates navigation. Once in a suitable position, the forceps can capture the appendage tissue. For details, see Figure 99.7. The second part of the system is the ligator or hollow suture (see Figure 99.8). The system is preloaded with a 0.012 inch support wire to provide mechanical support and allow fluoroscopic visualization. The suture can then be tightened to close the LAA. If the occlusion result

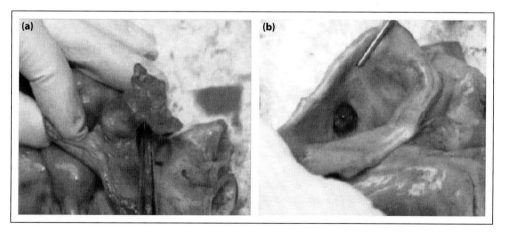

Figure 99.5   **(See color insert.)** (a,b) The first in vitro examination of the Occlutech™ device demonstrates a good fixation and adaption to the tissue.

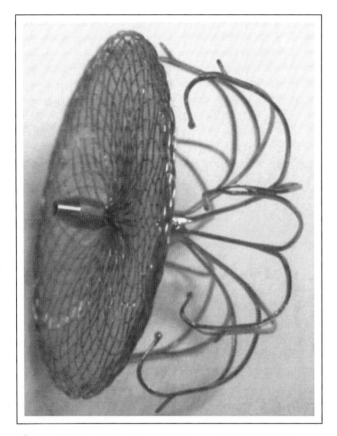

Figure 99.6 The endocardial closure device by Lifetech.

is not satisfactory, or in case complex anatomy is encountered, the first suture can be used as a guide for the application of more proximal sutures.

So far, this procedure was performed in four dogs. There was successful navigation, identification, and LAA capture

in all cases, as well as complete and secure closure of the LAA. Left lateral thoracotomy was performed in two cases to confirm the ligation (Figure 99.9). Unfortunately, there are no details available about the current status on human implantations or trials.

AtriCure™

Another device design for epicardial LAA occlusion is the AtriClip system by AtriCure. Its main component is a self-closing clip with two nitinol springs, two titanium tubes, and two polycarbonate elastomers covered with a polyester mesh. The clip is designed to apply uniform pressure over the entire length of the two branches and the polyester mesh serves as a matrix for epithelial tissue growth. The clip is available in four sizes ranging from 35 to 50 mm and a small thoracotomy has to be performed to place it around the LAA. The clip was evaluated in a trial in which 71 patients were enrolled. Seventy patients underwent cardiac surgery and concomitant clip placement and also bipolar radiofrequency pulmonary vein isolation was performed. In one patient, the LAA was too small for clip placement. During the procedure, the successful occlusion of the left atrial appendage was confirmed by TEE in 95.7% of the patients. Figure 99.10 shows the clip right after placement and on a CT scan.

There was no clip replacement necessary during surgery and also no device- or procedure-related complications. At the 3 month follow-up of 60 patients, the successful closure rate was 98.4% and no TIA or stroke occurred.[1]

Conclusion

Though high rates of technical success have been demonstrated with currently available left atrial appendage closure

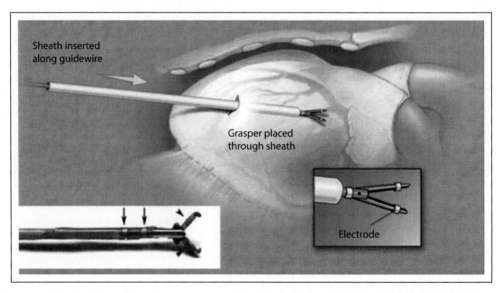

Figure 99.7 (**See color insert.**) The AEGIS system.

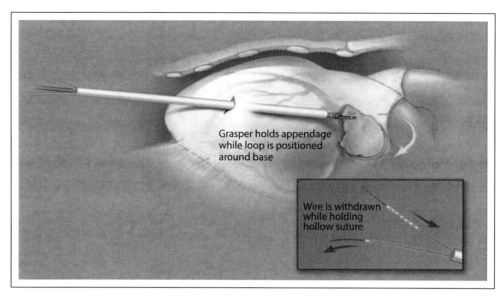

Figure 99.8 (**See color insert.**) The second part of the AEGIS system, the ligator or hollow suture.

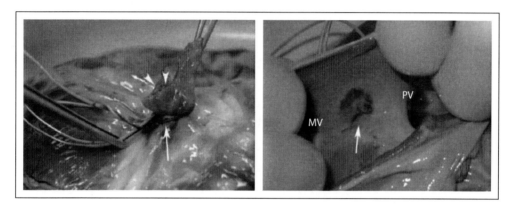

Figure 99.9 (**See color insert.**) Thoracotomy findings after LAA closure with the hollow suture.

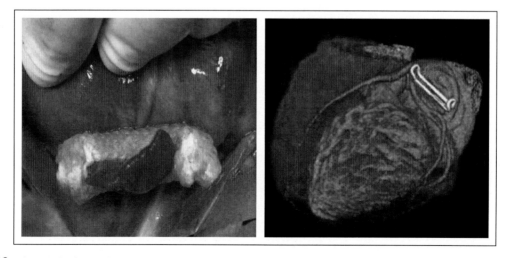

Figure 99.10 (**See color insert.**) The AtriClip system right after placement and on a CT scan.

devices and one device has been shown to be noninferior to anticoagulation with warfarin, further technological improvements can be made, particularly to facilitate reliable device delivery and assure optimal positioning minimizing the risk of appendage injury, thrombus formation, and incomplete closure. This has stimulated ongoing rapid developments with promising new concepts for left atrial appendage closure. Many new devices are undergoing preclinical and first human trials. Further data will clarify the merits of these novel technologies.

Reference

1. Ailawadi G, Gerdisch MW, Harvey RL, Hooker RL, Damiano RJ Jr, Salamon T et al. Exclusion of the left atrial appendage with a novel device: Early results of a multicenter trial. *J Thorac Cardiovasc Surg* 2011;142(5):1002–9, 1009.e1.

100

Extracorporeal ventricular assist devices

Johannes Wilde and Gerhard C. Schuler

An introducing case

A 22-year-old athletic man is admitted to the coronary care unit with chest pain on inspiration and progressive dyspnea and orthopnea. On examination, he is tachycardiac, hypotensive, tachypneic, and has loud rales, elevated jugular venous pressure, and peripheral edema.

Along with unspecific T-wave inversions in the electrocardiogram, echocardiography reveals a dilated left ventricle with severely reduced contractility. The diagnosis of acute viral myocarditis is confirmed by magnetic resonance imaging and myocardial biopsies. Laboratory findings include elevation of troponine, b-type natriuretic peptide, transaminases, and lactate levels in the arterial blood gas. In cardiogenic shock, he is admitted to the intensive care unit and started on diuretic and catecholamine treatment.

After a few hours of treatment, lactate levels are still high and hemodynamics as well as respiratory function have not improved. Invasive hemodynamic monitoring reveals a high pulmonary wedge pressure (32 mmHg), a low cardiac index of 1.2 L/kg/min and a very high systemic resistance coinciding with a mean arterial pressure of 55 mmHg despite high levels of catecholamine dosing and fluid supplementation.

The decision is made to use a mechanical assist device to stabilize the patient's circulation and hopefully restore organ function. An extracorporeal membrane oxygenation (ECMO) device is implanted. Within 1 h of ECMO therapy, the patient's state of consciousness improves. Lactate levels are falling and normalizing within 6 h. In addition, respiratory function improves such that mechanical ventilation is no longer required and renal function likewise improves. Rapid weaning of catecholamine therapy becomes possible. Four days later, the ECMO device can be weaned and explanted; the patient is discharged to ambulant care at day 27 with stable cardiopulmonary function and a normalized left ventricular contractility.

Therapeutic options in cardiogenic shock

Acute heart failure and development of cardiogenic shock represent entities of cardiac disease with persistent high mortality and a difficult approach of medical therapy.[1,2] The only sufficient and prognostic relevant intervention is to overcome the etiological cause of cardiogenic shock as soon as possible—if at all possible, for example, by percutaneous interventional revascularization in acute myocardial infarction or by cardiothoracic surgery in severe acute mitral regurgitation.[3]

Most of the possible medical interventions addressing the symptoms of shock and aiming to maintain a sufficient circulatory support will either not effect or even enhance the vicious circle of shock progression by promoting various cascades of inflammation and vasomotor dysregulation instead of stabilizing patient's hemodynamics.[4,5]

Furthermore, a number of underlying causes cannot be overcome by a single intervention and the main therapeutic goal is to gain time for myocardial recovery or otherwise for transplant evaluation.

With that purpose, a number of surgically or percutaneous implantable cardiac assist devices have been established to relieve either one ventricle or the heart in total from the burden of increased pre- and afterload coinciding with a decreased contractility and an increased myocardial oxygen demand, either following acute ischemia or due to acute myocarditis and decompensated dilatory heart disease.

In contrast to surgically implantable devices merely designed for mid- to long-term therapy in acute or chronic heart failure (bridge-to-transplant or destination therapy), percutaneous assist devices aim to stabilize the patient within a few hours. Usually, the hemodynamic support needs to be continued for several days allowing a bridge-to-recovery or a bridge-to-transplant strategy according to an underlying disease. A strategy of using a surgically implantable assist device for long-term support after stabilizing and evaluating a patient on a percutaneous assist device might be considered in selected cases.

Any cardiac assist device is employed to recover sufficient cardiac output, facilitate ventricular unloading, and reduce pulmonary congestion. In an acute setting, a percutaneous assist device is preferable because of a rather simple implantation procedure to be carried out in the catheter lab with low complication rates leading to an immediate and effective restoration of circulation and organ perfusion to gain time for recovery or decision making, especially in cases with unclear neurological outcome (e.g., after cardiopulmonary resuscitation). Easy handling and the prevention of common adverse effects as critical limb ischemia, bleeding complications, or hemolysis are important criteria of choice.

The veno-arterial ECMO represents a percutaneous extracorporeal total cardiopulmonary bypass involving an oxygenator to replace lung function in critical illness. The percutaneous left ventricular (LV) assist devices TandemHeart™ and Impella are intended for effective univentricular unloading, affecting gas exchange by tapering the congestion. All three devices provide a continuous flow. In contrast, the principle of intra-aortic counterpulsation generated by the intra-aortic balloon pump (IABP) facilitates a shift of intra-aortic pressure curves to a higher mean arterial pressure and a significant reduction of ventricular afterload. By this method, small augmentation of cardiac output is achieved.[6]

Veno-arterial ECMO: A total cardiopulmonary bypass

The ECMO device provides the highest degree of circulatory support among the percutaneous cardiac assist devices due to its ability to exercise a proposed volume of up to 6 L/min (depending on cannula size). The device features a centrifugal pump and a gas exchange membrane having been miniaturized remarkably to allow for transport purposes between hospitals as well as for stationary care on an intensive care unit. Two systems currently represent this last generation of ECMO or extracorporeal lifesupport (c): Lifebridge® (Lifebridge Medizintechnik AG, Ampfing, Germany) and CardioHelp® (Maquet GmbH und Co. KG, Rastatt, Germany).

An extra-long inflow cannula placed into the right atrium ranges from 18 to 31 French though a 21 French cannula will be effective in most cases. The diameter of arterial outflow cannula positioned into the descending aorta via femoral artery is limited by the peripheral vascular status and can be chosen between 15 and 22 French. The arterial outflow cannula is the flow-limiting module within the cardiopulmonary bypass. The diameter should be chosen as wide as possible but small enough to avoid critical vascular complications.

The implantation procedure consists of an arterial and a venous femoral puncture in Seldinger technique—either ipsilateral or contralateral. Alternatively, the venous access can be taken by cannulating the internal jugular vein; a

surgical approach utilizes arterial access to the axillary artery conducting a more efficient coronary and cerebral perfusion. The positioning of the venous cannula can be monitored by transesophageal echocardiography or with less time and effort on fluoroscopy, according to the local setting. After insertion, both cannulae are connected to the crystalloid-primed, air-evacuated bypass system implementing the circuit subsequently.

The use of an antegrade 6 French metal-reinforced bypass sheath to the superficial femoral artery can overcome the problem of critical limb ischemia almost completely (Figures 100.1 and 100.2).

Another common adverse effect of ECMO therapy is the risk of bleeding and hemolysis. The large intraluminal surface of the extracorporeal circulation provokes a pronounced

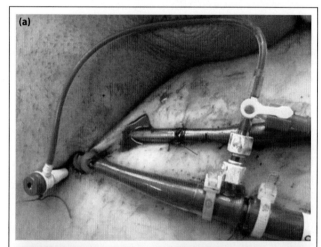

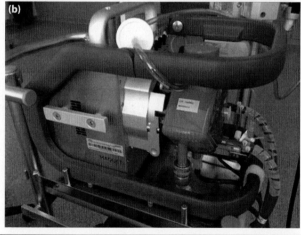

Figure 100.1 **(See color insert.)** (a) Puncture site of a femoro-femoral ECMO device in the right groin from medial to lateral: venous inflow cannula in the common femoral vein, arterial outflow cannula in the common femoral artery, antegrade access sheath in the superficial femoral artery for distal perfusion oft the right leg supplied by a little bypass from the arterial ECMO outflow cannula. (b) CardioHelp core unit with the centrifugal pump and the red-colored gas exchange membrane (Courtesy of Maquet GmbH und Co. KG, Rastatt, Germany).

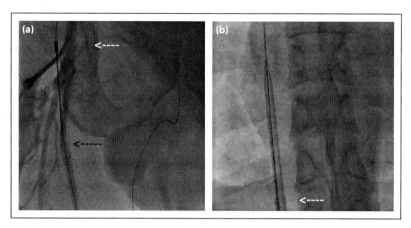

Figure 100.2   (a) A contrast radiography of the right-femoral ECMO puncture site: venous access sheath to the common femoral vein (medial) and arterial access sheath to the common femoral artery (lateral) as indicated by the white arrow. Puncture of the superficial femoral artery with a needle and wired in distal direction for introduction of the 6 French metal-reinforced access sheath for antegrade perfusion of the right leg (black arrow). Incidentally, the image displays a urinary catheter containing a temperature probe. (b) Venous ECMO inflow cannula introduced into the right atrium mounted on a dilatator. The arrow indicates the position of the radiodense end of the cannula after removal of the dilatator at the outlet of inferior caval vein to acknowledge the nonvisible inflow tract of the cannula within the right atrium.

activation of coagulation and complement system within the first 2 h of treatment, leading to a remarkable consumption of coagulation factors such as factors X–XIII, V, VII, prekallikrein, antithrombin III, protein C/S, plasminogen, and platelets. Complement activation triggers hemolysis and severe inflammatory response syndrome.[7,8] To suppress hypercoagulation and activation of the downstream complement cascades, it is recommended to maintain an activated clotting time of 180 s or more. Nevertheless, it remains a difficult balance to avoid both thrombus formation within the bypass modules and severe bleeding, respectively.

Current innovation provides different coatings of the intraluminal bypass layer (e.g., heparin–albumin coating, phosphorylcholine, polymers) to increase hemocompatibility of the extracorporeal bypass material and to attenuate the activation of complement and coagulation components, thereby allowing to reduce systemic heparin doses administered with up to 30 days of continuous ECMO.[7]

Frequent monitoring and substitution of platelet levels, antithrombin III, fibrinogen, and hemoglobin/hematocrit are recommended. Well-trained nursing and medical personnel are required to observe and handle ECMO therapy with all its intricacy and potential side effects. It has to be stated that veno-arterial ECMO is not a contraindication to prone positioning in severe pulmonary comorbidity with competent and experienced staff.

TandemHeart: A percutaneous extracorporeal left ventricular assist device

The TandemHeart system (CardiacAssist, Pittsburgh, PA, USA) provides powerful augmentation of LV output

up to 4 or 5 L/min almost competing with ECMO device (Figure 100.3). The principle of cardiac assistance differs considerably as TandemHeart is a true LV-assist device creating a bypass between the left atrium and the descending aorta. The implantation procedure requires advanced expertise and takes longer since a transseptal puncture and

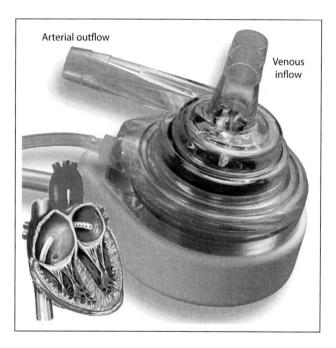

Arterial outflow

Venous inflow

Figure 100.3   (See color insert.) The centrifugal pump of the TandemHeart system. The venous inflow tract of the pump is connected to the venous inflow cannula, which is introduced into the left atrium after transseptal puncture. (Figure modified after CardiacAssist Inc., Pittsburgh, Pennsylvania, USA.)

dilatation of the interatrial septum are necessary to promote a 21 French inflow cannula of 62 or 72 cm of length for left atrial drainage. The outflow cannula is placed into the descending aorta via the common femoral artery using 15 or 17 French devices according to constitution and vascular state allowing a flow of 4 or 5 L/min, respectively. Inflow and outflow cannula are connected to a centrifugal pump after evacuation of any air within the circuit. An alternative strategy to use the TandemHeart device as a right ventricular assist device can be achieved by positioning the inflow cannula into the right atrium and a long outflow cannula into the main pulmonary artery.[9,10]

Although the FDA approval suggests use up to 6 h only; the TandemHeart device has been successfully used for more than 1 week. Adverse effects comprise critical limb ischemia and thrombus formation, especially along the inflow cannula in the left atrium. Effective anticoagulation by continuous heparin treatment is therefore recommended. Hemolysis and coagulation cascade activation appears to be a pressing but less of a problem in TandemHeart as compared to ECMO.

Impella: A percutaneous catheter-based left ventricular assist device

The active percutaneous LV-assist device Impella (Abiomed, Danvers, MA, USA) requires a single arterial access to the femoral or brachial artery to insert the catheter-mounted 12 French Impella 2.5 or the 14 French Impella CP™ pump system. The terminal pigtail catheter unit is introduced into the left ventricle across the aortic valve along with the small inlet area. A micro-axial pump with a rotational performance of 50,000 rounds per minute aspirates blood from the left ventricle and ejects via an outlet area lying in the ascending aorta. Flow capacity is up to 2.5 L/min with Impella 2.5 and 4 L/min with Impella CP. A surgically implantable 5 L/min version requiring femoral or axillary cutdown is also available (Figure 100.4).

IABP: The concept of intra-aortic counterpulsation

The intra-aortic counterpulsation by a 9.5 French intra-ortic ballon pump (IABP) has been considered as a first-line mechanical assistance in profound cardiac shock for many years. This does not constitute a true ventricular assist device since it does not contribute significantly to cardiac output. The concept of IABP refers to an early-diastolic augmentation by inflating the helium balloon, thereby raising mean arterial blood pressure and improving coronary and cerebral

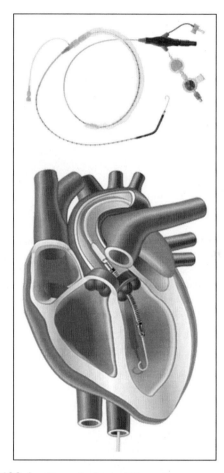

Figure 100.4 **(See color insert.)** The catheter-mounted Impella 2.5 device placed in the left ventricle across the aortic valve. (Figure modified after Abiomed Inc., Danvers, Massachusetts, USA.)

perfusion, and to a decrease of end-diastolic aortic pressure by rapid balloon deflation. The achieved intra-aortic volume reduction by 40 mL immediately at the beginning of systole results in a marked reduction of ventricular afterload. Consequently, stroke volume increases and the isovolumetric contractility phase shortens and ventricular systolic pressure, ventricular preload, and myocardial oxygen consumption are reduced.[6] Fiber-optic intra-aortic pressure sensing and real-time detection of the electrocardiogram ensure synchronization with the cardiac cycle (Figure 100.5).

Evidence and choice of device

However favorable the IABP concept appears, registry data supporting the use of IABP in cardiogenic shock complicating myocardial infarction, stem from the era before routine early percutaneous coronary intervention (PCI).[11] A meta-analysis from 2009 observed a higher mortality in patients treated with IABP in cardiogenic shock after primary PCI.[12] Similarly, the IABP-SHOCK-II trial published

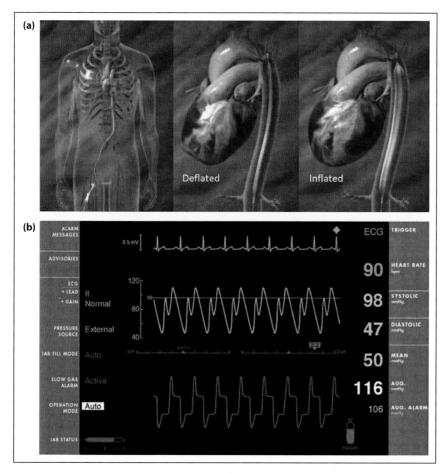

Figure 100.5 (**See color insert.**) (a) Position of the IABP device within the descending aorta. (b) Early-diastolic augmentation (116 mmHg) on balloon inflation immediately following the systolic peak (98 mmHg) before rapid balloon deflation facilitates a decrease of end-diastolic aortic pressure (47 mmHg). (Figure modified after Maquet GmbH und Co. KG, Rastatt, Germany.)

in 2012 did not show any benefit for IABP support in cardiogenic shock complicating myocardial infarction after early revascularization with respect to 30 day mortality.[2] Since patients with mechanical complications of myocardial infarction such as ventricular septal defect or papillary muscle rupture had not been included in the trial hemodynamic considerations, a small case series may still suggest a benefit for short-term IABP bridging in this particular subgroup of patients.[13]

ECMO, TandemHeart, and Impella generate active flow and sufficiently restore cardiac output to establish superior hemodynamic parameters compared to IABP.[14–19] As yet, no mortality effects have been demonstrated other than observational data suggesting lower mortality rates with TandemHeart or ECMO than estimated.[20–23]

The only contraindication to all four percutaneous assist devices is severe aortic regurgitation. Peripheral occlusive artery disease or bleeding disorders remain relative contraindications in certain conditions.

According to the literature, mortality approaches 50% in cardiogenic shock treated with fluids and inotropics/vasopressors without any mechanical assistance.[1,2] Active hemodynamic support by a percutaneous assist device offers some benefit to the cohort with a fatal outcome. There is also potential harm to the cohort with a favorable outcome by bleeding or ischemic complications.[24] Therefore, mechanical assistance is not generally recommended as a first-line therapy in cardiogenic shock, but should be considered in refractory circulatory insufficiency characterized by a growing need for vasopressors, persistently elevated or even rising lactate levels, renal dysfunction, and progressive multiorgan dysfunction.[25,26] Precise scoring systems and algorithms to stratify the individual patient's risk and to determine a time schedule of treatment are lacking. It is therefore important to revise the therapy response every few hours and escalate the hemodynamic support to a mechanical component where necessary.[23] Goals for therapy are a mean arterial pressure of at least 60 mmHg and a mixed venous oxygen saturation of 70%. To reach those, biventricular dysfunction or severe pulmonary comorbidity would possibly favor ECMO therapy, while TandemHeart and Impella can be an option in acute univentricular dysfunction.[27] Extended indications for percutaneous mechanical cardiac assistance refer to patient's transfer between hospitals, postcardiotomy shock, or elective high-risk percutaneous interventions.[28,29]

References

1. Goldberg RJ, Spencer FA, Gore JM et al. Thirty-year trends (1975–2005) in the magnitude of, management of, and hospital death rates associated with cardiogenic shock in patients with acute myocardial infarction: A population-based perspective. *Circulation* 2009;119(9):1211–9.

2. Thiele H, Zeymer U, Neumann FJ et al. Intraaortic balloon support for myocardial infarction with cardiogenic shock. *N Engl J Med* 2012;367(14):1287–96.

3. Hochman JS, Sleeper LA, White HD et al. One-year survival following early revascularization for cardiogenic shock. *JAMA* 2001;285:190–2.

4. Reynolds HR, Hochman JS. Cardiogenic shock: Current concepts and improving outcomes. *Circulation* 2008;294:448–54.

5. Samuels LE, Kaufman MS, Thomas MP et al. Pharmacological criteria for ventricular assist device insertion following postcardiotomy shock: Experience with the Abiomed BVS system. *J Card Surg* 1999;14:288–93.

6. Weber KT, Janicki JS. Intraaortic balloon counterpulsation. A review of physiological principles, clinical results, and device safety. *Ann Thorac Surg* 1974;17(6):602–36.

7. McILwain B, Timpa J, Kurundkar AR et al. Plasma concentrations of inflammatory cytokines rise rapidly during ECMO-related SIRS due to the release of pre-formed stores in the intestine. *LabInvest* 2010;90(1):128–39.

8. Urlesberger B, Zobel G, Rödl S et al. Activation of the clotting system: Heparin-coated versus non coated systems for extracorporeal circulation. *Int J Artif Organs* 1997;20(12):708–12.

9. Prutkin JM, Strote JA, Stout KK. Percutaneous right ventricular assist device as support for cardiogenic shock due to right ventricular infarction. *J Invasive Cardiol* 2008;20(7):E215–E216.

10. Kiernan MS, Krishnamurthy B, Kapur NK. Percutaneous right ventricular assist via the internal jugular vein in cardiogenic shock complicating an acute inferior myocardial infarction. *J Invasive Cardiol* 2010;22(2):E23–E26.

11. Sanborn TA, Sleeper LA, Bates ER et al. Impact of thrombolysis, intra-aortic balloon pump counter-pulsation, and their combination in cardiogenic shock complicating acute myocardial infarction: A report from the SHOCK trial registry. Should we emergently vascularize occluded coronaries for cardiogenic shock? *J Am Coll Cardiol* 2000;36(3 Suppl A):1123–9.

12. Sjauw KD, Engstrom AE, Vis MM et al. A systematic review and meta-analysis of intra-aortic balloon pump therapy in ST-elevation myocardial infarction: Should we change the guidelines? *Eur Heart J* 2009;30(4):459–68.

13. Thiele H, Lauer B, Hambrecht R et al. Short- and long-term hemodynamic effects of intra-aortic balloon support in ventricular septal defect complicating acute myocardial infarction. *Am J Cardiol* 2003;92(4):450–4.

14. Thiele H, Sick P, Boudriot E et al. Randomized comparison of intra-aortic balloon support with a percutaneous left ventricular assist device in patients with revascularized acute myocardial infarction complicated by cardiogenic shock. *Eur Heart J* 2005;26(13):1276–83.

15. Burkhoff D, Cohen H, Brunckhorst C et al. A randomized multicenter clinical study to evaluate the safety and efficacy of the TandemHeart percutaneous ventricular assist device versus conventional therapy with intraaortic balloon pumping for treatment of cardiogenic shock. *Am Heart J* 2006;152(3):469–8.

16. Seyfarth M, Sibbing D, Bauer I et al. A randomized clinical trial to evaluate the safety and efficacy of a percutaneous left ventricular assist device versus intra-aortic balloon pumping for treatment of cardiogenic shock caused by myocardial infarction. *J Am Coll Cardiol* 2008;52(19):1584–8.

17. Manzo-Silberman S, Fichet J, Mathonnet A et al. Percutaneous left ventricular assistance in post cardiac arrest shock: Comparison of intra aortic blood pump and Impella Recover LP2.5. *Resuscitation* 2013;84(5):609–15.

18. Thiele H, Lauer B, Hambrecht R et al. Reversal of cardiogenic shock by percutaneous left atrial-to-femoral arterial bypass assistance. *Circulation* 2001;104:2917–22.

19. Valgimigli M, Steendijk P, Serruys P et al. Use of Impella Recover LP 2.5 left ventricular assist device during high-risk percutaneous coronary interventions: Clinical, haemodynamic and biochemical findings. *EuroIntervention* 2006;2:91–100.

20. Kar B, Gregoric ID, Basra SS et al. The percutaneous ventricular assist device in severe refractory cardiogenic shock. *J Am Coll Cardiol* 2011;57(6):688–96.

21. Tsao NW, Shih CM, Yeh JS et al. Extracorporeal membrane oxygenation-assisted primary percutaneous intervention may improve survival of patients with acute myocardial infarction complicated by profound cardiogenic shock. *J Crit Care* 2012;27(5):530.e1–11.

22. Sakamoto S, Taniguchi N, Nakajima S et al. Extracorporeal life support for cardiogenic shock or cardiac arrest due to acute coronary syndrome. *Ann Thorac Surg* 2012;94:1–7.

23. Sheu JJ, Tsai TH, Lee FJ et al. Early extracorporeal membrane oxygenator-assisted primary percutaneous intervention improved 30-day clinical outcomes in patients with ST-segment elevation myocardial infarction complicated with profound cardiogenic shock. *Crit Care Med* 2010;38:1810–7.

24. Cheng JM, den Uil CA, Hoeks SE et al. Percutaneous left ventricular assist devices vs. intra-aortic balloon pump counterpulsation for treatment of cardiogenic shock: A meta-analysis of controlled trials. *Eur Heart J* 2009;30(17):2102–8.

25. O'Gara PT, Kushner FG, Ascheim DD, et al. 2013 ACCF/AHA guideline for the management of ST-elevation myocardial infarction: A report of the American College of Cardiology Foundation/American Heart Association Task Force on Practice Guidelines. *J Am Coll Cardiol* 2013;61(4):e78–140.

26. Steg PG, James SK, Atar D et al. ESC Guidelines for the management of acute myocardial infarction in patients presenting with ST-segment elevation. *Eur Heart J* 2012;33(20):2569–619.

27. Lamarche Y, Cheung A, Ignaszewski A, et al. Comparative outcomes in cardiogenic shock patients managed with Impella microaxial pump or extracorporeal life support. *J Thorac Cardiovasc Surg* 2011;142(1):60–5.

28. Jaroszewski DE, Kleisli T, Staley L et al. A traveling team concept to expedite the transfer and management of unstable patients in cardiopulmonary shock. *J Heart Lung Transplant* 2011;30(6):618–23.

29. Beurtheret S, Mordant P, Paoletti X et al. Emergency circulatory support in refractory cardiogenic shock patients in remote institutions: A pilot study (the cardiac-RESCUE program). *Eur Heart J* 2013;34(2):112–20.

101

Left ventricular partitioning with the cardiokinetics device

I. Bozdag-Turan, S. Kische, R. Goekmen Turan, C. A. Nienaber, and H. Ince

Introduction

In this chapter, we summarize a novel percutaneous ventricular restoration therapy (PVRT) to treat patients with left ventricular dysfunction and anteroapical regional wall motion abnormalities after a myocardial infarction (MI). Heart failure is a common, disabling, and lethal disorder carrying a heavy socioeconomic burden. Its prevalence in industrialized nations has reached epidemic levels and continues to rise. Despite advances over the past 30 years, the prognosis for patients admitted to hospitals with heart failure remains poor, with a 5 year mortality that is nearly 50% worse than that for patients with breast and colon cancer.[1,2]

Coronary artery disease is the leading cause of death in men and women today, causing >425,000 deaths annually, and it is estimated that 785,000 people will have an acute myocardial infarction (AMI) in the next 12 months. Cardiac performance after MI is compromised by ventricular remodeling, which represents a major cause of late infarct-related chronic heart failure and death.[2,3] Although conventional drug therapy may delay remodeling, there is no basic therapeutic regimen available for preventing or even reversing this process. By the use of interventional therapeutics, recanalization of the occluded infarct-related artery is possible, thereby improving or normalizing coronary blood flow. However, despite adequate reperfusion of infarcted tissue, the viability of the infarcted myocardium cannot, or can inadequately improve in most of these patients, especially when a left ventricular anteroapical aneurysm is present.

The ventricular partitioning device (VPD) (Cardiokinetix, Menlo Park, CA, USA) is a new medical device, which is deployed in the left ventricle (LV) of patients with anteroapical regional wall motion abnormalities following an MI to partition the ventricle and segregate the dysfunctional region. The VPD implant is delivered percutaneously from the femoral artery using standard techniques for left heart catheterization. It is hypothesized that the VPD will reduce LV volumes, decrease myocardial wall stress and, hence, improve LV hemodynamics.

Ventricular partitioning device

Device description and function

A catheter-mediated intraventricular implant (VPD) has been developed (Cardiokinetix) to partition the LV cavity for the treatment of patients with regional wall motion abnormalities, which are associated with post-left anterior descending (LAD) coronary artery infarction, dilated left ventricle, and systolic dysfunction. The VPD, also known as the Parachute™ device, is a partitioning membrane deployed within the aneurysmal LV. This novel device partitions an enlarged, scarred ventricle into a dynamic and a static chamber. The static chamber is the portion of LV volume, which is distal to the device and is excluded from the circulation. Stresses placed on the partitioned myocardium and the forces previously transmitted to the apical segment are decreased both in diastole and in systole, reducing the forces responsible for LV dilation. In addition to this regional unloading, the reduction in the size of the dynamic chamber results in a decrease in the myocardial stress in the normal myocardium via the Laplace's law, providing a global unloading of the ventricle.

The implantation was performed using local anesthesia. A 14 F sheath was placed using a femoral arterial access. Potentially active coronary ischemia was ruled out by a recent coronary angiography. Preimplantation, right heart catheterization was performed via the left femoral vein revealing a pulmonary artery systolic pressure of 25 mmHg and a mean pulmonary capillary wedge pressure of 5 mmHg.

Mechanism of the Parachute

The Parachute implant partitions the damaged muscle, isolating the nonfunctional muscle segment from the functional segment, which decreases the overall volume.

By reducing the overall volume of the left ventricle with the Parachute, the required pressure to fill the left ventricle is lowered. High filling pressures result in fluid retention in the lungs—pulmonary edema—causing shortness of breath.

When the Parachute partitions the damaged muscle, the functional segment performs better during each heartbeat. The increased performance is due to the viable heart muscle being properly stretched. Prior to the Parachute procedure, the damaged heart wall was being stretched since it had the least amount of resistance, but unfortunately could not contract because the muscle was nonfunctional. Because the Parachute is anchored into the functioning heart muscle, the torsional contraction a normal heart performs during each beat is translated down to the apex through the device. Because the Parachute is anchored into functioning heart muscle, the implant now contracts during each beat, which results in blood being ejected from the apex. Patients who experience heart failure when the heart has remodeled or enlarged, take on a round shape of the LV instead of the natural conical shape. With a round shape and malfunctioning apex, blood will settle in the apex of the heart. When the Parachute is implanted, the apex now has a conical shape and contracts to allow blood to circulate more closely to a normal-functioning left ventricle.[3,4]

Device system components

The system consists of three components: (1) an access system, (2) a delivery system, and (3) the VPD (Figure 101.1a, b, and c). The access system includes a guide catheter (14–16 F) and a dilator, and their purpose is to provide access to the apical region, often the LV. The delivery catheter has a central lumen that provides a channel for the torque shaft, at the distal end of which is a screw that engages the VPD. This catheter is used to deliver the collapsed VPD to the apex of the LV in preparation for its deployment. The inner lumen on the torque shaft provides a channel for inflating and deflating a balloon located just proximal to the engagement screw. When inflated, the balloon is designed to push against the struts of the device, ensuring that the struts engage the tissue of the LV wall. The VPD is composed of a self-expanding nitinol frame, an expanded polytetrafluoroethylene (ePTFE) occlusive membrane, and a distal atraumatic (pebax polymer) foot. The nitinol frame is shaped like an umbrella with 16 struts. The tip of each strut ends in a 2 mm anchor. Upon expansion of the VPD by the delivery catheter balloon, these anchors engage the tissue, stabilize the device, and prevent dislodgment and migration after the device is detached from the delivery

catheter. After the device is expanded, the occlusive membrane provides a barrier to seal off the static chamber on the distal side of the device. The distal atraumatic foot is radiopaque and provides a contact point between the apex of the LV and the VPD. The expanded nominal diameter of the device used in the trial was either 75 or 85 mm. To determine the device size, the cross section of the ventricular chamber was measured 3.5 cm proximal to the apex on the initial ventriculogram. For an apical length of 62 mm and a diameter of 40 mm, we found the 85 mm device to be appropriate (an oversizing of 30–50% for implantation is recommended).[1,2,5]

Case report

We present a patient in whom a Parachute was implanted after being screened according to echocardiographic and 3D cardiac CT parameters and in whom 3 and 6 month follow-up was available. A 68-year-old man with a history of anterior MI and subsequent development of LV anteroapical wall motion abnormalities was admitted in our hospital. He reported dyspnea on heavy exertion. His past surgical history included coronary bypass graft surgery and ICD implantation. Clinically, the patient had refractory class II–III NYHA (New York Heart Association) heart failure despite aggressive medical treatment. ECG showed sinus rhythm and right bundle branch block with deep Q-waves (V1 to V6), elevated ST segments in leads V1 to V4 and terminal T-wave depression. The patient was screened first by echocardiographic criteria: (I) ejection fraction (EF) 40%, (II) LV dilatation (LVEDD >56 mm and LVESD >38 mm), (III) anteroapical regional wall motion abnormalities (akinetic/dyskinetic), and (IV) LV apex diameter (LVAD) = 4.0 × 5.0 cm. Echocardiography revealed a dilated LV (65 mm) with anteroapical wall motion abnormalities, no apical thrombus, and calculated LVEF of 27% (by Simpson biplane formula). End-systolic volume index (ESVI) was 76.8 mL/m². LVAD was 4.5 × 5 cm (Figure 101.1a). A 3D cardiac CT demonstrated appropriate architecture and geometry with trabeculation of the LV (Figure 101.2a). To determine the functional status, we assessed NYHA classification and the standard 6 min walk test by two independent and blinded cardiologists before and 3 months after device implantation. Additionally, testing the change in quality of life was performed using Minnesota Living with Heart Failure Questionnaire. Potential active coronary ischemia was ruled out by coronary angiography.

The implantation was performed under local anesthesia via the right femoral artery. The collapsed implant was attached to the delivery catheter, and advanced retrogradely through the guide catheter across the aortic valve and positioned in the LV apex. Echocardiography was performed to assess appropriate positioning. The device was expanded using compliant balloon dilatation. Control

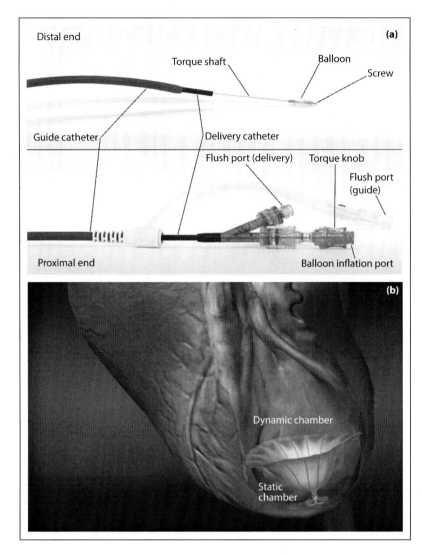

Figure 101.1 (**See color insert.**) (a) Access and delivery system for VPD (description in text). (b) The VPD positioned in the aneurysmal apex of the LV. The device has 16 nitinol struts that insert into the endocardium and is covered by an ePTFE membrane. The VPD partitions the ventricle into dynamic and static chambers.

echocardiography demonstrated that the Parachute was positioned correctly at the apex, with no residual leak between the walls of the LV and the device. LV end-diastolic pressure decreased immediately from 16 to 12 mmHg. The total procedure time was 62 min, and fluoroscopy time 10 min. The postimplantation course was uneventful, and the patient was discharged from the hospital after 2 days. The patient was discharged on aspirin, fosinopril, carvedilol, hydrochlorothiazide, and simvastatin, with the addition of low-dose warfarin (target international normalized ratio of 2.0) for 3 months. There was an increase of global LVEF, and a decrease of LVEDV and LVESV at 3 and 6 months after the Parachute implantation, compared with baseline parameters. Moreover, we found a decrease of NYHA class and NT-ProBNP 3 and 6 months after implantation compared with baseline. Furthermore, a significant improvement of the 6 min walk test and quality of life were observed 3 and 6 months after device implantation compared with baseline.[6] On discharge and 3 months after

the Parachute implantation, repeat echocardiographic and 3D cardiac CT examinations showed that the implant was in good position and there was no leak between the static and dynamic components of the LV chamber (Figures 101.1b and 101.2b). The ECG at rest, on exercise, and 24 h Holter ECG revealed no rhythm disturbances. There was no inflammatory response or myocardial reaction (normal white blood cell count, C-reactive protein [CRP], creatine phosphokinase [CPK]) on discharge, and 3–6 months after the implantation.

In conclusion, the combination of percutaneous LV volume reduction by the Parachute implantation and standard medical therapy may be an important option to consider in the treatment of patients with anteroapical wall motion abnormalities. There is also a need for adequate screening of potential candidates for the Parachute implantation. In this context, specific echocardiographic and 3D cardio CT criteria may serve as tools for a timely selection of candidates[6] (Figure 101.3).

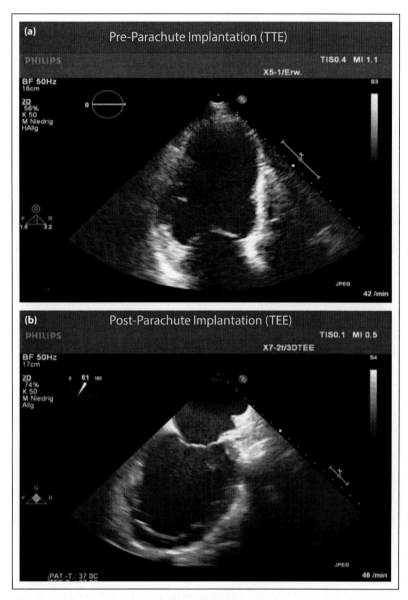

Figure 101.2 (a) LV dilatation with antero-apical wall motion abnormalities in transthoracic echocardiography (pre-Parachute implantation). (b) the Parachute device in two-chamber view on TEE (post-Parachute implantation).

Preclinical and clinical studies

The concept of restoring the LV geometry to improve its contractility has been proposed for many years in the surgical field. Several surgical approaches have been advocated to achieve LV volume reduction. In this context, partial left ventriculectomy (Batista procedure), cardiomyoplasty, and surgical ventricular remodeling (Dor procedure) represent an evolution of the same concept. Recent surgical trials (RESTORE and STICH) have shown that these attempts at reducing the LV volumes in order to improve its function have mixed effects on the functional capacity and the quality of life, and no effects on mortality reduction.[2]

Recently, a more generalized approach to mechanically correct the LV geometry has been proposed with the use of prosthetic devices. The correction can be performed acutely (Myosplint device) or in a slower fashion through a reduction in wall stress and containing further LV dilatation (CorCap Cardiac Support Device). Using these devices, a sustained decrease of LV volumes and improvement of global EF over long-term follow-up has been documented, although in a limited number of patients.

The invasiveness of the existing surgical alternatives and their still unclear clinical benefits have stimulated recent developments of alternative forms of treatment, including totally percutaneous techniques. The Parachute represents a promising modality to treat patients suffering from IHF after anterior/apical infarction. The concept of this device is a surgical one. In fact, placement of a Parachute is aimed at excluding the infarcted dyskinetic area and restoring, from the inside, the LV geometry and function by reducing the intracardiac volume and optimizing the ventricular wall stress.

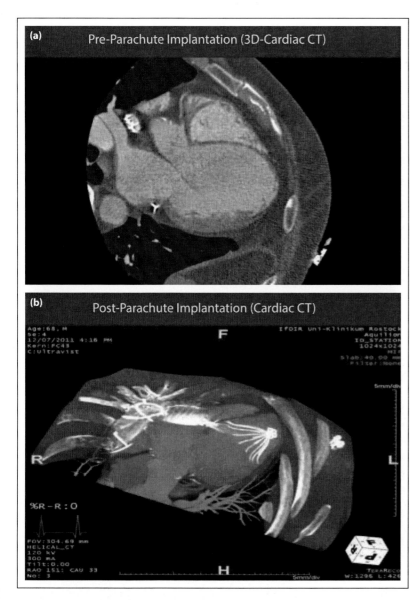

(a) Pre-Parachute Implantation (3D-Cardiac CT)

(b) Post-Parachute Implantation (Cardiac CT)

Figure 101.3 (a) LV dilatation with antero-apical regional wall motion abnormalities (pre-Parachute implantation. (b) Parachute device (post-Parachute implantation) on 3D cardiac CT.

Preclinical studies in an animal model of MI have indicated that the VPD implant has beneficial short- and medium-term effects on LV function, as measured by a decrease in LV volumes and end-diastolic pressure, increased cardiac output, and improvement in EF. Histopathological analysis, performed 6 months after implantation, showed that the luminal surface of the VPD was covered by organized thrombus and a smooth lining. The inflammatory response was focal and mild consisting of histiolymphocytic infiltrate surrounding the anchors and some portions of the graft with an occasional giant cell. Furthermore, recently published clinical studies showed that the percutaneous implantation of the Parachute ventricular partitioning device is safe and feasible and leads to improvement of cardiac function, clinical symptoms, as well as quality of life.[1–7]

How to identify patients for the Parachute device implantation

A three-stage evaluation was adopted in a series of patients referred for a Parachute ventricular partitioning device ("Parachute"). Patients with ischemic cardiomyopathy who meet the following criteria are considered suitable for a Parachute implantation.

1. Clinical evaluation criteria
   a. Documented anterior MI within the previous 3 months
   b. NYHA II–III
2. Echocardiographic, anatomical, and functional criteria
   a. EF <40%
   b. Anteroapical regional wall motion abnormalities

    c. Left ventricule apex diameter = 4.0 × 5.0 cm

    d. LV dilatation (left ventricular end-diastolic diameter [LVEDD] >56 mm, left ventricular end-systolic diameter [LVESD] >38 mm).

3. 3D cardiac computerized tomography

    a. Architecture

    b. Geometry

    c. Trabeculation of the left ventricule

After an initial clinical evaluation, step 2 screening was performed according to echocardiographic functional (LVEF <40%, apical/anterior akinesia/dyskinesia) and anatomical criteria (diameter of LV apex [LVAD] = 4.0 × 5.0 cm, LV dilatation). Patients meeting the echocardiographic criteria were selected for 3D cardiac CT (architecture, geometry, and trabeculation of the left ventricule) and eventually treated with the Parachute.[7]

Protocol for medications before and after device implantation

Four days prior to the procedure, all patients were placed on antiplatelet therapy consisting of 100 mg/day of aspirin. During the procedure, patients received intravenous boluses of unfractionated heparin to maintain the activated clotting time higher than 250 s. At the time of the implantation and on discharge, all patients also received optimal therapy for chronic heart failure consisting of an angiotensin-converting enzyme inhibitor/angiotensin receptor blocker, beta-blocker, and diuretic. In addition, patients were required to continue on the 100 mg/day of aspirin and oral anticoagulation for 12 months, postprocedure with a target INR of 2.0–3.0.

Conclusion

Parachute implantation represents a new frontier in the treatment of ischemic heart failure by LV geometrical remodeling. This procedure mimics previously proposed surgical strategies. In fact, with the Parachute, interventional cardiologists dedicated to the percutaneous treatment of structural heart disease have broken the boundaries between catheter-based intervention and surgery. For this reason, a preprocedure holistic evaluation of the LV function and geometry should be advocated to define the feasibility of the cardiac chambers remodeling.

Preclinical and clinical studies have demonstrated that the Parachute implant is safe and feasible in ischemic heart failure patients. Although the feasibility of the procedure can be optimized by adopting a strict selection protocol, the real benefits of our institutional screening strategy should be evaluated in the future with controlled trials comparing the effects of different preprocedure selection modalities and their results at long-term follow-up and in larger cohorts.

References

1. Sharkey H, Nikolic S, Khairkhahan A, Dae M. Left ventricular apex occluder; Description of a ventricular partitioning device. *EuroIntervention* 2006;2:125–7.
2. Jones RH, Velazquez EJ, Michler RE et al. Coronary bypass surgery with or without surgical ventricular reconstruction. *N Engl J Med* 2009;360:1705–17.
3. Otasevic P, Sagic D, Antonic Z, Nikolic S, Khairakhan A, Radovancevic B et al. First-in-man implantation of left ventricular partitioning device in a patient with chronic heart failure: Twelve-month follow-up. *J Card Fail* 2007;6:517–20.
4. Sagic D, Otasevic P, Sievert H, Elsasser A, Mitrovic V, Gradinac S. Percutaneous implantation of the left ventricular partitioning device for chronic heart failure: A pilot study with 1-year follow-up. *Eur J Heart Fail* 2010;6:600–6.
5. Nikolic S, Khairkhahan A, Ryu M, Champsaur G, Breznock E, Dae M. Percutaneous implantation of an intraventricular device for the treatment of heart failure: Experimental results and proof of concept. *J Card Fail* 2009;15:790–7.
6. Bozdag-Turan I, Bermaoui B, Turan RG, Paranskaya L, D'Ancona G, Kische S et al. Left ventricular partitioning device in a patient with chronic heart failure: Short-term clinical follow-up. *Int J Cardiol* 2013;163;e1–3.
7. Bozdag-Turan I, Bermaoui B, Paranskaya L, Turan R, D'Ancona G, Kische S et al. Challenges in patient selection for the parachute device implantation. *Catheter Cardiovasc Interv* 2013;82(5):E718–25.

102

Implantable assist devices for heart failure treatment

Saibal Kar and Takashi Matsumoto

Heart transplantation is the treatment of choice for end-stage heart failure (HF) patients resistant to any medical therapies. The International Society for Heart and Lung Transplantation reported that between 3600 and 3850 heart transplantations have been registered worldwide every year in the last few decades.[1] Advances in immunosuppression therapy have improved the survival of patients undergoing heart transplantation. However, there are still several limitations to heart transplantation. Many HF patients are not eligible for transplant due to their age or other comorbidities, and the supply of donor organs is not adequate. The death rate of recipients on the heart waiting list was 170 per 1000 patient-years at risk in 2008.[1] Therefore, the interest in the use of the left ventricular assist device (LVAD) has been increasing over the past few years. In 2009, the proportion of recipients who were bridged to heart transplantation with LVAD exceeded 30% for the first time.[1]

This chapter describes the currently available types of full hemodynamic support LVADs (the first-, second-, and third-generation LVADs), and also the partial hemodynamic support LVADs, focusing on their system, clinical use, and outcomes.

First-generation LVAD

The HeartMate VE (Thoratec Corporation, Pleasanton, CA, USA) and Novacor (World Heart Corporation, Oakland, CA, USA) were the commonly and routinely used implantable first-generation LVAD.

The HeartMate VE has a pulsatile pump driven by an electronic motor using a percutaneous power and control unit. The pump is implanted below the diaphragm in either an intraperitoneal position or preperitoneal pocket. An inflow cannula is placed in the left ventricular apex, and an outflow graft is passed over the diaphragm to the ascending aorta. The HeartMate VE can be operated in either fixed-rate (partial support) or automatic mode (full

support), and it can produce 76 mL stroke volume. In the Randomized Evaluation of Mechanical Assistance for the Treatment of Congestive Heart Failure (REMATCH) trial, 129 patients with end-stage HF were randomized to LVAD therapy or optimal medical therapy (OMT).[2] The frequency of serious adverse events was 2.35 (95% confidence interval, 1.86–2.95) times higher in the device group compared to the medical therapy group, with a high event rate of infection, bleeding, and malfunction of the device. However, LVAD therapy demonstrated a significant survival benefit (1-year survival rate; 52% vs. 25%, 2 year survival rate; 23% vs. 8%). Based on the REMATCH trial results, the HeartMate VE became the first LVAD to receive the Food and Drug Administration (FDA) approval for "destination therapy (DT)."

The Novacor has a pump drive unit, which can produce a maximal stroke volume of 70 mL. The pump unit is implanted in the left upper quadrant of the abdomen, and an inflow cannula is placed in the left ventricular apex and an outflow graft to the ascending aorta. In the Investigation of Nontransplant-Eligible Patients Who Are Inotrope Dependent (INTrEPID) trial, a prospective nonrandomized study comparing Novacor with OMT, the LVAD therapy showed improved survival rate at 6 months (46% vs. 22%) and 12 months (27% vs. 11%).[3] While overall adverse events rates were higher in the OMT group, cerebrovascular accidents were more common in the LVAD group (62% vs. 11% of OMT patients). The FDA approved the Novacor for "bridge-to-transplant (BTT)" therapy.

Second-generation LVAD

The second-generation LVAD has a continuous-flow rotary pump, which is a smaller, quieter, and more durable pump compared with the first-generation pulsatile LVAD. This design reduces the invasiveness of the LVAD implantation, resulting in the reduction of procedural complications such as bleeding and infection. The HeartMate II (Thoratec) and the Jarvik 2000 (Jarvik Heart, NY, USA) are the most common implantable second-generation LVADs.

The HeartMate II consists of an internal axial-flow blood pump with a percutaneous power and control unit, which can produce up to 10 L/min at a rotation speed of 8000–15,000 rpm. The pump has a volume of 63 mL and a weight of 390 g (in comparison, the first-generation LVAD HeartMate XVE had a volume of 450 mL and a weight of 1250 g). The pump was implanted preperitoneally or within the abdominal musculature. Comparing the aforementioned LVADs, 200 patients ineligible for transplantation were randomized in a 2:1 ratio to the continuous or pulsatile device.[4] The actuarial survival rates at 2 years significantly improved with the HeartMate II (58% vs. 24% for HeartMate XVE, $p = 0.008$). Also, the HeartMate II had a lower replacement and sepsis rate compared with HeartMate XVE (event rate of 0.06 vs. 0.51 per patient year and event rate of 0.39 vs. 1.11 per patient year). However, the rate of stroke and bleeding was not significantly different. The HeartMate II is the only continuous-flow LVAD approved for both BTT and DT use by the FDA.

The Jarvik 2000, which has a volume of 25 mL and a weight of 90 g, is small enough to be implanted through the left ventricular wall, thereby allowing direct inflow into the pump. A maximum flow of 6–7 L/min can be generated with a rotation speed of 8000–12,000 rpm. The outflow graft can be connected to either the ascending or descending aorta. In a retrospective study of 102 patients with the Jarvik 2000,[5] the mean support time was 159 days for 83 "BTT" patients, and 551 days for 19 "DT" patients. The freedom from system failure at 4 years was 95%. Although the Jarvik 2000 can be used as "BTT" application in the United States, it obtained the CE mark for both "BTT" and "DT" in the EU.

Third-generation LVAD

The technical feature of the third-generation LVAD is that the moving impeller does not have any mechanical contact within the pump. This unique mechanism is achieved with the magnetic and/or hydrodynamic suspension technology to suspend the moving impeller for contact-free rotation, and has the potential advantage to reduce hemolysis and improve device durability. There are several manufacturers of third-generation LVADs, such as the VentrAssist (Ventracor, Sydney, Australia), the HVAD (HeartWare, FL, USA), the DuraHeart (Terumo Heart Inc., MI, USA), and the INCOR (Berlin Heart AG, Berlin, Germany). The INCOR and DuraHeart have a magnetic suspension, the VentrAssist has a hydrodynamic suspension, and the HVAD has a hybrid hydromagnetic suspension. All of those third-generation LVADs received the CE mark, and

are commercially available in European countries. In the United States, the FDA approved the HVAD as a "BTT" application (other third-generation LVADs are an investigational device in the United States, and pivotal clinical trials are ongoing). I also believe the Berlin heart is also FDA approved.

The HVAD has a centrifugal blood pump, which is 50 mL in volume and 160 g in weight. The impeller is the only moving part inside the pump, and can generate a maximum flow of 10 L/min. A short inflow cannula is inserted into the LV, and the outflow graft connects the pump to the ascending aorta. The ADVANCE trial compared 499 BTT patients in the Interagency Registry for Mechanical Assisted Circulatory Support (INTERMACS) with 140 BTT patients with HVAD.[6] The INTERMACS policy did not allow disclosure of the types of LVADs implanted. The primary endpoint (180 day freedom from death from the original LVAD implanted or from explantation for heart transplantation or clinical recovery) was achieved in 90.7% of the HVAD patients and 90.1% of control patients, which established the noninferiority of the HVAD ($p < 0.001$; 15% noninferiority margin). And in the HVAD patients both the 6 min walk test and quality of life were significantly improved at 6 month follow-up. The adverse events were not compared; sepsis occurred in 11%, stroke in 13%, and bleeding requiring surgery in 14% of patients with HVAD. The HVAD received FDA approval for "BTT" use in 2012.

Partial hemodynamic support LVAD

LVAD (full hemodynamic support type) therapy has become the accepted treatment of choice for end-stage HF patients. As stated above, the size of device has become smaller, and the device durability has improved. However, one major concern is that full hemodynamic support LVAD implantation still needs major surgical procedures with a sternotomy and cardiopulmonary bypass.

The Synergy Pocket Micro-Pump (CircuLite, NJ, USA) is a small blood pump (the size of an AA battery), which generates a flow of 2.5–3.0 L/min (Figure 102.1). This device provides partial hemodynamic support. The implantation of the blood pump requires an off-pump right-sided minithoracotomy, with the inflow cannula placed in the left atrium and the outflow cannula connected to the right subclavian artery. The first clinical use of the Synergy Micro-Pump as a bridge to heart transplantation was reported in 2008,[7] and the acute and chronic hemodynamic effects were reported in 2009.[8] In the latter study, the Synergy Micro-Pump achieved acute hemodynamic improvement; cardiac output and cardiac index significantly increased the day

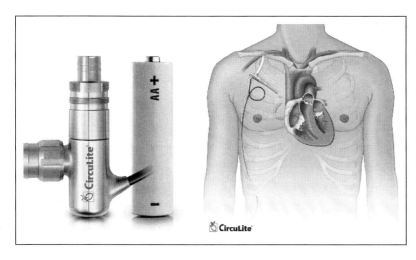

Figure 102.1 (**See color insert.**) Synergy Pocket Micro-Pump.

after implantation compared with baseline (from 3.8 to 6.3 L/min, from 2.0 to 3.3 L/min/m², respectively), while mean blood pressure was maintained. At 10 weeks after the implantation, the improved cardiac index was maintained and mean blood pressure was significantly increased from baseline (from 67 to 80 mmHg). The Synergy Micro-Pump received the CE mark in 2012, and the US pivotal clinical trial is ongoing.

Conclusions

With the limitation of heart transplantation and an increasing interest for mechanical hemodynamic support, LVADs have developed rapidly and dramatically. For advanced HF patients, LVAD (full hemodynamic support type) therapy has become the treatment of choice as both "bridge to heart transplantation" and "destination therapy." And, more recently, a partial hemodynamic support LVAD has emerged as a new therapeutic option. Further development of a smaller pump with sufficient flow volume and also implantation techniques may improve clinical outcomes of end-stage HF patients.

References

1. Stehlik J, Edwards LB, Kucheryavaya AY et al. The Registry of the International Society for Heart and Lung Transplantation: Twenty-Eighth Adult Heart Transplant Report—2011. *J Heart Lung Transplant* 2011;30:1078–94.
2. Rose EA, Gelijns AC, Moskowitz AJ et al. Long-term use of a left ventricular assist device for end-stage heart failure. *N Engl J Med* 2001;345:1435–43.
3. Rogers JG, Butler J, Lansman SL et al. Chronic mechanical circulatory support for inotrope-dependent heart failure patients who are not transplant candidates: Results of the INTrEPID Trial. *J Am Coll Cardiol* 2007;50:741–7.
4. Slaughter MS, Rogers JG, Milano CA et al. Advanced heart failure treated with continuous-flow left ventricular assist device. *N Engl J Med* 2009;361:2241–51.
5. Siegenthaler MP, Frazier OH, Beyersdorf F et al. Mechanical reliability of the Jarvik 2000 Heart. *Ann Thorac Surg* 2006;81:1752–8.
6. Aaronson KD, Slaughter MS, Miller LW et al. Use of an intrapericardial, continuous-flow, centrifugal pump in patients awaiting heart transplantation. *Circulation* 2012;125:3191–200.
7. Meyns B, Rega F, Ector J et al. Partial left ventricular support implanted through minimal access surgery as a bridge to cardiac transplant. *J Thorac Cardiovasc Surg* 2009;137:243–5.
8. Meyns B, Klotz S, Simon A et al. Proof of concept: Hemodynamic response to long-term partial ventricular support with the Synergy pocket micro-pump. *J Am Coll Cardiol* 2009;54:79–86.

103

Devices for hemodynamic monitoring

Wen-Loong Yeow, Neal Eigler, and Saibal Kar

Introduction

In the United States, heart failure occurs in about 5.7 million people and leads to about 55,000 deaths per year. Within 5 years of diagnosis, about half have died. The estimated annual health care and lost productivity national cost is $34.4 billon. Reducing heart failure (HF) hospitalization is part of the national heart prevention program. Daily self-reporting of symptoms and weights via telemonitoring, a proposed preventive strategy, has not been conclusively shown to be an effective method of reducing hospitalization or death. A likely explanation is that weight gain is a late sign of heart failure and a more sensitive method may be an implantable hemodynamics monitor. This chapter focuses on monitoring devices that are currently in use, such as transthoracic impedance, or have been or are currently being investigated in clinical trials.

OptiVol fluid status monitoring system

The OptiVol Fluid Status Monitoring system (Medtronic, Mounds View, MN, USA), currently incorporated into specific implantable cardioverter-defibrillator (ICD) and cardiac resynchronization therapy (CRT) devices, offers an insight into the patient's daily fluid status by monitoring the intrathoracic impedance. Principally, when thoracic fluid increases, electrical current conductance is increased and impedance is decreased. The impedance is measured from a right ventricular coil to a device that can monitor a patient's change from baseline and, hence, any trends; this allows clinicians to deduce the patient's fluid status and prescribe the necessary treatments.

The impedance is automatically measured at a preset interval and retrieved at follow-up. The results are presented as two trends: a daily impedance graph with a slowly adapting reference trend starting 34 days postimplant and an OptiVol fluid index graph of the daily difference between daily and reference impedance.[1] The daily graph

may indicate severity of the fluid accumulation while the index may indicate an event like cardiac decompensation once the trend crosses a clinician programmable threshold.

Apart from pulmonary edema, declining impedance may also be due to pulmonary consolidation, pleural effusion, fluid around the can, or hypervolemia. Rising impedance may indicate hypovolemia, positive pressure ventilation, or pneumothorax.

The initial validation study was the Medtronic Impedance Diagnostics in Heart Failure Trial (MID-HeFT), an observational study of 34 patients with New York Heart Association functional class (NYHA FC) III or IV with prior HF hospitalization to assess hemodynamics correlation and efficacy.[1] Impedance reduction began about 15 days before worsening of symptoms and 18 days before hospitalization. Correlation between impedance and pulmonary capillary wedge pressure ($r = -0.61$, $p < 0.001$) and inpatient net fluid loss ($r = -0.70$, $p < 0.001$) was good. Crossing a fluid index threshold of 60 Ω days was 77% sensitive for detecting HF admission within 30 days. However, there was 1.5 false positive (crossing fluid index threshold without HF admission within 30 days) per patient-year.

Compared to weight gain, crossing a fluid index threshold of 60 Ω days was significantly more sensitive (76% vs. 23%, $p < 0.0001$) and had a lower false positive per patient-year (1.9 vs. 4.3, $p < 0.0001$) for predicting HF hospitalization, emergency department, and clinic visits.[2] In addition, the frequency and duration of these crossings was associated with higher rates of HF hospitalization.[3]

An audible alert feature informing the patient that the fluid index threshold had been crossed was assessed by two nonrandomized studies. In the first study, the adjusted sensitivity and positive predictive value (PPV) was both 60% (95% CI 46–73) for HF deterioration within 2 weeks of an alert.[4] In the second study, HF hospitalization within 2 weeks was lower with the alert feature ON versus OFF (7% vs. 20%, $p < 0.001$), as well as combined cardiac death and HF hospitalization ($p = 0.007$) and with a false-positive rate per patient-year of only 0.25.[5]

However in the Diagnostic Outcome Trial in Heart Failure (DOT-HF), a randomized, controlled trial, an alert ON versus OFF group had similar combined rates of mortality and HF hospitalization (29% vs. 20%, $p = 0.063$), but led to increased HF hospitalization (HR = 1.79; 95% CI, 1.08–2.95; $p = 0.022$).[6] Also the alert ON versus OFF group had a higher number of outpatient clinic visits (250 vs. 84, $p < 0.0001$) where 46% occurred as a follow-up for audible alert (instead of clinical symptoms or signs). The trial was stopped early; only 335 out of the planned 2400 patients were randomized and in a *post hoc* futility analysis, a positive trial would have been unlikely.

The modest sensitivity and PPV were confirmed in a separate study of 501 patients.[7] The first 6 months was double-blinded (study phase 1) and thereafter, it was an open-label audible alert ON (study phase II/III) study with 371 patients. For predicting HF hospitalizations within 1 month of crossing the fluid index threshold, the *post hoc* sensitivity and PPV improved, but remained low from 29% to 66% and from 5% to 38% for study phase I and II/III, respectively.

Prediction of HF hospitalization with combined criteria was increased by 5.5-fold in a nonrandomized study of 694 patients (hazard ratio 5.5, 95% CI of 3.4–8.8, $p < 0.0001$).[8] The criteria included fluid index >100 Ω days or two of the following: long atrial fibrillation (AF) period, rapid ventricular rate during AF, index ≥60 Ω days, low patient activity, high heart rate at night, low heart rate variability, low CRT pacing, or ICD shocks.

An ongoing prospective randomized trial comparing an event-triggered wireless physician alert to standard of care for the reduction in heart failure and deaths will hopefully strengthen the role of this function.[9] Meanwhile, crossing the fluid index threshold has a moderate sensitivity and PPV for HF hospitalization, and the alert ON feature has not demonstrated a clear clinical benefit. Although better than daily weight, this function must be used in conjunction with other tools to manage a patient and the search for a single tool has led to strong interest in direct pressure monitoring.

Chronicle system

The Chronicle implantable hemodynamic monitor (IHM) system (Chronicle; Medtronic) consists of a modified pacemaker lead with a unipolar passive fixation tip, sensor, and a can.[10] The lead is implanted in the right ventricular outflow tract and the pressure transducer is located 2.8 cm from its tip. The pacemaker-like can is the memory unit and contains a lithium-manganese dioxide power source.

The sensor is able to measure heart rate, right ventricular diastolic pressure (RVDP), right ventricular systolic pressure (RVSP), maximal rate of pressure increase or decrease (max ±dP/dt), and estimated pulmonary artery diastolic

(ePAD) pressure.[10] Preejection interval (time from R-wave to max +dP/dt) and systolic time interval (time to max −dP/dt) are also calculated. The data from an external pressure reference device, carried by the patient at all times, corrects the absolute pressure recordings at interrogation.

Correlation with pressures from right heart catheterization during rest, Valsalva, and exercise were good; the baseline and 1 year correlation coefficients for RVSP was 0.96 and 0.94, RVDP was 0.96 and 0.83, and for ePADP was 0.87 and 0.87, respectively.[10]

In the Chronicle Offers Management to Patients with Advanced Signs and Symptoms of Heart Failure (COMPASS-HF) trial, a randomized, single-blinded, parallel controlled trial, the clinical efficacy, safety, and durability of the device was assessed.[11] A total of 274 patients with NYHA FC of III or IV were implanted with the device and were then randomized to hemodynamic assisted medical therapy or control groups. After 6 months, the hemodynamics were made accessible to the control group. Results were uploaded at least weekly from the home monitor through a telephone line and adjustments of medications were made with phone calls.

The 6 month freedom from system-related complications was 91.5%; 23 out of 24 complications were related to the lead and the other was due to premature battery failure. There were 40 additional hospitalization days from device- or procedure-related complications. The 6-month primary efficacy endpoint of visits to hospitals, emergency departments, or urgent clinic requiring intravenous therapy was reduced by 21% ($p = 0.33$). In a retrospective analysis, there was a 36% ($p = 0.03$) reduction of hospitalization alone.

As the primary efficacy endpoint was not met, the 2007 FDA's Circulatory System Devices Panel voted against its approval.[12]

The subsequent Reducing Decompensation Events Utilizing Intracardiac Pressures in Patients with Chronic Heart Failure (REDUCEhf) trial did not show improved efficacy either.[13] This was a prospective, single-blinded, randomized trial to evaluate the safety of combining an implantable hemodynamic monitoring system with a single-chamber ICD in patients that met class I indication for ICD. Enrollment was stopped early (the sponsor determined that a timely remanufacturing of the pressure-sensing lead, which demonstrated long-term failure from the previous studies, was not possible); 400 out of the planned 1300 patients were randomized to hemodynamic guided therapy or control group for 12 months. The 6 month freedom from system-related complications was 90.5%; these problems were related to the pressure lead, defibrillator lead, device, and indeterminate issues. The heart failure event rate of 0.48 per patients per year in the device arm was similar to the control arm (HR 0.99, CI 0.61–1.61, $p = 0.98$).

In the context of pressure-sensing lead issues and an incomplete study outcome, the Chronicle IHM system has been put on hold. These studies have, however, provided important study design clues to future hemodynamic monitoring device trials.

CardioMEMS system

The CardioMEMS Heart Failure Sensor (CardioMEMS, Atlanta, GA, USA) comprises a 15 mm × 3 mm silicone covered hermetically fused silica capsule containing an inductor coil and pressure-sensitive capacitor (Figure 103.1). At either end of the capsule is a nitinol wire loop designed to maintain device position in a vessel after deployment. The delivery system is advanced into a lower pulmonary artery via a 12 Fr percutaneous venous access and released by pulling on a tether wire. The sensor resonates at a specific frequency, which shifts with changes in pulmonary pressure. The interrogation device powers up the sensor and translates the resonant shifts into a pressure waveform.

In the feasibility study of 12 patients with NYHA FC III or IV, there was good correlation between the sensor and right heart catheterization for baseline and follow-up (median 62 days) pulmonary artery systolic pressure ($r^2 = 0.9$ and $r^2 = 0.94$, respectively) and diastolic pressure ($r^2 = 0.88$ and $r^2 = 0.48$).[14] All patients were on warfarin after the implant.

The CardioMEMS Heart Sensor Allows Monitoring of Pressure to Improve Outcomes in NYHA class III Heart Failure Patients (CHAMPION) trial was a prospective single-blinded trial to evaluate the efficacy and safety of hemodynamic guided therapy in patients with recent admissions for heart failure.[15] Overall, 550 patients were randomized after implantation to guided therapy ($n = 270$) and control ($n = 280$) group. All patients sent their data at least weekly. Patients continued their warfarin therapy while the others were initiated on aspirin (and clopidogrel for the first month).

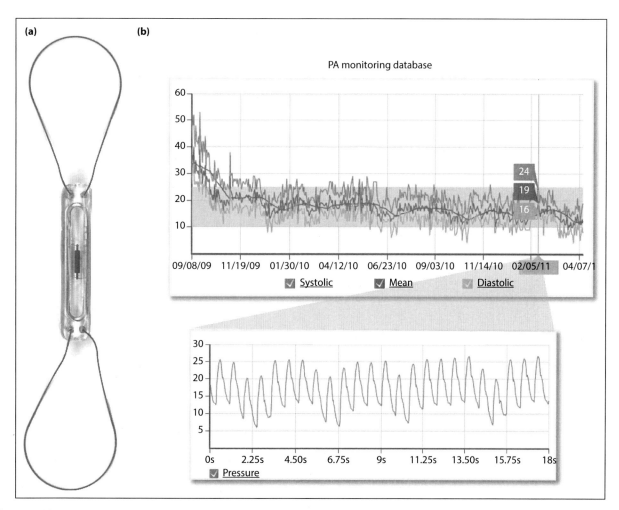

Figure 103.1   (**See color insert.**) (a) CardioMEMS sensor consisting of a battery-free inductor coil and pressure-sensitive capacitor. The nitinol wire loops maintain the device position in a ~10 mm vessel, ensuring unobstructed flow around sensor. (b) High-fidelity pulmonary artery pressure trend with specific waveform. This information is displayed on a secure website accessed by clinicians. (Reproduced with permission from CardioMEMS Inc, Atlanta, Georgia.)

There was no pressure sensor failure and freedom from device-related or system-related complications was 98.6%. Neither were there episodes of pulmonary infarction, embolism, nor removal of device. The rate of hospitalization at 6 months was reduced by 28% ($p = 0.0002$) and was reduced in both patients with preserved and reduced systolic function (ejection fraction <40%). At a mean follow-up of 15 months, the rate of hospitalization was reduced by 37% ($p < 0.0001$). Survival rates at 6 months were similar.

Despite the success of the trial, the FDA advisory panel expressed concerns about treatment bias toward the device from support mechanisms involving advisory contact between company nursing and other staff to the physicians involved. As a result, the panel voted against device effectiveness and approval.[16]

ImPressure system

The ImPressure monitoring system (ImPressure, Remon Medical Technologies, Caesarea, Israel; now Boston Scientific, Natick, MA, USA) is a battery-powered pressure-sensing module in a $15 \times 3 \times 2.4$ mm titanium case with a low-power control chip.[17] Self-expanding articulated nitinol anchors (17.5–28 mm proximal and 12.5–22.5 distal) stabilize the implant in the pulmonary artery. A pulmonary angiogram is required to identify a suitable anatomical landing site based on the anchor dimensions. To deliver the device, a 10 Fr percutaneous venous access is necessary. Aspirin and clopidogrel are prescribed for 1 month.

The interrogating device awakens the implant and 10 s of pressure waveforms are stored. Following pressure conversion, the pulmonary artery diastolic pressure can be displayed to the patient. The physician accesses the data through custom software.

The Pulmonary Artery Pressure by Implantable Device Responding to Ultrasonic Signal II (PAPIRUS II) trial was a prospective, observational, open-label registry in patients with NYHA FC III or IV.[17] A total of 40 patients were enrolled; 9 (23%) were excluded due to unsuitable PA anatomy and 31 underwent successful implant. Only 23 patients were able to perform daily home measurements. By 6 months, there was only one faulty sensor and correlations with a Millar pressure catheter (PMS Instruments, Maidenhead, UK) were good; the offset was 1.7 mmHg.

The Monitoring Pulmonary Artery Pressure by Implanted Device Responding to Ultrasonic Signal (PAPIRUS III) trial was a continuation of the PAPIRUS II trial. Continued pressure readings were collected for another 24 months. However, the results of this study have not been published and it seems further studies with this device are on hold. There are some obvious limitations with this device; the life of the battery is unknown and pulmonary artery size and anatomy requirements limit potential patients.

HeartPOD system

The HeartPOD (St. Jude Medical, CRMD, Sylmar, CA, USA) heart failure management system is a physician-directed, patient self-management system, guided by left atrial pressure (LAP) measurement.

The system consists of an implant and a Patient Advisory Module (PAM), a hand-held device (Figure 103.2).[18] The implant comprises a distal sensor module, lead, and an implantable communications module (ICM). The sensor module has a sensing diaphragm exposed to the left atrial blood volume and proximal/distal retention anchors for atrial septal fixation. The 3 mm sensor diaphragm senses the LAP, core temperature, and intracardiac electrogram

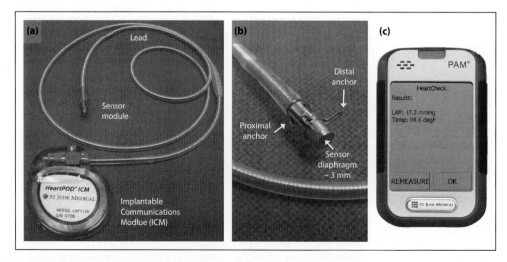

Figure 103.2 (a) HeartPOD system. (b) The sensor module. (c) Patient Advisory Module (PAM) checks LAP, and through DynamicRx feature, instructs patients to take their physician-directed medications and practice lifestyle changes based on the LAP. (The HeartPOD, PAM, and DynamicRx system are not for sale and are available for investigational use only in the United States.)

(IEGM). Within the sensor module is a hermetic titanium enclosure with four custom piezoresistive strain gauges, integrated circuitry, enclosed in a helium/argon atmosphere.

Transseptal access is required to deliver and position the sensor on the intra-atrial septum. Various methods of transseptal access can be used. An inferior approach with a Brockenbrough needle and dilator technique will require a femoral access so that the ICM can be placed in a subcutaneous pocket just above the lower rectus abdominus (now abandoned) or the lead can be transferred to exit from a subclavian/axillary vein. For direct prepectoral implant, an Agilis NxT Steerable Introducer (St. Jude Medical, Maple Grove, MN, USA) or La Crosse Transseptal Set (St. Jude Medical, St. Paul, MN, USA) can be used.[19]

Once transseptal access is achieved, an 11 Fr lead delivery sheath is placed across the septum.[18] LAP is then obtained and is correlated with simultaneous pulmonary wedge pressure. The sensor and lead are then advanced just enough so that the distal anchors are in the left atrium. The sheath and lead are pulled back together until the distal anchors are against the septum and then the sheath is pulled back, unsheathing the proximal anchors. Once the anchors are secure, the sheath is removed; the lead is connected to the ICM and secured in a subcutaneous pocket.

To interrogate the sensor, the PAM is placed <5 cm from the ICM. When the ICM is an antenna coil, the PAM with 128 kHz radiofrequency can power the sensor up.[19] The digitally encoded LAP and atrial waveform are recorded at 200 Hz for 15 s. With multiple preprogrammed algorithms, the PAM can interpret and compensate for various situations, such as rejecting excessive waveform changes with coughing and arrhythmias, informing the patient to remeasure LAP if there is <5 s of continuous waveform, adjust scaling errors, and sensor offset drift.

The PAM is initially calibrated to match catheter measurements at implant. Noninvasive calibration is performed at scheduled visits. The patient is required to perform forceful exhalation into a specifically designed mouthpiece attachment to the PAM, achieving airway pressure ≥40 mmHg for 8 s.[19] After 5 s, cardiac pressure and airway pressure should equalize, any inequality represents an offset error and is used to recalibrate the sensor.

The stored data are uploaded at follow-up and are used to formulate a treatment plan, which is then loaded onto PAM. Through the DynamicRx feature, the patient will be instructed on their medication dose and any other recommendations titrated to their LAP.[20]

The Hemodynamically Guided Home Self-Therapy in Severe Heart Failure Patients (HOMEOSTASIS) trial was a prospective, observational, open-label registry of 40 patients with NYHA FC III or IV and recent intravenous therapy for heart failure.[21] In the first 3 months after implant, treatment was clinically driven, and thereafter, therapy was pressure guided. Over the initial 12 months follow-up, there were significant improvements in LAP, frequency of elevated pressure (>25 mmHg), and NYHA FC. Although there were 9 deaths (3 from acute decompensated heart failure, 3 from other cardiac causes, and 3 noncardiac), none were device or study related. Sensor malfunction occurred in 4 patients (3 patients had successful reimplantation and 1 declined).

Additional patients were enrolled and a total of 84 patients were reported in regard to their long-term sensor performance.[19] Correlation with simultaneous pulmonary wedge pressure was good at 3 and 12 months ($r = 0.98$, mean difference 0.8 ± 4.0 mmHg). At 2 and 4 years, freedom from device failure was 95% and 88%, respectively.

The Left Atrial Pressure Monitoring to Optimize Heart Failure Therapy (LAPTOP-HF) trial, a randomized open-label study for patients with NYHA FC III and recent heart failure hospitalization, is underway (ClinicalTrials.gov number, NCT01121107). Patient with LAP monitoring system will be compared to patents with standard clinical care assisted with PAM as a reminder of their medication schedule. To monitor the LAP, either a standalone HeartPOD system or the Promote LAP system, which combines LAP monitoring with ICD or CRT-D in eligible patients, will be used.

As the only LAP monitoring device with a tailored treatment regime, this device holds great promise in patient care akin to self-blood glucose monitoring.

Summary

Although thoracic impedance monitoring is available, sensitivity and specificity in predicting HF hospitalization are modest. Its use in combination with other parameters seems to improve its accuracy; however, it remains to be vigorously tested. The HeartPOD LAP monitoring device with PAM is the last remaining direct pressure monitoring system in clinical trials and may make or break the role of hemodynamic devices in outpatient heart failure management.

Note: The above information is correct at the time of submission for publication.

References

1. Yu CM, Wang L, Chau E et al. Intrathoracic impedance monitoring in patients with heart failure: Correlation with fluid status and feasibility of early warning preceding hospitalization. *Circulation* 2005;112:841–8.
2. Abraham WT, Compton S, Haas G et al. Intrathoracic impedance vs daily weight monitoring for predicting worsening heart failure events: Results of the Fluid Accumulation Status Trial (FAST). *Congest Heart Fail* 2011;17:51–5.
3. Small RS, Wickemeyer W, Germany R et al. Changes in intrathoracic impedance are associated with subsequent risk of hospitalizations for acute decompensated heart failure: Clinical utility of implanted device monitoring without a patient alert. *J Card Fail* 2009;15:475–81.

4. Vollmann D, Nägele H, Schauerte P et al. Clinical utility of intrathoracic impedance monitoring to alert patients with an implanted device of deteriorating chronic heart failure. *Eur Heart J* 2007;28:1835–40.

5. Catanzariti D, Lunati M, Landolina M et al. Monitoring intrathoracic impedance with an implantable defibrillator reduces hospitalizations in patients with heart failure. *Pacing Clin Electrophysiol* 2009;32:363–70.

6. van Veldhuisen DJ, Braunschweig F, Conraads V et al. Intrathoracic impedance monitoring, audible patient alerts, and outcome in patients with heart failure. *Circulation* 2011;124:1719–26.

7. Conraads VM, Tavazzi L, Santini M, el al. Sensitivity and positive predictive value of implantable intrathoracic impedance monitoring as a predictor of heart failure hospitalizations: The SENSE-HF trial. *Eur Heart J* 2011;32:2266–73.

8. Whellan DJ, Ousdigian KT, Al-Khatib SM et al. Combined heart failure device diagnostics identify patients at higher risk of subsequent heart failure hospitalizations: Results from PARTNERS HF (Program to Access and Review Trending Information and Evaluate Correlation to Symptoms in Patients With Heart Failure) study. *J Am Coll Cardiol* 2010;55:1803–10.

9. Brachmann J, Böhm M, Rybak K, Klein G et al. Fluid status monitoring with a wireless network to reduce cardiovascular-related hospitalizations and mortality in heart failure: Rationale and design of the OptiLink HF Study. *Eur J Heart Fail* 2011;13:796–804.

10. Magalski A, Adamson P, Gadler F et al. Continuous ambulatory right heart pressure measurements with an implantable hemodynamic monitor: A multicenter, 12-month follow-up study of patients with chronic heart failure. *J Card Fail* 2002;8:63–70.

11. Bourge RC, Abraham WT, Adamson PB et al. Randomized controlled trial of an implantable continuous hemodynamic monitor in patients with advanced heart failure: The COMPASS-HF study. *J Am Coll Cardiol* 2008;51:1073–9.

12. U.S. Food and Drug Administration, Circulatory System Devices Panel. Chronicle Implantable Hemodynamic Monitor System premarket approval (P0500032) decision March 1, 2007. Accessed July 3, 2013 from http://www.fda.gov/AdvisoryCommittees/Committees MeetingMaterials/MedicalDevices/MedicalDevicesAdvisoryCommittee/ CirculatorySystemDevicesPanel/ucm125140.htm.

13. Adamson PB, Gold MR, Bennett T et al. Continuous hemodynamic monitoring in patients with mild to moderate heart failure: Results of The Reducing Decompensation Events Utilizing Intracardiac Pressures in Patients With Chronic Heart Failure (REDUCEhf) trial. *Congest Heart Fail* 2011;17:248–54.

14. Verdejo HE, Castro PF, Concepción R et al. Comparison of a radiofrequency-based wireless pressure sensor to swan-ganz catheter and echocardiography for ambulatory assessment of pulmonary artery pressure in heart failure. *J Am Coll Cardiol* 2007;50:2375–82.

15. Abraham WT, Adamson PB, Bourge RC et al. Wireless pulmonary artery haemodynamic monitoring in chronic heart failure: A randomised controlled trial. *Lancet* 2011;377:658–66.

16. Loh JP, Barbash IM, Waksman R. Overview of the 2011 food and drug administration circulatory system devices panel of the medical devices advisory committee meeting on the cardioMEMS champion heart failure monitoring system. *J Am Coll Cardiol* 2013; 61:1571–6.

17. Hoppe UC, Vanderheyden M, Sievert H et al. Chronic monitoring of pulmonary artery pressure in patients with severe heart failure: Multicentre experience of the monitoring Pulmonary Artery Pressure by Implantable device Responding to Ultrasonic Signal (PAPIRUS) II study. *Heart* 2009;95:1091–7.

18. Ritzema J, Melton I, Richards M et al. Direct left atrial pressure monitoring in ambulatory heart failure patients: Initial experience with a new permanent implantable device. *Circulation* 2007;116:2952–9.

19. Troughton RW, Ritzema J, Eigler NL et al. Direct left atrial pressure monitoring in severe heart failure: Long-term sensor performance. *J Cardiovasc Transl Res* 2011;4:3–13.

20. Abraham WT. Disease management: Remote monitoring in heart failure patients with implantable defibrillators, resynchronization devices, and haemodynamic monitors. *Europace* 2013;15(Suppl 1): i40–i46.

21. Ritzema J, Troughton R, Melton I et al. Physician-directed patient self-management of left atrial pressure in advanced chronic heart failure. Hemodynamically Guided Home Self-Therapy in Severe Heart Failure Patients (HOMEOSTASIS) Study Group. *Circulation* 2010 Mar 9;121:1086–95.

104

Neurohumoral remodeling for treatment of hypertension and heart failure

Stefan Bertog, Laura Vaskelyte, Ilona Hofmann, Jennifer Franke, Sameer Gafoor, and Horst Sievert

Introduction

Though no official definition for the term "neurohumoral remodeling" exists, it is commonly used to describe the manipulation of the neurohumoral axis and thereby the hormonal milieu to achieve an improvement in physiologic parameters. This can be achieved by the administration of medications, for example, sympatholytic agents such as beta-blockers and is, therefore, not strictly limited to the use of percutaneous or surgical methods. However, in the remainder of this chapter, it will be discussed in the context of catheter-based or minimally invasive techniques only.

Why is it worth exploring catheter-based or minimally invasive neurohumoral remodeling? Though a number of well-studied antihypertensive medications are available and have been demonstrated to have a favorable impact on major adverse cardiovascular and cerebral events, some patients' blood pressure remains suboptimally controlled despite multiple antihypertensive agents.

Depending on the definition and population studied, in high-income countries the prevalence of resistant hypertension ranges between 2% and 34%.[1–5] Importantly, the risk of major adverse cardiovascular and cerebral events is higher in patients with resistant hypertension than in patients with nonresistant hypertension.[4] Therefore, alternative treatment options are needed. Similar to hypertension, there have been major breakthroughs in the pharmacological treatment of congestive heart failure in recent decades. However, some patients remain symptomatic despite traditional multidrug regimens. Frequently, these patients are found to have a high sympathetic drive associated with a high mortality.[6,7] Reduction in overall sympathetic and, in particular, renal sympathetic tone beyond that achieved with beta-blockers may have a favorable impact on hemodynamic parameters in heart failure patients. Hence, both resistant hypertension and heart failure are conditions that may benefit from alternative catheter-based or minimally invasive methods of neurohumoral remodeling discussed in the following text.

It is important to first review the role of the kidney and the renal sympathetic nervous system in the regulation of the overall sympathetic tone and blood pressure control before we discuss the techniques used to interrupt renal sympathetic nerve fibers.

The kidney has a pivotal role in blood pressure control by the mechanism of pressure natriuresis. By this principle, it adjusts the amount of sodium and water excretion according to an intrinsically set blood pressure goal. Any volume load or increase in peripheral vascular resistance will, after a transient increase in blood pressure, lead to natriuresis and diuresis until the intrinsically set blood pressure goal is reestablished. This mechanism occurs largely independent of external influences and is elegantly demonstrated in an animal model of kidney cross-transplantation. If the kidneys of a hypertensive rat model are transplanted into a normotensive rat and vice versa, the hypertensive rat will become normotensive and the normotensive rat hypertensive.[8] This concept appears to translate into human physiology, as it has been demonstrated that hypertensive recipients of a kidney from a normotensive donor may normalize the blood pressure after transplantation and that normotensive recipients of a kidney from hypertensive donors or donors with a family history of hypertension are more likely to have severe hypertension after transplantation.[9–12] If the kidney is isolated from all external influences by denervation and maintenance of a constant plasma catecholamine and cortisol level, any increase in renal perfusion pressure leads to natriuresis and diuresis.[13,14] These findings lend support to the hypothesis that the kidneys have an intrinsically set blood pressure goal and are the primary determinant of blood pressure, irrespective of the host. Moreover, by the principle of pressure natriuresis, the kidneys can maintain an intrinsic blood pressure goal irrespective of external influences. However, the kidneys' goal can be manipulated by external influences. One such influence is the renal sympathetic nervous system.

Renal sympathetic nervous system: From microanatomy to molecular pathways

The kidneys receive sympathetic nerve signals from the central nervous system via *efferent* fibers and send signals to the central nervous system via *afferent* fibers.

Efferent sympathetic fibers

Signals from the cortex, limbic system, hypothalamus, and baroreceptors are integrated in autonomic brain stem centers and transmitted via efferent sympathetic fibers in the spinal cord to the intermediolateral column where they are relayed to presynaptic fibers that exit the spinal cord at Th10-L2. Within the splanchnic nerve, these fibers course to prevertebral ganglia where they are, once again, relayed in the celiac, superior mesenteric, and inferior mesenteric ganglion to postsynaptic fibers that course alongside the renal vasculature (predominantly within the adventitia) to the kidneys where they supply every aspect of the kidney, including the tubular epithelial cells, juxtaglomerular apparatus, and vasculature.

Renal sympathetic fibers have been described in direct proximity to the adluminal membrane of the tubular epithelial cells.[15,16] Norepinephrine is released and activates α-1b and β-1 receptors. Alpha-1b receptor stimulation causes activation[17] while β-1 receptor stimulation causes inhibition of the Na/K-ATPase[18] with an overall neutral effect. However, together with norepinephrine, neuropeptide Y is released activating the Na/K-ATPase.[19] The net effect is Na/K-ATPase stimulation thereby causing sodium retention and a blood pressure increase.[19] Tubular epithelial α-1b receptor activation stimulates intracellular phospholipase C leading to increased intracellular calcium concentration activating calcium/calmodulin-dependent calcineurin. Calcineurin activates the Na/K ATPase by dephosphorylation.[20]

Sympathetic nerve fibers adjacent to the granular cells of the juxtaglomerular apparatus release norepinephrine activating β-1 receptors. This causes G-protein-coupled activation of phosphodiesterase generating cyclic AMP. Cyclic AMP activates renin release from the cytoplasmic granules of the granular cells (modified smooth muscle cells). Renin causes activation of the renin–angiotensin–aldosterone system generating the potent vasoconstrictor angiotensin II and stimulating the production of mineralocorticoids leading to sodium and water retention. The former and latter will elevate the blood pressure. Angiotensin II enhances norepinephrine release at sympathetic nerve

terminals increasing the sympathetic tone.[21] It also causes vascular remodeling and left ventricular hypertrophy.

Finally, norepinephrine is released from nerve fiber endings in the surrounding vascular smooth muscle cells. This causes stimulation of α-1a receptors, activating phospholipase C that releases inositol triphosphate from phospholipids. Inositol triphosphate causes calcium release from the sarcoplasmic reticulum. Calcium binds to the contractile apparatus leading to vascular smooth muscle contraction and vasoconstriction.

There appears to be a graded response to activation of efferent sympathetic fibers. With lower-frequency stimulation, first, renin release is enhanced.[22] With higher frequencies, sodium reabsorption occurs. Vasoconstriction requires the highest frequency.[23]

Afferent sympathetic fibers

Afferent nerve fibers send information on pressure in the urinary collecting system and vasculature, and ionic composition of the interstitial fluid to the central nervous system. An increase in hydrostatic pressure in the renal pelvis or ureter and in renal venous pressure (or compression of the kidney) causes activation of mechanoreceptors. There are two types of chemoreceptors. The R1 receptors are activated in response to renal ischemia (e.g., by occlusion of the renal artery or hypoxemia) and the R2 receptors by changes in the interstitial fluid composition. It is important to note that the activation of afferent fibers, via its effect on autonomic centers in the brain stem, causes an increase of the overall sympathetic tone. In addition, a reno-renal reflex has been described whereby (in a rat model) afferent renal nerve stimulation exerts an inhibitory effect on the efferent sympathetic nerve activity of the contralateral kidney, leading to contralateral diuresis and natriuresis.[24] This may perhaps maintain overall fluid balance in case of unilateral obstruction to urine flow.

Pivotal animal experiments of renal denervation

Hypertension

One of the earliest experiments demonstrating the role of the renal sympathetic nerve fibers was performed on a dog model. Explantation of the kidneys followed by reimplantation into the same dog essentially causes bilateral renal sympathetic denervation. This is followed by natriuresis and diuresis.[25] Similarly, transection of the splanchnic nerves causes natriuresis[26] and a blood pressure reduction whereas splanchnic nerve stimulation causes an increase in blood pressure.[27,28] Finally, in a spontaneously hypertensive rat model characterized by increased renal sympathetic nerve activity[29] that develops hypertension within several weeks after birth and eventually cardiovascular and cerebrovascular disease,[29,30] the development and magnitude and of hypertension can be delayed or attenuated by bilateral renal sympathetic denervation.[30–32] These experiments lend support to the hypothesis that renal sympathetic nerve activity has an important role in the development of hypertension and that renal sympathetic denervation may delay or attenuate the development of hypertension. Moreover, experiments with the spontaneously hypertensive stroke-prone rat have demonstrated a marked delay in the occurrence of strokes.[33] This suggests that renal denervation may not only reduce the blood pressure but perhaps has a favorable effect on important cardiovascular endpoints associated with high blood pressure.

Congestive heart failure

Renal denervation has been reported in an animal model (Wistar rats) of myocardial infarction followed by heart failure. In animals that underwent renal denervation prior to coronary artery ligation, lower left ventricular end-diastolic pressure and left ventricular end-diastolic and end-systolic diameters were measured, compared to controls that did not undergo renal denervation prior to coronary ligation.[34] In addition, if prior renal denervation was performed, a higher dP/dt was noted indicating improved contractile reserve. Likewise, in Wistar rats with myocardial infarctions, hemodynamic parameters and BNP levels in those with renal denervation after the infarction were more favorable than in controls with a myocardial infarction but no renal denervation.[35] Moreover, sodium excretion was more pronounced and the ejection fraction higher if renal denervation was performed. These experiments support the hypothesis that the sympathetic nerve tone may cause unfavorable remodeling after myocardial infarctions and that remodeling may be ameliorated with prior renal denervation. It is possible that the mechanism underlying this beneficial effect is, at least in part, the result of the attenuated effect of renal sympathetic nerve signals to the tubuloepithelial cells. For example, experimental salt loading in an dog model of high-output heart failure (caused by an arteriovenous fistula) is followed by more pronounced natriuresis in those dogs that were subjected to prior renal denervation.[36] Similar findings have been reported in the Sprague Dawley rat model of heart failure (due to coronary ligation), liver cirrhosis (due to common bile duct ligation), and nephrotic syndrome (due to adriamycin injection). Salt loading is followed by more pronounced natriuresis in animals that underwent prior renal denervation.[37] On a molecular level, it has been shown that renal tubular Na/K/2Cl transporters located predominantly in the apical membrane of the thick ascending limb of the loop of Henle are more actively expressed in an animal model of heart failure possibly enhancing sodium retention. Prior renal denervation attenuates the expression of Na/K/2Cl transporters, thereby promoting natriuresis.[38]

Human experience with catheter-based renal denervation

Hypertension

First-in-man experience has demonstrated that renal denervation causes the desired physiologic changes, namely, a reduction in renal and overall sympathetic nerve activity. It has been shown that, in addition to a blood pressure reduction, renal denervation causes a reduction in muscle sympathetic tone and in total body norepinephrine spillover (by 28–42%),[39] both surrogates for overall sympathetic nerve activity. In addition, it is accompanied by a 47–75% reduction in renal norepinephrine spillover[39,40] a measure of renal sympathetic nerve activity, and by a 50% reduction in plasma renin levels.[39]

The blood pressure lowering effect of renal denervation has been shown in two main trials: Symplicity-1 (catheter-based renal sympathetic denervation for resistant hypertension—a multicenter safety and proof-of-principle cohort study)[40] and Symplicity HTN-2 (renal sympathetic denervation in patients with treatment-resistant hypertension).[41] Symplicity-1 was a nonrandomized safety and feasibility study with enrollment of 45 patients documented to have resistant hypertension defined as a blood pressure above goal despite treatment with at least three antihypertensive medications, ideally including a diuretic.[40] At 6 and 9 month follow-up, a statistically significant 22/11 mmHg and 24/11 mmHg office blood pressure reduction occurred, respectively. This difference remained significant after censoring of patients whose blood pressure medications were intensified. The response rate, defined as a systolic blood pressure reduction of at least 10 mmHg, was 87%. In addition, there was a significant, albeit less pronounced, 11 mmHg reduction in systolic ambulatory blood pressure in patients (total of 12) who underwent a 30 day follow-up. Angiographic follow-up at 14–30 days in 18 patients did not reveal any renal artery stenoses. Likewise, at 6 months, magnetic resonance angiography did not show any significant renal artery stenosis. However, in one patient progression of atherosclerotic plaque remote from the treatment site was reported. Importantly, there were no major procedural complications with the exception of one access-related pseudoaneurysm that did not require surgical intervention and one guide catheter-induced renal artery dissection treated with renal artery stenting.

Subsequently, Symplicity HTN-2 was performed.[41] One hundred and six patients with resistant hypertension underwent randomization to either renal denervation or conventional therapy. Primary endpoint was the change in systolic office blood pressure at 6 month follow-up. There was a significant 32/12 mmHg blood pressure reduction at 6 months (statistically significant both, for systolic and diastolic blood pressures). Importantly, there was no significant blood pressure reduction in the control group treated with conventional antihypertensive medications. Similar to Symplicity-1, there was a somewhat less pronounced but significant 11/7 mmHg reduction in ambulatory blood pressure at 6 months in those 20 patients who underwent 24 h blood pressure follow-up. A significant blood pressure response (defined identically to Symplicity-1) occurred in 84% of patients. Renal artery imaging was performed in 43 patients at 6 month follow-up (37 patients with Duplex ultrasonography, the remainder with CT- or magnetic resonance angiography) and no renal artery stenosis related to the treatment site was identified (progression of an atherosclerotic plaque remote from the treatment site was seen but did not require treatment).

A registry of 153 patients including Symplicity-1 patients[42] was used to assess the durability of the favorable blood pressure response described in both Symplicity trials. This showed that the blood pressure reduction was durable up to at least 24 months after the procedure.[42] In those 18 patients who underwent 24 month follow-up, the blood pressure reduction was 32/14 mmHg (statistically significant). In this registry, a renal artery stenosis was reported remote from the treatment site (in the proximal renal artery) treated with renal artery stenting. The aforementioned data are limited to the use of the Symplicity catheter, a steerable catheter with a single radio-frequency electrode that requires application of radio-frequency energy to the renal artery in a spiral, circumferential manner with 4–8 ablations (2 min each).

A number of other catheters have been designed, some of which have undergone human studies. The EnligHTN denervation system (St. Jude Medical, St. Paul, MN, USA) consists of a catheter with a basket-like tip housing four unipolar radio-frequency electrodes that can be expanded, establishing renal artery wall contact. Similar to the Symplicity catheter, 4–8 ablations are performed. To date, the results of one nonrandomized study, EnligHTN I (safety and efficacy study of renal artery ablation in resistant hypertension patients) have been published.[43] Forty-six patients underwent renal denervation with a 6-month office and ambulatory blood pressure reduction similar to that achieved in the Symplicity trials (26/10 and 10/6 mmHg (n = 44), respectively) with a similar (80%) responder rate (defined as an office systolic blood pressure reduction of ≥10 mmHg).

The Vessix device (Boston Scientific, Natick, MA, USA) is a balloon-tipped catheter with spirally arranged (4–6, depending on balloon size used) electrodes that can be delivered over a 0.014 inch guide wire into the renal arteries via an 8F guide sheath. Unique features are bipolar electrodes that allow delivery of lower energy levels (approximately 1 W) and the availability of smaller sizes that can be used in smaller (≥3 mm) accessory renal arteries. Preliminary results of REDUCE-HTN (treatment of resistant hypertension using a radio-frequency percutaneous transluminal angioplasty catheter) in 41 patients demonstrated significant blood pressure reductions, including four patients with accessory renal arteries (20/11 mmHg reduction in 6 month office blood pressure).

Similar to the Vessix system, the Covidien OneShot catheter (Covidien, Dublin, Ireland) is a balloon-tipped catheter advanced over a 0.014 inch guide wire into the renal arteries. Attached to the catheter in a spiral fashion is a unipolar radio-frequency electrode that emits 25 W of radio-frequency energy. The balloon catheter is perfused by saline exiting the balloon via several irrigation pores thereby providing cooling during the radio-frequency energy application. Preliminary data presented at CSI (Congenital and Structural Intervention)-Frankfurt 2013, showed a significant blood pressure reduction in eight treated patients (mean 31 mmHg reduction in systolic office blood pressure).

The Paradise technology (Recor Medical, Ronconcoma, NY, USA) is a balloon-tipped catheter delivered into the renal arteries over a 0.014 inch guide wire, via a 6 F guide catheter. Saline solution is used to perfuse the balloon, providing cooling during the circumferential ultrasound energy application. A significant blood pressure reduction of 36/17 mmHg occurred in eight patients who underwent a 3 month follow-up (REDUCE study).[44]

A recent meta-analysis of 12 studies including 561 patients using the radio-frequency energy Symplicity catheter (Medtronic, Minneapolis, MN, USA), ultrasound energy Recor system (Recor Medical, Menlo Park, CA, USA), or conventional radio-frequency energy catheters used for ablation of cardiac arrhythmias, demonstrated a significant mean blood pressure reduction of 29/11 mmHg at 6-month follow-up in controlled studies and of 25/11 mmHg in uncontrolled studies.[45] Importantly, though a significant and pronounced blood pressure reduction had been observed in most published studies, some investigators report less pronounced or absent responses.[46]

There are a number of limitations that apply to currently published studies; among others, a potential placebo and Hawthorne effect and investigator bias stand out. Only randomized controlled trials with a sham group will allow elimination of some of these potential sources of error. To this effect, a number of randomized controlled studies are enrolling patients. Symplicity HTN-3 (Renal Denervation in Patients with Uncontrolled Hypertension, www.clinicaltrials.gov: NCT01418261) is an ongoing randomized trial very similar in design to Symplicity HTN-2 with the important exception that patients in the control group will undergo a sham procedure. A total of 530 patients are expected to be enrolled.

Heart failure

Heart failure with reduced left ventricular systolic function

Beneficial effects after renal denervation in patients with chronic heart failure could be expected on theoretical grounds based on the notion that sympathetic nerve over-activity in heart failure patients is associated with increased mortality and on the beneficial effects seen after treatment with beta-receptor blockers and inhibitors of the renin–angiotensin–aldosterone system. However, concerns in patients whose hemodynamics may be marginal and dependent on an increased sympathetic drive for inotropic stimulation are warranted. Hence, Davies et al. (REACH-Pilot trial, renal artery denervation in chronic heart failure) have recently studied seven patients with systolic heart failure (the majority due to ischemic cardiomyopathy) in NYHA class III or IV despite optimal medical management with angiotensin conversion enzyme inhibitors or angiotensin receptor blockers, beta-blockers, and spironolactone who have undergone renal denervation. The primary goal was to assess the safety of renal denervation in this patient group. In all seven patients, the procedure was performed successfully without complications. Patients reported subjectively to feel better at follow-up and the 6 min walk distance at 6 months improved significantly (by 27 m). There was a trend toward a blood pressure reduction at follow-up. In four patients, loop diuretics were discontinued due to significant improvements in peripheral edema. In two patients, beta-blocker and angiotensin receptor blocker therapy were reduced and in one increased, respectively. Importantly, there was no heart failure decompensation in either of the patients. This suggests that renal denervation may be safe in patients with chronic systolic heart failure. Though the patients reported a subjective symptomatic improvement and the 6 min walking distance increased significantly, a definitive statement regarding the efficacy of renal denervation for heart failure would be premature. The REACH trial, planned to enroll 100 patients with an ejection fraction of <40% and NYHA class II or higher, will examine a change in heart failure symptoms (Kansas City Cardiomyopathy Questionnaire, NYHA class), peak exercise oxygen consumption, 6-min walking distance, and major adverse events 12 months after renal denervation. Patients will be randomized to renal denervation or a sham procedure.

Heart failure with preserved left ventricular ejection fraction

A change in diastolic parameters and left ventricular muscle mass in patients with hypertension, some of whom carried the diagnosis of heart failure with preserved ejection fraction has recently been demonstrated. Forty-six patients with resistant hypertension underwent renal denervation after which a significant reduction in interventricular septal thickness, left ventricular mass index, E/E′, and isovolumetric relaxation time was observed.[47] This suggests an improvement in left ventricular diastole and, perhaps, a role of renal denervation in patients with diastolic heart failure. In this context, two clinical trials specifically examining patients with diastolic heart failure merit attention, the DIASTOLE trial (denervation of the renal sympathetic nerves in heart failure with normal LV ejection fraction, www.clinicaltrials.gov, NCT01583881) and RDT-PEF (renal denervation in heart failure with preserved ejection fraction, www.clinicaltrials.gov, NCT01840059). In the former, approximately 30 patients will be randomized to renal denervation in addition to usual medical management versus medical management alone. The primary goal is the assessment of diastolic parameters such as E/E′ 12 months after renal denervation. In addition, clinical endpoints (e.g., overall mortality, hospitalization, and walking distance), a number of physiologic parameters such as left ventricular end-diastolic pressure and relaxation, and natriuretic peptide levels and structural changes (e.g., left ventricular and atrial volumes and left ventricular mass) will be assessed. In the latter, similar enrollment of 40 patients with diastolic heart failure is anticipated with randomization to renal denervation in addition to the usual medical management versus medical management. Primary outcomes will include a change in symptoms (Minnesota Living with Heart Failure Questionnaire), peak exercise oxygen consumption, biomarkers such as BNP, E/E′, left ventricular mass, and left atrial volume index.

One might ask: Why do we include renal denervation in structural cardiac interventions? It is true that we do not use a catheter in the heart to cause a change in cardiac structure. However, as described above, a number of potentially favorable changes occur to the heart as a result of the placement of a catheter into a remote site, the renal arteries. These changes, namely, a reduction in cardiac muscle mass and diastolic parameters (not to mention changes that may occur at a molecular level), though as subtle as they seem, may have equally important prognostic implications to changes that are caused by direct catheter-induced structural changes.

References

1. Gupta AK, Nasothimiou EG, Chang CL, Sever PS, Dahlof B, Poulter NR. Baseline predictors of resistant hypertension in the Anglo-Scandinavian Cardiac Outcome Trial (ASCOT): A risk score to identify those at high-risk. *J Hypertens* 2011;29(10):2004–13.
2. Cushman WC, Ford CE, Cutler JA, Margolis KL, Davis BR, Grimm RH et al. Success and predictors of blood pressure control in diverse North American settings: The antihypertensive and lipid-lowering treatment to prevent heart attack trial (ALLHAT). *J Clin Hypertens (Greenwich)* 2002;4(6):393–404.

3. Jamerson K, Weber MA, Bakris GL, Dahlof B, Pitt B, Shi V et al. Benazepril plus amlodipine or hydrochlorothiazide for hypertension in high-risk patients. *N Engl J Med* 2008;359(23):2417–28.

4. Daugherty SL, Powers JD, Magid DJ, Tavel HM, Masoudi FA, Margolis KL et al. Incidence and prognosis of resistant hypertension in hypertensive patients. *Circulation* 2012;125(13):1635–42.

5. Egan BM, Zhao Y, Axon RN, Brzezinski WA, Ferdinand KC. Uncontrolled and apparent treatment resistant hypertension in the United States, 1988 to 2008. *Circulation* 2011;124(9):1046–58.

6. Cohn JN, Levine TB, Olivari MT, Garberg V, Lura D, Francis GS et al. Plasma norepinephrine as a guide to prognosis in patients with chronic congestive heart failure. *N Engl J Med* 1984;311(13):819–23.

7. Rector TS, Olivari MT, Levine TB, Francis GS, Cohn JN. Predicting survival for an individual with congestive heart failure using the plasma norepinephrine concentration. *Am Heart J* 1987;114(1 Pt 1):148–52.

8. Rettig R. Does the kidney play a role in the aetiology of primary hypertension? Evidence from renal transplantation studies in rats and humans. *J Hum Hypertens* 1993;7(2):177–80.

9. Curtis JJ, Luke RG, Dustan HP, Kashgarian M, Whelchel JD, Jones P et al. Remission of essential hypertension after renal transplantation. *N Engl J Med* 1983;309(17):1009–15.

10. Guidi E, Bianchi G, Rivolta E, Ponticelli C, Quarto di Palo F, Minetti L et al. Hypertension in man with a kidney transplant: Role of familial versus other factors. *Nephron* 1985;41(1):14–21.

11. Guidi E, Menghetti D, Milani S, Montagnino G, Palazzi P, Bianchi G. Hypertension may be transplanted with the kidney in humans: A long-term historical prospective follow-up of recipients grafted with kidneys coming from donors with or without hypertension in their families. *J Am Soc Nephrol* 1996;7(8):1131–8.

12. Strandgaard S, Hansen U. Hypertension in renal allograft recipients may be conveyed by cadaveric kidneys from donors with subarachnoid haemorrhage. *Br Med J* 1986;292(6527):1041–4.

13. Roman RJ, Cowley AW, Jr. Characterization of a new model for the study of pressure-natriuresis in the rat. *Am J Physiol* 1985;248(2 Pt 2):F190–8.

14. Roman RJ, Cowley AW, Jr. Abnormal pressure-diuresis-natriuresis response in spontaneously hypertensive rats. *Am J Physiol* 1985;248(2 Pt 2):F199–205.

15. Barajas L, Liu L. The renal nerves in the newborn rat. *Pediatr Nephrol* 1993;7(5):657–66.

16. Muller J, Barajas L. Electron microscopic and histochemical evidence for a tubular innervation in the renal cortex of the monkey. *J Ultrastruct Res* 1972;41(5):533–49.

17. Gill JR, Jr., Casper AG. Effect of renal alpha-adrenergic stimulation on proximal tubular sodium reabsorption. *Am J Physiol* 1972;223(5):1201–5.

18. Gill JR, Jr., Casper AG. Depression of proximal tubular sodium reabsorption in the dog in response to renal beta adrenergic stimulation by isoproterenol. *J Clin Invest* 1971;50(1):112–8.

19. Ohtomo Y, Meister B, Hokfelt T, Aperia A. Coexisting NPY and NE synergistically regulate renal tubular Na+, K(+)-ATPase activity. *Kidney Int* 1994;45(6):1606–13.

20. Bertorello AM, Aperia A, Walaas SI, Nairn AC, Greengard P. Phosphorylation of the catalytic subunit of Na+, K(+)-ATPase inhibits the activity of the enzyme. *Proc Natl Acad Sci USA* 1991;88(24):11359–62.

21. Zimmerman BG, Gomer SK, Liao JC. Action of angiotensin on vascular adrenergic nerve endings: Facilitation of norepinephrine release. *Fed Proc* 1972;31(4):1344–50.

22. La Grange RG, Sloop CH, Schmid HE. Selective stimulation of renal nerves in the anesthetized dog. Effect on renin release during controlled changes in renal hemodynamics. *Circ Res* 1973;33(6):704–12.

23. Koepke JP, DiBona GF. Functions of the renal nerves. *Physiologist* 1985;28(1):47–52.

24. Kopp UC, Olson LA, DiBona GF. Renorenal reflex responses to mechano- and chemoreceptor stimulation in the dog and rat. *Am J Physiol* 1984;246(1 Pt 2):F67–77.

25. Quinby WC. The function of the kidney when deprived of its nerves. *J Exp Med* 1916;23(4):535–48.

26. Bernard C. Lecons sur les proprietes et les alterations pathologiques des liquides de l'Organisme. Paris: *Bailliers et Fils* 1859;2:170–1.

27. Kottke FJ, Kubicek WG, Visscher MB. The production of arterial hypertension by chronic renal artery-nerve stimulation. *Am J Physiol* 1945;145:38–47.

28. Kubicek WG, Kottke FJ, Laker DJ, Visscher MB. Renal function during arterial hypertension produced by chronic splanchnic nerve stimulation in the dog. *Am J Physiol* 1953;174(3):397–400.

29. Thoren P, Ricksten SE. Recordings of renal and splanchnic sympathetic nervous activity in normotensive and spontaneously hypertensive rats. *Clin Sci* 1979; 57(Suppl 5):197s–9s.

30. Abramczyk P, Zwolinska A, Oficjalski P, Przybylski J. Kidney denervation combined with elimination of adrenal-renal portal circulation prevents the development of hypertension in spontaneously hypertensive rats. *Clin Exp Pharmacol Physiol* 1999;26(1):32–4.

31. Norman RA, Jr., Dzielak DJ. Spontaneous hypertension is primarily the result of sympathetic overactivity and immunologic dysfunction. *Proc Soc Exp Biol Med* 1986;182(4):448–53.

32. Norman RA Jr, Dzielak DJ. Role of renal nerves in onset and maintenance of spontaneous hypertension. *Am J Physiol* 1982;243(2):H284–8.

33. Ikeda H, Shino A, Nagaoka A. Effects of chemical sympathectomy on hypertension and stroke in stroke-prone spontaneously hypertensive rats. *Eur J Pharmacol* 1979;53(2):173–9.

34. Nozawa T, Igawa A, Fujii N, Kato B, Yoshida N, Asanoi H et al. Effects of long-term renal sympathetic denervation on heart failure after myocardial infarction in rats. *Heart Vessels* 2002;16(2):51–6.

35. Hu J, Ji M, Niu C, Aini A, Zhou Q, Zhang L et al. Effects of renal sympathetic denervation on post-myocardial infarction cardiac remodeling in rats. *PLoS One* 2012;7(9):e45986.

36. Villarreal D, Freeman RH, Johnson RA, Simmons JC. Effects of renal denervation on postprandial sodium excretion in experimental heart failure. *Am J Physiol* 1994; 266(5 Pt 2):R1599–604.

37. DiBona GF. Role of the renal nerves in renal sodium retention and edema formation. *Trans Am Clin Climatol Assoc* 1990;101:38–44; discussion 5.

38. Torp M, Brond L, Nielsen JB, Nielsen S, Christensen S, Jonassen TE. Effects of renal denervation on the NKCC2 cotransporter in the thick ascending limb of the loop of Henle in rats with congestive heart failure. *Acta Physiol (Oxf)* 2012;204(3):451–9.

39. Schlaich MP, Sobotka PA, Krum H, Lambert E, Esler MD. Renal sympathetic-nerve ablation for uncontrolled hypertension. *N Engl J Med* 2009;361(9):932–4.

40. Krum H, Schlaich M, Whitbourn R, Sobotka PA, Sadowski J, Bartus K et al. Catheter-based renal sympathetic denervation for resistant hypertension: A multicentre safety and proof-of-principle cohort study. *Lancet* 2009;373(9671):1275–81.

41. Esler MD, Krum H, Sobotka PA, Schlaich MP, Schmieder RE, Bohm M. Renal sympathetic denervation in patients with treatment-resistant hypertension (The Symplicity HTN-2 Trial): A randomised controlled trial. *Lancet* 2010;376(9756):1903–9.

42. Catheter-based renal sympathetic denervation for resistant hypertension: Durability of blood pressure reduction out to 24 months. *Hypertension* 2011;57(5):911–7.

43. Worthley SG, Tsioufis CP, Worthley MI, Sinhal A, Chew DP, Meredith IT et al. Safety and efficacy of a multi-electrode renal sympathetic denervation system in resistant hypertension: The EnligHTN I trial. *Eur Heart J* 2013;34(28):2132–40.

44. Mabin T, Sapoval M, Cabane V, Stemmett J, Iyer M. First experience with endovascular ultrasound renal denervation for the treatment of resistant hypertension. *EuroIntervention* 2012;8(1):57–61.

45. Davis MI, Filion KB, Zhang D, Eisenberg MJ, Afilalo J, Schiffrin EL et al. Effectiveness of renal denervation therapy for resistant hypertension: A systematic review and meta-analysis. *J Am Coll Cardiol* 2013;62(3):231–41.

46. Persu A, Azizi M, Burnier M, Staessen JA. Residual effect of renal denervation in patients with truly resistant hypertension. *Hypertension* 2013;62(3):450–2.

47. Brandt MC, Mahfoud F, Reda S, Schirmer SH, Erdmann E, Bohm M et al. Renal sympathetic denervation reduces left ventricular hypertrophy and improves cardiac function in patients with resistant hypertension. *J Am Coll Cardiol* 2012;59(10):901–9.

105

Catheter retrieval of intracardiac masses

Brian J. deGuzman, Albert K. Chin, and Lishan Aklog

Introduction

Disease states that present as intracardiac masses encompass a very broad spectrum of pathology. Taken as a whole, this multitude of processes are commonly encountered in clinical practice, but each individual disease state taken separately accounts for relatively small numbers of patients seen in the clinical setting. Because of this, the treatment of masses found in the cardiac chambers that do not have standardized algorithms and optimal management is not well described. Regardless of the primary disease, intracardiac masses pose significant risk to patients and require urgent treatment. This chapter will outline the current status of the management of such disease states, with particular focus on catheter-based treatment and new technology that may simplify this approach, adding to the treatment armamentarium available to physicians managing these difficult situations.

Etiology

Intracardiac masses can occur from a large variety of pathologic processes. Cardiac tumors are rare, but often present as a mass in one of the chambers of the heart. Of the primary cardiac tumors, 70% are benign and 30% malignant, the most common of these being myxoma.[1] They are usually pedunculated, polypoid masses of 4–6 cm in size that present secondary to obstruction of venous drainage across the atrioventricular valves or to pulmonary, systemic, or paradoxical embolization.[1] Diagnosis is usually made with transthoracic or transesophageal echocardiography, but can also be made with computerized tomography (CT), magnetic resonance imaging (MRI), or cine angiography during cardiac chamber investigation. Management historically has been formal surgical resection via median sternotomy, with cardiopulmonary bypass and direct resection of the tumor from its anatomical attachment with appropriate margins, if possible. Typically, this carries a mortality rate of less than 3%.[1] Other tumors that can

present with intracardiac components include but are not limited to fibroelastomas, fibromas, rhabdomyomas, and right atrial extension of infradiaphragmatic tumors such as renal, adrenal, and hepatic tumors.[1] As with myxoma, the intracardiac component of these types of tumors can be responsible for hemodynamic compromise secondary to obstruction of normal blood flow, as well as pulmonary, paradoxical, or systemic embolization. Embolization can occur from thrombus that forms on the tumor surface or from fragmentation and dislodgement of the tumor material itself.

Intracardiac masses are often the result of thrombus formation, which again can originate from a wide variety of pathologic processes. Thrombus formation can occur *de novo* within a chamber of the heart in an area of myocardial hypokinesis or akinesis. These wall motion abnormalities result in stagnation of blood in that area and subsequent clot formation if Virchow's triad is met, namely, hypercoagulability, stasis of blood, and endothelial injury. Uncommonly, thrombus originating in the ileofemoral system or the inferior vena cava (IVC) may propagate into the right atrium.[2]

Indwelling vascular catheters

Indwelling vascular catheters such as peripherally inserted central catheter (PICC) lines, dialysis catheters, and port-type catheters can also serve as a nidus for thrombus formation. These catheters typically are placed peripherally, but with a common anatomic placement goal with the tip of the catheter in proximity to the superior vena caval–right atrial junction. The mechanism of thrombus formation can be explained by the continuous mechanical trauma to the vascular or cardiac endothelium by the catheter tip during each cardiac cycle.[3] The catheter also disrupts the laminar flow causing localized blood stasis and the hypercoagulability of the underlying disease state will often satisfy Virchow's triad resulting in thrombus formation. Furthermore, with dialysis catheters, high blood flow rates during hemodialysis causes additional endothelial damage and can also activate the coagulation cascade resulting in thrombus formation. Indwelling catheters can result in related right atrial thrombus formation in up to 6% of patients and, as many patients remain asymptomatic, the incidence of right atrial thrombus may be even higher.[4] In fact, Ducatman et al. reported that up to 29% of hemodialysis (HD) patients with a permanent catheter were found to have intramural thrombi based on postmortem examination.[5]

Management of catheter-associated right atrial thrombus is not well defined, however, and it has been suggested that the appropriate treatment should be determined by the size of the thrombus.[6] Ghani et al. concluded that a thrombus measuring less than 2 cm should be treated with anticoagulation for 2 weeks prior to catheter removal alone.[7] Once a clot presents in the right atrium, the prognosis is poor without active thrombectomy. A review of the literature involving patients with right atrial thrombus found that the condition was uniformly fatal without treatment, while a 50% mortality rate was observed when either anticoagulation or thrombolytic therapy was administered as primary treatment and when surgical extraction was performed, the mortality rate was reduced to 14%.[8]

These poor outcomes are likely due to the most serious complication of a large right atrial thrombus, that is, pulmonary embolism. Other published series examining free-floating right atrial clots suggest that mortality rates from this complication can reach as high as 45%.[9–11] Because of the excessive risk of embolization and mortality, it is suggested that if the thrombus is larger than 2 cm, an immediate surgical thrombectomy should be considered along with concomitant removal of the catheter.[6,12] Furthermore, findings of lower mortality in surgically treated groups by Negulescu et al. suggest that patients with thrombi larger than 2 cm should undergo open, direct thrombectomy in the absence of any contraindication for surgery.[13–15] Candidacy for surgery with large intracardiac thrombus is generally based on extent and severity of comorbid diseases and should be considered carefully as this approach can carry an operative mortality risk of up to 23%.[16] Because of the lack of clear, consensual clinical data, no current guidelines regarding the management of intracardiac catheter-related thrombus are available.

Intracardiac device leads

Intracardiac thrombus formation can also be associated with permanently implanted pacemaker leads. Recently, an autopsy study reported right atrial pacemaker lead thrombosis in 14% of the patients at 4 years after implantation.[17] With the current number of implanted leads around 5 million worldwide and 1.2 million new leads being implanted annually,[18] this complication is likely to become more common; however, the diagnostic and therapeutic strategies to treat lead-related thrombus remain ambiguous.

Native valves, prosthetic valves, and implanted devices

Thrombus formation can also occur on prosthetic valves and septal occlusion devices.[19,20] Mobile clot formation on these prosthetic devices is rare. Diagnostic algorithms vary and treatment options as well as outcomes are not well defined.

Infected vegetations occur within the heart on both native and prosthetic valves and present as intracardiac masses. Infective endocarditis occurs by invasion of the endothelial surface cardiac structures by microorganisms, including bacteria, fungus, rickettsia, chlamydia, and virus. Although this process commonly affects heart valves, it can also affect the atrial or ventricular myocardium, shunts (patent ductusarteriosis [PDA]), and septal defects (ventricularseptal defect [VSD]). Intact endothelium is resistant to infection, but injury to heart valve endothelium leads to deposition of platelets and fibrin complex that are receptive to bacterial colonization. Bacteremia commonly originates from oral mucosa or the genitourinary, or gastrointestinal tract, but can occur from any source that creates hematogenous releases of microorganisms. Subsequently, fibronectin binds bacteria to the platelet–fibrin complex, initiating a vegetation that can then grow, shed organisms, fragment, or embolize. Tricuspid vegetations are large due to the low pressure in right heart chambers, allowing them to grow extensively, and may be in excess of 2 cm.[21] Pulmonary emboli, often septic, occur in 75% of patients with active tricuspid valve endocarditis (TVE).[22] Embolized vegetations are on occasion seen floating free in the right ventricle or pulmonary artery, or maybe entrapped in the tricuspid chordal apparatus during diagnostic imaging. The finding of typical echocardiographic features involving right heart structures in the presence of positive blood cultures with a typical organism should be regarded as diagnostic of right-sided endocarditis. Among the various valves, the tricuspid valve is the most frequently affected, occurring in 60–70% of cases.[23] In one study, the main predictors of death in right-sided infective endocarditis in intravenous drug abusers were vegetation size (>20 mm) and fungal etiology.[24] One well-accepted operative indication for TVE in the active stage is tricuspid valve vegetations >20 mm, which persist after recurrent pulmonary emboli, with or without concomitant right heart failure.[25]

Treatment

The vast majority of intracardiac masses are currently treated with either pharmacologic therapy, including both systemic anticoagulation and thrombolytic therapy, or open surgical intervention requiring median sternotomy and cardiopulmonary bypass. Both of these treatment algorithms have significant risk associated with them. Furthermore, systemic anticoagulation and thrombolysis

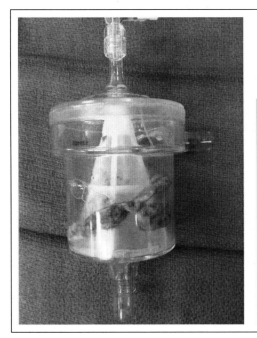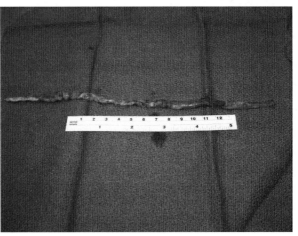

Figure 105.1   **(See color insert.)** A large, chronic thrombus removed from the right atrium via vacuum-assisted catheter retrieval concomitantly with PICC line removal.

will not be effective in many of these disease states as they are not thrombotic in nature. Further still, even thrombotic intracardiac masses have often progressed beyond the early, acute stage of clot formation and have become partially or completely organized with fibrin deposition (Figure 105.1). Once that process has occurred, these mature, fibrotic clots are no longer responsive to either anticoagulation or thrombolysis, resulting in unpredictable and often ineffective results. These treatment options also carry the risk of major bleeding complications with systemic anticoagulation ranging from 1% to 19% and thrombolytic therapy from 9% to 22% with an intracranial bleeding risk for 3–5% of which most are fatal.[26,27] These treatment options also require significant resource utilization with prolonged hospitalization, ICU utilization, and in the case of catheter-directed thrombolysis, multiple visits to the procedural suite. Also, many patients found with intracardiac masses have a contraindication to either systemic anticoagulation or thrombolytic treatment, or are at high risk for traditional surgical intervention.

Medical therapy

Currently, regarding benign or malignant tumors that present as intracardiac masses, there is no role for medical management unless the patient is not a candidate for surgical tumor removal. Medical therapy in these instances should be limited to anticoagulation to prevent thrombus formation while awaiting resection, antibiotic therapy if infectious complications occur prior to removal, or

palliative care in the event the patient is not an appropriate candidate for resection of the tumor.

Medical treatment of venous thromboembolism was instituted in 1960 with the first randomized clinical trial evaluating the efficacy of anticoagulation in patients with pulmonary embolism.[28] This treatment has subsequently been extrapolated and used to treat thrombus that presents as a cardiac mass. Anticoagulation therapy does not typically resolve existent thrombus, but prevents its propagation, and may reduce the incidence and mortality rate of pulmonary embolism.

Streptokinase, urokinase, and recombinant tissue plasminogen activator (rTPA) are compounds available for fibrinolytic therapy. All three agents convert plasminogen to plasmin, with subsequent enzymatic degradation of fibrin clot. Studies on the efficacy of the three available fibrinolytic agents demonstrate no difference in clot resolution after 24 h.[29] The positive effect of thrombolytic agents is partially offset by their potential for major bleeding complications, including intracerebral hemorrhage. The risk of hemorrhage during fibrinolytic therapy varies between 6% and 20%.[30] Several therapeutic approaches are possible in patients with cardiac thrombi. Fibrinolysis is generally efficient, but exposes the patient to the risk of migration of the intracavity thrombus, with occasionally deleterious evolution.[31,32] Heparin treatment alone has been proposed as an alternative when the other two techniques are contraindicated. If there is no contraindication for systemic thrombolytic therapy and thrombi are demonstrated in multiple cardiac chambers, entailing a higher risk of surgical intervention, thrombolytic therapy is sometimes recommended.

However, the duration and infusion rate are important determinants of successful and uncomplicated lysis. Low dose and long time infusion should be chosen to avoid fragmentation of thrombi and related complications. Because of limited available data treating intracardiac thrombi pharmacologically, assessment in a randomized study is required to define the appropriate therapeutic strategy.

Medical therapy for vegetations that present as cardiac masses essentially consists of appropriate antibiotic treatment for a culture-positive bacterium or for coverage of the suspected organism. Anticoagulation may also be appropriate to prevent thrombus formation or propagation on the vegetation. Thrombolytic medications have no role in the treatment of these intracardiac lesions.

Surgical therapy

Intracardiac tumor masses are generally treated with surgical resection as the most appropriate therapy. Generally accepted indications for operation include the diagnosis of myxoma or other tumor, the presence of obstructive physiology, or embolic symptoms. If left untreated, death usually occurs within 1–2 years after onset of obstructive symptoms with up to 10% of patients expiring from embolic complications prior to surgical intervention.[1] The natural history of patients with constitutional symptoms alone that do not undergo resection is unknown. When surgical management is undertaken, the objective is to perform complete resection with adequate margin, under direct vision, and in an *en bloc* fashion when possible. This technique usually results only in a small defect in the myocardial wall; however, on occasion, large defects result, necessitating more extensive repair with autologous or xenograft material. Resections of these tumors are substantial procedures, necessitating a median sternotomy, cardiopulmonary bypass, and cardioplegic arrest. Right atrial tumors are resected through the right atrium under direct vision. Tumor manipulation during the procedure should be avoided to prevent embolization, with every effort being made to remove the tumor intact. In the case of benign myxoma, operative mortality is less than 3% with as many as 30–75% of familial tumors recurring.[1] Because of the high mortality rates of right atrial thrombi that are larger than 2 cm in size from pulmonary embolism, it has been suggested that once discovered, a similar approach should be considered and surgical resection be undertaken urgently; however, clear guidelines have yet to be fully elucidated.[9,10,33] If a patient has significant comorbidities and surgical intervention has been deemed inappropriate because of excessive risk, then other treatment options can be considered.

Surgical treatment of infective endocarditis presenting as an intracardiac mass is indicated in the presence of congestive heart failure due to valve dysfunction, uncontrolled infection, persistent bacteremia despite appropriate antibiotic administration, fungal endocarditis, and large vegetation of greater than 10 mm in size because of increased risk for embolization. The rationale behind surgical management is excision of all infected vegetation material and nonviable cardiac tissue followed by repair or replacement of underlying structures. When these present as mobile, pedunculated masses this can often be accomplished by simple excision of the vegetation itself from its attachment without damaging the valvular apparatus with any microscopic residual vegetation effectively treated with further antibiotic therapy. Surgical resection of intracardiac vegetations also require median sternotomy, cardiopulmonary bypass, and cardioplegic arrest which carry an operative mortality of 15–20% and have a 5 year survival of 70–80% for native valve disease.[34]

Catheter therapy

A variety of devices have been devised for a percutaneous approach to thrombectomy and extraction of undesirable intravascular material (UIM). Although these devices were neither designed for nor intended to be used to remove intracardiac masses they are worth discussing to understand the evolution of current techniques used to extract intracardiac masses.

Greenfield developed a suction tip catheter for pulmonary embolectomy in 1971.[35] The catheter was previously available in the form of a 10 F steerable catheter with either a 5-mm- or a 7-mm-diameter cupped tip. Percutaneous entry was performed in either the femoral or jugular vein, and embolectomy conducted under fluoroscopic guidance. Vacuum was established by means of a syringe to aspirate a portion of the embolus into the cup, whereupon sustained vacuum was maintained as the catheter was withdrawn to remove the clot. Multiple passes of the suction cup catheter were applied until improvements in the pulmonary artery pressure and cardiac output denoted a successful clinical result. A series of 46 patients undergoing Greenfield suction pulmonary embolectomy between 1970 and 1992 demonstrated an overall success rate of 76%, with a 1 month survival rate of 70%.[36] Conventional straight catheter sheaths may be employed for percutaneous embolectomy.

An approach termed the "Meyerovitz technique" applies vacuum via a connected 60 cc syringe to a readily available 8 F or 9 F coronary guiding catheter without distal side holes that has been advanced through a 10 F introducer sheath.[37] However, this technique typically returns limited volumes of clot during extraction due to the small caliber of the guiding catheters used.

Multiple catheter designs address venous thromboembolism via clot fragmentation. Peripheral angioplasty balloon catheters have been applied to restore patency in intraluminal occlusion. Dilatation of thrombus in large-caliber vessels may result in significant distal embolization; therefore, balloon angioplasty may be combined with wall stent placement to decrease recurrent embolism resulting from dislodgement of balloon-dilated endoluminal thrombus. This technique is obviously not applicable to intracardiac pathology, but does highlight an approach commonly taken to use any and all technology to achieve a mechanical endovascular solution to a mechanical endovascular problem.

Another approach to fragmentation therapy utilizes manual rotation of a pigtail catheter to disrupt the clot, with concomitant site-specific thrombolytic injection to augment the mechanical therapy.[38] The 5 F pigtail catheter is ensheathed in a coaxial 5.5 F introducer sheath. This device seeks to recanalize an occluded vessel, without retrieval of disrupted segments. Treated patients are subjected to distal embolization that may potentially be clinically significant. Another specialized catheter fragmentation device by Amplatz applies high-speed rotation of a distal impeller on a 7 F catheter to draw the clot toward the impeller, resulting in disintegration of the thrombus into tiny particles. Microthrombi generated by this system are not removed from the circulation but instead intentionally embolized downstream. The smaller clot fragments generated by the Amplatz impeller is an improvement over pigtail embolectomy; however, the presence of circulating microhemolytic fragments may be of concern, particularly if a substantial volume of debris is generated. Clot fragmentation coupled with embolic removal has a theoretic edge over fragmentation alone. An 11 F Aspirex device integrating high-speed rotation of a distally situated spiral with vacuum capability is undergoing clinical trials to evaluate its effectiveness in pulmonary arteries between 6 and 14 mm in diameter.[39] This device combination of mechanical thrombolysis with vacuum removal addresses organized thrombus and seeks the removal of fragmentation by-products.

Another approach to clot fragmentation is catheter rheolysis. This class of therapeutic catheter utilizes a multilumen catheter with separate injection and retrieval ports. High-pressure fluid infusion through one or more injection ports serves to fragment thrombus upon contact. Infusion through the injection port or ports create a Venturi effect, establishing a pressure differential between the injection and retrieval ports that create a backflow through the retrieval lumen for removal of thrombus fragments and infused fluid. Rheolytic catheters are sized in the 6 F to 7 F range, and were not designed to be used in vessels greater than 12 mm in diameter.[38] Their application in massive pulmonary embolisms has been described in small clinical series, with resultant limited effectiveness.[38] Although there is significant knowledge of these devices being used to treat venous thromboembolic disease, including pulmonary embolism, there is only anecdotal information on use of these types of devices in the setting of intracardiac masses as first-line treatment as catheter-based therapy.

Chartier and colleagues have reported a small experience using a catheter-based technique as a primary approach to manage intracardiac thrombus. Their technique involves snaring the mass within the cardiac chamber and then "dragging" or moving the specimen caudally into the IVC. Following this maneuver, a vena caval filter is deployed cephalad to the clot. Once the IVC filter is open, providing protection from distal embolization, the clot is released in the vascular space below the filter. The clot theoretically would then be trapped by the IVC filter, preventing pulmonary embolization.[40,41] In their most recent report, they treated four patients with this technique with a procedural success rate of 25% and a procedural 50% mortality rate.[42]

What we have learned from both catheter-based treatment and surgical therapy regarding these diseases is that these masses are often large in size ranging from 1 to 30 cm in length and up to 2–4 cm in diameter (Figure 105.2); that complete or substantial removal is desired, in order to effectively remove these larger masses a large-bore catheter is required; and that using a large-bore catheter can result in significant potential for blood loss during the retrieval procedure. Because of the aforementioned issues, there are clearly inherent limitations of current instrumentation and techniques and, therefore, catheter retrieval of intracardiac masses is rarely attempted. Most of the typical tools available such as small-bore aspiration catheters, snares, and balloon catheters are not specifically designed with the intent of removing large-sized masses from the vasculature or cardiac chambers. Not only do they have significant design limitations for removing large endovascular masses, but they must also be used with caution because of the procedural risk of fragmentation that may result in subsequent embolization and poor outcomes.

A simplified approach to the *en bloc* removal of undesirable intravascular material (UIM) including large intracardiac masses has been developed and is currently in clinical use. The authors noted that during open surgical embolectomy, it is often possible to perform removal of a large mass of organized thrombus when a vacuum-powered extraction device is inserted into the main pulmonary artery to engage a clot and remove the material *en bloc* or substantially *en bloc*. The concept of using suction as a mechanical

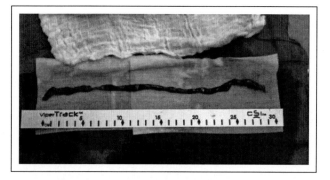

Figure 105.2 **(See color insert.)** A large pulmonary embolism in transit removed using AngioVac catheter retrieval techniques.

extraction force to retrieve pulmonary emboli in the open setting gave way to using suction as the extraction force to retrieve an intracardiac mass in a catheter-based setting.

Blood flow established by venous drainage during extracorporeal circulation can generate significant negative vacuum pressure that can be used to pull UIM such as tumor, thrombus, vegetations, or other compressible masses into a drainage cannula and the extracorporeal circuit. Once the UIM is removed from the body it is then trapped by an in-line filter connected to the extracorporeal circuit so that the cleansed blood can be returned to the patient. In this case, the venous drainage cannula acts as a retrieval catheter. In other cases, if an excessively large caliber of the material or noncompressibility prevents its introduction into the venous drainage cannula, the device can serve as an extraction tool. In these instances, the UIM may be grasped by the cannula tip under vacuum, held firmly in place with negative pressure and extracted by removing the device from the vasculature.

The mechanics of thrombectomy elucidated using these techniques in the open surgical setting and the flow dynamics of extracorporeal circulation suggested a possible technique of percutaneous venous extraction. An extracorporeal circuit may be established containing a large-bore cannula connected to an outflow line, an in-line filter, a centrifugal pump, and an inflow line connected to a percutaneous reinfusion cannula. The distal end of the venous outflow cannula is fitted with a balloon-activated funnel-shaped tip that allows for enhanced engagement of the UIM and for compression of the material to allow a mass larger than the internal diameter of the cannula to be reshaped into a smaller diameter for transit into the cannula and circuit. The venous drainage cannula is advanced into proximity of an intracardiac mass, while an inflow cannula is inserted percutaneously into a separate venous site for blood return. Activation of the centrifugal pump creates a unidirectional flow that not only

creates a vacuum at the funnel tip of the drainage cannula to extract UIM, but simultaneously provides the driving force for reinfusion of filtered blood volume back to the patient to eliminate blood loss, maintain circulating blood volume, and keep hemodynamics stable. Vascular access for insertion of both the extraction cannula and the reinfusion cannula can be accomplished either percutaneously or by surgical cutdown in either internal jugular or femoral vessels. The technique establishes a venous-to-venous bypass circulation without oxygenation, powered by a compact centrifugal pump generating a flow rate up to 6 L/min.

The sizes of both outflow and inflow cannulae are maximized to accommodate the large size of many of these intracardiac masses and to optimize flow rates and kinetic energy to facilitate removal. Previous suction thrombectomy devices were small bore and typically extracted the clot in piecemeal fashion with multiple catheter insertions and removals and with shed blood neither filtered nor reinfused, therefore, being lost. Small-bore aspiration catheters typically rely on hand-held syringe aspiration to create suction forces to remove debris. This technique may cause concern as the suction forces can be excessive as well as unpredictable. If a 60 cc syringe is used during catheter aspiration through a small-bore device, 5 pounds of force applied to the plunger will result in pressure at the tip approaching −250 mmHg. Using a centrifugal pump and a large-bore (25 F) cannula to create suction offers a more predictable and gentle alternative (Figures 105.3 and 105.4). At 6 L/min of flow, the approximate pressure in the cannula is approximately −145 mmHg, but importantly maintains a positive pressure within the vascular chamber. Therefore, this technique provides adequate suction to remove intracardiac masses while minimizing potential damage to cardiac structures, including valvular apparatus. And while syringe aspiration catheter systems lose the blood shed during that process, the use of a vascular drainage cannula mated to an

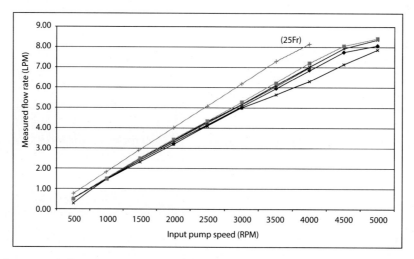

Figure 105.3 Large-bore cannula flow rates based on centrifugal pump speed in revolutions per minute (RPM). LPM, liters per minute.

Pump speed (RPM)	Flow rate (LPM)	Cannula pressure (mmHg)	Vessel pressure (mmHg)	Distance to clot (cm)	Comments
0	0	0	0	11	
1000	1.45	0	0	11	
1500	2.4	−1	0	11	
2000	3.27	−33	0	11	
2500	4.25	−62	−2	<11	Moving slowly
3000	5.2	−100	−2	<11	
3500	6.16	−145	3	<11	Advanced to 5 cm, clot captured

Figure 105.4 Negative pressure measurements in a large-bore (22 F) cannula relative to fluid flow rate. RPM, revolutions per minute; LPM, liters per minute.

extracorporeal circulatory system provides a mechanism to filter the shed blood and return it to the patient thereby avoiding exsanguination.

Elements of the funnel drainage cannula and extracorporeal circuit used to extract intracardiac masses are shown in Figures 105.5 and 105.6. The funnel cannula (AngioVac® cannula, Angiodynamics, Latham, New York) contains a 22 F body with distal fingers that are balloon expandable to generate a maximal funnel diameter of 48 F. The funnel drainage cannula is connected to ½ inch tubing that leads to the in-line filter with a 150 cc capacity and a 140 micron filter pore size. The centrifugal pump is downstream of the filter, and connected to the reinfusion line and cannula, completing the extracorporeal circuit. In preparation for the establishment of an extracorporeal bypass, a loading dose of intravenous heparin is administered to the patient and a continuous infusion or intermittent boluses are given to maintain the patient's activated clotting time (ACT) at 250 s or greater. Prior to use, the circuit is primed with normal saline, yielding a closed system that accomplishes vacuum extraction, filtering, and reinfusion in concurrent fashion. With use of the Rotaflow centrifugal pump

(MAQUET Cardiovascular, Wayne, NJ, USA), priming of the circuit requires approximately 500 cc of saline; however, any currently available centrifugal pump can be used. Venous access is established via the femoral or jugular approach, and through the introducer sheath, a standard guide wire is advanced to the site of the target cardiac mass. The AngioVac cannula obturator can accommodate up to a 0.0038 inch guide wire. A 26 F introducer sheath (Gore® DrySeal Sheath, W.L. Gore & Associates, Medical Products Division, Flagstaff, AZ, USA) is inserted in the femoral or jugular venous access site and the drainage cannula fitted with its internal tapered obturator is advanced over the previously placed guide wire to position the funnel tip to approximate the UIM. The obturator is removed from the drainage cannula, the cannula connected to the outflow limb of the circuit, and the balloon inflated with 1:1 saline/contrast mix to a pressure of 1–2 atmospheres to expand the balloon and open the funnel tip of the AngioVac cannula. The centrifugal pump is activated prior to advancement of the funnel cannula toward the mass. The rotational speed of the pump is increased in increments of 500 mL/min until flow rates are optimized (maximized) to generate maximal suction pressure as well as kinetic energy of the blood flow path. Once this is accomplished, the AngioVac is advanced toward the mass and extraction occurs. Once the mass has been engaged at the tip of the AngioVac, pump velocity is maintained and as the mass is compressed and extracted through the cannula and filtered from the blood, flow will then be reestablished at previous optimized rates. Blood flow rate, which is monitored via an in-line flow probe and displayed on the pump console, generally increases as the RPMs of the pump are increased. A sudden drop to zero flow may be a signal that a large mass has become seated in the funnel in which case the device can be withdrawn thereby extracting the UIM. If the diameter and density of a mass prevents its passage through the venous drainage cannula, the cannula may be removed from the body and its lumen cleared externally and re-introduced if necessary. Following suction removal

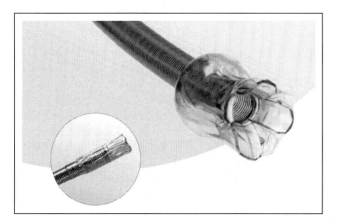

Figure 105.5 The AngioVac funnel drainage cannula used to extract intracardiac masses.

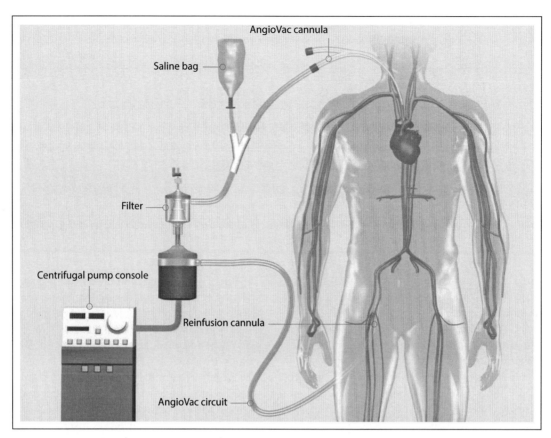

Figure 105.6   (**See color insert.**) The extracorporeal circuit and filter system used with the AngioVac funnel drainage cannula.

of a mass, echocardiographic images and occasionally a completion chamber injection is performed to evaluate the completeness of thrombus extraction. Visual confirmation of the removal of a mass can also be obtained by examining the filter that is transparent. Subsequently, a mass can be removed from the filter and sent for appropriate pathologic or microbiologic examination.

Endovascular extraction with the funnel cannula is not only a negative-pressure phenomena but also a flow-directed process. The centrifugal pump generates both sufficient flow to perform suction extraction of an intracardiac mass at one end of the circuit as well as vascular reinfusion at the opposite end of the circuit. The balloon situated at the funnel portion of the drainage cannula not only serves to expand the funnel for engagement of UIM but also to allow for compression of a mass so that a large mass can enter into a lumen smaller than its original size. As kinetic energy imparted on the UIM via blood flow facilitates its extraction, to optimize mass removal, it is important to enhance the flow past the UIM if possible. This is done by reinfusing blood on the opposite side of the UIM within the vasculature relative to the tip of the suction cannula. This allows for increased blood flow velocity against a mass being retrieved and in a sense "flushing" it toward the drainage cannula. Therefore, choice of access sites for

suction and reinfusion can be procedurally important to create this hydrodynamic advantage.

Clinical experience

Other than Chartier's experience retrieving intracardiac masses using catheter-based techniques,[42] data specific to these diseases have been scarce. In a more recent review of *Catheter-Based Therapies for Massive Pulmonary Embolism*, Todoran and Sobieszczyk initially described the AngioVac embolectomy catheter as a novel embolectomy system approved by the FDA for removal of UIM.[43] At that time, clinical experience with the system was limited. Subsequently, Todoran reported the first clinical use of the device in December 2009 for the successful removal of an intracardiac mass. In that report, they described the first true *en bloc* removal of an infected intracardiac vegetation using a catheter-based technique.[44] At their institution, a 53-year-old male who had previously undergone valve replacement and implantable cardiac defibrillator (ICD) implantation returned 4 years after his operation with sepsis from infection of his pacemaker system, which was promptly removed. However, an infected mass in the right atrium remained, which was removed successfully

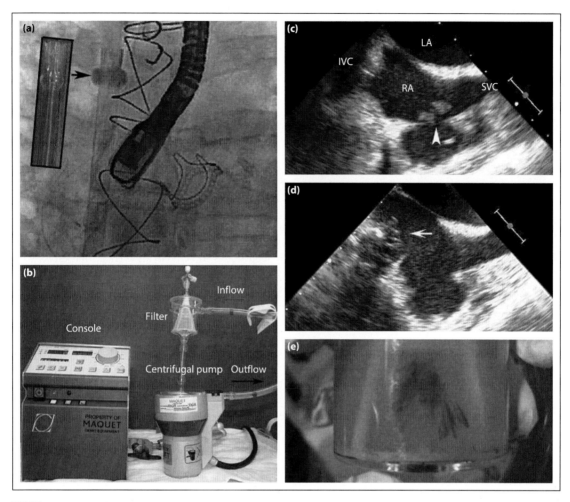

Figure 105.7   **(See color insert.)** Use of the AngioVac platform to remove an infected right atrial vegetation. (a) Insertion of AngioVac cannula under fluoroscopic guidance with the balloon tip inflated (arrow). (b) The circuit consists of a console, filter, centrifugal pump, and standard bypass tubing. The aspirated blood from the AngioVac cannula (inflow) is filtered and then returned to the patient (outflow). (c) TEE demonstrates right atrial mass (arrowhead) before extraction. RA, right atrium; LA, left atrium; SVC, superior vena cava; IVC, inferior vena cava. (d) TEE of the right atrium after mass extraction with the cannula (arrow) in the inferior vena cava. (e) Filter is shown containing the extracted vegetation. (Adapted from Todoran TM, Sobieszczyk P. *Progr Cardiovasc Dis* 2010;52:429–37.)

by a percutaneous catheter-based removal system (Figure 105.7). The patient's fever resolved 48 h after fibrin sheath extraction, and he had no further sequelae from his endocarditis 6 months after the procedure.

Also during the early phase of clinical use, Dudiy et al. reported a case of catheter-based removal of a large right atrial thrombus.[45] They describe a 55-year-old Jehovah's Witness with a history of complete heart block treated with permanent pacemaker/defibrillator implantation and several revisions. The patient had lead remnants in the distal superior vena cava (SVC) and two epicardial leads. The preoperative work-up including trans-esophageal echocardiogram (TEE) and three-dimensional computerized tomography revealed a large, mobile clot in the right atrium that tracked up to the SVC and prolapsed into the right ventricle (Figure 105.8). Catheter-based treatment with the AngioVac system was performed via a right femoral

approach. Once the flows were optimized and the cannula advanced to the mass, the mass was no longer visualized on TEE and there was no flow indicating that the mass was trapped at the tip of the cannula. The cannula was removed from the vasculature under active suction thereby extracting the mass while maintaining the advantage of reinfusion of the shed blood through the reinfusion cannula, minimizing blood loss during the procedure. The patient was hemodynamically stable throughout the procedure. The retrieved mass was a 7.3 cm × 1.4 cm × 0.7 cm soft but organized piece of material consistent with a chronic thrombus (Figure 105.9). The TEE showed no residual mass either in right atrial (RA) or right ventricular (RV) and no emboli in the pulmonary arteries and the follow-up CTA revealed no mass in the right heart.

Sakhuja et al. were the first to report the use of this novel catheter-based technology to remove not only intracardiac

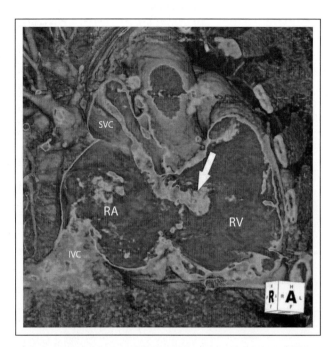

Figure 105.8   (**See color insert.**) A large, mobile mass in the right atrium that tracked up to the superior vena cava and prolapsed into the right ventricle seen on three-dimensional computerized tomography. (Adapted from Todoran TM et al. *J Vasc Interv Radiol* 2011;22(9).)

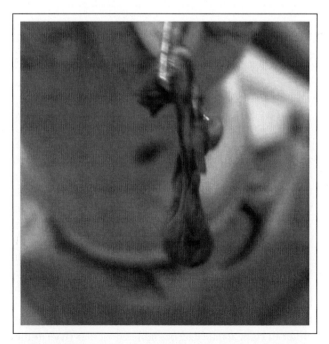

Figure 105.9   (**See color insert.**) Thrombus removed from the same patient using the AngioVac device. (Adapted from Todoran TM et al. *J Vasc Interv Radiol* 2011;22(9).)

masses but also right atrial vegetations associated with central venous catheters or pacemaker leads, valvular vegetations, vena caval obstruction from intravascular thrombus or tumor, and massive pulmonary embolism with contraindications to thrombolytic therapy.[46] In their series of 14 patients, material was aspirated in 86% of patients with a 79% procedural success rate. There was one procedure-associated pericardial effusion requiring treatment and no procedure-associated symptomatic pulmonary emboli or deaths. These results led the authors to conclude that catheter-based intervention for these intracardiac masses and other vascular pathology with the AngioVac device appears safe and may be an effective therapy for this group of patients.

Pillai and Subramanian described using catheter-based techniques to remove an intracardiac mass with a hybrid approach.[47] Also using the AngioVac catheter-based system, they were able to remove an intracardiac mass safely, avoiding a potentially high-risk surgical procedure likely reducing the patient's morbidity, mortality, and length of hospitalization.

Catheter-based therapy has also recently been applied to the treatment of native tricuspid valvular endocarditis (Figures 105.10 through 105.12) and refractory active prosthetic valve endocarditis.[48] Divekar and Fernandez reported the use of an aspiration catheter system for transcatheter therapy of refractory active rigxht-sided endocarditis on a bioprosthetic valve in a high-risk surgical patient as a bridge to surgical intervention. Catheter-based techniques were used here to remove large infective vegetations from a pulmonic valve prosthesis. By debulking the bioburden on the biological valve implant, they were able to relieve refractory sepsis in their patient and effectively bridge him to surgery, which previously was not an option (Figures 105.13 through 105.16).

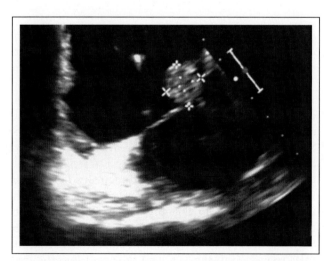

Figure 105.10   Infected tricuspid valve endocarditis vegetation.

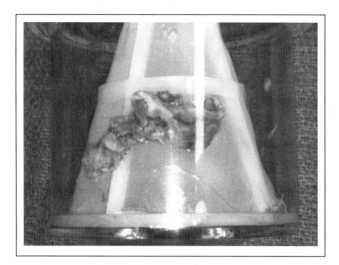

Figure 105.11 (**See color insert.**) Tricuspid valve vegetation after percutaneous catheter retrieval.

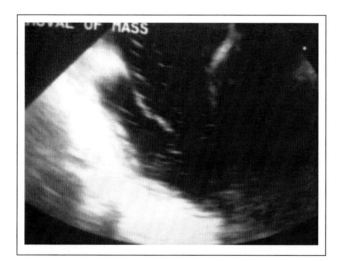

Figure 105.12 Intact tricuspid valve after catheter extraction.

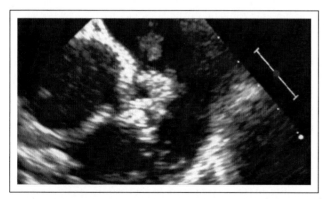

Figure 105.13 Infective endocarditis on a prosthetic valve implant. (Adapted from Pillai JB et al. *Innovations* 2012; 7(1):59–61.)

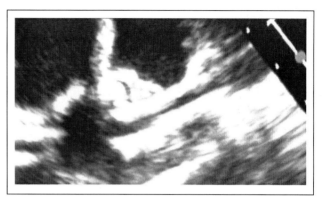

Figure 105.14 An AngioVac device traversing the infected prosthetic while on suction. (Adapted from Pillai JB et al. *Innovations* 2012;7(1):59–61.)

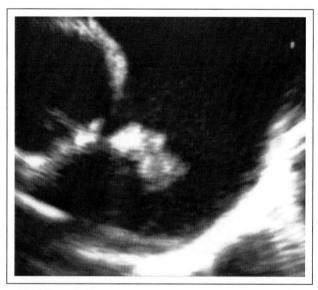

Figure 105.15 Postprocedural debrided prosthetic valve. (Adapted from Pillai JB et al. *Innovations* 2012;7(1):59–61.)

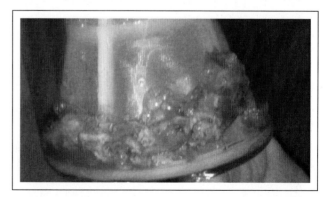

Figure 105.16 (**See color insert.**) Infected vegetation within the filter trap. (Adapted from Pillai JB et al. *Innovations* 2012;7(1):59–61.)

In the setting of large lead vegetations presenting as intracardiac masses, Patel et al. reported a small series of patients involving percutaneous extraction of large vegetations (>2 cm) from ICD/pacing leads using the AngioVac cannula in patients with infective endocarditis using this catheter-based treatment.[49] They successfully treated three patients (with intracardiac masses that measured 1.5 cm × 4 cm, 3 cm × 2 cm, and 3.5 cm × 1.7 cm) utilizing the AngioVac system to debulk lead vegetations. Using this technique, catheter-based treatment may significantly reduce the incidence of septic pulmonary embolism at the time of lead removal associated with vegetations.

Percutaneous septal occlusion devices are known to serve as a nidus for thrombus formation and development of an intracardiac masses. Previously, these would be treated with anticoagulation, thrombolytics, or surgical resection. In a report by Sievert et al., a large right atrial thrombus originating from a patent foramen ovale (PFO) closure device was resistant to anticoagulation and antiplatelet therapy.[50] A full 8 months subsequent to implantation of the device, the 20 by 20 mm intracardiac chronic thrombus was removed *en bloc* (Figure 105.17) using the AngioVac catheter technique. The procedure was performed percutaneously, thereby avoiding open surgical intervention.

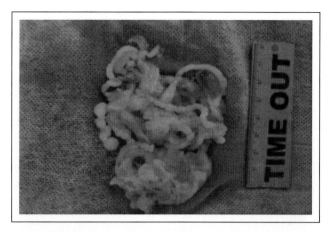

Figure 105.18   (**See color insert.**) An intracardiac tumor removed percutaneously using flow-directed catheter retrieval (AngioVac).

These same percutaneous catheter techniques have also been used to remove tumors presenting as intracardiac masses. To date, these cases have included primary cardiac myxoma, metastatic intracardiac sarcoma (Figure 105.18), adrenal cell carcinoma with intracaval and cardiac extension, hepatic tumor with supradiaphragmatic extension, and renal cell tumor with caval extension and intracardiac embolization.[51]

To date the worldwide experience utilizing the AngioVac cannula to treat UIM has surpassed 700 total cases with catheter-based retrieval of intracardiac masses totaling approximately 250 (Figure 105.19). The anatomic spectrum of disease that has been treated with the AngioVac device is extensive and includes ileofemoral deep vein thrombosis, inferior vena caval thrombus, pulmonary embolism, IVC filter thrombus, intracardiac masses as discussed above, extract arterial thrombus from the aorta, and even to thrombectomize the extracardiac conduit of a Fontan patient. The AngioVac cannula has been shown to be effective with some amount of UIM being aspirated in approximately 95% of cases and with 90% of cases resulting in complete removal of the UIM as intended by the physician. With a 1% conversion rate, a 0.9% complication rate, and a 0.14% mortality rate, the device appears to be safe for use in this clinical setting as well. Furthermore, no patients were found to have hemolysis, thrombocytopenia, or significant anemia postprocedure.

Although the echocardiographic characteristics that predict a high success for catheter-based retrieval using this device have not been defined, the current experience suggests that a heterogeneous, pedunculated, mobile mass is best suited for this technique. Heterogeneity suggests that the mass is compressible and would likely pass easily through the device and circuit. A pedunculated mass by definition has a stalk that would likely be easy to break or shear during the retrieval process for easy removal. Mobility of a mass would also facilitate entrance into the

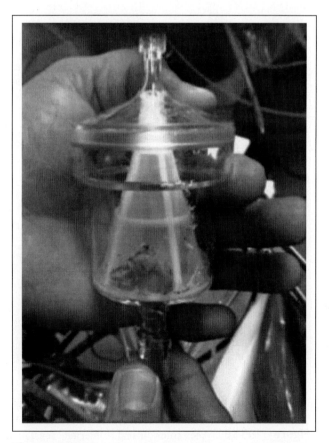

Figure 105.17   (**See color insert.**) A right atrial thrombus retrieved from a PFO closure device. (Adapted from Patel N et al. *J Card Surg* 2013;20:1–4.)

Patients	700+
Mean age	54
Gender	52% Male 48% Female
Primary location of UIM™	PA 20% RA 35% Ileofem/IVC 43% Other 2%
Material aspirated	97%
Procedural success	91%
Conversion to open	1%
Complications	0.9% 2 wire perfs, 1 iliac vein perf, 1 RA perf, 1 tricuspid chord rupture, 1 IVC perf
Procedural mortality	0.14% 1 RA perf, poor pt selection

Figure 105.19 Current clinical experience utilizing the AngioVac cannula to percutaneously remove undesirable intravascular material (UIM). PA, pulmonary artery; RA, right atrium; Ileofem/IVC, ileofemoral vein/inferior vena cava; perf, perforation.

flow path of the blood entering into the drainage cannula and once that kinetic energy has been applied, separation of a mass from the attachment point can occur.

Discussion

Intracardiac masses are not infrequently encountered in clinical practice and result from a broad spectrum of diseases, including thrombus, tumor, and vegetation. Historically, these have been treated with either medical or surgical approaches depending on the primary disease process, the size of the mass, and other comorbid factors that may affect the risk–benefit ratio. Many intracardiac masses tend to be unresponsive to thrombolytic therapy because either the primary disease process is not thrombotic in nature or because the thrombus is mature and not susceptible to thrombolysis. If the mass is of thrombotic origin, dissolution is a function of the amount of interaction achieved between the pharmacologic agent with the mass and what percentage of the mass is acute, fresh thrombus without significant fibrin deposition. Likewise, effective treatment of intracardiac masses of infectious etiology depends on the antimicrobial sensitivity of the organism and penetration of the medication into the infected mass.

It is generally accepted, however, that tumors, refractory thrombus, resistant infective endocarditis, and masses larger than 2 cm in size undergo surgical treatment unless significant contraindications exist for operative resection. Certainly, left untreated, these specific situations result in significant morbidity and mortality with traditional medical and surgical options also carrying significant risk. Because of this and other factors, optimal treatment algorithms have not been defined and guidelines for therapy do not exist.

Catheter-based techniques to remove intracardiac masses have been reported, but experience is limited.

Anecdotal information suggests that attempts have been made to employ embolectomy balloon catheters, snare-type devices, and small-bore aspiration catheters in attempts to percutaneously remove intracardiac masses. And although the proliferation of instrumentation in the catheterization field continues, few devices have been specifically designed or developed for endovascular and intracardiac extraction of the large masses associated with these types of diseases. Presently available percutaneous devices are limited by their small size relative to the large size of many of these masses. For example, the luminal cross-sectional area of a 7 F catheter is equal to 3 mm², which encompasses 0.5% of the surface area of a 30 mm diameter mass with a cross-sectional area of 615 mm². This means that a 7 F catheter approaching a mass of that size contacts only 0.5% of the cross-sectional area of the mass on a single pass. An impractical number of catheter passes would be required to remove the mass and would require it be done in piecemeal fashion.

Percutaneous interventional devices utilizing mechanical or rheolytic fragmentation may be of benefit, but would carry a significant risk of fragmentation or embolization of an intracardiac mass, likely resulting in the inability to retrieve a mass and poor outcomes.

The large-bore funnel cannula and the extracorporeal circulatory system of the AngioVac platform effectively removes large intracardiac masses via vacuum and kinetic energy. It provides high-flow blood drainage that facilitates *en bloc* removal of UIM and intracardiac masses such as tumor, thrombus, and vegetations. Once the mass enters the drainage cannula, it is removed from the body through the circuit where the in-line filter removes the mass from the system. A funnel-shaped cannula tip allows for improved engagement of UIM utilizing vacuum forces generated by flow. The funnel shape also facilitates removal of the UIM by conforming and compressing a mass utilizing both negative pressure and kinetic energy, so that much larger specimen can be removed through a cannula with a smaller internal diameter. Bench-top tests and clinical experience indicate that optimal flow rates must be present to generate vacuum and kinetic energy sufficient to remove large masses. In some of the procedures that yielded little or no material extraction, this was likely due to a combination of lack of sufficient flow rates, firm adherence of the UIM to the endocardial surface, and presence of a non-compressible mass. An advanced degree of fibrotic attachment associated with some intracardiac masses may result in the inability to dislodge the material using vacuum. The centrifugal pump provides the negative pressure to remove the mass as well as the drive force to reinfuse the cleansed blood. Because reinfusion of shed blood occurs simultaneous to removal, hemodynamic stability is maintained and blood loss is minimized. The large conduit size also ensures low shear stress in the flow path thereby minimizing the potential for hemolysis during vacuum extraction. Suction therapy is conducted by a centrifugal pump, which generates typical flow rates up to 5 L/min through the 22 F cannula and large circuit tubing diameter. At this flow rate and cannula size, laminar flow is maintained in the extracorporeal circuit, providing atraumatic passage for circulating cellular components. The filter chamber is transparent to provide immediate visual feedback to corroborate echocardiographic or angiographic evidence of complete removal. Once retrieval has been accomplished, a mass can be removed from the filter for further pathologic examination and all blood in the circuit can be returned to the patient.

Percutaneous catheter retrieval of intracardiac masses using this technique has been shown to be both safe and effective with appropriate patient selection being important for procedural success. Intracardiac masses that exhibit heterogeneity, that are pedunculated, and that appear freely mobile have been positive predictors of AngioVac extraction.

Conclusion

Treatment of large intracardiac masses continues to be a challenging area of clinical management. Current medical and surgical options have demonstrated only modest clinical outcomes and are often associated with significant risk. Furthermore, large intracardiac masses pose an immediate threat to patients and require urgent intervention, typically open surgical resection, to avoid a life-threatening complication.

Catheter-based treatment of intracardiac masses appears to be entering a new era with more effective therapy than previously available for clinical use. Removal of UIM using a large-diameter funnel tip cannula and extracorporeal circulation allows for removal of masses from the cardiac chambers that previously required open surgical resection.

This can be done percutaneously in multiple settings, including the operating room, hybrid suite, cardiac catheterization lab, or interventional radiology. The procedure is intuitive in nature and therefore does not require extensive additional training for technical proficiency or clinical success. Absolute contraindications to the percutaneous technique are limited, applying to patients with severe arterial or venous disease that would compromise vascular access to an intracardiac mass.

Further clinical experience will delineate additional associated techniques and define best patient selection criteria for optimal application of vacuum extraction with the AngioVac funnel cannula. The guidelines for catheter-based intervention to treat intracardiac masses remains poorly defined; however, early clinical results have been promising using the AngioVac suction cannula with extracorporeal circulation. It appears to offer a safe and effective treatment option to manage diseases that result in intracardiac mass. Continued research into this and other catheter retrieval approaches for intracardiac masses and any UIM is certainly warranted.

References

1. http://ctsnet.org/index.php?n = Main.CardiacTumors.
2. Khurana A, Tak T. Venous thromboembolic disease presenting as inferior vena cava thrombus extending into the right atrium. *Clin Med Res* 2004;2(2):125–7.
3. Forauer AR, Theoharis C. Histologic changes in the human vein wall adjacent to indwelling central venous catheters. *J Vasc Interv Radiol* 2003;14(9 Pt 1):1163–8.
4. Timsit JF, Farkas JC, Boyer JM, Martin JB, Misset B, Renaud B et al. Central vein catheter-related thrombosis in intensive care patients: Incidence, risks factors, and relationship with catheter-related sepsis. *Chest* 1998;114(1):207–13.
5. Ducatman BS, McMichan JC, Edwards WD. Catheter-induced lesions of the right side of the heart. A one-year prospective study of 141 autopsies. *JAMA* 1985;253(6):791–5.
6. Stavroulopoulos A, Aresti V, Zounis C. Right atrial thrombi complicating haemodialysis catheters. A meta-analysis of reported cases and a proposal of a management algorithm. *Nephrol Dial Transplant* 2012;27(7):2936–44.
7. Ghani MK, Boccalandro F, Denktas AE, Barasch E. Right atrial thrombus formation associated with central venous catheters utilization in hemodialysis patients. *Intensive Care Med* 2003;29(10):1829–32.
8. Armstrong W, Feigenbaum H, Dillon J. Echocardiographic detection of right atrial thromboembolism. *Chest* 1985;87(6):801–6.
9. Kurisu S, Inoue I, Kawagoe T, Ishihara M, Shimatani Y, Hata T et al. Right atrial thrombosis as a complication of arrhythmogenic right ventricular cardiomyopathy. *Intern Med* 2006;45(7):457–60.
10. European Working Group on Echocardiography. The European Cooperative Study on the clinical significance of right heart thrombi. *Eur Heart J* 1989;10:1046–59.
11. Ludovic C, Jérôme B, Maxence D, Philippe A, Jean-Paul B, Jean-Jacques B et al. Free-floating thrombi in the right heart diagnosis, management, and prognostic indexes in 38 consecutive patients. *Circulation* 1999;99:2779–83.
12. Kinney EL, Wright RJ. Efficacy of treatment of patients with echocardiographically detected right-sided heart thrombi: A meta-analysis. *Am Heart J* 1989;118(3):569–73.

13. Nasir H, Paul ES, Mourad HS, Erwin VK, Mubeenkhan M, Devang K. Sanghavi et al. Large right atrial thrombus associated with central venous catheter requiring open heart surgery. *Case Rep Med* 2012;2012:1–4.

14. Negulescu O, Coco M, Croll J, Mokrzycki MH. Large atrial thrombus formation associated with tunneled cuffed hemodialysis catheters. *Clin Nephrol* 2003;59(1):40–6.

15. van Laecke S, Dhondt A, de Sutter J, Vanholder, R. Right atrial thrombus in an asymptomatic hemodialysis patient with malfunctioning catheter and patent foramen ovale. *Hemodialysis Int* 2005;9(3):236–40.

16. Rose PS, Punjabi NM, Pearse DB. Treatment of right heart thromboemboli. *Chest* 2002;121(3):806–14.

17. Novak M, Dvorak P, Kamaryt P, Slana B, Lipoldova J. Autopsy and clinical context in deceased patients with implanted pacemakers and defibrillators: Intra-cardiac findings near their leads and electrodes. *Europace* 2009;11:1510–6.

18. Wood MA, Ellenbogen KA. Cardiology patient page cardiac pacemakers from the patient's perspective. *Circulation* 2002;105:2136–213.

19. Roudaut R, Serri K, Lafitte S. Thrombosis of prosthetic heart valves: Diagnosis and therapeutic considerations. *Heart* 2007;93(1):137–42.

20. Krumsdorf U, Ostermayer S, Billinger K, Trepels T, Zadan E, Horvath E et al. Incidence and clinical course of thrombus formation on atrial septal defect and patient foramen ovale closure devices in 1,000 consecutive patients. *J Am Coll Cardiol* 2004;43:302–9.

21. Moss R, Munt B. Injection drug use and right sided endocarditis. *Heart* 2003;89:577–81.

22. http://ctsnet.org/index.php?n=Main.Endocarditis.

23. Miro JM, del Rio A, Mestres CA. Infective endocarditis and cardiac surgery in intravenous drug abusers and HIV-1 infected patients. *Cardiol Clin* 2003;21:167–84.

24. Martin-Davila P, Navas E, Fortun J, Moya JL, Cobo J, Pintado V et al. Analysis of mortality and risk factors associated with native valve endocarditis in drug users: The importance of vegetation size. *Am Heart J* 2005;150:1099–106.

25. Habib G, Hoen B, Tornos P, Thuny F, Prendergast B, Vilacosta I et al. Guidelines on the prevention, diagnosis, and treatment of infective endocarditis (new version 2009): The Task Force on the Prevention, Diagnosis, and Treatment of Infective Endocarditis of the European Society of Cardiology. *Eur Heart J* 2009;30:2369–413.

26. Levine MN, Raskob G, Beyth RJ, Kearon C, Schulman S. Hemorrhagic complications of anticoagulant treatment. The Seventh ACCP Conference on Antithrombotic and Thrombolytic Therapy. *Chest* 2004;126:287S–310S.

27. Todd JL, Tapson VF. Recent advances in chest medicine thrombolytic therapy for acute pulmonary embolism: A critical appraisal. *Chest* 2009;135(5):1321–9.

28. Barritt D, Jordan S. Anticoagulant drugs in the treatment of pulmonary embolism: A controlled trial. *Lancet* June 1960;275 (7138):1309–12.

29. Almoosa, K. Is thrombolytic therapy effective for pulmonary embolism? *Am Fam Physician* 2002;65:1097–102.

30. Harris T, Meek S. When should we thrombolyse patients with pulmonary embolism? A systematic review of the literature. *Emerg Med J* 2005;22(11):766–71.

31. Mangin L, Tremel F, Cracowski JL, Chavanon O, Mallion JM, Baguet JP. Pulmonary embolism with right intra-auricular thrombus: Fatal outcome during fibrinolysis. *Presse Med* 2002;31:1454–57.

32. Nishi I, Ishimitsu T, Ishizu T, Ueno Y, Suzuki A, Seo Y et al. Peripartum cardiomyopathy and biventricular thrombi. *Circ J* 2002;9:863–65.

33. Chapoutot L, Nazeyrollas P, Metz D, Maes D, Maillier B, Jennesseaux C et al. Floating right heart thrombi and pulmonary embolism: Diagnosis, outcome and therapeutic management. *Cardiology* 1996;87:169–74.

34. Prendergast BD, Tornos P. Valvular heart disease: Changing concepts in disease management surgery for infective endocarditis who and when? *Circulation* 2010;121:1141–52.

35. Greenfield L, Bruce T, Nichols N. Transvenous pulmonary embolectomy by catheter device. *Ann Surg* 1971;174(6):881–6.

36. Greenfield L, Proctor M, Williams D, Wakefield T. Long-term experience with transvenous catheter pulmonary embolectomy. *J Vasc Surg* 1993;18(3):450–8.

37. Goldhaber S. Integration of catheter thrombectomy into our armamentarium to treat acute pulmonary embolism. *Chest* 1998;114: 1237–8.

38. Schmitz-Rode T, Jannsens U, Schild H, Basche S, Hanrath P, Gunther R. Fragmentation of massive pulmonary embolism using a pigtail rotation catheter. *Chest* 1998;114:1427–36.

39. Kuchar, N. Catheter embolectomy for acute pulmonary embolism. *Chest* 2007;132:657–63.

40. Loubeyre C, Chartier L, Beregi JP, Asseman P, Coullet JM, Bauchart JJ et al. How should pulmonary embolism associated with mobile right atrial thrombus be treated? Is there a place for interventional cardiology? *Eur Heart J* 1995;16(suppl):268.

41. Beregi JP, Aumégeat V, Loubeyre C, Coullet JM, Asseman P, Debaecker-Steckelorom C et al. Right atrial thrombi: Percutaneous mechanical thrombectomy. *Cardiovasc Intervent Radiol* 1997;20:142–5.

42. Chartier L, Béra J, Delomez M, Asseman P, Beregi J-P, Bauchart J-J et al. Free-floating thrombi in the right heart; diagnosis, management, and prognostic indexes in 38 consecutive patients. *Circulation* 1999;99:2779–83.

43. Todoran TM, Sobieszczyk P. Catheter-based therapies for massive pulmonary embolism. *Progr Cardiovasc Dis* 2010;52:429–37.

44. Todoran TM, Sobieszczyk PS, Levy MS, Perry TE, Shook DC, Kinlay S et al. Percutaneous extraction of right atrial mass using the angio-Vac aspiration system. *J Vasc Interv Radiol* 2011;22(9):1345–7.

45. Dudiy Y, Kronzon I, Cohen HA, Ruiz CE. Vacuum thrombectomy of large right atrial thrombus. *Catheter Cardiovasc Interv* 2011;79(2):001–004.

46. Sakhuja R, Gandhi R, Rogers RK, Margey RJP, Jaff MR, Schainfeld R. A novel endovenous approach for treatment of massive central venous or pulmonary arterial thrombus, mass, or vegetation: The angiovac suction cannula and circuit. *J Am Coll Cardiol* 2011;57:E1535.

47. Pillai JB, DeLaney ER, Patel NC, Subramanian VA. Hybrid minimally invasive extraction of atrial clot avoids redo sternotomy in Jehovah's witness. *Innovations* 2012;7(1):59–61.

48. Divekar AA, Scholz T, Fernandez JD. Novel percutaneous transcatheter intervention for refractory active endocarditis as a bridge to surgery-angiovac aspiration system. *Catheter Cardiovasc Interv* 2013;81(6):1008–12.

49. Patel N, Azemi T, Zaeem F, Underhill D, Gallagher R, Hagberg R et al. Vacuum assisted vegetation extraction for the management of large lead vegetations. *J Card Surg* 2013;20:1–4.

50. Wunderlich N, Franke J, deGuzman B, Sievert H. A novel technique to remove a right atrial thrombotic mass attached to a patent foramen ovale closure device. *Catheter Cardiovasc Interv* 2014; 83(6):1022.

51. Brown RJ, Uhlman MA, Fernandez JD, Collins T, Brown JA. Novel use of AngioVac system to prevent pulmonary embolism during radical nephrectomy with inferior vena cava thrombectomy. *Curr Urol* 2013;7:34–6.

106

How to avoid and manage major complications

Howaida El Said and Andras Bratincsak

Incidence and severity of complications

Although congenital cardiac catheterization has made tremendous progress in the last 10 years, complications or *adverse events are still common.*

Initial retrospective studies conducted in the 1990s reported an incidence rate of 15–20%. Despite the development of safer techniques, likely due to the ever-increasing applications of interventional procedures, the rate of complications did not change substantially. In the latest and so far largest prospective multicenter study, *adverse events occurred in about 16% of the cases*, ranging from 8% to 18%, depending on the participating center.[1] That means that even when implementing the best practices and protocols to improve patient outcome, every interventional cardiologist who enters the catheterization suite should be prepared for complications.

Obviously, not all complications are life threatening and their potential deleterious effects on patients depends on the extent and severity of the adverse event. The cumulative incidence of 16% accounts for simple technical complications, which do not pose any harm to the patients such as an uncomplicated balloon rupture, and catastrophic adverse events such as stroke, vessel dissection, or death. For standardization, the adverse events have been stratified based on their severity (Table 106.1).[1] Minimal and minor adverse events (level 1 and 2) are not life threatening and do not pose any permanent harm to the patient; however, moderate, major, and catastrophic complications could be life threatening and are grouped as high-severity adverse events (HSAE). In this chapter, we will primarily focus on HSAE or major complications.

Risk stratification of catheterization procedures based on adverse events

Based on the difference in the incidence and severity of complications, congenital cardiac *catheterization procedures*

Table 106.1 Severity of adverse events

Level of severity	Definition	Example
1 (no harm)	No harm to the patient, no change in condition, no intervention, may have required monitoring	Equipment problem Balloon rupture
2 (minor)	Transient change in patient's condition, not life threatening, returns to normal, requiring monitoring or minor intervention (holding medication, ordering lab test)	Nonsustained arrhythmia Groin hematoma Minor bleeding
3 (moderate)	Transient change in patient's condition that may be life threatening if not treated, returns to normal after treatment, requiring monitoring and intervention (medication, ICU transfer, catheter intervention)	Sustained arrhythmia with hemodynamic consequences Vascular damage requiring intervention Transfusion due to bleeding
4 (major)	Change in condition that is life threatening if not treated, may be permanent change, may require ICU admit, hospital re-admit, invasive monitoring, intubation, cardioversion, invasive procedure, or catheter intervention	Stroke Hypotension requiring CPR Malignant arrhythmia requiring multiple treatments Surgical intervention
5 (catastrophic)	Death, emergent surgery, ECMO	Vessel tear requiring surgery

Table 106.2	Risk stratification of catheterization procedures			
Procedure type	Risk category 1	Risk category 2	Risk category 3	Risk category 4
Diagnostic	Age >1 year	Age >1 month and <1 year	Age <1 month	
Balloon valvuloplasty		Pulmonary valve, age >1 month	Pulmonary valve, age <1 month Aortic valve, age >1 month	Aortic valve, age <1 month
Balloon angioplasty		Aorta <8 atm RVOT	Aorta >8 atm Pulmonary artery, <4 vessels Pulmonary artery, >4 vessels, <8 atm Systemic artery, vein, surgical shunt, or AP collateral	Pulmonary artery, >4 vessels Pulmonary vein
Stent placement		Systemic vein	Aorta RVOT Systemic artery	Pulmonary artery Pulmonary vein Surgical shunt AP collateral VSD
Stent redilation		Aorta Atrial septum RVOT Systemic artery Systemic vein	Pulmonary artery Pulmonary vein	VSD
Device or coil closure	L-SVC Venous collateral	ASD or PFO PDA Fontan fenestration AP collateral	Coronary fistula Fontan baffle leak Surgical shunt	Perivalvular leak VSD
Other	Myocardial biopsy	Foreign body retrieval, snare Transseptal procedure	Balloon atrial septostomy Recanalization of occluded or jailed vessel	Atrial septum dilation and stent Atretic valve perforation Cath <4 days after surgery

were stratified according to the innate risk to the procedure (Table 106.2).[2] Risk stratification of procedures can further guide operators in preparation for the catheterization.

Most complications occur during interventional procedures (22%), somewhat less during diagnostic cases (14%), and the least during endomyocardial biopsies (3.3%).[1–4] Age and weight is an important predictor as well. There are certain hemodynamic measures that pose vulnerability and, therefore, could lead to complications. These hemodynamic characteristics are for patients with single ventricles: end-diastolic pressure (EDP) >18 mmHg, saturation <78%, mixed venous saturation <50%, main pulmonary artery (MPA) mean pressure >17 mmHg, and for patients without single ventricles: EDP >18 mmHg, saturation <95%, mixed venous saturation <60%, and MPA systolic pressure >45 mmHg.[2] Among the potential causes, multivariate analysis identified independent predictors of adverse events (Table 106.3).

Anticipation

There is nothing wrong with being obsessive-compulsive in this business. When asked to do a catheterization, the interventional cardiologist should first confirm that the procedure is indicated and indeed the best thing for the patient. It is possible that the patient would be better served with a different intervention or even with surgery. Once it is confirmed that a cardiac catheterization is the optimal procedure to pursue, ask yourself: *Am I prepared*

Table 106.3	Independent predictors of adverse events		
Characteristic	OR (odds ratio)	95% CI	*p* value
Risk category 2	2.0	1.0–3.8	0.04
Risk category 3	4.9	2.7–9.0	<0.001
Risk category 4	4.8	2.5–9.2	<0.001
Hemodynamic vulnerability variables 1 of 4	1.8	1.2–2.8	0.01
Hemodynamic vulnerability variables >1 of 4	2.0	1.2–3.3	0.008
Age <1 year	1.5	1.0–2.2	0.05

for the worst case scenario? Always have a backup plan for complications! Do not do an intervention without surgical support!

Preparation

There is a list of things that enhance the safety of catheterizations, and this list starts way before the procedure itself. Following these steps may help you to avoid some of the complications:

1. Know your patient: read the medical records, talk to the family, and discuss with patient's primary cardiologist and with the cardiac surgeon prior to an intervention. There can never be too much communication!
2. Weekly meetings are very useful for a quick overview of the cases for the following week. The meeting should involve the fellow and head technician and nurse. This will assure that you have what you need prior to the procedure. Choose a day of the week that works for your team and stick to it every week. This should be a brief 15-min meeting.
3. Preadmission: Consider preadmission for the following circumstances:
   a. Newborns or patients with polycythemia that may need hydration when NPO
   b. Patients with impaired ventricular function that may need inotrope support
   c. Patients with impaired renal function that may need hydration or acetylcysteine to avoid contrast-related complications
   d. Patients that are on warfarin and need anticoagulation with heparin, for example, patients with mechanical mitral valve
4. Think about your case the day before. If you are training a fellow, plan to meet with him or her the day before to discuss the case. This is a good time to review the available imaging studies. Walk through the procedure step by step. Start with the overall aim, then discuss access, equipment, and devices to be used, and go through the different scenarios. Ask yourself: What can go wrong with this case? Discuss those in detail, as that will keep you aware of what not to do and if it happens you will be prepared.
5. Day of the procedure: Discuss the cases with your head technician and nurse to assure that all anticipated equipment, catheters, stents, devices, and imaging are available.
6. Go through the consent with the family in detail. Have a routine and say everything that could happen. For example:
   a. Start by telling the family what their patient has and what you are planning to do. Draw the heart and explain in detail.
   b. Go through all the potential risks using simple terms: bleeding, thrombosis, infection, arrhythmias,

perforation of a vessel or the heart, clot formation and embolus, and stroke. Also review procedure specific complications: vessel tear, device embolization, need for transfusion, and death. It sounds harsh, but it is necessary.
7. Just before the case: Review all previous studies again such as last CXR, ECG, echocardiogram, and angiograms.

Preprocedure checklist

In order to fly an airplane, the pilot has to go through an aviation checklist. Previous reports have recommended using a similar checklist to improve operating room safety. "Time out" prior to the procedure is mandated by every medical center. In addition, recently a *checklist* was developed by Gordon and colleagues[5] that *enhances safety* of both diagnostic and interventional catheterization procedures (Table 106.4).

Venous and arterial access

To avoid access-related complications, follow the guidelines below:

1. Access is key. There are several sites for access. We will go through the most common.
   a. Femoral access:
      i. Try to avoid accessing the artery with a sheath whenever possible. Think whether you really need a sheath in the artery.
      ii. Place a quick cath in the artery first and change out to a sheath later in the case to decrease the amount of time the sheath is in the artery
      iii. Use the Seldinger technique without a syringe to avoid injury of the posterior part of the vessel. Access the vessel on the way in, not on the way out.[6] If you need a syringe use a slip tip not a luer lock.
      iv. Use the shortest needle possible based on the patient's weight.
      v. Use a Micropuncture kit (Cook Medical, Bloomington, IN, USA); the wire used has a relatively long floppy tip that allows the wire to go into the vessel rather than go through it.
      vi. Avoid wire mismatch at all costs; if you need to, you can use the micropuncture sheath and dilator (Cook Medical) to size up the wire before using a larger sheath.
      vii. Access the vein first.
      viii. In newborns, you can use a short butterfly needle. When you first introduce the butterfly, leave the tubing on without a syringe. When you get blood flash back, have your nurse attach a 3 mm slip tip syringe to the tubing and draw

Table 106.4 Preprocedural checklist

1.	Confirm that all team members have introduced themselves by name and role.		
2.	Confirm patient's name, procedure, purpose of the procedure, and any planned intervention.		
3.	Confirm that consents have been signed.		
4.	Is the patient going to be admitted after the procedure?		If yes, will they need higher level of care? Will ICU bed be needed? Will the patient need to be left with central access or an arterial line?
5.	Does the patient have allergies to medications or latex?		
6.	Will antibiotics be given?		
7.	Will heparin be given?		
8.	Anticipate critical events and major potential complications!	Interventional cardiologist:	What are the critical steps? How long will the case take? Is there a potential need for blood and if so has it been ordered? Is there special equipment required and if so is it available?
		Anesthesia:	Are there any patient-specific risks? Is additional access needed?
		Nursing and technicians:	Are there patient or equipment issues?
9.	If patient is intubated, check endotracheal tube under fluoroscopy.		
10.	Position the patient and check yourself the position of the feet prior to draping the patient.		

back gently while you manipulate the butterfly to get the best blood return. Then cut the tubing as close as possible to the hub. At that point, you are well lined up with the vessel and you can introduce your micropuncture wire. You may need to manipulate the butterfly a bit to get in. Lifting the needle tip helps separate the anterior part of the vessel and allows entry into the vessel with the wire.

b. *Jugular access:* Use the right internal jugular if possible rather than the left. Position the patient and palpate to find the entry point, then use ultrasound to confirm the entry site to avoid low or high entry.

c. *Umbilical access:* Use fluoroscopy to confirm wire position prior to placing the sheath in the umbilical vein. You may use the umbilical artery, but beware of the sharp turn of the artery and do not place a sheath.

2. Give heparin for all your procedures, as you cannot anticipate how long the case is going to take. We delay giving heparin in biopsy cases until the biopsy is done. Check activated clotting time (ACT) every hour or more frequently if patient has a coagulation problem.

3. After the procedure:
a. Appropriate pressure should be applied after removal of the sheath. Feel the pulses in the foot while holding pressure. You should apply just enough pressure to stop the bleeding, but not to stop the distal pulse.
b. For children less than 2 years of age or weight <10 kg, apply pressure dressing lightly and remove after 2–3 h.

Despite the best effort, *access-related complications* are still common; however, major complications only rarely occur (Table 106.5). HSAE may happen more often in infants or small children (<10 kg), children with multiple previous catheterizations or heart surgeries, after a prolonged puncture time, or when obtaining access in an unplanned vessel.[7] Postprocedural monitoring is paramount to recognize these complications as early as possible.

Anesthesia

HSAE related to *sedation and anesthesia* usually could be prevented by vigilant monitoring (Table 106.5). Airway and respiratory control could be essential in certain cases. The anesthesiologist should be involved in the planning and management of every single case.

Certain complications can be difficult to avoid: in these cases, the anesthesiologist together with the operator should be prepared to handle the major complications.

Electricity

Conduction problems and arrhythmias are among the most common adverse events in catheterization. The severity can range from simple premature atrial or ventricular contractions that happen in almost every single case, over transient arrhythmias to sustained ventricular tachycardia or a complete atrioventricular (AV) block requiring rather timely intervention or even cardio-pulmonary resuscitation (CPR).

Table 106.5   How to avoid and handle major complications[6]

Major complications		How to avoid	How to treat
Access related	Bleeding	Appropriate pressure, pressure dressing for appropriate time, bed rest for 6 h after arterial puncture.	Hold manual pressure for 10–20 min, apply appropriate pressure dressing, bed rest.
	Hematoma		Early detection, compress hematoma for 10 min to allow for it to diffuse. Replace pressure dressing, bed rest.
	Subcutaneous bleed (third space accumulation)		Leeches may be used to relieve compartment syndrome.
	Retroperitoneal hematoma	Identify cases in which puncture site of the vessel not the skin was high and hold above the inguinal ligament as well in those cases.	Early detection with CT scan if suspected. Observe for signs of deterioration. NPO. Vascular repair and evacuation if necessary.
	Thrombosis	Lidocaine subcutaneous around arterial sheath to relax the vessel. Allow sheath to bleed back briefly prior to removal. Appropriate pressure to the vessel (not to hard), feel pulse in the foot while compressing. Pressure dressing for <3 h for patients less than 2 years of age. Start low-dose heparin 10 µg/kg/h without checking PT/PTT if foot is cool and pulse is felt.	If pulse is not felt, start therapeutic heparin for 24 h. If no resolution in 24 h, then do ultrasound and give low-dose tPA. 0.05 µg/kg/h for the first hour as a test dose 0.1 µg/kg/h for 4–6 more hours. Stop before if pulses are felt and start therapeutic heparin. Keep heparin for 24 h after pulse is regained. May repeat 12 h later after checking fibrinogen. Do not allow fibrinogen to drop below 150 mg/dL.[8]
	Vessel tear	Avoid deep skin cut with scalpel. Avoid wire mismatch. Do not use force. Dilate up the vessel using smaller-size dilator if needed prior to insertion of the sheath. Take out sheath slowly. If sheath feels tight, give lidocaine subcutaneous first and very slowly with slow steady pull in increments remove the sheath. Do not use force.	Pressure and observation. May need to have surgery (may be difficult due to patient size).
	Pseudoaneurysm	Avoid posterior vessel puncture (obtain access on the way in). Appropriate pressure during sheath removal. Use more caution when patient is on aspirin and plavix or has vasculitis.	Early detection. Try compression "flattening the pseudoaneurym" while barely feeling the pulse. Ultrasound with Doppler if >1 cm would try ultrasound-guided compression or thrombin injection.
	AV fistula	Avoid through and through access of artery and vein. Avoid puncturing the vein and artery in close proximity. Avoid prolonged access of artery and vein on the same side. Appropriate pressure during sheath removal.	Early detection. Local prolonged compression. Ultrasound localization of the fistula with selective compression at the exact connection between the vessels.
Anesthesia related	Airway obstruction	Monitor saturation and end-tidal CO_2 and proper management of ETT with suction	Reintubation, tube reposition, positive pressure ventilation.
	Acidosis	Follow arterial blood pressure during the procedure.	Sodium bicarbonate, hyperventilation.
	Hypoxia	Monitor saturation and proper management of ETT with suction, and so on	Oxygen, airway management.
	Low cardiac output	Avoid sedation or anesthetics that cause myocardial depression and peripheral vasodilatation.	Inotrope support (dopamine, milrinone, epinephrine).
	Hypothermia (low COP/acidosis)	Heating pad. Temperature probe. Warm flush if possible.	

(continued)

Table 106.5 (continued) How to avoid and handle major complications[6]

Major complications		How to avoid	How to treat
	Malignant hyperthermia	Autonomic dominate disorder. Reaction to halothane and succinyl choline with hyperthermia and rigidity.	Dantrium (start at 1 mg/kg and increase to 10 mg/kg).
	Peripheral nerve injury (brachial plexus)	Proper arm positioning. Avoid overextension or abduction of the arms.	Usually reversible.
Infection	Infection	Sterile conditions should be followed. Antibiotic prophylaxis for 24 h with device/stent placement or prolonged procedures. Fever that starts after or lasts beyond 12 h should be worked up. Patients that are in the ICU prior to cath are at higher risk.	Early recognition. 3–5 blood cultures are drawn and antibiotics started pending cultures. Implanted device may need to be removed in resistant cases.
CNS complications	Air embolus	Fluid-filled catheter. Passive bleed back of the sheath (air can be trapped in the hub). Do not aspirate when a wire is in the sheath. CO_2 should be used in balloon catheters not air. Injector pointing down during injection.	If air is collected in a chamber, then direction of the catheter to this area with suction of the air can be performed. If it has dispersed, than there is not much you can do at this point.
	Thrombus, stroke	Heparin 100 µg/kg/h. Keep ACT at 250–280, check hourly. Flush long sheaths frequently. Hydrate especially with polycythemia.	Therapeutic heparin and possibly tPa.
	Wire perforation of vessels	Do not place wire in the carotid. Monitor wire in the jugular vein.	If vein will likely stop spontaneously. Consult neuroradiology.
General hemodynamic complications	Pulmonary edema	Monitor IV fluid and contrast given.	Diurese.
	Pulmonary hemorrhage	Avoid implanting large stents to severely stenotic pulmonary vessels. Gentle manipulation of wires, catheters, and sheaths in branch pulmonary arteries.	Increase PEEP, prolonged ventilation, transfusion.
	Pulmonary hypertensive crisis	Anticipate patients with reactive pulmonary bed and elevated PVR.	Oxygen, diuresis, iNO readily available.
	Hypotension	Avoid procedures that cause prolonged mitral or tricuspid regurgitation.	NS, LR, packed red blood cells, dopamine, epinephrine.
	Cardiac arrest		CPR.
	Hypercyanotic spell	Use light sedation or anxiolytic prior to procedure.	Oxygen, morphine, epinephrine.
Angiography complication	Myocardial stain	Large catheter with multiple holes. Test injection. Lower pressure for intracavity injections.	
	Allergic reaction (hypotension, bronchospasm)	Awareness of the possibility. Premedication in suspected or known cases of allergy.	Antihistaminic (benadryl 1–1.5 mg/kg), steroids (decadron 0.5 mg/kg), epinephrine (0.1 mcg/kg), IV fluids and manage bronchospasm.

Category	Complication	How to avoid	Management
	Renal toxicity/CNS toxicity	Caution in valuable/predisposed cases. Avoid too much contrast in a short time. Maximum contrast for ionic 4 mg/kg; for non-ionic 8–10 mg/kg. With larger doses, give a dose of lasix (0.5 mg) and IV fluid. Fenoldopam before and after the cath (0.03–0.1 mcg/kg/min).	IV fluid and diuretics. Hemodialysis.
Electricity	Asystole Bradycardia	Echo for EF, avoid hypoxia, avoid prolonged iatrogenic AV valve regurgitation, obtain blood gas frequently, careful coronary angiography/intervention.	Atropine, isoproterenol, epinephrine, pacing, CPR.
	AV block	Awareness of underlying CHD: ccTGA, DILV, AVSD, heterotaxy. Careful device selection and positioning with ASD or VSD closure.	Pacing, atropine, isoproterenol, CPR.
	Atrial flutter Supraventricular tachycardia	Review of medications.	Digoxin, sotalol, DC cardioversion. Adenosine, esmolol, DC cardioversion.
	Ventricular tachycardia	Review of medications, ICD, necessity of the procedure.	Lidocaine, amiodarone.
	Ventricular fibrillation		Defibrillation.
	Pacemaker or ICD malfunction	Awareness of programming, device interrogation within 30 days of the procedure.	Programmer and magnet in cath lab.
Balloon atrial septostomy	Balloon rupture/air embolism	Ensure that balloon is deaerated. Controlled jerk of the catheter and avoid follow through.	Catastrophic event (prevention is the only therapy).
	Injury to mitral valve, pulmonary vein, or IVC	Have a clear understanding of where that balloon is. May use echo guidance to better visualize mitral valve and pulmonary vein.	
Pulmonary valve balloon	Annulus disruption	Accurate measurement of annulus. Balloon/annulus ratio not to exceed 1.5. Awareness of the dysplastic valve (small annulus, no poststenotic dilation).	Tape effusion. Autotransfuse. Surgery. May try covered stent.
	Tricuspid valve injury	Cross the valve with a balloon wedge when possible. Use a short balloon (infants 2 cm, older children 3 cm).	Damage is done, surgical correction if severe or hemodynamically significant.
	RVOT perforation	Cross with a soft floppy tipped wire (e.g., Wholey wire). For tight stenosis, use JR catheter to direct the wire away from RVOT.	Early recognition of wrong wire position prior to introducing the catheter or balloon. Withdraw wire and tap effusion. If not controlled, it is a surgical emergency.
Aortic valve balloon	Aortic regurgitation	Avoid valve perforation with use of floppy tipped wire. Avoid overdilation. Be happy with some residual stenosis and minimal or no regurgitation. Avoid dilation of mild aortic regurgitation with no LVH.	Mild to moderate regurgitation is well tolerated in hypertrophied ventricle. May need ECMO or urgent surgery if not tolerated.
	Stunned ventricle	Inotropic support prior to dilation.	
	"Hooded coronary" with ischemia postdilation	Recognition of this rare association and do not dilate the valve.	Surgical emergency. Likely needs ECMO.

(continued)

Table 106.5 (continued) How to avoid and handle major complications[6]

Major complications		How to avoid	How to treat
Pulmonary artery balloon	Wire perforation of distal vessel/ pulmonary hemorrhage or hemoptysis	Use appropriate wire with a soft tip and avoid inadvertently pushing the wire in.	Usually self-limited. Tape pleural effusion. Pull wire slightly out of the opening, but still in the vessel. May need to tamponade with a balloon.
	Vessel rupture	Avoid overdilation. For postoperative >6 months can go up to 50% of normal vessel. For congenital stenosis use only 10% more than normal vessel. For fresh postsurgical cases, dilation should only be done within the first 2 weeks or after the first 6–8 weeks (sutures are still intact in the first 2 weeks, healing occurs at 6–8 weeks).	Do not lose wire position. Tamponade with the same balloon. Covered stent if available.
	Balloon rupture and loss of fragments	Do not exceed burst atmospheres for balloon. Beware of calcification.	Do not lose wire position as the fragment is likely to still be on the wire. Pass snare over the wire to retrieve.
Pulmonary artery stent	Balloon rupture with incomplete inflation of the stent	Avoid Palmaz stents with sharp edges. Use BIB balloon or balloon shorter than the stent.	Forceful injection of saline rather than contrast. Use pressure injector to inject 50% more than filling volume of the balloon. Be prepared to deal with a torn balloon as above.
	Slippage of the stent over the balloon	Cover the stent as it passes through the hub of the sheath. Do not extrude the stent from the sheath if the marks are not centered.	
	Coronary compression	Beware of the proximity of the RCA to the origin of the LPA in TOF and variants. Test the vessel with balloon only and injection of the aortic root prior to placement of the stent.	Place a wire in the coronary to prop it open. Chest compression may flatten the stent some. Consider coronary stent placement. Alert the operating room.
	Bronchial compression	Beware of the proximity of the left bronchus to the LPA when the geometry of the region has been altered by an arch repair as in Norwood. Consider CT scan prior to intervention to better understand their relationship.[9]	Surgical removal of the stent if significant compression.
	Reperfusion injury	Avoid complete relief of the stenosis if very tight (stage it). Distribute the wealth and dilate various segments especially with high PA pressure.	Medical management with mechanical ventilation and diuretics usually suffices.
Coarctation balloon/stent	Aortic dissection	Do not exceed the size of the smallest adjacent normal aorta or more than 3× the stenotic segment. Superstiff wire with a long floppy tip. Wire in the subclavian artery. Shortest balloon possible. Use BIB balloon when possible.	Place a stent, preferably a covered one.
	Vessel rupture		Inflate the balloon to tamponade the vessel. Place a covered stent. Surgical emergency if not controlled.
	Aortic aneurysm		Covered stent or surgical correction.

	Complication	Avoidance	Management
Pericardial effusion	Exaggerated vagal response	IV hydration for 24 h after the procedure.	IV fluids.
	Pericardial tamponade	Avoid stiff wires. Gentle catheter manipulation.	Early detection and echo confirmation. Tap effusion and if needed autotransfuse.
PDA closure	Residual leak/hemolysis	Do not leave the lab with a residual jet.	IV fluid. Try to closure residual leak. Surgery.
	Embolization (especially with coils)	Use appropriate coil or device for the shape and size of the PDA. Avoid free-hand delivery of coils in larger PDAs. Avoid undersizing of the device (PDA may distensible), balloon size if not sure.	Snare the embolized coil or device.
ASD closure	Embolization	Appropriate sizing and visualization prior to release.	Snare if in an appropriate site. Surgery may be preferred to avoid injury of valves.
	Erosion	Avoid over- or undersizing. True cause unknown. Make family aware as it can happen up to many months to 2 years after the procedure.	Surgical emergency.
	Heart block	Avoid oversizing of the device. Be cautious with an absent inferior rim.	Change to a smaller device if still in the lab. Steroids and observation. Remove device if not reversed.
Coronary fistula	Ischemia due to occlusion of important side branches	Adequate assessment of branches with a balloon angio catheter if needed.	
	Thrombosis of dilated coronary artery after closure	Gentle handling of the vessel, avoid roughing it back, place on anticoagulation, even Coumadin in large fistulae.	
Endomyocardial biopsy	Cardiac perforation	Take biopsy from interventricular septum or the apex. Avoid biting from the same site.	Tap effusion and autotransfuse. Surgical emergency if not controlled.
	TV injury	Use a long sheath with a curve. Use a balloon wedge catheter to position the long sheath. RV angiogram prior to biopsy.	

Even in the catheterization laboratory, the most common cause of *bradycardia* and *asystole* is hypoxia of the myocardium. Myocardial hypoxia should be prevented by careful preprocedural evaluation (echocardiogram assessing left ventricle [LV] function) and careful monitoring during the catheterization, avoiding prolonged compromised cardiac output. Procedures involving coronary arteries should follow meticulous techniques to avoid air/thrombus embolization or obstruction of the coronary arteries.

Atrioventricular block may occur in any patient if the AV node or the His bundle is damaged. Special attention should be taken during device closure of atrial septal defects (ASDs)and perimembranous ventricular septal defects (VSDs). It is paramount to be aware of conditions prone to AV block (ccTGA [congenitally corrected transposition of the great arteries], double inlet left ventricle/L-transposition of the great arteries [DILV/L-TGA], atrioventricular septal defect [AVSD] with straddling tricuspid valve, heterotaxy with left isomerism) and be prepared to "treat" the AV block by right ventricular (RV) pacing or administration of drugs improving AV conduction (Table 106.5).

Tachyarrhythmias may be well tolerated in a consciously sedated patient with two ventricles and normal LV systolic function or could be lethal in a patient with a single ventricle and poor systolic function; therefore, almost any tachyarrhythmia may pose a risk of HSAE (Table 106.5). An electrophysiologist should be involved in the discussion and appropriate planning of the procedure in patients with a history of SVT or VT requiring medical therapy. The anesthesiologist should be well aware of the situation and be prepared for drug administration and or cardioversion or defibrillation. Timely, which sometimes means immediate, attention to an arrhythmia could prevent further hemodynamic deterioration and potentially fatal complications.

While *pacemakers and ICDs* could be an advantage during the procedure, ensuring appropriate heart rate and terminating life-threatening arrhythmias, they could also increase the complexity of a case and even provide inappropriate or undesired therapy at times.

Every patient with a device should have an interrogation within a month prior to the catheterization and the operator should review the programming prior to the procedure. If there is an inappropriate therapy that compromises data collection or poses risk to the patient, a magnet should be readily available to cease ICD therapy or provide pacing of the programmed chamber. A programmer is also very helpful to change certain parameters during catheterization or after the use of a magnet.

Complications during interventional procedures

Specific complications related to certain *interventional procedures* are detailed in Table 106.5.

References

1. Bergersen L, Marshall A, Gauvreau K et al. Adverse event rates in congenital cardiac catheterization—A multi-center experience. *Catheter Cardiovasc Interv* 2010;75:389–400.
2. Bergersen L, Gauvreau K, Foerster SR et al. Catheterization for Congenital Heart Disease Adjustment for Risk Method (CHARM). *J Am Coll Cardiol Cardiovasc Interv* 2011;4:1037–46.
3. Daly KP, Marshall AC, Vincent JA et al. Endomyocardial biopsy and selective coronary angiography are low-risk procedures in pediatric heart transplant recipients: Results of a multicenter experience. *J Heart Lung Transplant* 2012;31:398–409.
4. Holzer RJ, Gauvreau K, Kreutzer J et al. Balloon angioplasty and stenting of branch pulmonary arteries: adverse events and procedural characteristics: Results of a multi-institutional registry. *Circ Cardiovasc Interv* 2011;4:287–96.
5. Gordon BM, Lam T, Bahjri K, Hashmi A, Kuhn MA. Utility of preprocedure checklists in the cardiac catheterization laboratory. *Abstract at SCAI 2012 Meeting.* Society for Cardiovascular Angiography and Interventions, May 9–12, 2012, Las Vegas, USA.
6. Mullins CE. *Cardiac Catheterization in Congenital Heart Disease: Pediatric and Adult.* Malden, MA: Blackwell Futura; 2006.
7. Roushdy AM, Abdelmonem N, El Fiky AA. Factors affecting vascular access complications in children undergoing congenital cardiac catheterization. *Cardiol Young* 2012;22:136–44.
8. Bratincsak A, El-Said HG, Moore JW. Low dose tissue plasminogen activator treatment for vascular thrombosis following cardiac catheterization in children—A single center experience. *Catheter Cardiovasc Interv* 2013;82:782–5.
9. Ferandos C, El-Said H, Hamzeh R, Moore JW. Adverse impact of vascular stent "mass effect" on airways. *Catheter Cardiovasc Interv* 2009;74:132–6.

Index

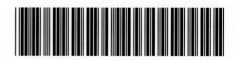